S A U N D E R S

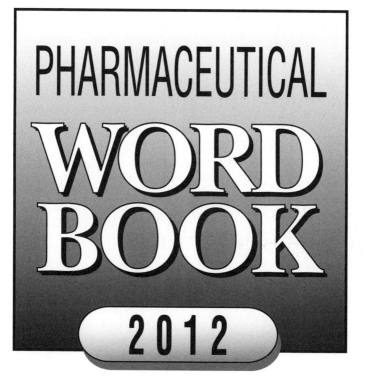

PHARMACEUTICAL
WORD
BOOK

2012

ELLEN DRAKE, CMT, FAAMT
RANDY DRAKE, MS

SAUNDERS

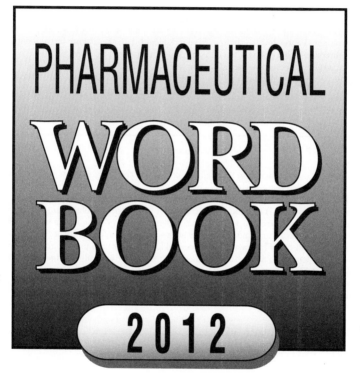

PHARMACEUTICAL
WORD
BOOK

2012

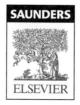

SAUNDERS

ELSEVIER

SAUNDERS
ELSEVIER

3251 Riverport Lane
Maryland Heights, Missouri 63043

SAUNDERS PHARMACEUTICAL WORD BOOK 2012 ISBN: 978-1-4377-0997-1

Notice

Knowledge and best practice in this field are constantly changing. As new research and experience broaden our knowledge, changes in practice, treatment, and drug therapy may become necessary or appropriate. Readers are advised to check the most current information provided (i) on procedures featured or (ii) by the manufacturer of each product to be administered, to verify the recommended dose or formula, the method and duration of administration, and contraindications. It is the responsibility of the practitioner, relying on his or her own experience and knowledge of the patient, to make diagnoses, to determine dosages and the best treatment for each individual patient, and to take all appropriate safety precautions. To the fullest extent of the law, neither the Publisher nor the Authors assume any liability for any injury and/or damage to persons or property arising out or related to any use of the material contained in this book.

The Publisher

Previous editions copyrighted 2011, 2010, 2009, 2008, 2007, 2006, 2005, 2004, 2003, 2002, 2001, 2000, 1999, 1998, 1997, 1996, 1995, 1994, 1992

ISSN: 1072-7779
ISBN: 978-1-4377-0997-1

Printed in the United States of America

Last d

Contents

Preface

This is a professional medical reference. It was written *by* medical professionals *for* medical professionals. It has been published by the world's largest publisher of professional medical references. You can rely on the information in this book.

The *Saunders Pharmaceutical Word Book* series has been compiled primarily with the medical transcriptionist in mind, although it will certainly appeal to coders, quality assurance personnel, nurses, ward clerks, students of all allied health professions—anyone who has a need for a quick, easy-to-use drug reference that gives more information than just the spelling. Even physicians may find it useful to get quick information on medications their patients may be using for conditions outside their specialty. The "Notes on Using the Text" will show you the format of generic and brand name entries, explain the variety of information this book contains, and give tips on how to find that information.

We think you will find this edition more complete and more valuable than ever; however, no book is ever perfect. Although we have tried to be as accurate and comprehensive as possible, we certainly welcome your comments regarding additions, inconsistencies, or inaccuracies. Please send them to us via e-mail at the address below, or via regular mail to Elsevier Saunders, 3251 Riverport Lane, Maryland Heights, MO 63043. We welcome your suggestions.

Authors' e-mail address:
  authors@spwb.com
Authors' web site:
  spwb.com

ELLEN DRAKE, CMT, FAAMT
RANDY DRAKE, MS
Atlanta, Georgia

Notes on Using the Text

The purpose of the *Saunders Pharmaceutical Word Book* is to provide the medical transcriptionist (as well as medical record administrators and technicians, coders, nurses, ward clerks, court reporters, legal secretaries, medical assistants, allied health students, physicians, and even pharmacists) a quick, easy-to-use reference that gives not only the correct spellings and capitalizations of drugs, but the designated uses of those drugs, the cross-referencing of brand names to generics, and the usual methods of administration (e.g., capsule, IV, cream). The indication of the preferred nonproprietary (generic) names and the agencies adopting these names (e.g., USAN, USP) should be particularly useful to those writing for publication. The reader will also find various trademarked or proprietary names (e.g., Spansule, Dosepak) that are not drugs but are closely associated with the packaging or administration of drugs.

There are four different ways to refer to drugs. One of these ways is not the name of the drug itself but the class to which it belongs—aminoglycosides, for example. Inexperienced transcriptionists sometimes confuse these classes with the names of drugs. We have included over 350 drug classes in the main list, with a brief description of the therapeutic use and/or method of action common to drugs in the class. Beyond a class description, each drug has three names. The first is the *chemical name*, which describes its chemical composition and how the molecules are arranged. It is often long and complex, sometimes containing numbers, Greek letters, italicized letters, and hyphens between elements. This name is rarely used in dictation except in research hospitals and sometimes in the laboratory section when the blood or urine is examined for traces of the drug. The second name for a drug is the *nonproprietary* or *generic name*. This is a name chosen by the discovering manufacturer or agency and submitted to a nomenclature committee (the United States Adopted Names Council, for example). The name is simpler than the chemical name but often reflects the chemical entity. It is arrived at by using guidelines provided by the nomenclature committee—beta-blockers must end in "olol," for example—and must be unique. There is increasing emphasis on the adoption of the same nonproprietary name by various nomenclature committees worldwide (see the list on page xi). The third name for a drug is the *trade* or *brand name*. There may be several trade names for the same generic drug, each marketed by a different company. These are the ones that are advertised and may have unusual capitalization.

The international and British spellings of generic drugs are cross-referenced to the American spellings, and vice versa. Occasionally there will be three different spellings—one American, one international, and another British—which are all cross-referenced to each other. Other special features that may be useful, especially for students, are the commonly used prescribing abbreviations and the sound-alike lists that are found in the appendices. The Therapeutic Drug Levels and Most Prescribed Drugs appendices will be useful as well.

This information was compiled using a variety of sources including direct communication with over 500 drug companies. The orphan entries are taken directly from the latest list issued by the FDA. When sources differed, we ranked our sources as to reliability and went with what we thought was the most reliable source. We recognize that there may be several published ways in which to type a single drug, but we have chosen to use only one of those ways. In the instance of internal capitalization (e.g., pHisoHex), it should be recognized that in most instances it is acceptable to type such words with initial capitalization only (Phisohex).

How the Book Is Arranged

While other pharmaceutical references have separate listings for brand names and generics, or put entries into separate sections by body system or therapeutic use, we have chosen to list all entries in one comprehensive alphabetical listing. Therefore, it is not necessary to know if the term sought is a brand name, a generic, a drug class, a chemotherapy protocol, approved or investigational, or slang; what it's used for; or which body system it affects. If it's given to a patient, it's in "the list." In addition to strict pharmaceuticals, we have included other "consumable" products, such as *in vitro* testing kits, radiographic contrast and other imaging agents, wound dressings, etc.

All entries are in alphabetical order by word. Initial numbers, chemical prefixes (*N*-, *p*-, L-, D-, etc.), and punctuation (prime, hyphens, etc.) are ignored. For example, L-dopa would be alphabetized under "dopa," but levodopa under "levo."

We have indicated brand names with initial capital letters unless an unusual combination of capitals and lowercase has been designated by the manufacturer (e.g., pHisoHex, ALternaGEL). Generic names are rendered in lowercase. Where the same name can be either generic or brand, both have been included.

The general format of a *generic* entry is:

entry council(s) *designated use* [other references] dosages 🔊 sound-alike(s)

| #1 | #2 | #3 | #4 | #5 | #6 |

1. The name of the drug (in bold).
2. The various agencies that have approved the name, shown in small caps, which may be any or all of the following:

   USAN   United States Adopted Name Council
   USP   United States Pharmacopeial Convention
   NF   National Formulary
   FDA   U.S. Food and Drug Administration
   INN   International Nonproprietary Name (a project of the World Health Organization)
   BAN   British Approved Name
   JAN   Japanese Accepted Name

3. The indications, sometimes referred to as the drug's "designated use," "approved use," or "therapeutic action." This is provided only for official FDA-approved names or other names for the same substance (e.g., the British name of an official U.S. generic). This entry is always in italics.
4. The entry in brackets is one of four cross-references:

   see: refers the reader to the "official" name(s).
   now: for an older generic name no longer used, refers reader to the current official name(s).
   also: a substance that has two or more different names, each officially recognized by one of the above groups, will cross-reference the other name(s).
   q.v.   Latin for *quod vide*; which see. Used exclusively for abbreviations, it invites the reader to turn to the reference in parentheses.

   If there is more than one cross-reference, alternate names will follow the order of the above agency list; i.e., U.S. names, then international names, then British and Japanese names. The first cross-reference will always be to the approved U.S. name, unless the entry itself is the U.S. name.
5. Dosage information, including the delivery form(s), is given for medications that may be dispensed generically. No dosage information appears for drugs dispensed only under the brand name. Some drugs may be available in more than one strength, indicated by a comma in the dosage field:

   erythromycin stearate USP, BAN *macrolide antibiotic* 250, 500 mg oral

   A semicolon in the dosage field separates different delivery forms, such as:

   nitroglycerin USP *coronary vasodilator; antianginal; antihypertensive* [also: glyceryl trinitrate] 0.3, 0.4, 0.6 mg sublingual; 2.5, 6.5, 9 mg oral; 5 mg/mL injection; 0.1, 0.2, 0.4, 0.6 mg/hr. transdermal; 2% topical

   (Note that some delivery forms come in multiple strengths.)
6. Sound-alike drugs follow the "ear" icon. Listen again to make sure you've found the drug actually being dictated.

The general format for a *brand name* entry is:

Entry ⓒ form(s) ℞/OTC *designated use* [generics] dosages ② sound-alike(s)
| #1 | #2 | #3 | #4 | #5 | #6 | #7 | #8 |

1. The drug name (in bold), which almost always starts with a capital letter.
2. If a brand is not marketed in the U.S., an icon designates the country where it is available. Canadian brands are designated by ⓒ, European brands by ⓔ.
3. The form of administration; e.g., tablets, capsules, syrup. (Sometimes these words are slurred by the dictator, causing confusion regarding the name.)
4. The ℞ or OTC status. A few drugs may be either ℞ or OTC depending on strength or various state laws.
5. The designated use in italics as for generics. These are more complete or less complete as supplied by the individual drug companies.
6. The brackets that follow contain the generic names of the active ingredients to which the reader may refer for further information.
7. Dosage information follows the generics. For multi-ingredient drugs, a bullet separates the dosages of each ingredient, listed in the same order as the generics. For example,

> **Fiorinal** capsules ℞ *barbiturate sedative; analgesic; antipyretic* [butalbital; aspirin; caffeine] 50•325•40 mg

shows a three-ingredient product containing 50 mg butalbital, 325 mg aspirin, and 40 mg caffeine.

Some drugs may have more than one strength, indicated by a comma in the dosage field:

> **Norpace** capsules ℞ *antiarrhythmic* [disopyramide phosphate] 100, 150 mg

A semicolon in the dosage field separates either different products listed together, such as:

> **Pred Mild; Pred Forte** eye drop suspension ℞ *corticosteroidal anti-inflammatory* [prednisolone acetate] 0.12%; 1%

or different delivery forms:

> **Phenergan** tablets, suppositories, injection ℞ *antihistamine; sedative; antiemetic; motion sickness relief* [promethazine HCl] 12.5, 25, 50 mg; 12.5, 25 mg; 25, 50 mg/mL

(Note that all three delivery forms of Phenergan come in multiple strengths.)

Liquid delivery forms show the strength per usual dose where appropriate. Thus injectables and drops are usually shown per milliliter (mL), with oral liquids and syrups shown per 5 mL or 15 mL.

The ≟ symbol indicates that dosage information has not been supplied by the manufacturer for one or more ingredients.

The ≛ symbol is used when a value *cannot* be given because the generic entry refers to multiple ingredients.

8. Sound-alike drugs follow the "ear" icon.

Experimental, Investigational, and Orphan Drugs

Before a drug can be advertised or sold in the United States, it must first be approved for marketing by the U.S. Food and Drug Administration. With a few exceptions, FDA approval is contingent solely upon the manufacturer demonstrating that the proposed drug is both safe and effective.

To provide such proof, the manufacturer undertakes a series of tests. Preclinical (before human) research is done through computer simulation, then *in vitro* (L. "in glass," meaning laboratory) tests, then in animals. In most cases neither the public nor the general medical community hears about "experimental drugs" in this stage of testing. Neither are they listed in this reference.

If safety and efficacy are successfully demonstrated during the preclinical stage, an Investigational New Drug (IND) application is filed with the FDA. There are three phases of clinical trials, designated Phase I, Phase II, and Phase III. After each phase, the FDA will review the findings and approve or deny further testing.

An orphan drug is a drug or biological product for the diagnosis, treatment, or prevention of a rare disease or condition. A rare disease is one that affects fewer than 200,000 persons or for which there is no reasonable expectation that the cost of development will be recovered through U.S. sales of the product. Federal subsidies are provided to the manufacturer for the development of orphan drugs.

A Brief Note on the Transcription of Drugs

Many references are available describing several acceptable ways to transcribe drug information when dictated. We offer the following only as brief guidelines.

The generally accepted style today for the transcription of medical reports for hospital and doctors' office charts (see the American Medical Association *Manual of Style*[1] for publications) is to capitalize the initial letter of brand name drugs and lowercase generic name drugs. The institution may also designate that brand name drugs with unusual capitalization may be typed with initial capital letter only, or typed using the manufacturer's scheme.

The Institute for Safe Medication Practices (ISMP) has issued a list of *Error-Prone Abbreviations, Symbols, and Dose Designations* that should be avoided in prescribing instructions. The Joint Commission has mandated a graduated implementation of the ISMP list and has placed certain ISMP abbreviations in a "Do Not Use" list, directing healthcare organizations to add at least three more abbreviations to the Joint Commission's list. This mandate essentially means that each institution may have its own "Do Not Use" list that differs from other institutions. For that reason, it may be simpler for medical transcriptionists and MTSOs to simply adopt the entire ISMP list as a "Do Not Use" list, assuming, of course, that doing so is acceptable to the originator or client.

Because many of the abbreviations on the ISMP "error-prone" list are Latin or pseudo-Latin abbreviations, many MTs have chosen to translate all Latin abbreviations into English, although this practice is by no means universal. In fact, in its discussion of drug-related terminology, *The Book of Style for Medical Transcription*[2] provides a list of Latin abbreviations for which it says "do not translate." If Latin dosing and dosage abbreviations are used, they should be transcribed in lowercase with periods.

Commas are omitted between the drug name, the dosage, and the instructions for purposes of simplification. Items in a series may be separated by either commas (if no internal commas are used) or semicolons. A simple series might be typed:

Procardia, nitroglycerin sublingual, and Tolinase

or

Procardia 10 mg 3 times a day, nitroglycerin 0.4 mg p.r.n., and Tolinase 250 mg twice a day.

or

Procardia 10 mg t.i.d., nitroglycerin 0.4 mg p.r.n., and Tolinase 250 mg b.i.d.

A more complex or lengthy list of medications, or a list with internal commas, may require the use of semicolons to separate the items in a series. The use of numerals, even for numbers less than ten, is recommended to make dosing information stand out. When two numbers are adjacent to each other, write out one number and use a numeral for the other (e.g., Tylenol No. 3 one q. 4–6 h. p.r.n.). Occasionally, physicians may dictate the number of pills or capsules to be dispensed. When they do, the number should be set off by commas as it is for oxycodone with APAP in this example:

Vigamox 0.5% 1 drop OS; EconoPred 1% 1 drop OS (shake well); atropine 1% 1 drop OS 3 days only (each 5 minutes apart, given at 9 a.m., 1 p.m., 5 p.m., and 9 p.m.); and oxycodone with APAP 5/325, #5, no refills, 1 tablet every 4-6 hours p.r.n. ["#5, no refills" could also be placed in parentheses]

The typing of chemicals with superscripts or subscripts, italics, small capitals, and Greek letters often presents a problem to the transcriptionist. In general, Greek letters are written out (alpha-, beta-, gamma-, etc.). Italics and small capitals are written as standard letters followed by a hyphen (dl-alpha-tocopherol, L-dopa).

When typing nonproprietary (generic) isotope names, element symbols should be included with the name. It may appear to be redundant, but it is the correct form. Therefore, we would type sodium pertechnetate Tc 99m, iodohippurate sodium I 131, or sodium iodide I 125. Occasionally the physician may simply dictate isotopes such as Tc 99m, iodine 131 or I 131, or sodium iodide I 125, and unless he is indicating a trademarked name, it should be typed with a space, no hyphen, and no superscript. This reference indicates proper capitalization, spacing, and hyphenation of isotope entries.

Other combinations of letters and numbers are usually written without spaces or hyphens (OKT1, OKT3, T101, SC1), but this is a complex subject and is dealt with extensively in the AMA *Manual of Style*.

---

[1] AMA *Manual of Style: A Guide for Authors and Editors*, 10th ed. New York: Oxford Press; 2007.

[2] *The Book of Style for Medical Transcription*, 3rd ed. Modesto, California: Association for Healthcare Documentation Integrity (formerly AAMT); 2008.

A (vitamin A) [q.v.]

A and D ointment OTC *moisturizer; emollient* [fish liver oil (vitamins A and D); cholecalciferol; lanolin]

A and D Medicated ointment (discontinued 2008) OTC *diaper rash treatment* [zinc oxide; vitamins A and D]

A & D softgels OTC *vitamin supplement* [vitamins A and D] 10 000•400 U

A1cNOW+ fingerstick test kit for professional use ℞ *in vitro diagnostic aid for glycosylated hemoglobin levels* ⧈ Acanya; A.C.N.

A1cNOW Selfcheck fingerstick test kit for home use OTC *in vitro diagnostic aid for glycosylated hemoglobin levels*

A-200 shampoo (discontinued 2011) OTC *pediculicide for lice* [pyrethrins; piperonyl butoxide] 0.33%•4%

AA (arachadonic acid) [q.v.]

AABP Otic Solution ear drops ℞ *anesthetic; analgesic* [benzocaine; antipyrine; acetic acid; polycosanol] 1.4%•5.4%•0.01%•0.01%

AAD (adaptive aerosol delivery) system [see: I-neb AAD; Prodose AAD]

a-(3-aminophthalimido) glutaramide *investigational (orphan) agent for multiple myeloma*

abacavir succinate USAN *antiviral nucleoside reverse transcriptase inhibitor for HIV infection*

abacavir sulfate USAN *antiviral nucleoside reverse transcriptase inhibitor (NRTI) for HIV infection*

abacavir sulfate & lamivudine *nucleoside reverse transcriptase inhibitor (NRTI) combination for HIV and AIDS* 60•30 mg oral

abacavir sulfate & lamivudine & zidovudine *nucleoside reverse transcriptase inhibitor (NRTI) combination for HIV and AIDS* 300•150•300 mg oral

abafilcon A USAN *hydrophilic contact lens material*

abamectin USAN, INN *antiparasitic*

abanoquil INN, BAN

abaperidone INN

abarelix USAN *GnRH antagonist to suppress LH and FSH, leading to the cessation of testosterone production (medical castration, androgen ablation); treatment for prostate cancer*

abatacept *selective T-cell co-stimulation modulator for rheumatoid arthritis (RA) and juvenile idiopathic arthritis*

Abbo-Pac (trademarked packaging form) *unit dose package*

Abbott TestPack Plus hCG-Urine Plus test kit for professional use ℞ *in vitro diagnostic aid; urine pregnancy test* [monoclonal antibody-based enzyme immunoassay]

ABC to Z tablets (discontinued 2008) OTC *vitamin/mineral/iron supplement* [multiple vitamins & minerals; iron (as ferrous fumarate); folic acid; biotin] ±•18•0.4•0.03 mg

abciximab USAN, INN *monoclonal antibody to glycoprotein (GP) IIb/IIIa receptors; antithrombotic/antiplatelet agent for PTCA and acute arterial occlusive disorders*

ABE (antitoxin botulism equine) [see: botulism equine antitoxin, trivalent]

abecarnil INN *anxiolytic*

Abelcet suspension for IV infusion ℞ *systemic polyene antifungal for aspergillosis and other resistant fungal infections (orphan)* [amphotericin B lipid complex (ABLC)] 100 mg/20 mL

Abelmoschus moschatus *medicinal herb* [see: ambrette]

abetimus INN

abetimus sodium USAN *investigational (NDA filed, orphan) oligonucleotide immunosuppressant for systemic lupus erythematosus–associated nephritis*

Abilify tablets, oral solution, IM injection ℞ *antipsychotic for schizophrenia and manic episodes of a bipolar disorder; adjunctive treatment for major depression* [aripiprazole] 2, 5, 10, 15, 20, 30 mg; 1 mg/mL; 7.5 mg/mL

Abilify Discmelt (orally disintegrating tablets) ℞ *antipsychotic for schizophrenia and manic episodes of a bipolar disorder; adjunctive treatment for major depression* [aripiprazole] 10, 15 mg

abiraterone acetate *testosterone antagonist antineoplastic for late-stage metastatic prostate cancer*

Ablavar IV injection ℞ *parenteral gadolinium-based contrast agent (GBCA) for vascular enhancement in magnetic resonance angiography (MRA)* [gadofosveset trisodium] 244 mg/mL

ABLC (amphotericin B lipid complex) [q.v.]

ablukast USAN, INN *antiasthmatic; leukotriene antagonist*

ablukast sodium USAN *antiasthmatic; leukotriene antagonist*

abobotulinumtoxin A *neurotoxin complex derived from* Clostridium botulinum; *treatment for cervical dystonia (orphan) and facial wrinkles; also used for achalasia, Frey syndrome, palmar hyperhidrosis, and Tourette syndrome* [also: botulinum toxin, type A]

abortifacients *a class of agents that stimulate uterine contractions sufficient to produce uterine evacuation*

ABPP (aminobromophenylpyrimidinone) [see: bropirimine]

Abraxane suspension of albumin-bound microspheres for IV infusion ℞ *antineoplastic for metastatic breast cancer; investigational (Phase III) for non–small cell lung cancer (NSCLC)* [paclitaxel; human albumin] 100• 900 mg/dose

Abreva cream OTC *antiviral for cold sores and fever blisters* [docosanol] 10%

abrineurin USAN *treatment for amyotrophic lateral sclerosis (ALS)*

Abrus precatorius *medicinal herb* [see: precatory bean]

absinthe; absinthites; absinthium *medicinal herb* [see: wormwood]

absorbable cellulose cotton [see: cellulose, oxidized]

absorbable collagen sponge [see: collagen sponge, absorbable]

absorbable dusting powder [see: dusting powder, absorbable]

absorbable gelatin film [see: gelatin film, absorbable]

absorbable gelatin sponge [see: gelatin sponge, absorbable]

absorbable surgical suture [see: suture, absorbable surgical]

Absorbase ointment OTC *nontherapeutic base for compounding various dermatological preparations* [water-in-oil emulsion of cholesterolized petrolatum and purified water]

absorbent gauze [see: gauze, absorbent]

Absorbine Antifungal Foot aerosol powder (discontinued 2007) OTC *antifungal* [miconazole nitrate; alcohol 10%] 2%

Absorbine Footcare spray liquid (discontinued 2008) OTC *antifungal* [tolnaftate] 1%

Absorbine Jr. liniment, topical liquid OTC *mild anesthetic; antipruritic; counterirritant* [menthol] 1.27%, 4%; 1.4%

Absorbine Jr. Back Patch transdermal patch OTC *mild anesthetic; antipruritic; counterirritant* [menthol] 5%

Absorbine Jr. Extra Strength topical liquid OTC *mild anesthetic; antipruritic; counterirritant* [menthol] 4%

Absorbine Jr. Ultra Strength transdermal patch, topical spray OTC *mild anesthetic; antipruritic; counterirritant* [menthol] 6,5%; 12%

Abstral sublingual tablets ℞ *transmucosal narcotic analgesic for chronic pain in opioid-tolerant cancer patients* [fentanyl (as citrate)] 100, 200, 300, 400, 600, 800 mcg ② epiestriol

Abthrax *investigational (NDA filed, orphan) treatment for inhalational anthrax poisoning* [raxibacumab]

abunidazole INN

ABV (Adriamycin, bleomycin, vinblastine) *chemotherapy protocol for Kaposi sarcoma*

ABV (Adriamycin, bleomycin, vincristine) *chemotherapy protocol for Kaposi sarcoma*

ABVD (Adriamycin, bleomycin, vinblastine, dacarbazine) *chemotherapy protocol for Hodgkin lymphoma*

AC (Adriamycin, cisplatin) *chemotherapy protocol for bone sarcoma*

AC; A-C (Adriamycin, cyclophosphamide) *chemotherapy protocol for breast cancer, endometrial cancer, and pediatric neuroblastoma* [also known as: CY/A]

AC/paclitaxel (Adriamycin, cyclophosphamide; paclitaxel), sequential *chemotherapy protocol for breast cancer*

ACA125 *investigational (orphan) agent for epithelial ovarian cancer*

acacia NF, JAN *suspending agent; emollient; demulcent*

acacia (Acacia senegal; A. verek) gum *medicinal herb for colds, cough, periodontal disease, and wound healing*

acadesine USAN, INN, BAN *platelet aggregation inhibitor; investigational (NDA filed) for injury caused by stroke*

acamprosate INN

acamprosate calcium GABA/*taurine analogue for the treatment of alcoholism*

acamylophenine [see: camylofin]

Acanthopanax senticosus medicinal herb [see: eleuthero]

Acanya gel ℞ *antibiotic and keratolytic for acne* [clindamycin phosphate; benzoyl peroxide] 1.2%•2.5% ⍰ A1cNOW; A.C.N.

acaprazine INN

acarbose USAN, INN, BAN *antidiabetic agent for type 2 diabetes; alpha-glucosidase inhibitor that delays the digestion of dietary carbohydrates* 25, 50, 100 mg oral

ACAT (acylCoA transferase) inhibitors *a class of antihyperlipidemics that lower serum cholesterol levels* ⍰ ACT

Accolate film-coated tablets ℞ *leukotriene receptor antagonist (LTRA) for prevention and chronic treatment of asthma* [zafirlukast] 10, 20 mg ⍰ Equilet

Accretropin injection ℞ *growth hormone for children and adults with congenital or endogenous growth hormone*

deficiency, short bowel syndrome, or AIDS-wasting syndrome; for children with Turner syndrome, Prader-Willi syndrome, or renal-induced growth failure [somatropin] 5 mg (15 IU) per mL

Accu-Chek Advantage reagent strips for home use OTC *in vitro diagnostic aid for blood glucose*

AccuHist oral drops OTC *decongestant; antihistamine; for children 6–36 months* [pseudoephedrine HCl; chlorpheniramine maleate] 9•0.8 mg/mL

AccuHist DM Pediatric oral drops ℞ *antitussive; antihistamine; decongestant; for children 1–24 months* [dextromethorphan hydrobromide; brompheniramine maleate; pseudoephedrine HCl] 4•1•15 mg/mL

AccuHist DM Pediatric syrup (discontinued 2007) OTC *decongestant; antihistamine; antitussive; expectorant; for children 2–11 years* [dextromethorphan hydrobromide; pseudoephedrine HCl; brompheniramine maleate; guaifenesin] 5•30•2•50 mg/5 mL

AccuHist PDX oral drops ℞ *antitussive; antihistamine; decongestant; for children 6–36 months* [dextromethorphan hydrobromide; chlorpheniramine maleate; pseudoephedrine HCl] 3•0.8•9 mg/mL

AccuHist PDX syrup ℞ *antitussive; antihistamine; decongestant; expectorant* [dextromethorphan hydrobromide; brompheniramine maleate; phenylephrine HCl; guaifenesin] 5•2•5•50 mg/5 mL

AccuNeb solution for inhalation ℞ *sympathomimetic bronchodilator for children 2–12 years* [albuterol sulfate] 0.021%, 0.042% (0.63, 1.25 mg/3 mL)

Accu-Pak (trademarked packaging form) *unit dose blister pack*

Accupep HPF powder OTC *enteral nutritional therapy for GI impairment*

Accupril film-coated tablets ℞ *angiotensin-converting enzyme (ACE) inhibitor for hypertension; adjunctive treat-*

ment for congestive heart failure (CHF) [quinapril HCl] 5, 10, 20, 40 mg

Accurbron syrup (discontinued 2008) ℞ antiasthmatic; bronchodilator [theophylline; alcohol 7.5%] 150 mg/15 mL

Accuretic film-coated tablets ℞ combination angiotensin-converting enzyme (ACE) inhibitor and diuretic for hypertension [quinapril HCl; hydrochlorothiazide] 10•12.5, 20•12.5, 20•25 mg

Accutane capsules (discontinued 2009) ℞ keratolytic for severe recalcitrant cystic acne [isotretinoin] 10, 20, 40 mg ⊡ AK-Ten

Accuzyme ointment ℞ proteolytic enzyme for débridement of necrotic tissue; vulnerary [papain; urea] 830 000 IU/g•10%

Accuzyme spray (discontinued 2009) ℞ proteolytic enzyme for débridement of necrotic tissue; vulnerary [papain; urea] 830 000 IU/g•10%

Accuzyme SE spray ℞ proteolytic enzyme for débridement of necrotic tissue; vulnerary [papain; urea] 650 000 IU/g•10%

ACD solution (acid citrate dextrose; anticoagulant citrate dextrose) [see: anticoagulant citrate dextrose solution]

ACD whole blood [see: blood, whole]

ACe (Adriamycin, cyclophosphamide) chemotherapy protocol for breast cancer

ACE (Adriamycin, cyclophosphamide, etoposide) chemotherapy protocol for small cell lung cancer (SCLC) [also known as: CAE]

ACE inhibitors (angiotensin-converting enzyme inhibitors) [q.v.]

acebrochol INN

aceburic acid INN

acebutolol USAN, INN, BAN antihypertensive; antiadrenergic (beta-blocker); antiarrhythmic [also: acebutolol HCl]

acebutolol HCl JAN antihypertensive (beta-blocker); antiarrhythmic for premature ventricular contractions (PVCs);

also used for ventricular tachycardia [also: acebutolol] 200, 400 mg oral

acecainide INN antiarrhythmic [also: acecainide HCl]

acecainide HCl USAN investigational (orphan) antiarrhythmic [also: acecainide]

acecarbromal INN CNS depressant; sedative; hypnotic

aceclidine USAN, INN cholinergic

aceclofenac INN, BAN

acedapsone USAN, INN, BAN antimalarial; antibacterial; leprostatic

acediasulfone sodium INN

acedoben INN

acefluranol INN, BAN

acefurtiamine INN

acefylline clofibrol INN

acefylline piperazine INN [also: acepifylline]

aceglaton JAN [also: aceglatone]

aceglatone INN [also: aceglaton]

aceglutamide INN antiulcerative [also: aceglutamide aluminum]

aceglutamide aluminum USAN, JAN antiulcerative [also: aceglutamide]

ACEIs (angiotensin-converting enzyme inhibitors) [q.v.]

acellular pertussis vaccine [see: diphtheria & tetanus toxoids & acellular pertussis (DTaP) vaccine, adsorbed]

acemannan USAN, INN hydrogel wound dressing

acemetacin INN, BAN, JAN

acemethadone [see: methadyl acetate]

aceneuramic acid INN

acenocoumarin [see: acenocoumarol]

acenocoumarol NF, INN [also: nicoumalone]

Aceon tablets ℞ angiotensin-converting enzyme (ACE) inhibitor for hypertension and stable coronary artery disease (CAD) [perindopril erbumine] 2, 4, 8 mg ⊡ Aczone; Ocean

aceperone INN ⊡ aspirin; azaperone; Easprin; esuprone

Acephen suppositories OTC analgesic; antipyretic [acetaminophen] 120, 325, 650 mg ⊡ Asaphen; Ucephan

acephenazine dimaleate [see: aceto-phenazine maleate]

acepifylline BAN [also: acefylline piperazine]

acepromazine INN, BAN *veterinary sedative* [also: acepromazine maleate]

acepromazine maleate USAN *veterinary sedative* [also: acepromazine]

aceprometazine INN

acequinoline INN

acerola *(Malpighia glabra; M. punicifolia)* fruit *natural dietary source of vitamin C* ☑ azarole

acesulfame INN, BAN

Aceta tablets, elixir (discontinued 2008) OTC *analgesic; antipyretic* [acetaminophen] 325, 500 mg; 120 mg/5 mL ☑ ICE-T; Iosat

Aceta with Codeine tablets ℞ *narcotic analgesic; antitussive; antipyretic* [codeine phosphate; acetaminophen] 30•300 mg

Acetadote IV injection ℞ *antidote to severe acetaminophen overdose (orphan); also used to prevent contrast media nephrotoxicity* [acetylcysteine] 20% in 30 mL single-dose vials

Aceta-Gesic tablets (discontinued 2007) OTC *analgesic; antipyretic; antihistamine; sleep aid* [acetaminophen; phenyltoloxamine citrate] 325•30 mg

p-**acetamidobenzoic acid** [see: acedoben]

6-acetamidohexanoic acid [see: acexamic acid]

4-acetamidophenyl acetate [see: diacetamate]

acetaminocaproic acid [see: acexamic acid]

acetaminophen USP *analgesic; antipyretic* [also: paracetamol] 80, 325, 500 mg oral; 160, 166.6 mg/5 mL oral; 120, 325, 650 mg rectal

acetaminophen & butalbital *analgesic; barbiturate sedative* 300•50 mg oral

acetaminophen & caffeine & butalbital *analgesic; barbiturate sedative* 300•40•50, 325•40•50, 500•40•50 mg oral

acetaminophen & caffeine & butalbital & codeine phosphate *barbiturate sedative; narcotic analgesic and antitussive* 325•40•50•30 mg oral

acetaminophen & caffeine & dihydrocodeine bitartrate *narcotic analgesic and antitussive* 712.8•60•32 mg

acetaminophen & codeine *narcotic analgesic; narcotic antitussive* 300•15, 300•30, 300•60 mg oral; 30•12 mg/5 mL oral

acetaminophen & hydrocodone bitartrate *analgesic; narcotic antitussive* 325•5, 325•7.5, 325•10, 500•2.5, 500•5, 500•10, 650•7.5, 650•10, 750•7.5, 750•10 mg oral; 325•10, 500•7.5 mg/15 mL oral

acetaminophen & isometheptene mucate & dichloralphenazone *cerebral vasoconstrictor and analgesic for vascular and tension headaches; "possibly effective" for migraine headaches* 325•65•100 mg oral

acetaminophen & oxycodone HCl *narcotic analgesic* 325•7.5, 325•10, 500•7.5, 650•10 mg oral

acetaminophen & pentazocine HCl *narcotic agonist-antagonist analgesic; antipyretic* 650•25 mg oral

acetaminophen & propoxyphene napsylate *narcotic analgesic; withdrawn from the market in 2010 due to safety concerns* 500•100, 650•100 mg oral

acetaminophen & tramadol HCl *central analgesic for acute pain* 37.5•325 mg oral

acetaminophenol (N-acetyl-*p*-aminophenol) [see: acetaminophen]

acetaminosalol INN

acetanilid (or acetanilide) NF

acetannin [see: acetyltannic acid]

acetarsol INN, BAN [also: acetarsone]

acetarsone NF [also: acetarsol]

acetarsone salt of arecoline [see: drocarbil]

Acetasol ear drops ℞ *antibacterial; antifungal; antiseptic* [acetic acid; benzethonium chloride] 2%•0.02%

Acetasol HC ear drops ℞ *corticosteroidal anti-inflammatory; antibacterial; antifungal; acidifying agent* [hydrocortisone; acetic acid; benzethonium chloride] 1%•2%•0.02%

Acetavance injection (name changed to **Ofirmev** upon marketing release in 2010)

acetazolamide USP, INN, BAN, JAN *carbonic anhydrase inhibitor; diuretic for edema and glaucoma; anticonvulsant for centrencephalic epilepsies; treatment for acute mountain sickness* 125, 250, 500 mg oral; 500 mg injection

acetazolamide sodium USP, JAN *carbonic anhydrase inhibitor; diuretic; anticonvulsant; antiglaucoma; treatment for acute mountain sickness* 500 mg base/vial injection

acetcarbromal [see: acecarbromal]

acet-dia-mer-sulfonamide (sulfacetamide, sulfadiazine & sulfamerazine) [q.v.]

acetergamine INN

Acetest reagent tablets for professional use (discontinued 2008) ℞ *in vitro diagnostic aid for acetone (ketones) in the urine or blood*

acetiamine INN

acetic acid NF, JAN *acidifying agent* 0.25%

acetic acid, aluminum salt [see: aluminum acetate]

acetic acid, calcium salt [see: calcium acetate]

acetic acid, diluted NF *bladder irrigant*

acetic acid, ethyl ester [see: ethyl acetate]

acetic acid, glacial USP, INN *acidifying agent*

acetic acid, potassium salt [see: potassium acetate]

acetic acid, sodium salt trihydrate [see: sodium acetate]

acetic acid, zinc salt dihydrate [see: zinc acetate]

Acetic Acid 2% and Aluminum Acetate Otic ear drops ℞ *antibacterial; antifungal; antiseptic; astringent* [acetic acid; aluminum acetate] 2%• ?

acetic acid & antipyrine & benzocaine & polycosanol *analgesic; anesthetic* 0.01%•5.4%•1.4%•0.01% otic drops

acetic acid & hydrocortisone *acidifying agent; corticosteroid; anti-inflammatory* 2%•1% otic solution

acetic acid 5-nitrofurfurylidenehydrazide [see: nihydrazone]

Acetic Acid Otic ear drops ℞ *antibacterial; antifungal; antiseptic* [acetic acid; benzethonium chloride] 2%•0.02%

aceticyl [see: aspirin]

acetilum acidulatum [see: aspirin]

acetiromate INN

acetohexamide USAN, USP, INN, BAN, JAN *sulfonylurea antidiabetic that stimulates insulin secretion in the pancreas*

acetohydroxamic acid (AHA) USAN, USP, INN *urease enzyme inhibitor for chronic urea-splitting urinary infections*

acetol [see: aspirin]

acetomenaphthone BAN

acetomeroctol

acetone NF *solvent; antiseptic* ⑨ Istin

acetophen [see: aspirin]

acetophenazine INN *antipsychotic* [also: acetophenazine maleate]

acetophenazine maleate USAN, USP *antipsychotic* [also: acetophenazine]

p-acetophenetidide *(withdrawn from the market)* [see: phenacetin]

acetophenetidin *(withdrawn from the market)* [now: phenacetin]

acetorphine INN, BAN *enkephalinase inhibitor for acute diarrhea; investigational for opioid withdrawal and GERD*

acetosal [see: aspirin]

acetosalic acid [see: aspirin]

acetosalin [see: aspirin]

acetosulfone sodium USAN *antibacterial; leprostatic* [also: sulfadiasulfone sodium]

acetoxyphenylmercury [see: phenylmercuric acetate]

acetoxythymoxamine [see: moxisylyte]

acetphenarsine [see: acetarsone]

acetphenetidin (*withdrawn from the market*) [now: phenacetin]

acetphenolisatin [see: oxyphenisatin acetate]

acetrizoate sodium USP [also: sodium acetrizoate]

acetrizoic acid USP

acetryptine INN

acetsalicylamide [see: salacetamide]

acet-theocin sodium [see: theophylline sodium acetate]

aceturate USAN, INN *combining name for radicals or groups*

acetyl adalin [see: acetylcarbromal]

N-acetyl cysteine (NAC) *natural source of cysteine; promotes an increase in the endogenous antioxidant glutathione*

acetyl sulfisoxazole [see: sulfisoxazole acetyl]

***l*-acetyl-α-methadol (LAAM)** [see: levomethadyl acetate]

***p*-acetylaminobenzaldehyde thiosemicarbazone** [see: thioacetazone; thiacetazone]

acetylaminobenzene [see: acetanilid]

N-acetyl-*p*-aminophenol (APAP; NAPA) [see: acetaminophen]

acetylaniline [see: acetanilid]

acetylated polyvinyl alcohol *viscosity-increasing agent*

acetyl-bromo-diethylacetylcarbamide [see: acecarbromal]

acetylcarbromal [see: acecarbromal]

acetylcholine chloride USP, INN, BAN, JAN *cardiac depressant; cholinergic; miotic; peripheral vasodilator*

acetylcholinesterase (AChE) inhibitors *a class of drugs that alter acetylcholine neurotransmitters, used as a cognition adjuvant in Alzheimer dementia* [also called: cholinesterase inhibitors]

N-acetylcysteinate lysine *investigational (orphan) for cystic fibrosis*

acetylcysteine (N-acetylcysteine) USAN, USP, INN, BAN *mucolytic inhaler; antidote to severe acetaminophen overdose (orphan); investigational (orphan) for acute liver failure; also used to prevent contrast media nephrotoxicity* [also: *N*-acetyl-L-cysteine; NAC]

10%, 20% oral; 10%, 20% inhalation solution

acetylcysteine sodium *mucolytic inhaler* 10%, 20% inhalation

N-acetyl-D-glucosamine *natural remedy for osteoarthritis*

acetyldigitoxin (α-acetyldigitoxin) NF, INN

acetyldihydrocodeinone [see: thebacon]

N-acetyl-DL-leucine [see: acetylleucine]

acetylin [see: aspirin]

acetylkitasamycin JAN *antibacterial* [also: kitasamycin; kitasamycin tartrate]

acetyl-L-carnitine (ALC; ALCAR) *natural protector of neurologic and cardiac function; biologically active amino acid that transports fatty acids into the cellular mitochondria for increased energy output; acetylated form of L-carnitine*

N-acetyl-L-cysteine JAN *mucolytic inhaler* [also: acetylcysteine]

N-acetyl-L-cysteine salicylate [see: salnacedin]

acetylleucine (N-acetyl-DL-leucine) INN

acetylmethadol INN *narcotic analgesic* [also: methadyl acetate]

acetyloleandomycin [see: troleandomycin]

2-acetyloxybenzoic acid [see: aspirin]

acetylpheneturide JAN [also: pheneturide]

acetylphenylisatin [see: oxyphenisatin acetate]

N-acetyl-procainamide (NAPA) [see: acecainide HCl]

acetylpropylorvinol [see: acetorphine]

acetylresorcinol [see: resorcinol monoacetate]

acetylsal [see: aspirin]

N-acetylsalicylamide [see: salacetamide]

acetylsalicylate aluminum [see: aspirin aluminum]

acetylsalicylic acid (ASA) [now: aspirin]

acetylsalicylic acid, phenacetin & caffeine [see: APC]

acetylspiramycin JAN *macrolide antibiotic* [also: spiramycin]

acetylsulfamethoxazole JAN *broad-spectrum sulfonamide bacteriostatic* [also: sulfamethoxazole; sulphamethoxazole; sulfamethoxazole sodium]

acetyltannic acid USP

acetyltannin [see: acetyltannic acid]

acevaltrate INN

acexamic acid INN

AChE (acetylcholinesterase) inhibitors [q.v.]

Achillea millefolium medicinal herb [see: yarrow]

aciclovir INN, JAN *antiviral* [also: acyclovir]

acid acriflavine [see: acriflavine HCl]

acid alpha-glucosidase, human [see: alglucosidase alfa]

acid citrate dextrose (ACD) [see: anticoagulant citrate dextrose solution]

Acid Gone oral liquid OTC *antacid* [aluminum hydroxide; magnesium carbonate] 95•358 mg/15 mL

acid histamine phosphate [see: histamine phosphate]

Acid Jelly OTC *antibacterial; acidity modifier; moisturizer/lubricant* [acetic acid; oxyquinoline sulfate; ricinoleic acid; glycerin] 0.921%•0.025%• 0.7%•5%

Acid Mantle cream base (name changed to **A-Mantle** in 2007)

Acid Reducer 200 film-coated tablets OTC *histamine H_2 antagonist for episodic heartburn and acid indigestion* [cimetidine] 200 mg

acid sphingomyelinase *investigational (orphan) agent for Niemann-Pick disease type B*

acid trypaflavine [see: acriflavine HCl]

acidogen [see: glutamic acid HCl]

acidol HCl [see: betaine HCl]

Acidophilus capsules, wafers OTC *natural intestinal bacteria; probiotic; dietary supplement; fever blister treatment* [Lactobacillus acidophilus] >100 million CFU; 20 million CFU

acidophilus *(Lactobacillus acidophilus) natural bacteria for replenishment of normal flora in the gastrointestinal tract and vagina; not generally regarded as safe and effective as an antidiarrheal*

Acidophilus with Bifidus wafers OTC *natural intestinal bacteria; probiotic; dietary supplement* [Lactobacillus acidophilus; L. bifidus] 1 billion CFU total

acidulated phosphate fluoride (sodium fluoride & hydrofluoric acid) *dental caries preventative*

acidum acetylsalicylicum [see: aspirin]

Acid-X tablets (discontinued 2009) OTC *analgesic; antipyretic; antacid* [acetaminophen; calcium carbonate] 500•250 mg

acifran USAN, INN *antihyperlipoproteinemic* ② Isovorin

aciglumin [see: glutamic acid HCl]

acinitrazole BAN *veterinary antibacterial* [also: nithiamide; aminitrozole]

Aciphex enteric-coated delayed-release tablets ℞ *proton pump inhibitor for duodenal ulcers, erosive or ulcerative gastroesophageal reflux disease (GERD), H. pylori infection, and other gastroesophageal disorders* [rabeprazole sodium] 20 mg

acipimox INN, BAN

acistrate INN *combining name for radicals or groups*

acitemate INN

acitretin USAN, INN, BAN *second generation retinoid; retinoic acid analogue; systemic antipsoriatic*

acivicin USAN, INN *antineoplastic*

ackee *(Blighia sapida) fruit medicinal herb for colds, fever, edema, and epilepsy; not generally regarded as safe and effective as seeds and unripened fruit are highly toxic*

aclacinomycin A [now: aclarubicin]

aclantate INN

Aclaro PD emulsion ℞ *hyperpigmentation bleaching agent* [hydroquinone] 4%

aclarubicin USAN, INN, BAN *antibiotic antineoplastic* [also: aclarubicin HCl]

aclarubicin HCl JAN *antibiotic antineoplastic* [also: aclarubicin]

aclatonium napadisilate INN, BAN, JAN

aclidinium bromide *investigational (Phase III) long-acting inhaled anticholinergic for chronic obstructive pulmonary disease (COPD)*

Aclovate ointment, cream ℞ *corticosteroidal anti-inflammatory* [alclometasone dipropionate] 0.05%

A.C.N. tablets (discontinued 2008) OTC *vitamin supplement* [vitamins A, B₃, and C] 25 000 U•25 mg•250 mg ② A1cNOW; Acanya

Acne Clear gel OTC *keratolytic for acne* [benzoyl peroxide] 10%

Acne Lotion 10 OTC *antiseptic and keratolytic for acne* [colloidal sulfur] 10%

Acne Medication gel OTC *keratolytic for acne* [benzoyl peroxide] 10%

Acno lotion (discontinued 2009) OTC *antiseptic and keratolytic for acne* [sulfur] 3% ② A1cNOW; Acanya

Acno Cleanser topical liquid OTC *cleanser for acne* [isopropyl alcohol] 60%

Acnomel; Adult Acnomel cream OTC *antiseptic, antifungal, and keratolytic for acne* [sulfur; resorcinol; alcohol] 8%•2%•11%

Acnotex lotion OTC *antiseptic, antifungal, and keratolytic for acne* [sulfur; resorcinol; isopropyl alcohol] 8%•2%•20%

ACNU (1-(4-amino-2-methyl-5-pyrimidnyl)-methyl-3-(2-chloroethyl)-3-nitrosourea) [see: nimustin]

acodazole INN *antineoplastic* [also: acodazole HCl]

acodazole HCl USAN *antineoplastic* [also: acodazole]

Acomplia ⓔⓤⓡ (available in 7 European countries) *investigational (NDA filed) selective cannabinoid CB₁ blocker for smoking cessation, weight loss, increasing HDL, increasing insulin sensitivity, and decreasing C-reactive protein (CRP) levels* [rimonabant] 20 mg

aconiazide INN *investigational (orphan) agent for tuberculosis*

aconite *(Aconitum napellus)* plant and root *medicinal herb for fever, hypertension, and neuralgia; not generally regarded as safe and effective as it is highly toxic*

aconitine USP ② Akineton

acortan [see: corticotropin]

Acorus calamus *medicinal herb* [see: calamus]

acoxatrine INN

9-acridinamine monohydrochloride [see: aminacrine HCl]

acridinyl anisidide [see: amsacrine]

acridinylamine methanesulfon anisidide (AMSA) [see: amsacrine]

acridorex INN

acrids *a class of agents that have a pungent taste or cause heat and irritation when applied to the skin*

acriflavine NF

acriflavine HCl NF [also: acriflavinium chloride]

acriflavinium chloride INN [also: acriflavine HCl]

acrihellin INN

acrinol JAN [also: ethacridine lactate; ethacridine]

acrisorcin USAN, USP, INN *antifungal*

acrivastine USAN, INN, BAN *antihistamine*

acrocinonide INN

acronine USAN, INN *antineoplastic*

acrosoxacin BAN *antibacterial* [also: rosoxacin]

AcryDerm Strands wound dressing ℞ *high-exudate absorbent dressing for cavitated wounds*

ACT oral rinse OTC *dental caries preventative* [sodium fluoride; alcohol 7%] 0.05% ② AZT

ACT (actinomycin) [see: cactinomycin; dactinomycin]

Actaea alba; A. pachypoda; A. rubra *medicinal herb* [see: white cohosh]

Actaea racemosa *medicinal herb* [see: black cohosh]

actagardin INN

actaplanin USAN, INN, BAN *veterinary growth stimulant*

actarit INN

Actemra IV infusion ℞ *once-monthly interleukin-6 inhibitor for moderate to severe rheumatoid arthritis* [tocilizumab] 20 mg/mL

ACTH (adrenocorticotropic hormone) [see: corticotropin]

Acthar Gel [see: H.P. Acthar Gel]

ActHIB powder for injection ℞ *vaccine for* H. influenzae *type b (HIB) infections in children 2–18 months and invasive diseases caused by HIB infections in children 15–18 months* [Haemophilus influenzae b conjugate vaccine; tetanus toxoid] 10•24 mcg/0.5 mL 🔲 AK-Tob

ActHIB/Tripedia IM injection ℞ *vaccine for* H. influenzae *type b (HIB) infections in children younger than 5 months* [Haemophilus influenzae b conjugate vaccine; diphtheria & tetanus toxoids & acellular pertussis (DTaP) vaccine] 10 mcg•6.7 LfU•5 LfU•46.8 mcg per 0.5 mL

Acthrel IV infusion ℞ *diagnostic aid for adrenocorticotropic hormone (ACTH)-dependent Cushing syndrome (orphan)* [corticorelin ovine (as triflutate)] 100 mcg

ActiBath effervescent tablets OTC *moisturizer; emollient* [colloidal oatmeal] 20%

Acticin cream ℞ *parasiticide for scabies and lice; also used for papulopustular rosacea* [permethrin] 5%

Acticort 100 lotion ℞ *corticosteroidal anti-inflammatory* [hydrocortisone] 1%

Actidose with Sorbitol oral suspension OTC *adsorbent antidote for poisoning; reduces intestinal transit time* [activated charcoal; sorbitol] 25• $\underline{2}$ g/120 mL; 50• $\underline{2}$ g/240 mL

Actidose-Aqua oral suspension OTC *adsorbent antidote for poisoning* [activated charcoal] 25 g/120 mL, 50 g/240 mL

Actifed Cold & Allergy tablets OTC *decongestant; antihistamine* [phenylephrine HCl; chlorpheniramine maleate] 10•4 mg

Actigall capsules ℞ *naturally occurring bile acid for primary biliary cirrhosis (orphan); gallstone preventative and dissolving agent* [ursodiol] 300 mg

Actimid investigational (orphan) agent for multiple myeloma [a-(3-aminophthalimido) glutaramide]

Actimmune subcu injection ℞ *immunoregulator for chronic granulomatous disease (orphan) and severe malignant osteopetrosis (orphan); investigational (orphan) for renal cell carcinoma and pulmonary fibrosis* [interferon gamma-1b] 100 mcg (2 million IU)

actinium *element (Ac)*

actinomycin C BAN *antibiotic antineoplastic* [also: cactinomycin]

actinomycin D JAN *antibiotic antineoplastic* [also: dactinomycin]

actinoquinol INN *ultraviolet screen* [also: actinoquinol sodium]

actinoquinol sodium USAN *ultraviolet screen* [also: actinoquinol]

actinospectocin [see: spectinomycin]

Actiq "lollipops" ℞ *transmucosal narcotic analgesic for chronic pain in opioid-tolerant cancer patients* [fentanyl (as citrate)] 200, 400, 600, 800, 1200, 1600 mcg

actisomide USAN, INN *antiarrhythmic* 🔲 octazamide

Activase powder for IV infusion ℞ *tissue plasminogen activator (tPA) for acute myocardial infarction, acute ischemic stroke, or pulmonary embolism; investigational (orphan) for intraventricular hemorrhage with intracerebral hemorrhage* [alteplase] 50, 100 mg/vial (29, 58 million IU/vial)

Activase Cathflo [see: Cathflo Activase]

activated attapulgite [see: attapulgite, activated]

activated carbon

activated charcoal [see: charcoal, activated]

activated 7-dehydrocholesterol [see: cholecalciferol]

activated ergosterol [see: ergocalciferol]

activated prothrombin complex BAN

Activated Vegetable Charcoal capsules OTC *adsorbent antidote for poisoning* [activated charcoal] 260 mg

Activella film-coated tablets (in packs of 28) ℞ *a mixture of natural and synthetic hormones; hormone replacement therapy for postmenopausal symptoms* [estradiol; norethindrone acetate] 1•0.5, 0.5•0.1 mg

actodigin USAN, INN *cardiotonic*

Actonel film-coated tablets ℞ *bisphosphonate bone resorption inhibitor for Paget disease and corticosteroid-induced or age-related osteoporosis in men and women* [risedronate sodium] 5, 30, 35, 75, 150 mg

Actonel with Calcium monthly dosepak (28 film-coated tablets) ℞ *bisphosphonate bone resorption inhibitor for postmenopausal osteoporosis in women; calcium supplement* [risedronate sodium; calcium (as carbonate)] 35•0 mg × 4 tablets; 0•500 mg × 24 tablets

Actonel with Calcium weekly dosepak (7 film-coated tablets) (discontinued 2007) ℞ *bisphosphonate bone resorption inhibitor for postmenopausal osteoporosis in women; calcium supplement* [risedronate sodium; calcium (as carbonate)] 35•0 mg × 1 tablet; 0•500 mg × 6 tablets

ACTOplus met film-coated tablets ℞ *combination antidiabetic agent for type 2 diabetes that decreases hepatic glucose production and increases cellular response to insulin without increasing insulin secretion* [pioglitazone HCl; metformin HCl] 15•500, 15•850 mg

ACTOplus met XR film-coated extended-release tablets ℞ *combination antidiabetic agent for type 2 diabetes that decreases hepatic glucose production and increases cellular response to insulin without increasing insulin secretion* [pioglitazone (as HCl); metformin HCl] 15•1000, 30•1000 mg

Actos tablets ℞ *antidiabetic for type 2 diabetes that increases cellular response to insulin without increasing insulin secretion* [pioglitazone HCl] 15, 30, 45 mg

Act·O·Vial (trademarked packaging form) *vial system*

ACU·dyne ointment, perineal wash concentrate, prep solution, skin cleanser, prep swabs, swabsticks OTC *broad-spectrum antimicrobial* [povidone-iodine]

ACU·dyne Douche vaginal concentrate OTC *antiseptic/germicidal cleanser and deodorizer* [povidone-iodine]

Acular; Acular LS eye drops ℞ *nonsteroidal anti-inflammatory drug (NSAID) for allergic conjunctivitis, cataract extraction, and corneal refractive surgery* [ketorolac tromethamine] 0.5%; 0.4%

Acular PF eye drops (discontinued 2009) ℞ *nonsteroidal anti-inflammatory drug (NSAID) for allergic conjunctivitis, cataract extraction, and corneal refractive surgery* [ketorolac tromethamine] 0.5%

Acurox *investigational (NDA filed) immediate-release opioid analgesic for moderate-to-severe pain; incorporates abuse-deterrent technology to prevent its conversion to a street drug* [oxycodone HCl; niacin]

AcuTect ℞ *radiopharmaceutical diagnostic aid for acute venous thrombosis* [technetium Tc 99m apcitide]

Acuvail eye drops ℞ *nonsteroidal anti-inflammatory drug (NSAID) for allergic conjunctivitis, cataract extraction, and corneal refractive surgery* [ketorolac tromethamine] 0.45%

acycloguanosine [see: acyclovir]

acyclovir USAN, USP, BAN *oral antiviral for herpes simplex virus type 2 (HSV-2, genital herpes), herpes zoster (shingles), and adult-onset varicella (chickenpox); prophylaxis of viral infections in immunocompromised patients* [also: aciclovir] 200, 400, 800 mg oral; 200/5 mL oral

acyclovir & hydrocortisone *antiviral for herpes simplex; corticosteroidal anti-inflammatory* 5%•1% topical

acyclovir redox [see: redox-acyclovir]

acyclovir sodium USAN *parenteral antiviral for herpes simplex virus types 1 and 2 (HSV-1 and HSV-2), herpes simplex encephalitis, and neonatal HSV infections; prophylaxis of viral infections in immunocompromised patients* 50 mg/mL injection

acylCoA transferase (ACAT) inhibitors *a class of antihyperlipidemics that lower serum cholesterol levels*

acylpyrin [see: aspirin]

Aczone gel ℞ *antibacterial for acne vulgaris* [dapsone] 5% ⊠ Aceon; Ocean

AD (Adriamycin, dacarbazine) *chemotherapy protocol for bone and soft tissue sarcoma*

A+D Zinc Oxide cream OTC *diaper rash treatment* [dimethicone; zinc oxide] 1%•10%

ADA (adenosine deaminase) [see: pegademase bovine; pegademase]

Adacel IM injection ℞ *active immunizing agent for diphtheria, tetanus, and pertussis; Tdap (tetanus predominant) booster vaccine used in adults and children ≥ 11 years* [diphtheria toxoid; tetanus toxoid; detoxified pertussis toxins] 2 LfU•5 LfU•2.5 mcg per 0.5 mL dose

adafenoxate INN

Adagen IM injection ℞ *adenosine deaminase (ADA) enzyme replacement for severe combined immunodeficiency disease (orphan)* [pegademase bovine] 250 U/mL

Adalat capsules (discontinued 2008) ℞ *calcium channel blocker for angina* [nifedipine] 10, 20 mg

Adalat CC film-coated sustained-release tablets ℞ *calcium channel blocker for hypertension; also used for anal fissures and Raynaud phenomenon* [nifedipine] 30, 60, 90 mg

adalimumab INN *recombinant human immunoglobulin G1 (rhIgG1); tumor necrosis factor-alpha (TNF-α) blocker;* *DMARD for moderate to severe rheumatoid arthritis (RA), psoriatic arthritis, and ankylosing spondylitis; immunostimulant for Crohn disease*

adamantanamine [see: amantadine]

adamantanamine HCl [see: amantadine HCl]

adamexine INN

adapalene USAN, INN, BAN *synthetic retinoid analogue for topical treatment of acne* 0.1% topical

Adapettes solution (discontinued 2009) OTC *rewetting solution for hard contact lenses*

Adapettes Especially for Sensitive Eyes solution OTC *rewetting solution for soft contact lenses*

adaprolol maleate USAN *ophthalmic antihypertensive (beta-blocker)*

adaptive aerosol delivery (AAD) system [see: I-neb AAD; Prodose AAD]

adatanserin INN *anxiolytic; antidepressant* [also: adatanserin HCl]

adatanserin HCl USAN *anxiolytic; antidepressant* [also: adatanserin]

AdatoSil 5000 intraocular injection ℞ *retinal tamponade for retinal detachment* [polydimethylsiloxane] 10, 15 mL

Adavite tablets (discontinued 2008) OTC *vitamin supplement* [multiple vitamins; folic acid; biotin] ≜•400•35 mcg ⊠ Advate

Adavite-M tablets (discontinued 2008) OTC *vitamin/mineral/iron supplement* [multiple vitamins & minerals; iron; folic acid; biotin] ≜•27 mg•0.4 mg•30 mcg

ADC (antibody-drug conjugate) [q.v.]

ADC with Fluoride pediatric oral drops (discontinued 2008) ℞ *vitamin supplement; dental caries preventative* [vitamins A, C, and D; fluoride] 1500 U•35 mg•400 U•0.5 mg per mL

Adcetris IV infusion ℞ *antineoplastic for Hodgkin lymphoma and anaplastic large cell lymphoma (ALCL)* [brentuximab vedotin] 50 mg/vial

Adcirca film-coated tablets ℞ *selective vasodilator for pulmonary arterial hypertension (orphan)* [tadalafil] 20 mg

Adderall tablets (discontinued 2011) ℞ *CNS stimulant for attention-deficit/ hyperactivity disorder (ADHD), narcolepsy, and obesity* [amphetamine aspartate; amphetamine sulfate; dextroamphetamine sulfate; dextroamphetamine saccharate] 5, 7.5, 10, 12.5, 15, 20, 30 mg total amphetamines (25% of each)

Adderall XR capsules containing extended-release spheres ℞ *once-daily CNS stimulant for attention-deficit/hyperactivity disorder (ADHD)* [amphetamine aspartate; amphetamine sulfate; dextroamphetamine sulfate; dextroamphetamine saccharate] 5, 10, 15, 20, 25, 30 mg total amphetamines (25% of each)

adder's mouth *medicinal herb* [see: chickweed]

adder's tongue (Erythronium americanum) bulb and leaves *medicinal herb used as an emetic, antiscrofulous agent, and emollient*

ADD-Vantage (trademarked delivery device) *intravenous drug admixture device*

ADE (ara-C, daunorubicin, etoposide) *chemotherapy protocol for acute myelocytic leukemia (AML)*

adefovir dipivoxil USAN *nucleotide analogue reverse transcriptase inhibitor for chronic hepatitis B virus (HBV) infection*

ADEKs caplets (discontinued 2011) OTC *vitamin/mineral supplement* [multiple vitamins & minerals; folic acid; biotin] ≐•200•50 mcg ⍰ Adoxa; Edex; Iodex

ADEKs pediatric oral drops (discontinued 2008) OTC *vitamin/mineral supplement* [multiple vitamins & minerals; biotin] ≐•15 mcg ⍰ Adoxa; Edex; Iodex

adelmidrol INN

ademetionine INN

adenazole [see: tocladesine]

adenine USP, JAN *amino acid*

adenine arabinoside (ara-A) [see: vidarabine]

adeno-associated viral vector containing the gene for human coagulation Factor IX *investigational (orphan) agent for moderate to severe hemophilia*

adeno-associated viral-based vector cystic fibrosis gene therapy *investigational (orphan) for cystic fibrosis*

Adenocard IV injection ℞ *antiarrhythmic for paroxysmal supraventricular tachycardia* [adenosine] 3 mg/mL

Adenoscan IV infusion ℞ *cardiac diagnostic aid; cardiac stressor; adjunct to thallium 201 myocardial perfusion scintigraphy* [adenosine] 3 mg/mL

adenosine USAN, BAN *antiarrhythmic for paroxysmal supraventricular tachycardia; also used as a diagnostic aid for coronary artery disease; investigational (orphan) for brain tumors* 3 mg/mL injection

adenosine deaminase (ADA) [see: pegademase bovine; pegademase]

adenosine monophosphate (AMP) [see: adenosine phosphate]

adenosine phosphate USAN, INN, BAN *nutrient; treatment for varicose veins and herpes infections*

adenosine triphosphatase (ATPase) *investigational (Phase III) injection for acute treatment of paroxysmal supraventricular tachycardia (PSVT)*

adenosine triphosphate (ATP) disodium JAN

S-adenosyl-L-methionine (SAMe) *natural amino acid derivative used to treat depression and protect the liver from toxic overload; regenerates liver function and restores hepatic glutathione levels when taken with B vitamins; investigational (orphan) for AIDS-related myelopathy*

adenovirus-based vector Factor VIII complementary DNA to somatic cells *investigational (orphan) agent for hemophilia A*

adenovirus-mediated herpes simplex virus-thymidine kinase gene *investigational (orphan) agent for malignant glioma*

5'-adenylic acid [see: adenosine phosphate]

adepsine oil [see: mineral oil]

adhesive bandage [see: bandage, adhesive]

adhesive tape [see: tape, adhesive]

adibendan INN

adicillin INN, BAN

adimolol INN

adinazolam USAN, INN, BAN *antidepressant; sedative*

adinazolam mesylate USAN *antidepressant*

Adipex-P capsules, tablets ℞ *anorexiant; CNS stimulant* [phentermine HCl] 37.5 mg

adiphenine INN *smooth muscle relaxant* [also: adiphenine HCl]

adiphenine HCl USAN *smooth muscle relaxant* [also: adiphenine]

adipiodone INN, JAN *parenteral radiopaque contrast medium* [also: iodipamide]

adipiodone meglumine JAN *parenteral radiopaque contrast medium (49.42% iodine)* [also: iodipamide meglumine]

aditeren INN

aditoprim INN

Adlea topical liquid *investigational highly purified natural product used during surgery to block pain receptors* [capsaicin]

adnephrine [see: epinephrine]

Adolph's Salt Substitute OTC *salt substitute; electrolyte replenisher* [potassium chloride] 64 mEq K/5 g; 35 mEq K/5 g

adosopine INN

Adoxa film-coated tablets ℞ *tetracycline antibiotic* [doxycycline (as monohydrate)] 50, 75, 100, 150 mg ⊘ ADEKs; Edex; Iodex

adozelesin USAN, INN *antineoplastic*

Adprin-B coated tablets (discontinued 2007) OTC *analgesic; antipyretic; antiinflammatory; antirheumatic* [aspirin (buffered with calcium carbonate, magnesium oxide, and magnesium carbonate)] 325, 500 mg

ADR (Adriamycin) [see: Adriamycin; doxorubicin HCl]

adrafinil INN

adrenal [see: epinephrine]

adrenal cortical steroids *a class of steroid hormones that stimulate the adrenal cortex*

Adrenalin Chloride nose drops ℞ *nasal decongestant* [epinephrine (as HCl)] 0.1% (1 mg/mL or 1:1000)

Adrenalin Chloride solution for inhalation (discontinued 2009) ℞ *sympathomimetic bronchodilator and vasopressor for bronchial asthma* [epinephrine (as HCl)] 1:100, 1:1000 (10, 1 mg/mL)

Adrenalin Chloride subcu, IV, IM or intracardiac injection ℞ *sympathomimetic bronchodilator and vasopressor for bronchial asthma, bronchospasm, and COPD* [epinephrine (as HCl)] 1:1000 (1 mg/mL)

adrenaline BAN *vasoconstrictor; sympathomimetic bronchodilator; topical antiglaucoma agent; vasopressor for shock; emergency treatment of anaphylaxis* [also: epinephrine]

adrenaline bitartrate [see: epinephrine bitartrate]

adrenaline HCl [see: epinephrine HCl]

adrenalone USAN, INN *ophthalmic adrenergic*

adrenamine [see: epinephrine]

adrenergic agonists *a class of bronchodilators that relax the bronchial muscles, reducing bronchospasm; a class of cardiac agents that increase myocardial contractility, causing a vasopressor effect to counteract shock (inadequate tissue perfusion)* [also called: sympathomimetics]

adrenine [see: epinephrine]

adrenochromazone [see: carbazochrome salicylate]

adrenochrome [see: carbazochrome salicylate]

adrenochrome guanylhydrazone mesilate JAN

adrenochrome monoaminoguanidine sodium methylsulfonate

[see: adrenochrome guanylhydrazone mesilate]

adrenochrome monosemicarbazone sodium salicylate [see: carbazochrome salicylate]

adrenocorticotrophin [see: corticotropin]

adrenocorticotropic hormone (ACTH) [see: corticotropin]

adrenone [see: adrenalone]

AdreView IV injection ℞ *radioactive diagnostic aid for the detection of metastatic pheochromocytoma or neuroblastoma (orphan)* [iobenguane sulfate I 123] 74 MBq/mL (2 mCi/mL)

Adriamycin PFS (preservative-free solution) IV injection ℞ *anthracycline antibiotic antineoplastic* [doxorubicin HCl] 2 mg/mL

Adriamycin RDF (rapid dissolution formula) powder for IV injection ℞ *anthracycline antibiotic antineoplastic* [doxorubicin HCl] 10, 20, 50, 150 mg/vial

Adria-Oncoline Chemo-Pin (trademarked delivery form)

adrogolide INN

adrogolide HCl USAN *dopamine D_1 receptor agonist for Parkinson disease*

Adrucil IV injection ℞ *antimetabolite antineoplastic for colorectal (orphan), esophageal (orphan), breast, stomach, and pancreatic cancers; investigational (orphan) for glioblastoma multiforme; also used for several other cancers* [fluorouracil] 50 mg/mL

ADS (azodisal sodium) [now: olsalazine sodium]

adsorbed diphtheria toxoid [see: diphtheria toxoid, adsorbed]

Adsorbocarpine eye drops ℞ *antiglaucoma agent; direct-acting miotic* [pilocarpine HCl] 1%, 2%, 4%

Adsorbonac eye drops (discontinued 2010) OTC *corneal edema-reducing agent* [sodium chloride (hypertonic saline solution)] 2%, 5%

ADT (trademarked dosage form) *alternate-day therapy* ② ACT; AZT

Adult Acnomel [see: Acnomel]

Advagraf ⑪ extended-release form of **Prograf** (approved in Europe) *investigational (NDA filed) once-daily immunosuppressant for liver, kidney, and heart transplants* [tacrolimus]

Advair Diskus 100/50; Advair Diskus 250/50; Advair Diskus 500/50 inhalation powder in a metered-dose inhaler ℞ *combination corticosteroidal anti-inflammatory and bronchodilator for chronic asthma and chronic obstructive pulmonary disease (COPD) with chronic bronchitis and/or emphysema* [fluticasone propionate; salmeterol (as xinafoate)] 100•50 mcg; 250•50 mcg; 500•50 mcg

Advair HFA 45/21; Advair HFA 115/21; Advair HFA 230/21 inhalation aerosol in a metered-dose inhaler ℞ *combination corticosteroidal anti-inflammatory and bronchodilator for chronic asthma* [fluticasone propionate; salmeterol (as xinafoate)] 45•21 mcg; 115•21 mcg; 230•21 mcg

Advance test stick for home use OTC *in vitro diagnostic aid; urine pregnancy test*

"Advanced" or "Advanced Formula" products [see also under product name]

Advanced Care Cholesterol Test kit for home use OTC *in vitro diagnostic aid for cholesterol in the blood*

Advanced D5000 softgels OTC *vitamin D supplement* [vitamin D] 5000 U

Advanced Ear Health Formula caplets OTC *dietary lipotropic; vitamin/calcium supplement* [choline; inositol; multiple B vitamins; vitamin C; calcium; bioflavonoids] 111•111•≛• 100•200 mg

Advanced Eye Relief eye drops OTC *moisturizer/lubricant* [propylene glycol; glycerin] 1%•0.3%

Advanced Eye Relief Redness Instant Relief; Advanced Eye Relief Redness Maximum Relief eye drops OTC *decongestant; vasoconstrictor* [naphazoline HCl] 0.012%; 0.03%

Advanced-RF Natal Care tablets (discontinued 2009) ℞ *vitamin/mineral/calcium/iron supplement; stool softener* [multiple vitamins & minerals; calcium; iron; folic acid; docusate sodium] ± • 200 • 90 • 1 • 50 mg

Advantage 24 vaginal gel OTC *spermicidal contraceptive (for use with a diaphragm)* [nonoxynol 9] 3.5% ⊠ ADD-Vantage

Advantage Invisible Acne Patch topical liquid OTC *keratolytic* [salicylic acid] 2%

Advate powder for IV injection ℞ *systemic hemostatic; antihemophilic for the prevention and control of bleeding in classical hemophilia (hemophilia A) and von Willebrand disease (orphan)* [antihemophilic factor VIII, recombinant] 250, 500, 1000, 1500, 2000, 3000 U/vial ⊠ Adavite

Advera oral liquid OTC *enteral nutritional therapy for HIV and AIDS patients* [lactose-free formula] 240 mL

Advia Centaur HBc IgM test kit for professional use (discontinued 2008) ℞ *in vitro diagnostic aid to detect IgM antibodies to hepatitis B core (HBc) antigen*

Advicor caplets ℞ *combination treatment for hypercholesterolemia and mixed dyslipidemia: HMG-CoA reductase inhibitor to lower LDL and total cholesterol plus niacin to raise HDL and lower triglycerides* [lovastatin; extended-release niacin] 20 • 500, 20 • 750, 20 • 1000, 40 • 1000 mg

Advil tablets, Liqui-Gels (liquid-filled gelcaps) OTC *analgesic; antiarthritic; antipyretic; nonsteroidal anti-inflammatory drug (NSAID) for mild to moderate pain, migraine headaches, and primary dysmenorrhea* [ibuprofen] 200 mg

Advil, Children's oral suspension OTC *analgesic; antipyretic; nonsteroidal anti-inflammatory drug (NSAID) for minor aches and pains* [ibuprofen] 100 mg/5 mL

Advil, Children's; Advil Junior Strength chewable tablets (discontinued 2009) OTC *analgesic; antipyretic; nonsteroidal anti-inflammatory drug (NSAID) for minor aches and pains* [ibuprofen] 50 mg; 100 mg

Advil Allergy Sinus caplets OTC *decongestant; antihistamine; analgesic; antipyretic* [pseudoephedrine HCl; chlorpheniramine maleate; ibuprofen] 30 • 2 • 200 mg

Advil Cold & Sinus Liqui-gels (liquid-filled gelcaps), caplets OTC *decongestant; analgesic; antipyretic* [pseudoephedrine HCl; ibuprofen] 30 • 200 mg

Advil Migraine liquid-filled capsules OTC *analgesic; antipyretic; nonsteroidal anti-inflammatory drug (NSAID) for mild to moderate pain of migraine headaches* [ibuprofen] 200 mg

Advil Pediatric Drops oral suspension OTC *analgesic; antipyretic; nonsteroidal anti-inflammatory drug (NSAID) for minor aches and pains* [ibuprofen] 40 mg/mL

Advil PM capsules, caplets OTC *analgesic; antipyretic; antihistaminic sleep aid* [ibuprofen; diphenhydramine citrate] 200 • 25 mg; 200 • 38 mg

AEDs (anti-epileptic drugs) [see: anticonvulsants]

AEGR-733 *investigational (Phase III, orphan) novel antihyperlipidemic for homozygous familial hypercholesterolemia*

A-E-R pads OTC *emollient; astringent* [hamamelis water (witch hazel)] 50%

AeroBid; AeroBid-M oral inhalation aerosol ℞ *corticosteroidal anti-inflammatory for chronic asthma* [flunisolide] 250 mcg/dose ⊠ EryPed

AeroCaine aerosol solution (discontinued 2007) OTC *anesthetic; antiseptic* [benzocaine; benzethonium chloride] 13.6% • 0.5% ⊠ argon; Ircon

AeroChamber (trademarked delivery device) *aerosol holding chamber*

Aerofreeze topical spray OTC *refrigerant anesthetic* [trichloromonofluoromethane; dichlorodifluoromethane] ⊠ OraVerse

Aerohist extended-release tablets ℞ *antihistamine; anticholinergic to dry*

mucosal secretions [chlorpheniramine maleate; methscopolamine nitrate] 8•2.5 mg

AeroHist Plus extended-release caplets ℞ *decongestant; antihistamine; anticholinergic to dry mucosal secretions* [phenylephrine HCl; chlorpheniramine maleate; methscopolamine nitrate] 20•8•2.5 mg

AeroKid syrup ℞ *decongestant; antihistamine; anticholinergic to dry mucosal secretions* [phenylephrine HCl; chlorpheniramine maleate; methscopolamine nitrate] 10•4•1.25 mg/5 mL

Aerolate Sr.; Aerolate Jr.; Aerolate III timed-action capsules ℞ *antiasthmatic; bronchodilator* [theophylline] 260 mg; 130 mg; 65 mg

Aerolizer (trademarked delivery device) *oral inhaler for encapsulated dry powder*

Aeropin *investigational (orphan) for cystic fibrosis* [heparin, 2-O-desulfated]

Aeroseb-Dex aerosol spray ℞ *corticosteroidal anti-inflammatory* [dexamethasone] 0.01%

aerosol OT [see: docusate sodium]

aerosolized pooled immune globulin [see: globulin, aerosolized pooled immune]

AeroSpan oral inhalation aerosol ℞ *corticosteroidal anti-inflammatory for chronic asthma* [flunisolide hemihydrate] 80 mcg/dose ☒ erizepine

Aerotrol (trademarked delivery form) *inhalation aerosol* ☒ Urotrol

AeroTuss 12 oral suspension ℞ *antitussive* [dextromethorphan tannate] 30 mg/5 mL ☒ Artiss

AeroZoin topical spray OTC *skin protectant; antiseptic* [benzoin; isopropyl alcohol 44.8%] 30% ☒ Orasone; Ureacin

Aesculus hippocastanum; A. californica; A. glabra medicinal herb [see: horse chestnut]

Aethusa cynapium medicinal herb [see: dog poison]

aethylis chloridum [see: ethyl chloride]

afalanine INN

Afeditab CR extended-release tablets ℞ *calcium channel blocker for hypertension; also used for anal fissures and Raynaud phenomenon* [nifedipine] 30, 60 mg

Afinitor tablets ℞ *once-daily antineoplastic for advanced renal cell carcinoma, subependymal giant cell astrocytoma (SGCA) secondary to tuberous sclerosis complex (TSC), and pancreatic neuroendocrine tumors* [everolimus] 2.5, 5, 10 mg

aflibercept *vascular endothelial growth factor (VEGF) inhibitor; investigational (NDA filed) angiogenesis inhibitor for various solid tumors, wet age-related macular degeneration (AMD), central retinal vein occlusion (CRVO), and diabetic macular edema (DME)* [also known as: VEGF Trap (for cancer); VEGF Trap-Eye (for macular degeneration)]

afloqualone INN, JAN

Afluria suspension for IM injection in prefilled syringes ℞ *seasonal influenza virus types A and B vaccine for patients* ≥ 6 months [influenza split-virus vaccine (preservative free)] 0.5 mL/dose

Afluria suspension for IM injection in multidose vials ℞ *seasonal influenza virus types A and B vaccine for patients* ≥ 6 months [influenza split-virus vaccine (with thiomersal preservative)] 0.5 mL/dose (mercury 24.5 mcg/dose)

afovirsen INN *antisense antiviral*

afovirsen sodium USAN *antisense antiviral*

AFP-Scan *investigational (orphan) for diagnostic aid for AFP-producing tumors, hepatoblastoma, and hepatocellular carcinoma* [monoclonal antibodies to human alpha-fetoprotein (AFP), murine, radiolabeled with technetium Tc 99m]

A-Free Prenatal tablet OTC *prenatal vitamin/mineral/calcium/iron supplement* [multiple vitamins & minerals; calcium; iron (as ferrous fumarate); folic acid; biotin] ± •333•9•0.27•0.01 mg

Afrezza *investigational (NDA filed) orally inhaled, ultra rapid–acting insulin for diabetes* [insulin]

African ginger *medicinal herb* [see: ginger]

African pepper; African red pepper *medicinal herb* [see: cayenne]

Afrin 12-Hour Original nasal spray, pump spray OTC *nasal decongestant* [oxymetazoline HCl] 0.05%

Afrin All Night No-Drip; Afrin No-Drip 12-Hour; Afrin No-Drip 12-Hour Extra Moisturizing; Afrin No-Drip 12-Hour Severe Congestion with Menthol nasal spray OTC *nasal decongestant* [oxymetazoline HCl] 0.05%

Afrin Children's Pump Mist nasal spray (discontinued 2007) OTC *nasal decongestant* [phenylephrine HCl] 0.25%

Afrin Extra Moisturizing nasal spray OTC *nasal decongestant* [oxymetazoline HCl] 0.05%

Afrin Moisturizing Saline Mist solution (discontinued 2008) OTC *nasal moisturizer* [sodium chloride (saline solution)] 0.64%

Afrin Severe Congestion with Menthol nasal spray OTC *nasal decongestant* [oxymetazoline HCl] 0.05%

Afrin Sinus nasal spray OTC *nasal decongestant* [oxymetazoline HCl] 0.05%

Afrin Sinus with Vapornase; Afrin No-Drip Sinus with Vapornase nasal spray (discontinued 2008) OTC *nasal decongestant* [oxymetazoline HCl] 0.05%

Aftate for Athlete's Foot spray powder, spray liquid OTC *antifungal* [tolnaftate] 1%

Aftate for Jock Itch spray powder OTC *antifungal* [tolnaftate] 1%

afurolol INN

A/G Pro tablets OTC *dietary supplement* [protein hydrolysate; multiple vita-

mins & minerals; multiple amino acids] 542• ± mg ⍰ AKPro

agalsidase alfa USAN *investigational (NDA filed, orphan) enzyme replacement therapy for Fabry disease*

agalsidase beta *enzyme replacement therapy for Fabry disease (orphan)*

agalsidase beta & ceramide trihexosidase (CTH) *investigational (orphan) enzyme replacement therapy for Fabry disease*

aganodine INN

agar NF, JAN *suspending agent* ⍰ Icar

agar-agar [see: agar]

Agathosma betulina *medicinal herb* [see: buchu]

agave (*Agave americana*) plant *medicinal herb used as an antiseptic, diuretic, and laxative and for jaundice and liver disease, pulmonary tuberculosis, and syphilis; also used to combat putrefactive bacteria in the stomach and intestines*

age cross-link breakers *a class of investigational antiaging compounds that break age-mediated bonds between proteins*

Agenerase capsules, oral solution (discontinued 2008) ℞ *protease inhibitor antiviral for HIV infection* [amprenavir; vitamin E] 50 mg•36 U; 15 mg•46 U per mL

Aggrastat IV infusion ℞ *platelet aggregation inhibitor for acute coronary syndrome, unstable angina, myocardial infarction, and cardiac surgery* [tirofiban HCl] 50, 250 mcg/mL

aggregated albumin [see: albumin, aggregated]

aggregated radio-iodinated I 131 serum albumin [see: albumin, aggregated iodinated I 131 serum]

Aggrenox dual-release capsules ℞ *platelet aggregation inhibitor to reduce the risk of stroke* [dipyridamole (extended release); aspirin (immediate release)] 200•25 mg

aglepristone INN

agofollin [see: estradiol]

agomelatine *agonist to melatonin MT$_1$ and MT$_2$ receptors and antagonist to serotonin 5-HT$_{2c}$ receptors; investigational (Phase III) oral treatment for major depressive disorder (MDD)*

Agoral oral liquid OTC *stimulant laxative* [sennosides] 25 mg/15 mL ⊡ Aquoral

Agriflu suspension for IM injection in prefilled syringes ℞ *seasonal influenza virus types A and B vaccine for patients* ≥ *18 years* [influenza split-virus vaccine (preservative free)] 0.5 mL/dose

agrimony *(Agrimonia eupatoria)* plant *medicinal herb for diarrhea, gastroenteritis, jaundice, kidney stones, liver disorders, mucous membrane inflammation with discharge; also used topically as an astringent and antiseptic*

agrimony, hemp *medicinal herb* [see: hemp agrimony]

Agropyron repens medicinal herb [see: couch grass]

Agrylin capsules ℞ *thrombolytic and antiplatelet agent for essential thrombocytopenia (orphan); investigational (orphan) for thrombocytosis and polycythemia vera* [anagrelide HCl] 0.5 mg

ague tree *medicinal herb* [see: sassafras]

agurin [see: theobromine sodium acetate]

AHA (acetohydroxamic acid) [q.v.]

AHA (alpha hydroxy acids) [see: glycolic acid]

AH-chew D chewable tablets ℞ *nasal decongestant* [phenylephrine HCl] 10 mg

AH-chew D oral suspension (discontinued 2010) ℞ *nasal decongestant* [phenylephrine tannate] 10 mg/5 mL

AH-chew Ultra chewable tablets ℞ *decongestant; antihistamine; anticholinergic to dry mucosal secretions* [phenylephrine HCl; chlorpheniramine maleate; methscopolamine nitrate] 10•2•1.25 mg

AH-chew Ultra Tannate oral suspension ℞ *decongestant; antihistamine; anticholinergic to dry mucosal secretions* [phenylephrine tannate; chlorpheniramine tannate; methscopolamine nitrate] 10•2•1.5 mg/5 mL

AHF (antihemophilic factor) [q.v.]

AHG (antihemophilic globulin) [see: antihemophilic factor]

A-Hydrocort IV or IM injection ℞ *corticosteroid; anti-inflammatory* [hydrocortisone sodium succinate] 100, 250, 500, 1000 mg/vial

AIIRAs (angiotensin II receptor antagonists) [q.v.]

air, compressed [see: air, medical]

air, medical USP *medicinal gas*

Airacof oral liquid ℞ *narcotic antitussive; antihistamine; sleep aid; decongestant* [codeine phosphate; diphenhydramine HCl; phenylephrine HCl] 7.5•12.5•7.5 mg/5 mL ⊡ Ercaf

Airet solution for inhalation ℞ *sympathomimetic bronchodilator* [albuterol sulfate] 0.083%

AI-RSA *investigational (orphan) agent for autoimmune uveitis*

ajmaline JAN

Akarpine eye drops (discontinued 2009) ℞ *antiglaucoma agent; direct-acting miotic* [pilocarpine HCl] 1%, 2%, 4%

AKBeta eye drops ℞ *antiglaucoma agent (beta-blocker)* [levobunolol HCl] 0.25%, 0.5%

AK-Con eye drops ℞ *decongestant; vasoconstrictor* [naphazoline HCl] 0.1%

AK-Dilate eye drops ℞ *decongestant; vasoconstrictor; mydriatic* [phenylephrine HCl] 2.5%, 10%

AK-Fluor antecubital venous injection ℞ *ophthalmic diagnostic agent* [fluorescein] 10%, 25%

Akineton IV or IM injection (discontinued 2009) ℞ *anticholinergic; antiparkinsonian* [biperiden lactate] 5 mg/mL ⊡ aconitine

Akineton tablets ℞ *anticholinergic; antiparkinsonian* [biperiden HCl] 2 mg ⊡ aconitine

aklomide USAN, INN, BAN *coccidiostat for poultry* ⊡ iogulamide

AK-NaCl eye drops, ophthalmic ointment OTC *corneal edema-reducing*

agent [sodium chloride (hypertonic saline solution)] 5%

Akne-Mycin ointment ℞ *antibiotic for acne* [erythromycin] 2%

AK-Pentolate eye drops ℞ *mydriatic; cycloplegic* [cyclopentolate HCl] 1%

AK-Poly-Bac ophthalmic ointment ℞ *antibiotic* [polymyxin B sulfate; bacitracin zinc] 10 000•500 U/g

AKPro eye drops (discontinued 2009) ℞ *antiglaucoma agent* [dipivefrin HCl] 0.1% ⃠ A/G Pro

AK-Rinse ophthalmic solution (discontinued 2010) OTC *extraocular irrigating solution* [sterile isotonic solution]

AK-Spore eye drops ℞ *antibiotic* [polymyxin B sulfate; neomycin sulfate; gramicidin] 10 000 U•1.75 mg•0.025 mg per mL ⃠ Exubera

AK-Spore ophthalmic ointment ℞ *antibiotic* [polymyxin B sulfate; neomycin sulfate; bacitracin zinc] 10 000 U•5 mg•400 U per g ⃠ Exubera

AK-Spore H.C. ophthalmic ointment (discontinued 2009) ℞ *corticosteroidal anti-inflammatory; antibiotic* [hydrocortisone; neomycin sulfate; bacitracin zinc; polymyxin B sulfate] 1%•0.35%•400 U/g•10 000 U/g

AK-Sulf eye drops, ophthalmic ointment ℞ *antibiotic* [sulfacetamide sodium] 10% ⃠ Ocusulf

AK-Ten ophthalmic gel ℞ *anesthetic for ocular procedures* [lidocaine HCl] 3.5% ⃠ Accutane

AK-Tob eye drops ℞ *aminoglycoside antibiotic* [tobramycin] 0.3%

AK-Tracin ophthalmic ointment (discontinued 2009) ℞ *bactericidal antibiotic* [bacitracin] 500 U/g

Akwa Tears eye drops (discontinued 2010) OTC *moisturizer/lubricant* [polyvinyl alcohol] 1.4%

Akwa Tears ophthalmic ointment (discontinued 2010) OTC *moisturizer/lubricant* [white petrolatum; mineral oil]

al12 lotion, topical foam OTC *moisturizer; emollient* [ammonium lactate] 12%

ALA (alpha lipoic acid) *natural antioxidant* [q.v.]

ALA; 5-ALA HCl [see: aminolevulinic acid HCl]

alacepril INN, JAN

Alacol syrup, oral drops ℞ *decongestant; antihistamine; drops for children 2–5 years* [phenylephrine HCl; brompheniramine maleate] 5•2 mg/5 mL; 1•0.4 mg/mL

Alacol DM syrup, oral drops (discontinued 2010) ℞ *antitussive; antihistamine; decongestant* [dextromethorphan hydrobromide; brompheniramine maleate; phenylephrine HCl] 10•2•5 mg/5 mL; 5•1•2.5 mg/2.5 mL

Ala-Cort cream, lotion ℞ *corticosteroidal anti-inflammatory* [hydrocortisone] 1%

Alacramyn (name changed to **Anascorp** upon marketing release in 2011)

alafosfalin INN, BAN

Alagesic LQ oral solution ℞ *barbiturate sedative; analgesic; antipyretic* [butalbital; acetaminophen; caffeine] 50•325•40 mg/15 mL

Alahist AC oral liquid ℞ *narcotic antitussive; decongestant* [codeine phosphate; phenylephrine HCl] 10•7.5 mg/5 mL

Alahist DHC oral liquid ℞ *narcotic antitussive; decongestant* [dihydrocodeine bitartrate; phenylephrine HCl] 3•7.5 mg/5 mL

Alahist DM oral liquid ℞ *antitussive; antihistamine; decongestant* [dextromethorphan hydrobromide; brompheniramine maleate; phenylephrine HCl] 15•4•7.5 mg/5 mL

Alahist IR caplets ℞ *antihistamine* [dexbrompheniramine maleate] 2 mg

Alahist LQ oral liquid ℞ *decongestant; antihistamine; sleep aid* [phenylephrine HCl; diphenhydramine HCl] 7.5•25 mg/5 mL

Alamag oral suspension OTC *antacid* [aluminum hydroxide; magnesium hydroxide] 225•200 mg/5 mL

Alamag Plus oral suspension OTC *antacid; antiflatulent* [aluminum hydroxide; magnesium hydroxide; simethicone] 225•200•25 mg/5 mL

Alamast eye drops ℞ *mast cell stabilizer for allergic conjunctivitis* [pemirolast potassium] 0.1%

alamecin USAN *antibacterial*

alanine (L-alanine) USAN, USP, INN *nonessential amino acid; symbols: Ala, A*

alanine nitrogen mustard [see: melphalan]

alanosine INN

alaproclate USAN, INN *antidepressant*

Ala-Quin cream ℞ *corticosteroidal anti-inflammatory; antifungal; antibacterial* [hydrocortisone; clioquinol] 0.5%•3% ⊚ Alcaine; Aloquin; Elocon; elucaine

Ala-Scalp lotion ℞ *corticosteroidal anti-inflammatory* [hydrocortisone] 2%

Alaseb T shampoo OTC *antiseborrheic; antipsoriatic; keratolytic; antiseptic* [sulfur; salicylic acid; coal tar] 2%•2%•1%

AlaSTAT lab test for professional use ℞ *test for allergic reaction to latex* ⊚ Elestat

Alasulf vaginal cream ℞ *broad-spectrum antibiotic; antiseptic; moisturizer/lubricant* [sulfanilamide; aminacrine HCl; allantoin] 15%•0.2%•2% ⊚ alusulf

alatrofloxacin mesylate USAN *broad-spectrum fluoroquinolone antibiotic*

Alavert orally disintegrating tablets OTC *nonsedating antihistamine for allergic rhinitis; also used for chronic idiopathic urticaria* [loratadine] 10 mg

Alavert Children's syrup OTC *nonsedating antihistamine for allergic rhinitis* [loratadine] 5 mg/5 mL

Alavert D-12 Hour, Allergy & Sinus extended-release tablets OTC *nonsedating antihistamine; decongestant* [loratadine; pseudoephedrine HCl] 5•120 mg

Alaway eye drops OTC *antihistamine and mast cell stabilizer for allergic conjunctivitis* [ketotifen (as fumarate)] 0.025%

alazanine triclofenate INN

Albafort capsules OTC *vitamin/iron supplement* [ferrous fumarate; desiccated liver; vitamins B_{12} and C; folic acid] 384•240•0.015•100•0.8 mg

Albalon eye drops (discontinued 2009) ℞ *decongestant; vasoconstrictor; moisturizer/lubricant* [naphazoline HCl; polyvinyl alcohol] 0.1%•1.4%

Albatussin capsules ℞ *antitussive; decongestant; expectorant* [carbetapentane citrate; phenylephrine HCl; guaifenesin] 25•10•400 mg

Albatussin oral liquid OTC *antitussive; decongestant; antihistamine; sleep aid* [dextromethorphan hydrobromide; phenylephrine HCl; pyrilamine maleate] 15•5•12.5 mg/5 mL

Albatussin SR extended-release capsules (discontinued 2007) ℞ *antitussive; antihistamine; sleep aid; decongestant; expectorant* [dextromethorphan hydrobromide; pyrilamine maleate; phenylephrine HCl; potassium guaiacolsulfonate] 40•25•20•600 mg

Albay subcu or IM injection (discontinued 2010) ℞ *venom sensitivity testing (subcu); venom desensitization therapy (IM)* [extracts of honeybee, yellow jacket, yellow hornet, white-faced hornet, mixed vespid, and wasp venom] ⊚ Eye-Lube-A

albendazole USAN, INN, BAN *anthelmintic for neurocysticercosis (tapeworm) and cestode-induced hydatid cyst disease (orphan)*

albendazole oxide INN, BAN

Albenza Tiltab (film-coated tablets) ℞ *anthelmintic for neurocysticercosis (tapeworm) and cestode-induced hydatid cyst disease (orphan)* [albendazole]

Alberta Lens ℞ *contact lens* [sulfocon B]

albiglutide *investigational (Phase III) glucagon-like peptide-1 (GLP-1) for type 2 diabetes*

Albolene topical liquid OTC *therapeutic skin cleanser*

Albright solution (sodium citrate and citric acid) *urine alkalizer; compounding agent*

albucid [see: sulfacetamide]

albumin, aggregated USAN *lung imaging aid (with technetium Tc 99m)*

albumin, aggregated iodinated I 131 serum USAN, USP *radioactive agent*

albumin, chromated Cr 51 serum USAN *radioactive agent*

albumin, human USP *blood volume expander for shock, burns, and hypoproteinemia* 5%, 25% injection

albumin, iodinated (^{125}I) human serum INN *radioactive agent; blood volume test* [also: albumin, iodinated I 125 serum]

albumin, iodinated (^{131}I) human serum INN, JAN *radioactive agent; intrathecal imaging agent; blood volume test* [also: albumin, iodinated I 131 serum]

albumin, iodinated I 125 USP *radioactive agent; blood volume test*

albumin, iodinated I 125 serum USAN, USP *radioactive agent; blood volume test* [also: iodinated (^{125}I) human serum albumin]

albumin, iodinated I 131 USP *radioactive agent; intrathecal imaging agent; blood volume test*

albumin, iodinated I 131 serum USAN, USP *radioactive agent; intrathecal imaging agent; blood volume test* [also: iodinated (^{131}I) human serum albumin]

albumin, normal human serum [now: albumin, human]

Albuminar-5; Albuminar-25 IV infusion ℞ *blood volume expander for shock, burns, and hypoproteinemia* [human albumin] 5%; 25%

Albunex injection ℞ *ultrasound heart imaging agent* [human albumin, sonicated] 5%

Albustix reagent strips for professional use ℞ *in vitro diagnostic aid for albumin (protein) in the urine*

Albutein 5%; Albutein 25% IV infusion ℞ *blood volume expander for shock, burns, and hypoproteinemia* [human albumin] 5%; 25%

albuterol USAN, USP *sympathomimetic bronchodilator* [also: salbutamol] 90 mcg inhalation

Albuterol HFA inhalation aerosol with a CFC-free propellant (discontinued 2007) ℞ *sympathomimetic bronchodilator* [albuterol] 90 mcg/dose

albuterol sulfate USAN, USP *sympathomimetic bronchodilator* [also: salbutamol sulfate] 2, 4, 8 mg oral; 2 mg/5 mL oral; 0.021%, 0.042%, 0.083%, 0.5% (0.63, 1.25, 2.5, 5 mg/3 mL) inhalation solution

albuterol sulfate & ipratropium bromide *bronchodilator combination for bronchospasm, emphysema, and chronic obstructive pulmonary disease (COPD)* 0.083%●0.017% (3●0.5 mg/dose) inhaler

albutoin USAN, INN *anticonvulsant*

ALC (acetyl-L-carnitine) [q.v.]

alcaftadine *antihistamine for allergic conjunctivitis*

Alcaine Drop-Tainers (eye drops) ℞ *topical anesthetic* [proparacaine HCl] 0.5% ☒ Ala-Quin; Aloquin; Elocon; elucaine

alcanna *medicinal herb* [see: henna (*Alkanna*)]

ALCAR (acetyl-L-carnitine) [q.v.]

Alcare foam OTC *antiseptic* [ethyl alcohol] 62% ☒ Allegra

Alchemilla xanthochlora; A. vulgaris *medicinal herb* [see: lady's mantle]

alclofenac USAN, INN, BAN, JAN *anti-inflammatory*

alclometasone INN, BAN *topical corticosteroidal anti-inflammatory* [also: alclometasone dipropionate]

alclometasone dipropionate USAN, USP, JAN *topical corticosteroidal anti-inflammatory* [also: alclometasone] 0.05% topical

alcloxa USAN, INN *astringent; keratolytic* [also: aluminum chlorohydroxy allantoinate]

Alco-Gel OTC *antiseptic for instant sanitation of hands* [ethyl alcohol] 60%

alcohol USP *topical anti-infective/anti-septic; astringent; solvent; a widely abused "legal street drug" used to produce euphoria* [also: ethanol]

alcohol, dehydrated USP *antidote* [also: ethanol, dehydrated]

alcohol, diluted NF *solvent*

alcohol, rubbing USP, INN *rubefacient*

5% Alcohol and 5% Dextrose in Water; 10% Alcohol and 5% Dextrose in Water IV infusion R *for caloric replacement and rehydration* [dextrose; alcohol] 5%•5%; 10%•5%

Alcon Saline Especially for Sensitive Eyes solution (discontinued 2010) OTC *rinsing/storage solution for soft contact lenses* [sodium chloride (preserved saline solution)]

Alcortin A gel R *corticosteroidal anti-inflammatory; antimicrobial; emollient* [hydrocortisone; iodoquinol; aloe polysaccharides] 2%•1%•1%

alcuronium chloride USAN, INN, BAN, JAN *skeletal muscle relaxant*

Aldactazide tablets R *antihypertensive; diuretic* [spironolactone; hydrochlorothiazide] 25•25, 50•50 mg

Aldactone film-coated tablets R *antihypertensive; potassium-sparing diuretic for essential hypertension, hypokalemia, congestive heart failure, severe heart failure, cirrhosis of the liver, and nephrotic syndrome; also used for female hirsutism* [spironolactone] 25, 50, 100 mg

Aldara cream R *immunomodulator for external genital and perianal warts (condylomata acuminata), actinic keratoses, and superficial basal cell carcinoma (sBCC)* [imiquimod] 5% in 250 mg single-use packets

alder, spotted *medicinal herb* [see: witch hazel]

alder, striped *medicinal herb* [see: winterberry; witch hazel]

alder buckthorn; European black alder *medicinal herb* [see: buckthorn]

alderlin [see: pronethalol]

aldesleukin USAN, INN, BAN *immunostimulant; biological response modifier; antineoplastic for metastatic melanoma* *and renal cell carcinoma (orphan); investigational (orphan) for immunodeficiency diseases, acute myelogenous leukemia (AML), and non-Hodgkin lymphoma*

aldesulfone sodium INN *antibacterial; leprostatic* [also: sulfoxone sodium]

Aldex AN chewable tablets R *antihistamine; sleep aid* [doxylamine succinate] 5 mg

Aldex CT chewable caplets OTC *decongestant; antihistamine; sleep aid* [phenylephrine HCl; diphenhydramine HCl] 5•12.5 mg

Aldex DM Tannate oral suspension R *antitussive; antihistamine; sleep aid; decongestant* [dextromethorphan hydrobromide; pyrilamine maleate; phenylephrine HCl] 15•16•5 mg/5 mL

Aldex GS DM tablets R *antitussive; decongestant; expectorant* [dextromethorphan hydrobromide; pseudoephedrine HCl; guaifenesin] 15•30•190 mg

aldioxa USAN, INN, JAN *astringent; keratolytic*

Aldoclor-150; Aldoclor-250 film-coated tablets (discontinued 2007) R *combination central antiadrenergic and diuretic for hypertension* [methyldopa; chlorothiazide] 150•250 mg; 250•250 mg

aldocorten [see: aldosterone]

Aldoril 15; Aldoril 25; Aldoril D30; Aldoril D50 film-coated tablets (discontinued 2007) R *combination central antiadrenergic and diuretic for hypertension* [methyldopa; hydrochlorothiazide] 250•15 mg; 250•25 mg; 500•30 mg; 500•50 mg

aldosterone INN, BAN

Aldurazyme powder for IV infusion R *enzyme replacement therapy for mucopolysaccharidosis I (MPS I) (orphan)* [laronidase] 2.9 mg/vial

alefacept USAN *immunosuppressant; recombinant human LFA-3/IgG1 (leukocyte function–associated antigen, type 3/immunoglobulin G1) fusion protein for chronic plaque psoriasis*

aleglitazar *peroxisome proliferator–activated receptor (PPAR)–alpha and –gamma agonist; investigational (Phase III) once-daily oral antidiabetic to control blood glucose levels, lower triglycerides, and raise HDL*

alemcinal USAN, INN *motilin agonist to stimulate gastrointestinal peristaltic action*

alemtuzumab *humanized monoclonal antibody (huMAb); antineoplastic for B-cell chronic lymphocytic leukemia (B-CLL; orphan); investigational (Phase III) cerebral anti-inflammatory for multiple sclerosis*

Alenaze-D; Alenaze-D NR oral liquid ℞ *decongestant; antihistamine* [phenylephrine HCl; brompheniramine maleate] 7.5•2 mg/5 mL; 7.5•4 mg/5 mL

alendronate sodium USAN *bisphosphonate bone resorption inhibitor for Paget disease and corticosteroid-induced or age-related osteoporosis in men and women; investigational (orphan) for bone manifestations of Gaucher disease and pediatric osteogenesis imperfecta* 5, 10, 35, 40, 70, 75 mg oral

alendronic acid INN, BAN

Alenic Alka chewable tablets (discontinued 2007) OTC *antacid* [aluminum hydroxide; magnesium trisilicate] 80•20 mg

Alenic Alka oral liquid OTC *antacid* [aluminum hydroxide; magnesium carbonate] 31.7•137.3 mg/5 mL

Alenic Alka, Extra Strength chewable tablets (discontinued 2007) OTC *antacid* [aluminum hydroxide; magnesium carbonate] 160•105 mg

alentemol INN *antipsychotic; dopamine agonist* [also: alentemol hydrobromide]

alentemol hydrobromide USAN *antipsychotic; dopamine agonist* [also: alentemol]

alepride INN

Alesse tablets (in packs of 28) ℞ *monophasic oral contraceptive* [levonorgestrel; ethinyl estradiol] 0.1 mg•20 mcg × 21 days; counters × 7 days

alestramustine INN

aletamine HCl USAN *antidepressant* [also: alfetamine]

Aletris farinosa *medicinal herb* [see: star grass]

Aleurites moluccana; A. cordata *medicinal herb* [see: tung seed]

Aleve tablets, capsules, gelcaps OTC *analgesic; nonsteroidal anti-inflammatory drug (NSAID) for osteoarthritis, rheumatoid arthritis, juvenile arthritis, ankylosing spondylitis, primary dysmenorrhea, bursitis/tendinitis, and other mild to moderate pain* [naproxen (as sodium)] 200 mg (220 mg) ℞ Aluvia; ELF; olive

Aleve Cold & Sinus; Aleve Sinus & Headache extended-release caplets OTC *decongestant; analgesic; antipyretic* [pseudoephedrine HCl; naproxen sodium] 120•220 mg

alexidine USAN, INN *antibacterial* ℞ aloxidone

alexitol sodium INN, BAN

alexomycin USAN *veterinary growth promoter for poultry and swine*

alfacalcidol (1α-hydroxycholecalciferol; 1α-hydroxyvitamin D₃) INN, BAN, JAN *vitamin D precursor (converted to calcifediol in the body); calcium regulator for treatment of hypocalcemia and osteodystrophy from chronic renal dialysis*

alfadex INN

alfadolone INN [also: alphadolone]

alfalfa (Medicago sativa) leaves and flowers *medicinal herb for anemia, appetite stimulation, arthritis, atherosclerosis, blood cleansing, diabetes, hemorrhages, kidney cleansing, lowering cholesterol levels, nausea, pituitary disorders, and peptic ulcers*

alfaprostol USAN, INN, BAN *veterinary prostaglandin*

alfaxalone INN, JAN [also: alphaxalone]

Alfenta IV or IM injection (discontinued 2011) ℞ *narcotic analgesic; primary anesthetic for surgery* [alfentanil HCl] 500 mcg/mL ℞ Alphanate

alfentanil INN, BAN *narcotic analgesic* [also: alfentanil HCl]

alfentanil HCl USAN *narcotic analgesic; primary anesthetic for surgery* [also: alfentanil] 500 mcg/mL injection

Alferon N intralesional injection ℞ *immunomodulator and antiviral for condylomata acuminata; investigational (Phase III) cytokine for HIV, AIDS, and ARC* [interferon alfa-n3] 5 million IU/mL

alfetamine INN *antidepressant* [also: aletamine HCl]

alfetamine HCl [see: aletamine HCl]

alfuzosin INN, BAN *alpha$_1$-adrenergic blocker for hypertension and benign prostatic hyperplasia (BPH)* [also: alfuzosin HCl]

alfuzosin HCl USAN *alpha$_1$-adrenergic blocker for hypertension and benign prostatic hyperplasia (BPH)* [also: alfuzosin] 10 mg oral

algeldrate USAN, INN *antacid*

algestone INN *anti-inflammatory* [also: algestone acetonide]

algestone acetonide USAN, BAN *anti-inflammatory* [also: algestone]

algestone acetophenide USAN *progestin*

algin [see: sodium alginate]

alginic acid NF, BAN *tablet binder and emulsifying agent*

alginic acid, sodium salt [see: sodium alginate]

alglucerase USAN, INN, BAN *glucocerebrosidase enzyme replacement for Gaucher disease type I (orphan)*

alglucosidase alfa *exogenous source of the acid alpha-glucosidase enzyme; enzyme replacement therapy for patients with Pompe disease (glycogenosis type 2; glycogen storage disease type II; GSDII) (orphan)*

alibendol INN

alicaforsen sodium USAN, INN *anti-inflammatory; antisense inhibitor of intercellular adhesion molecule 1 (ICAM-1)*

aliconazole INN

alidine dihydrochloride [see: anileridine]

alidine phosphate [see: anileridine]

alifedrine INN

aliflurane USAN, INN *inhalation anesthetic*

Align Daily Probiotic Supplement capsules OTC *natural probiotic supplement* [Bifidobacterium infantis 35624] 4 mg (10^9 live cultures)

alimadol INN

alimemazine INN *phenothiazine antihistamine; antipruritic* [also: trimeprazine tartrate; trimeprazine; alimemazine tartrate]

alimemazine tartrate JAN *phenothiazine antihistamine; antipruritic* [also: trimeprazine tartrate; alimemazine; trimeprazine]

Alimentum ready-to-use oral liquid OTC *hypoallergenic infant food* [casein protein formula]

Alimentum Advance ready-to-use oral liquid OTC *hypoallergenic infant food with omega-3 and omega-6 fatty acids* [casein protein formula; iron; docosahexaenoic acid (DHA); arachidonic acid (AA)]

Alimta powder for IV infusion ℞ *antineoplastic for malignant pleural mesothelioma (orphan) and non–small cell lung cancer (NSCLC)* [pemetrexed disodium] 100, 500 mg ⑨ Elimite

Alinia tablets, powder for oral suspension ℞ *antiprotozoal for pediatric diarrhea due to* Cryptosporidium parvum *and* Giardia lamblia *infections (orphan)* [nitazoxanide] 500 mg; 100 mg/5 mL

alinidine INN, BAN

alipamide USAN, INN, BAN *diuretic; antihypertensive*

alisactide [see: alsactide]

aliskiren hemifumarate *direct renin inhibitor for hypertension*

alisobumal [see: butalbital]

alisporivir *investigational cyclophilin inhibitor for hepatitis C virus infections*

alitame USAN *sweetener*

alitretinoin USAN, INN *second-generation retinoid; topical treatment of cutaneous lesions of Kaposi sarcoma (orphan); oral treatment of chronic eczema; investigational (Phase III, orphan) oral treatment for acute promy-*

elocytic leukemia (APL); investigational (orphan) to prevent retinal detachment

alizapride INN

Alka-Mints chewable tablets OTC *antacid* [calcium carbonate] 850 mg

Alkanna tinctoria medicinal herb [see: henna]

Alka-Seltzer; Alka-Seltzer Lemon Lime effervescent tablets OTC *antacid; analgesic; antipyretic* [sodium bicarbonate; citric acid; aspirin; phenylalanine] 1700•1000•325•9 mg

Alka-Seltzer, Extra Strength effervescent tablets OTC *antacid; analgesic; antipyretic* [sodium bicarbonate; citric acid; aspirin] 1985•1000•500 mg

Alka-Seltzer, Original effervescent tablets OTC *antacid; analgesic; antipyretic* [sodium bicarbonate; citric acid; aspirin] 1916•1000•325 mg

Alka-Seltzer Gold effervescent tablets OTC *antacid* [sodium bicarbonate; potassium bicarbonate; citric acid] 1050•344•1000 mg

Alka-Seltzer Heartburn Relief effervescent tablets OTC *antacid* [sodium bicarbonate; citric acid; phenylalanine] 1940•1000•5.6 mg

Alka-Seltzer Plus Cold effervescent tablets OTC *decongestant; antihistamine; analgesic; antipyretic* [phenylephrine bitartrate; chlorpheniramine maleate; aspirin] 7.8•2•325 mg

Alka-Seltzer Plus Cold & Cough effervescent tablets, oral liquid (discontinued 2010) OTC *antitussive; antihistamine; decongestant; analgesic; antipyretic* [dextromethorphan hydrobromide; chlorpheniramine maleate; phenylephrine HCl; acetaminophen] 10•2•5•250 mg; 10•2•5•325 mg/10 mL

Alka-Seltzer Plus Cold & Cough Liqui-Gels (liquid-filled gelcaps) OTC *antitussive; antihistamine; decongestant; analgesic; antipyretic* [dextromethorphan hydrobromide; chlorpheniramine maleate; phenylephrine HCl; acetaminophen] 10•2•30•325 mg

Alka-Seltzer Plus Cold Medicine Liqui-Gels (liquid-filled gelcaps) OTC *decongestant; antihistamine; analgesic; antipyretic* [pseudoephedrine HCl; chlorpheniramine maleate; acetaminophen] 30•2•325 mg

Alka-Seltzer Plus Day Cold oral liquid OTC *antitussive; decongestant; analgesic; antipyretic* [dextromethorphan hydrobromide; phenylephrine HCl; acetaminophen] 10•5•325 mg/10 mL

Alka-Seltzer Plus Day & Night Cold effervescent tablets OTC *antitussive; decongestant; analgesic; antipyretic; antihistamine/sleep aid added* PM [dextromethorphan hydrobromide; phenylephrine HCl; acetaminophen; doxylamine succinate added PM] 10•5•250 mg AM; 10•5•250•6.25 mg PM

Alka-Seltzer Plus Day & Night Cold Liqui-Gels (liquid-filled gelcaps) OTC *antitussive; analgesic; antipyretic; decongestant added* AM; *antihistamine/sleep aid added* PM [dextromethorphan hydrobromide; acetaminophen; phenylephrine HCl added AM; doxylamine succinate added PM] 10•325•5 mg AM; 15•325•6.25 mg PM

Alka-Seltzer Plus Day Non-Drowsy Cold Liqui-Gels (liquid-filled gelcaps), oral liquid OTC *antitussive; decongestant; analgesic; antipyretic* [dextromethorphan hydrobromide; phenylephrine HCl; acetaminophen] 10•5•325 mg; 10•5•325 mg/10 mL

Alka-Seltzer Plus Fast Crystal Packs powder for oral solution OTC *decongestant; antihistamine; analgesic; antipyretic* [phenylephrine HCl; chlorpheniramine maleate; acetaminophen] 10•4•650 mg

Alka-Seltzer Plus Flu effervescent tablets OTC *antitussive; antihistamine; analgesic; antipyretic* [dextromethorphan hydrobromide; chlorpheniramine maleate; aspirin] 15•2•500 mg

Alka-Seltzer Plus Mucus & Congestion effervescent tablets, Liqui-

Gels (liquid-filled gelcaps) OTC *antitussive; expectorant* [dextromethorphan hydrobromide; guaifenesin] 10•200 mg

Alka-Seltzer Plus Night Cold Liqui-Gels (liquid-filled gelcaps) OTC *antitussive; antihistamine; sleep aid; analgesic; antipyretic* [dextromethorphan hydrobromide; doxylamine succinate; acetaminophen] 15•6.25•325 mg

Alka-Seltzer Plus Night Cold oral liquid OTC *antitussive; decongestant; antihistamine; sleep aid; analgesic; antipyretic* [dextromethorphan hydrobromide; phenylephrine HCl; doxylamine succinate; acetaminophen] 10•5•6.25•325 mg/10 mL

Alka-Seltzer Plus Night-Time Cold effervescent tablets OTC *antitussive; decongestant; antihistamine; sleep aid; analgesic; antipyretic* [dextromethorphan hydrobromide; phenylephrine HCl; doxylamine succinate; acetaminophen] 10•5•6.25•250 mg

Alka-Seltzer Plus Regular Seltzer Multi-Symptom Cold Relief; Alka-Seltzer Plus Sparkling Original Cold Formula effervescent tablets OTC *decongestant; antihistamine; analgesic; antipyretic* [phenylephrine HCl; chlorpheniramine maleate; acetaminophen] 5•2•250 mg

Alka-Seltzer Plus Sinus effervescent tablets OTC *decongestant; analgesic; antipyretic* [phenylephrine HCl; aspirin] 5•250 mg

Alka-Seltzer PM effervescent tablets (discontinued 2009) OTC *antihistaminic sleep aid; analgesic; antipyretic* [diphenhydramine citrate; aspirin] 38•325 mg

Alka-Seltzer Wake-Up Call effervescent tablets (discontinued 2009) OTC *analgesic; antipyretic; anti-inflammatory* [aspirin; caffeine] 500•65 mg

Alka-Seltzer with Aspirin effervescent tablets OTC *antacid; analgesic; antipyretic* [sodium bicarbonate; citric acid; aspirin] 1700•1200•325, 1900•1000•325, 1900•1000•500 mg

alkavervir (Veratrum viride alkaloids)

Alkavite extended-release tablets OTC *vitamin/mineral supplement for alcohol-related deficiencies* [multiple vitamins & minerals; calcium carbonate; iron sulfate; folic acid; biotin] ≛•68.5•60•1•0.03 mg

Alkeran film-coated tablets, powder for IV infusion ℞ *nitrogen mustard-type alkylating antineoplastic for multiple myeloma (orphan) and ovarian cancer; investigational (orphan) for metastatic melanoma; also used for breast and testicular cancers and bone marrow transplantation* [melphalan] 2 mg; 50 mg

alkyl aryl sulfonate *surfactant/wetting agent*

alkylamines *a class of antihistamines*

alkylbenzyldimethylammonium chloride [see: benzalkonium chloride]

alkyldimethylbenzylammonium chloride [see: benzalkonium chloride]

alkylpolyaminoethylglycine JAN

alkylpolyaminoethylglycine HCl JAN

All Day Allergy Children's chewable tablets OTC *nonsedating antihistamine for allergic rhinitis* [cetirizine HCl] 10 mg

All Day Allergy-D extended-release tablets OTC *nonsedating antihistamine and decongestant for allergic rhinitis* [cetirizine HCl; pseudoephedrine HCl] 5•120 mg

Allanderm-T ointment OTC *proteolytic enzyme for débridement of necrotic tissue; vulnerary* [trypsin; Peruvian balsam; castor oil] 90 U•87 mg•788 mg per g

AllanEnzyme ointment ℞ *proteolytic enzyme for débridement of necrotic tissue; vulnerary* [papain; urea] 830 000 U/g•10% (note: one of two products with the same name)

AllanEnzyme ointment ℞ *proteolytic enzyme for débridement of necrotic tissue; vulnerary; wound deodorant* [papain; urea; chlorophyllin copper complex] 521 700 U/g•10%•0.5%

(note: one of two products with the same name)

AllanEnzyme spray ℞ *proteolytic enzyme for débridement of necrotic tissue; vulnerary* [papain; urea] 830 000 IU/g•10%

AllanfillEnzyme spray ℞ *proteolytic enzyme for débridement of necrotic tissue; vulnerary; wound deodorant* [papain; urea; chlorophyllin copper complex] ≥ 521 700 U/g•10%•0.5%

AllanHist PDX oral drops ℞ *antitussive; antihistamine; decongestant; for children 1–24 months* [dextromethorphan hydrobromide; brompheniramine maleate; pseudoephedrine HCl] 3•1•12.5 mg/mL

allantoin USAN, BAN *topical vulnerary; moisturizer; investigational (orphan) for skin blistering and erosions associated with inherited epidermolysis bullosa*

AllanVan-DM B.I.D. oral suspension ℞ *antitussive; antihistamine; sleep aid; decongestant* [dextromethorphan tannate; pyrilamine tannate; phenylephrine tannate] 25•30•12.5 mg/5 mL

AllanVan-S B.I.D. oral suspension ℞ *decongestant; antihistamine; sleep aid* [phenylephrine tannate; pyrilamine tannate] 12.5•30 mg/5 mL

Allbee C-800 caplets OTC *vitamin supplement* [multiple B vitamins; vitamins C and E; folic acid; biotin] ≛• 800•45•0.4•0.3 mg

Allbee C-800 plus Iron film-coated tablets (discontinued 2008) OTC *vitamin/iron supplement* [iron (as ferrous fumarate); multiple B vitamins; vitamins C and E; folic acid] 27 mg•≛• 800 mg•45 U•0.4 mg

Allbee with C caplets OTC *vitamin supplement* [multiple B vitamins; vitamin C; folic acid; biotin] ≛• 300•0.4•0.3 mg

Allbee-T tablets (discontinued 2008) OTC *vitamin supplement* [multiple B vitamins; vitamin C] ≛•500 mg

Allegra capsules (discontinued 2007) ℞ *nonsedating antihistamine for allergic rhinitis and chronic idiopathic urti-caria* [fexofenadine HCl] 60 mg ⍰ agar; Alcare; Icar

Allegra film-coated tablets, oral suspension OTC *nonsedating antihistamine for allergic rhinitis and chronic idiopathic urticaria* [fexofenadine HCl] 60, 180 mg; 30 mg/5 mL ⍰ agar; Alcare; Icar

Allegra Allergy, Children's; Allegra Hives, Children's oral suspension OTC *nonsedating antihistamine for allergic rhinitis and hives* [fexofenadine HCl] 30 mg/5 mL ⍰ agar; Alcare; Icar

Allegra ODT (orally disintegrating tablets) OTC *nonsedating antihistamine for allergic rhinitis* [fexofenadine HCl] 30 mg ⍰ agar; Alcare; Icar

Allegra-D 12-Hour; Allegra-D 24-Hour dual-release film-coated tablets OTC *nonsedating antihistamine; decongestant* [fexofenadine HCl (immediate release); pseudoephedrine HCl (extended release)] 60•120 mg; 180•240 mg ⍰ agar; Alcare; Icar

allegron [see: nortriptyline]

Allent sustained-release capsules ℞ *decongestant; antihistamine* [pseudoephedrine HCl; brompheniramine maleate] 120•12 mg

AllePak Dose Pack tablets ℞ *anticholinergic to dry mucosal secretions; decongestant added* AM; *antihistamine added* PM [methscopolamine nitrate; pseudoephedrine HCl added AM; chlorpheniramine maleate added PM] 2.5•120 mg AM; 2.5•8 mg PM

Aller-Chlor tablets, syrup OTC *antihistamine* [chlorpheniramine maleate] 4 mg; 2 mg/5 mL

Allerest tablets OTC *decongestant; antihistamine* [pseudoephedrine HCl; chlorpheniramine maleate] 30•2 mg

Allerest PE tablets OTC *decongestant; antihistamine* [phenylephrine HCl; chlorpheniramine maleate] 10•4 mg

Allerfrim film-coated tablets, syrup (discontinued 2010) OTC *decongestant; antihistamine* [pseudoephedrine HCl; triprolidine HCl] 60•2.5 mg; 60•2.5 mg/10 mL

Allergan Enzymatic tablets (discontinued 2010) OTC *enzymatic cleaner for soft contact lenses* [papain]

Allergan Hydrocare [see: Hydrocare]

Allergen Ear Drops ℞ *anesthetic; analgesic* [benzocaine; antipyrine] 1.4%•5.4%

allergenic extracts *a class of agents derived from various biological sources containing antigens that possess immunologic activity*

allergenic extracts (aqueous, glycerinated, or alum-precipitated) *over 900 allergens available for diagnosis of and desensitization to specific allergies*

Allergy tablets OTC *antihistamine* [chlorpheniramine maleate] 4 mg

Allergy DN tablets ℞ *anticholinergic to dry mucosal secretions; decongestant added* AM; *antihistamine added* PM [methscopolamine nitrate; pseudoephedrine HCl added AM; chlorpheniramine maleate added PM] 2.5•120 mg AM; 2.5•8 mg PM

Allergy Relief tablets OTC *antihistamine* [chlorpheniramine maleate] 4 mg

Allergy Relief & Nasal Decongestant extended-release caplets OTC *nonsedating antihistamine; decongestant* [loratadine; pseudoephedrine sulfate] 10•240 mg

Allergy-Time tablets OTC *antihistamine* [chlorpheniramine maleate] 4 mg

AllerMax caplets, oral liquid OTC *antihistamine; sleep aid* [diphenhydramine HCl] 50 mg; 12.5 mg/5 mL

Allermist (name changed to **Veramyst** upon marketing release in 2007)

AllerTan oral suspension (discontinued 2009) ℞ *decongestant; antihistamine; sleep aid* [phenylephrine tannate; chlorpheniramine tannate; pyrilamine tannate] 15•8•12.5 mg/5 mL

AlleRx oral suspension ℞ *decongestant; antihistamine* [phenylephrine tannate; chlorpheniramine tannate] 7.5•3 mg/5 mL ☑ Alrex

AlleRx DF tablets ℞ *antihistamine; anticholinergic to dry mucosal secretions* [chlorpheniramine maleate;

methscopolamine nitrate] 4•2.5 mg AM; 8•2.5 mg PM

AlleRx Dose Pack controlled-release tablets ℞ *anticholinergic to dry mucosal secretions; decongestant added* AM; *antihistamine added* PM [methscopolamine nitrate; pseudoephedrine HCl added AM; chlorpheniramine maleate added PM] 2.5•120 mg AM; 2.5•8 mg PM

AlleRx-D controlled-release caplets (discontinued 2007) ℞ *decongestant; anticholinergic to dry mucosal secretions* [pseudoephedrine HCl; methscopolamine nitrate] 120•2.5 mg

alletorphine BAN, INN

Allfen C extended-release caplets (discontinued 2007) ℞ *antitussive; expectorant* [carbetapentane citrate; guaifenesin] 5•1000 mg

Allfen CDX oral liquid ℞ *narcotic antitussive; expectorant* [codeine phosphate; guaifenesin] 20•200 mg/5 mL

Allfen DM sustained-release tablets ℞ *antitussive; expectorant* [dextromethorphan hydrobromide; guaifenesin] 58•1000 mg

Allfen Jr. tablets (discontinued 2008) ℞ *expectorant* [guaifenesin] 400 mg

all-heal *medicinal herb* [see: mistletoe; valerian]

Alli capsules OTC *lipase inhibitor for weight loss in overweight adults* ≥ 18 *years* [orlistat] 60 mg

Allium cepa *medicinal herb* [see: onion]

Allium porrum *medicinal herb* [see: leek]

Allium sativum *medicinal herb* [see: garlic]

All-Nite oral liquid OTC *antitussive; antihistamine; sleep aid; decongestant; analgesic; antipyretic* [dextromethorphan hydrobromide; doxylamine succinate; acetaminophen; alcohol 10%] 30•12.6•1000 mg/30 mL

All-Nite Children's Cold/Cough Relief oral liquid (discontinued 2007) OTC *antitussive; antihistamine; decongestant; for children 6–11 years* [dextromethorphan hydrobromide; chlorpheniramine maleate; pseudoephedrine HCl] 15•2•30 mg/15 mL

allobarbital USAN, INN *hypnotic*

allobarbitone [see: allobarbital]

alloclamide INN

allocupreide sodium INN

AlloMap lab test for professional use ℞ *blood test for heart transplant rejection markers*

allomethadione INN [also: aloxidone]

allopurinol USAN, USP, INN, BAN, JAN *xanthine oxidase inhibitor for gout and hyperuricemia; antineoplastic adjunct for reducing uric acid levels following chemotherapy for leukemia, lymphoma, and solid-tumor malignancies (orphan); investigational for angina* 100, 300 mg oral

allopurinol riboside *investigational (orphan) agent for Chagas disease and for cutaneous and visceral leishmaniasis*

allopurinol sodium *antineoplastic adjunct for reducing uric acid levels following chemotherapy for leukemia, lymphoma, and solid tumor malignancies (orphan); investigational (orphan) for ex vivo preservation of organs for transplant* 500 mg injection

Allovectin-7 *investigational (Phase III, orphan) for invasive and metastatic melanoma* [HLA-B7/beta2M DNA lipid complex]

Allpyral subcu or IM injection ℞ *allergenic sensitivity testing (subcu); allergenic desensitization therapy (IM)* [allergenic extracts, alum-precipitated]

Allres DS Tannate oral suspension (discontinued 2010) ℞ *antitussive; antihistamine; decongestant* [dextromethorphan hydrobromide; chlorpheniramine maleate; pseudoephedrine HCl] 30•4•30 mg/5 mL

Allres Pd oral suspension (discontinued 2010) ℞ *antitussive; decongestant* [carbetapentane citrate; pseudoephedrine HCl] 7.5•30 mg/5 mL

allspice *(Eugenia pimenta; Pimenta dioica; P. officinalis)* unripe fruit and leaves *medicinal herb for diarrhea and gas; also used as a purgative and tonic*

all-*trans*-retinoic acid (ATRA) [see: tretinoin]

allyl isothiocyanate USAN, USP

allylamines *a class of antifungals*

allylbarbituric acid [now: butalbital]

allylestrenol INN, JAN [also: allyloestrenol]

allyl-isobutylbarbituric acid [see: butalbital]

allylisopropylmalonylurea [see: aprobarbital]

4-allyl-2-methoxyphenol [see: eugenol]

N-allylnoretorphine [see: alletorphine]

N-allylnoroxymorphone HCl [see: naloxone HCl]

allyloestrenol BAN [also: allylestrenol]

allylprodine INN, BAN

5-allyl-5-*sec*-butylbarbituric acid [see: talbutal]

allylthiourea INN

allylpropymal [see: aprobarbital]

Almacone chewable tablets, oral liquid OTC *antacid; antiflatulent* [aluminum hydroxide; magnesium hydroxide; simethicone] 200•200•20 mg; 200•200•20 mg/5 mL

Almacone II oral liquid OTC *antacid; antiflatulent* [aluminum hydroxide; magnesium hydroxide; simethicone] 400•400•40 mg/5 mL

almadrate sulfate USAN, INN *antacid*

almagate USAN, INN *antacid*

almagodrate INN

almasilate INN, BAN

Almebex Plus B$_{12}$ oral liquid OTC *vitamin supplement* [multiple B vitamins]

almecillin INN

almestrone INN

alminoprofen INN, JAN

almitrine INN, BAN *respiratory stimulant* [also: almitrine mesylate]

almitrine mesylate USAN *respiratory stimulant* [also: almitrine]

almokalant INN *antiarrhythmic*

almond *(Prunus amygdalus)* kernels *medicinal herb used as a demulcent, emollient, and pectoral*

almond oil NF *emollient and perfume; oleaginous vehicle*

almotriptan USAN, INN *vascular seroto-nin 5-HT$_{1B/1D/1F}$ receptor agonist for the acute treatment of migraine*

almotriptan malate USAN *vascular serotonin 5-HT$_{1B/1D/1F}$ receptor agonist for the acute treatment of migraine*

almoxatone INN

alnespirone INN

alniditan dihydrochloride USAN *serotonin 5-HT$_{1D}$ agonist for migraine*

Alnus glutinosa *medicinal herb* [see: black alder]

Alocril *eye drops* ℞ *mast cell stabilizer for allergic conjunctivitis* [nedocromil sodium] 2%

Alodox Convenience Kit *tablets* ℞ *tetracycline antibiotic* [doxycycline (as hyclate)] 20 mg

aloe USP

aloe (*Aloe vera* and more than 500 other species) *leaves and juice medicinal herb for burns, hemorrhoids, insect bites, and scalds; also used as a deodorant and to aid digestion and limit scarring; not generally regarded as safe and effective as a cathartic*

Aloe Grande *lotion* OTC *moisturizer; emollient; skin protectant* [vitamins A and E; aloe] 3333.3•50• $\frac{2}{}$ U/g

Aloe Vesta *cloth* OTC *emollient/protectant* [dimethicone; aloe]

Aloe Vesta *lotion* OTC *emollient/protectant* [dimethicone; aloe vera gel] 3%• $\frac{2}{}$

Aloe Vesta *ointment* OTC *antifungal; emollient/protectant* [miconazole nitrate; aloe] 2%• $\frac{2}{}$

Aloe Vesta *spray* OTC *emollient/protectant* [petrolatum; aloe extract] 36%• $\frac{2}{}$

Aloe Vesta Perineal *solution* OTC *emollient/protectant* [propylene glycol; aloe vera gel]

alofilcon A USAN *hydrophilic contact lens material*

alogliptin *investigational (NDA filed) dipeptidyl peptidase-4 (DPP-4) inhibitor oral antidiabetic that enhances the function of the body's incretin system to increase insulin production in the pan-creas and reduce glucose production in the liver*

aloin BAN ⑳ ellaOne

Alomide *Drop-Tainers (eye drops)* ℞ *mast cell stabilizer for vernal kerato-conjunctivitis (orphan)* [lodoxamide tromethamine] 0.1%

alonacic INN

alonimid USAN, INN *sedative; hypnotic*

Alophen *enteric-coated tablets* OTC *stimulant laxative* [bisacodyl] 5 mg

Aloprim *powder for IV infusion* ℞ *antineoplastic adjunct for reducing uric acid levels following chemotherapy for leukemia, lymphoma, and solid-tumor malignancies (orphan); investigational (orphan) for ex vivo preservation of organs for transplant* [allopurinol sodium] 500 mg

Aloquin *gel* ℞ *antimicrobial; emollient* [iodoquinol; aloe] 1.25%•1% ⑳ Ala-Quin; Alcaine; Elocon; elucaine

Alor 5/500 *tablets (discontinued 2009)* ℞ *narcotic analgesic; antipyretic* [hydrocodone bitartrate; aspirin] 5•500 mg

Alora *transdermal patch* ℞ *estrogen replacement therapy for the treatment of postmenopausal symptoms and prevention of postmenopausal osteoporosis* [estradiol] 25, 50, 75, 100 mcg/day

aloracetam INN

alosetron INN, BAN *antiemetic; serotonin 5-HT$_3$ receptor antagonist for diarrhea-predominant irritable bowel syndrome (IBS) in women* [also: alosetron HCl] ⑳ Elestrin

alosetron HCl USAN *antiemetic; serotonin 5-HT$_3$ receptor antagonist for diarrhea-predominant irritable bowel syndrome (IBS) in women (base=89%)* [also: alosetron]

alovudine USAN, INN *antiviral*

Aloxi *capsules (discontinued 2010)* ℞ *antiemetic to prevent chemotherapy-induced and postoperative nausea and vomiting* [palonosetron (as HCl)] 0.5 mg ⑳ I-L-X; Olux

Aloxi *IV injection* ℞ *antiemetic to prevent chemotherapy-induced and postoperative nausea and vomiting* [palonosetron (as HCl)] 0.05 mg/mL ⑨ I-L-X; Olux

aloxidone BAN [also: allomethadione] ⑨ alexidine

aloxiprin INN, BAN

aloxistatin INN

Aloysiatriphylla **spp.** *medicinal herb* [see: lemon verbena]

alozafone INN

alpertine USAN, INN *antipsychotic*

alpha amylase (α-amylase) USAN *anti-inflammatory*

alpha fetoprotein, recombinant human (rhAFP) *investigational (orphan) for myasthenia gravis*

alpha hydroxy acids (AHA) [see: glycolic acid]

alpha interferon-2A [see: interferon alfa-2A]

alpha interferon-2B [see: interferon alfa-2B]

alpha interferon-N1 [see: interferon alfa-N1]

alpha interferon-N3 [see: interferon alfa-N3]

Alpha Keri Moisturizing Soap bar OTC *therapeutic skin cleanser*

Alpha Keri Shower & Bath OTC *bath emollient*

Alpha Keri Therapeutic Bath Oil (name changed to **Alpha Keri Shower & Bath** in 2008)

alpha lipoic acid (ALA) *natural antioxidant that is both fat- and water-soluble and readily crosses cell membranes; used in the treatment of AIDS, diabetes, liver ailments, oxidative stress injuries, and various cancers*

d-**alpha tocopherol** *fat-soluble vitamin; antioxidant; platelet aggregation inhibitor; topical emollient (relative potency: 100%) [see also: vitamin E]*

dl-**alpha tocopherol** *fat-soluble vitamin; antioxidant; platelet aggregation inhibitor; topical emollient (relative potency: 74%) [see also: vitamin E]*

d-**alpha tocopheryl acetate** *fat-soluble vitamin; antioxidant; platelet aggregation inhibitor; topical emollient (relative potency: 91%) [see also: vitamin E]*

dl-**alpha tocopheryl acetate** *fat-soluble vitamin; antioxidant; platelet aggregation inhibitor; topical emollient (relative potency: 67%) [see also: vitamin E]*

d-**alpha tocopheryl acid succinate** *fat-soluble vitamin; antioxidant; platelet aggregation inhibitor; topical emollient (relative potency: 81%) [see also: vitamin E]*

dl-**alpha tocopheryl acid succinate** *fat-soluble vitamin; antioxidant; platelet aggregation inhibitor; topical emollient (relative potency: 60%) [see also: vitamin E]*

alpha$_1$ PI (alpha$_1$-proteinase inhibitor) [q.v.]

alpha$_1$-acid glycoprotein *investigational (orphan) antidote to tricyclic antidepressant and cocaine overdose*

alpha$_1$-adrenergic blockers *a class of agents that block the alpha$_1$ adrenergic receptors, used for the treatment of hypertension and benign prostatic hyperplasia (BPH) also called: antiadrenergics*

alpha$_1$-antitrypsin, recombinant (rAAT) *investigational (orphan) for alpha$_1$-antitrypsin deficiency in the ZZ phenotype population, cystic fibrosis, and to delay the progression of emphysema and chronic obstructive pulmonary disease*

alpha$_1$-antitrypsin, transgenic human *investigational (Phase II, orphan) for emphysema secondary to alpha$_1$-antitrypsin deficiency*

alpha$_1$-proteinase inhibitor (alpha$_1$ PI) *enzyme replacement therapy for hereditary alpha$_1$ PI deficiency, which leads to progressive panacinar emphysema (orphan)*

alphacemethadone [see: alphacetylmethadol]

alphacetylmethadol BAN, INN

alpha-chymotrypsin [see: chymotrypsin]

alpha-cypermethrin BAN

α-D-galactopyranose [see: galactose]

alpha-D-galactosidase *digestive enzyme*

alphadolone BAN [also: alfadolone]

alpha-estradiol [see: estradiol]
alpha-estradiol benzoate [see: estradiol benzoate]
alpha-ethyltryptamine (alpha-EtT) *a hallucinogenic street drug chemically related to MDMA* [see also: MDMA; alpha-methyltryptamine]
alphafilcon A USAN *hydrophilic contact lens material*
alpha-galactosidase A [see: agalsidase alfa; agalsidase beta]
Alphagan P eye drops ℞ *selective alpha₂ agonist for open-angle glaucoma and ocular hypertension; investigational (orphan) for anterior ischemic optic neuropathy* [brimonidine tartrate] 0.1%, 0.15%
alpha-glucosidase, human acid [see: alglucosidase alfa]
alpha-glucosidase inhibitors *a class of antidiabetic agents for type 2 diabetes that delay the digestion of dietary carbohydrates*
17 alpha-hydroxyprogesterone; 17 alpha-progesterone (17P) *naturally occurring progesterone; hormone therapy to prevent preterm births*
17 alpha-hydroxyprogesterone caproate *synthetic progesterone; hormone therapy to prevent preterm birth in women with a history of spontaneous preterm delivery* [also: hydroxyprogesterone caproate]
alpha-hypophamine [see: oxytocin]
alpha-L-iduronidase [now: laronidase]
alpha-melanocyte stimulating hormone *investigational (orphan) agent for the prevention and treatment of acute renal failure due to ischemia*
alphameprodine INN, BAN
alphamethadol INN, BAN
alpha-methyldopa [now: methyldopa]
alpha-methyltryptamine (alpha-MeT) *a hallucinogenic street drug chemically related to MDMA* [see also: MDMA; alpha-ethyltryptamine]
Alphanate powder for IV injection ℞ *systemic hemostatic; antihemophilic for the prevention and control of bleeding in classical hemophilia (hemophilia A) and*

von Willebrand disease (orphan) [antihemophilic factor concentrate, human] (actual number of AHF units is indicated on the vial) ⃟ Alfenta
AlphaNine SD powder for IV infusion ℞ *systemic hemostatic; antihemophilic for factor IX deficiency (hemophilia B; Christmas disease) (orphan)* [factor IX, human, solvent/detergent treated] ≥ 150 U/vial (actual number of units is indicated on the vial)
alpha-phenoxyethyl penicillin, potassium [see: phenethicillin potassium]
alphaprodine INN, BAN [also: alphaprodine HCl]
alphaprodine HCl USP [also: alphaprodine]
Alpharadin *investigational (Phase III) radioactive antineoplastic for bone metastases of hormone-refractory prostate cancer* [radium-233]
alphasone acetophenide [now: algestone acetonide]
alphaxalone BAN [also: alfaxalone]
alpidem USAN, INN, BAN *anxiolytic*
Alpinia officinarum; A. galanga *medicinal herb* [see: galangal]
Alpinia oxyphylla; A. fructus *medicinal herb* [see: bitter cardamom]
Alpinia speciosa *medicinal herb for edema, fungal infections, hypertension, and thrombosis*
alpiropride INN
alprafenone INN
alprazolam USAN, USP, INN, BAN, JAN *benzodiazepine anxiolytic; sedative; treatment for panic disorders and agoraphobia* 0.25, 0.5, 1, 2, 3 mg oral
Alprazolam Intensol oral drops ℞ *benzodiazepine anxiolytic; sedative* [alprazolam] 1 mg/mL
Alprazolam ODT (orally disintegrating tablets) ℞ *benzodiazepine anxiolytic; sedative* [alprazolam] 0.25, 0.5, 1, 2 mg
alprenolol INN, BAN *antiadrenergic (beta-blocker)* [also: alprenolol HCl]
alprenolol HCl USAN, JAN *antiadrenergic (beta-blocker)* [also: alprenolol]

alprenoxime HCl USAN *antiglaucoma agent*

alprostadil USAN, USP, INN, BAN, JAN *vasodilator for erectile dysfunction; platelet aggregation inhibitor; investigational (orphan) for peripheral arterial occlusive disease*

alprostadil alfadex BAN

alprostadil lipid emulsion *vasodilator; platelet aggregation inhibitor; investigational (orphan) for acute respiratory distress syndrome (ARDS) and ischemic ulcerations due to peripheral arterial disease*

alrestatin INN *aldose reductase enzyme inhibitor* [also: alrestatin sodium]

alrestatin sodium USAN *aldose reductase enzyme inhibitor* [also: alrestatin]

Alrex eye drop suspension ℞ *corticosteroidal anti-inflammatory for seasonal allergic conjunctivitis* [loteprednol etabonate] 0.2% ☒ AlleRx

alsactide INN

alseroxylon JAN *antihypertensive; rauwolfia derivative*

Alsuma subcu injection ℞ *vascular serotonin receptor agonist for the acute treatment of migraine and cluster headaches* [sumatriptan (as succinate)] 6 mg/0.5 mL dose

Altabax ointment ℞ *antibiotic for impetigo caused by* Staphylococcus aureus *and* Streptococcus pyogenes *infections* [retapamulin] 1%

Altacaine eye drops ℞ *topical anesthetic* [tetracaine HCl] 0.5%

Altace capsules ℞ *antihypertensive; angiotensin-converting enzyme (ACE) inhibitor; treatment for myocardial infarction (MI), congestive heart failure (CHF), and stroke* [ramipril] 1.25, 2.5, 5, 10 mg

Altafed syrup OTC *decongestant; antihistamine* [pseudoephedrine HCl; triprolidine HCl] 30•1.25 mg/5 mL

Altafrin eye drops ℞ *decongestant; vasoconstrictor; mydriatic* [phenylephrine HCl] 2.5%, 10%

altanserin INN *serotonin antagonist* [also: altanserin tartrate]

altanserin tartrate USAN *serotonin antagonist* [also: altanserin]

altapizone INN

Altarussin syrup OTC *expectorant* [guaifenesin] 100 mg/5 mL

Altarussin-PE oral liquid OTC *decongestant; expectorant* [pseudoephedrine HCl; guaifenesin] 60•200 mg/10 mL

Altaryl Children's Allergy oral liquid OTC *antihistamine; sleep aid* [diphenhydramine HCl] 12.5 mg/5 mL

Altastaph *investigational (orphan) prophylaxis against* S. aureus *infections in low birthweight neonates* [Staphylococcus aureus immune globulin, human]

Altavera film-coated tablets (in packs of 28) ℞ *monophasic oral contraceptive* [levonorgestrel; ethinyl estradiol] 150•30 mcg × 21 days; counters × 7 days

Altazine eye drops OTC *decongestant; vasoconstrictor* [tetrahydrozoline HCl] 0.05% ☒ Ilotycin

Altazine Irritation Relief eye drops (discontinued 2011) OTC *decongestant; astringent* [tetrahydrozoline HCl; zinc sulfate] 0.05%•0.25%

Altazine Moisture Relief eye drops (discontinued 2011) OTC *decongestant; vasoconstrictor; moisturizer/lubricant* [tetrahydrozoline HCl; polyethylene glycol 400; povidone] 0.05%•1%•1%

alteconazole INN

alteplase USAN, INN, BAN, JAN *tissue plasminogen activator (tPA) for acute myocardial infarction, acute ischemic stroke, or pulmonary embolism; investigational (orphan) for intraventricular hemorrhage with intracerebral hemorrhage*

alteratives *a class of agents that produce gradual beneficial changes in the body, usually by improving nutrition, without having any marked specific effect*

ALternaGEL oral liquid OTC *antacid* [aluminum hydroxide gel] 600 mg/5 mL

Althaea officinalis *medicinal herb* [see: marsh mallow]

althiazide USAN *antihypertensive* [also: altizide]

altinicline INN

altinicline maleate USAN *nicotinic acetylcholine receptor agonist*

altizide INN *antihypertensive* [also: althiazide]

Altoprev extended-release tablets ℞ *HMG-CoA reductase inhibitor for hyperlipidemia, mixed dyslipidemia, atherosclerosis, and the prevention and treatment of coronary heart disease (CHD)* [lovastatin] 10, 20, 40, 60 mg

altoqualine INN

Altracin *investigational (orphan) antibiotic for pseudomembranous enterocolitis* [bacitracin]

altrenogest USAN, INN, BAN *veterinary progestin*

altretamine USAN, INN, BAN *antineoplastic for advanced ovarian adenocarcinoma (orphan)*

altumomab USAN, INN *monoclonal antibody to carcinoembryonic antigen (CEA)*

altumomab pentetate USAN *monoclonal antibody to carcinoembryonic antigen (CEA)* [also: indium In 111 altumomab pentetate]

Aludrox oral suspension OTC *antacid; antiflatulent* [aluminum hydroxide; magnesium hydroxide; simethicone] 307•103• ≟ mg/5 mL

alukalin [see: kaolin]

alum, ammonium USP *topical astringent*

alum, potassium USP *topical astringent* [also: aluminum potassium sulfate]

alum root (*Geranium maculatum*) *medicinal herb used as an astringent, hemostatic, and antiseptic*

alumina & magnesia USP *antacid*

aluminopara-aminosalicylate calcium (**alumino *p*-aminosalicylate calcium**) JAN

aluminosilicic acid, magnesium salt hydrate [see: silodrate]

aluminum *element* (Al)

aluminum, micronized *astringent*

aluminum acetate USP *topical astringent; Burow solution*

aluminum aminoacetate [see: dihydroxyaluminum aminoacetate]

aluminum ammonium sulfate dodecahydrate [see: alum, ammonium]

aluminum bismuth oxide [see: bismuth aluminate]

aluminum carbonate, basic USAN, USP *antacid*

aluminum chlorhydroxide [now: aluminum chlorohydrate]

aluminum chlorhydroxide alcohol soluble complex [now: aluminum chlorohydrex]

aluminum chloride USP *topical astringent for hyperhidrosis* 20% topical

aluminum chloride, basic [see: aluminum sesquichlorohydrate]

aluminum chloride hexahydrate [see: aluminum chloride]

aluminum chloride hydroxide hydrate [see: aluminum chlorohydrate]

aluminum chlorohydrate USAN *anhidrotic*

aluminum chlorohydrex USAN *topical astringent*

aluminum chlorohydrol propylene glycol complex [now: aluminum chlorohydrex]

aluminum chlorohydroxy allantoinate JAN *astringent; keratolytic* [also: alcloxa]

aluminum clofibrate INN, BAN, JAN

aluminum dihydroxyaminoacetate [see: dihydroxyaluminum aminoacetate]

aluminum flufenamate JAN

aluminum glycinate, basic [see: dihydroxyaluminum aminoacetate]

aluminum hydroxide gel USP *antacid* 320, 450, 600 mg/5 mL oral

aluminum hydroxide gel, dried USP, JAN *antacid*

aluminum hydroxide glycine [see: dihydroxyaluminum aminoacetate]

aluminum hydroxide hydrate [see: algeldrate]

aluminum hydroxychloride [now: aluminum chlorohydrate]

aluminum magnesium carbonate hydroxide dihydrate [see: almagate]

aluminum magnesium hydroxide carbonate hydrate [see: hydrotalcite]

aluminum magnesium hydroxide oxide sulfate [see: almadrate sulfate]

aluminum magnesium hydroxide oxide sulfate hydrate [see: almadrate sulfate]

aluminum magnesium hydroxide sulfate [see: magaldrate]

aluminum magnesium hydroxide sulfate hydrate [see: magaldrate]

aluminum monostearate NF, JAN

aluminum oxide

Aluminum Paste ointment OTC *occlusive skin protectant* [metallic aluminum] 10%

aluminum phosphate gel USP *(disapproved for use as an antacid in 1989)*

aluminum potassium sulfate JAN *topical astringent* [also: alum, potassium]

aluminum potassium sulfate dodecahydrate [see: alum, potassium]

aluminum sesquichlorohydrate USAN *anhidrotic*

aluminum silicate, natural JAN

aluminum silicate, synthetic JAN

aluminum sodium carbonate hydroxide [see: dihydroxyaluminum sodium carbonate]

aluminum subacetate USP *topical astringent*

aluminum sulfate USP *anhidrotic*

aluminum sulfate hydrate [see: aluminum sulfate]

aluminum zirconium glycine tetrachloro hydrate complex [see: aluminum zirconium tetrachlorohydrex gly]

aluminum zirconium glycine trichloro hydrate complex [see: aluminum zirconium trichlorohydrex gly]

aluminum zirconium octachlorohydrate USP *anhidrotic*

aluminum zirconium octachlorohydrex gly USP *anhidrotic*

aluminum zirconium pentachlorohydrate USP *anhidrotic*

aluminum zirconium pentachlorohydrex gly USP *anhidrotic*

aluminum zirconium tetrachlorohydrate USP *anhidrotic*

aluminum zirconium tetrachlorohydrex gly USAN, USP *anhidrotic*

aluminum zirconium trichlorohydrate USP *anhidrotic*

aluminum zirconium trichlorohydrex gly USAN, USP *anhidrotic*

Alupent inhalation aerosol powder (discontinued 2008) ℞ *sympathomimetic bronchodilator* [metaproterenol sulfate] 0.65 mg/dose

Alupent solution for inhalation (discontinued 2009) ℞ *sympathomimetic bronchodilator* [metaproterenol sulfate] 0.4%, 0.6%, 5%

Alustra cream ℞ *hyperpigmentation bleaching agent* [hydroquinone; tretinoin (in a base containing glycolic acid and vitamins C and E)] 4% • 0.1%

alusulf INN ☑ Alasulf

Alu-Tab film-coated tablets (discontinued 2008) OTC *antacid* [aluminum hydroxide gel] 500 mg

Aluvia cream ℞ *moisturizer; emollient; keratolytic* [urea] 40% ☑ Aleve; ELF; olive

alvameline INN

alverine INN, BAN *anticholinergic* [also: alverine citrate]

alverine citrate USAN, NF *anticholinergic* [also: alverine]

Alvesco inhalation aerosol ℞ *once-daily corticosteroidal anti-inflammatory for persistent asthma* [ciclesonide] 80, 160 mcg/activation

alvimopan *peripherally acting opioid receptor antagonist for postoperative ileus (POI); restores normal bowel function after surgery*

alvircept sudotox USAN, INN *antiviral*

Alwextin *investigational (orphan) vulnerary for skin blistering and erosions associated with inherited epidermolysis bullosa* [allantoin]

Alzhemed *investigational (Phase III) amyloid-beta antagonist to reduce plaque* *formation in Alzheimer disease* [tramiprosate]

amabevan [see: carbarsone]

amacetam HCl [now: pramiracetam HCl]

amacetam sulfate [now: pramiracetam sulfate]

amadinone INN *progestin* [also: amadinone acetate]

amadinone acetate USAN *progestin* [also: amadinone]

amafolone INN, BAN

amalgucin ② imiloxan

Amanita muscaria **mushrooms** *a species that produces muscarine and ibotenic acid, a psychotropic substance ingested as a street drug*

amanozine INN

amantadine INN, BAN *antiviral for influenza A virus; dopaminergic antiparkinson agent* [also: amantadine HCl]

amantadine HCl USAN, USP, JAN *antiviral for influenza A infections; dopaminergic antiparkinson agent* [also: amantadine] 100 mg oral; 50 mg/5 mL oral

amantanium bromide INN

A-Mantle cream OTC *nontherapeutic base for compounding various dermatological preparations*

amantocillin INN

amara; amargo *medicinal herb* [see: quassia]

amaranth (*Amaranthus* **spp.**) leaves and flowers *medicinal herb for diarrhea, dysentery, excessive menstruation, and nosebleeds*

amaranth (**FD&C Red No. 2**) USP

amargo; amara *medicinal herb* [see: quassia]

amarsan [see: acetarsone]

Amaryl tablets ℞ *once-daily sulfonylurea antidiabetic that stimulates insulin secretion in the pancreas* [glimepiride] 1, 2, 4 mg

Amazing Spiderman Gummies, The OTC *vitamin/mineral supplement* [multiple vitamins and minerals; folic acid; biotin] ± • 100 • 22.5 mcg

ambamustine INN

ambasilide INN *antiarrhythmic*

ambazone INN, BAN ② ampyzine

ambenonium chloride USP, INN, BAN, JAN *anticholinesterase muscle stimulant for myasthenia gravis*

ambenoxan INN, BAN

amber; amber touch-and-heal *medicinal herb* [see: St. John wort]

Ambi 10 bar (discontinued 2008) OTC *therapeutic skin cleanser* ② AMPA

Ambi 10PEH/4CPM caplets OTC *decongestant; antihistamine* [phenylephrine HCl; chlorpheniramine maleate] 10 • 4 mg

Ambi 10PEH/4CPM/20DM caplets ℞ *decongestant; antihistamine; antitussive* [phenylephrine HCl; chlorpheniramine maleate; dextromethorphan hydrobromide] 10 • 4 • 20 mg

Ambi 10PEH/400GFN caplets ℞ *decongestant; expectorant* [phenylephrine HCl; guaifenesin] 10 • 400 mg

Ambi 10PEH/400GFN/20DM caplets ℞ *decongestant; expectorant; antitussive* [phenylephrine HCl; guaifenesin; dextromethorphan hydrobromide] 10 • 400 • 20 mg

Ambi 20DM/4CPM caplets ℞ *antitussive; antihistamine* [dextromethorphan hydrobromide; chlorpheniramine maleate] 20 • 4 mg

Ambi 40PSE/400GFN; Ambi 60PSE/400GFN caplets ℞ *decongestant; expectorant* [pseudoephedrine HCl; guaifenesin] 40 • 400 mg; 60 • 400 mg

Ambi 40PSE/400GFN/20DM; Ambi 60PSE/400GFN/20DM caplets ℞ *decongestant; expectorant; antitussive* [pseudoephedrine HCl; guaifenesin; dextromethorphan hydrobromide] 40 • 400 • 20 mg; 60 • 400 • 20 mg

Ambi 60/580 caplets ℞ *decongestant; expectorant* [pseudoephedrine HCl; guaifenesin] 60 • 580 mg ② AMPA

Ambi 60/580/30 extended-release caplets ℞ *decongestant; expectorant; antitussive* [pseudoephedrine HCl; guaifenesin; dextromethorphan hydrobromide] 60 • 580 • 30 mg ② AMPA

Ambi 60PSE/4CPM caplets OTC *decongestant; antihistamine* [pseudoephedrine HCl; chlorpheniramine maleate] 60•4 mg

Ambi 60PSE/4CPM/20DM caplets ℞ *decongestant; antihistamine; antitussive* [pseudoephedrine HCl; chlorpheniramine maleate; dextromethorphan hydrobromide] 60•4•20 mg

Ambi 80/700/40; Ambi 80/780/40 extended-release caplets (discontinued 2007) ℞ *decongestant; expectorant; antitussive* [pseudoephedrine HCl; guaifenesin; dextromethorphan hydrobromide] 80•700•40 mg; 80•780•40 mg ② AMPA

Ambi 1000/5 caplets ℞ *expectorant; antitussive* [guaifenesin; carbetapentane citrate] 1000•5 mg ② AMPA

Ambi 1000/55 extended-release tablets ℞ *expectorant; antitussive* [guaifenesin; dextromethorphan hydrobromide] 1000•55 mg ② AMPA

ambicromil INN, BAN *prophylactic antiallergic* [also: probicromil calcium]

ambicromil calcium [see: probicromil calcium]

Ambien film-coated tablets ℞ *imidazopyridine sedative and hypnotic for the short-term treatment of insomnia* [zolpidem tartrate] 5, 10 mg

Ambien CR controlled-release bilayered tablets ℞ *imidazopyridine sedative and hypnotic for the short-term treatment of insomnia* [zolpidem tartrate] 6.25, 12.5 mg

Ambifed; Ambifed-G caplets ℞ *decongestant; expectorant* [pseudoephedrine HCl; guaifenesin] 30•400 mg; 20•400 mg

Ambifed CD; Ambifed CDX caplets ℞ *narcotic antitussive; decongestant; expectorant* [codeine phosphate; pseudoephedrine HCl; guaifenesin] 10•30•400 mg; 20•30•400 mg

Ambifed-G DM extended-release caplets ℞ *antitussive; decongestant; expectorant* [dextromethorphan hydrobromide; pseudoephedrine HCl; guaifenesin] 20•20•400, 30•60•1000 mg

AmBisome powder for IV infusion ℞ *systemic polyene antifungal for cryptococcal meningitis, visceral leishmaniasis, and histoplasmosis (orphan)* [amphotericin B lipid complex (ABLC)] 50 mg/vial

ambomycin USAN, INN *antineoplastic*

ambrette (Abelmoschus moschatus) seeds and oil *medicinal herb for gastric cancer, gonorrhea, hysteria, and respiratory disorders; also used as a fragrance in cosmetics and a flavoring in alcoholic beverages, bitters, and coffees; not generally regarded as safe and effective for medicinal uses*

ambrisentan *endothelin 1 (ET1) receptor antagonist (ERA); vasodilator for pulmonary arterial hypertension (PAH)*

ambroxol INN [also: ambroxol HCl]

ambroxol HCl JAN [also: ambroxol]

ambruticin USAN, INN *antifungal*

ambucaine INN

ambucetamide INN, BAN

ambulatory ara-C + DNR (daunorubicin) *chemotherapy protocol for acute myelocytic leukemia (AML)*

ambuphylline USAN *diuretic; smooth muscle relaxant* [also: bufylline]

ambuside USAN, INN, BAN *diuretic*

ambuterol [see: mabuterol]

ambutonium bromide BAN

ambutoxate [see: ambucaine]

amcinafal USAN, INN *anti-inflammatory*

amcinafide USAN, INN *anti-inflammatory*

amcinonide USAN, USP, INN, BAN, JAN *topical corticosteroidal anti-inflammatory* 0.1% topical

amdinocillin USAN, USP *aminopenicillin antibiotic* [also: mecillinam]

amdinocillin pivoxil USAN *antibacterial* [also: pivmecillinam; pivmecillinam HCl]

amdoxovir USAN *nucleoside analog antiviral*

Amdry-D extended-release caplets ℞ *decongestant; anticholinergic to dry mucosal secretions* [pseudoephedrine HCl; methscopolamine nitrate] 120•2.5 mg

ameban [see: carbarsone]

amebarsone [see: carbarsone]

amebicides *a class of drugs that kill amoebae*

amebucort INN

amechol [see: methacholine chloride]

amedalin INN *antidepressant* [also: amedalin HCl] 🄐 imidoline; omidoline

amedalin HCl USAN *antidepressant* [also: amedalin]

amediplase INN

ameltolide USAN, INN, BAN *anticonvulsant*

amenozine [see: amanozine]

Amerge film-coated tablets ℞ (available OTC in Europe as **Triptan**) *vascular serotonin 5-HT$_{1D}$ receptor agonist for the acute treatment of migraine* [naratriptan (as HCl)] 1, 2.5 mg

Americaine ointment, anorectal ointment, aerosol spray (discontinued 2007) OTC *anesthetic* [benzocaine] 20%

Americaine Anesthetic Lubricant gel (discontinued 2007) ℞ *anesthetic lubricant for upper GI procedures* [benzocaine] 20%

Americaine First Aid ointment OTC *anesthetic* [benzocaine] 20%

American angelica *medicinal herb* [see: angelica]

American aspen *medicinal herb* [see: poplar]

American centaury (*Sabatia angularis*) plant *medicinal herb used as a bitter tonic, emmenagogue, febrifuge, and vermifuge*

American elder *medicinal herb* [see: elderberry]

American elm *medicinal herb* [see: slippery elm]

American foxglove *medicinal herb* [see: feverweed]

American ginseng (*Panax quinquefolia*) *medicinal herb* [see: ginseng]

American hellebore (*Veratrum viride*) [see: hellebore]

American ivy (*Parthenocissus quinquefolia*) bark and twigs *medicinal herb used as an alterative, astringent, and expectorant*

American nightshade *medicinal herb* [see: pokeweed]

American pepper; American red pepper *medicinal herb* [see: cayenne]

American saffron *medicinal herb* [see: safflower]

American valerian *medicinal herb* [see: lady's slipper]

American vegetable tallow tree; American vegetable wax *medicinal herb* [see: bayberry]

American woodbine *medicinal herb* [see: American ivy]

Americet tablets ℞ *barbiturate sedative; analgesic; antipyretic* [butalbital; aspirin; caffeine] 50•325•40 mg

americium *element* (Am)

Amerifed oral liquid (discontinued 2007) OTC *decongestant; antihistamine* [pseudoephedrine HCl; chlorpheniramine maleate] 80•4 mg/5 mL

Amerigel lotion, ointment OTC *emollient; diaper rash treatment*

Amerituss AD oral liquid (discontinued 2007) ℞ *antitussive; antihistamine; decongestant* [dextromethorphan hydrobromide; chlorpheniramine maleate; phenylephrine HCl] 30•6•20 mg/10 mL

amesergide USAN, INN *serotonin antagonist; antidepressant*

ametantrone INN *antineoplastic* [also: ametantrone acetate]

ametantrone acetate USAN *antineoplastic* [also: ametantrone]

ametazole BAN [also: betazole HCl; betazole]

A-Methapred powder for injection ℞ *corticosteroid; anti-inflammatory; immunosuppressant* [methylprednisolone sodium succinate] 40, 125 mg/vial

amethocaine BAN *topical anesthetic* [also: tetracaine]

amethocaine HCl BAN *local anesthetic* [also: tetracaine HCl]

amethopterin [now: methotrexate]

Amevive powder for IM injection ℞ *immunosuppressant for chronic plaque psoriasis* [alefacept] 15 mg/dose

amezepine INN

amezinium metilsulfate INN, JAN

amfebutamone INN *aminoketone anti-depressant; non-nicotine aid to smoking cessation* [also: bupropion HCl; bupropion]

amfebutamone HCl [see: bupropion HCl]

amfecloral INN, BAN *anorectic* [also: amphecloral]

amfenac INN, BAN *anti-inflammatory* [also: amfenac sodium]

amfenac sodium USAN, JAN *anti-inflammatory* [also: amfenac]

amfepentorex INN

amfepramone INN *anorexiant* [also: diethylpropion HCl; diethylpropion]

amfepramone HCl *anorexiant* [see: diethylpropion HCl]

amfetamine INN *CNS stimulant* [also: amphetamine sulfate; amphetamine]

amfetaminil INN

amfilcon A USAN *hydrophilic contact lens material*

amflutizole USAN, INN *gout suppressant*

amfodyne [see: imidecyl iodine]

amfomycin INN *antibacterial* [also: amphomycin]

amfonelic acid USAN, INN, BAN *CNS stimulant*

amibiarson [see: carbarsone]

Amicar tablets, syrup ℞ *systemic hemostatic to control excessive bleeding* [aminocaproic acid] 500, 1000 mg; 250 mg/mL ② Omacor

amicarbalide INN, BAN

amicibone INN

amicloral USAN *veterinary food additive*

amicycline USAN, INN *antibacterial*

amidantel INN, BAN

amidapsone USAN, INN *antiviral for poultry*

Amidate IV injection ℞ *rapid-acting nonbarbiturate general anesthetic* [etomidate] 2 mg/mL

amidefrine mesilate INN *adrenergic* [also: amidephrine mesylate; amidephrine]

amidephrine BAN *adrenergic* [also: amidephrine mesylate; amidefrine mesilate]

amidephrine mesylate USAN *adrenergic* [also: amidefrine mesilate; amidephrine]

amidofebrin [see: aminopyrine]

amidol [see: dimepheptanol]

amidone HCl [see: methadone HCl]

amidopyrazoline [see: aminopyrine]

amidopyrine [now: aminopyrine]

amidotrizoate sodium [see: diatrizoate sodium]

amidotrizoic acid JAN *radiopaque contrast medium* [also: diatrizoic acid]

amiflamine INN

amifloverine INN

amifloxacin USAN, INN, BAN *broad-spectrum fluoroquinolone antibiotic*

amifloxacin mesylate USAN *broad-spectrum fluoroquinolone antibiotic*

amifostine USAN, INN, BAN *chemoprotective agent for cisplatin and paclitaxel chemotherapy* (orphan); *treatment for moderate to severe xerostomia following postoperative radiation therapy* (orphan); *investigational* (orphan) *for cyclophosphamide-induced granulocytopenia* 500 mg injection

Amigesic film-coated tablets, film-coated caplets, capsules ℞ *analgesic; antipyretic; anti-inflammatory; antirheumatic* [salsalate] 500 mg; 750 mg; 500 mg

amiglumide INN

amikacin USP, INN, BAN *aminoglycoside antibiotic; investigational* (orphan) *for bronchopulmonary* Pseudomonas aeruginosa *infections in cystic fibrosis patients*

amikacin sulfate USAN, USP, JAN *aminoglycoside antibiotic* 50, 250 mg/mL injection

amikhelline INN ② Amoclan

Amikin IV or IM injection, pediatric injection ℞ *aminoglycoside antibiotic* [amikacin sulfate] 250 mg/mL; 50 mg/mL

amilomer INN

amiloride INN, BAN *antihypertensive; potassium-sparing diuretic* [also: amiloride HCl]

amiloride HCl USAN, USP *antihypertensive; potassium-sparing diuretic for* *congestive heart failure; investigational (orphan) inhalant for cystic fibrosis; also used for lithium-induced polyuria* [also: amiloride] 5 mg oral

amiloxate USAN *ultraviolet B sunscreen*

aminacrine BAN *topical antiseptic* [also: aminacrine HCl; aminoacridine]

aminacrine HCl USAN *vaginal antiseptic* [also: aminoacridine; aminacrine]

aminarsone [see: carbarsone]

amindocate INN

amine resin [see: polyamine-methylene resin]

amineptine INN

Aminess 5.2% IV infusion ℞ *nutritional therapy for renal failure* [multiple essential amino acids]

Aminess N film-coated tablets ℞ *nutritional therapy for dialysis patients* [multiple essential amino acids]

aminicotin [see: niacinamide]

aminitrozole INN *veterinary antibacterial* [also: nithiamide; acinitrazole]

2-amino-2-deoxyglucose [see: glucosamine]

aminoacetic acid JAN *nonessential amino acid; urologic irrigant; symbols:* Gly, G [also: glycine]

aminoacridine INN *topical antiseptic* [also: aminacrine HCl; aminacrine]

aminoacridine HCl [see: aminacrine HCl]

9-aminoacridine monohydrochloride [see: aminacrine HCl]

p-**aminobenzenearsonic acid** [see: arsanilic acid]

p-**aminobenzenesulfonamide** [see: sulfanilamide]

p-**aminobenzene-sulfonylacetylimide** [see: sulfacetamide]

aminobenzoate potassium USP *water-soluble vitamin; analgesic; "possibly effective" for scleroderma and other skin diseases and Peyronie disease* 500 mg oral

aminobenzoate sodium USP *analgesic*

p-**aminobenzoic acid** [see: aminobenzoic acid]

aminobenzoic acid (4-aminobenzoic acid) USP *water-soluble vitamin; ultra-*violet screen; "possibly effective" for scleroderma and other skin diseases and Peyronie disease*

aminobenzylpenicillin [see: ampicillin]

γ-**amino-β-hydroxybutyric acid** JAN

Aminobrain Forte capsules OTC *vitamin/mineral/amino acid supplement* [multiple B vitamins and minerals; vitamin E; folic acid; gingko biloba] ≟•15 U•400 mcg•60 mg

aminobromophenylpyrimidinone (ABPP) [see: bropirimine]

γ-**aminobutyric acid (GABA)** JAN *inhibitory neurotransmitter*

aminocaproic acid USAN, USP, INN, BAN *systemic hemostatic; investigational (orphan) topical treatment for traumatic hyphema of the eye* [also: ∈-aminocaproic acid] 500 mg oral; 250 mg/mL oral; 250 mg/mL injection

∈-**aminocaproic acid** JAN *systemic hemostatic* [also: aminocaproic acid]

aminocardol [see: aminophylline]

Amino-Cerv vaginal cream ℞ *emollient; antifungal; anti-inflammatory* [urea; sodium propionate; methionine; cystine; inositol] 8.34%•0.5%•0.83%•0.35%•0.83%

aminodeoxykanamycin [see: bekanamycin]

2-aminoethanethiol [see: cysteamine]

2-aminoethanethiol HCl [see: cysteamine HCl]

2-aminoethanol [see: monoethanolamine]

aminoethyl nitrate (2-aminoethyl nitrate) INN

amino-ethyl-propanol [see: ambuphylline]

aminoethylsulfonic acid JAN [also: taurine]

Aminofen; Aminofen Max tablets OTC *analgesic; antipyretic* [acetaminophen] 325 mg; 500 mg

aminoform [see: methenamine]

2-aminoglutaramic acid [see: glutamine]

aminoglutethimide USP, INN, BAN *adrenal steroid inhibitor; antisteroidal antineoplastic*

aminoglycosides *a class of bactericidal antibiotics effective against gram-negative organisms* (also called: "mycins")

aminoguanidine monohydrochloride [see: pimagedine HCl]

6-aminohexanoic acid [see: aminocaproic acid]

aminohippurate sodium USP *diagnostic aid for renal function* [also: *p*-aminohippurate sodium] 20% injection

p-aminohippurate sodium JAN *renal function test* [also: aminohippurate sodium]

aminohippuric acid (p-aminohippuric acid) USP

aminohydroxypropylidene diphosphonate (APD) [see: pamidronate disodium]

aminoisobutanol [see: ambuphylline]

aminoisometradine [see: methionine]

aminoketones *a class of oral antidepressants*

5-aminolevulinic acid HCl (5-ALA HCl) USAN *photosensitizer for photodynamic therapy of precancerous actinic keratoses of the face and scalp (for use with the* BLU-U Blue Light Photodynamic Therapy Illuminator*)*

aminometradine INN, BAN

Amino-Min-D capsules (discontinued 2008) OTC *calcium/mineral supplement* [calcium (as carbonate); multiple minerals; vitamin D] 250 mg•±•100 U

aminonat [see: protein hydrolysate]

Amino-Opti-C sustained-release tablets OTC *vitamin C supplement with multiple bioflavonoids* [vitamin C; lemon bioflavonoids; rose hips; rutin; hesperidin] 1000•250•?•?•? mg

aminopenicillins *a subclass of penicillins (q.v.)*

aminopentamide sulfate [see: dimevamide]

aminophenazone INN [also: aminopyrine]

aminophenazone cyclamate INN

p-aminophenylarsonic acid [see: arsanilic acid]

aminophylline USP, INN, BAN, JAN *smooth muscle relaxant; bronchodilator* (theophylline=79%) 100, 200 mg oral; 25 mg/mL injection

aminopromazine INN [also: proquamezine]

aminopterin sodium INN, BAN *antifolate antineoplastic*

4-aminopyridine (4-AP) [see: fampridine, dalfampridine]

aminopyrine NF, JAN [also: aminophenazone]

aminoquin naphthoate [see: pamaquine naphthoate]

aminoquinol INN

aminoquinoline [see: aminoquinol]

4-aminoquinoline [see: chloroquine phosphate]

8-aminoquinoline [see: primaquine phosphate]

aminoquinuride INN

aminorex USAN, INN, BAN *anorectic*

aminosalicylate calcium USP [also: calcium para-aminosalicylate]

aminosalicylate potassium USP

aminosalicylate sodium (p-aminosalicylate sodium) USP *bacteriostatic; tuberculosis retreatment agent; investigational (orphan) for Crohn disease*

aminosalicylic acid (4-aminosalicylic acid; p-aminosalicylic acid) USP *antibacterial; tuberculostatic (orphan); investigational (orphan) for ulcerative colitis*

5-aminosalicylic acid (5-ASA) [see: mesalamine]

aminosalyle sodium [see: aminosalicylate sodium]

aminosidine *investigational (orphan) agent for tuberculosis,* Mycobacterium avium *complex (MAC), and visceral leishmaniasis*

aminosidine sulfate [see: paromomycin sulfate]

21-aminosteroids *a class of potent antioxidants that can protect against oxygen radical–mediated lipid peroxidation and progressive neuronal degeneration* *following brain or spinal trauma, sub-arachnoid hemorrhage, or stroke* [also called: lazaroids]

aminosuccinic acid [see: aspartic acid]

Aminosyn 3.5% (5%, 7%, 8.5%, 10%); Aminosyn II 3.5% (5%, 7%, 8.5%, 10%, 15%); Aminosyn-PF 7% (10%) IV infusion ℞ *total parenteral nutrition (except 3.5%); peripheral parenteral nutrition (all)* [multiple essential and nonessential amino acids] ⊡ amanozine

Aminosyn 3.5% M; Aminosyn II 3.5% M IV infusion ℞ *peripheral parenteral nutrition* [multiple essential and nonessential amino acids; electrolytes]

Aminosyn 7% (8.5%) with Electrolytes; Aminosyn II 7% (8.5%, 10%) with Electrolytes IV infusion ℞ *total parenteral nutrition; peripheral parenteral nutrition* [multiple essential and nonessential amino acids; electrolytes] ⊡ amanozine

Aminosyn II 3.5% in 5% (25%) Dextrose; Aminosyn II 4.25% in 10% (20%, 25%) Dextrose; Aminosyn II 5% in 25% Dextrose IV infusion ℞ *total parenteral nutrition (except 3.5% in 5%); peripheral parenteral nutrition (not 20% and 25%)* [multiple essential and nonessential amino acids; dextrose]

Aminosyn II 3.5% M in 5% Dextrose; Aminosyn II 4.25% M in 10% Dextrose IV infusion ℞ *total parenteral nutrition (4.25% in 10% only); peripheral parenteral nutrition (both)* [multiple essential and nonessential amino acids; electrolytes; dextrose]

Aminosyn-HBC 7% IV infusion ℞ *nutritional therapy for high metabolic stress* [multiple branched-chain essential and nonessential amino acids; electrolytes]

Aminosyn-RF 5.2% IV infusion ℞ *nutritional therapy for renal failure* [multiple essential amino acids]

aminothiazole INN

aminotrate phosphate [see: trolnitrate phosphate]

aminoxaphen [see: aminorex]

Aminoxin enteric-coated tablets OTC *vitamin B$_6$ supplement* [pyridoxal-5'-phosphate] 20 mg

aminoxytriphene INN

aminoxytropine tropate HCl [see: atropine oxide HCl]

Amio-Aqueous investigational (orphan) *antiarrhythmic for incessant ventricular tachycardia* [amiodarone]

amiodarone USAN, INN, BAN *antiarrhythmic for acute ventricular tachycardia and fibrillation (orphan)*

amiodarone HCl *ventricular antiarrhythmic for acute ventricular tachycardia and fibrillation (orphan)* 200, 400 mg oral; 50 mg/mL injection

amiperone INN ⊡ Empirin

amiphenazole INN, BAN

amipizone INN ⊡ ampyzine

amipramidine [see: amiloride HCl]

amiprilose INN *synthetic monosaccharide anti-inflammatory* [also: amiprilose HCl]

amiprilose HCl USAN *synthetic monosaccharide anti-inflammatory* [also: amiprilose]

amiquinsin INN *antihypertensive* [also: amiquinsin HCl]

amiquinsin HCl USAN *antihypertensive* [also: amiquinsin]

amisometradine NF, INN, BAN

amisulpride INN

amiterol INN ⊡ Emetrol

amithiozone [see: thioacetazone; thiacetazone]

amitivir USAN, INN *influenza vaccine* ⊡ emitefur

Amitiza softgels ℞ *selective chloride channel activator to increase fluid secretion in the small intestine for the treatment of chronic idiopathic constipation in adults and irritable bowel syndrome with constipation (IBS-C) in women* [lubiprostone] 8, 24 mcg

amitraz USAN, INN, BAN *scabicide*

44   amitriptyline

amitriptyline (AMT) INN, BAN *tricyclic antidepressant* [also: amitriptyline HCl]

amitriptyline HCl USP, JAN *tricyclic antidepressant* [also: amitriptyline] 10, 25, 50, 75, 100, 150 mg oral

amitriptylinoxide INN

amixetrine INN ⊡ amogastrin

AmLactin cream, lotion OTC *moisturizer; emollient* [ammonium lactate] 12%

AmLactin AP cream (discontinued 2009) OTC *local anesthetic; moisturizer; emollient* [pramoxine HCl; lactic acid] 1%•12%

AmLactin Foot Cream Therapy OTC *moisturizer; emollient* [ammonium lactate; potassium lactate; sodium lactate]

AmLactin XL lotion OTC *moisturizer; emollient* [ammonium lactate; potassium lactate; sodium lactate]

amlexanox USAN, INN, JAN *anti-inflammatory for aphthous ulcers; topical histamine and leukotriene inhibitor*

amlintide USAN *antidiabetic for type 1 diabetes* [see also: pramlintide acetate]

amlodipine INN, BAN *antianginal; antihypertensive; calcium channel blocker* [also: amlodipine besylate]

amlodipine besylate USAN *antianginal; antihypertensive; calcium channel blocker* [also: amlodipine] 2.5, 5, 10 mg oral

amlodipine besylate & benazepril HCl *combination angiotensin-converting enzyme (ACE) inhibitor and calcium channel blocker for hypertension* 2.5•10, 5•10, 5•20, 5•40, 10•20, 10•40 mg

amlodipine maleate USAN *antianginal; antihypertensive*

ammi (*Ammi majus; A. visnaga*) dried ripe fruits *medicinal herb for angina, bronchial asthma, diabetes, diuresis, kidney and bladder stones, psoriasis, respiratory diseases, and vitiligo*

ammoidin [see: methoxsalen]

[¹³N] ammonia [see: ammonia N 13]

ammonia [see: ammonia spirit, aromatic]

ammonia N 13 USAN, USP *radioactive diagnostic aid for cardiac and liver imaging* 30–300 mCi/8 mL injection

ammonia solution, strong NF *solvent; source of ammonia* [also: ammonia water]

ammonia spirit, aromatic USP *respiratory stimulant*

ammonia water JAN *solvent; source of ammonia* [also: ammonia solution, strong]

ammoniated mercury [see: mercury, ammoniated]

ammonio methacrylate copolymer NF *coating agent*

ammonium alum [see: alum, ammonium]

ammonium benzoate USP

ammonium carbonate NF *source of ammonia*

ammonium chloride USP, JAN *urinary acidifier; diuretic; expectorant* 486, 500 mg oral; 5 mEq/mL (26.75%) injection

ammonium 2-hydroxypropanoate [see: ammonium lactate]

ammonium ichthosulfonate [see: ichthammol]

ammonium lactate (lactic acid neutralized with ammonium hydroxide) USAN *antipruritic; emollient for xerosis* 12% topical

ammonium mandelate USP

ammonium molybdate USP *dietary molybdenum supplement; additive to IV solutions for total parenteral nutrition* (54% elemental molybdenum) 46 mcg/mL (25 mcg/mL Mo) injection

ammonium molybdate tetrahydrate [see: ammonium molybdate]

ammonium phosphate NF *pharmaceutic aid*

ammonium salicylate NF

ammonium tetrathiomolybdate *investigational (orphan) for Wilson disease*

ammonium valerate NF

Ammonul IV infusion ℞ *adjunctive therapy (rescue agent) to prevent and treat hyperammonemia due to urea* cycle enzymopathy (orphan) [sodium benzoate; sodium phenylacetate] 101•100 mg/mL

ammophyllin [see: aminophylline]

Amnaranthus **spp.** *medicinal herb* [see: amaranth]

Amnesteem capsules ℞ *keratolytic for severe recalcitrant cystic acne* [isotretinoin] 10, 20, 40 mg

AMO Endosol; AMO Endosol Extra ophthalmic solution (discontinued 2008) ℞ *intraocular irrigating solution* [sodium chloride (balanced saline solution)]

AMO Vitrax intraocular injection (discontinued 2010) ℞ *viscoelastic agent for ophthalmic surgery* [hyaluronate sodium] 30 mg/mL

amobarbital USP, INN, JAN *sedative; hypnotic; anticonvulsant; also abused as a street drug* [also: amylobarbitone]

amobarbital sodium USP, JAN *hypnotic; sedative; anticonvulsant; also abused as a street drug*

amocaine chloride [see: amolanone HCl]

amocarzine INN

Amoclan powder for oral suspension ℞ *aminopenicillin antibiotic plus synergist* [amoxicillin; clavulanate potassium] 200•28.5, 400•57 mg/5 mL ⟳ amikhelline

amodiaquine USP, INN, BAN *antiprotozoal*

amodiaquine HCl USP *antimalarial*

amogastrin INN, JAN ⟳ amixetrine

amolanone INN

amolanone HCl [see: amolanone]

amonafide INN *antineoplastic*

amoproxan INN

amopyroquine INN

amorolfine USAN, INN, BAN *antimycotic*

Amorphophallus konjac *medicinal herb* [see: glucomannan]

Amosan powder OTC *oral antibacterial* [sodium peroxyborate monohydrate]

amoscanate INN

amosulalol INN [also: amosulalol HCl]

amosulalol HCl JAN [also: amosulalol]

amotriphene [see: aminoxytriphene]

amoxapine USAN, USP, INN, BAN, JAN *tricyclic antidepressant* 25, 50, 100, 150 mg oral

amoxecaine INN

Amoxicilin Pulsys oral *investigational (NDA filed) once-daily aminopenicillin antibiotic for tonsillitis and pharyngitis due to streptococcal infections* [amoxicillin]

amoxicillin USAN, USP, JAN *aminopenicillin antibiotic* [also: amoxicilline; amoxycillin] 125, 200, 250, 400, 500, 875 mg oral; 125, 200, 250 mg/5 mL oral

amoxicillin & clavulanate potassium *aminopenicillin antibiotic plus synergist* 200•28.5, 250•125, 400•57, 500•125, 875•125, 1000•62.5 mg oral; 200•28.5, 250•62.5, 400•57, 600•42.9 mg/5 mL oral

amoxicillin sodium USAN *aminopenicillin antibiotic*

amoxicillin trihydrate [see: amoxicillin]

amoxicilline INN *aminopenicillin antibiotic* [also: amoxicillin; amoxycillin]

amoxicllin & clarithromycin & omeprazole *combination aminopenicillin and macrolide antibiotic plus a gastric antisecretory* 500•500•20 mg oral

Amoxil chewable tablets (discontinued 2008) ℞ *aminopenicillin antibiotic* [amoxicillin] 200, 400 mg

Amoxil film-coated caplets, capsules ℞ *aminopenicillin antibiotic* [amoxicillin] 875 mg; 500 mg

Amoxil powder for oral suspension, pediatric oral drops (discontinued 2009) ℞ *aminopenicillin antibiotic* [amoxicillin] 125, 200 mg/5 mL; 50 mg/mL

amoxycillin BAN *aminopenicillin antibiotic* [also: amoxicillin; amoxicilline]

amoxydramine camsilate INN [also: amoxydramine camsylate]

amoxydramine camsylate [also: amoxydramine camsilate]

AMP; A₅MP (adenosine monophosphate) [see: adenosine phosphate]

AMPA (α-amino-3-hydroxy-5-methyl-4-isoxazolepropionic acid) ☒ Ambi

ampakines *a class of drugs that modulate neurotransmitters by affecting the AMPA-glutamate receptors (AMPA-GluR) in the brain, enhancing cognition and memory; investigational treatment for Alzheimer and other dementias*

amperozide INN, BAN *antipsychotic*

Amphadase solution for injection ℞ *adjuvant to increase the absorption and dispersion of injected drugs, hypodermoclysis, and subcutaneous urography; investigational (NDA filed) agent to clear vitreous hemorrhage; also used for diabetic retinopathy* [hyaluronidase (bovine)] 150 U/mL

amphecloral USAN *anorectic* [also: amfecloral]

amphenidone INN

amphetamine BAN *CNS stimulant; often abused as a street drug, which causes strong psychic dependence* [also: amphetamine sulfate; amfetamine]

d-amphetamine [see: dextroamphetamine]

(+)-amphetamine [see: dextroamphetamine]

l-amphetamine [see: levamphetamine]

(−)-amphetamine [see: levamphetamine]

amphetamine aspartate *CNS stimulant*

amphetamine complex (resin complex of amphetamine & dextroamphetamine) [q.v.]

amphetamine phosphate, dextro [see: dextroamphetamine phosphate]

Amphetamine Salt Combo tablets ℞ *CNS stimulant mixture for attention-deficit/hyperactivity disorder (ADHD)* [amphetamine aspartate; amphetamine sulfate; dextroamphetamine sulfate; dextroamphetamine saccharate] 5, 10, 20, 30 mg total amphetamines (25% of each)

amphetamine succinate, levo [see: levamphetamine succinate]

amphetamine sulfate USP *CNS stimulant; often abused as a street drug,* which causes strong psychic dependence [also: amfetamine; amphetamine]

amphetamine sulfate, dextro [see: dextroamphetamine sulfate]

amphetamines *a class of CNS stimulants that includes amphetamine, dextroamphetamine, levamphetamine, methamphetamine, and their salts*

amphetamines, mixed (equal parts amphetamine aspartate, amphetamine sulfate, dextroamphetamine sulfate, and dextroamphetamine saccharate) *CNS stimulant for attention-deficit/hyperactivity disorder (ADHD), narcolepsy, and obesity; also abused as a street drug, which causes strong psychic dependence* [5, 10, 15, 20, 25, 30 mg oral]

Amphocin powder for IV infusion (discontinued 2008) ℞ *systemic polyene antifungal* [amphotericin B deoxycholate] 50 mg/vial

amphocortrin [see: amphomycin]

Amphojel tablets OTC *antacid* [aluminum hydroxide gel] 300, 600 mg

amphomycin USAN, BAN *antibacterial* [also: amfomycin]

amphotalide INN

Amphotec powder for IV infusion ℞ *systemic polyene antifungal for invasive aspergillosis* [amphotericin B cholesteryl sulfate] 50, 100 mg/vial

amphotericin B USP, INN, BAN, JAN *polyene antifungal*

amphotericin B cholesteryl sulfate *systemic polyene antifungal for invasive aspergillosis*

amphotericin B deoxycholate *systemic polyene antifungal* 50 mg injection

amphotericin B lipid complex (ABLC) *systemic polyene antifungal for meningitis, leishmaniasis, histoplasmosis, and other invasive infections* (orphan)

ampicillin USAN, USP, INN, BAN, JAN *aminopenicillin antibiotic* 250, 500 mg oral

ampicillin sodium USAN, USP, JAN *aminopenicillin antibiotic* 125, 250, 500 mg, 1, 2, 10 g injection

ampicillin sodium & sulbactam sodium *aminopenicillin antibiotic plus synergist* 1•0.5, 2•1, 10•5 g injection

ampiroxicam INN, BAN

Amplicor Chlamydia test kit for professional use ℞ *in vitro diagnostic aid for* Chlamydia trachomatis [DNA amplification test]

Amplicor HIV-1 Monitor test kit for professional use ℞ *in vitro diagnostic aid for HIV-1 in blood* [polymerase chain reaction (PCR) test]

Amplicor MTB test kit for professional use ℞ *in vitro diagnostic aid for* Mycobacterium *tuberculosis* [polymerase chain reaction (PCR) test]

Ampligen *investigational (Phase III, orphan) RNA synthesis inhibitor and immunomodulator for AIDS, renal cell carcinoma, metastatic melanoma, and chronic fatigue syndrome* [poly I: poly C12U]

amprenavir USAN, INN *protease inhibitor antiviral for HIV infection*

amprocidum [see: amprolium]

amprolium USAN, INN, BAN *coccidiostat for poultry*

amprotropine phosphate

Ampyra film-coated extended-release tablets ℞ *potassium-channel blocker to improve walking with multiple sclerosis* [dalfampridine] 10 mg

ampyrimine INN ⍰ embramine; imipramine

ampyzine INN *CNS stimulant* [also: ampyzine sulfate] ⍰ amipizone

ampyzine sulfate USAN *CNS stimulant* [also: ampyzine]

amquinate USAN, INN *antimalarial*

amrinone INN, BAN *cardiotonic* [also: inamrinone]

amrinone lactate [now: inamrinone lactate]

Amrix extended-release capsules ℞ *once-daily skeletal muscle relaxant* [cyclobenzaprine HCl] 15, 30 mg

amrubicin INN

AMSA; *m*-AMSA (acridinylamine methanesulfon anisidide) [see: amsacrine]

amsacrine USAN, INN, BAN *investigational (NDA filed, orphan) antineoplastic for acute adult leukemias (AML, APL, and ALL) and lymphomas*

Amsidyl *investigational (NDA filed, orphan) antineoplastic for acute adult leukemias (AML, APL, and ALL) and lymphomas* [amsacrine]

amsonate INN, BAN *combining name for radicals or groups*

AMT (amitriptyline HCl) [q.v.]

amtolmetin guacil INN

Amturnide tablets ℞ *once-daily combination direct renin inhibitor, calcium channel blocker, and diuretic for hypertension* [aliskiren (as hemifumarate); amlodipine besylate; hydrochlorothiazide] 150•5•12.5, 300•5•12.5, 300•5•25, 300•10•12.5, 300•10•25 mg

Amvaz tablets (discontinued 2007) ℞ *antianginal; antihypertensive; calcium channel blocker* [amlodipine] 2.5, 5, 10 mg

Amvisc; Amvisc Plus intraocular injection ℞ *viscoelastic agent for ophthalmic surgery* [hyaluronate sodium] 12 mg/mL; 16 mg/mL

amyl alcohol, tertiary [see: amylene hydrate]

amyl nitrite USP, JAN *coronary vasodilator; antianginal; also abused as a euphoric street drug and sexual stimulant* 0.3 mL inhalant

amylase *digestive enzyme (digests carbohydrates)* [100 IU/mg in pancrelipase; 25 IU/mg in pancreatin]

amylase [see: alpha amylase]

amylene hydrate NF *solvent*

amylin *a naturally occurring neuroendocrine hormone synthesized in the pancreas in the postprandial period* [see: amlintide; pramlintide acetate]

amylmetacresol INN, BAN

amylobarbitone BAN *sedative; hypnotic; anticonvulsant* [also: amobarbital]

amylocaine BAN

amylopectin sulfate, sodium salt
[see: sodium amylosulfate]

amylosulfate sodium [see: sodium amylosulfate]

Amytal Sodium powder for injection ℞ *sedative; hypnotic; anxiolytic; anticonvulsant; also abused as a street drug* [amobarbital sodium]

Amyvid injection *investigational (NDA filed) radioactive contrast agent to visualize beta-amyloid plaques on PET scans, which is used to detect Alzheimer disease* [florbetapir F 18]

anabolic steroids *a class of hormones derived from or closely related to testosterone that increase anabolic (tissue-building) and decrease catabolic (tissue-depleting) processes*

anacetrapib *investigational (NDA filed) antihyperlipidemic; cholesterol ester transfer protein (CETP) inhibitor that raises HDL cholesterol and decreases plaque formation in the arteries*

Anacin caplets, tablets OTC *analgesic; antipyretic; anti-inflammatory* [aspirin; caffeine] 400•32 mg; 400•32, 500•32 mg ℞ Enzone; inosine; Unasyn

Anacin Advanced Headache tablets OTC *analgesic; antipyretic; anti-inflammatory* [acetaminophen; aspirin; caffeine] 250•250•65 mg

Anacin Aspirin Free film-coated tablets OTC *analgesic; antipyretic* [acetaminophen] 500 mg

Anacin P.M., Aspirin Free film-coated caplets OTC *antihistaminic sleep aid; analgesic; antipyretic* [diphenhydramine HCl; acetaminophen] 25•500 mg

Anadrol-50 tablets ℞ *anabolic steroid for anemia; also abused as a street drug* [oxymetholone] 50 mg ℞ Inderal

anafebrina [see: aminopyrine]

Anafranil capsules ℞ *tricyclic antidepressant for obsessive-compulsive disorders* [clomipramine HCl] 25, 50, 75 mg

anagestone INN *progestin* [also: anagestone acetate]

anagestone acetate USAN *progestin* [also: anagestone]

anagrelide INN *antithrombotic/antiplatelet agent* [also: anagrelide HCl]

anagrelide HCl USAN *antithrombotic/antiplatelet agent for essential thrombocythemia (orphan); investigational (orphan) for thrombocytosis and polycythemia vera* [also: anagrelide] 0.5, 1 mg oral

anakinra USAN, INN *interleukin-1 receptor antagonist (IL-1ra); nonsteroidal anti-inflammatory drug (NSAID) for rheumatoid arthritis*

analeptics *a class of central nervous system stimulants used to maintain or improve alertness*

Analgesia Creme OTC *analgesic* [trolamine salicylate] 10%

Analgesic Balm OTC *analgesic; mild anesthetic; antipruritic; counterirritant* [methyl salicylate; menthol]

Analgesic Balm-GRX OTC *analgesic; mild anesthetic; antipruritic; counterirritant* [methyl salicylate; menthol] 14%•6%

Analgesic Creme Rub OTC *analgesic* [trolamine salicylate] 10%

analgesics *a class of drugs that relieve pain or reduce sensitivity to pain without causing loss of consciousness*

analgesine [see: antipyrine]

Analpram-E 2.5% anorectal cream ℞ *corticosteroidal anti-inflammatory; local anesthetic* [hydrocortisone acetate; pramoxine] 2.5%•1%

Analpram-HC anorectal cream, lotion ℞ *corticosteroidal anti-inflammatory; local anesthetic* [hydrocortisone acetate; pramoxine] 1%•1%, 2.5%•1%; 2.5%•1%

AnaMantle HC; AnaMantle HC 2.5% cream ℞ *corticosteroidal anti-inflammatory; anesthetic* [hydrocortisone acetate; lidocaine] 0.5%•3%; 2.5%•3%

Anamirta cocculus; A. paniculata *medicinal herb* [see: levant berry]

ananain *investigational (orphan) proteolytic enzymes for debridement of severe burns*

Ananas comosus medicinal herb [see: pineapple]

Anaphalis margaritacea; Gnaphalium polycephalum; G. uliginosum medicinal herb [see: everlasting]

anaphrodisiacs *a class of agents that reduce sexual desire or potency*

Anaplex-DM Cough syrup ℞ *antitussive; antihistamine; decongestant* [dextromethorphan hydrobromide; brompheniramine maleate; pseudoephedrine HCl] 30•4•60 mg/5 mL

Anaplex DMX oral suspension (discontinued 2010) ℞ *antitussive; antihistamine; decongestant* [dextromethorphan tannate; brompheniramine tannate; pseudoephedrine tannate] 60•8•90 mg/5 mL

Anaplex HD oral liquid (discontinued 2009) ℞ *narcotic antitussive; antihistamine; decongestant* [hydrocodone bitartrate; brompheniramine maleate; pseudoephedrine HCl] 1.7•2•30 mg/5 mL

Anaprox; Anaprox DS film-coated tablets ℞ *analgesic; nonsteroidal antiinflammatory drug (NSAID) for osteoarthritis, rheumatoid arthritis, juvenile arthritis, ankylosing spondylitis, primary dysmenorrhea, bursitis/tendinitis, and other mild to moderate pain* [naproxen (as sodium)] 250 mg (275 mg); 500 mg (550 mg)

anarel [see: guanadrel sulfate]

anaritide INN, BAN *antihypertensive; diuretic* [also: anaritide acetate]

anaritide acetate USAN *antihypertensive; diuretic; investigational (orphan) for acute renal failure and renal transplants*

Anascorp powder for IV infusion ℞ *treatment for venomous scorpion stings (orphan)* [centruoides (scorpion) immune F(ab′)2, equine] 120 mg

Anaspaz tablets ℞ *GI/GU antispasmodic; antiparkinsonian; anticholinergic "drying agent" for allergic rhinitis and hyperhidrosis* [hyoscyamine sulfate] 0.125 mg

anastrozole USAN, INN, BAN *aromatase inhibitor; estrogen antagonist; antineoplastic for advanced breast cancer; also used as an adjunct to testosterone replacement therapy for postandropausal symptoms* 1 mg oral

Anatrast oral/rectal paste ℞ *radiopaque contrast medium for esophageal imaging (oral) or defecography (rectal)* [barium sulfate] 100%

Anatrofin brand name for stenbolone acetate, an anabolic steroid abused as a street drug ⑨ Entrophen

anatumomab mafenatox INN

Anavar brand name for oxandrolone, an anabolic steroid abused as a street drug

anaxirone INN

anayodin [see: chiniofon]

anazocine INN

anazolene sodium USAN, INN *blood volume and cardiac output test* [also: sodium anoxynaphthonate]

Anbesol topical liquid, oral gel OTC *mucous membrane anesthetic; antipruritic; counterirritant; antiseptic* [benzocaine; phenol; alcohol 70%] 6.3%•0.5%

Anbesol, Baby; Anbesol Jr. oral gel OTC *mucous membrane anesthetic* [benzocaine] 7.5%; 10%

Anbesol, Maximum Strength topical liquid, oral gel OTC *mucous membrane anesthetic* [benzocaine; alcohol 50%] 20%

Anbesol Cold Sore Therapy oral ointment OTC *mucous membrane anesthetic; vulnerary; antipruritic/counterirritant; emollient* [benzocaine; allantoin; camphor; petrolatum] 20%•1%•3%•65%

ancarolol INN

Ancef powder or frozen premix for IV or IM injection (discontinued 2007) ℞ *first-generation cephalosporin antibiotic* [cefazolin sodium] 0.5, 1, 5, 10 g

ancestim USAN, INN *recombinant-methionyl human stem cell factor (r-met-HuSCF); hematopoietic growth factor*

Ancet topical liquid OTC *soap-free therapeutic skin cleanser*

anchusa medicinal herb [see: henna (Alkanna)]

ancitabine INN [also: ancitabine HCl] ☒ enocitabine

ancitabine HCl JAN [also: ancitabine]

Ancobon capsules ℞ *systemic antifungal* [flucytosine] 250, 500 mg

ancrod USAN, INN, BAN *anticoagulant enzyme derived from the venom of the Malayan pit viper; investigational (orphan) for cardiopulmonary bypass in heparin-intolerant patients; investigational (Phase III) for acute ischemic stroke*

Andehist DM NR oral drops (discontinued 2007) ℞ *antitussive; antihistamine; decongestant; for children 1–24 months* [dextromethorphan hydrobromide; carbinoxamine maleate; pseudoephedrine HCl] 4•1•15 mg/mL

Andehist DM NR syrup (discontinued 2010) ℞ *antitussive; antihistamine; decongestant* [dextromethorphan hydrobromide; brompheniramine maleate; pseudoephedrine HCl] 15•4•45 mg/5 mL

Andehist NR oral drops (discontinued 2007) ℞ *decongestant; antihistamine* [pseudoephedrine HCl; carbinoxamine maleate] 15•1 mg/mL

Andehist NR syrup (discontinued 2010) ℞ *decongestant; antihistamine* [pseudoephedrine HCl; brompheniramine maleate] 45•4 mg/5 mL

andolast INN

andrachne *(Andrachne aspera; A. cordifolia; A. phyllanthoides)* root *medicinal herb for eye inflammation; not generally regarded as safe and effective*

Androcur *investigational (orphan) antiandrogen for severe hirsutism* [cyproterone acetate]

Androderm transdermal patch (for nonscrotal area) ℞ *androgen for hypogonadism or testosterone deficiency in men; hormone replacement therapy (HRT) for postandropausal symptoms* [testosterone] 2.5, 5 mg/day (12.2, 24.3 mg total)

AndroGel single-use packets, metered-dose pump ℞ *androgen for hypogonadism or testosterone deficiency in men;* *hormone replacement therapy (HRT) for postandropausal symptoms; investigational (Phase II, orphan) for AIDS-wasting syndrome* [testosterone; alcohol 67%] 1% (25, 50 mg/pkt.); 1%, 1.62% (12.5, 20.25 mg/pump)

Androgel-DHT *investigational (Phase III) transdermal testosterone replacement therapy for postandropausal symptoms; investigational (Phase II, orphan) for AIDS-wasting syndrome* [dihydrotestosterone]

androgens *a class of sex hormones responsible for the development of the male sex organs and secondary sex characteristics*

Androgyn [see: depAndrogyn]

Android capsules (discontinued 2007) ℞ *androgen for hypogonadism or testosterone deficiency in men, delayed puberty in boys, and metastatic breast cancer in women; hormone replacement therapy for postandropausal symptoms; also abused as a street drug* [methyltestosterone] 10 mg ☒ EndaRoid; Inderide

Andropogon citratus *medicinal herb* [see: lemongrass]

androstanazole [now: stanozolol]

androstane [see: androstanolone; stanolone]

androstanolone INN *anabolic steroid; investigational (orphan) for AIDS-wasting syndrome* [also: stanolone]

androtest P [see: testosterone propionate]

Androvite for Men tablets OTC *vitamin/mineral/iron supplement* [multiple vitamins & minerals; iron (as amino acid chelate); folic acid] ≛•3•0.07 mg

Androxy tablets ℞ *oral androgen for hypogonadism or testosterone deficiency in men, delayed puberty in boys, and metastatic breast cancer in women; hormone replacement therapy (HRT) for postandropausal symptoms* [fluoxymesterone] 10 mg ☒ Ondrox

anecortave INN *angiostatic steroid* [also: anecortave acetate]

anecortave acetate USAN *angiostatic steroid* [also: anecortave]

AneCream cream ℞ *anesthetic* [lidocaine HCl] 4%

Anectine IV or IM injection, Flo-Pack (powder for injection) ℞ *muscle relaxant; anesthesia adjunct* [succinylcholine chloride] 20 mg/mL; 500, 1000 mg

Anemagen OB gelcaps (discontinued 2008) ℞ *vitamin/calcium/iron supplement* [multiple vitamins; calcium; ferrous fumarate; folic acid] ≜•200•27•1 mg

Anemone patens medicinal herb [see: pasque flower]

anertan [see: testosterone propionate]

Anestacon oral jelly ℞ *mucous membrane anesthetic* [lidocaine HCl] 2%

Anestafoam topical foam OTC *anesthetic* [lidocaine HCl] 4%

anesthesin [see: benzocaine]

anesthetics *a class of agents that abolish the sensation of pain*

anesthrone [see: benzocaine]

anethaine [see: tetracaine HCl]

anethole NF *flavoring agent*

anetholtrithion JAN

Anethum foeniculum medicinal herb [see: fennel]

Anethum graveolens medicinal herb [see: dill]

aneurine HCl [see: thiamine HCl]

Anexsia; Anexsia 5/500; Anexsia 7.5/650; Anexsia 10/660 tablets (discontinued 2009) ℞ *narcotic analgesic; antipyretic* [hydrocodone bitartrate; acetaminophen] 5•325, 7.5•325 mg; 5•500 mg; 7.5•650 mg; 10•660 mg

Anextuss extended-release tablets (discontinued 2008) ℞ *antitussive; decongestant; expectorant* [dextromethorphan hydrobromide; phenylephrine HCl; guaifenesin] 60•40•600 mg

angelica *(Angelica atropurpurea)* root *medicinal herb for appetite stimulation, bronchial disorders, colds, colic, cough, exhaustion, gas, heartburn, and rheumatism; also used as a tonic*

Angelica levisticum medicinal herb [see: lovage]

Angelica polymorpha; A. sinensis; A. dahurica medicinal herb [see: dong quai]

Angeliq film-coated tablets (in packs of 28) ℞ *monophasic oral contraceptive* [drospirenone; estradiol] 0.5•1 mg 🔢 one.click

Angiomax powder for IV injection ℞ *anticoagulant thrombin inhibitor for percutaneous coronary intervention (PCI), percutaneous transluminal coronary angioplasty (PTCA), or heparin-induced thrombocytopenia (HIT); used with aspirin therapy* [bivalirudin] 250 mg/vial

angiotensin 1-7 *investigational (orphan) agent for myelodysplastic syndrome and neutropenia due to bone marrow transplantation*

angiotensin II INN

angiotensin amide USAN, NF, BAN *vasoconstrictor* [also: angiotensinamide]

angiotensin receptor blockers (ARBs); angiotensin II receptor antagonists (AIIRAs) *a class of antihypertensives that reduce the vasoconstricting effects of angiotensin II by blocking the angiotensin receptor sites in the vascular smooth muscles* [compare to: angiotensin-converting enzyme inhibitors; renin inhibitors]

angiotensinamide INN *vasoconstrictor* [also: angiotensin amide]

angiotensin-converting enzyme inhibitors (ACEIs) *a class of antihypertensives that reduce the vasoconstricting effects of angiotensin II by blocking the enzyme (kininase II) that converts angiotensin I to angiotensin II* [compare to: angiotensin II receptor antagonists; renin inhibitors]

anhidrotics *a class of agents that reduce or suppress perspiration* [also called: anidrotics; antihydrotics]

anhydrohydroxyprogesterone [now: ethisterone]

anhydrous lanolin [see: lanolin, anhydrous]

anidoxime USAN, INN, BAN *analgesic*

anidrotics *a class of agents that reduce or suppress perspiration* [also called: anhidrotics; antihydrotics]

anidulafungin USAN, INN *echinocandin antifungal for candidemia of the internal organs, esophageal candidiasis, and other serious fungal infections*

anilamate INN

anileridine USP, INN, BAN *narcotic analgesic*

anileridine HCl USP *narcotic analgesic*

anilopam INN *analgesic* [also: anilopam HCl]

anilopam HCl USAN *analgesic* [also: anilopam]

Animal Shapes Children's Chewable Vitamins OTC *vitamin supplement* [multiple vitamins; folic acid; hydrogenated oil] ≟•300 mcg

Animal Shapes + Iron chewable tablets OTC *vitamin/iron supplement* [multiple vitamins; iron (as ferrous fumarate); folic acid] ≟•15•0.3 mg

Animi-3 capsules ℞ *dietary supplement; lipid lowering agent* [omega-3 fatty acids (eicosapentaenoic acid and docosahexaenoic acid); vitamin B_6; vitamin B_{12}; folic acid; phytosterols] 500•12.5•0.5•1•200 mg (35 mg EPA; 350 mg DHA)

anion exchange resin [see: polyamine-methylene resin]

anipamil INN

aniracetam USAN, INN *mental performance enhancer*

anirolac USAN, INN *anti-inflammatory; analgesic*

anisacril INN

anisatil USAN *combining name for radicals or groups* ⍰ inositol

anise (Pimpinella anisum) oil and seeds *medicinal herb for colic, convulsions, cough, gas, intestinal cleansing, iron-deficiency anemia, mucous discharge, promoting expectoration, and psoriasis; also used as an antibacterial, antimicrobial, and antiseptic* ⍰ Uni-Ace

anise oil NF ⍰ Anusol; Enisyl; Enseal; Unisol

anise root; sweet anise *medicinal herb* [see: sweet cicely]

anisindione NF, INN, BAN *indanedione-derivative anticoagulant*

anisopirol INN

anisopyradamine [see: pyrilamine maleate]

anisotropine methylbromide USAN, JAN *anticholinergic; peptic ulcer adjunct* [also: octatropine methylbromide] 50 mg oral

anisoylated plasminogen streptokinase activator complex (APSAC) [see: anistreplase]

anisperimus INN

anistreplase USAN, INN, BAN *fibrinolytic; thrombolytic enzyme for acute myocardial infarction*

Anisum officinarum; A. vulgare *medicinal herb* [see: anise]

anitrazafen USAN, INN *topical anti-inflammatory*

anodynes *a class of agents that lessen or relieve pain*

anodynine [see: antipyrine]

anodynon [see: ethyl chloride]

anorectics *a class of central nervous system stimulants that suppress the appetite* [also called: anorexiants; anorexigenics]

anorexiants *a class of central nervous system stimulants that suppress the appetite* [also called: anorectics; anorexigenics]

anorexigenics *a class of central nervous system stimulants that suppress the appetite* [also called: anorexiants; anorectics]

anovlar [see: norethindrone & ethinyl estradiol]

anoxomer USAN *antioxidant; food additive*

anoxynaphthonate sodium [see: anazolene sodium]

anpirtoline INN

Ansaid film-coated tablets (discontinued 2010) ℞ *analgesic; nonsteroidal anti-inflammatory drug (NSAID) for osteoarthritis and rheumatoid arthritis* [flurbiprofen] 50, 100 mg ansamycin [see: rifabutin]

ansoxetine INN

Answer One-Step; Answer Plus; Answer Quick & Simple test kit for home use OTC *in vitro diagnostic aid; urine pregnancy test*

Answer Ovulation test kit for home use OTC *in vitro diagnostic aid to predict ovulation time*

Antabuse tablets ℞ *deterrent to alcohol consumption* [disulfiram] 250 mg

Antacid chewable tablets OTC *antacid; calcium supplement* [calcium (as carbonate)] 200 mg (500 mg)

Antacid oral suspension OTC *antacid* [aluminum hydroxide; magnesium hydroxide] 225•200 mg/5 mL

antacids *a class of drugs that neutralize gastric acid*

antafenite INN

Antara capsules ℞ *antihyperlipidemic for primary hypercholesterolemia, hypertriglyceridemia, and mixed dyslipidemia; also used for hyperuricemia* [fenofibrate] 43, 130 mg

antastan [see: antazoline HCl]

antazoline INN, BAN [also: antazoline HCl]

antazoline HCl USP [also: antazoline]

antazoline phosphate USP *antihistamine*

antazoline phosphate & naphazoline HCl *topical ocular antihistamine and decongestant* 0.5%•0.05%

antazonite INN

antelmycin INN *anthelmintic* [also: anthelmycin]

anterior pituitary

anthelmintics *a class of drugs effective against parasitic infections* [also called: vermicides; vermifuges]

anthelmycin USAN *anthelmintic* [also: antelmycin]

Anthemis nobilis medicinal herb [see: chamomile]

anthiolimine INN

Anthoxanthum odoratum medicinal herb [see: sweet vernal grass]

anthracyclines *a class of antibiotic antineoplastics*

anthralin USP *topical antipsoriatic* [also: dithranol] 1% topical

anthramycin USAN *antineoplastic* [also: antramycin]

anthraquinone of cascara [see: cascara sagrada]

anthrax test [see: Rapid Anthrax Test]

anthrax vaccine *active bacterin derived from an attenuated strain of* Bacillus anthracis

Anthriscus cerefolium medicinal herb [see: chervil]

anti-A blood grouping serum USP *in vitro blood testing*

antiadrenergics *a class of agents that block the alpha$_1$ adrenergic receptors in the sympathetic nervous system, used for the treatment of hypertension and benign prostatic hyperplasia (BPH)* [also called: sympatholytics; alpha$_1$-adrenergic blockers]

antiandrogens *a class of hormonal antineoplastics*

antib [see: thioacetazone; thiacetazone]

anti-B blood grouping serum USP *in vitro blood testing*

anti-B4-blocked ricin [see: ricin (blocked) ...]

antibason [see: methylthiouracil]

AntibiOtic ear drops ℞ *corticosteroidal anti-inflammatory; antibiotic* [hydrocortisone; neomycin sulfate; polymyxin B sulfate] 1%•5 mg•10 000 U per mL

Antibiotic Ear Solution ℞ *corticosteroidal anti-inflammatory; antibiotic* [hydrocortisone; neomycin sulfate; polymyxin B sulfate] 1%•5 mg•10 000 U per mL

Antibiotic Ear Suspension ℞ *corticosteroidal anti-inflammatory; antibiotic* [hydrocortisone; neomycin sulfate; polymyxin B sulfate] 1%•5 mg•10 000 U per mL

antibiotics *a class of agents that destroy or arrest the growth of micro-organisms*

antibody-drug conjugate (ADC) *a class of agents that are a combination of a targeted monoclonal antibody vehicle (T-MAV; q.v.) and a cytotoxic* drug (effector molecule); the T-MAV delivers the drug directly to its target, usually a cancerous tumor

antibromics a class of agents that mask undesirable or offensive odors [also called: deodorants]

anti-C blood grouping serum [see: blood grouping serum, anti-C]

anti-c blood grouping serum [see: blood grouping serum, anti-c]

anticholinergics a class of agents that block parasympathetic nerve impulses, producing antiemetic, antinausea, and antispasmodic effects; also used to dry mucosal secretions

anticoagulant citrate dextrose (ACD) solution USP anticoagulant for storage of whole blood and during cardiac surgery

anticoagulant citrate phosphate dextrose adenine solution USP anticoagulant for storage of whole blood

anticoagulant citrate phosphate dextrose solution USP anticoagulant for storage of whole blood

anticoagulant heparin solution USP anticoagulant for storage of whole blood

anticoagulant sodium citrate solution USP anticoagulant for plasma and for blood for fractionation

anticoagulants a class of therapeutic agents that inhibit or inactivate blood clotting factors

anticonvulsants a class of drugs that prevent seizures by suppressing abnormal neuronal discharges in the central nervous system [also called: anti-epileptic drugs (AEDs)]

anti-D antibodies [see: $Rh_O(D)$ immune globulin]

antidopaminergics a class of antiemetic drugs

antidotes a class of drugs that counteract the effects of toxic doses of other drugs or toxic substances

anti-E blood grouping serum [see: blood grouping serum, anti-E]

anti-e blood grouping serum [see: blood grouping serum, anti-e]

antiemetics a class of agents that prevent or alleviate nausea and vomiting [also called: antinauseants]

antienite INN

antiepilepsirine [now: ilepcimide]

anti-epileptic drugs (AEDs) a class of drugs that prevent seizures by suppressing abnormal neuronal discharges in the central nervous system [also called: anticonvulsants]

antiestrogen [see: tamoxifen citrate]

antiestrogens a class of hormonal antineoplastics

antifebriles a class of agents that relieve or reduce fever [also called: antipyretics; antithermics; febricides; febrifuges]

antifebrin [see: acetanilide]

antifolic acid [see: methotrexate]

antiformin, dental JAN [also: sodium hypochlorite, diluted]

anti–growth and differentiation factor 8 antibody, recombinant human (anti-GDF8) investigational (orphan) for Duchenne and Becker muscular dystrophies

antihemophilic factor (AHF; FVIII) USP systemic hemostatic; antihemophilic for the prevention and control of bleeding in classical hemophilia (hemophilia A) and von Willebrand disease (orphan)

Antihemophilic Factor (Porcine) Hyate:C powder for IV injection ℞ antihemophilic to correct coagulation deficiency [antihemophilic factor VIII:C] 400–700 porcine units/vial

antihemophilic factor, human [now: antihemophilic factor]

antihemophilic factor, recombinant (rFVIII) antihemophilic for treatment of hemophilia A and presurgical prophylaxis for hemophiliacs (orphan)

antihemophilic factor A [see: antihemophilic factor]

antihemophilic factor B [see: factor IX complex]

antihemophilic globulin (AHG) [see: antihemophilic factor]

antihemophilic human plasma [now: plasma, antihemophilic human]

antihemophilic plasma, human
[now: plasma, antihemophilic human]
antiheparin [see: protamine sulfate]
antihistamines *a class of drugs that counteract the effect of histamine*
antihydrotics *a class of agents that reduce or suppress perspiration* [also called: anhidrotics; anidrotics]
antihyperlipidemic agents *a class of drugs that lower serum lipid levels* [also called: antilipemics]
anti-inhibitor coagulant complex *antihemophilic to correct factor VIII deficiency and coagulation deficiency*
anti-interferon-gamma Fab from goats *investigational (orphan) immunologic for corneal allograft rejection*
Anti-Itch cream OTC *poison ivy treatment* [diphenhydramine HCl; zinc acetate] 2%•0.1%
Anti-Itch gel (discontinued 2007) OTC *poison ivy treatment* [camphor; alcohol 37%] 0.45%
antilipemics *a class of drugs that lower serum lipid levels* [also called: antihyperlipidemics]
Antilirium IV or IM injection (discontinued 2008) ℞ *cholinergic to reverse anticholinergic overdose; investigational (orphan) for Friedreich and other inherited ataxias; also used for delirium tremens and Alzheimer disease* [physostigmine salicylate] 1 mg/mL
antilithics *a class of agents that prevent the formation of stone or calculus* [see also: litholytics]
antilymphocyte immunoglobulin BAN
antimelanoma antibody XMMME-001-DTPA 111 indium *investigational (orphan) imaging aid for systemic and nodal melanoma metastasis*
antimelanoma antibody XMMME-001-RTA *investigational (orphan) agent for stage III melanoma*
antimony *element (Sb)*
antimony potassium tartrate USP *antischistosomal*
antimony sodium tartrate USP, JAN *antischistosomal*

antimony sodium thioglycollate USP
antimony sulfide [see: antimony trisulfide colloid]
antimony trisulfide colloid USAN *pharmaceutic aid*
antimonyl potassium tartrate [see: antimony potassium tartrate]
antimuscarinics *a class of anticholinergic agents*
anti-MY9-blocked ricin [see: ricin (blocked) ...]
antinauseants *a class of agents that prevent or alleviate nausea and vomiting* [also called: antiemetics]
antineoplastics *a class of chemotherapeutic agents capable of selective action on neoplastic (abnormally proliferating) tissues*
antineoplastons *a class of naturally occurring peptides that suppress cancer oncogenes and stimulate the body's cancer suppressor genes*
Antioxidant Formula tablets OTC *vitamin/mineral supplement* [vitamins A, C, and E; multiple minerals] 5000 U•250 mg•200 U• ±
anti-pellagra vitamin [see: niacin]
antiperiodics *a class of agents that prevent periodic or intermittent recurrence of symptoms, as in malaria*
anti-pernicious anemia principle [see: cyanocobalamin]
antiphlogistics *a class of agents that reduce inflammation and fever*
antipsychotics *a class of psychotropic agents that are used to treat schizophrenia and other psychiatric illnesses; further classified as conventional (typical) antipsychotics and novel (atypical) antipsychotics* [q.v.]
antipyretics *a class of agents that relieve or reduce fever* [also called: antifebriles; antithermics; febricides; febrifuges]
antipyrine USP, JAN *analgesic; investigational (orphan) diagnostic agent to determine hepatic drug metabolizing activity* [also: phenazone]
Antipyrine and Benzocaine Otic ear drops ℞ *anesthetic; analgesic* [benzocaine; antipyrine] 1.4%•5.4%

antipyrine & benzocaine & polycosanol & acetic acid *analgesic; anesthetic* 5.4%•1.4%•0.01%•0.01% otic drops

N-antipyrinylnicotinamide [see: nifenazone]

antirabies serum (ARS) USP *passive immunizing agent*

anti-Rh antibodies [see: Rh$_O$(D) immune globulin]

anti-Rh typing serums [now: blood grouping serums]

antiscorbutic vitamin [see: ascorbic acid]

antiscorbutics *a class of agents that are sources of vitamin C and are effective in the prevention or relief of scurvy*

antiscrofulous herbs *a class of agents that counteract scrofuloderma (tuberculous cervical lymphadenitis)*

antisense 20-mer phosphorothiolate oligonucleotide *investigational (orphan) agent for renal cell carcinoma*

antisense drugs *a class of antiviral drugs that interfere with the replication of viral protein*

Antiseptic Wound & Skin Cleanser topical liquid OTC *antiseptic wound and skin cleanser* [benzethonium chloride] 0.1%

antiseptics *a class of agents that inhibit the growth and development of microorganisms, usually on a body surface, without necessarily killing them* [see also: disinfectants; germicides]

Antispas IM injection (discontinued 2008) ℞ *gastrointestinal anticholinergic/antispasmodic for irritable bowel syndrome (IBS)* [dicyclomine HCl] 10 mg/mL

Antispasmodic elixir ℞ *GI/GU anticholinergic/antispasmodic; sedative* [atropine sulfate; scopolamine hydrobromide; hyoscyamine sulfate; phenobarbital] 0.0194•0.0065•0.1037•16.2 mg/5 mL

antispasmodics *a class of agents that relieve spasms or cramps, usually of gastrointestinal tract or blood vessels*

antisterility vitamin [see: vitamin E]

anti-T lymphocyte immunotoxin XMMLY-H65-RTA [now: zolimomab aritox]

anti-tac, humanized; SMART anti-tac [now: daclizumab]

anti-tap-72 immunotoxin *investigational (orphan) for metastatic colorectal adenocarcinoma*

antithermics *a class of agents that relieve or reduce fever* [also called: antifebriles; antipyretics; febricides; febrifuges]

antithrombin III (AT-III) INN, BAN *agent for thrombosis and pulmonary emboli of congenital AT-III deficiency (orphan); investigational (Phase III, orphan) for heparin deficiency in patients undergoing surgical or obstetrical procedures and for AT-III-dependent heparin resistance*

antithrombin III, human [see: antithrombin III]

antithrombin III, recombinant human (rhATIII) [see: antithrombin III]

antithrombin III concentrate [see: antithrombin III]

antithymocyte globulin (ATG) *treatment for aplastic anemia; passive immunizing agent to prevent allograft rejection of renal transplants (orphan); investigational (orphan) for other solid organ and bone marrow transplants; investigational (orphan) for myelodysplastic syndrome (MDS)*

antithymocyte serum [see: antithymocyte globulin]

antitoxin botulism equine (ABE) [see: botulism equine antitoxin, trivalent]

antitoxins *a class of drugs used for passive immunization that consist of antibodies which combine with toxins to neutralize them*

anti–transforming growth factor B1,2,3 *investigational (orphan) for idiopathic pulmonary fibrosis* [compare: monoclonal antibody to transforming growth factor beta 1]

α₁-antitrypsin [see: alpha₁-antitrypsin]

antituberculous agents *a class of antibiotics, divided into primary and retreatment agents*

Antitussive Hydrocodone Bitartrate and Homatropine Methylbromide tablets ℞ *narcotic antitussive; anticholinergic* [hydrocodone bitartrate; homatropine methylbromide] 5•1.5 mg

antitussives *a class of drugs that prevent or relieve cough*

antivenin (Crotalidae) polyvalent (equine) USP *passive immunizing agent for pit viper (rattlesnake, copperhead, and cottonmouth moccasin) bites*

antivenin (Crotalidae) polyvalent immune Fab (equine) *investigational (orphan) treatment for pit viper (rattlesnake, copperhead, and cottonmouth moccasin) bites*

antivenin (Crotalidae) polyvalent immune Fab (ovine) *treatment for pit viper (rattlesnake, copperhead, and cottonmouth moccasin) bites (orphan)*

antivenin (Crotalidae) purified (avian) *investigational (orphan) treatment for pit viper (rattlesnake, copperhead, and cottonmouth moccasin) bites*

antivenin (Latrodectus mactans) (equine) USP *passive immunizing agent for black widow spider bites* ≥ 6000 U/vial

antivenin (Micrurus fulvius) (equine) USP *passive immunizing agent for coral snake bites* injection

antivenins *a class of drugs used for passive immunization against or treatment for venomous bites and stings*

Antivert; Antivert/25; Antivert/50 tablets ℞ *anticholinergic; antihistamine; antivertigo agent; motion sickness preventative* [meclizine HCl] 12.5 mg; 25 mg; 50 mg

Antivipmyn *investigational (orphan) treatment for pit viper (rattlesnake, copperhead, and cottonmouth moccasin) bites* [antivenin (Crotalidae) polyvalent immune Fab (equine)]

antivirals *a class of drugs effective against viral infections*

antixerophthalmic vitamin [see: vitamin A]

Antizol injection ℞ *antidote to methanol or ethylene glycol poisoning (orphan)* [fomepizole] 1 g/mL ⊡ Entsol

antler (deer and elk) *natural remedy for aging, energy, hormone balancing, impotence, infertility, and longevity*

antrafenine INN

antramycin INN *antineoplastic* [also: anthramycin]

Antrizine tablets ℞ *anticholinergic; antihistamine; antivertigo agent; motion sickness preventative* [meclizine HCl] 12.5 mg

Antrocol elixir ℞ *gastrointestinal anticholinergic/antispasmodic; sedative* [atropine sulfate; phenobarbital] 0.195•16 mg/5 mL

Antrypol (available only from the Centers for Disease Control and Prevention) (discontinued 2011) ℞ *antiparasitic for African trypanosomiasis and onchocerciasis* [suramin sodium]

antrypol [see: suramin sodium]

Anturane tablets, capsules (discontinued 2009) ℞ *uricosuric for gout* [sulfinpyrazone] 100 mg; 200 mg ⊡ Intron A

Anturol gel *investigational (NDA filed) urinary antispasmodic for overactive bladder* [oxybutynin chloride]

Anucort HC rectal suppositories ℞ *corticosteroidal anti-inflammatory* [hydrocortisone acetate] 25 mg

Anu-Med rectal suppositories OTC *temporary relief of hemorrhoidal symptoms* [phenylephrine HCl] 0.25%

Anumed HC rectal suppositories ℞ *corticosteroidal anti-inflammatory* [hydrocortisone acetate] 10 mg

Anusol anorectal ointment (name changed to **Tucks** in 2006) ⊡ anise oil; Enisyl; Enseal; Unisol

Anusol-HC anorectal cream ℞ *corticosteroidal anti-inflammatory* [hydrocortisone] 2.5%

Anusol-HC rectal suppositories ℞ *corticosteroidal anti-inflammatory* [hydrocortisone acetate] 25 mg

Anzemet film-coated tablets, IV injection ℞ *antiemetic to prevent nausea and vomiting following chemotherapy or surgery; also used to prevent radiation-induced nausea and vomiting* [dolasetron mesylate] 50, 100 mg; 20 mg/mL

Aosept + Aodisc solution + tablet OTC *two-step chemical disinfecting system for soft contact lenses* [hydrogen peroxide–based] ☒ Azopt

AP (Adriamycin, Platinol) *chemotherapy protocol for ovarian, endometrial, and thyroid cancer and mesothelioma*

AP-1903 *investigational (orphan) agent for graft-versus-host disease*

Apacet chewable tablets, drops (discontinued 2008) OTC *analgesic; antipyretic* [acetaminophen] 80 mg; 100 mg/mL

apafant USAN, INN *platelet activating factor antagonist for allergies, asthma, and acute pancreatitis*

apalcillin sodium USAN, INN *antibacterial*

Apap film-coated tablets OTC *analgesic; antipyretic* [acetaminophen] 325, 500 mg

APAP (N-acetyl-*p*-aminophenol) [see: acetaminophen]

Apap 500 oral liquid OTC *analgesic; antipyretic* [acetaminophen] 500 mg/5 mL

Apap Infant's Drops (discontinued 2011) OTC *analgesic; antipyretic* [acetaminophen] 100 mg/mL

Apap Plus tablets OTC *analgesic; antipyretic* [acetaminophen; caffeine] 500•65 mg

Apatate with Fluoride pediatric oral liquid (discontinued 2008) ℞ *vitamin supplement; dental caries preventative* [vitamins B_1, B_6, and B_{12}; fluoride] 15•0.5•0.025•0.5 mg/5 mL

apaxifylline USAN, INN *selective adenosine A_1 antagonist for cognitive deficits*

apazone USAN *anti-inflammatory* [also: azapropazone]

APC (aspirin, phenacetin & caffeine) *(withdrawn from market)*

apcitide [see: technetium Tc 99m apcitide]

APD (aminohydroxypropylidene diphosphonate) [see: pamidronate disodium]

APE (aminophylline, phenobarbital, ephedrine)

Apep *investigational (orphan) antineoplastic for non-Hodgkin lymphoma* [mitoguazone]

aperients *a class of agents that have a mild purgative or laxative effect* [see also: aperitives]

aperitives *a class of agents that stimulate the appetite or have a mild purgative or laxative effect* [see also: aperients]

Apetigen oral liquid OTC *vitamin/amino acid supplement* [multiple B vitamins; L-lysine HCl] ± •206.33 mg ☒ aptocaine; Opti-gen

Apetigen-Plus oral liquid OTC *vitamin/iron supplement* [multiple B vitamins; iron (as ferrous gluconate)] ± •4.17 mg/5 mL

Apetigen-Plus tablets OTC *vitamin/iron supplement* [multiple B vitamins; vitamin C; iron (as ferrous gluconate)] ± •225•10 mg

Apetil oral liquid (discontinued 2008) OTC *vitamin/mineral supplement* [multiple B vitamins; multiple minerals] ☒ Epitol

ApexiCon ointment ℞ *corticosteroidal anti-inflammatory* [diflorasone diacetate] 0.05%

ApexiCon E cream ℞ *corticosteroidal anti-inflammatory; emollient* [diflorasone diacetate] 0.05%

aphrodisiacs *a class of agents that arouse or increase sexual desire or potency*

Aphrodyne tablets ℞ *alpha$_2$-adrenergic blocker for impotence and orthostatic hypotension; sympatholytic; mydriatic; may have aphrodisiac activity; no FDA-sanctioned indications* [yohimbine HCl] 5.4 mg ☒ avridine

Aphthaid *investigational (orphan) for severe aphthous stomatitis in terminally*

immunocompromised patients [lactic acid]

Aphthasol oral paste ℞ anti-inflammatory for aphthous ulcers; topical histamine and leukotriene inhibitor [amlexanox] 5% ② efetozole

apicillin [see: ampicillin]

apicycline INN

Apidra subcu or IV injection in vials and **OptiClik** cartridges ℞ antidiabetic; rapid-onset, short-acting insulin analogue for diabetes [insulin glulisine, human (rDNA)] 100 IU/mL; 300 U/3 mL

Apidra SoloSTAR prefilled self-injector ℞ antidiabetic; rapid-onset, short-acting insulin analogue for diabetes [insulin glulisine, human (rDNA)] 300 U/3 mL

apiquel fumarate [see: aminorex]

Apium graveolens medicinal herb [see: celery]

apixaban factor Xa coagulation inhibitor; investigational (Phase III) antithrombotic for deep vein thrombosis (DVT), venous thromboembolism (VTE), and stroke prevention

APL 400-020 V-Beta DNA vaccine investigational (orphan) agent for cutaneous T-cell lymphoma

Aplenzin extended-release tablets ℞ aminoketone antidepressant for major depressive disorder (MDD) [bupropion (as hydrobromide)] 174, 348, 522 mg

Aplidin investigational (orphan) antineoplastic for multiple myeloma [plitidepsin]

Apligraf ℞ living skin construct for diabetic foot ulcers and pressure sores [graftskin]

Aplisol intradermal injection ℞ tuberculosis skin test [tuberculin purified protein derivative (PPD)] 5 U/0.1 mL

aplonidine HCl [see: apraclonidine HCl]

Apocynum androsaemifolium medicinal herb [see: dogbane]

apodol [see: anileridine HCl]

Apokyn subcu injection ℞ dopamine agonist for hypomobility episodes of late-stage Parkinson disease (orphan) [apomorphine HCl] 10 mg/mL ② Opcon

apolipoproteinA-I Milano (ApoA-I Milano) a naturally occurring component of high-density lipoprotein (HDL); investigational (Phase III) for reversing plaque buildup in arteries

Apomate investigational (orphan) radiodiagnostic aid to assess the rejection status of heart and lung transplants [technetium Tc 99m rh-Annexin V]

apomorphine BAN dopamine D_1 agonist for Parkinson disease [also: apomorphine HCl]

apomorphine HCl USP dopamine D_1 agonist for hypomobility episodes of late-stage Parkinson disease (orphan) [also: apomorphine]

apovincamine INN

appetizers a class of agents that stimulate the appetite [see also: aperitives]

APPG (aqueous penicillin G procaine) [see: penicillin G procaine]

apple *(Pyrus malus)* fruit medicinal herb for constipation and diarrhea, dysentery, fever, heart ailments, scurvy, and warts ② IPOL

apple, ground medicinal herb [see: chamomile]

apple, hog; Indian apple; May apple medicinal herb [see: mandrake]

Appli-Kit (trademarked device) ointment and adhesive dosage covers

Appli-Ruler (trademarked device) OTC dose-determining pads

Appli-Tape (trademarked device) OTC dosage covers

Apra, Children's elixir OTC analgesic; antipyretic [acetaminophen] 160 mg/ 5 mL

apraclonidine INN, BAN topical adrenergic for glaucoma [also: apraclonidine HCl]

apraclonidine HCl USAN topical adrenergic for glaucoma [also: apraclonidine] 0.5% eye drops

apramycin USAN, INN, BAN antibacterial

Aprela investigational (Phase III) treatment for postmenopausal osteoporosis *and vasomotor symptoms* [bazedoxifene; conjugated estrogens]

aprepitant USAN *neurokinin NK$_1$ receptor antagonist; antiemetic for chemotherapy-induced and postoperative nausea and vomiting*

Apresazide 25/25; Apresazide 50/50; Apresazide 100/50 capsules (discontinued 2007) ℞ *antihypertensive; vasodilator; diuretic* [hydralazine HCl; hydrochlorothiazide] 25•25 mg; 50•50 mg; 100•50 mg

Apresoline tablets ℞ *antihypertensive; vasodilator* [hydralazine HCl] 10, 25, 50, 100 mg

Apri tablets (in packs of 28) ℞ *monophasic oral contraceptive* [desogestrel; ethinyl estradiol] 0.15 mg•30 mcg × 21 days; counters × 7 days

apricot (Prunus armeniaca) fruit, seeds, and kernel oil *medicinal herb for asthma, constipation, cough, eye inflammation, hemorrhage, infertility, spasm, and vaginal infections; not generally regarded as safe and effective as apricot kernel ingestion causes cyanide poisoning*

apricot kernel water JAN

aprikalim INN *antianginal*

aprindine USAN, INN, BAN *antiarrhythmic*

aprindine HCl USAN, JAN *antiarrhythmic*

Apriso enteric-coated granules in extended-release capsules ℞ *anti-inflammatory for active ulcerative colitis, proctosigmoiditis, and proctitis* [mesalamine (5-aminosalicylic acid)] 375 mg

aprobarbital NF, INN *sedative*

Aprodine tablets, syrup OTC *decongestant; antihistamine* [pseudoephedrine HCl; triprolidine HCl] 60•2.5 mg; 60•2.5 mg/10 mL

aprofene INN

aprosulate sodium INN

aprotinin USAN, INN, BAN, JAN *protease inhibitor; systemic hemostatic for coronary artery bypass graft (CABG) surgery (orphan)*

A.P.S. (aspirin, phenacetin & salicylamide) [q.v.]

APSAC (anisoylated plasminogen streptokinase activator complex) [see: anistreplase]

aptazapine INN *antidepressant* [also: aptazapine maleate]

aptazapine maleate USAN *antidepressant* [also: aptazapine]

aptiganel HCl USAN *NMDA ion channel blocker for stroke and traumatic brain injury*

Aptivus softgels, oral solution ℞ *antiretroviral for HIV-1 infections; must be used with* **Norvir** (ritonavir) [tipranavir disodium] 250 mg; 100 mg/mL

aptocaine INN, BAN

apyron [see: magnesium salicylate]

Aqua Glycolic Face; Aqua Glycolic Hand & Body lotion OTC *moisturizer; emollient; exfoliant* [glycolic acid; hyaluronic acid]

AquaBalm cream (discontinued 2008) OTC *moisturizer; emollient*

Aqua-Ban enteric-coated tablets OTC *diuretic* [ammonium chloride; caffeine] 325•100 mg

Aqua-Ban, Maximum Strength tablets OTC *diuretic* [pamabrom] 50 mg

Aqua-Ban Plus enteric-coated tablets OTC *diuretic; iron supplement* [ammonium chloride; caffeine; ferrous sulfate] 650•200•6 mg

Aquabase ointment OTC *nontherapeutic base for compounding various dermatological preparations* ② Equipoise

Aquacare cream, lotion OTC *moisturizer; emollient; keratolytic* [urea] 10%

Aquachloral Supprettes (suppositories) (discontinued 2009) ℞ *nonbarbiturate sedative and hypnotic* [chloral hydrate] 324, 648 mg

aquaday [see: menadione]

AquADEKs softgels OTC *vitamin/mineral supplement* [multiple vitamins & minerals; coenzyme Q10; folic acid; biotin] ≟•10•0.2•0.1 mg ② Ocudox

AquADEKs Pediatric oral liquid OTC *vitamin/mineral supplement* [multiple vitamins & minerals; coenzyme Q10; biotin] ≐•2•0.015 mg

Aqua-E oral liquid OTC *vitamin supplement* [vitamin E] 20 U/mL

aquakay [see: menadione]

AquaMEPHYTON IM or subcu injection (discontinued 2007) ℞ *coagulant to correct anticoagulant-induced prothrombin deficiency; vitamin K supplement* [phytonadione] 2, 10 mg/mL

Aquanil lotion OTC *moisturizer; emollient*

Aquanil Cleanser lotion OTC *soap-free therapeutic skin cleanser*

Aquaphilic ointment OTC *nontherapeutic base for compounding various dermatological preparations*

Aquaphilic with Carbamide ointment OTC *base for compounding various dermatological preparations; moisturizer; emollient* [urea] 10%, 20%

Aquaphor; Aquaphor Healing ointment OTC *nontherapeutic base for compounding various dermatological preparations*

Aquasol A IM injection ℞ *vitamin deficiency therapy* [vitamin A] 50 000 U/mL ☒ Ixel

Aquasol E oral drops OTC *vitamin supplement* [vitamin E (as *dl*-alpha tocopherol acetate)] 15 U/0.3 mL ☒ Ixel

Aquatab C tablets (discontinued 2010) ℞ *antitussive; decongestant; expectorant* [carbetapentane citrate; phenylephrine HCl; guaifenesin] 30•10•400 mg

Aquatab D extended-release tablets (discontinued 2007) ℞ *decongestant; expectorant* [pseudoephedrine HCl; guaifenesin] 75•1200 mg

Aquatab D Dose Pack sustained-release tablets (discontinued 2007) ℞ *decongestant; expectorant* [pseudoephedrine HCl; guaifenesin] 60•600 mg

Aquatab DM tablets, syrup (discontinued 2007) ℞ *antitussive; expectorant* [dextromethorphan hydrobromide; guaifenesin] 60•1200 mg; 10•200 mg/5 mL

Aquatensen tablets (discontinued 2008) ℞ *antihypertensive; diuretic* [methyclothiazide] 5 mg

Aquavan (name changed to **Lusedra** upon marketing release in 2008) ☒ Ocufen

Aquavit-E oral drops OTC *vitamin supplement* [vitamin E (as *dl*-alpha tocopheryl acetate)] 15 U/0.3 mL ☒ Ocuvite

aqueous penicillin G procaine (APPG) [see: penicillin G procaine]

Aquilegia vulgaris medicinal herb [see: columbine]

aquinone [see: menadione]

Aquoral throat spray ℞ *saliva substitute* [lipid-based formula] ☒ Agoral

ara-A (adenine arabinoside) [see: vidarabine]

ara-AC (azacytosine arabinoside) [see: fazarabine]

arabinofuranosylcytosine [see: cytarabine]

9-β-D-arabinofuranosylguanine (ara-G) *antineoplastic*

arabinogalactans *a class of dietary fiber used as an immune booster; stimulates macrophages, increases levels of natural killer (NK) cells, interferon-gamma (IFN-γ), tumor necrosis factor-alpha (TNF-α), and interleukin-1 beta (IL-1 β)* [see also: larch]

arabinoluranosylcytosine HCl [see: cytarabine HCl]

arabinosyl cytosine [see: cytarabine]

ara-C (cytosine arabinoside) [see: cytarabine]

ara-C + ADR (Adriamycin) *chemotherapy protocol for acute myelocytic leukemia* [also known as: ara-C + doxorubicin]

ara-C + DNR (daunorubicin); ara-C + DNR, ambulatory *chemotherapy protocol for acute myelocytic leukemia (AML)* [also known as: DA]

arachadonic acid (AA) *natural omega-6 fatty acid*

arachis oil [see: peanut oil]

Aracmyn *investigational (orphan) treatment for black widow spider bites* [*Latrodectus* immune F(ab)2]

ara-cytidine [see: cytarabine]

ara-G (9-β-D-arabinofuranosylguanine) *antineoplastic* ⚗ ARC; Eryc

Aralast NP powder for IV infusion ℞ *enzyme replacement therapy for hereditary alpha₁-proteinase inhibitor deficiency, which leads to progressive panacinar emphysema* [alpha$_1$-proteinase inhibitor] ≥ 16 mg/mL (400, 800 mg/vial)

Aralen Phosphate film-coated tablets ℞ *antimalarial; amebicide* [chloroquine phosphate] 500 mg

Aralia racemosa medicinal herb [see: spikenard]

Aralia spp. medicinal herb [see: ginseng]

Aramine IV, subcu or IM injection (discontinued 2009) ℞ *vasopressor for acute hypotensive shock, anaphylaxis, or traumatic shock* [metaraminol bitartrate] 10 mg/mL (1%)

Aranelle tablets (in packs of 28) ℞ *triphasic oral contraceptive* [norethindrone; ethinyl estradiol] ⚗ Urea Nail
Phase 1 (7 days): 0.5 mg•35 mcg;
Phase 2 (9 days): 1 mg•35 mcg;
Phase 3 (5 days): 0.5 mg•35 mcg;
Counters (7 days)

Aranesp IV or subcu injection, prefilled syringes ℞ *erythropoiesis-stimulating agent (ESA); recombinant human erythropoietin for anemia associated with chronic renal failure or chemotherapy for nonmyeloid malignancies* [darbepoetin alfa] 25, 40, 60, 100, 200, 300, 500 mcg/mL; 25, 40, 60, 100, 150, 200, 300, 500 mcg/dose

Aranesp SureClick prefilled self-injector ℞ *hematopoietic; recombinant erythropoietin analogue for anemia associated with chronic renal failure* [darbepoetin alfa]

aranidipine INN

aranotin USAN, INN *antiviral*

araprofen INN

Arava film-coated tablets ℞ *immunomodulator for rheumatoid arthritis (RA)* [leflunomide] 10, 20, 100 mg

ARBs (angiotensin II receptor blockers) [see: angiotensin II receptor antagonists]

arbaprostil USAN, INN *gastric antisecretory*

arbekacin INN

arberry medicinal herb [see: uva ursi]

Arbinoxa tablets, oral liquid ℞ *antihistamine for allergic rhinitis* [carbinoxamine maleate] 4 mg; 4 mg/5 mL

arbutamine INN, BAN *cardiac stressor for diagnosis of coronary artery disease* [also: arbutamine HCl]

arbutamine HCl USAN *cardiac stressor for diagnosis of coronary artery disease* [also: arbutamine]

Arbutus uva ursi medicinal herb [see: uva ursi]

ARC ointment OTC *emollient; astringent* [petrolatum; zinc oxide] 28.5%• 9.14%

Arcalyst subcu injection ℞ *immunosuppressant for cryopyrin-associated periodic syndromes (CAPS), including familial cold autoinflammatory syndrome (FCAS) and Muckle-Wells syndrome (MWS); investigational (Phase II) for chronic gout* [rilonacept] 220 mg/dose

Arcapta Neohaler powder in capsules for use in a **Neohaler** oral inhalation device ℞ *once-daily maintenance bronchodilator to improve pulmonary airflow in patients with COPD* [indacaterol (as maleate)] 75 mcg/dose

archangel medicinal herb [see: angelica]

arcitumomab USAN *investigational (orphan) imaging agent for detection of recurrent or metastatic thyroid cancers*

arclofenin USAN, INN *hepatic function test*

Arcobee with C caplets (discontinued 2008) OTC *vitamin supplement* [multiple B vitamins; vitamin C] ≛•300 mg

Arctium lappa; A. majus; A. minus medicinal herb [see: burdock]

Arctostaphylos uva ursi medicinal herb [see: uva ursi]

ardacin INN

ardeparin sodium USAN, INN *a low molecular weight heparin–type anticoagulant and antithrombotic for the prevention of deep vein thrombosis (DVT) following knee replacement surgery*

arecoline acetarsone salt [see: drocarbil]

arecoline hydrobromide NF

Aredia powder for IV infusion ℞ *bisphosphonate bone resorption inhibitor for the prevention and treatment of postmenopausal osteoporosis; also used for bone metastases of breast cancer* [pamidronate disodium] 30, 90 mg/vial

Arestin sustained-release microspheres for subgingival injection ℞ *tetracycline antibiotic for periodontitis* [minocycline (as HCl)] 1 mg

arfalasin INN

arfendazam INN

arformoterol tartrate *long-acting beta$_2$ agonist; sympathomimetic bronchodilator for chronic obstructive pulmonary disease (COPD), bronchitis, and emphysema* (base=68%)

argatroban USAN, INN, JAN *anticoagulant for heparin-induced thrombocytopenia (HIT) and thrombosis syndrome (HITTS); prevention of HIT or HITTS in percutaneous coronary intervention (PCI)* 50, 125, 250 mg/vial injection

Argesic-SA tablets ℞ *analgesic; antiinflammatory* [salsalate] 500 mg

argimesna INN

Arginaid Extra oral liquid OTC *enteral nutritional treatment for wound healing* [whey protein formula]

L-argininamide [see: iseganan HCl]

arginine (L-arginine) USP, INN *nonessential amino acid; ammonia detoxicant; diagnostic aid for pituitary function; symbols: Arg, R*

arginine butanoate [see: arginine butyrate]

arginine butyrate (L-arginine butyrate) USAN *investigational (orphan)* for beta-hemoglobinopathies, beta-thalassemia, and sickle cell disease

arginine deiminase, pegylated *investigational (orphan) treatment for hepatocellular carcinoma and invasive malignant melanoma*

arginine glutamate (L-arginine L-glutamate) USAN, BAN, JAN *ammonia detoxicant*

arginine HCl USAN, USP, JAN *ammonia detoxicant; diagnostic aid for pituitary (growth hormone) function*

L-arginine monohydrochloride [see: arginine HCl]

8-L-arginine vasopressin [see: vasopressin]

8-arginineoxytocin [see: argiprestocin]

8-L-argininevasopressin tannate [see: argipressin tannate]

argipressin INN, BAN *antidiuretic* [also: argipressin tannate]

argipressin tannate USAN *antidiuretic* [also: argipressin]

argiprestocin INN

argon *element (Ar)* ⊡ AeroCaine; Ircon

argyn [see: silver protein, mild]

Aricept film-coated tablets ℞ *cognition adjuvant for Alzheimer dementia; also used for vascular dementia, post-stroke aphasia, and memory improvement in multiple sclerosis patients* [donepezil HCl] 5, 10, 23 mg ⊡ Orasept

Aricept oral drops (discontinued 2010) ℞ *cognition adjuvant for Alzheimer dementia; also used for vascular dementia, post-stroke aphasia, and memory improvement in multiple sclerosis patients* [donepezil HCl] 1 mg/mL ⊡ Orasept

Aricept transdermal patch *investigational (NDA filed) cognition adjuvant for Alzheimer dementia* [donepezil HCl]

Aricept ODT (orally disintegrating tablets) ℞ *cognition adjuvant for Alzheimer dementia; also used for vascular dementia, post-stroke aphasia, and memory improvement in multiple sclerosis patients* [donepezil HCl] 5, 10 mg

Aridex Pediatric oral drops (discontinued 2007) ℞ *antitussive; antihistamine; decongestant* [carbetapentane citrate; carbinoxamine maleate; phenylephrine HCl] 4•1•2 mg/mL

Aridex-D pediatric oral drops (discontinued 2007) ℞ *decongestant; antihistamine* [phenylephrine HCl; carbinoxamine maleate] 2•1 mg/mL

Aridol inhalation powder ℞ *mucolytic for bronchiectasis and cystic fibrosis (orphan)* [mannitol] 10, 20, 40 mg

arildone USAN, INN *antiviral*

Arimidex film-coated tablets ℞ *aromatase inhibitor; estrogen antagonist; antineoplastic for advanced breast cancer; also used as an adjunct to testosterone replacement therapy for postandropausal symptoms* [anastrozole] 1 mg

aripiprazole USAN *novel (atypical) quinolinone antipsychotic for schizophrenia and manic episodes of a bipolar disorder; adjunctive treatment for major depression; dopamine D_2 and serotonin $5\text{-}HT_1$ and $5\text{-}HT_2$ agonist*

Aristocort tablets (discontinued 2008) ℞ *corticosteroid; anti-inflammatory* [triamcinolone] 1, 2, 4, 8 mg

Aristolochia clematitis *medicinal herb* [see: birthwort]

Aristospan Intra-articular injection ℞ *corticosteroidal anti-inflammatory* [triamcinolone hexacetonide] 20 mg/mL

Aristospan Intralesional injection ℞ *corticosteroidal anti-inflammatory* [triamcinolone hexacetonide] 5 mg/mL

Arixtra subcu injection in prefilled syringes ℞ *selective factor Xa inhibitor; antithrombotic for prevention of deep vein thrombosis (DVT) and acute pulmonary embolism (PE) following abdominal or orthopedic surgery; investigational (NDA filed) for acute coronary syndrome (ACS)* [fondaparinux sodium] 2.5 mg/0.5 mL, 5 mg/0.4 mL, 7.5 mg/0.6 mL, 10 mg/0.8 mL

Arm-A-Med (trademarked packaging form) *single-dose plastic vial*

Arm-A-Vial (trademarked packaging form) *single-dose plastic vial*

armodafinil *analeptic for excessive daytime sleepiness due to narcolepsy (orphan), obstructive sleep apnea, or shift work sleep disorder (SWSD); investigational (Phase III) for jet lag; isomer of modafinil*

Armoracia rusticana; A. lapathiofolia *medicinal herb* [see: horseradish]

Armour Thyroid tablets ℞ *natural thyroid replacement for hypothyroidism or thyroid cancer* [thyroid, desiccated (porcine)] 15, 30, 60, 90, 120, 180, 240, 300 mg

arnica (Arnica montana; A. cordifolia; A. fulgens) flowers *medicinal herb used as a topical counterirritant and vulnerary for acne, bruises, rashes, and other dermal lesions; not generally regarded as safe and effective taken internally as it is highly toxic*

arnolol INN

arofylline USAN *phosphodiesterase IV inhibitor for asthma*

Aromasin tablets ℞ *aromatase inhibitor; antihormonal antineoplastic for advanced breast cancer in postmenopausal women (orphan)* [exemestane] 25 mg

aromatase inhibitors *a class of antihormonal antineoplastics which block the conversion of androgens to estrogens, effectively depriving hormone-dependent tumors of estrogen in postmenopausal women*

aromatic ammonia spirit [see: ammonia spirit, aromatic]

aromatic cascara fluidextract [see: cascara fluidextract, aromatic]

aromatic cascara sagrada [see: cascara fluidextract, aromatic]

aromatic elixir NF *flavored and sweetened vehicle*

aromatics *a class of agents that have an agreeable odor and stimulating qualities; also, substances with a specific molecular structure in organic chemistry*

aronixil INN

arotinolol INN [also: arotinolol HCl]

arotinolol HCl JAN [also: arotinolol]

arprinocid USAN, INN, BAN *coccidiostat*

arpromidine INN

Arranon IV infusion ℞ *antineoplastic for T-cell acute lymphoblastic leukemia (T-ALL; orphan) and T-cell lympho-*

blastic lymphoma (T-LBL; orphan)
[nelarabine] 5 mg/mL

arrow wood; Indian arrow wood; Indian arrow *medicinal herb* [see: wahoo]

ARS (antirabies serum) [q.v.]

arsambide [see: carbarsone]

arsanilic acid INN, BAN *immunomodulator*

arseclor [see: dichlorophenarsine HCl]

arsenic *element (As)* ② Orazinc

arsenic acid, sodium salt [see: sodium arsenate]

arsenic trioxide (AsO₃) JAN *antineoplastic for acute promyelocytic leukemia (orphan); investigational (orphan) for other leukemias, multiple myeloma, myelodysplastic syndromes, liver cancer, and malignant glioma*

arsenobenzene [see: arsphenamine]

arsenobenzol [see: arsphenamine]

arsenphenolamine [see: arsphenamine]

Arsobal (available only from the Centers for Disease Control) (discontinued 2011) ℞ *investigational anti-infective for trypanosomiasis* [melarsoprol]

arsphenamine USP

arsthinenol [also: arsthinol]

arsthinol INN [also: arsthinenol]

arteflene USAN, INN *antimalarial*

artegraft USAN *arterial prosthetic aid*

artemether INN *natural herbal drug for malaria; a derivative of* artemisinin

Artemisia absinthium medicinal herb [see: wormwood]

Artemisia annua medicinal herb [see: sweet wormwood]

Artemisia dracunculus medicinal herb [see: tarragon]

Artemisia vulgaris medicinal herb [see: mugwort]

artemisinin INN *natural herbal drug for malaria; a compound derivative of the sweet wormwood plant, Artemisia annua*

artemotil INN

artenimol INN

arterenol [see: norepinephrine bitartrate]

artesunate INN *antimalarial; investigational (NDA filed, orphan) rectal suppositories for emergency treatment of malaria*

Artha-G tablets OTC *analgesic; anti-inflammatory* [salsalate] 750 mg

ArthriCare, Double Ice gel (discontinued 2008) OTC *mild anesthetic; antipruritic; counterirritant* [menthol; camphor] 4%•3.1%

ArthriCare, Odor Free rub (discontinued 2008) OTC *mild anesthetic; antipruritic; counterirritant; analgesic* [menthol; methyl nicotinate; capsaicin] 1.25%•0.25%•0.025%

ArthriCare Triple Medicated gel (discontinued 2008) OTC *mild anesthetic; antipruritic; counterirritant* [methyl salicylate; menthol; methyl nicotinate] 30%•1.5%•0.7%

"Arthritis Formula"; "Arthritis Strength" products [see under product name]

Arthritis Hot Creme OTC *analgesic; mild anesthetic; antipruritic; counterirritant* [methyl salicylate; menthol] 15%•10%

Arthritis Pain Formula caplets OTC *analgesic; antipyretic; anti-inflammatory; antirheumatic* [aspirin (buffered with magnesium hydroxide and aluminum hydroxide)] 500 mg

Arthropan IM injection (discontinued 2007) ℞ *analgesic; antipyretic; anti-inflammatory; antirheumatic* [choline salicylate] 870 mg/5 mL

Arthrotec film-coated tablets ℞ *analgesic; nonsteroidal anti-inflammatory drug (NSAID) for osteoarthritis, rheumatoid arthritis, and ankylosing spondylitis with a coating to protect gastric mucosa* [diclofenac sodium (enteric-coated core); misoprostol (coating)] 50•0.2, 75•0.2 mg

articaine INN *amide local anesthetic for dentistry* [also: carticaine]

articaine HCl USAN *amide local anesthetic for dentistry* [also: articaine; carticaine]

articaine HCl & epinephrine bitartrate *local anesthetic; vasoconstrictor* 4%•≜ injection

artichoke (Cynara scolymus) flower heads *medicinal herb for albuminuria, bile stimulation, diabetes, diuresis, dyspepsia, jaundice, liver diseases, and postoperative anemia*

Articoat bandages OTC *antimicrobial dressings*

Articulose L.A. IM injection ℞ *corticosteroid; anti-inflammatory* [triamcinolone diacetate] 40 mg/mL

Artificial Tears eye drops OTC *moisturizer/lubricant*

Artificial Tears ophthalmic ointment OTC *ocular moisturizer/lubricant* [white petrolatum; mineral oil; lanolin]

Artificial Tears Plus eye drops OTC *moisturizer/lubricant* [polyvinyl alcohol] 1.4%

artilide INN *antiarrhythmic* [also: artilide fumarate]

artilide fumarate USAN *antiarrhythmic* [also: artilide]

Artiss topical liquid, powder for topical liquid ℞ *kit to adhere autologous skin grafts to wounds from burns; the sealant and thrombin are mixed just before applying to the graft, and it "sets" in about 60 seconds* [fibrin sealant, human; thrombin, human] 96–125 mg/mL; 2.5–6.5 IU/mL ⊡ AeroTuss

Arzerra IV infusion ℞ *monoclonal antibody antineoplastic for chronic lymphocytic leukemia (CLL)* [ofatumumab] 20 mg/mL ⊡ OraSure

Arzol Silver Nitrate topical swab ℞ *antiseptic* [silver nitrate; potassium nitrate] 75%•25%

arzoxifene INN *selective estrogen receptor modulator (SERM) for breast cancer, uterine fibroids, endometriosis, and dysfunctional uterine bleeding* [also: arzoxifene HCl]

arzoxifene HCl USAN *selective estrogen receptor modulator (SERM) for breast cancer, uterine fibroids, endometriosis, and dysfunctional uterine bleeding;* *investigational (Phase III) for postmenopausal osteoporosis* [also: arzoxifene]

AS-013 [see: prostaglandin E₁ enol ester]

⁷⁴As [see: sodium arsenate As 74]

5-ASA (5-aminosalicylic acid) [see: mesalamine]

ASA (acetylsalicylic acid) [see: aspirin]

ASA-404 *antiangiogenic antineoplastic; investigational (Phase III) for lung cancer; investigational (Phase II) for prostate and ovarian cancers*

Asacol; Asacol HD delayed-release caplets ℞ *anti-inflammatory for active ulcerative colitis, proctosigmoiditis, and proctitis* [mesalamine (5-aminosalicylic acid)] 400 mg; 800 mg ⊡ Isocal; Os-Cal

asafetida; asafoetida (Ferula assafoetida; F. foetida; F. rubricaulis) gum resin from dried roots and rhizomes *medicinal herb for abdominal tumors, amenorrhea, asthma, colic, convulsions, corns and calluses, edema; also used as an expectorant; not generally regarded as safe and effective in children as it may induce methemoglobinemia*

asafoetida *medicinal herb* [see: asafetida]

Asarum canadense *medicinal herb* [see: wild ginger]

ASC Lotionized topical liquid OTC *disinfectant/antiseptic; medicated cleanser for acne* [triclosan] 0.3%

Asclepias geminata *medicinal herb* [see: gymnema]

Asclepias syriaca *medicinal herb* [see: milkweed]

Asclepias tuberosa *medicinal herb* [see: pleurisy root]

Asclera injection ℞ *polyethylene glycol monododecyl ether* [polidocanol] 0.5%, 1%

Ascocaps capsules (discontinued 2010) OTC *vitamin C supplement* [ascorbic acid] 500 mg

Ascocid granules for oral solution OTC *vitamin supplement* [vitamin C (as calcium ascorbate)] 4 g/tsp.

Ascomp with Codeine capsules ℞ *barbiturate sedative; narcotic analgesic; antipyretic* [butalbital; codeine phosphate; aspirin; caffeine] 50•30•325•40 mg

Ascor L 500 injection ℞ *vitamin C supplement* [ascorbic acid] 500 mg/mL ⊡ ozagrel

ascorbic acid (L-ascorbic acid; vitamin C) USP, INN, BAN, JAN *water-soluble vitamin; antiscorbutic; urinary acidifier; topical sunscreen* 250, 500, 1000, 1500 mg oral; 240 mg/tsp. oral; 500 mg/5 mL oral; 500 mg/mL injection

L-ascorbic acid, monosodium salt [see: sodium ascorbate]

L-ascorbic acid 6-palmitate [see: ascorbyl palmitate]

ascorbyl gamolenate INN, BAN

ascorbyl palmitate NF *antioxidant*

Ascriptin caplets OTC *analgesic; antipyretic; anti-inflammatory; antirheumatic* [aspirin (buffered with magnesium hydroxide, aluminum hydroxide, and calcium carbonate)] 500 mg

Ascriptin; Ascriptin A/D coated caplets (discontinued 2008) OTC *analgesic; antipyretic; anti-inflammatory; antirheumatic* [aspirin (buffered with magnesium hydroxide, aluminum hydroxide, and calcium carbonate)] 500 mg; 325 mg

asenapine *novel (atypical) serotonin 5-HT$_{2A}$ and dopamine D$_2$ receptor antagonist; antipsychotic for schizophrenia and manic episodes of a bipolar disorder*

aseptichrome [see: merbromin]

ash, bitter *medicinal herb* [see: quassia; wahoo]

ash, mountain; American mountain ash; European mountain ash *medicinal herb* [see: mountain ash]

ash, poison *medicinal herb* [see: fringe tree]

Asimina triloba *medicinal herb* [see: pawpaw]

Asmalix elixir (discontinued 2008) ℞ *antiasthmatic; bronchodilator* [theophylline] 80 mg/15 mL

Asmanex Twisthaler (powder for oral inhalation) ℞ *corticosteroidal anti-inflammatory for chronic asthma; not indicated for acute attacks* [mometasone furoate] 200 mcg/adult dose, 100 mcg/pediatric dose

AsmaPred Plus oral solution ℞ *corticosteroid; anti-inflammatory* [prednisolone; alcohol 1.8%] 15 mg/5 mL

AsO$_3$ (arsenic trioxide) [q.v.]

asobamast INN, BAN

asocainol INN

Aspalathus linearis; A. contaminata; Borbonia pinifolia *medicinal herb* [see: red bush tea]

asparaginase (L-asparaginase) USAN, JAN *antineoplastic adjunct for acute lymphocytic leukemia* [also: colaspase]

asparagine (L-asparagine) *nonessential amino acid; symbols: Asn, N* ⊡ esproquine

L-asparagine amidohydrolase [see: asparaginase]

asparagus (*Asparagus officinalis*) roots, seeds *medicinal herb for acne, constipation, contraception, edema, neuritis, parasites, rheumatism, stimulating hair growth, and toothache*

aspartame USAN, NF, INN, BAN *sweetener*

L-aspartate potassium JAN

aspartic acid (L-aspartic acid) USAN, INN *nonessential amino acid; symbols: Asp, D*

L-aspartic acid insulin [see: insulin aspart]

aspartocin USAN, INN *antibacterial*

aspen, European *medicinal herb* [see: black poplar]

aspen poplar; American aspen; quaking aspen *medicinal herb* [see: poplar]

Aspercreme; Aspercreme with Aloe cream OTC *analgesic* [trolamine salicylate] 10%

Aspercreme Max Roll-On topical liquid OTC *mild anesthetic; antipruritic; counterirritant* [menthol] 16%

Aspercreme Rub lotion OTC *analgesic* [trolamine salicylate] 10%

Aspergillus oryase **proteinase** [see: asperkinase]

Aspergum chewing gum tablets (discontinued 2009) OTC *analgesic; antipyretic; anti-inflammatory; antirheumatic* [aspirin] 227.5 mg

asperkinase

asperlin USAN *antibacterial; antineoplastic*

Asperula odorata medicinal herb [see: sweet woodruff]

aspidium *(Dryopteris filix-mas)* plant *medicinal herb for bloody nose, menorrhagia, worm infections including tapeworm and ringworm, and wound healing; not generally regarded as safe and effective for internal use as it is highly toxic*

aspidosperma USAN

aspirin USP, BAN, JAN *analgesic; antipyretic; anti-inflammatory; antirheumatic* 325, 500, 650, 975 mg oral; 120, 200, 300, 600 mg suppositories ◙ aceperone; azaperone; Easprin; esuprone

aspirin, buffered USP *analgesic; antipyretic; anti-inflammatory; antirheumatic* 325, 500 mg oral

aspirin aluminum NF, JAN

aspirin & butalbital & caffeine *analgesic; barbiturate sedative* 325•50•40 mg oral

aspirin & caffeine & butalbital & codeine phosphate *analgesic; barbiturate sedative; narcotic antitussive* 325•40•50•30 mg oral

aspirin & codeine phosphate *antipyretic; analgesic; narcotic antitussive* 15•325 mg oral

aspirin & codeine phosphate & carisoprodol *narcotic analgesic; skeletal muscle relaxant* 325•16•200 mg oral

aspirin & dipyridamole *platelet aggregation inhibitor; coronary vasodilator* 25•200 mg

aspirin DL-**lysine** JAN *analgesic; antipyretic*

Aspirin Free Excedrin caplets, geltabs OTC *analgesic; antipyretic* [acetaminophen; caffeine] 500•65 mg

Aspirin Low Dose chewable tablets OTC *analgesic; antipyretic; anti-inflammatory* [aspirin] 81 mg

aspirin & oxycodone HCl *narcotic analgesic* 325•4.8355 mg oral

Aspirin with Codeine No. 3 and No. 4 tablets ℞ *narcotic antitussive; analgesic; antipyretic* [codeine phosphate; aspirin] 30•325 mg; 60•325 mg

ASPIRINcheck urine test kit for professional use ℞ *in vitro diagnostic aid for antiplatelet metabolites of aspirin*

Aspirin-Free Pain Relief tablets, caplets (discontinued 2008) OTC *analgesic; antipyretic* [acetaminophen] 325, 500 mg; 500 mg

AspirLow enteric-coated tablets OTC *analgesic; antipyretic; anti-inflammatory* [aspirin] 81 mg ◙ Isuprel

aspogen [see: dihydroxyaluminum aminoacetate]

aspoxicillin INN, JAN

Asprimox Extra Protection for Arthritis Pain tablets, caplets (discontinued 2008) OTC *analgesic; antipyretic; anti-inflammatory; antirheumatic* [aspirin (buffered with aluminum hydroxide, magnesium hydroxide, and calcium carbonate)] 325 mg

aspro [see: aspirin]

astatine *element (At)*

Astelin nasal spray in a metered-dose pump ℞ *antihistamine and mast cell stabilizer for allergic and vasomotor rhinitis* [azelastine (as HCl)] 0.1% (125 mcg/spray)

astemizole USAN, INN, BAN *antiallergic; second-generation piperidine antihistamine*

Astepro nasal spray in a metered-dose pump ℞ *antihistamine and mast cell stabilizer for allergic rhinitis* [azelastine (as HCl)] 0.15% (187.6 mcg/spray)

astifilcon A USAN *hydrophilic contact lens material*

astragalus *(Astragalus membranaceus)* root *medicinal herb for cancer, chronic fatigue, and Epstein-Barr syndrome; also used to strengthen the* *immune system, especially after chemotherapy and HIV treatments*

Astramorph PF (preservative free) IV, IM, or subcu injection ℞ *narcotic analgesic* [morphine sulfate] 0.5, 1 mg/mL

astringents *a class of agents that contract tissue, reducing secretions or discharges* [see also: hemostatics; styptics]

AstrinGyn topical solution ℞ *hemostatic to control superficial bleeding from skin biopsies, cervical biopsies, colposcopy, etc.* [ferric subsulfate] 259 mg/g

Astroglide vaginal gel OTC *moisturizer/lubricant* [glycerin; propylene glycol]

astromicin INN *antibacterial* [also: astromicin sulfate]

astromicin sulfate USAN, JAN *antibacterial* [also: astromicin]

AT-III (antithrombin III) [q.v.]

Atacand tablets ℞ *angiotensin receptor blocker (ARB) for hypertension and heart failure* [candesartan cilexetil] 4, 8, 16, 32 mg

Atacand HCT 16-12.5; Atacand HCT 32-12.5; Atacand HCT 32-25 tablets ℞ *combination angiotensin receptor blocker (ARB) and diuretic for hypertension* [candesartan cilexetil; hydrochlorothiazide] 16•12.5; 32•12.5 mg; 32•25 mg

atamestane INN *aromatase inhibitor*

ataprost INN

ataquimast INN

atarvet [see: acepromazine]

atazanavir sulfate *azapeptide protease inhibitor; antiretroviral for HIV-1 infection*

Atelvia delayed-release tablets ℞ *once-weekly bisphosphonate bone resorption inhibitor for corticosteroid-induced or age-related osteoporosis in men and women* [risedronate sodium] 35 mg

atenolol USAN, INN, BAN, JAN *antianginal; antihypertensive; beta-blocker; treatment for acute myocardial infarction; also used to prevent migraine headaches* 25, 50, 100 mg oral

atenolol & chlorthalidone *combination beta-blocker and diuretic for hypertension* 50•25, 100•25 mg oral

atevirdine INN *antiviral* [also: atevirdine mesylate] ② etofuradine

atevirdine mesylate USAN *non-nucleoside reverse transcriptase inhibitor (NNRTI) antiviral* [also: atevirdine]

ATG (antithymocyte globulin) [q.v.]

Atgam IV infusion ℞ *treatment for aplastic anemia; immunizing agent to prevent allograft rejection of renal transplants* [antithymocyte globulin, equine] 50 mg/mL

athyromazole [see: carbimazole]

atipamezole USAN, INN, BAN *alpha$_2$-receptor antagonist*

atiprimod dihydrochloride USAN *immunomodulator; anti-inflammatory; antiarthritic*

atiprimod dimaleate USAN *immunomodulator; anti-inflammatory; antiarthritic*

atiprosin INN *antihypertensive* [also: atiprosin maleate]

atiprosin maleate USAN *antihypertensive* [also: atiprosin]

Ativan IV or IM injection ℞ *benzodiazepine anxiolytic; preanesthetic sedative; anticonvulsant* [lorazepam] 2, 4 mg/mL

atizoram USAN, INN

atlafilcon A USAN *hydrophilic contact lens material*

ATnativ *investigational (orphan) agent for congenital AT-III deficiency in patients undergoing surgical or obstetrical procedures* [antithrombin III]

atolide USAN, INN *anticonvulsant*

Atolone tablets (discontinued 2008) ℞ *corticosteroid; anti-inflammatory* [triamcinolone] 4 mg

atomoxetine HCl *selective norepinephrine reuptake inhibitor; non-stimulant treatment for attention-deficit/hyperactivity disorder (ADHD); also used for nocturnal enuresis; investigational (orphan) for Tourette syndrome* 10, 18, 25, 40, 60, 80, 100 mg oral

Atopiclair cream OTC *moisturizer; emollient*

atorolimumab INN

atorvastatin calcium USAN *HMG-CoA reductase inhibitor for hypercholesterolemia, dysbetalipoproteinemia, hypertriglyceridemia, mixed dyslipidemia, and the prevention of cardiovascular disease and stroke in high-risk patients* (10, 20, 40, 80 mg available in Canada)

atosiban USAN, INN *oxytocin antagonist* ⊡ etazepine

atovaquone USAN, INN, BAN *antimalarial; antiprotozoal for AIDS-related* Pneumocystis *pneumonia (orphan); investigational (orphan) for AIDS-related* Toxoplasma gondii *encephalitis*

atovaquone & chloroguanide HCl *combination antiprotozoal and dihydrofolate reductase inhibitor for malaria* 250•100 mg oral

ATP (adenosine triphosphate) [see: adenosine triphosphate disodium]

ATPase (adenosine triphosphatase) [q.v.]

ATPase (adenosine triphosphatase) inhibitors *a class of gastric antisecretory agents that inhibit the ATPase "proton pump" within the gastric parietal cell* [also called: proton pump inhibitors; substituted benzimidazoles]

ATRA (all-*trans*-retinoic acid) [see: tretinoin]

atracurium besilate INN *skeletal muscle relaxant; nondepolarizing neuromuscular blocker; adjunct to anesthesia* [also: atracurium besylate]

atracurium besylate USAN, BAN *skeletal muscle relaxant; nondepolarizing neuromuscular blocker; adjunct to anesthesia* [also: atracurium besilate] 10 mg/mL injection

Atralin gel ℞ *keratolytic for acne* [tretinoin] 0.05% ⊡ iotrolan

atrasentan HCl USAN *endothelin-A (EtA; ETA; ETₐ) receptor antagonist*

atreleuton USAN *5-lipoxygenase inhibitor for asthma*

Atridox controlled-release gel for subgingival injection ℞ *antibiotic for periodontal disease* [doxycycline hyclate] 10%

Atrigel (trademarked dosage form) *sustained-release gel*

Atrigel Depot (trademarked dosage form) *sustained-release subcu injection*

atrimustine INN

atrinositol INN

Atripla film-coated caplets ℞ *antiretroviral combination therapy for HIV-1 infection in adults* [efavirenz; emtricitabine; tenofovir disoproxil fumarate] 600•200•300 mg

atromepine INN

Atropa belladonna medicinal herb [see: belladonna]

AtroPen auto-injector (automatic IM injection device) ℞ *antidote for organophosphorous or carbamate insecticides* [atropine sulfate] 0.5, 1, 2 mg/ 0.7 mL dose

atropine USP, BAN *anticholinergic*

Atropine Care eye drops ℞ *mydriatic; cycloplegic* [atropine sulfate] 1%

atropine methonitrate INN, BAN *anticholinergic* [also: methylatropine nitrate]

atropine methylnitrate [see: methylatropine nitrate]

atropine oxide INN *anticholinergic* [also: atropine oxide HCl]

atropine oxide HCl USAN *anticholinergic* [also: atropine oxide]

atropine propionate [see: prampine]

atropine sulfate USP, JAN GI/GU *antispasmodic; antiparkinsonian; bronchodilator; cycloplegic; mydriatic; antidote to insecticide poisoning* [also: atropine sulphate] 0.4, 0.6 mg oral; 1% eye drops; 0.05, 0.1, 0.3, 0.4, 0.5, 0.8, 1 mg/mL injection

atropine sulphate BAN GI/GU *antispasmodic; antiparkinsonian; bronchodilator; cycloplegic; mydriatic* [also: atropine sulfate]

Atropine-1 eye drops (discontinued 2010) ℞ *mydriatic; cycloplegic* [atropine sulfate] 1%

Atrosept sugar-coated tablets ℞ *urinary antibiotic; analgesic; antispas-

modic; acidifier [methenamine; phenyl salicylate; atropine sulfate; methylene blue; hyoscyamine sulfate; benzoic acid] 40.8•18.1•0.03•5.4•0.03•4.5 mg

Atrovent inhalation aerosol (discontinued 2008) ℞ *anticholinergic bronchodilator for bronchospasm, emphysema, and chronic obstructive pulmonary disease (COPD); antisecretory for rhinorrhea* [ipratropium bromide] 18 mcg/dose

Atrovent nasal spray ℞ *anticholinergic bronchodilator for bronchospasm, emphysema, and chronic obstructive pulmonary disease (COPD); antisecretory for rhinorrhea* [ipratropium bromide] 0.03%, 0.06% (21, 42 mcg/dose)

Atrovent HFA inhalation aerosol with a CFC-free propellant ℞ *anticholinergic bronchodilator for bronchospasm, emphysema, and chronic obstructive pulmonary disease (COPD)* [ipratropium bromide] 17 mcg/dose

ATryn powder for IV infusion ℞ *agent for the prevention of perioperative and peripartum thromboembolic events in patients with hereditary antithrombin deficiency* [antithrombin III, recombinant] 1750 IU

A/T/S topical solution, gel ℞ *antibiotic for acne* [erythromycin; alcohol 66%–92%] 2% ② oats

Attain oral liquid OTC *enteral nutritional therapy* [lactose-free formula] ② 8 in 1

attapulgite, activated USP *suspending agent; GI adsorbent*

Attenuvax powder for subcu injection ℞ *measles vaccine* [measles virus vaccine, live attenuated] 0.5 mL

Atuss DS oral suspension ℞ *antitussive; antihistamine; decongestant* [dextromethorphan hydrobromide; chlorpheniramine maleate; pseudoephedrine HCl] 30•4•30 mg/5 mL

Atuss DS Tannate oral suspension ℞ *antitussive; antihistamine; decongestant* [dextromethorphan tannate; chlorpheniramine tannate; pseudoephedrine tannate] 60•8•60 mg/5 mL

Atuss HD dual-release capsules (discontinued 2009) ℞ *narcotic antitussive; antihistamine; decongestant* [hydrocodone bitartrate (immediate release); chlorpheniramine maleate (extended release); pseudoephedrine HCl (extended release)] 5•2•30 mg

Atuss HS oral suspension (discontinued 2009) ℞ *narcotic antitussive; antihistamine; decongestant* [hydrocodone tannate; chlorpheniramine tannate; pseudoephedrine tannate] 10•8•60 mg/5 mL

Atuss HX dual-release capsules (discontinued 2011) ℞ *narcotic antitussive; expectorant* [hydrocodone bitartrate (extended release); guaifenesin (immediate release)] 5•100 mg

"atypical" antipsychotics [see: novel antipsychotics]

¹⁹⁸Au [see: gold Au 198]

augmented betamethasone dipropionate *topical corticosteroid*

Augmentin film-coated tablets, chewable tablets, powder for oral suspension ℞ *aminopenicillin antibiotic plus synergist* [amoxicillin; clavulanate potassium] 250•125, 500•125, 875•125 mg; 400•57 mg; 125•31.25, 250•62.5, 400•57 mg/5 mL

Augmentin ES-600 powder for oral suspension ℞ *aminopenicillin antibiotic plus synergist* [amoxicillin; clavulanate potassium] 600•42.9 mg/5 mL

Augmentin XR extended-release film-coated tablets ℞ *aminopenicillin antibiotic plus synergist* [amoxicillin; clavulanic acid] 1000•62.5 mg

augmerosen *investigational (NDA filed, orphan) antineoplastic for malignant melanoma; investigational (Phase III, orphan) for multiple myeloma and chronic lymphocytic leukemia (CLL)*

Auralgan ear drops ℞ *anesthetic and analgesic for acute otitis media and the removal of cerumen* [benzocaine; antipyrine; acetic acid; polycosanol] 1.4%•5.4%•0.01%•0.01%

auranofin USAN, INN, BAN, JAN *antirheumatic (29% gold)*

aureoquin [now: quinetolate]

Auriculin *investigational (orphan) for acute renal failure and renal transplants* [anaritide acetate]

Auro Ear Drops OTC *cerumenolytic to emulsify and disperse ear wax* [carbamide peroxide] 6.5% ⑨ E-R-O Ear Drops

Auro-Dri ear drops OTC *antiseptic; astringent* [boric acid] 2.75% ⑨ Ear-Dry

Auroguard Otic ear drops ℞ *anesthetic; analgesic* [benzocaine; antipyrine] 1.4%•5.4%

Aurolate IM injection ℞ *antirheumatic* [gold sodium thiomalate] 50 mg/mL ⑨ Oralet

aurolin [see: gold sodium thiosulfate]

auropin [see: gold sodium thiosulfate]

aurosan [see: gold sodium thiosulfate]

aurothioglucose USP *antirheumatic (50% gold)* 50 mg/mL injection

aurothioglycanide INN

aurothiomalate disodium [see: gold sodium thiomalate]

aurothiomalate sodium [see: gold sodium thiomalate]

Australian tea tree *medicinal herb* [see: tea tree oil]

Autohaler (delivery device) *breath-activated metered-dose inhaler*

auto-injector (delivery device) *automatic IM injection device*

Autoject2 (trademarked delivery device) *prefilled glass syringe*

autologous DNP-conjugated tumor vaccine *investigational (Phase III, orphan) theraccine for postsurgical stage III malignant melanoma*

autologous DNP-modified tumor vaccine *investigational (Phase III, orphan) theraccine for adjuvant treatment of ovarian cancer*

autologous incubated macrophage *investigational (orphan) agent to improve motor and sensory outcome in spinal cord injury*

autolymphocyte therapy (ALT) *investigational (orphan) for metastatic renal cell carcinoma*

autoprothrombin I [see: factor VII]

autoprothrombin II [see: factor IX]

autumn crocus (*Colchicum autumnale; C. speciosum; C. vernum*) plant and corm *medicinal herb for edema, gonorrhea, gout, prostate enlargement, and rheumatism; not generally regarded as safe and effective as it is highly toxic because of its colchicine content*

AVA (anthrax vaccine, adsorbed) [q.v.]

Avage cream ℞ *retinoid pro-drug; adjuvant treatment for facial wrinkles, hyper- and hypopigmentation, and benign lentigines* [tazarotene] 0.1%

Avail tablets (discontinued 2008) OTC *vitamin/mineral/iron supplement* [multiple vitamins & minerals; iron; folic acid] ≚•18•0.4 mg

Avalide tablets ℞ *combination angiotensin receptor blocker (ARB) and diuretic for hypertension* [irbesartan; hydrochlorothiazide] 150•12.5, 300•12.5, 300•25 mg

avanafil *phosphodiesterase type 5 (PDE-5) inhibitor; investigational (NDA filed) fast-acting selective vasodilator for erectile dysfunction (ED)*

Avandamet film-coated tablets ℞ *antidiabetic combination for type 2 diabetes that decreases hepatic glucose production and increases cellular response to insulin without increasing insulin secretion* [rosiglitazone maleate; metformin HCl] 2•500, 2•1000, 4•500, 4•1000 mg

Avandaryl tablets ℞ *antidiabetic combination for type 2 diabetes that increases cellular response to insulin and stimulates insulin secretion in the pancreas* [rosiglitazone maleate; glimepiride] 4•1, 4•2, 4•4, 8•2, 8•4 mg

Avandia film-coated tablets ℞ *antidiabetic for type 2 diabetes that increases cellular response to insulin without increasing insulin secretion* [rosiglitazone maleate] 2, 4, 8 mg

Avapro tablets ℞ *angiotensin receptor blocker (ARB) for hypertension; treat-*

ment to delay the progression of diabetic nephropathy [irbesartan] 75, 150, 300 mg

Avar gel ℞ *antibiotic and keratolytic for acne* [sulfacetamide sodium; sulfur] 10%•5%

Avar Cleanser; Avar LS Cleanser topical liquid ℞ *antibiotic and keratolytic for acne* [sulfacetamide sodium; sulfur] 10%•5%; 10%•2%

Avar Green gel (tinted for "color correction") (discontinued 2008) ℞ *antibiotic and keratolytic for acne* [sulfacetamide sodium; sulfur] 10%•5%

Avar-e Emollient; Avar-e Green; Avar-e LS cream (Green is tinted for "color correction") ℞ *antibiotic and keratolytic for acne* [sulfacetamide sodium; sulfur] 10%•5%; 10%•5%; 10%•2%

avasimibe USAN, INN *acylCoA transferase (ACAT) inhibitor for hyperlipidemia and atherosclerosis*

Avastin IV infusion ℞ *antineoplastic; angiogenesis inhibitor for glioblastoma, metastatic renal and colorectal cancer, and non–small cell lung cancer; investigational (Phase III) for prostate, pancreatic, and ovarian cancers* [bevacizumab] 25 mg/mL

Aveeno lotion OTC *moisturizer; emollient* [colloidal oatmeal] 1%

Aveeno Anti-Itch cream (discontinued 2009) OTC *poison ivy treatment* [calamine; pramoxine HCl] 3%•1%

Aveeno Baby lotion OTC *moisturizer; emollient* [dimethicone] 1.2%

Aveeno Cleansing bar (discontinued 2010) OTC *soap-free therapeutic skin cleanser* [colloidal oatmeal] 51%

Aveeno Cleansing for Acne-Prone Skin bar (discontinued 2010) OTC *medicated cleanser for acne* [salicylic acid; colloidal oatmeal]

Aveeno Daily Moisturizing lotion OTC *moisturizer; emollient* [dimethicone] 1.25%

Aveeno Moisturizing cream OTC *moisturizer; emollient* [colloidal oatmeal] 1%

Aveeno Oilated Bath packets (discontinued 2010) OTC *bath emollient* [colloidal oatmeal; mineral oil] 43%• ²⁄₂

Aveeno Regular Bath packets OTC *bath emollient* [colloidal oatmeal] 100%

Aveeno Shave gel OTC *moisturizer; emollient* [oatmeal flour]

Aveeno Shower & Bath oil OTC *bath emollient* [colloidal oatmeal] 5%

Avelox film-coated tablets, IV infusion ℞ *broad-spectrum fluoroquinolone antibiotic* [moxifloxacin (as HCl)] 400 mg; 400 mg/bag ⓘ Euflex; I-Valex

Avena sativa medicinal herb [see: oats]

Aventyl HCl Pulvules (capsules) ℞ *tricyclic antidepressant* [nortriptyline HCl] 25 mg

avertin [see: tribromoethanol]

avian flu vaccine [see: influenza virus vaccine, H5N1]

Aviane tablets (in packs of 28) ℞ *monophasic oral contraceptive* [levonorgestrel; ethinyl estradiol] 0.1 mg• 20 mcg × 21 days; counters × 7 days ⓘ Iophen

avicatonin INN

Avidoxy; Avidoxy DK (defense kit) film-coated caplets ℞ *broad-spectrum tetracycline antibiotic for severe acne; the "kit" includes a 2% salicylic acid wash and a sunscreen* [doxycycline (as monohydrate)] 100 mg ⓘ Efudex

avilamycin USAN, INN, BAN *antibacterial*

avinar [see: uredepa]

Avinza dual-release (immediate- plus extended-release) capsules ℞ *once-daily narcotic analgesic for treatment of chronic pain* [morphine sulfate] 30, 45, 60, 75, 90, 120 mg

Avita cream, gel ℞ *keratolytic for acne* [tretinoin] 0.025%

Avitene Hemostat nonwoven dressing (discontinued 2010) ℞ *topical hemostat for surgery* [microfibrillar collagen hemostat]

avitriptan fumarate USAN *serotonin 5-HT₁ agonist for migraine*

avizafone INN, BAN

avobenzone USAN, INN *sunscreen*

avocado *(Persea americana; P. gratissima) fruit and seed medicinal herb for diarrhea, dysentery, inducing menstruation, lowering total cholesterol and improving overall lipid profile, promoting hair growth, and stimulating wound healing; also used as an aphrodisiac*

avocado sugar extract *natural weight-loss agent used to diminish carbohydrate cravings* [see also: D-mannoheptulose]

Avodart softgels ℞ *treatment for benign prostatic hyperplasia (BPH); also used to prevent prostate cancer* [dutasteride] 0.5 mg

Avolean capsules OTC *natural weight-loss agent used to diminish carbohydrate cravings* [avocado sugar extract] 50 mg ☒ Iophylline

Avonex single-dose vials and prefilled syringes for IM injection ℞ *immunomodulator for relapsing remitting multiple sclerosis (orphan); investigational (orphan) for non-A, non-B hepatitis, juvenile rheumatoid arthritis, Kaposi sarcoma, brain tumors, and various other cancers* [interferon beta-1a] 30 mcg (6.6 MIU)

avoparcin USAN, INN, BAN *glycopeptide antibiotic*

Avosil ointment OTC *analgesic; anti-inflammatory* [sodium salicylate] 2%

avridine USAN, INN *antiviral* ☒ Aphrodyne

Award ℞ *hydrophilic contact lens material* [hilafilcon A]

axamozide INN

Axanum tablets *investigational (NDA filed) combination nonsteroidal anti-inflammatory drug (NSAID) and proton pump inhibitor for osteoarthritis, rheumatoid arthritis, and ankylosing spondylitis* [naproxen; aspirin]

axerophthol [see: vitamin A]

Axert tablets ℞ *vascular serotonin receptor agonist for the acute treatment of migraine* [almotriptan malate] 6.25, 12.5 mg

axetil USAN, INN *combining name for radicals or groups*

Axid Pulvules (capsules); oral liquid ℞ *histamine H_2 antagonist for gastric and duodenal ulcers and gastroesophageal reflux disease (GERD); also used to prevent NSAID-induced gastric ulcers* [nizatidine] 150 mg; 15 mg/mL

Axid AR ("acid reducer") tablets OTC *histamine H_2 antagonist for acid indigestion and heartburn* [nizatidine] 75 mg

Axiron topical solution in a metered-dose pump ℞ *androgen for hypogonadism or testosterone deficiency in men; hormone replacement therapy (HRT) for postandropausal symptoms* [testosterone] 30 mg/1.5 mL pump

axitinib *investigational (Phase III) vascular endothelial growth factor (VEGF) receptor inhibitor for metastatic renal cell carcinoma (RCC); investigational (Phase II) for hepatocellular carcinoma*

axitirome USAN, INN *antihyperlipidemic*

Axona oral powder packets ℞ *once-daily dietary supplement to induce hyperketonemia for the management of mild-to-moderate Alzheimer disease; source of medium-chain triglycerides (MCT)* [caprylidene] 40 g (20 g MCT)

Axsain cream OTC *counterirritant; analgesic for muscle and joint pain* [capsaicin] 0.25%

Aygestin tablets ℞ *synthetic progestin for amenorrhea, abnormal uterine bleeding, and endometriosis* [norethindrone acetate] 5 mg

Ayr Mentholated Vapor Inhaler OTC *antiseptic; mild anesthetic; antipruritic; counterirritant; emollient* [eucalyptus oil; menthol; lavender oil]

Ayr Saline nasal mist, nose drops, nasal gel OTC *nasal moisturizer* [sodium chloride (saline solution)] 0.65%

5-AZA (5-azacitidine) [see: azacitidine]

5-aza-2'-deoxycytidine *investigational (orphan) for acute leukemia*

azabon USAN, INN *CNS stimulant* ☒ Isopan

azabuperone INN

azacitidine (5-AZA; 5-AZC) USAN, INN *demethylating antineoplastic for myelodysplastic syndrome (orphan);*

also used for acute lymphocytic leuke-mia and acute myelogenous leukemia

azaclorzine INN *coronary vasodilator* [also: azaclorzine HCl]

azaclorzine HCl USAN *coronary vaso-dilator* [also: azaclorzine]

azaconazole USAN, INN *antifungal* ⑨ isoconazole

azacosterol INN *avian chemosterilant* [also: azacosterol HCl]

azacosterol HCl USAN *avian chemosterilant* [also: azacosterol]

AZA-CR [see: azacitidine]

Azactam powder for IV or IM injec-tion ℞ *monobactam bactericidal anti-biotic* [aztreonam] 0.5, 1, 2 g

azacyclonol INN, BAN [also: azacyclo-nol HCl]

azacyclonol HCl NF [also: azacyclonol]

5-azacytosine arabinoside (ara-AC) [see: fazarabine]

5-aza-2′-deoxycytidine *investigational (orphan) for acute leukemia*

Azadirachta indica medicinal herb [see: neem tree]

azaftozine INN

azalanstat dihydrochloride USAN *hypolipidemic*

azaline B [now: prazarelix acetate]

azalomycin INN, BAN

azaloxan INN *antidepressant* [also: aza-loxan fumarate]

azaloxan fumarate USAN *antidepres-sant* [also: azaloxan]

azamethiphos BAN

azamethonium bromide INN, BAN

azamulin INN ⑨ azumolene

azanator INN *bronchodilator* [also: azanator maleate]

azanator maleate USAN *bronchodilator* [also: azanator]

azanidazole USAN, INN, BAN *antiproto-zoal*

azaperone USAN, INN, BAN *antipsy-chotic* ⑨ aceperone; aspirin; Easprin; esuprone

azapetine BAN ⑨ Aseptone; isobutane

azapetine phosphate [see: azapetine]

azaprocin INN ⑨ isoprazone

azapropazone INN, BAN *anti-inflam-matory* [also: apazone]

azaquinzole INN ⑨ isoconazole

azaribine USAN, INN, BAN *antipsoriatic*

azarole USAN *immunoregulator* ⑨ acerola

Azasan tablets ℞ *immunosuppressant for organ transplantation and rheuma-toid arthritis* [azathioprine] 25, 50, 75, 100 mg

azaserine USAN, INN *antifungal*

azasetron INN

AzaSite eye drops ℞ *macrolide antibi-otic for bacterial conjunctivitis* [azithro-mycin] 1%

azaspirium chloride INN

azaspirones *a class of anxiolytics*

azastene

azatadine INN, BAN *piperidine antihista-mine for allergic rhinitis and chronic urticaria* [also: azatadine maleate]

azatadine maleate USAN, USP *piperi-dine antihistamine for allergic rhinitis and chronic urticaria* [also: azatadine]

azatepa INN *antineoplastic* [also: azetepa]

azathioprine USAN, USP, INN, BAN, JAN *immunosuppressant for organ trans-plantation and rheumatoid arthritis; investigational (orphan) graft-versus-host (GVH) disease of the oral mucosa* 50 mg oral

azathioprine sodium USP *immunosup-pressant for organ transplantation and rheumatoid arthritis* 100 mg injection

5-AZC (5-azacitidine) [see: azacitidine]

Azdone tablets ℞ *narcotic analgesic; antipyretic* [hydrocodone bitartrate; aspirin] 5•500 mg

azdU (3′-azido-2′,3′-dideoxyuridine) [see: azidouridine]

azelaic acid USAN, INN *topical antimicro-bial and keratolytic for acne and rosacea*

azelastine INN, BAN *peripherally selec-tive phthalazinone antihistamine for allergic and vasomotor rhinitis; mast cell stabilizer; antiasthmatic* [also: azel-astine HCl]

azelastine HCl USAN, JAN *peripherally selective phthalazinone antihistamine and mast cell stabilizer for allergic and vaso-motor rhinitis and allergic conjunctivi-*

tis; antiasthmatic (base=91%) [also: azelastine] 0.5% eye drops; 0.1% nasal spray

Azelex cream ℞ *antimicrobial and keratolytic for inflammatory acne vulgaris* [azelaic acid] 20%

azelnidipine INN

azepexole INN, BAN

azephine [see: azapetine phosphate]

azepinamide [see: glypinamide]

azepindole USAN, INN *antidepressant*

azetepa USAN, BAN *antineoplastic* [also: azatepa]

azetirelin INN

azficel-T *autologous cell dermal filler for moderate to severe nasolabial folds*

azidamfenicol INN, BAN

3′-azido-2′,3′-dideoxyuridine (azdU) [see: azidouridine]

azidoamphenicol [see: azidamfenicol]

azidocillin INN, BAN

azidothymidine (AZT) [now: zidovudine]

azidouridine (azdU) *investigational (orphan) antiviral for HIV and AIDS*

Azilect tablets ℞ *once-daily monoamine oxidase B (MAO-B) inhibitor for Parkinson disease* [rasagiline] 0.5, 1 mg

azilsartan medoxomil *angiotensin receptor blocker (ARB) for hypertension*

azimexon INN

azimilide dihydrochloride USAN *investigational (NDA filed) antiarrhythmic and antifibrillatory*

azintamide INN

azinthiamide [see: azintamide]

azipramine INN *antidepressant* [also: azipramine HCl]

azipramine HCl USAN *antidepressant* [also: azipramine]

aziridinyl benzoquinone [see: diaziquone]

azithromycin USAN, USP, INN, BAN *macrolide antibiotic* 250, 500, 600 mg oral; 1 g/pkt. oral; 100, 200 mg/5 mL oral; 500 mg injection ⊘ astromicin

azlocillin USAN, INN, BAN *penicillin antibiotic*

azlocillin sodium USP *penicillin antibiotic*

Azmacort oral inhalation aerosol ℞ *corticosteroidal anti-inflammatory for chronic asthma; not indicated for chronic attacks* [triamcinolone acetonide] 75 mcg/dose

Azo Standard tablets ℞ *urinary tract analgesic for relief of pain, burning, urgency, and frequency due to mucosal irritation from surgery, catheterization, endoscopic procedures, or trauma; adjunct to antibacterial agents for urinary tract infection (UTI)* [phenazopyridine HCl] 97.5 mg

Azo Test Strips reagent strips for home use OTC *in vitro diagnostic aid for urinary tract infections*

azoconazole [now: azaconazole]

azodisal sodium (ADS) [now: olsalazine sodium]

"azoles" *a class of fungicides that include all with generic names ending in "azole," such clotrimazole, fluconazole, etc.*

azolimine USAN, INN *diuretic*

Azopt eye drop suspension ℞ *carbonic anhydrase inhibitor for glaucoma* [brinzolamide] 1% ⊘ Aosept

Azor tablets ℞ *combination calcium channel blocker and angiotensin receptor blocker (ARB) for hypertension* [amlodipine (as besylate); olmesartan medoxomil] 5•20, 5•40, 10•20, 10•40 mg

azosemide USAN, INN, JAN *diuretic*

Azo-Standard tablets OTC *urinary tract analgesic for relief of pain, burning, urgency, and frequency due to mucosal irritation from surgery, catheterization, endoscopic procedures, or trauma; adjunct to antibacterial agents for urinary tract infection (UTI)* [phenazopyridine HCl] 95 mg

Azostix reagent strips for professional use ℞ *in vitro diagnostic aid to estimate the amount of BUN in whole blood*

Azo-Sulfisoxazole tablets (discontinued 2008) ℞ *urinary anti-infective; urinary analgesic* [sulfisoxazole; phenazopyridine HCl] 500•50 mg

azotomycin USAN, INN *antibiotic antineoplastic*

azovan blue BAN *blood volume test* [also: Evans blue]

azovan sodium [see: Evans blue]

AZT (azathioprine) [q.v.]

AZT (azidothymidine) [now: zidovudine]

AZT (azithromycin) [q.v.]

aztreonam USAN, USP, INN, BAN, JAN *monobactam bactericidal antibiotic; inhalation therapy for* Pseudomonas aeruginosa *infections in cystic fibrosis patients (orphan)* 0.5, 1, 2 g/vial injection

azulene sulfonate sodium JAN [also: sodium gualenate]

Azulfidine tablets ℞ *anti-inflammatory for ulcerative colitis; also used for ankylosing spondylitis, Crohn disease, and regional enteritis* [sulfasalazine] 500 mg

Azulfidine EN-tabs enteric-coated delayed-release tablets ℞ *anti-inflammatory for ulcerative colitis, rheumatoid arthritis (RA), and juvenile rheumatoid arthritis (JRA); also used for ankylosing spondylitis, Crohn disease, and regional enteritis* [sulfasalazine] 500 mg

azumolene INN *skeletal muscle relaxant* [also: azumolene sodium] 🔟 azamulin

azumolene sodium USAN *skeletal muscle relaxant* [also: azumolene]

azure A carbacrylic resin [see: azuresin]

azuresin NF, BAN

Azurette tablets (in packs of 28) ℞ *biphasic oral contraceptive* [desogestrel; ethinyl estradiol]
Phase 1 (21 days): 0.15 mg•20 mcg;
Phase 2 (5 days): 0•10 mcg;
Counters (2 days)

1,4-B (1,4-butanediol) *a precursor to gamma hydroxybutyrate (GHB); a formerly legal alternative to GHB, now also illegal (Schedule I)* [see: gamma hydroxybutyrate (GHB)]

B Complex + C timed-release tablets (discontinued 2008) OTC *vitamin supplement* [multiple B vitamins; vitamin C] ≛•500 mg

B Complex Plus B-12 tablets OTC *vitamin supplement* [multiple B vitamins; protease (as papain)] ≛•10 mg

B Complex with C and B-12 injection ℞ *parenteral vitamin supplement* [multiple vitamins]

B Complex with Vitamin B-12 tablets OTC *vitamin supplement* [multiple B vitamins; folic acid] ≛•400 mcg

B Complex-50 sustained-release tablets (discontinued 2008) OTC *vitamin supplement* [multiple B vitamins; folic acid; biotin] ≛•400•50 mcg

B Complex-150 sustained-release tablets (discontinued 2008) OTC *vitamin supplement* [multiple B vitamins; folic acid; biotin] ≛•400•150 mcg

B & O Supprettes No. 15A; B & O Supprettes No. 16A suppositories ℞ *narcotic analgesic* [belladonna extract; opium] 16.2•30 mg; 16.2•60 mg

B vitamins [see: vitamin B]

B₁ (vitamin B₁) [see: thiamine HCl]

B₂ (vitamin B₂) [see: riboflavin]

B₂-400 capsules OTC *vitamin supplement* [vitamin B₂] 400 mg

B₃ (vitamin B₃) [see: niacin; niacinamide]

B₅ (vitamin B₅) [see: calcium pantothenate]

B₆ (vitamin B₆) [see: pyridoxine HCl]

B₈ (vitamin B₈) [see: adenosine phosphate]

B-12 tablets OTC *vitamin supplement* [vitamin B₁₂] 1500 mcg

B₁₂ (vitamin B₁₂) [see: cyanocobalamin]

B₁₂ₐ (vitamin B₁₂ₐ) [see: hydroxocobalamin]

B_{12b} (vitamin B_{12b}) [see: hydroxocobalamin]

B-50 tablets OTC *vitamin supplement* [multiple B vitamins; folic acid; biotin] ±•100•50 mcg

B-100 Ultra B Complex tablets OTC *vitamin supplement* [multiple B vitamins; folic acid; biotin] ±•100•100 mcg

B_c (vitamin B_c) [see: folic acid]

B_t (vitamin B_t) [see: carnitine]

Babee Teething oral lotion OTC *mucous membrane anesthetic; antiseptic* [benzocaine; cetalkonium chloride] 2.5%•0.02%

baby brain I (cyclophosphamide, vincristine, cisplatin, etoposide) *chemotherapy protocol for pediatric brain tumors* [also known as: COPE]

Baby D Drops oral drops OTC *vitamin D supplement* [cholecalciferol (vitamin D₃)] 400 U/0.03 mL

Baby Vitamin oral drops OTC *vitamin supplement* [multiple vitamins]

Baby Vitamin with Iron oral drops OTC *vitamin/iron supplement* [multiple vitamins; iron (as ferrous sulfate)] ±•10 mg/mL

BabyBIG powder for IV infusion ℞ *treatment for infant botulism type A or B (orphan)* [botulism immune globulin (BIG)] 100 mg/vial

Babylax [see: Fleet Babylax]

Baby's Bliss Gripe Water oral drops OTC *natural product to relieve colic, stomach cramps, hiccups, and gas in infants* [ginger; fennel; sodium bicarbonate; fructose]

BAC (benzalkonium chloride) [q.v.]

bacampicillin INN, BAN *aminopenicillin antibiotic* [also: bacampicillin HCl]

bacampicillin HCl USAN, USP, JAN *aminopenicillin antibiotic* [also: bacampicillin]

bachelor's buttons *medicinal herb* [see: cornflower; feverfew; tansy; buttercup]

Bacid capsules OTC *probiotic; dietary supplement; fever blister treatment; not generally regarded as safe and effective as an antidiarrheal* [Lactobacillus acidophilus] ≥ 500 million CFU

Baci-IM powder for IM injection ℞ *bactericidal antibiotic* [bacitracin] 50 000 U

bacillus Calmette-Guérin (BCG) vaccine [see: BCG vaccine]

bacitracin USP, INN, BAN, JAN *bactericidal antibiotic; investigational (orphan) for pseudomembranous enterocolitis* 500 U/g topical; 500 U/g ophthalmic; 50 000 U/vial injection

bacitracin zinc USP, BAN *bactericidal antibiotic*

bacitracin zinc & neomycin sulfate & polymyxin B sulfate *topical antibiotic* 400 U•5 mg•10 000 U per g ophthalmic

bacitracin zinc & polymyxin B sulfate *topical antibiotic* 500•10 000 U/g ophthalmic

bacitracins zinc complex [see: bacitracin zinc]

Backache Maximum Strength Relief film-coated caplets OTC *analgesic; antirheumatic* [magnesium salicylate] 467 mg

Back-Pack (trademarked packaging form) *unit-of-use package*

baclofen (L-baclofen) USAN, USP, INN, BAN, JAN *skeletal muscle relaxant for intractable spasticity due to multiple sclerosis or spinal cord injury (orphan); investigational (orphan) for trigeminal neuralgia, cerebral palsy, spinal cord disease, and dystonia* 10, 20 mg oral

bacmecillinam INN

Bacmin tablets ℞ *vitamin/mineral/iron supplement* [multiple vitamins & minerals; iron (as ferrous fumarate); folic acid; biotin] ±•27•1•0.15 mg

bactericidal and permeability-increasing (BPI) protein, recombinant *investigational (Phase III, orphan) treatment for meningococcemia*

bacteriostatic sodium chloride [see: sodium chloride]

Bacteriostatic Sodium Chloride Injection ℞ *IV diluent* [sodium chloride (normal saline solution)] 0.9% (normal)

Bacti-Cleanse topical liquid OTC *soap-free therapeutic skin cleanser* [benzalkonium chloride]

Bactigen B Streptococcus-CS slide test for professional use ℞ *in vitro diagnostic aid for Group B streptococcal antigens in vaginal and cervical swabs*

Bactigen Meningitis Panel slide test for professional use ℞ *in vitro diagnostic aid for* H. influenzae, N. meningitidis, *and* S. pneumoniae *in various fluids* [latex agglutination test]

Bactigen Salmonella-Shigella slide test for professional use ℞ *in vitro diagnostic aid for salmonella and shigella* [latex agglutination test]

Bactine Antiseptic Anesthetic topical liquid, topical spray OTC *anesthetic; antiseptic* [lidocaine HCl; benzalkonium chloride] 2.5%•0.13%

Bactine Hydrocortisone; Maximum Strength Bactine cream OTC *corticosteroidal anti-inflammatory* [hydrocortisone] 0.5%; 1%

Bactine Pain Relieving Cleansing Spray OTC *anesthetic; antiseptic* [lidocaine HCl; benzalkonium chloride] 2.5%•0.13%

Bactine Pain Relieving Cleansing Wipes (discontinued 2008) OTC *anesthetic; antiseptic* [pramoxine HCl; benzalkonium chloride] 1%•0.13%

BactoShield aerosol foam, solution OTC *broad-spectrum antimicrobial; germicidal* [chlorhexidine gluconate; alcohol 4%] 4%

BactoShield 2 solution OTC *broad-spectrum antimicrobial; germicidal* [chlorhexidine gluconate; alcohol 4%] 2%

Bactrim; Bactrim DS tablets ℞ *broad-spectrum sulfonamide antibiotic* [sulfamethoxazole; trimethoprim] 400•80 mg; 800•160 mg

Bactrim IV infusion (discontinued 2010) ℞ *broad-spectrum sulfonamide antibiotic* [sulfamethoxazole; trimethoprim] 400•80 mg/5 mL

Bactrim Pediatric oral suspension (discontinued 2010) ℞ *broad-spectrum sulfonamide antibiotic* [sulfamethoxazole; trimethoprim] 200•40 mg/5 mL

Bactroban cream ℞ (available OTC in Canada) *antibiotic* [mupirocin (as calcium)] 2%

Bactroban ointment ℞ *antibiotic for impetigo* [mupirocin] 2%

Bactroban Nasal ointment in single-use tubes ℞ *antibiotic for iatrogenic methicillin-resistant* Staphylococcus aureus (MRSA) *infections* [mupirocin (as calcium)] 2%

Bagshawe protocol, modified *chemotherapy protocol for gestational trophoblastic neoplasm* [see: CHAMOCA]

bakeprofen INN

baker's yeast *natural source of protein and B-complex vitamins*

BAL (British antilewisite) [now: dimercaprol]

BAL in Oil deep IM injection ℞ *chelating agent for arsenic, gold, and mercury poisoning; adjunct to lead poisoning* [dimercaprol in peanut oil] 10% ☒ bolenol

Balacall DM syrup ℞ *antitussive; antihistamine; decongestant* [dextromethorphan hydrobromide; brompheniramine maleate; phenylephrine HCl] 10•2•5 mg/5 mL

Balacet 325 film-coated caplets (discontinued 2010) ℞ *narcotic analgesic; antipyretic; all products containing propoxyphene were withdrawn from the market in 2010 due to safety concerns* [propoxyphene napsylate; acetaminophen] 100•325 mg

balafilcon A USAN *hydrophilic contact lens material*

balaglitazone *investigational (Phase III) peroxisome proliferator–activated receptor (PPAR) agonist for type 2 diabetes*

Balamine DM syrup, oral drops (discontinued 2007) ℞ *antitussive; antihistamine; decongestant; drops for children 1–18 months* [dextromethorphan hydrobromide; carbinoxamine male-

ate; pseudoephedrine HCl] 12.5•4•
60 mg/5 mL; 3.5•2•25 mg/mL

Balanced B-50; Balanced B-100
tablets OTC *vitamin supplement* [multiple B vitamins; folic acid; biotin]
±•400•50 mcg; ±•100•100 mcg

balipramine BAN [also: depramine]

balm *medicinal herb* [see: lemon balm]

balm, eye; eye root *medicinal herb*
[see: goldenseal]

balm, mountain *medicinal herb* [see:
yerba santa]

balm, squaw; squaw mint *medicinal herb* [see: pennyroyal]

**balm of Gilead (*Populus balsamifera;
P. candicans*)** buds *medicinal herb
used as an antiscorbutic, balsamic,
diuretic, stimulant, and vulnerary*

Balmex ointment, cream OTC *astringent; moisturizer; emollient* [zinc oxide]
11.3%

Balmex Baby powder OTC *diaper rash
treatment* [zinc oxide; Peruvian balsam; cornstarch]

Balmex Emollient lotion OTC *moisturizer; emollient*

balmony *medicinal herb* [see: turtlebloom]

Balneol lotion OTC *corticosteroidal anti-inflammatory* [hydrocortisone] 0.25%
Ⓩ bolenol

Balneol for Her vaginal lotion OTC
corticosteroidal anti-inflammatory
[hydrocortisone] 0.25%

Balneol Hygienic Cleansing lotion
OTC *emollient/protectant* [mineral oil;
lanolin]

Balneol Perianal Cleansing lotion
(name changed to **Balneol Hygienic
Cleansing** in 2008)

Balnetar bath oil OTC *antipsoriatic;
antipruritic; emollient* [coal tar] 2.5%

balsalazide INN, BAN *gastrointestinal
anti-inflammatory for ulcerative colitis*
[also: balsalazide disodium]

balsalazide disodium USAN *gastrointestinal anti-inflammatory for ulcerative
colitis* [also: balsalazide] 750 mg oral

balsalazide sodium [see: balsalazide
disodium]

balsalazine [see: balsalazide disodium;
balsalazide]

balsam apple; balsam pear *medicinal
herb* [see: bitter melon]

balsam Peru [see: peruvian balsam;
balsam tree]

balsam poplar *medicinal herb* [see:
balm of Gilead]

balsam tree *medicinal herb* [see: Peruvian balsam]

balsamics; balsams *a class of agents
that soothe or heal; balms; also, certain
resinous substances of vegetable origin*

Balsamodendron myrrha *medicinal
herb* [see: myrrh]

balsan [see: peruvian balsam]

Baltussin HC oral liquid (discontinued 2007) Ⅸ *narcotic antitussive;
antihistamine; decongestant* [hydrocodone bitartrate; chlorpheniramine
maleate; phenylephrine HCl] 5•4•
10 mg/10 mL

Balziva tablets (in packs of 28) Ⅸ
monophasic oral contraceptive [norethindrone; ethinyl estradiol] 0.4 mg•
35 mcg × 21 days; counters × 7 days

bamaluzole INN

bambermycin INN, BAN *antibacterial
antibiotic* [also: bambermycins]

bambermycins USAN *antibacterial antibiotic* [also: bambermycin]

bambuterol INN, BAN

bamethan INN, BAN *vasodilator* [also:
bamethan sulfate]

bamethan sulfate USAN, JAN *vasodilator* [also: bamethan]

bamifylline INN, BAN *bronchodilator*
[also: bamifylline HCl] Ⓩ pimefylline

bamifylline HCl USAN *bronchodilator*
[also: bamifylline]

bamipine INN, BAN

bamnidazole USAN, INN *antiprotozoal*
(*Trichomonas*)

Banadyne-3 topical solution OTC
mucous membrane anesthetic; antipruritic; counterirritant; antiseptic [lidocaine;
menthol; alcohol 45%] 4%•1%

Banalg lotion OTC *analgesic; mild anesthetic; antipruritic; counterirritant* [methyl salicylate; camphor; menthol] 4.9%•2%•1%

Banalg Hospital Strength lotion OTC *analgesic; mild anesthetic; antipruritic; counterirritant* [methyl salicylate; menthol] 14%•3%

Bancap HC capsules (discontinued 2008) ℞ *narcotic analgesic; antipyretic* [hydrocodone bitartrate; acetaminophen] 5•500 mg

bandage, adhesive USP *surgical aid*

bandage, gauze USP *surgical aid*

Banflex IV or IM injection ℞ *skeletal muscle relaxant; analgesic; anticholinergic* [orphenadrine citrate] 30 mg/mL

banocide [see: diethylcarbamazine citrate]

Banophen caplets, capsules OTC *antihistamine; sleep aid* [diphenhydramine HCl] 25 mg

Banophen Allergy; Banophen Children's Allergy oral liquid OTC *antihistamine; sleep aid* [diphenhydramine HCl] 12.5 mg/5 mL

Banzel film-coated tablets, oral suspension ℞ *triazole anticonvulsant; adjunctive therapy for Lennox-Gastaut syndrome (orphan)* [rufinamide] 200, 400 mg; 40 mg/mL ☑ Panasal

bapineuzumab *investigational (Phase III) monoclonal antibody against amyloid plaque in the brain, used to treat mild-to-moderate Alzheimer disease*

Baptisia tinctoria medicinal herb [see: wild indigo]

baquiloprim INN, BAN

Baraclude film-coated tablets, oral solution ℞ *nucleoside reverse transcriptase inhibitor (NRTI); antiviral for chronic hepatitis B virus (HBV) infection* [entecavir] 0.5, 1 mg; 0.05 mg/mL

Barbados aloe *medicinal herb* [see: aloe]

barbenyl [see: phenobarbital]

barberry (Berberis vulgaris) bark *medicinal herb for bacteria-associated diarrhea, blood cleansing, cough, fever, indigestion, jaundice, liver disorders, sciatica, and sore throat*

barberry, California *medicinal herb* [see: Oregon grape]

barbexaclone INN

Barbidonna; Barbidonna No. 2 tablets (discontinued 2008) ℞ *GI/GU anticholinergic/antispasmodic; sedative* [atropine sulfate; scopolamine hydrobromide; hyoscyamine hydrobromide; phenobarbital] 0.025•0.0074•0.1286•16 mg; 0.025•0.0074•0.1286•32 mg

barbiphenyl [see: phenobarbital]

barbital NF, INN, JAN [also: barbitone]

barbital, soluble [now: barbital sodium]

barbital sodium NF, INN [also: barbitone sodium]

barbitone BAN [also: barbital]

barbitone sodium BAN [also: barbital sodium]

barbiturates *a class of sedative/hypnotics that produce a wide range of mood alteration; often abused as addictive street drugs*

bardana *medicinal herb* [see: burdock]

Baricon powder for oral suspension ℞ *radiopaque contrast medium for gastrointestinal imaging* [barium sulfate] 98% ☑ Paracaine; Puregon

Baridium tablets ℞ *urinary tract analgesic for the relief of pain, burning, urgency, and frequency due to mucosal irritation from surgery, catheterization, endoscopic procedures, or trauma; adjunct to antibacterial agents for urinary tract infection (UTI)* [phenazopyridine HCl] 100 mg ☑ Perdiem; Prodium; Pyridium

barium *element (Ba)* ☑ broom

barium hydroxide lime USP *carbon dioxide absorbent*

barium sulfate USP, JAN *oral/rectal radiopaque contrast medium for gastrointestinal imaging*

barley (Hordeum vulgare) juice powder *medicinal herb for anemia, arthritis, blood cleansing, boils, bronchitis, cancer, metal poisoning, poor circulation, and reducing total and LDL cholesterol and increasing HDL cholesterol*

barley malt soup extract *bulk laxative*

barmastine USAN, INN *antihistamine*

BarnesHind Saline for Sensitive Eyes solution (discontinued 2010) OTC *rinsing/storage solution for soft contact lenses* [sodium chloride (preserved saline solution)]

barnidipine INN ② pranidipine

Barobag powder for oral/rectal suspension ℞ *radiopaque contrast medium for gastrointestinal imaging* [barium sulfate] 95%

Baro-cat oral suspension ℞ *radiopaque contrast medium for gastrointestinal imaging* [barium sulfate] 1.5%

Baros effervescent granules (discontinued 2009) ℞ *adjunct to gastrointestinal imaging* [sodium bicarbonate; tartaric acid] 460•420 mg/g

Barosma betulina; B. cenulata; B. serratifolia medicinal herb [see: buchu]

barosmin [see: diosmin]

Barosperse powder for oral/rectal suspension ℞ *radiopaque contrast medium for gastrointestinal imaging* [barium sulfate] 95%

Barosperse, Liquid oral suspension ℞ *radiopaque contrast medium for gastrointestinal imaging* [barium sulfate] 60%

Bar-test tablets ℞ *radiopaque contrast medium for gastrointestinal imaging* [barium sulfate] 650 mg

barucainide INN

BAS (benzyl analogue of serotonin) [see: benanserin HCl]

base [def.] *The active part of a compound. In* naproxen sodium, *for example, the base is* naproxen. [compare to: salt]

basic aluminum acetate [see: aluminum subacetate]

basic aluminum aminoacetate [see: dihydroxyaluminum aminoacetate]

basic aluminum carbonate [see: aluminum carbonate, basic]

basic aluminum chloride [see: aluminum sesquichlorohydrate]

basic aluminum glycinate [see: dihydroxyaluminum aminoacetate]

basic bismuth carbonate [see: bismuth subcarbonate]

basic bismuth gallate [see: bismuth subgallate]

basic bismuth nitrate [see: bismuth subnitrate]

basic bismuth potassium bismuthotartrate [see: bismuth potassium tartrate]

basic bismuth salicylate [see: bismuth subsalicylate]

basic fibroblast growth factor (bFGF) [see: ersofermin]

basic fuchsin [see: fuchsin, basic]

basic zinc acetate [see: zinc acetate, basic]

basifungin USAN, INN *antifungal*

basil (Ocimum basilicum) leaves *medicinal herb for colds, headache, indigestion, insect and snake bites, and whooping cough*

basiliximab USAN *immunosuppressant; IL-2 receptor antagonist for the prevention of acute rejection of renal transplants (orphan)*

basswood; bast tree *medicinal herb* [see: linden tree]

bastard hemp *medicinal herb* [see: hemp nettle]

bastard saffron *medicinal herb* [see: safflower]

batanopride INN *antiemetic* [also: batanopride HCl]

batanopride HCl USAN *antiemetic* [also: batanopride]

batebulast INN

batelapine INN *antipsychotic* [also: batelapine HCl]

batelapine maleate USAN *antipsychotic* [also: batelapine]

batilol INN

batimastat USAN, INN *antineoplastic; matrix metalloproteinase (MMP) inhibitor*

batoprazine INN ② butaperazine

batroxobin INN, JAN

batyl alcohol [see: batilol]

batylol [see: batilol]

baxitozine INN

bay; bay laurel; bay tree; Indian bay; sweet bay *medicinal herb* [see: laurel]

bay, holly; red bay; white bay
medicinal herb [see: magnolia]

bayberry (Myrica cerifera) bark,
berries, root bark *medicinal herb for
cholera, diarrhea, dysentery, glands,
goiter, indigestion, jaundice, excessive
menstruation, scrofuloderma, and uterine hemorrhage; not generally regarded
as safe and effective because of its high
tannin content*

Baycadron elixir ℞ *corticosteroidal
anti-inflammatory* [dexamethasone]
0.5 mg/5 mL

Bayer Arthritis Regimen delayed-
release enteric-coated tablets OTC
*analgesic; antipyretic; anti-inflamma-
tory; antirheumatic* [aspirin] 500 mg

**Bayer Aspirin, Genuine; Maximum
Bayer Aspirin** film-coated tablets,
film-coated caplets OTC *analgesic;
antipyretic; anti-inflammatory; antirheumatic* [aspirin] 325 mg; 500 mg

Bayer Aspirin Regimen delayed-
release enteric-coated tablets and
caplets OTC *analgesic; antipyretic; anti-
inflammatory; antirheumatic* [aspirin]
81, 325 mg

Bayer Back & Body Pain caplets
OTC *analgesic; antipyretic; anti-inflammatory; antirheumatic* [aspirin; caf-
feine] 500•32.5 mg

Bayer Children's Aspirin chewable
tablets OTC *analgesic; antipyretic; anti-
inflammatory* [aspirin] 81 mg

Bayer Muscle & Joint Cream OTC
*analgesic; mild anesthetic; antipruritic;
counterirritant* [methyl salicylate;
menthol; camphor] 30%•10%•4%

**Bayer Nutritional Science Vital &
Sharp Mind** softgels OTC *vitamin/
EFA/herbal supplement* [multiple B
vitamins; docosahexaenoic acid
(DHA); gingko biloba extract; folic
acid] $\pm$•170•180•0.2 mg

Bayer Plus caplets OTC *analgesic; antipyretic; anti-inflammatory; antirheumatic* [aspirin (buffered with calcium
carbonate, magnesium carbonate,
and magnesium oxide)] 500 mg

Bayer PM Aspirin Plus Sleep Aid
caplet OTC *analgesic; antipyretic; anti-
inflammatory; antirheumatic; antihistaminic sleep aid* [aspirin; diphenhydramine HCl] 500•25 mg

Bayer Quick Release Crystals oral
powder OTC *analgesic; antipyretic;
anti-inflammatory* [aspirin; caffeine]
850•65 mg/pkt.

Bayer Select Backache caplets OTC
*analgesic; antipyretic; anti-inflamma-
tory; antirheumatic* [magnesium sali-
cylate] 580 mg

Bayer Timed Release, 8-Hour caplets
OTC *analgesic; antipyretic; anti-inflammatory; antirheumatic* [aspirin] 650 mg

**Bayer Women's Aspirin Plus Cal-
cium** caplets OTC *analgesic; antipyretic; anti-inflammatory; antirheumatic;
calcium supplement* [aspirin; calcium]
81•300 mg

BayGam IM injection (name changed
to **GamaSTAN S/D** in 2007)

BayHep B IM injection (name
changed to **HyperHEP B S/D** in
2007)

BayRab IM injection (name changed
to **HyperRab S/D** in 2007)

BayRho-D Full Dose IM injection in
prefilled syringes (name changed to
HyperRHO S/D Full Dose in 2008)

BayTet IM injection (discontinued
2010) ℞ *passive immunizing agent for
post-exposure tetanus prophylaxis in
patients with incomplete or uncertain
pre-exposure immunization with tetanus
toxoids* [tetanus immune globulin,
solvent/detergent treated] 250 IU

bazedoxifene *second-generation selective
estrogen receptor modulator (SERM);
investigational (NDA filed) for the prevention and treatment of postmenopausal osteoporosis*

bazinaprine INN

B$_c$ (vitamin B$_c$) [see: folic acid]

BC Allergy, Sinus, Headache oral
powder OTC *decongestant; antihistamine; analgesic; antipyretic* [pseudo-
ephedrine HCl; chlorpheniramine

maleate; acetaminophen] 60•4•650 mg/pkt.

BC Arthritis Strength oral powder OTC *analgesic; antipyretic; anti-inflammatory* [aspirin; salicylamide; caffeine] 742•222•38 mg

BC Fast Pain Relief; BC Fast Pain Relief Arthritis oral powder OTC *analgesic; antipyretic; anti-inflammatory* [aspirin; caffeine] 845•65 mg/pkt.; 1000•65 mg/pkt.

B-C with Folic Acid tablets (discontinued 2008) ℞ *vitamin supplement* [multiple B vitamins; vitamin C; folic acid] ±•500•0.5 mg

B-C with Folic Acid Plus tablets (discontinued 2008) ℞ *hematinic; vitamin/mineral/iron supplement* [multiple vitamins & minerals; iron (as ferrous fumarate); folic acid; biotin] ±•27•0.8•0.15 mg

BCAA (branched-chain amino acids) [see: isoleucine; leucine; valine]

BCAD 2 powder OTC *enteral nutritional therapy for maple syrup urine disease (MSUD)* 1 lb./can

BCAVe; B-CAVe (bleomycin, CCNU, Adriamycin, Velban) *chemotherapy protocol for Hodgkin lymphoma* ☒ PCV

BCG Vaccine powder for multiple dermal puncture device ℞ *active bacterin for tuberculosis prevention* [BCG vaccine, Tice strain] 50 mg (1–8 × 10⁸ CFU)

BCG vaccine (bacillus Calmette-Guérin) USP *active bacterin for tuberculosis prevention; antineoplastic for urinary bladder cancer*

BCNU (bis-chloroethyl-nitroso-urea) [see: carmustine]

B-Complex elixir (discontinued 2008) OTC *vitamin supplement* [multiple B vitamins]

B-Complex and B-12 tablets (discontinued 2008) OTC *vitamin supplement* [multiple B vitamins; protease] ±• 10 mg

B-Complex with B-12 tablets (discontinued 2008) OTC *vitamin supplement* [multiple B vitamins]

B-Complex/Vitamin C caplets (discontinued 2008) OTC *vitamin supplement* [multiple B vitamins; vitamin C] ±•300 mg

BCOP (BCNU, cyclophosphamide, Oncovin, prednisone) *chemotherapy protocol* ☒ BEACOPP; PCP

BCVPP (BCNU, cyclophosphamide, vinblastine, procarbazine, prednisone) *chemotherapy protocol for Hodgkin lymphoma*

B-D glucose chewable tablets OTC *blood glucose elevating agent for hypoglycemia* [glucose] 5 g

BDNF (brain-derived neurotrophic factor) [see: methionyl neurotropic factor, brain-derived]

BDO (1,4-butanediol) *a precursor to gamma hydroxybutyrate (GHB); a formerly legal alternative to GHB, now also illegal (Schedule I)* [see: gamma hydroxybutyrate (GHB)]

BDP (beclomethasone dipropionate) [q.v.]

BDP Nasal HFA dry nasal aerosol *investigational (NDA filed) dry powder delivery form of a corticosteroidal anti-inflammatory for seasonal or perennial rhinitis* [beclomethasone dipropionate (BDP)] 320 mcg/actuation

BEACOPP; BEACOPP escalated (bleomycin, etoposide, Adriamycin, cyclophosphamide, Oncovin, procarbazine, prednisone) [with filgrastim hematopoietic] *chemotherapy protocol for Hodgkin lymphoma* ☒ BCOP; PCP

bean herb *medicinal herb* [see: summer savory]

bean trefoil *medicinal herb* [see: buckbean]

Beano oral liquid, tablets OTC *digestive aid* [alpha-D-galactosidase enzyme]

bearberry *medicinal herb* [see: uva ursi]

beard, old man's *medicinal herb* [see: fringe tree; woodbine]

Bear-E-Yum CT oral suspension ℞ *radiopaque contrast medium for gastrointestinal imaging* [barium sulfate] 1.5%

Bear-E-Yum GI oral suspension ℞ *radiopaque contrast medium for gastrointestinal imaging* [barium sulfate] 60%

bear's grape *medicinal herb* [see: uva ursi]

bear's weed *medicinal herb* [see: yerba santa]

bearsfoot *medicinal herb* [see: hellebore]

Beaumont root *medicinal herb* [see: Culver root]

beaver tree *medicinal herb* [see: magnolia]

Bebulin VH powder for IV infusion ℞ *systemic hemostatic; antihemophilic for factor IX deficiency (hemophilia B; Christmas disease) (orphan)* [factor IX complex (factors II, IX, and X), human, heat treated] (actual number of units is indicated on the vial)

becanthone HCl USAN *antischistosomal* [also: becantone]

becantone INN *antischistosomal* [also: becanthone HCl]

becantone HCl [see: becanthone HCl]

becaplermin USAN *recombinant platelet-derived growth factor B for diabetic foot and leg ulcers*

beciparcil INN

beclamide INN, BAN

becliconazole INN

beclobrate INN, BAN

beclometasone INN *corticosteroidal inhalant for asthma; intranasal steroid* [also: beclomethasone dipropionate; beclomethasone; beclometasone dipropionate]

beclometasone dipropionate JAN *corticosteroidal inhalant for asthma; intranasal steroid* [also: beclomethasone dipropionate; beclomethasone; beclometasone]

beclomethasone BAN *corticosteroidal anti-inflammatory for chronic asthma* [also: beclomethasone dipropionate; beclomethasone; beclometasone dipropionate]

beclomethasone dipropionate (BDP) USAN, USP *corticosteroidal anti-inflammatory for chronic asthma and rhinitis; investigational (Phase III, orphan) oral treatment for intestinal graft vs. host disease* [also: beclometasone; beclomethasone; beclometasone dipropionate]

beclotiamine INN

Beconase AQ nasal spray ℞ *corticosteroidal anti-inflammatory for seasonal or perennial rhinitis* [beclomethasone dipropionate] 0.042% (42 mcg/dose)

bectumomab USAN *monoclonal antibody IgG$_{2a}$ to B cell, murine* [also: technetium Tc 99m bectumomab]

bedstraw (Galium aparine; G. verum) plant *medicinal herb used as an antispasmodic, aperient, diaphoretic, diuretic, and vulnerary*

bee balm *medicinal herb* [see: lemon balm]

bee pollen *natural remedy for anemia, bodily weakness, cerebral hemorrhage, colitis, constipation, enteritis, and weight loss; also used as an anti-aging agent and prenatal nutritional supplement; not generally regarded as safe and effective because of widespread allergic reactions*

bee venom (derived from Apis mellifera) *natural remedy for arthritis and multiple sclerosis, and for hyposensitization of persons highly sensitive to bee stings*

beechwood creosote [see: creosote carbonate]

beef tallow JAN

Beelith film-coated tablets OTC *vitamin/magnesium supplement* [vitamin B$_6$; magnesium (as oxide)] 20•362 mg

bee's nest plant *medicinal herb* [see: carrot]

beeswax, white JAN [also: wax, white]

beeswax, yellow JAN [also: wax, yellow]

Bee-Zee tablets OTC *vitamin/zinc supplement* [multiple vitamins; zinc; folic acid; biotin] ±•22.5•0.4•0.3 mg

befiperide INN

Be-Flex Plus capsules (discontinued 2011) ℞ *antihistamine; sleep aid; analgesic; antipyretic* [phenyltoloxamine citrate; acetaminophen; salicylamide] 20•300•200 mg

befloxatone INN

befunolol INN [also: befunolol HCl] ② pafenolol

befunolol HCl JAN [also: befunolol]

befuraline INN ② bufrolin

behenyl alcohol [see: docosanol]

behepan [see: cyanocobalamin]

bekanamycin INN *antibiotic* [also: bekanamycin sulfate]

bekanamycin sulfate JAN *antibiotic* [also: bekanamycin]

belarizine INN

belatacept *CTLA-4 fusion protein; immunosuppressant to prevent kidney transplant rejection*

belfosdil USAN, INN *antihypertensive; calcium channel blocker*

Belganyl (available only from the Centers for Disease Control) (discontinued 2011) ℞ *antiparasitic for African trypanosomiasis and onchocerciasis* [suramin sodium]

belimumab *human monoclonal antibody to B-lymphocyte stimulator (BLyS) protein for active systemic lupus erythematosus (SLE)*

Bellacane elixir (discontinued 2008) ℞ *GI/GU anticholinergic/antispasmodic; sedative* [atropine sulfate; scopolamine hydrobromide; hyoscyamine sulfate; phenobarbital] 0.0194•0.0065•0.1037•16.2 mg/5 mL ② bulaquine; Polocaine

Bellacane tablets (discontinued 2008) ℞ *GI/GU anticholinergic/antispasmodic; sedative* [hyoscyamine sulfate; phenobarbital] 0.125•15 mg ② bulaquine; Polocaine

Bellacane SR sustained-release tablets (discontinued 2008) ℞ *GI/GU anticholinergic/antispasmodic; sedative; analgesic* [belladonna alkaloids; phenobarbital; ergotamine tartrate] 0.2•40•0.6 mg

belladonna *(Atropa belladonna)* leaves, tops, and berries *medicinal herb used as an antispasmodic, calmative, diaphoretic, diuretic, and narcotic* ② Paladin

belladonna alkaloids *a class of GI/GU anticholinergic/antispasmodics that includes atropine sulfate, scopolamine hydrobromide, hyoscyamine hydrobromide, and hyoscyamine sulfate*

belladonna alkaloids & phenobarbital *GI/GU anticholinergic/antispasmodic; sedative* 0.13•16.2 mg oral

belladonna extract USP *GI/GU anticholinergic/antispasmodic; antiparkinsonian; respiratory antisecretory* 27–33 mg/100 mL oral

Bellahist-D LA sustained-release caplets ℞ *decongestant; antihistamine; anticholinergic to dry mucosal secretions* [phenylephrine HCl; chlorpheniramine maleate; hyoscyamine sulfate; atropine sulfate; scopolamine hydrobromide] 20•8•0.19•0.04•0.01 mg

Bellamine tablets (discontinued 2009) ℞ *GI/GU anticholinergic/antispasmodic; sedative; analgesic* [belladonna alkaloids; phenobarbital; ergotamine tartrate] 0.2•40•0.6 mg

Bell/ans tablets OTC *antacid* [sodium bicarbonate] 520 mg

Bellatal tablets ℞ *long-acting barbiturate sedative, hypnotic, and anticonvulsant* [phenobarbital] 16.2 mg

Bellergal-S tablets (discontinued 2008) ℞ *GI/GU anticholinergic/antispasmodic; sedative; analgesic* [belladonna extract; phenobarbital; ergotamine tartrate] 0.2•40•0.6 mg

Bellis perennis *medicinal herb* [see: wild daisy]

bells, May *medicinal herb* [see: lily of the valley]

beloxamide USAN, INN *antihyperlipoproteinemic*

beloxepin USAN *norepinephrine uptake inhibitor for depression*

Bel-Phen-Ergot SR sustained-release tablets (discontinued 2009) ℞ *GI/GU anticholinergic/antispasmodic; sed-*

ative; analgesic [belladonna alkaloids; phenobarbital; ergotamine tartrate] 0.2•40•0.6 mg

bemarinone INN *cardiotonic; positive inotropic; vasodilator* [also: bemarinone HCl]

bemarinone HCl USAN *cardiotonic; positive inotropic; vasodilator* [also: bemarinone]

bemegride USP, INN, BAN, JAN

bemesetron USAN, INN *antiemetic*

bemetizide INN, BAN

Beminal 500 tablets (discontinued 2008) OTC *vitamin supplement* [multiple B vitamins; vitamin C] ≜•500 mg

bemitradine USAN, INN *antihypertensive; diuretic*

bemoradan USAN, INN *cardiotonic*

benactyzine INN, BAN

benactyzine HCl *mild antidepressant; anticholinergic*

Benadryl IV or IM injection ℞ *antihistamine; motion sickness preventative; sleep aid* [diphenhydramine HCl] 50 mg/mL

Benadryl; Benadryl 2% cream, spray OTC *antihistamine* [diphenhydramine HCl] 1%; 2%

Benadryl Allergy Liqui-Gels (liquid-filled gelcaps), Kapseals (sealed capsules), Ultratabs (tablets), chewable tablets OTC *antihistamine; sleep aid* [diphenhydramine HCl] 25 mg; 25 mg; 25 mg; 12.5 mg

Benadryl Allergy & Cold caplets OTC *decongestant; antihistamine; sleep aid; analgesic* [phenylephrine HCl; diphenhydramine HCl; acetaminophen] 5•12.5•325 mg

Benadryl Allergy Plus Sinus Headache caplets OTC *decongestant; antihistamine; sleep aid; analgesic; antipyretic* [phenylephrine HCl; diphenhydramine HCl; acetaminophen] 5•12.5•325 mg

Benadryl Allergy Quick Dissolve Strips (orally disintegrating film) OTC *antihistamine; sleep aid* [diphenhydramine HCl] 25 mg

Benadryl Children's Allergy oral liquid OTC *antihistamine; sleep aid* [diphenhydramine HCl] 12.5 mg/5 mL

Benadryl Children's Allergy Fastmelt (orally disintegrating tablets) OTC *antihistamine; sleep aid* [diphenhydramine citrate] 19 mg

Benadryl Children's Allergy & Sinus oral liquid OTC *decongestant; antihistamine; sleep aid* [pseudoephedrine HCl; diphenhydramine citrate] 30•19 mg/5 mL

Benadryl Children's Anti-Itch gel OTC *poison ivy treatment* [camphor] 0.45%

Benadryl Decongestant Allergy film-coated tablets OTC *decongestant; antihistamine; sleep aid* [pseudoephedrine HCl; diphenhydramine HCl] 60•25 mg

Benadryl Itch Relief spray, cream, stick OTC *antihistamine; astringent* [diphenhydramine HCl; zinc acetate] 2%•0.1%

Benadryl Itch Relief, Children's spray, cream OTC *antihistamine; astringent* [diphenhydramine HCl; zinc acetate] 1%•0.1%

Benadryl Itch Stopping Gel; Benadryl Itch Stopping Gel Children's Formula OTC *antihistamine; astringent* [diphenhydramine HCl; zinc acetate] 2%•1%; 1%•1%

Benadryl Itch Stopping Spray OTC *antihistamine; astringent* [diphenhydramine HCl; zinc acetate; alcohol] 1%•0.1%•73.6%, 2%•0.1%•73.5%

Benadryl Severe Allergy & Sinus Headache caplets OTC *decongestant; antihistamine; sleep aid; analgesic; antipyretic* [phenylephrine HCl; diphenhydramine HCl; acetaminophen] 5•25•325 mg

Benadryl-D Allergy & Sinus tablets OTC *decongestant; antihistamine; sleep aid* [phenylephrine HCl; diphenhydramine HCl] 10•25 mg

Benadryl-D Children's Allergy & Sinus oral liquid OTC *decongestant;*

antihistamine; sleep aid [pseudoephedrine HCl; diphenhydramine HCl] 30•12.5 mg

benafentrine INN

benanserin HCl

benapen [see: benethamine penicillin]

benaprizine INN anticholinergic [also: benapryzine HCl; benapryzine]

benapryzine BAN anticholinergic [also: benapryzine HCl; benaprizine]

benapryzine HCl USAN anticholinergic [also: benaprizine; benapryzine]

benaxibine INN ☑ pinoxepin

benazepril INN, BAN angiotensin-converting enzyme (ACE) inhibitor for hypertension [also: benazepril HCl]

benazepril HCl USAN angiotensin-converting enzyme (ACE) inhibitor for hypertension; also used for heart failure, nondiabetic nephropathy, and the prevention of recurrent stroke [also: benazepril] 5, 10, 20, 40 mg oral

benazepril HCl & amlodipine besylate antihypertensive; calcium channel blocker; angiotensin-converting enzyme (ACE) inhibitor 10•2.5, 10•5, 20•5, 20•10 mg

benazepril HCl & hydrochlorothiazide combination angiotensin-converting enzyme (ACE) inhibitor and diuretic for hypertension 5•6.25, 10•12.5, 20•12.5, 20•25 mg oral

benazeprilat USAN, INN antihypertensive; angiotensin-converting enzyme (ACE) inhibitor

bencianol INN

bencisteine INN

benclonidine INN

Bencort lotion ℞ keratolytic and corticosteroidal anti-inflammatory for acne [benzoyl peroxide; hydrocortisone] 5%•0.5% ☑ Penecort

bencyclane INN [also: bencyclane fumarate]

bencyclane fumarate JAN [also: bencyclane]

bendacalol mesylate USAN antihypertensive

bendamustine HCl INN purine analogue; alkylating antineoplastic for

chronic lymphocytic leukemia (orphan) and non-Hodgkin lymphoma (orphan); derivative of mechlorethamine HCl

bendazac USAN, INN, BAN, JAN anti-inflammatory

bendazol INN

benderizine INN

bendrofluazide BAN diuretic; antihypertensive [also: bendroflumethiazide]

bendroflumethiazide USP, INN diuretic; antihypertensive [also: bendrofluazide]

bendroflumethiazide & nadolol combination diuretic and beta-blocker for hypertension 5•40, 5•80 mg oral

bendroflumethiazide & rauwolfia serpentina antihypertensive; diuretic; peripheral antiadrenergic 4•50 mg oral

Benefiber chewable tablets OTC dietary fiber supplement [guar gum] 1 g fiber

Benefiber; Benefiber for Children powder for oral solution OTC dietary fiber supplement [guar gum] 1.5 g fiber/tsp.

Benefiber Drink Mix; Benefiber Sticks powder for oral solution OTC dietary fiber supplement [guar gum] 3 g fiber/packet

Benefiber Plus Calcium chewable tablets, powder for oral solution OTC dietary fiber/calcium supplement [guar gum; calcium] 1 g fiber•100 mg; 3 g fiber•300 mg per tsp.

Benefiber Plus Heart Health caplets, powder for oral solution OTC dietary fiber/vitamin B supplement [guar gum; vitamins B_6 and B_{12}; folic acid] 1 g fiber•0.23 mg•0.67 mcg•44.7 mcg; 1.5 g fiber•0.35 mg•1 mcg•67 mg per tsp.

Benefiber Ultra caplets OTC dietary fiber supplement [guar gum] 1 g fiber

BeneFin investigational (Phase III, orphan) angiogenesis inhibitor for the treatment of solid tumors [squalamine lactate (shark cartilage powder)]

BeneFIX powder for IV infusion ℞ systemic hemostatic; antihemophilic for factor IX deficiency (hemophilia B; Christmas disease) (orphan) [factor

IX, recombinant] 250, 500, 1000, 2000 U/vial

Beneprotein powder for oral liquid OTC *dietary protein supplement* [100% whey protein] 6 g protein/dose

benethamine penicillin INN, BAN

benexate INN

benexate HCl JAN

benfluorex Ⓔ INN *antidiabetic; weight-loss aid*

benfosformin INN

benfotiamine INN, JAN *lipophilic form of vitamin B₁ (thiamine)* [compare: thiamine; thiamine HCl]

benfurodil hemisuccinate INN

bengal gelatin [see: agar]

Ben-Gay Original ointment OTC *analgesic; mild anesthetic; antipruritic; counterirritant* [methyl salicylate; menthol] 18.3%•16%

Ben-Gay Patch OTC *mild anesthetic; antipruritic; counterirritant* [menthol] 1.4%

Ben-Gay Regular Strength cream OTC *analgesic; mild anesthetic; antipruritic; counterirritant* [methyl salicylate; menthol] 15%•10%

Ben-Gay Ultra Strength cream OTC *analgesic; mild anesthetic; antipruritic; counterirritant* [methyl salicylate; menthol; camphor] 30%•10%•4%

Ben-Gay Vanishing Scent gel OTC *mild anesthetic; antipruritic; counterirritant* [menthol; camphor] 3%• ⅟2

benhepazone INN

Benicar film-coated tablets ℞ *angiotensin receptor blocker (ARB) for hypertension* [olmesartan medoxomil] 5, 20, 40 mg ② Penecare

Benicar HCT film-coated tablets ℞ *combination angiotensin receptor blocker (ARB) and diuretic for hypertension* [olmesartan medoxomil; hydrochlorothiazide] 20•12.5, 40• 12.5, 40•25 mg

benidipine INN

Benlysta powder for IV infusion ℞ *monthly treatment for active systemic lupus erythematosus (SLE)* [belimumab] 120, 400 mg/vial

benmoxin INN

benolizime INN

Benoquin cream (discontinued 2010) ℞ *depigmenting agent for vitiligo* [monobenzone] 20%

benorilate INN [also: benorylate]

benorterone USAN, INN *antiandrogen*

benorylate BAN [also: benorilate]

benoxafos INN

benoxaprofen USAN, INN, BAN *anti-inflammatory; analgesic*

benoxinate HCl USP *topical ophthalmic anesthetic* [also: oxybuprocaine; oxybuprocaine HCl]

benoxinate HCl & fluorescein sodium *topical ophthalmic anesthetic; corneal disclosing agent* 0.4%•0.25% eye drops

benpenolisin INN

benperidol USAN, INN, BAN *antipsychotic*

benproperine INN [also: benproperine phosphate]

benproperine phosphate JAN [also: benproperine]

benrixate INN

Bensal HP ointment ℞ *antifungal; keratolytic* [benzoic acid; salicylic acid] 6%•3%

bensalan USAN, INN *disinfectant*

benserazide USAN, INN, BAN *decarboxylase inhibitor; antiparkinsonian adjunct* [also: benserazide HCl]

benserazide HCl JAN *decarboxylase inhibitor; antiparkinsonian adjunct* [also: benserazide]

Benson's Bottom Paint cream, ointment OTC *diaper rash treatment*

bensuldazic acid INN, BAN

Bensulfoid cream (discontinued 2009) OTC *antiseptic and keratolytic for acne* [colloidal sulfur; resorcinol; alcohol] 8%•2%•12%

bensylyte HCl [see: phenoxybenzamine HCl]

Ben-Tann oral suspension (discontinued 2009) ℞ *antihistamine; sleep aid* [diphenhydramine tannate] 25 mg/5 mL

bentazepam USAN, INN *sedative*

bentemazole INN

bentiamine INN
bentipimine INN
bentiromide USAN, INN, BAN, JAN *diagnostic aid for pancreas function*
bentonite NF, JAN *suspending agent*
bentoquatam USAN *topical skin protectant for allergic contact dermatitis and poison ivy exposure*
Bentyl capsules, tablets, syrup, IM injection ℞ *gastrointestinal anticholinergic/antispasmodic for irritable bowel syndrome (IBS)* [dicyclomine HCl] 10 mg; 20 mg; 10 mg/5 mL; 10 mg/mL
benurestat USAN, INN *urease enzyme inhibitor*
Benz 42 ℞ *hydrophilic contact lens material* [hefilcon A]
Benza topical solution OTC *antiseptic* [benzalkonium chloride] 1:750
Benzac 5; Benzac 10 gel ℞ *keratolytic and antiseptic for acne* [benzoyl peroxide; alcohol] 5%•12%; 10%•12%
Benzac AC 2½; Benzac W 2½; Benzac W 5; Benzac W 10 gel (discontinued 2008) ℞ *keratolytic for acne* [benzoyl peroxide] 2.5%; 2.5%; 5%; 10%
Benzac AC 5; Benzac AC 10 gel ℞ *keratolytic for acne* [benzoyl peroxide] 5%; 10%
Benzac AC Wash 2½ topical liquid (discontinued 2008) ℞ *keratolytic for acne* [benzoyl peroxide] 2.5%
Benzac AC Wash 5; Benzac W Wash 5; Benzac AC Wash 10; Benzac W Wash 10 topical liquid ℞ *keratolytic for acne* [benzoyl peroxide] 5%; 5%; 10%; 10%
BenzaClin gel ℞ *antibiotic and keratolytic for acne* [clindamycin phosphate; benzoyl peroxide] 1%•5%
Benzagel Wash gel ℞ *keratolytic and antiseptic for acne* [benzoyl peroxide; alcohol] 10%•14%
benzaldehyde NF *flavoring agent*
benzalkonium chloride (BAC) NF, INN, BAN, JAN *preservative; bacteriostatic antiseptic; surfactant/wetting agent* 17% topical

Benzamine (trademarked ingredient) *antioxidant; a proprietary blend of the nutritional supplements aminobenzoic acid, vitamin E, and alpha lipoic acid (ALA); also known as* **Primorine**
Benzamycin gel ℞ *antibiotic and keratolytic for acne* [erythromycin; benzoyl peroxide; alcohol] 3%•5%•20%
benzaprinoxide INN
benzarone INN
benzathine benzylpenicillin INN *natural penicillin antibiotic* [also: penicillin G benzathine; benzathine penicillin; benzylpenicillin benzathine]
benzathine penicillin BAN *natural penicillin antibiotic* [also: penicillin G benzathine; benzathine benzylpenicillin; benzylpenicillin benzathine]
benzathine penicillin G [see: penicillin G benzathine]
benzatropine INN *antiparkinsonian; anticholinergic* [also: benztropine mesylate; benztropine]
benzazoline HCl [see: tolazoline HCl]
benzbromaron JAN *uricosuric* [also: benzbromarone]
benzbromarone USAN, INN, BAN *uricosuric* [also: benzbromaron]
benzchinamide [see: benzquinamide]
benzchlorpropamide [see: beclamide]
Benzedrex inhaler ℞ *nasal decongestant* [propylhexedrine] 250 mg
BenzEFoam aerosol foam ℞ *keratolytic for acne* [benzoyl peroxide] 5.3%
benzene ethanol [see: phenylethyl alcohol]
benzene hexachloride, gamma [now: lindane]
benzeneacetic acid, sodium salt [see: sodium phenylacetate]
benzenebutanoic acid, sodium salt [see: sodium phenylbutyrate]
1,3-benzenediol [see: resorcinol]
benzenemethanol [see: benzyl alcohol]
benzestrofol [see: estradiol benzoate]
benzestrol USP, INN, BAN
benzethacil [see: penicillin G benzathine]
benzethidine INN, BAN

benzethonium chloride USP, INN, BAN, JAN *topical anti-infective; preservative*

benzetimide INN *anticholinergic* [also: benzetimide HCl]

benzetimide HCl USAN *anticholinergic* [also: benzetimide]

benzfetamine INN *CNS stimulant; anorexiant* [also: benzphetamine HCl; benzphetamine]

benzhexol BAN *anticholinergic; antiparkinsonian* [also: trihexyphenidyl HCl; trihexyphenidyl]

N-benzhydryl-N-methylpiperazine [see: cyclizine HCl]

benzilone bromide [see: benzilonium bromide]

benzilonium bromide USAN, INN, BAN *anticholinergic*

2-benzimidazolepropionic acid [see: procodazole]

benzimidazoles, substituted *a class of gastric antisecretory agents that inhibit the ATPase "proton pump" within the cell* [also called: proton pump inhibitors; ATPase inhibitors]

benzin, petroleum JAN

benzindamine HCl [see: benzydamine HCl]

benzindopyrine INN *antipsychotic* [also: benzindopyrine HCl]

benzindopyrine HCl USAN *antipsychotic* [also: benzindopyrine]

benzinoform [see: carbon tetrachloride]

benziodarone INN, BAN

Benziq; Benziq LS gel ℞ *keratolytic for acne* [benzoyl peroxide] 5.25%; 2.75%

Benziq Wash soap ℞ *keratolytic for acne* [benzoyl peroxide] 5.25%

benzisoxazoles *a class of novel (atypical) antipsychotic agents*

benzmalecene INN

benzmethoxazone [see: chlorthenoxazine]

benznidazole INN

benzoaric acid [see: ellagic acid]

benzoate & phenylacetate [see: sodium benzoate & sodium phenylacetate]

benzobarbital INN

benzocaine USP, INN, BAN *topical anesthetic; mucous membrane anesthetic; nonprescription diet aid* [also: ethyl aminobenzoate] 5% topical

benzocaine & polycosanol & acetic acid & antipyrine *anesthetic; analgesic* 1.4%•0.01%•0.01%•5.4% otic drops

benzoclidine INN

benzoctamine INN, BAN *sedative; muscle relaxant* [also: benzoctamine HCl]

benzoctamine HCl USAN, INN *sedative; muscle relaxant* [also: benzoctamine]

Benzodent oral ointment OTC *mucous membrane anesthetic* [benzocaine] 20%

benzodepa USAN, INN *antineoplastic*

benzodiazepine HCl [see: medazepam HCl]

benzodiazepines *a class of nonbarbiturate sedative/hypnotics and anticonvulsants*

benzododecinium chloride INN

benzogynestryl [see: estradiol benzoate]

benzoic acid USP, JAN *antifungal; urinary acidifier*

benzoic acid, phenylmethyl ester [see: benzyl benzoate]

benzoic acid, potassium salt [see: potassium benzoate]

benzoic acid, sodium salt [see: sodium benzoate]

benzoin USP, JAN *topical protectant*

Benzoin Compound tincture OTC *skin protectant; antiseptic* [benzoin; aloe; alcohol 74–80%]

benzol [see: benzene ...]

benzonatate USP, INN, BAN *antitussive* 100, 150, 200 mg oral

benzophenone

benzopyrrolate [see: benzopyrronium]

benzopyrronium bromide INN

benzoquinamide HCl *post-anesthesia antiemetic*

benzoquinone amidoinohydrazone thiosemicarbazone hydrate [see: ambazone]

benzoquinonium chloride

benzorphanol [see: levophenacylmorphan]

Benz-O-Sthetic aerosol spray, gel OTC *anesthetic* [benzocaine] 20%

benzosulfinide [see: saccharin]

benzosulphinide sodium [see: saccharin sodium]

benzothiazepines *a class of calcium channel blockers*

benzothiozon [see: thioacetazone; thiacetazone]

benzotript INN

benzoxiquine USAN, INN *antiseptic/disinfectant*

benzoxonium chloride INN

benzoyl *p*-aminosalicylate (B-PAS) [see: benzoylpas calcium]

benzoyl peroxide USAN, USP *keratolytic* 2.5%, 4%, 4.5%, 5%, 5.75%, 6.5%, 7%, 8%, 8.5%, 10% topical

benzoyl peroxide & clindamycin phosphate *keratolytic and lincosamide antibiotic for acne* 5%•1% topical

benzoyl peroxide & erythromycin *keratolytic and antibiotic for acne* 5%• 3% topical

m-benzoylhydratropic acid [see: ketoprofen]

benzoylmethylecgonine [see: cocaine]

benzoylpas calcium USAN, USP *antibacterial; tuberculostatic* [also: calcium benzamidosalicylate]

benzoylsulfanilamide [see: sulfabenzamide]

benzoylthiamindisulfide [see: bisbentiamine]

benzoylthiaminmonophosphate [see: benfotiamine]

benzphetamine BAN *CNS stimulant; anorexiant* [also: benzphetamine HCl; benzfetamine]

benzphetamine chloride [see: benzphetamine HCl]

benzphetamine HCl NF *CNS stimulant; anorexiant* [also: benzfetamine; benzphetamine] 25, 50 mg oral

benzpiperylon [see: benzpiperylone]

benzpiperylone INN

benzpyrinium bromide NF, INN

benzquercin INN

benzquinamide USAN, INN, BAN *postanesthesia antinauseant and antiemetic*

benzthiazide USP, INN, BAN *diuretic; antihypertensive*

benztropine BAN *anticholinergic; antiparkinsonian* [also: benztropine mesylate; benzatropine]

benztropine mesylate USP *anticholinergic; antiparkinsonian* [also: benzatropine; benztropine] 0.5, 1, 2 mg oral; 1 mg/mL injection

benztropine methanesulfonate [see: benztropine mesylate]

benzydamine INN, BAN *analgesic; antipyretic; anti-inflammatory* [also: benzydamine HCl]

benzydamine HCl USAN, JAN *analgesic; antipyretic; anti-inflammatory; investigational (orphan) radioprotectant for oral mucosa following radiation therapy for head and neck cancer* [also: benzydamine]

benzydroflumethiazide [see: bendroflumethiazide]

benzyl alcohol NF, INN, JAN *antimicrobial agent; antiseptic; local anesthetic*

benzyl analogue of serotonin (BAS) [see: benanserin HCl]

benzyl antiserotonin [see: benanserin HCl]

benzyl benzoate USP, JAN

benzyl carbinol [see: phenylethyl alcohol]

S-benzyl thiobenzoate [see: tibenzate]

benzylamide [see: beclamide]

benzylamines *a class of antifungals structurally related to the allylamines*

N-benzylanilinoacetamidoxime [see: cetoxime]

2-benzylbenzimidazole [see: bendazol]

benzyldimethyltetradecylammonium chloride [see: miristalkonium chloride]

benzyldodecyldimethylammonium chloride [see: benzododecinium chloride]

benzylhexadecyldimethylammonium [see: cetalkonium]

benzylhexadecyldimethylammonium chloride [see: cetalkonium chloride]

benzylhydrochlorothiazide JAN

p-benzyloxyphenol [see: monoben-
zone]

benzylpenicillin INN, BAN *natural
penicillin antibiotic; investigational
(orphan) for penicillin hypersensitivity
assessment*

benzylpenicillin benzathine JAN *natural penicillin antibiotic* [also: penicillin G benzathine; benzathine benzylpenicillin; benzathine penicillin]

benzylpenicillin potassium BAN, JAN
natural penicillin antibiotic [also: penicillin G potassium]

benzylpenicillin procaine *natural
penicillin antibiotic* [see: penicillin G
procaine]

benzylpenicillin sodium BAN *natural
penicillin antibiotic* [also: penicillin G
sodium]

benzylpenicilloic acid [see: benzyl-
penicillin]

benzylpenicilloyl polylysine USP
diagnostic aid for penicillin sensitivity

benzylpenilloic acid [see: benzylpeni-
cillin]

benzylsulfamide INN

benzylsulfanilamide [see: benzylsul-
famide]

**BEP (bleomycin, etoposide, Plati-
nol)** *chemotherapy protocol for testicular cancer, germ cell tumors, and adenocarcinoma* [also known as: PEB]

bepafant INN

bepanthen [see: panthenol]

beperidium iodide INN

bephene oxinaphthoate [see: bephenium hydroxynaphthoate]

bephenium embonate [see: bephenium hydroxynaphthoate]

bephenium hydroxynaphthoate
USP, INN, BAN

bepiastine INN

bepotastine besilate *selective histamine
H_1 antagonist for allergic conjunctivitis*

Bepreve eye drops ℞ *mast cell stabilizer
for allergic conjunctivitis* [bepotastine
(as besilate)] 1.5%

bepridil INN, BAN *vasodilator; antianginal; calcium channel blocker* [also:
bepridil HCl]

bepridil HCl USAN *vasodilator; antianginal; calcium channel blocker* [also:
bepridil]

beractant USAN *pulmonary surfactant
for neonatal respiratory distress syndrome or respiratory failure (orphan)*

beraprost USAN, INN *platelet aggregation inhibitor; peripheral vasodilator;
prostacyclin analogue; investigational
(orphan) for pulmonary arterial hypertension (PAH)*

beraprost sodium USAN *platelet aggregation inhibitor*

berberine chloride JAN

berberine sulfate JAN

berberine tannate JAN

Berberis vulgaris *medicinal herb* [see:
barberry]

berculon A [see: thioacetazone; thia-
cetazone]

berefrine USAN, INN *mydriatic*

bergamot, scarlet *medicinal herb* [see:
Oswego tea]

bergamot, wild *medicinal herb* [see:
wild bergamot]

**bergamot oil (*Citrus aurantium; C.
bergamia*)** fruit peel *medicinal herb
used in conjunction with long-wave UV
light therapy for psoriasis and vitiligo; not
generally regarded as safe and effective
because of its photosensitizing properties*

bergenin JAN

Berinert-P (name changed to **Cinryze**
upon marketing approval in 2008)

berkelium *element (Bk)* ▣ brooklime

berlafenone INN

bermastine [see: barmastine]

bermoprofen INN

Berocca tablets (discontinued 2008)
℞ *vitamin supplement* [multiple B
vitamins; vitamin C; folic acid] ± •
500•0.5 mg

Berocca Plus tablets (discontinued
2008) ℞ *hematinic; vitamin/mineral/
iron supplement* [multiple vitamins &
minerals; iron (as ferrous fumarate);
folic acid; biotin] ± •27•0.8•0.15 mg

Berri-Freez gel OTC *mild anesthetic; antipruritic; counterirritant* [menthol] 3.5%

bertosamil INN

beryllium *element (Be)*

berythromycin USAN, INN *antiamebic; antibacterial*

besifloxacin *broad-spectrum fluoroquinolone antibiotic; topical treatment for bacterial conjunctivitis*

besigomsin INN

besilate INN *combining name for radicals or groups* [also: besylate]

besipirdine INN *cognition enhancer for Alzheimer disease* [also: besipiridine HCl]

besipirdine HCl USAN *cognition enhancer for Alzheimer disease* [also: besipiridine]

Besivance eye drop suspension ℞ *broad-spectrum fluoroquinolone antibiotic for bacterial conjunctivitis* [besifloxacin (as HCl)] 0.6%

besulpamide INN

besunide INN

besylate USAN *combining name for radicals or groups* [also: besilate]

beta alethine *investigational (orphan) antineoplastic and immunostimulant multiple myeloma and metastatic melanoma*

beta blockers (β-blockers) *a class of cardiac agents characterized by their antihypertensive, antiarrhythmic, and antianginal actions; a class of topical antiglaucoma agents* [also called: beta-adrenergic antagonists]

beta carotene USAN, USP *vitamin A precursor* [also: betacarotene] 15 mg (25 000 IU) oral

beta cyclodextrin (β-cyclodextrin) [now: betadex]

Beta XMA cream OTC *moisturizer; emollient* [aloe]

betacarotene INN *vitamin A precursor* [also: beta carotene]

betacetylmethadol INN, BAN

betadex USAN, INN *sequestering agent*

beta-D-galactosidase *digestive enzyme* [see: tilactase]

beta-D-galactosidase [see: lactase enzyme]

Betadine aerosol, gauze pads, lubricating gel, cream, ointment, skin cleanser, foam, solution, swab, swabsticks OTC *broad-spectrum antimicrobial* [povidone-iodine] 5%; 10%; 5%; 5%; 10%; 7.5%; 7.5%; 10%; 10%; 10%

Betadine shampoo OTC *broad-spectrum antimicrobial for dandruff* [povidone-iodine] 7.5%

Betadine 5% Sterile Ophthalmic Prep solution ℞ *broad-spectrum antimicrobial for eye surgery* [povidone-iodine] 5%

Betadine First Aid Antibiotics Plus Moisturizer ointment (discontinued 2008) OTC *antibiotic* [polymyxin B sulfate; bacitracin zinc] 10 000•500 IU/g

Betadine Medicated vaginal gel (discontinued 2008) OTC *antiseptic/germicidal cleanser and deodorant* [povidone-iodine] 10%

Betadine Medicated vaginal suppositories OTC *antiseptic/germicidal cleanser and deodorant* [povidone-iodine] 10%

Betadine Medicated Douche; Betadine Medicated Disposable Douche; Betadine Premixed Medicated Disposable Douche vaginal solution OTC *antiseptic/germicidal cleanser and deodorant* [povidone-iodine] 10%

Betadine Plus First Aid Antibiotics and Pain Reliever ointment (discontinued 2008) OTC *antibiotic; anesthetic* [polymyxin B sulfate; bacitracin zinc; pramoxine HCl] 10 000 IU• 500 IU•10 mg per g

Betadine PrepStick swab OTC *broad-spectrum antimicrobial* [povidone-iodine] 10%

Betadine PrepStick Plus swab OTC *broad-spectrum antimicrobial* [povidone-iodine; alcohol] 10%• ²

beta-estradiol [see: estradiol]

beta-estradiol benzoate [see: estradiol benzoate]

betaeucaine HCl [now: eucaine HCl]

Betagan Liquifilm eye drops ℞ *antiglaucoma agent (beta-blocker)* [levobunolol HCl] 0.25%, 0.5%

Betagen ointment, solution (discontinued 2008) OTC *broad-spectrum* *antimicrobial* [povidone-iodine] 1%; 10% 🔲 butacaine

Betagen surgical scrub OTC *broad-spectrum antimicrobial* [povidone-iodine] 7.5% 🔲 butacaine

beta-glucocerebrosidase [see: alglucerase]

betahistine INN, BAN *vasodilator* [also: betahistine HCl; betahistine mesilate]

betahistine HCl USAN *vasodilator; treatment for vertigo due to Meniere syndrome* [also: betahistine; betahistine mesilate]

betahistine mesilate JAN *vasodilator* [also: betahistine HCl; betahistine]

beta-hypophamine [see: vasopressin]

betaine HCl USP *electrolyte replenisher for homocystinuria (orphan)*

Betaject 3 (trademarked delivery device) *automatic subcutaneous self-injector for* **Betaseron**

beta-lactams *a class of antibiotics*

beta-lactone [see: propiolactone]

betameprodine INN, BAN

betamethadol INN, BAN

betamethasone USAN, USP, INN, BAN, JAN *corticosteroidal anti-inflammatory*

betamethasone acetate USP, JAN *corticosteroidal anti-inflammatory*

betamethasone acetate & betamethasone sodium phosphate *corticosteroidal anti-inflammatory* 3•3 mg/mL injection

betamethasone acibutate INN, BAN *corticosteroidal anti-inflammatory*

betamethasone benzoate USAN, USP, BAN *topical corticosteroidal anti-inflammatory*

betamethasone dipropionate USAN, USP, BAN, JAN *topical corticosteroidal anti-inflammatory* (base=78%)

betamethasone dipropionate, augmented *topical corticosteroidal anti-inflammatory* 0.05% topical

betamethasone dipropionate & clotrimazole *corticosteroidal anti-inflammatory; broad-spectrum antifungal* 0.05%•1% topical

betamethasone sodium phosphate USP, BAN, JAN *corticosteroidal anti-inflammatory*

betamethasone sodium phosphate & betamethasone acetate *corticosteroidal anti-inflammatory* 3•3 mg/mL injection

betamethasone valerate USAN, USP, BAN, JAN *topical corticosteroidal anti-inflammatory; mousse for scalp psoriasis* 0.1% topical

betamicin INN *antibacterial* [also: betamicin sulfate]

betamicin sulfate USAN *antibacterial* [also: betamicin]

betamipron INN

betanaphthol NF

betanidine INN *antihypertensive* [also: bethanidine sulfate; bethanidine; betanidine sulfate]

betanidine sulfate JAN *antihypertensive* [also: bethanidine sulfate; betanidine; bethanidine]

Betapace tablets ℞ *antiarrhythmic (beta-blocker) for life-threatening ventricular arrhythmias (orphan)* [sotalol HCl] 80, 120, 160, 240 mg

Betapace AF tablets ℞ *antiarrhythmic (beta-blocker) for atrial fibrillation or atrial flutter* [sotalol HCl] 80, 120, 160 mg

betaprodine INN, BAN

beta-propiolactone [see: propiolactone]

beta-pyridylcarbinol [see: nicotinyl alcohol]

BetaRx *investigational (orphan) antidiabetic for type 1 patients on immunosuppression* [porcine islet preparation, encapsulated]

Betasept topical liquid OTC *broad-spectrum antimicrobial; germicidal* [chlorhexidine gluconate; alcohol 4%] 4%

Betaseron powder for subcu injection ℞ *immunomodulator for relapsing-remitting multiple sclerosis (orphan); investigational (orphan) for AIDS* [interferon beta-1b] 0.25 mg (8 MIU)

Extavia powder for subcu injection ℞ *immunomodulator for relapsing-remit-*

ting multiple sclerosis (orphan) [interferon beta-1b] 0.25 mg (8 MIU)/dose

BetaTan oral suspension (discontinued 2010) ℞ *antitussive; antihistamine; decongestant* [carbetapentane tannate; brompheniramine tannate; phenylephrine tannate] 30•4•7.5 mg/5 mL

Betathine *investigational (orphan) antineoplastic and immunostimulant for multiple myeloma and metastatic melanoma* [beta alethine]

Beta-Val cream, lotion ℞ *corticosteroidal anti-inflammatory* [betamethasone valerate] 0.1%

BetaVent syrup ℞ *antitussive; expectorant* [carbetapentane citrate; guaifenesin] 20•100 mg/5 mL

betaxolol INN, BAN *topical antiglaucoma agent; beta-blocker for hypertension; antianginal* [also: betaxolol HCl]

betaxolol HCl USAN, USP *topical antiglaucoma agent; beta-blocker for hypertension; antianginal* [also: betaxolol] 10, 20 mg oral; 0.5% eye drops

Betaxon eye drops (discontinued 2009) ℞ *antiglaucoma agent (beta-blocker)* [levobetaxolol HCl] 0.5% ☑ butikacin

betazole INN [also: betazole HCl; ametazole]

betazole HCl USP [also: betazole; ametazole]

betazolium chloride [see: betazole HCl]

betel nut *(Areca catechu)* leaves and quids (a mixture of tobacco, powdered or sliced areca nut, and slaked lime wrapped in a *Piper betel* leaf) *medicinal herb used as a digestive aid and mild stimulant; not generally regarded as safe and effective as it causes leukoplakia and oral cancer*

beth root *medicinal herb* [see: birthroot]

bethandidine sulfate *investigational (orphan) prevention and treatment of primary ventricular fibrillation*

bethanechol chloride USP, BAN, JAN *cholinergic urinary stimulant for postsurgical and postpartum urinary retention* 5, 10, 25, 50 mg oral

bethanidine BAN *antihypertensive* [also: bethanidine sulfate; betanidine; betanidine sulfate]

bethanidine sulfate USAN *antihypertensive; investigational (orphan) agent for the prevention and treatment of primary ventricular fibrillation* [also: betanidine; bethanidine; betanidine sulfate]

betiatide USAN, INN, BAN *pharmaceutic aid*

Betimol eye drops ℞ *antiglaucoma agent (beta-blocker)* [timolol hemihydrate] 0.25%, 0.5%

Betonica officinalis medicinal herb [now: *Stachys officinalis*] [see: betony]

betony (Stachys officinalis) plant *medicinal herb for anxiety, delirium, diarrhea, fever, jaundice, liver and spleen sclerosis, migraine headache, mouth or throat irritation, nervousness, palpitations, and toothache; also used as a purgative and emetic agent* ☑ biotin; Bitin; butane

Betoptic Drop-Tainers (eye drops) (discontinued 2010) ℞ *antiglaucoma agent (beta-blocker)* [betaxolol HCl] 0.5%

Betoptic S Drop-Tainers (eye drop suspension) ℞ *antiglaucoma agent (beta-blocker)* [betaxolol HCl] 0.25%

betoxycaine INN

betoxycaine HCl [see: betoxycaine]

betula oil [see: methyl salicylate]

Betula spp. medicinal herb [see: birch]

Betuline lotion OTC *analgesic; mild anesthetic; antipruritic; counterirritant* [methyl salicylate; camphor; menthol]

bevacizumab *recombinant humanized monoclonal antibody to vascular endothelial growth factor (VEGF); angiogenesis inhibitor for brain, colorectal, renal, and non–small cell lung cancers; investigational (Phase III) for prostate, pancreatic, and ovarian cancers*

bevantolol INN, BAN *antianginal; antihypertensive; antiarrhythmic* [also: bevantolol HCl]

bevantolol HCl USAN *antianginal; antihypertensive; antiarrhythmic* [also: bevantolol]

bevonium methylsulphate BAN [also: bevonium metilsulfate]

bevonium metilsulfate INN [also: bevonium methylsulphate]

bexarotene USAN, INN *synthetic retinoid analogue antineoplastic for cutaneous T-cell lymphoma (orphan)*

bexlosteride USAN, INN *antineoplastic 5α-reductase inhibitor for prostate cancer*

Bexxar Dosimetric Package IV infusion ℞ *first of two steps in the radiotherapeutic treatment of non-Hodgkin lymphoma (NHL)* [tositumomab; iodine I 131 tositumomab] 450•35 mg (5 mCi of radiation)

Bexxar Therapeutic Package IV infusion ℞ *second of two steps in the radiotherapeutic treatment of non-Hodgkin lymphoma (orphan)* [tositumomab; iodine I 131 tositumomab] 450•35 mg (delivers 65–75 cGy of radiation)

Beyaz film-coated tablets (in packs of 28) ℞ *monophasic oral contraceptive; iron supplement* [drospirenone; ethinyl estradiol; folic acid (as levomefolate calcium)] 3 mg•20 mcg•451 mcg × 24 days; 0•0•451 mcg × 4 days

bezafibrate USAN, INN, BAN, JAN *antihyperlipidemic*

bezitramide INN, BAN

bezomil INN *combining name for radicals or groups*

bFGF (basic fibroblast growth factor) [see: ersofermin]

B.F.I. Antiseptic powder OTC *antiseptic* [bismuth-formic-iodide] 16%

BHA (butylated hydroxyanisole) [q.v.]

BHAPs (bisheteroarylpiperazines) *a class of antiviral drugs*

BHT (butylated hydroxytoluene) [q.v.]

bialamicol INN, BAN *antiamebic* [also: bialamicol HCl]

bialamicol HCl USAN *antiamebic* [also: bialamicol]

biallylamicol [see: bialamicol]

biantrazole [now: losoxantrone HCl]

biapenem USAN, INN *antibacterial*

Biavax II powder for subcu injection (discontinued 2009) ℞ *rubella and mumps vaccine* [rubella & mumps virus vaccine, live; neomycin] 1000 U•20 000 U•25 mcg/0.5 mL dose

Biaxin Filmtabs (film-coated tablets), granules for oral suspension ℞ *macrolide antibiotic* [clarithromycin] 250, 500 mg; 125, 250 mg/5 mL

Biaxin XL film-coated extended-release tablets ℞ *once-daily macrolide antibiotic* [clarithromycin] 500 mg

bibapcitide USAN *glycoprotein (GP) IIb/IIIa receptor antagonist; investigational (Phase III) diagnostic imaging aid for deep vein thrombosis*

bibenzonium bromide INN, BAN

bibrocathin [see: bibrocathol]

bibrocathol INN

bicalutamide USAN, INN, BAN *antiandrogen antineoplastic for prostate cancer* 50 mg oral

bicalutamide + LHRH-A (bicalutamide, leuprolide acetate [Lupron Depot injection]) *chemotherapy protocol for prostate cancer*

bicalutamide + LHRH-A (goserelin acetate [Zoladex subcu implant] or leuprolide) *chemotherapy protocol for prostate cancer*

Bicarsim; Bicarsim Forte tablets OTC *antiflatulent* [simethicone] 80 mg; 125 mg

Bichloracetic Acid topical liquid ℞ *cauterant; keratolytic* [dichloroacetic acid] 10 mL

bicifadine INN *analgesic* [also: bicifadine HCl]

bicifadine HCl USAN *analgesic* [also: bicifadine]

Bicillin C-R; Bicillin C-R 900/300 Tubex (cartridge-needle unit) for deep IM injection ℞ *natural penicillin antibiotic* [penicillin G benzathine; penicillin G procaine] 300 000•300 000, 600 000•600 000; 900 000•300 000 U

Bicillin L-A Tubex (cartridge-needle unit) for deep IM injection ℞ *natural penicillin antibiotic* [penicillin G benzathine] 600 000, 1 200 000, 2 400 000 U

biciromab USAN, INN, BAN *monoclonal antibody to fibrin*

Bicitra oral solution (discontinued 2009) ℞ *urinary alkalinizing agent* [sodium citrate; citric acid] 500•334 mg/5 mL

biclodil INN *antihypertensive; vasodilator* [also: biclodil HCl]

biclodil HCl USAN *antihypertensive; vasodilator* [also: biclodil]

biclofibrate INN

biclotymol INN

BiCNU powder for IV injection ℞ *nitrosourea-type alkylating antineoplastic for brain tumors, multiple myeloma, Hodgkin disease and non-Hodgkin lymphomas* [carmustine] 100 mg/dose

bicozamycin INN

Bicozene cream (discontinued 2011) OTC *anesthetic; antifungal* [benzocaine; resorcinol] 6%•1.67% ⧅ pecazine

bicyclomycin [see: bicozamycin]

bidCAP (trademarked dosage form) *twice-daily capsule*

Bidex-A extended-release tablets ℞ *antitussive; expectorant* [dextromethorphan hydrobromide; guaifenesin] 25•600 mg ⧅ Pediox

Bidex-DMI tablets (discontinued 2009) OTC *antitussive; expectorant* [dextromethorphan hydrobromide; guaifenesin] 20•400 mg/10 mL

Bidhist extended-release tablets (discontinued 2009) ℞ *antihistamine* [brompheniramine maleate] 6 mg

Bidhist-D extended-release tablets ℞ *decongestant; antihistamine* [pseudoephedrine HCl; brompheniramine maleate] 45•6 mg ⧅ PD-Hist D

BiDil film-coated tablets ℞ *vasodilator combination for heart failure in black patients* [hydralazine HCl; isosorbide dinitrate] 37.5•20 mg

bidimazium iodide INN, BAN

bidisomide USAN, INN *antiarrhythmic*

Biebrich scarlet red [see: scarlet red]

Biebrich scarlet-picroaniline blue

bietamiverine INN

bietamiverine HCl [see: bietamiverine]

bietaserpine INN

bifemelane INN [also: bifemelane HCl]

bifemelane HCl JAN [also: bifemelane]

bifepramide INN

bifeprofen INN

bifeprunox *dopamine agonist; investigational (NDA filed) novel (atypical) antipsychotic for schizophrenia; investigational (Phase III) for bipolar disorder*

BiferaRx film-coated tablets ℞ *hematinic* [iron; vitamin B$_{12}$; folic acid] 28•0.025•1 mg

Bifidobacterium lactis *natural intestinal bacteria; probiotic; dietary supplement*

Bifidobacterium longum infantis **35624** *natural intestinal bacteria; probiotic; dietary supplement; investigational (orphan) agent for pediatric Crohn disease*

Bifidobacterium sp. *natural intestinal bacteria; probiotic; dietary supplement* [see also: lactic acid bacteria]

bifluranol INN, BAN

bifonazole USAN, INN, BAN, JAN *antifungal*

Big Shot B-12 tablets (discontinued 2008) OTC *vitamin B$_{12}$ supplement* [cyanocobalamin] 5 mg

Bignonia sempervirens *medicinal herb* [see: gelsemium]

biguanides *a class of antidiabetic agents that decrease hepatic glucose production and increase cellular response to insulin*

bilastine INN

bilberry (Myrtilli fructus; Vaccinium myrtillus) *fruit medicinal herb for cold hands and feet, diarrhea, edema, increasing microvascular blood flow, gastroenteritis, mucous membrane inflammation, night blindness, and varicose veins* ⧅ Bluboro

bile acid sequestrants *a class of antihyperlipidemic agents*

bile acids, conjugated *investigational (orphan) for steatorrhea in short bowel syndrome*

bile acids, oxidized [see: dehydrocholic acid]

bile salts BAN *digestive enzymes; laxative*

BiliCheck (breath analyzer device) *in vitro diagnostic aid for infant jaundice*

Bili-Labstix reagent strips (discontinued 2008) OTC *in vitro diagnostic aid for multiple urine products*

Biltricide film-coated tablets ℞ *anthelmintic for schistosomiasis (liver flukes); investigational (orphan) for neurocysticercosis* [praziquantel] 600 mg

bimakalim INN

bimatoprost *topical prostamide analogue; antihypertensive for glaucoma and ocular hypertension; used cosmetically to grow, thicken, and darken eyelashes*

bimazol [see: carbimazole]

bimethadol [see: dimepheptanol]

bimethoxycaine lactate

bimosiamose disodium USAN *anti-inflammatory for asthma, psoriasis, and reperfusion injury following transplants or coronary revascularization*

bindarit USAN, INN *antirheumatic; investigational (orphan) for lupus nephritis*

bindazac [see: bendazac]

binedaline INN ⑨ *pinadoline*

binetrakin USAN, INN *immunomodulator for gastrointestinal carcinoma and rheumatoid arthritis*

binfloxacin USAN, INN *veterinary antibacterial*

binifibrate INN ⑨ *ponfibrate*

biniramycin USAN, INN *antibacterial antibiotic*

binizolast INN

binodaline [see: binedaline]

binospirone INN *anxiolytic* [also: binospirone mesylate]

binospirone mesylate USAN *anxiolytic* [also: binospirone]

Bio Glob ophthalmic strips OTC *corneal disclosing agent* [fluorescein sodium] 1 mg

Bio T Pres; Bio T Pres Pediatric oral liquid ℞ *antitussive; decongestant; expectorant* [dextromethorphan hydrobromide; phenylephrine HCl; guaifenesin] 10•5•200 mg/5 mL; 5•2.5•75 mg/5 mL

bioallethrin BAN *pediculicide*

Biobrane wound dressing OTC *nylon fabric matrix bound to a silicon film*

Biobrane-L light adherence wound dressing OTC *nylon fabric matrix bound to a silicon film*

Biobron SF oral liquid OTC *antitussive; decongestant; expectorant* [dextromethorphan hydrobromide; phenylephrine HCl; guaifenesin] 15•10•350 mg/5 mL

Biocef capsules, powder for oral suspension (discontinued 2007) ℞ *first-generation cephalosporin antibiotic* [cephalexin] 500 mg; 250 mg/5 mL

Bioclate powder for IV injection (discontinued 2008) ℞ *systemic hemostatic; antihemophilic for the prevention and control of bleeding in classic hemophilia (hemophilia A) and von Willebrand disease (orphan)* [antihemophilic factor concentrate, recombinant] 250, 500, 1000 IU

Biocult-GC culture paddles for professional use ℞ *in vitro diagnostic aid for Neisseria gonorrhoeae*

Biodine Topical solution OTC *broad-spectrum antimicrobial* [povidone-iodine] 1%

bioflavonoids (vitamin P) *a class of more than 4000 natural substances with widespread biological activity, including anthelmintic, antimicrobial, antimalarial, antineoplastic, antioxidant, anti-inflammatory, and antiviral activity; historically named "vitamin P"*

Bioflex tablets OTC *vitamin C supplement with multiple bioflavonoids and herbs* [vitamin C; citrus bioflavonoids; rutin; hesperidin; hawthorn berry extract; horse chestnut extract; witch hazel extract] 500•50•40•25•25•25•25 mg

BioGaia oral concentrate OTC *natural intestinal bacteria; probiotic; dietary supplement* [Lactobacillus reuteri] 100 million U/5 drops

biogastrone [see: carbenoxolone]

Biogil oral liquid ℞ *antitussive; decongestant; expectorant* [dextromethorphan hydrobromide; phenylephrine

HCl; guaifenesin] 15•10•300 mg/5 mL ⊡ Bo-Cal

BioGtuss oral liquid ℞ *antitussive; decongestant; expectorant* [dextromethorphan hydrobromide; phenylephrine HCl; guaifenesin] 15•10•300 mg/5 mL

Biohist-LA sustained-release tablets (discontinued 2007) ℞ *decongestant; antihistamine* [pseudoephedrine HCl; chlorpheniramine maleate] 120•12 mg

biological indicator for dry-heat sterilization USP *sterilization indicator*

biological indicator for ethylene oxide sterilization USP *sterilization indicator*

biological indicator for steam sterilization USP *sterilization indicator*

Biomide 750 tablets ℞ *vitamin/mineral supplement* [vitamin B₃; multiple minerals; folic acid] 750•≛•0.5 mg

Bion Tears eye drops OTC *moisturizer/lubricant* [hydroxypropyl methylcellulose] 0.3%

Bionect cream, gel, topical spray ℞ *wound healing agent for skin irritations, dermal ulcers, wounds, and burns* [hyaluronate sodium] 0.2%

Bionel; Bionel Pediatric oral liquid OTC *antitussive; decongestant; expectorant* [dextromethorphan hydrobromide; pseudoephedrine HCl; guaifenesin] 15•30•200 mg/5 mL; 5•15•50 mg/5 mL

bioral [see: carbenoxolone]

Bio-Rescue *investigational (orphan) chelating agent for acute iron poisoning* [dextran; deferoxamine]

bioresmethrin INN

bios I [see: inositol]

bios II [see: biotin]

Biosafe HbA1c (hemoglobin A1c) test kit for home use OTC *in vitro diagnostic aid for glycemic control*

Biosafe PSA (prostate-specific antigen) test kit for home use OTC *in vitro diagnostic aid for prostate function*

Biosafe Total Cholesterol (only) test kit for home use OTC *in vitro diagnostic aid for hypercholesterolemia*

Biosafe Total Cholesterol Panel (includes HDL, LDL, and triglycerides) test kit for home use OTC *in vitro diagnostic aid for hypercholesterolemia and hypertriglyceridemia*

Biosafe TSH (thyroid-stimulating hormone) test kit for home use OTC *in vitro diagnostic aid for thyroid function*

biosimilar [def.] *a generic version of a biological medicine, such as a monoclonal antibody; for example,* **Reditux** *contains biosimilar* **rituximab** *and sells for half the price of the original drug,* **Rituxan** (note: "biosimilar" is the official European term; the official U.S. term is "follow-on protein product")

Biospec DMX oral liquid OTC *antitussive; expectorant* [dextromethorphan hydrobromide; guaifenesin] 15•25 mg/5 mL

Biosynject *investigational (orphan) for newborn hemolytic disease and ABO blood incompatibility of organ or bone marrow transplants* [trisaccharides A and B]

biosynthetic human parathyroid hormone (1-34) [see: teriparatide]

BioTears gelcaps OTC *nutritional support to increase tear production for symptomatic relief of chronic dry eyes* [vitamins A, B₆, C, D₃, and E; magnesium (from sulfate); omega-3 and -6 EFAs; mucopolysaccharides; turmeric; lactoferrin] 500 U•4 mg•50 mg•25 U•16 U•10 mg•401 mg•125 mg•50 mg•5 mg ⊡ bitters

Biotect Plus oral liquid OTC *vitamin/mineral/iron supplement* [multiple vitamins & minerals; iron] ≛•3.33 mg/5 mL

Biotene Dry Mouth toothpaste OTC *dental caries preventative* [sodium monofluorophosphate]

Bioténe with Calcium mouthwash OTC

biotexin [see: novobiocin]

BioThrax IM injection ℞ *anthrax immunization* [anthrax vaccine (*Bacillus anthracis*)] 83 kDa ⑦ Bite Rx

Bio-Throid capsules ℞ *natural thyroid replacement for hypothyroidism or thyroid cancer* [thyroid, desiccated (porcine)] 7.5, 15, 30, 60, 90, 120, 150, 180, 240 mg

biotin USP, INN, JAN *B complex vitamin; vitamin H* ⑦ betony; Bitin; butane

Biotin Forte tablets (discontinued 2008) OTC *vitamin supplement* [multiple B vitamins; vitamin C; folic acid; biotin] ± • 200 • 0.8 • 3 mg, ± • 100 • 0.8 • 5 mg

BioTropin *investigational (orphan) for cachexia due to AIDS* [somatropin]

Biotuss oral liquid (discontinued 2009) ℞ *antitussive; decongestant; expectorant* [dextromethorphan hydrobromide; phenylephrine HCl; guaifenesin] 15 • 10 • 300 mg/5 mL

Bio-Tussi oral liquid OTC *antitussive; decongestant; expectorant* [dextromethorphan hydrobromide; phenylephrine HCl; guaifenesin] 10 • 5 • 200 mg/5 mL

BIP (bleomycin, ifosfamide, Platinol) [with mesna rescue] *chemotherapy protocol for cervical cancer*

bipenamol INN *antidepressant* [also: bipenamol HCl]

bipenamol HCl USAN *antidepressant* [also: bipenamol]

biperiden USP, INN, BAN, JAN *anticholinergic; antiparkinsonian*

biperiden HCl USP, BAN, JAN *anticholinergic; antiparkinsonian*

biperiden lactate USP, BAN, JAN *anticholinergic; antiparkinsonian*

biphasic insulin [see: insulin, biphasic]

biphenamine HCl USAN *topical anesthetic; antibacterial; antifungal* [also: xenysalate]

Biphenox tablets OTC *analgesic; antipyretic; antihistamine; sleep aid* [acetaminophen; phenyltoloxamine citrate] 325 • 30 mg

biprofenide [see: bifepramide]

birch (*Betula* spp.) bark and leaves *medicinal herb for bladder problems, blood cleansing, and eczema*

birch oil, sweet [see: methyl salicylate]

bird flu vaccine [see: influenza virus vaccine, H5N1]

bird lime *medicinal herb* [see: mistletoe]

bird pepper *medicinal herb* [see: cayenne]

bird's nest root *medicinal herb* [see: carrot]

biricodar dicitrate USAN *multi-drug–resistance inhibitor*

biriperone INN

birthroot (*Trillium erectum*; *T. grandiflorum*; *T. pendulum*) plant *medicinal herb for insect and snake bites, stimulating menses and diaphoresis, and stopping bleeding after childbirth; also used as an antiseptic and astringent*

birthwort (*Aristolochia clematitis*) root and flowering plant *medicinal herb used as a diaphoretic, emmenagogue, febrifuge, oxytocic, and stimulant*

Bisac-Evac enteric-coated tablets, suppositories OTC *stimulant laxative* [bisacodyl] 5 mg; 10 mg

bisacodyl USP, INN, BAN, JAN *stimulant laxative* 5 mg oral; 10 mg suppositories

bisacodyl tannex USAN *stimulant laxative*

Bisa-Lax enteric-coated tablets, suppositories OTC *stimulant laxative* [bisacodyl] 5 mg; 10 mg

bisantrene INN *antineoplastic* [also: bisantrene HCl]

bisantrene HCl USAN *antineoplastic* [also: bisantrene]

bisaramil INN

bisatin [see: oxyphenisatin acetate]

bisbendazole INN

bisbentiamine INN, JAN

bisbutiamine [see: bisbutitiamine]

bisbutitiamine JAN

bis-chloroethyl-nitrosourea (BCNU) [see: carmustine]

bisdequalinium diacetate JAN

bisfenazone INN

bisfentidine INN

bis(4-fluorophenyl)phenylacetamide *investigational (orphan) for sickle cell disease*

bisheteroarylpiperazines (BHAPs) *a class of antiviral drugs*

bishop's wort *medicinal herb* [see: nutmeg; betony]

bishydroxycoumarin [now: dicumarol]

bisibutiamine JAN [also: sulbutiamine]

Bismatrol chewable tablets, oral liquid OTC *antidiarrheal; antinauseant* [bismuth subsalicylate] 262 mg; 87.33, 175 mg/5 mL

bismucatebrol [see: bibrocathol]

Bismuth chewable tablets OTC *antidiarrheal; antinauseant* [bismuth subsalicylate] 262 mg

bismuth *element (Bi)*

bismuth, milk of USP *antacid; astringent*

bismuth aluminate USAN

bismuth betanaphthol USP

bismuth carbonate USAN

bismuth carbonate, basic [see: bismuth subcarbonate]

bismuth citrate USP

bismuth cream [see: bismuth, milk of]

bismuth gallate, basic [see: bismuth subgallate]

bismuth glycollylarsanilate BAN [also: glycobiarsol]

bismuth hydroxide [see: bismuth, milk of]

bismuth hydroxide nitrate oxide [see: bismuth subnitrate]

bismuth magma [now: bismuth, milk of]

bismuth magnesium aluminosilicate JAN

bismuth oxycarbonate [see: bismuth subcarbonate]

bismuth potassium tartrate NF

bismuth sodium triglycollamate USP

bismuth subcarbonate USAN, JAN *antacid; GI adsorbent*

bismuth subcitrate potassium *antacid; GI adsorbent*

bismuth subgallate USAN, USP *antacid; GI adsorbent; systemic deodorizer for ostomy and incontinence odors*

bismuth subnitrate USP, JAN *skin protectant*

bismuth subsalicylate (BSS) USAN, JAN *antiperistaltic; antacid; GI adsorbent*

bisnafide dimesylate USAN *antineoplastic; DNA and RNA synthesis inhibitor*

bisobrin INN *fibrinolytic* [also: bisobrin lactate] ☒ buspirone

bisobrin lactate USAN *fibrinolytic* [also: bisobrin]

Bisolvon *investigational (orphan) agent for keratoconjunctivitis sicca of Sjögren syndrome* [bromhexine HCl]

bisoprolol USAN, INN, BAN *beta-blocker for hypertension*

bisoprolol fumarate USAN, JAN *beta-blocker for hypertension* 5, 10 mg oral

bisoprolol fumarate & hydrochlorothiazide *combination beta-blocker and diuretic for hypertension* 2.5•6.25, 5•6.25, 10•6.25 mg oral

bisorcic INN

bisoxatin INN, BAN *laxative* [also: bisoxatin acetate]

bisoxatin acetate USAN *laxative* [also: bisoxatin]

bisphosphonates *a class of calcium-regulating agents that inhibit normal and abnormal bone resorption; investigational to reduce the risk for breast and colon cancer*

bispyrithione magsulfex USAN *antibacterial; antidandruff; antifungal*

bistort (Polygonum bistorta) root *medicinal herb for bleeding, cholera, cuts, diarrhea, dysentery, gum disease (mouthwash), and hemorrhoids*

bis-tropamide [now: tropicamide]

Bi-Tann DP oral suspension ℞ *decongestant; antihistamine* [pseudoephedrine tannate; dexchlorpheniramine tannate] 75•5 mg/2.5 mL

Bite Rx solution OTC *astringent wet dressing (Burow solution) for insect bites* [aluminum acetate] 0.5% ☒ BioThrax

bithionol NF, INN, BAN, JAN *anti-infective for paragonimiasis and fascioliasis (available only from the Centers for Disease Control and Prevention)* bithionolate sodium USAN *topical anti-infective* [also: sodium bitionolate]

bithionoloxide INN

Bitin (available only from the Centers for Disease Control) (discontinued 2011) ℞ *anti-infective for paragonimiasis and fascioliasis* [bithionol] ⑨
betony; biotin; butane

bitipazone INN

bitolterol INN, BAN *sympathomimetic bronchodilator* [also: bitolterol mesylate; bitolterol mesilate]

bitolterol mesilate JAN *sympathomimetic bronchodilator* [also: bitolterol mesylate; bitolterol]

bitolterol mesylate USAN *sympathomimetic bronchodilator* [also: bitolterol; bitolterol mesilate]

bitoscanate INN

bitter ash *medicinal herb* [see: quassia; wahoo]

bitter ash; bitter quassia; bitter wood *medicinal herb* [see: quassia]

bitter buttons *medicinal herb* [see: tansy]

bitter cardamom (*Alpinia fructus; A. oxyphylla*) *medicinal herb for dementia, excessive water loss, and gastric lesions*

bitter cucumber *medicinal herb* [see: bitter melon]

bitter dogbane *medicinal herb* [see: dogbane]

bitter grass *medicinal herb* [see: star grass]

bitter herb *medicinal herb* [see: centaury]

bitter melon (*Momordica charantia*) fruit, leaves, seeds, oil *medicinal herb used as an antimicrobial and hypoglycemic; also used to reduce fertility in both males and females, and can act as an abortifacient*

bitter quassia; bitter ash; bitter wood *medicinal herb* [see: quassia tree]

bitter tonics; bitters *a class of agents that have a bitter taste, used as tonics, alteratives, or appetizers*

bitter wintergreen *medicinal herb* [see: pipsissewa]

bitter wood; bitter ash; bitter quassia *medicinal herb* [see: quassia tree]

bitterroot; bitterwort *medicinal herb* [see: dogbane; gentian]

bitters; bitter tonics *a class of agents that have a bitter taste, used as tonics, alteratives, or appetizers* ⑨ BioTears

bittersweet herb; bittersweet twigs *medicinal herb* [see: bittersweet nightshade]

bittersweet nightshade (*Solanum dulcamara*) *medicinal herb for topical application on abrasions and felons; not generally regarded as safe and effective for internal use as it is highly toxic*

bitterweed *medicinal herb* [see: fleabane; horseweed]

bitterwort; bitterroot *medicinal herb* [see: gentian]

bivalirudin USAN *anticoagulant thrombin inhibitor for percutaneous coronary intervention (PCI), percutaneous transluminal coronary angioplasty (PTCA), or heparin-induced thrombocytopenia (HIT); used with aspirin therapy*

bizelesin USAN, INN *antineoplastic* ⑨
pecilocin

black alder (*Alnus glutinosa*) bark and leaves *medicinal herb used as an astringent, demulcent, emetic, hemostatic, and tonic*

black alder dogwood *medicinal herb* [see: buckthorn; cascara sagrada]

black birch *medicinal herb* [see: birch]

black cherry; poison black cherry *medicinal herb* [see: belladonna]

black choke *medicinal herb* [see: wild black cherry]

black cohosh (*Cimicifuga racemosa*) root and rhizome *medicinal herb for asthma, bronchitis, dysmenorrhea, dyspepsia, epilepsy, hypertension, hormone imbalance, lung disorders, menopause, rheumatism, snake bite, sore throat, St. Vitus dance, and tuberculosis*

black currant (*Ribes nigrum*) *medicinal herb* [see: currant]

black dogwood *medicinal herb* [see: buckthorn; cascara sagrada]

black elder *medicinal herb* [see: elderberry]

black false hellebore *(Veratrum niger)* [see: hellebore]

black ginger *medicinal herb* [see: ginger]

black hellebore *(Helleborus niger)* [see: hellebore]

black mulberry *(Morus nigra) medicinal herb* [see: mulberry]

black oak *(Quercus tinctoria) medicinal herb* [see: white oak]

black poplar *(Populus nigra; P. tremula)* buds *medicinal herb used as a diaphoretic, diuretic, expectorant, and vulnerary*

black root *medicinal herb* [see: Culver root]

black sanicle *medicinal herb* [see: sanicle]

black snakeroot *medicinal herb* [see: black cohosh; sanicle]

black walnut *(Juglans nigra)* hulls and leaves *medicinal herb for parasites, ringworm, skin rashes, and stopping lactation; also used as an external antiseptic*

black widow spider antivenin [see: antivenin *(Latrodectus mactans)*]

black willow *(Salix nigra) medicinal herb* [see: willow]

blackberry *(Rubus fructicosus; R. villosus)* berries, leaves, and root bark *medicinal herb for bleeding, cholera, diarrhea in children, dysentery, sinus drainage, and vomiting*

Black-Draught tablets, chewable tablets, granules OTC *stimulant laxative* [sennosides] 6 mg; 10 mg; 20 mg/5 mL

blackwort *medicinal herb* [see: comfrey]

bladder fucus; bladderwrack *medicinal herb* [see: kelp *(Fucus)*]

bladderpod *medicinal herb* [see: lobelia]

Blairex Lens Lubricant solution (discontinued 2010) OTC *rewetting solution for soft contact lenses*

Blairex Sterile Saline aerosol solution OTC *rinsing/storage solution for soft contact lenses* [sodium chloride (saline solution)]

blastomycin NF

blazing star *medicinal herb* [see: star grass]

blazing star *(Liatris scariosa; L. spicata; L. squarrosa)* root *medicinal herb used as a diuretic*

Blenoxane powder for IM, IV, subcu, or intrapleural injection (discontinued 2009) ℞ *glycopeptide antibiotic antineoplastic for Hodgkin and non-Hodgkin lymphomas, testicular and squamous cell carcinomas, and malignant pleural effusion (orphan); investigational (orphan) for pancreatic cancer* [bleomycin sulfate] 15, 30 U

bleomycin (BLM) INN, BAN *glycopeptide antibiotic antineoplastic* [also: bleomycin sulfate; bleomycin HCl] 🔟 paulomycin; peliomycin

bleomycin HCl JAN *glycopeptide antibiotic antineoplastic* [also: bleomycin sulfate; bleomycin]

bleomycin sulfate USAN, USP, JAN *glycopeptide antibiotic antineoplastic for Hodgkin and non-Hodgkin lymphomas, testicular and squamous cell carcinomas, and malignant pleural effusion (orphan); investigational (orphan) for pancreatic cancer* [also: bleomycin; bleomycin HCl] 15, 30 U injection

Bleph-10 eye drops, ophthalmic ointment ℞ *antibiotic* [sulfacetamide sodium] 10%

Blephamide eye drop suspension, ophthalmic ointment ℞ *corticosteroidal anti-inflammatory; antibiotic* [prednisolone acetate; sulfacetamide sodium] 0.2%•10%

blessed cardus; holy thistle *medicinal herb* [see: blessed thistle]

blessed thistle *(Cnicus benedictus)* plant *medicinal herb for blood cleansing, digestive disorders, headache, hormonal imbalance, lactation disorders, liver and gallbladder ailments, menstrual disorders, poor circulation, and strengthening heart and lungs*

Blighia sapida medicinal herb [see: ackee]

blind nettle *(Lamium album)* plant and flowers *medicinal herb used as an* *antispasmodic, astringent, expectorant, and styptic*

Blinx ophthalmic solution (discontinued 2010) OTC *extraocular irrigating solution* [sterile isotonic solution]

BlisterGard topical liquid OTC *skin protectant*

Blistex ointment OTC *antipruritic/counterirritant; mild local anesthetic; vulnerary* [camphor; phenol; allantoin] 0.5%•0.5%•1%

Blistik lip balm OTC *antipruritic/counterirritant; mild local anesthetic; skin protectant; sunscreen (SPF 10)* [camphor; phenol; allantoin; dimethicone; padimate O; oxybenzone] 0.5%•0.5%•1%•2%•6.6%•2.5%

Blis-To-Sol topical liquid OTC *antifungal; keratolytic* [tolnaftate] 1%

Blis-To-Sol topical powder OTC *antifungal* [zinc undecylenate] 12%

BLM (bleomycin) [q.v.]

Blocadren tablets ℞ *antihypertensive; antianginal; migraine preventative; beta-blocker* [timolol maleate] 5, 20 mg

blood, whole USP *blood replenisher*

blood, whole human [now: blood, whole]

blood cells, human red [now: blood cells, red]

blood cells, red USP *blood replenisher*

blood group specific substances A, B & AB USP *blood neutralizer*

blood grouping serum, anti-A [see: anti-A blood grouping serum]

blood grouping serum, anti-B [see: anti-B blood grouping serum]

blood grouping serum, anti-C USP *for in vitro blood testing*

blood grouping serum, anti-c USP *for in vitro blood testing*

blood grouping serum, anti-D USP *for in vitro blood testing*

blood grouping serum, anti-E USP *for in vitro blood testing*

blood grouping serum, anti-e USP *for in vitro blood testing*

blood mononuclear cells, allogenic peripheral *investigational (orphan) agent for pancreatic cancer*

blood staunch *medicinal herb* [see: fleabane; horseweed]

Blood Sugar Balance tablets OTC *dietary supplement* [multiple minerals and herbs]

blood volume expanders *a class of therapeutic blood modifiers used to increase the volume of circulating blood* [also called: plasma expanders]

bloodroot (Sanguinaria canadensis) root and rhizome *medicinal herb for diuresis, fever, inducing emesis, nasal polyps, rheumatism, sedation, skin cancer, stimulating menstrual flow, and warts; also used in toothpaste and mouthwash; not generally regarded as safe and effective for internal use*

BLP-25 liposome vaccine *investigational (Phase III) antineoplastic vaccine against MUC-1 for the treatment of non–small cell lung cancer*

Bluboro powder packets (discontinued 2008) OTC *astringent wet dressing (modified Burow solution)* [aluminum sulfate; calcium acetate] 🄍 bilberry

blue cohosh (Caulophyllum thalictroides) root *medicinal herb for cramps, epilepsy, induction of labor, menstrual flow stimulant, nerves, and chronic uterine problems*

blue curls *medicinal herb* [see: woundwort]

blue flag (Iris versicolor) root *medicinal herb used as a cathartic, diuretic, laxative, sialagogue, and vermifuge*

Blue Gel Muscular Pain Reliever gel OTC *mild anesthetic; antipruritic; counterirritant* [menthol]

blue ginseng *medicinal herb* [see: blue cohosh]

blue gum tree *medicinal herb* [see: eucalyptus]

Blue Ice gel OTC *mild anesthetic; antipruritic; counterirritant* [menthol] 2% 🄍 Boil-Ease

blue mountain tea *medicinal herb* [see: goldenrod]

blue pimpernel; blue skullcap *medicinal herb* [see: skullcap]

blue vervain (Verbena hastata) plant *medicinal herb for asthma, bladder and bowel disorders, bronchitis, colds, convulsions, cough, fever, insomnia, pulmonary tuberculosis, stomach upset, and worms*

blueberry *medicinal herb* [see: bilberry; blue cohosh]

bluebonnet; bluebottle *medicinal herb* [see: cornflower]

Blue-Emu spray OTC *mild anesthetic; antipruritic; counterirritant* [menthol] 2.5%

blue-green algae (Chloroplast membrane sulfolipids) *nutritional supplement for boosting the immune system*

bluensomycin INN *antibiotic*

BLU-U Blue Light PhotoDynamic Illuminator (device) *used with* **Levulan** (5-aminolevulinic acid HCl) *for photodynamic therapy of precancerous actinic keratoses of the face and scalp*

BMY-45622 *investigational (orphan) antineoplastic for ovarian cancer*

Bo-Cal tablets (discontinued 2008) OTC *calcium/magnesium supplement* [calcium; magnesium; vitamin D] 250 mg•125 mg•100 U

boceprevir *oral hepatitis C virus (HCV) protease inhibitor for chronic hepatitis C infections*

Bodi Kleen spray OTC *emollient/protectant* [trolamine lauryl sulfate]

Body Fortress Natural Amino tablets OTC *protein supplement* [protein; lactalbumin hydrolysate] 1.67•1.5 g

boforsin [see: colforsin]

bofumustine INN

bogbean; bog myrtle *medicinal herb* [see: buckbean]

Boil-Ease ointment OTC *anesthetic* [benzocaine] 20% ☐ Blue Ice

bolandiol INN *anabolic* [also: bolandiol dipropionate]

bolandiol dipropionate USAN, JAN *anabolic* [also: bolandiol]

bolasterone USAN, INN *anabolic steroid; also abused as a street drug*

bolazine INN

Boldea fragrans *medicinal herb* [see: boldo]

boldenone INN, BAN *veterinary anabolic steroid; also abused as a street drug* [also: boldenone undecylenate]

boldenone undecylenate USAN *veterinary anabolic steroid; also abused as a street drug* [also: boldenone]

boldo (Peumus boldus) plant and leaves *medicinal herb for bile stimulation, colds, constipation, digestive disorders, earache, edema, gallstones, gonorrhea, gout, liver disease, rheumatism, syphilis, and worms*

Boldu boldus *medicinal herb* [see: boldo]

bolenol USAN, INN *anabolic* ☐ BAL in Oil

bolmantalate USAN, INN, BAN *anabolic*

bolus alba [see: kaolin]

Bombay aloe *medicinal herb* [see: aloe]

bometolol INN

BOMP; CLD-BOMP (bleomycin, Oncovin, mitomycin, Platinol) *chemotherapy protocol for cervical cancer*

Bonamil Infant Formula with Iron powder, oral liquid OTC *total or supplementary infant feeding* 453 g; 384, 946 mL

bone ash [see: calcium phosphate, tribasic]

Bone Assure capsules OTC *vitamin/mineral/calcium supplement to maintain bone mineral density* [calcium (from bis-glycinate); magnesium (from oxide); zinc (from citrate); manganese (from citrate); trimethylglycine; multiple vitamins and minerals] 1000•320•12•3•100• ± per 6 capsules

Bone Meal tablets (discontinued 2008) OTC *calcium/phosphorus supplement* [calcium; phosphorus] 236•118 mg

bone powder, purified [see: calcium phosphate, tribasic]

Bonefos ⓒ capsules, IV infusion (available in Canada) *investigational (orphan) bisphosphonate bone resorption inhibitor for hypercalcemia and osteolysis of malignancy* [clodronate disodium tetrahydrate] 400 mg; 60 mg/mL

boneset *(Eupatorium perfoliatum)* plant *medicinal herb for chills, colds, constipation, dengue fever, edema, fever, flu, pneumonia, and rheumatism* ⚆ Panacet; poinsettia

Bone-Up capsules OTC *vitamin/mineral/ calcium supplement to maintain bone mineral density* [calcium (hydroxyapatite); protein; magnesium (oxide); zinc (monomethionine); manganese; glucosamine HCl; multiple vitamins and minerals] 1000•1000•600•10• 5•300• ≛ per 6 capsules

Bonine chewable tablets OTC *antiemetic; motion sickness preventative* [meclizine HCl] 25 mg

Bonine for Kids chewable tablets OTC *antiemetic; motion sickness preventative* [cyclizine HCl] 25 mg

Bonisara tablets ℞ *nutritional supplement for osteoporosis* [strontium gluconate; Ranamine (q.v.)] 680•30 mg

Boniva once-daily film-coated tablets (discontinued 2010) ℞ *bisphosphonate bone resorption inhibitor for the prevention and treatment of postmenopausal osteoporosis in women* [ibandronate (as sodium)] 2.5 mg

Boniva once-monthly film-coated tablets, once-quarterly IV injection in a prefilled syringe ℞ *bisphosphonate bone resorption inhibitor for the prevention and treatment of postmenopausal osteoporosis in women; also used for metastatic bone disease in breast cancer* [ibandronate (as sodium)] 150 mg; 5 mg

Bontril PDM tablets ℞ *CNS stimulant; anorexiant* [phendimetrazine tartrate] 35 mg

Bontril Slow Release capsules ℞ *CNS stimulant; anorexiant* [phendimetrazine tartrate] 105 mg

bookoo *medicinal herb* [see: buchu]

Boost oral liquid OTC *enteral nutritional therapy* [milk-based formula] 240 mL ⚆ Bucet

Boost Glucose Control oral liquid OTC *enteral nutritional therapy formulated for low blood glucose response* [milk-based formula] 8 oz.

Boost High Protein; Boost Kid Essentials; Boost Kid Essentials 1.5; Boost Kid Essentials 1.5 with Fiber; Boost Plus oral liquid OTC *enteral nutritional therapy* [lactose-free formula] 237–244 mL

Boostrix IM injection ℞ *active immunizing agent for tetanus, diphtheria, and pertussis; Tdap (tetanus predominant) booster vaccine used in adolescents and adults 10–64 years old* [diphtheria toxoid; tetanus toxoid; inactivated pertussis toxins] 2.5 LfU•5 LfU•8 mcg per 0.5 mL dose

bopindolol INN

boracic acid [see: boric acid]

borage *(Borago officinalis)* leaves *medicinal herb for bronchitis, colds, eye inflammation, hay fever, strengthening of heart, lactation stimulation, rashes, rheumatism, ringworm; not generally regarded as safe and effective* ⚆ Berocca

borax [see: sodium borate]

Borbonia pinifolia medicinal herb [see: red bush tea]

boric acid NF, JAN *acidifying agent; ophthalmic emollient; antiseptic; astringent* ⚆ BrachySeed

2-bornanone [see: camphor]

bornaprine INN, BAN

bornaprolol INN

bornelone USAN, INN *ultraviolet screen*

bornyl acetate USAN

borocaptate sodium B 10 USAN *antineoplastic; radioactive agent* [also: sodium borocaptate (^{10}B)]

Borocell *investigational (orphan) for boron neutron capture therapy (BNCT) for glioblastoma multiforme* [sodium monomercaptoundecahydro-closododecaborate]

Borofair Otic ear drops ℞ *antibacterial; antifungal; antiseptic; astringent* [acetic acid; aluminum acetate] 2%• ≛

Borofax Skin Protectant ointment OTC *astringent* [zinc oxide] 15%

boroglycerin NF

boron *element (B); trace mineral for enhancing mental acuity and improving alertness; not generally regarded as safe* *and effective as it is highly toxic if taken internally or absorbed through broken skin* ☒ bryony

bortezomib *proteasome inhibitor; antineoplastic for multiple myeloma (orphan) and mantle cell (non-Hodgkin) lymphoma; investigational for rheumatoid arthritis*

Bosatria *investigational (orphan) immunomodulator for asthma due to hypereosinophilic syndrome* [mepolizumab]

bosentan USAN, INN *endothelin receptor antagonist (ERA); vasodilator for pulmonary arterial hypertension (orphan); also used to prevent digital ulcers in systemic sclerosis*

Boston Advance Cleaner; Boston Cleaner solution OTC *cleaning solution for rigid gas permeable contact lenses*

Boston Advance Comfort Formula solution OTC *disinfecting/wetting/soaking solution for rigid gas permeable contact lenses*

Boston Conditioning Solution OTC *disinfecting/wetting/soaking solution for rigid gas permeable contact lenses*

Boston Rewetting Drops OTC *rewetting solution for rigid gas permeable contact lenses*

Boston Simplicity Multi-Action solution OTC *disinfecting/wetting/soaking solution for rigid gas permeable contact lenses*

bosutinib *investigational (Phase III) antineoplastic for Philadelphia chromosome–positive chronic myeloid leukemia (CML)*

Boswellia serrata medicinal herb [see: frankincense]

botiacrine INN

Botox powder for injection ℞ *neurotoxin complex for blepharospasm and strabismus of dystonia (orphan), cervical dystonia (orphan), axillary hyperhidrosis, upper limb spasticity, and chronic migraine headaches; investigational (orphan) for pediatric cerebral palsy* [onabotulinumtoxin A] 100, 200 U/vial

Botox Cosmetic powder for injection ℞ *neurotoxin complex for the temporary treatment of wrinkles* [onabotulinumtoxin A] 50, 100 U/vial

BottomBetter ointment (discontinued 2010) OTC *diaper rash treatment*

botulinum toxin, type A [now: abobotulinumtoxin A; incobotulinumtoxin A; onabotulinumtoxin A]

botulinum toxin, type B [now: rimabotulinumtoxin B]

botulinum toxin, type F *investigational (orphan) neurotoxin for cervical dystonia and essential blepharospasm*

botulism antitoxin USP *passive immunizing agent*

botulism equine antitoxin, trivalent *passive immunizing agent*

botulism immune globulin intravenous (BIG-IV) *treatment for infant botulism type A or B (orphan)*

Bounty Bears chewable tablets (discontinued 2008) OTC *vitamin supplement* [multiple vitamins; folic acid] ≛•0.3 mg

Bounty Bears Plus Iron chewable tablets (discontinued 2008) OTC *vitamin/iron supplement* [multiple vitamins; iron; folic acid] ≛•15•0.3 mg

bourbonal [see: ethyl vanillin]

bovactant BAN

bovine fibrin BAN

bovine superoxide dismutase (bSOD) [see: orgotein]

bower, virgin's *medicinal herb* [see: woodbine]

Bowman's root *medicinal herb* [see: Culver root]

box, mountain *medicinal herb* [see: uva ursi]

boxberry *medicinal herb* [see: wintergreen]

boxidine USAN, INN *antihyperlipoproteinemic*

Boyol salve OTC *anti-infective; anesthetic* [ichthammol; benzocaine] 10%• ≛

BP 4.25%; BP 5.25% soap ℞ *keratolytic for acne* [benzoyl peroxide] 4.25%; 5.25%

BP 7% Wash soap OTC *keratolytic for acne* [benzoyl peroxide] 7%

BP 8 Cough oral suspension (discontinued 2011) Ŗ *antitussive; decongestant; expectorant* [dextromethorphan hydrobromide; pseudoephedrine HCl; guaifenesin] 30•60•1000 mg

BP-50% topical emulsion Ŗ *moisturizer; emollient; keratolytic* [urea] 50%

BP Allergy Junior oral suspension Ŗ *antihistamine; decongestant* [chlorpheniramine tannate; phenylephrine tannate] 4•20 mg/5 mL

BP Cleansing Wash soap Ŗ *antibiotic and keratolytic for acne* [sulfacetamide sodium; sulfur] 10%•4%

BP Manuvite SP sustained-release caplets Ŗ *vitamin/mineral supplement* [vitamins B_6, B_{12}, and E; multiple minerals; folic acid; saw palmeto extract] 12.5 mg•250 mcg•92 U• ± •1 mg•320 mg

BP New Allergy DM oral suspension (discontinued 2010) Ŗ *antitussive; antihistamine; decongestant* [dextromethorphan tannate; brompheniramine tannate; phenylephrine tannate] 30•10•25 mg/5 mL

BP Poly-650 tablets Ŗ *analgesic; antipyretic; antihistamine; sleep aid* [acetaminophen; phenyltoloxamine citrate] 650•60 mg

BP Prenate tablets + capsules Ŗ *prenatal vitamin/mineral/calcium/iron/omega-3 supplement; stool softener* [multiple vitamins & minerals; calcium; iron (as carbonyl and ferrous gluconate); folic acid; docusate sodium + docosahexaenoic acid (DHA)] ± •100•30•1•75 mg (tablets) + 275 mg (capsules)

B-PAS (benzoyl para-aminosalicylate) [see: benzoylpas calcium]

BPD-MA (benzoporphyrin derivative) [see: verteporfin]

B-Plex tablets (discontinued 2008) Ŗ *vitamin supplement* [multiple B vitamins; vitamin C; folic acid] ± •500•0.5 mg

BPM PE DM syrup Ŗ *antihistamine; decongestant; antitussive* [brompheniramine maleate; phenylephrine HCl; dextromethorphan hydrobromide] 2•5•10 mg/5 mL

BPM Pseudo 6/45 extended-release tablets Ŗ *antihistamine; decongestant* [brompheniramine maleate; pseudoephedrine HCl] 6•45 mg

BrachySeed I-125 implants Ŗ *radioactive brachytherapy* [iodine I 125 ceramic beads] 0.19–0.65 mCi (7–24.1 MBq) ☑ boric acid

BrachySeed Pd-103 ceramic bead implants Ŗ *radioactive "seeds" for ultrasound-guided brachytherapy for adenocarcinoma of the prostate* [palladium Pd 103] 1.0–1.8 mCi (37–66.6 MBq)

brain-derived neurotrophic factor (BDNF) [see: methionyl neurotropic factor, brain-derived]

brallobarbital INN

bramble *medicinal herb* [see: blackberry]

BranchAmin 4% IV infusion Ŗ *nutritional therapy for high metabolic stress* [multiple branched-chain essential amino acids]

branched-chain amino acids (BCAA) *investigational (orphan) for amyotrophic lateral sclerosis* [see: isoleucine; leucine; valine]

brandy mint *medicinal herb* [see: peppermint]

Brasivol cream OTC *abrasive cleanser for acne* [aluminum oxide]

brasofensine maleate USAN *dopamine reuptake inhibitor*

Brassica alba *medicinal herb* [see: mustard]

Bravelle powder for subcu or IM injection Ŗ *follicle-stimulating hormone (FSH); ovulation stimulant for polycystic ovary disease (orphan) and assisted reproductive technologies (ART)* [urofollitropin] 75 IU ☑ Prefill

brazergoline INN

Breathe Free nasal spray OTC *nasal moisturizer* [sodium chloride (saline solution)] 0.65%

Breezee Mist Aerosol powder OTC *antifungal; mild anesthetic; antipruritic; anhidrotic* [undecylenic acid; menthol; aluminum chlorohydrate]

Breezee Mist Antifungal powder (discontinued 2007) OTC *antifungal for tinea pedis, tinea cruris, and tinea corporis* [miconazole nitrate] 2% (note: one of two products with the same name)

Breezee Mist Antifungal powder (discontinued 2007) OTC *antifungal* [tolnaftate] 1% (note: one of two products with the same name)

Breezee Mist Foot Powder OTC *absorbent; anhidrotic* [talc; aluminum chlorohydrate]

brefonalol INN

bremazocine INN

bremelanotide *investigational (Phase II) for erectile dysfunction*

brentuximab vedotin INN *antineoplastic for Hodgkin lymphoma and anaplastic large cell lymphoma (ALCL); an antibody-drug conjugate (ADC) of a chimeric IgG1 antibody to CD30 (brentuximab) with the antimitotic agent monomethyl auristatin E (MMAE; vedotin)*

brequinar INN *antineoplastic* [also: brequinar sodium]

brequinar sodium USAN *antineoplastic* [also: brequinar]

bretazenil USAN, INN *anxiolytic*

Brethine tablets, IV or subcu injection (discontinued 2009) ℞ *sympathomimetic bronchodilator for asthma and bronchospasm; also used as a tocolytic to stop preterm labor* [terbutaline sulfate] 2.5, 5 mg; 1 mg/mL

bretylium tosilate INN *antiadrenergic; antiarrhythmic* [also: bretylium tosylate]

bretylium tosylate USAN, BAN *antiadrenergic; antiarrhythmic* [also: bretylium tosilate] 500, 1000 mg/vial injection

Brevibloc; Brevibloc Double Strength IV infusion ℞ *antiarrhythmic; antihypertensive; beta-blocker; treatment for supraventricular tachycardia and intraoperative/postoperative tachycardia or hypertension; also used for unstable angina* [esmolol HCl] 10, 250 mg/mL; 20 mg/mL

Brevicon tablets (in Wallettes of 28) ℞ *monophasic oral contraceptive* [norethindrone; ethinyl estradiol] 0.5 mg•35 mcg × 21 days; counters × 7 days ② parvaquone

Brevital Sodium powder for IV injection ℞ *barbiturate general anesthetic* [methohexital sodium] 2.5 g

Brevoxyl Cleansing Lotion ℞ *keratolytic for acne* [benzoyl peroxide] 4%, 8%

Brevoxyl-4; Brevoxyl-8 gel ℞ *keratolytic for acne* [benzoyl peroxide] 4%; 8%

Brevoxyl-4 Acne Wash; Brevoxyl-8 Acne Wash topical liquid ℞ *keratolytic for acne* [benzoyl peroxide] 4%; 8%

brewer's yeast *natural source of protein and B-complex vitamins*

Bridion ⑩ (approved in Europe) *investigational (NDA filed) selective relaxation binding agent (SRBA) to reverse the effects of strong muscle relaxants, used for postanesthesia "stir-up"* [sugammadex]

Briellyn tablets (in packs of 28) ℞ *monophasic oral contraceptive* [norethindrone; ethinyl estradiol] 0.4 mg• 35 mcg

brifentanil INN *narcotic analgesic* [also: brifentanil HCl]

brifentanil HCl USAN *narcotic analgesic* [also: brifentanil]

Brigham tea; Brigham Young weed *medicinal herb* [see: ephedra]

Brik-Paks (trademarked delivery form) *ready-to-use liquid containers*

Brilinta tablets ℞ *twice-daily antiplatelet agent to prevent thrombotic events* [ticagrelor] 90 mg

brimonidine INN *ophthalmic alpha$_2$-adrenergic agonist for open-angle glaucoma and ocular hypertension* [also: brimonidine tartrate] ② bromindione

brimonidine tartrate USAN *selective alpha₂ agonist for open-angle glaucoma and ocular hypertension; investigational (orphan) for anterior ischemic optic neuropathy* [also: brimonidine] 0.2% eye drops

brinaldix [see: clopamide]

brinase INN [also: brinolase]

Brinavess injection *investigational (Phase III) selective ion channel blocker for the acute conversion of atrial fibrillation* [vernakalant]

brinazarone INN

brindoxime INN

brineurin [now: abrineurin]

brinolase USAN *fibrinolytic enzyme* [also: brinase]

brinzolamide USAN, INN *topical carbonic anhydrase inhibitor for glaucoma*

Bristoject (trademarked delivery form) *prefilled disposable syringe*

Brite Eyes II eye drops OTC *antioxidant and anti-glycation agent to prevent free radical damage in the lens; moisturizer/lubricant* [N-acetyl-L-carnitine; glycerin; carboxymethylcellulose sodium] 1%•1%•0.3%

British antilewisite (BAL) [now: dimercaprol]

British tobacco *medicinal herb* [see: coltsfoot]

brivudine INN

brobactam INN

brobenzoxaldine [see: broxaldine]

broclepride INN

brocresine USAN, INN, BAN *histidine decarboxylase inhibitor*

brocrinat USAN, INN *diuretic*

brodimoprim INN

brofaromine INN *reversible/selective MAO inhibitor*

Brofed oral liquid (discontinued 2007) ℞ *decongestant; antihistamine* [pseudoephedrine HCl; brompheniramine maleate] 60•8 mg/10 mL

brofezil INN, BAN

brofoxine USAN, INN *antipsychotic*

brolaconazole INN

brolamfetamine INN

Brolene eye drops *investigational (orphan) for* Acanthamoeba *keratitis* [propamidine isethionate] 0.1%

Brom 2 mg/PE 5 mg/DM 10 mg syrup ℞ *antihistamine; decongestant; antitussive* [brompheniramine maleate; phenylephrine HCl; dextromethorphan hydrobromide] 2•5•10 mg/5 mL

bromacrylide INN

bromadel [see: carbromal]

bromadoline INN *analgesic* [also: bromadoline maleate]

bromadoline maleate USAN *analgesic* [also: bromadoline]

Bromaline oral liquid OTC *decongestant; antihistamine* [pseudoephedrine HCl; brompheniramine maleate] 15•1 mg/5 mL

Bromaline DM oral liquid OTC *antitussive; antihistamine; decongestant* [dextromethorphan hydrobromide; brompheniramine maleate; pseudoephedrine HCl] 10•2•30 mg/10 mL

bromamid INN

Bromanate pediatric elixir (discontinued 2007) OTC *decongestant; antihistamine* [pseudoephedrine HCl; brompheniramine maleate] 30•2 mg/10 mL

Bromanate DM Cold & Cough elixir (discontinued 2007) OTC *antitussive; antihistamine; decongestant* [dextromethorphan hydrobromide; brompheniramine maleate; pseudoephedrine HCl] 5•1•15 mg/5 mL

bromanylpromide [see: bromamid]

Bromatan Plus oral suspension ℞ *antitussive; antihistamine; decongestant* [dextromethorphan tannate; dexchlorpheniramine tannate; pseudoephedrine tannate] 30•3.5•45 mg/5 mL

Bromatan-DM oral suspension (discontinued 2010) ℞ *antitussive; antihistamine; decongestant* [dextromethorphan tannate; brompheniramine tannate; phenylephrine tannate] 20•8•20 mg/5 mL

Bromatane DX syrup (discontinued 2007) ℞ *antitussive; antihistamine; decongestant* [dextromethorphan hydrobromide; brompheniramine maleate; pseudoephedrine HCl; alcohol 1%] 20•4•60 mg/10 mL

bromauric acid NF

bromazepam USAN, INN, BAN, JAN *benzodiazepine anxiolytic; minor tranquilizer* ② premazepam

bromazine INN *antihistamine* [also: bromodiphenhydramine HCl; bromodiphenhydramine] ② promazine

bromazine HCl [see: bromodiphenhydramine HCl]

brombenzonium [see: bromhexine HCl]

bromchlorenone USAN, INN *topical anti-infective*

Bromday eye drops ℞ *long-acting (once daily) nonsteroidal anti-inflammatory drug (NSAID) for pain and inflammation following cataract extraction surgery* [bromfenac (as sodium)] 0.09%

Bromdex D syrup ℞ *antitussive; antihistamine; decongestant* [dextromethorphan hydrobromide; brompheniramine maleate; pseudoephedrine HCl] 30•3•50 mg/5 mL

bromebric acid INN, BAN

bromelain JAN *anti-inflammatory; proteolytic enzymes* [also: bromelains]

bromelains USAN, INN, BAN *anti-inflammatory; proteolytic enzymes* [also: bromelain]

bromelin [see: bromelains]

bromerguride INN

Brometane-DX Cough syrup ℞ *antitussive; antihistamine; decongestant* [dextromethorphan hydrobromide; brompheniramine maleate; pseudoephedrine HCl] 10•2•30 mg/5 mL

brometenamine INN

bromethol [see: tribromoethanol]

Bromfed DM oral liquid ℞ *antitussive; antihistamine; decongestant* [dextromethorphan hydrobromide; brompheniramine maleate; pseudoephedrine HCl; alcohol 0.95%] 10•2•30 mg/5 mL

bromfenac INN *long-acting nonsteroidal anti-inflammatory drug (NSAID); analgesic; antipyretic* [also: bromfenac sodium]

bromfenac sodium USAN *long-acting nonsteroidal anti-inflammatory drug (NSAID); analgesic; antipyretic; ocular treatment following cataract extraction surgery; investigational (Phase III) treatment for dry eye syndrome* [also: bromfenac] 0.09% eye drops

Bromfenex extended-release capsules (discontinued 2008) ℞ *decongestant; antihistamine* [pseudoephedrine HCl; brompheniramine maleate] 120•12 mg

Bromfenex PD extended-release capsules (discontinued 2008) ℞ *decongestant; antihistamine* [pseudoephedrine HCl; brompheniramine maleate] 60•6 mg

bromhexine INN, BAN *expectorant; mucolytic* [also: bromhexine HCl] ② pramoxine

bromhexine HCl USAN, JAN *expectorant; mucolytic; investigational (orphan) for keratoconjunctivitis sicca of Sjögren syndrome* [also: bromhexine]

Bromhist-DM oral drops (discontinued 2010) ℞ *antitussive; antihistamine; decongestant; for children 1–24 months* [dextromethorphan hydrobromide; brompheniramine maleate; pseudoephedrine HCl] 4•1•15 mg/mL

Bromhist-DM Pediatric syrup ℞ *antitussive; decongestant; antihistamine; expectorant* [dextromethorphan hydrobromide; pseudoephedrine HCl; brompheniramine maleate; guaifenesin] 5•30•2•50 mg/5 mL

Bromhist-NR; Bromhist Pediatric oral drops ℞ *decongestant; antihistamine; for children 1–24 months* [pseudoephedrine HCl; brompheniramine maleate] 12.5•1 mg/mL; 15•1 mg/mL

Bromhist-PDX oral drops (discontinued 2010) ℞ *antitussive; antihistamine; decongestant; for children 1–24 months* [dextromethorphan hydrobromide;

brompheniramine maleate; pseudoephedrine HCl] 3•1•12.5 mg/mL

Bromhist-PDX syrup ℞ *antitussive;
decongestant; antihistamine; expectorant* [dextromethorphan hydrobromide; phenylephrine HCl; brompheniramine maleate; guaifenesin]
5•5•2•50 mg/5 mL

bromindione USAN, INN, BAN *anticoagulant* ② brimonidine

bromine *element (Br)*

bromisoval INN [also: bromisovalum;
bromvalerylurea; bromovaluree]

bromisovalum NF [also: bromisoval;
bromvalerylurea; bromovaluree]

2-bromo-α-ergocryptine [see: bro-
mocriptine]

bromocamphor [see: camphor, mono-
bromated]

bromociclen INN [also: bromocyclen]

bromocriptine USAN, INN, BAN *dopamine agonist for Parkinson disease; lactation inhibitor; treatment for acromegaly,
infertility, and hypogonadism; suppresses
increased postprandial blood sugar*

bromocriptine mesilate JAN *dopamine
agonist for Parkinson disease; lactation
inhibitor; treatment for acromegaly,
infertility, and hypogonadism; suppresses increased postprandial blood sugar*
[also: bromocriptine mesylate]

bromocriptine mesylate USAN, USP
*dopamine agonist for Parkinson disease;
lactation inhibitor; treatment for acromegaly, infertility, and hypogonadism;
suppresses increased postprandial blood
sugar in type 2 diabetes* [also: bromocriptine mesilate] 2.5, 5 mg oral

bromocyclen BAN [also: bromociclen]

bromodeoxyuridine [now: broxuri-
dine]

bromodiethylacetylurea [see: carbro-
mal]

bromodiphenhydramine BAN *antihistamine; sleep aid* [also: bromodiphenhydramine HCl; bromazine]

bromodiphenhydramine HCl USP
antihistamine; sleep aid [also: bromazine; bromodiphenhydramine]

bromofenofos INN

bromoform USP

bromofos INN

1-bromoheptadecafluorooctane
[see: perflubron]

bromoisovaleryl urea (BVU) [see:
bromisovalum]

bromophenol blue

bromophin [see: apomorphine HCl]

bromophos [see: bromofos]

bromopride INN

Bromo-Seltzer effervescent granules
OTC *antacid; analgesic; antipyretic*
[sodium bicarbonate; citric acid;
acetaminophen] 2781•2224•325
mg/dose

**bromotheophyllinate aminoisobu-
tanol** [see: pamabrom]

bromotheophyllinate pyranisamine
[see: pyrabrom]

bromotheophyllinate pyrilamine
[see: pyrabrom]

8-bromotheophylline [see: pamabrom]

bromovaluree [also: bromisovalum;
bromisoval; bromvalerylurea]

11-bromovincamine [see: brovinca-
mine]

**bromovinyl arabinosyluracil (BV-
araU)** [see: sorivudine]

bromoxanide USAN, INN *anthelmintic*

bromperidol USAN, INN, BAN, JAN
antipsychotic

bromperidol decanoate USAN, BAN
antipsychotic

Bromphenex DM oral liquid ℞ *antitussive; antihistamine; decongestant*
[dextromethorphan hydrobromide;
brompheniramine maleate; pseudoephedrine HCl] 30•4•60 mg/5 mL

Bromphenex HD oral liquid (discontinued 2009) ℞ *narcotic antitussive;
antihistamine; decongestant* [hydroco-
done bitartrate; brompheniramine
maleate; pseudoephedrine HCl] 1.7•
2•30 mg/5 mL

brompheniramine INN, BAN *alkylamine antihistamine* [also: brompheniramine maleate]

brompheniramine maleate USP
alkylamine antihistamine [also: brom-

pheniramine] 10 mg/mL injection; 1 mg/mL oral

brompheniramine maleate & phenylephrine HCl *antihistamine; decongestant* 6•7.5, 12•15 mg oral

brompheniramine maleate & phenylephrine HCl & dihydrocodeine bitartrate *antihistamine; decongestant; narcotic analgesic and antitussive* 4•7.5•3 mg oral

brompheniramine maleate & pseudoephedrine HCl *antihistamine; decongestant* 1•7.5, 4•60 mg/5 mL oral

brompheniramine maleate & pseudoephedrine HCl & hydrocodone bitartrate *antihistamine; decongestant; narcotic antitussive* 3•30•2.5 mg/5 mL oral

brompheniramine tannate *alkylamine antihistamine* 12 mg oral; 12 mg/5 mL oral

brompheniramine tannate & phenylephrine tannate *antihistamine; decongestant* 12•20 mg/5 mL oral

Bromplex HD oral liquid (discontinued 2009) ℞ *narcotic antitussive; antihistamine; decongestant* [hydrocodone bitartrate; brompheniramine maleate; pseudoephedrine HCl] 1.7•2•30 mg/5 mL

Brompton's Cocktail; Brompton's Mixture (refers to any oral narcotic/alcoholic solution containing morphine and either cocaine or a phenothiazine derivative) ℞ *prophylaxis for chronic, severe pain*

bromvalerylurea JAN [also: bromisovalum; bromisoval; bromovaluree]

Bronchial capsules (discontinued 2007) ℞ *antiasthmatic; bronchodilator; expectorant* [theophylline; guaifenesin] 150•90 mg

Bronchitol (name changed to **Aridol** upon marketing release in 2010)

Broncholate syrup ℞ *bronchodilator; decongestant; expectorant* [ephedrine HCl; guaifenesin] 12.5•200 mg/10 mL

Broncotron-D oral suspension ℞ *antitussive; decongestant; expectorant* [dextromethorphan hydrobromide; phenylephrine HCl; guaifenesin] 20•5•200 mg/5 mL

Brondelate elixir (discontinued 2007) ℞ *antiasthmatic; bronchodilator; expectorant* [theophylline; guaifenesin] 192•150 mg/15 mL

Bronkaid Dual Action caplets OTC *bronchodilator; decongestant; expectorant* [ephedrine sulfate; guaifenesin] 25•400 mg

Bronkids oral drops ℞ *antitussive; antihistamine; decongestant; for children 6–24 months* [dextromethorphan hydrobromide; chlorpheniramine maleate; phenylephrine HCl] 2.75•0.6•1.5 mg/mL

Bronkodyl capsules (discontinued 2008) ℞ *antiasthmatic; bronchodilator* [theophylline] 100, 200 mg

bronopol INN, BAN, JAN

Brontuss DX oral liquid OTC *antitussive; decongestant; expectorant* [dextromethorphan hydrobromide; phenylephrine HCl; guaifenesin] 20•10•200 mg/5 mL

brook bean *medicinal herb* [see: buckbean]

brooklime *(Veronica beccabunga)* plant *medicinal herb used as a diuretic, emmenagogue, and febrifuge* ⚕ berkelium

broom *(Cytisus scoparius)* plant and bloom *medicinal herb for inducing bowel evacuation, diuresis, and emesis; also used as a homeopathic remedy for arrhythmias, diphtheria, and head and throat congestion* ⚕ barium

broom, butcher's *medicinal herb* [see: butcher's broom]

broom, dyer's; green broom *medicinal herb* [see: dyer's broom]

broparestrol INN

broperamole USAN, INN *anti-inflammatory*

bropirimine USAN, INN *antineoplastic; antiviral*

broquinaldol INN

brosotamide INN

brosuximide INN

Brotapp oral liquid OTC *decongestant; antihistamine* [pseudoephedrine HCl; brompheniramine maleate] 15•1 mg/5 mL

Brotapp DM oral liquid OTC *antitussive; antihistamine; decongestant* [dextromethorphan hydrobromide; brompheniramine maleate; pseudoephedrine HCl] 10•2•30 mg/10 mL

brotianide INN, BAN

brotizolam USAN, INN, BAN, JAN *hypnotic*

Brovana inhalation solution for nebulization ℞ *twice-daily bronchodilator for chronic obstructive pulmonary disease (COPD), bronchitis, and emphysema* [arformoterol (as tartrate)] 15 mcg/2 mL dose

brovanexine INN

brovavir [see: sorivudine]

BrōveX oral suspension ℞ *antihistamine* [brompheniramine tannate] 12 mg/5 mL

BrōveX ADT oral suspension (discontinued 2011) ℞ *decongestant; antihistamine* [phenylephrine tannate; brompheniramine tannate] 10•12 mg/5 mL

BrōveX CB; BrōveX CBX caplets ℞ *narcotic antitussive; antihistamine* [codeine phosphate; brompheniramine maleate] 10•4 mg; 20•4 mg

BrōveX CT chewable tablets ℞ *antihistamine* [brompheniramine tannate] 12 mg

BrōveX D oral suspension (discontinued 2007) ℞ *decongestant; antihistamine* [phenylephrine tannate; brompheniramine tannate] 20•12 mg/5 mL

BrōveX PB caplets ℞ *decongestant; antihistamine* [phenylephrine HCl; brompheniramine maleate] 10•4 mg

BrōveX PB C; BrōveX PB CX caplets ℞ *narcotic antitussive; antihistamine; decongestant* [codeine phosphate; brompheniramine maleate;

phenylephrine HCl] 10•4•10 mg; 20•4•10 mg

BrōveX PB DM caplets ℞ *antitussive; antihistamine; decongestant* [dextromethorphan hydrobromide; brompheniramine maleate; phenylephrine HCl] 20•4•10 mg

BrōveX PD oral suspension ℞ *decongestant; antihistamine* [pseudoephedrine HCl; brompheniramine maleate] 30•6 mg/5 mL

BrōveX PEB DM oral liquid ℞ *antitussive; antihistamine; decongestant* [dextromethorphan hydrobromide; brompheniramine maleate; phenylephrine HCl] 20•4•10 mg/5 mL

BrōveX PSB oral liquid ℞ *decongestant; antihistamine* [pseudoephedrine HCl; brompheniramine maleate] 20•4 mg/5 mL

BrōveX PSB DM oral liquid ℞ *antitussive; antihistamine; decongestant* [dextromethorphan hydrobromide; brompheniramine maleate; pseudoephedrine HCl] 20•4•20 mg/5 mL

BrōveX SR extended-release capsules ℞ *decongestant; antihistamine* [pseudoephedrine HCl; brompheniramine maleate] 90•9 mg

brovincamine INN [also: brovincamine fumarate]

brovincamine fumarate JAN [also: brovincamine]

brown algae *medicinal herb* [see: kelp (*Laminaria*)]

brownwort *medicinal herb* [see: woundwort]

broxaldine INN

broxaterol INN

Broxine *investigational (NDA filed, orphan) radiosensitizer for primary brain tumors* [broxuridine]

broxitalamic acid INN

broxuridine INN *investigational (NDA filed, orphan) radiosensitizer for primary brain tumors*

broxyquinoline INN

brucine sulfate NF

bruisewort *medicinal herb* [see: comfrey; soapwort]

bryony *(Bryonia alba; B. dioica)* root *medicinal herb used as a pectoral and purgative; not generally regarded as safe and effective as root is poisonous in high doses (ingestion of as few as 40 berries can be fatal in adults, 15 in children)* ⊡ boron

bryostatin-1 *investigational (orphan) agent for esophageal cancer*

bSOD (bovine superoxide dismutase) [see: orgotein]

BSS (bismuth subsalicylate) [q.v.]

BSS; BSS Plus ophthalmic solution ℞ *intraocular irrigating solution* [sodium chloride (balanced saline solution)]

BTA Stat Test test kit for home use OTC *in vitro diagnostic aid for bladder tumor analytes in the urine* [rapid immunoassay (RIA)]

bucainide INN *antiarrhythmic* [also: bucainide maleate]

bucainide maleate USAN *antiarrhythmic* [also: bucainide]

bucco *medicinal herb* [see: buchu]

Bucet capsules (discontinued 2008) ℞ *barbiturate sedative; analgesic; antipyretic* [butalbital; acetaminophen] 50•650 mg ⊡ Boost

bucetin INN, BAN, JAN

buchu *(Agathosma betulina; Barosma betulina; B. cenulata; B. serratifolia)* leaves *medicinal herb for edema, gas, gout, inflammation, kidney and urinary tract infections, and prostatitis; also used as a douche for leukorrhea and vaginal yeast infections*

buciclovir INN

bucillamine INN, JAN

bucindolol INN, BAN *antihypertensive* [also: bucindolol HCl]

bucindolol HCl USAN *antihypertensive* [also: bucindolol]

buckbean *(Menyanthes trifoliata)* leaves *medicinal herb used as a tonic, cathartic, diuretic, anthelmintic, and emetic*

buckeye; California buckeye; Ohio buckeye *medicinal herb* [see: horse chestnut]

buckhorn brake *(Osmunda cinnamomea; O. regalis)* root *medicinal herb used as a demulcent and tonic*

Buckley's Chest Congestion oral liquid OTC *expectorant* [guaifenesin] 100 mg/5 mL

Buckley's Cough Mixture oral liquid OTC *antitussive* [dextromethorphan hydrobromide] 12.5 mg/5 mL

buckthorn *(Rhamnus cathartica; R. frangula)* bark and berries *medicinal herb for bleeding, bowel disorders, chronic constipation, fever, gallstones, lead poisoning, and liver disorders* [see also: cascara sagrada] ⊡ buquiterine

bucku *medicinal herb* [see: buchu]

bucladesine INN [also: bucladesine sodium]

bucladesine sodium JAN [also: bucladesine]

buclizine INN, BAN *antinauseant; antiemetic; anticholinergic; motion sickness relief* [also: buclizine HCl]

buclizine HCl USAN *antinauseant; antiemetic; anticholinergic; motion sickness relief* [also: buclizine]

buclosamide INN, BAN

bucloxic acid INN

bucolome INN, JAN

bucricaine INN

bucrilate INN *tissue adhesive* [also: bucrylate]

bucromarone USAN, INN *antiarrhythmic*

bucrylate USAN *tissue adhesive* [also: bucrilate]

bucumolol INN [also: bucumolol HCl]

bucumolol HCl JAN [also: bucumolol]

Budeprion SR sustained-release (12-hour) film-coated tablets ℞ *antidepressant for major depressive disorder (MDD); also used for attention-deficit/hyperactivity disorder (ADHD), neuropathic pain, and weight loss* [bupropion (as HCl)] 100, 150 mg

Budeprion XL sustained-release (24-hour) film-coated tablets ℞ *antidepressant for major depressive disorder (MDD); also used for attention deficit/hyperactivity disorder (ADHD), neuro-*

pathic pain, and weight loss [bupropion (as HCl)] 150, 300 mg

budesonide USAN, INN, BAN, JAN topical corticosteroidal anti-inflammatory; oral inhalation aerosol for chronic asthma; nasal aerosol for allergic rhinitis; rectal treatment for inflammatory bowel disease 3 mg oral; 80, 160, 250, 500, 1000 mcg/inhalation

budipine INN

budotitane INN

budralazine INN, JAN

bufenadine [see: bufenadrine]

bufenadrine INN

bufeniode INN

bufetolol INN [also: bufetolol HCl]

bufetolol HCl JAN [also: bufetolol]

bufexamac INN, BAN, JAN

bufezolac INN

buffered aspirin [see: aspirin, buffered]

Bufferin coated tablets, coated caplets OTC analgesic; antipyretic; anti-inflammatory; antirheumatic [aspirin (buffered with calcium carbonate, magnesium oxide, and magnesium carbonate)] 325, 500 mg

Bufferin AF Nite Time tablets (discontinued 2008) OTC antihistaminic sleep aid; analgesic; antipyretic [diphenhydramine HCl; acetaminophen] 30•500 mg

bufilcon A USAN hydrophilic contact lens material

buflomedil INN, BAN

bufogenin INN

buformin USAN, INN antidiabetic

bufrolin INN, BAN ☑ befuraline

bufuralol INN, BAN

bufylline BAN diuretic; smooth muscle relaxant [also: ambuphylline]

bugbane medicinal herb [see: hellebore; black cohosh]

bugleweed *(Lycopus virginicus)* plant medicinal herb for cough, excessive menses, nervous indigestion, and other nervous disorders

bugloss medicinal herb [see: borage]

Bugs Bunny Complete chewable tablets (discontinued 2008) OTC vitamin/mineral/calcium/iron supplement [multiple vitamins & minerals; calcium; iron; folic acid; biotin] ≞• 100•18•0.4•0.04 mg

Bugs Bunny Plus Iron chewable tablets (discontinued 2008) OTC vitamin/iron supplement [multiple vitamins; iron; folic acid] ≞•15•0.3 mg

Bugs Bunny with Extra C Children's chewable tablets (discontinued 2008) OTC vitamin supplement [multiple vitamins; folic acid] ≞•0.3 mg

bugwort medicinal herb [see: black cohosh]

buku medicinal herb [see: buchu]

bulaquine INN ☑ Bellacane

Bulk Forming Fiber Laxative film-coated tablets OTC bulk laxative; antidiarrheal [calcium polycarbophil] 625 mg

bulk-producing laxatives a subclass of laxatives that work by increasing the hydration and volume of stool to stimulate peristalsis; also form an emollient gel to ease the movement of stool through the intestines [see also: laxatives]

bull's foot medicinal herb [see: coltsfoot]

bumadizone INN

bumecaine INN

bumepidil INN

bumetanide USAN, USP, INN, BAN, JAN loop diuretic for congestive heart failure, hepatic cirrhosis, and renal disease; also used for adult nocturia 0.5, 1, 2 mg oral; 0.25 mg/mL injection

bumetrizole USAN, INN ultraviolet screen

Bumex tablets (discontinued 2009) ℞ loop diuretic [bumetanide] 0.5, 1, 2 mg

Buminate 5%; Buminate 25% IV infusion (discontinued 2011) ℞ blood volume expander for shock, burns, and hypoproteinemia [human albumin] 5%; 25%

bunaftine INN

bunamidine INN, BAN anthelmintic [also: bunamidine HCl]

bunamidine HCl USAN anthelmintic [also: bunamidine]

bunamiodyl INN [also: buniodyl]

bunamiodyl sodium [see: bunamiodyl; buniodyl]

bunaprolast USAN, INN *antiasthmatic; 5-lipoxygenase inhibitor*

bunapsilate INN *combining name for radicals or groups*

bunazosin INN [also: bunazosin HCl]

bunazosin HCl JAN [also: bunazosin]

bundlin [now: sedecamycin]

buniodyl BAN [also: bunamiodyl]

bunitrolol INN [also: bunitrolol HCl]

bunitrolol HCl JAN [also: bunitrolol]

bunolol INN *antiadrenergic (beta-receptor)* [also: bunolol HCl]

bunolol HCl USAN *antiadrenergic (beta-receptor)* [also: bunolol]

Bupap caplets ℞ *barbiturate sedative; analgesic; antipyretic* [butalbital; acetaminophen] 50•650 mg

buparvaquone INN, BAN

buphenine INN, BAN *peripheral vasodilator* [also: nylidrin HCl]

Buphenyl tablets, powder for oral solution ℞ *antihyperammonemic for urea cycle disorders (orphan); investigational (orphan) for various sickling disorders and spinal muscular atrophy* [sodium phenylbutyrate] 500 mg; 3 g/tsp., 8.6 g/tbsp.

bupicomide USAN, INN *antihypertensive*

bupivacaine INN, BAN *injectable local anesthetic* [also: bupivacaine HCl]

bupivacaine HCl USAN, USP, JAN *injectable local anesthetic* [also: bupivacaine] 0.25%, 0.5%, 0.75%

bupivacaine HCl & epinephrine *injectable local anesthetic; vasoconstrictor* 0.25%•1:200 000, 0.5%• 1:200 000, 0.75%•1:200 000

Bupivicaine Spinal injection ℞ *local anesthetic for obstetric use* [bupivacaine HCl; dextrose] 0.75%•8.25%

bupranol [see: bupranolol]

bupranolol INN [also: bupranolol HCl]

bupranolol HCl JAN [also: bupranolol]

Buprenex IV or IM injection ℞ *narcotic agonist-antagonist analgesic* [buprenorphine HCl] 0.3 mg/mL

buprenorphine INN, BAN *narcotic agonist-antagonist analgesic* [also: buprenorphine HCl]

buprenorphine HCl USAN, JAN *narcotic agonist-antagonist analgesic for inpatient treatment of opiate dependence (orphan)* [also: buprenorphine] 2, 8 mg oral; 0.3 mg/mL injection

bupropion BAN *aminoketone antidepressant; non-nicotine aid to smoking cessation* [also: bupropion HCl; amfebutamone]

bupropion HCl USAN *aminoketone antidepressant; non-nicotine aid to smoking cessation; also used for attention-deficit/hyperactivity disorder (ADHD), neuropathic pain, and weight loss* [also: amfebutamone; bupropion] 75, 100, 150, 200, 300 mg oral

bupropion hydrobromide *aminoketone antidepressant for major depressive disorder (MDD)*

buquineran INN, BAN

buquinolate USAN, INN *coccidiostat for poultry*

buquiterine INN

buramate USAN, INN *anticonvulsant; antipsychotic* ⑫ PowerMate

burdock (Arctium lappa; A. majus; A. minus) *root medicinal herb for arthritis, blood cleansing, dandruff, eczema, edema, fever, gout, kidney and lung disorders, rheumatism, skin diseases, and tumors; also used as an antimicrobial and diaphoretic*

burefrine [now: berefrine]

burnet (Pimpinella magna; P. saxifrage) *root medicinal herb used as an antispasmodic, astringent, carminative, diaphoretic, diuretic, stimulant, and stomachic* ⑫ Parnate

burning bush *medicinal herb* [see: fraxinella; wahoo]

Burn-O-Jel gel OTC *anesthetic* [lidocaine] 0.5%

burodiline INN

Burow solution [see: aluminum acetate]

Burow's Otic ear drops ℞ *antibacterial; antifungal; antiseptic; astringent* [acetic acid; aluminum acetate] 2%• ≟

burr seed; turkey burr seed; clot-bur; hareburr; hurr-burr; thorny burr *medicinal herb* [see: burdock]

burrage *medicinal herb* [see: borage]

buserelin INN, BAN *hormonal antineo-plastic; gonad-stimulating principle; luteinizing hormone-releasing hormone analogue* [also: buserelin acetate]

buserelin acetate USAN, JAN *hormonal antineoplastic; gonad-stimulating prin-ciple; luteinizing hormone-releasing hormone analogue* [also: buserelin]

BuSpar tablets (discontinued 2010) ℞ *nonsedating azaspirone anxiolytic* [buspirone HCl] 5, 15, 30 mg

buspirone INN, BAN *nonsedating aza-spirone anxiolytic* [also: buspirone HCl] ⑨ bisobrin

buspirone HCl USAN *nonsedating aza-spirone anxiolytic* [also: buspirone] 5, 7.5, 10, 15, 30 mg oral

busulfan USP, INN, JAN *alkylating anti-neoplastic for chronic myelogenous leu-kemia (CML); pretreatment for bone marrow or stem cell transplants (orphan); investigational (orphan) for neoplastic meningitis and primary brain malignancies* [also: busulphan]

Busulfex IV infusion ℞ *alkylating anti-neoplastic for chronic myelogenous leu-kemia (CML); pretreatment for bone marrow or stem cell transplants (orphan)* [busulfan] 6 mg/mL

busulphan BAN *alkylating antineoplastic* [also: busulfan]

butabarbital USP *sedative; hypnotic* [also: secbutobarbitone]

butabarbital sodium USP *sedative; hyp-notic* [also: secbutabarbital sodium]

butacaine INN, BAN [also: butacaine sulfate]

butacaine sulfate USP [also: butacaine]

butacetin USAN *analgesic; antidepressant*

butacetoluide [see: butanilicaine]

butaclamol INN *antipsychotic* [also: butaclamol HCl]

butaclamol HCl USAN *antipsychotic* [also: butaclamol]

butadiazamide INN

butafosfan INN, BAN

butalamine INN, BAN

butalbital USAN, USP, INN *barbiturate sedative*

butalbital & acetaminophen *barbi-turate sedative; analgesic; antipyretic* 50•300 mg oral

butalbital & acetaminophen & caf-feine *barbiturate sedative; analgesic; antipyretic* 50•300•40, 50•325•40, 50•500•40 mg oral

butalbital & acetaminophen & caf-feine & codeine phosphate *barbi-turate sedative; analgesic; narcotic antitussive* 50•325•40•30 mg oral

butalbital & aspirin & caffeine *anal-gesic; barbiturate sedative* 50•325•40 mg oral

butalbital & aspirin & caffeine & codeine phosphate *barbiturate sed-ative; analgesic; narcotic antitussive* 50•325•40•30 mg oral

Butalbital Compound tablets, cap-sules ℞ *barbiturate sedative; analgesic; antipyretic* [butalbital; aspirin; caf-feine] 50•325•40 mg

butalgin [see: methadone HCl]

butallylonal NF

butamben USAN, USP *topical anesthetic*

butamben picrate USAN *topical anes-thetic*

butamirate INN *antitussive* [also: buta-mirate citrate; butamyrate]

butamirate citrate USAN *antitussive* [also: butamirate; butamyrate]

butamisole INN *veterinary anthelmintic* [also: butamisole HCl]

butamisole HCl USAN *veterinary ant-helmintic* [also: butamisole]

butamiverine [see: butaverine]

butamoxane INN

butamyrate BAN *antitussive* [also: butamirate citrate; butamirate]

butane (n-butane) NF *aerosol propel-lant* ⑨ betony; biotin; Bitin

1,4-butanediol (1,4-B; BDO); butane-1,4-diol *precursor to gamma hydroxybutyrate (GHB); a formerly legal alternative to GHB, now also ille-gal (Schedule I)* [see: gamma hydroxy-butyrate (GHB)]

butanilicaine INN, BAN
butanixin INN
butanserin INN
butantrone INN
butaperazine USAN, INN *antipsychotic* ⊡ batoprazine
butaperazine maleate USAN *antipsychotic*
butaprost USAN, INN, BAN *bronchodilator*
butaverine INN
butaxamine INN *antidiabetic; antihyperlipoproteinemic* [also: butoxamine HCl; butoxamine]
butcher's broom *(Ruscus aculeatus)* rhizomes *medicinal herb for atherosclerosis, circulatory disorders, hemorrhoids, thrombosis, varicose veins, and venous insufficiency; not generally regarded as safe and effective*
butedronate tetrasodium USAN *bone imaging aid*
butedronic acid INN
butelline [see: butacaine sulfate]
butenafine *benzylamine antifungal*
butenafine HCl USAN *topical benzylamine antifungal*
butenemal [see: vinbarbital]
buteprate INN *former combining name for radicals or groups (name rescinded by the USAN)* [now: probutate]
buterizine USAN, INN *peripheral vasodilator*
butetamate INN [also: butethamate]
butethal NF [also: butobarbitone]
butethamate BAN [also: butetamate]
butethamine HCl NF
butethanol [see: tetracaine]
Butex Forte capsules ℞ *barbiturate sedative; analgesic; antipyretic* [butalbital; acetaminophen] 50•650 mg
buthalital sodium INN [also: buthalitone sodium]
buthalitone sodium BAN [also: buthalital sodium]
buthiazide USAN *diuretic; antihypertensive* [also: butizide]
Butibel tablets, elixir ℞ *GI/GU anticholinergic/antispasmodic; sedative* [belladonna extract; butabarbital sodium] 15•15 mg; 15•15 mg/5 mL

butibufen INN
butidrine INN
butikacin USAN, INN, BAN *antibacterial* ⊡ Betaxon
butilfenin USAN, INN *hepatic function test*
butinazocine INN
butinoline INN
butirosin INN *antibacterial antibiotic* [also: butirosin sulfate; butirosin sulphate]
butirosin sulfate USAN *antibacterial antibiotic* [also: butirosin; butirosin sulphate]
butirosin sulphate BAN *antibacterial antibiotic* [also: butirosin sulfate; butirosin]
Butisol Sodium tablets, elixir ℞ *sedative; hypnotic* [butabarbital sodium] 30, 50 mg; 30 mg/5 mL
butixirate USAN, INN *analgesic; antirheumatic*
butixocort INN
butizide INN *diuretic; antihypertensive* [also: buthiazide]
butobarbitone BAN [also: butethal]
butobendine INN
butoconazole INN, BAN *topical antifungal* [also: butoconazole nitrate]
butoconazole nitrate USAN, USP *topical antifungal* [also: butoconazole]
butocrolol INN
butoctamide INN [also: butoctamide semisuccinate]
butoctamide semisuccinate JAN [also: butoctamide]
butofilolol INN
butonate USAN, INN *anthelmintic*
butopamine USAN, INN *cardiotonic*
butopiprine INN
butoprozine INN *antiarrhythmic; antianginal* [also: butoprozine HCl] ⊡ batoprazine
butoprozine HCl USAN *antiarrhythmic; antianginal* [also: butoprozine]
butopyrammonium iodide INN
butopyronoxyl USP
butorphanol USAN, INN, BAN *analgesic; antitussive*

butorphanol tartrate USAN, USP, BAN, JAN *narcotic agonist-antagonist analgesic; antitussive* (base=68%) 10 mg nasal spray; 1, 2 mg/mL injection

butoxamine BAN *antidiabetic; antihyperlipoproteinemic* [also: butoxamine HCl; butaxamine]

butoxamine HCl USAN *antidiabetic; antihyperlipoproteinemic* [also: butaxamine; butoxamine]

2-butoxyethyl nicotinate [see: nicoboxil]

butoxylate INN

butoxyphenylacethydroxamic acid [see: bufexamac]

Butrans transdermal patch ℞ *narcotic agonist-antagonist analgesic* [buprenorphine HCl] 5, 10, 20 mcg/hr.

butriptyline INN, BAN *antidepressant* [also: butriptyline HCl]

butriptyline HCl USAN *antidepressant* [also: butriptyline]

butropium bromide INN, JAN

butterbur *(Petasites hybridus)* leaves and root *medicinal herb used as an analgesic for migraines and as an antispasmodic for asthma, cough, and gastrointestinal and urinary tract disorders; not generally regarded as safe and effective due to organ damage and carcinogenic properties*

buttercup *(Ranunculus acris; R. bulbosus; R. scleratus)* plant *medicinal herb used as an acrid, anodyne, antispasmodic, diaphoretic, and rubefacient*

butterfly weed *medicinal herb* [see: pleurisy root]

butternut *(Juglans cinerea)* bark, leaves, flowers *medicinal herb used as an anthelmintic, antiseptic, cathartic, cholagogue, and nervine*

butterweed *medicinal herb* [see: fleabane; horseweed]

butydrine [see: butidrine]

butyl alcohol NF *solvent*

butyl aminobenzoate (butyl p-aminobenzoate) [now: butamben]

butyl p-aminobenzoate picrate [see: butamben picrate]

butyl chloride NF

butyl 2-cyanoacrylate [see: enbucrilate]

butyl DNJ (deoxynojirimycin) [see: deoxynojirimycin]

butyl p-hydroxybenzoate [see: butylparaben]

butyl methoxydibenzoylmethane [see: avobenzone]

butyl nitrite; isobutyl nitrite *amyl nitrite substitutes, sold as euphoric street drugs, which produce a quick but short-lived "rush"* [see also: amyl nitrite; volatile nitrites]

butyl parahydroxybenzoate JAN *antifungal agent* [also: butylparaben]

p-butylaminobenzoyldiethylaminoethyl HCl JAN

butylated hydroxyanisole (BHA) NF, BAN *antioxidant*

butylated hydroxytoluene (BHT) NF, BAN *antioxidant*

α-butylbenzyl alcohol [see: fenipentol]

1-butylbiguanide [see: buformin]

N-butyl-deoxynojirimycin [see: deoxynojirimycin]

1,4-butylene glycol (1,4-BG) *precursor to gamma hydroxybutyrate (GHB); a formerly legal alternative to GHB, now also illegal (Schedule I)* [see: gamma hydroxybutyrate (GHB)]

1,5-(butylimino)-1,5-dideoxy-D-glucitol *investigational (orphan) for Fabry disease*

butylmesityl oxide [see: butopyronoxyl]

butylparaben NF *antifungal agent* [also: butyl parahydroxybenzoate]

butylphenamide

butylphenylsalicylamide [see: butylphenamide]

butylscopolamine bromide JAN

butynamine INN

butyrate propionate [see: probutate; buteprate]

butyrophenones *a class of dopamine receptor antagonists with conventional (typical) antipsychotic activity* [also called: phenylbutylpiperadines]

butyrylcholesterinase *investigational (orphan) agent for reduction and clear-*

ance of serum cocaine levels and post-surgical apnea

butyrylperazine [see: butaperazine]

O-butyrylthiamine disulfide [see: bisbutitiamine]

butyvinyl [see: vinylbital]

buzepide metiodide INN

BV-araU (bromovinyl arabinosyl-uracil) [see: sorivudine]

B-Vex D oral suspension (discontinued 2009) ℞ *decongestant; antihistamine* [phenylephrine tannate; bromphen-iramine tannate] 20•12 mg/5 mL

B-Vex PD oral suspension ℞ *decongestant; antihistamine* [pseudoephedrine tannate; brompheniramine tannate] 30•6 mg/5 mL

BVU (bromoisovaleryl urea) [see: bromisovalum]

BW 12C *investigational (orphan) agent for sickle cell disease*

Byclomine capsules, tablets (discontinued 2011) ℞ *gastrointestinal anticholinergic/antispasmodic for irritable bowel syndrome (IBS)* [dicyclomine HCl] 10 mg; 20 mg ⅌ picolamine

Bydureon Ⓔ extended-release injection *investigational (NDA filed) once-weekly antidiabetic for type 2 diabetes; investigational (Phase II) once-monthly dosing* [exenatide]

Byetta subcu injection in prefilled pen injector ℞ *antidiabetic for type 2 diabetes that improves the body's normal glucose-sensing mechanisms and slows gastric emptying* [exenatide] 5, 10 mcg/dose (250 mcg/mL)

Bystolic tablets ℞ *beta-blocker for hypertension* [nebivolol (as HCl)] 2.5, 5, 10, 20 mg

C (vitamin C) [see: ascorbic acid]

C & E softgels OTC *vitamin supplement* [vitamins C and E] 500•400 mg

C Factors "1000" Plus tablets OTC *vitamin C supplement with multiple bioflavonoids* [vitamin C; rose hips; citrus bioflavonoids; rutin; hesperidin] 1000•25•250•50•25 mg

C vitamin [see: ascorbic acid]

^{14}C urea *diagnostic aid for* H. pylori *in the stomach* [also: carbon C 14 urea]

C1-inhibitor, human (C1-INH) *serine proteinase inhibitor (serpin) to prevent acute attacks of angioedema in adolescents or adults with hereditary angioedema*

CA (cytarabine, asparaginase) *chemotherapy protocol for acute myelocytic leukemia (AML)*

^{45}Ca [see: calcium chloride Ca 45]

^{47}Ca [see: calcium chloride Ca 47]

cabastine INN

cabazitaxel *microtubule inhibitor antineoplastic for metastatic hormone-refractory prostate cancer (mHRPC)*

cabbage, cow *medicinal herb* [see: masterwort; white pond lily]

cabbage, meadow; swamp cabbage *medicinal herb* [see: skunk cabbage]

cabbage, water *medicinal herb* [see: white pond lily]

cabergoline USAN, INN *dopamine agonist for hyperprolactinemia* 0.5 mg oral

cabis bromatum [see: bibrocathol]

CABO (cisplatin, Abitrexate, bleomycin, Oncovin) *chemotherapy protocol for head and neck cancer*

cabufocon A USAN *hydrophobic contact lens material*

cabufocon B USAN *hydrophobic contact lens material*

cacao butter JAN *suppository base; emollient/protectant* [also: cocoa butter]

Cachexon *investigational (orphan) for AIDS-related cachexia* [L-glutathione, reduced]

cactinomycin USAN, INN *antibiotic antineoplastic* [also: actinomycin C]

cade oil [see: juniper tar]

cadexomer INN

cadexomer iodine USAN, INN, BAN *antiseptic; antiulcerative wound dressing*

cadmium *element* (Cd)

cadralazine INN, BAN, JAN

Ca-DTPA (calcium pentetate) [see: pentetate calcium trisodium]

Caduet film-coated tablets ℞ *combination calcium channel blocker and HMG-CoA reductase inhibitor for coronary artery disease (CAD), hypertension, chronic unstable angina, and hyperlipidemia* [amlodipine besylate; atorvastatin (as calcium)] 2.5•10, 2.5•20, 2.5•40, 5•10, 5•20, 5•40, 5•80, 10•10, 10•20, 10•40, 10•80 mg ⧄ Duet

CAE (cyclophosphamide, Adriamycin, etoposide) *chemotherapy protocol for small cell lung cancer (SCLC)* [also known as: ACE]

CAF (cyclophosphamide, Adriamycin, fluorouracil); CAF, dose dense *chemotherapy protocol for breast cancer*

cafaminol INN

Cafatine suppositories (discontinued 2008) ℞ *migraine-specific vasoconstrictor* [ergotamine tartrate; caffeine] 2•200 mg

Cafatine-PB tablets ℞ *migraine treatment; vasoconstrictor; anticholinergic; sedative* [ergotamine tartrate; caffeine; pentobarbital sodium; belladonna extract] 1•100•30•0.125 mg

Cafcit oral solution, injectable ℞ *analeptic; CNS stimulant for apnea of prematurity (orphan)* [caffeine citrate] 20 mg/mL

cafedrine INN, BAN

Cafergot suppositories (discontinued 2008) ℞ *migraine treatment; vasoconstrictor* [ergotamine tartrate; caffeine] 2•100 mg

Cafergot tablets ℞ *migraine treatment; vasoconstrictor* [ergotamine tartrate; caffeine] 1•100 mg

Caffedrine tablets OTC *CNS stimulant; analeptic* [caffeine] 200 mg

caffeic acid phenethyl ester (CAPE) *antimicrobial substance found in bee propolis*

caffeine USP, BAN, JAN *methylxanthine analeptic; CNS stimulant; diuretic; treatment for apnea of prematurity (orphan); potentiator of various NSAIDs* ⧄ C-Phen; Kuvan

caffeine citrate *methylxanthine analeptic; CNS stimulant for apnea of prematurity (orphan)* 10, 20 mg/mL oral; 10, 20 mg/mL injection

caffeine monohydrate [see: caffeine, citrated]

caffeine nut *medicinal herb* [see: kola nut]

caffeine & sodium benzoate *analeptic for respiratory depression due to an overdose of CNS depressants* 250 mg/mL injection

Cal Carb-HD powder for oral solution OTC *calcium supplement* [calcium carbonate] 2.5 g Ca/pkt.

Caladryl cream (discontinued 2007) OTC *antihistamine; astringent; antipruritic; emollient* [diphenhydramine HCl; calamine] 1%•8%

Caladryl lotion OTC *poison ivy treatment* [calamine; pramoxine HCl; alcohol 2.2%] 8%•1%

Caladryl Clear lotion OTC *poison ivy treatment* [pramoxine HCl; zinc acetate; alcohol 2%] 1%•0.1%

Calafol tablets ℞ *vitamin/calcium supplement* [vitamins B_6, B_{12}, and D; calcium; folic acid] 25 mg•425 mcg•400 U•400 mg•1.6 mg ⧄ clove oil

Calagel gel OTC *poison ivy treatment* [diphenhydramine HCl; zinc acetate; benzethonium chloride] 2%•0.215%•0.15%

calamine USP, JAN *topical protectant; antipruritic; astringent; poison ivy treatment* ⧄ Chlo-Amine; gallamine

Calamine, Phenolated lotion OTC *poison ivy treatment* [calamine; zinc oxide; phenol] 8%•8%•1%

Calamine Lotion OTC *poison ivy treatment* [calamine; zinc oxide] 6.97%• 6.97%

calamint (*Calamintha officinalis*) *medicinal herb* [see: summer savory]

Calamintha hortensis medicinal herb [see: summer savory]

Calamintha montana medicinal herb [see: winter savory]

calamus (*Acorus calamus*) rhizome *medicinal herb for anxiety, bad breath from smoking, colic, digestive disorders, fever, gas, irritated throat, and promoting wound healing; not generally regarded as safe and effective and is prohibited in the U.S. as a food additive or supplement*

Calamycin lotion OTC *antihistamine; astringent; anesthetic; antiseptic* [pyrilamine maleate; zinc oxide; calamine; benzocaine; chloroxylenol; alcohol 2%]

Calan film-coated tablets (discontinued 2009) ℞ *antianginal; antiarrhythmic; antihypertensive; calcium channel blocker* [verapamil HCl] 40, 80, 120 mg ⊡ Clenia; Gilenya; kaolin; khellin

Calan SR film-coated sustained-release tablets ℞ *antihypertensive; antianginal; antiarrhythmic; calcium channel blocker* [verapamil HCl] 120, 180, 240 mg

Calcarb 600 with Vitamin D tablets OTC *calcium supplement* [calcium (as carbonate); vitamin D] 600 mg•200 U

Cal-Carb Forte chewable tablets, caplets OTC *antacid; calcium supplement* [calcium (as carbonate)] 500 mg (1250 mg)

Cal-C-Caps capsules OTC *calcium supplement* [calcium (as citrate)] 180 mg (860 mg) ⊡ gelcaps

Cal-Cee tablets OTC *calcium supplement* [calcium (as citrate)] 250 mg (1150 mg) ⊡ Colace

Calcet film-coated tablets OTC *calcium supplement* [calcium; vitamin D] 150 mg•100 U ⊡ Glyset

Calcet Plus film-coated tablets OTC *vitamin/calcium/iron supplement* [multiple vitamins; calcium (as carbonate); iron (as ferrous fumarate); folic acid] ≛•152.8•18•0.8 mg

Calcibind powder for oral solution ℞ *antiurolithic to prevent stone formation in absorptive calciuria type I* [cellulose sodium phosphate] 300 g bulk pack

Calcibon oral suspension OTC *mineral supplement* [multiple minerals; vitamin D] ≛•66.67 U/5 mL ⊡ clozapine

CalciCaps tablets (discontinued 2008) OTC *calcium supplement* [calcium (as dibasic calcium phosphate, gluconate, and carbonate); vitamin D] 125 mg•67 U

CalciCaps with Iron tablets (discontinued 2008) OTC *calcium/iron supplement* [calcium (as dibasic calcium phosphate, gluconate, and carbonate); vitamin D; iron (as ferrous gluconate)] 125 mg•67 U•7 mg

Calci-Chew chewable tablets OTC *calcium supplement* [calcium (as carbonate)] 500 mg (1250 mg)

calcidiol [see: calcifediol]

calcifediol (**25-hydroxycholecalciferol; 25-hydroxyvitamin D₃**) USAN, USP, INN *vitamin D precursor (converted to calcitriol in the body); calcium regulator for treatment of metastatic bone disease or hypocalcemia associated with chronic renal dialysis*

calciferol [now: ergocalciferol]

Calciferol Drops for oral or IM administration OTC *vitamin supplement; vitamin deficiency therapy for refractory rickets, familial hypophosphatemia, and hypoparathyroidism* [ergocalciferol (vitamin D₂)] 8000 U/mL

Calcifolic-D wafers ℞ *vitamin/calcium supplement* [vitamins B₆, B₁₂, and D; calcium; folic acid] 10 mg•125 mcg•300 U•≛•1 mg

Calcijex injection ℞ *vitamin D therapy for hypoparathyroidism and hypocalce-*

mia of chronic renal dialysis [calcitriol] 1 mcg/mL

Calci-Mix capsules OTC *calcium supplement* [calcium (as carbonate)] 500 mg (1250 mg)

Calcionate syrup OTC *calcium supplement* [calcium (as glubionate)] 117 mg/5 mL (1.8 g/5 mL)

calcipotriene USAN *topical antipsoriatic* [also: calcipotriol] 0.005% topical

calcipotriol INN, BAN *topical antipsoriatic* [also: calcipotriene]

Calciquid syrup OTC *calcium supplement* [calcium (as glubionate)] 117 mg/5 mL (1.8 g/5 mL)

calcitonin (human) USAN, INN, BAN, JAN *calcium regulator for symptomatic Paget disease (osteitis deformans) (orphan)*

calcitonin (salmon) USAN, INN, BAN *calcium regulator for Paget disease (orphan), hypercalcemia, and postmenopausal osteoporosis* 200 IU/dose nasal spray

calcitonin gene-related peptide (CGRP) antagonists *investigational (Phase III) class of agents for migraine headaches*

calcitonin salmon (synthesis) JAN *synthetic analogue of calcitonin (salmon); calcium regulator* [also: salcatonin]

Cal-Citrate tablets, capsules OTC *calcium supplement* [calcium (as citrate)] 250 mg (1150 mg); 225 mg (1070 mg)

calcitriol (1α,25-dihydroxycholecalciferol; 1,25-hydroxyvitamin D$_3$; 1,25 [OH]$_2$D$_3$) USAN, INN, BAN, JAN *physiologically active form of vitamin D; calcium regulator for hypoparathyroidism and hypocalcemia due to chronic renal dialysis; topical treatment of plaque psoriasis* 0.25, 0.5 mcg oral; 1 mcg/mL oral; 1, 2 mcg injection

calcium *element* (Ca)

calcium, oyster shell [see: calcium carbonate]

Calcium 500 chewable tablets OTC *calcium supplement* [calcium; vitamin D] 500 mg•100 IU

Calcium 500+D; Calcium 600+D; Calcium 1000+D tablets, caplets OTC *calcium supplement* [calcium; vitamin D$_3$] 500 mg•400 IU; 600 mg•200 IU, 600 mg•400 IU; 1000 mg•800 IU

Calcium 600 tablets OTC *calcium supplement* [calcium (as carbonate)] 600 mg (1500 mg)

Calcium 600 with Vitamin D tablets OTC *calcium supplement* [calcium; vitamin D] 600 mg•200 IU, 600 mg•400 IU

Calcium 600-D tablets OTC *calcium supplement* [calcium; vitamin D] 600 mg•200 IU

calcium acetate USP, JAN *dietary calcium supplement (25% elemental calcium); buffering agent for hyperphosphatemia of end-stage renal disease (orphan)* 667 mg oral (169 mg Ca)

calcium alginate fiber *topical hemostatic*

calcium aminacyl B-PAS (benzoyl para-aminosalicylate) [see: benzoylpas calcium]

calcium 4-aminosalicylate trihydrate [see: aminosalicylate calcium]

calcium amphomycin [see: amphomycin]

Calcium Antacid chewable tablets OTC *antacid; calcium supplement* [calcium (as carbonate)] 300 mg (750 mg)

calcium antagonists *a class of coronary vasodilators that inhibit cardiac muscle contraction and slow cardiac electrical conduction velocity* [also called: calcium channel blockers; slow channel blockers]

calcium ascorbate (vitamin C) USP *water-soluble vitamin; antiscorbutic* 500 mg oral; 3256 mg/tsp. oral

calcium benzamidosalicylate INN, BAN *antibacterial; tuberculostatic* [also: benzoylpas calcium]

calcium benzoyl *p*-aminosalicylate (B-PAS) [see: benzoylpas calcium]

calcium benzoylpas [see: benzoylpas calcium]

calcium bis-dioctyl sulfosuccinate
[see: docusate calcium]

calcium bis-glycinate *dietary calcium supplement*

calcium bromide JAN

calcium carbimide INN [also: cyanamide]

calcium carbonate USP *antacid; dietary calcium supplement (40% elemental calcium); investigational (orphan) for hyperphosphatemia of end-stage renal disease* [also: precipitated calcium carbonate] 500, 600, 650, 1250, 1500 mg oral; 1250 mg/5 mL oral

Calcium Carbonate tablets OTC *calcium supplement* [calcium (as carbonate); vitamin D] 600 mg•200 IU

calcium carbonate, precipitated
[now: calcium carbonate]

calcium carbophil *bulk laxative*

calcium caseinate *dietary calcium supplement; infant formula modifier*

calcium channel blockers *a class of coronary vasodilators that inhibit cardiac muscle contraction and slow cardiac electrical conduction velocity* [also called: calcium antagonists; slow channel blockers]

calcium chloride USP, JAN *calcium replenisher*

calcium chloride Ca 45 USAN *radioactive agent*

calcium chloride Ca 47 USAN *radioactive agent*

calcium chloride dihydrate [see: calcium chloride]

calcium citrate USP *dietary calcium supplement (21% elemental calcium)* 0.95, 1.2 g oral; 3.6 g/5 mL oral

calcium citrate tetrahydrate [see: calcium citrate]

calcium clofibrate INN

calcium cyanamide [see: calcium carbimide]

calcium D-glucarate tetrahydrate [see: calcium saccharate]

calcium D-gluconate lactobionate monohydrate [see: calcium glubionate]

calcium dioctyl sulfosuccinate [see: docusate calcium]

calcium disodium edathamil [see: edetate calcium disodium]

calcium disodium edetate JAN *heavy metal chelating agent* [also: edetate calcium disodium; sodium calcium edetate; sodium calciumedetate]

Calcium Disodium Versenate IM, IV, or subcu injection ℞ *chelating agent for acute or chronic lead poisoning and lead encephalopathy* [edetate calcium disodium] 200 mg/mL

calcium dobesilate INN

calcium doxybensylate [see: calcium dobesilate]

calcium DTPA [see: pentetate calcium trisodium]

calcium edetate sodium [see: edetate calcium disodium]

calcium EDTA (ethylene diamine tetraacetic acid) [see: edetate calcium disodium]

calcium folinate INN, BAN, JAN *antianemic; folate replenisher; antidote to folic acid antagonists* [also: leucovorin calcium]

calcium glubionate USAN, INN *dietary calcium supplement (6.5% elemental calcium)*

calcium gluceptate USP *parenteral calcium replenisher* [also: calcium glucoheptonate]

calcium glucoheptonate INN *parenteral calcium replenisher* [also: calcium gluceptate]

calcium gluconate (calcium D-gluconate) USP *dietary calcium supplement (9% elemental calcium); investigational (orphan) wash for hydrofluoric acid burns* 500, 556, 650, 975, 1000 mg oral; 3.85 g/15 mL oral; 10% injection

calcium glycerinophosphate [see: calcium glycerophosphate]

calcium glycerophosphate NF, JAN

calcium hopantenate JAN

calcium hydroxide USP *astringent*

calcium hydroxide phosphate [see: calcium phosphate, tribasic]

calcium hydroxyapatite, microcrystalline *calcium supplement* 150 mg oral

calcium hydroxylapatite *subcutaneous collagen production stimulant for HIV-related facial lipoatrophy and moderate to severe facial wrinkles and folds; oral calcium supplement*

calcium hypophosphite NF

calcium iodide *expectorant*

calcium iodododocosanoate [see: iodobehenate calcium]

calcium lactate USP, JAN *dietary calcium supplement (13% elemental calcium)* 650, 770 mg oral

calcium lactate hydrate [see: calcium lactate]

calcium lactate pentahydrate [see: calcium lactate]

calcium lactobionate USP *dietary calcium supplement*

calcium lactobionate dihydrate [see: calcium lactobionate]

calcium lactophosphate NF

calcium L-aspartate JAN

calcium levofolinate [see: levoleucovorin calcium]

calcium levulate [see: calcium levulinate]

calcium levulinate USP *dietary calcium supplement*

calcium levulinate dihydrate [see: calcium levulinate]

Calcium & Magnesium tablets OTC *mineral supplement* [calcium; magnesium] 100•50 mg

Calcium/Magnesium tablets OTC *mineral supplement* [calcium; magnesium] 1000•500 mg

Calcium Magnesium Zinc film-coated caplets OTC *vitamin/mineral supplement* [calcium; magnesium; zinc; vitamin D] $\underline{?}$•$\underline{?}$•$\underline{?}$•200 IU

calcium mandelate USP

calcium MCHA (microcrystalline hydroxyapatite) [see: calcium hydroxyapatite, microcrystalline]

calcium oxide [see: lime]

calcium pangamate [now: dimethylglycine HCl]

calcium pantothenate (calcium D-pantothenate; vitamin B$_5$) USP, INN, JAN *water-soluble vitamin; coenzyme A precursor* [also: pantothenic acid] 100, 218, 545 mg oral

calcium pantothenate, racemic (calcium DL-pantothenate) USP *water-soluble vitamin; enzyme cofactor*

calcium para-aminosalicylate JAN [also: aminosalicylate calcium]

calcium phosphate, dibasic USP, JAN *dietary calcium supplement; tablet base*

calcium phosphate, monocalcium [see: calcium phosphate, dibasic]

calcium phosphate, tribasic NF *dietary calcium supplement (39% elemental calcium)* [also: durapatite; hydroxyapatite]

calcium polycarbophil USAN, USP *bulk laxative; antidiarrheal*

calcium polystyrene sulfonate JAN *ion exchange resin for hyperkalemia*

calcium polysulfide & calcium thiosulfate [see: lime, sulfurated]

calcium saccharate USP, INN *stabilizer*

calcium silicate NF *tablet excipient*

calcium sodium ferriclate INN *hematinic* [also: ferriclate calcium sodium]

calcium stearate NF, JAN *tablet and capsule lubricant*

calcium sulfate NF *tablet and capsule diluent*

calcium tetracemine disodium [see: edetate calcium disodium]

calcium trisodium pentetate INN, BAN *plutonium chelating agent* [also: pentetate calcium trisodium]

calcium 10-undecenoate [see: calcium undecylenate]

calcium undecylenate USAN *antifungal*

Calcium with Vitamin D tablets OTC *calcium supplement* [calcium; vitamin D] 1000 mg•400 IU

calciumedetate sodium [see: edetate calcium disodium]

Calcium-Folic Acid Plus D chewable wafers R *vitamin/mineral/calcium supplement* [multiple vitamins & minerals; calcium (as carbonate); folic acid] $\pm$•537•1 mg

Caldesene ointment OTC *moisturizer; emollient; astringent* [cod liver oil (vitamins A and D); zinc oxide; lanolin] ⊡ clodazon

Caldesene topical powder OTC *drying agent; astringent; emollient* [talc; zinc oxide] 81%●15% ⊡ clodazon

caldiamide INN *pharmaceutic aid* [also: caldiamide sodium]

caldiamide sodium USAN, BAN *pharmaceutic aid* [also: caldiamide]

Caldolor IV injection ℞ *analgesic; antipyretic; antiarthritic; nonsteroidal anti-inflammatory drug (NSAID)* [ibuprofen] 100 mg/mL

Calel D tablets (discontinued 2008) OTC *calcium supplement* [calcium carbonate; vitamin D] 500 mg●200 IU

Calendula officinalis medicinal herb [see: marigold]

calfactant USAN *surface-active extract of saline lavage of calf lungs, used for prevention of respiratory distress syndrome (RDS) in premature infants (orphan)*

Cal-G capsules OTC *calcium supplement* [calcium (as gluconate)] 50 mg (700 mg)

CAL-G; CALGB 8811; CALGB 9111 *chemotherapy protocol for acute lymphocytic leukemia (ALL)* [see: Larson regimen]

Cal-Gest chewable tablets OTC *calcium supplement* [calcium (as carbonate)] 200 mg (500 mg)

Calgonate wash *investigational (orphan) emergency treatment for hydrofluoric acid burns* [calcium gluconate]

California barberry *medicinal herb* [see: Oregon grape]

California buckthorn *medicinal herb* [see: buckthorn; cascara sagrada]

California false hellebore (Veratrum californicum) [see: hellebore]

californium *element (Cf)*

calioben [see: calcium iodobehenate]

Cal-Lac capsules OTC *calcium supplement* [calcium (as lactate)] 96 mg (500 mg)

Callergy Clear lotion OTC *local anesthetic; astringent; emollient* [pramoxine HCl; zinc oxide] 1%●0.1%

Calluna vulgaris medicinal herb [see: heather]

Calmasyn ointment OTC *astringent; mild anesthetic; antipruritic; counterirritant* [zinc oxide; menthol] 20%●0.45%

calmatives *a class of soothing agents that reduce excitement, nervousness, distress, or irritation* [also called: sedatives]

Calmol 4 rectal suppositories OTC *emollient; astringent* [cocoa butter; zinc oxide] 80%●10%

Calmoseptine ointment OTC *astringent; mild anesthetic; antipruritic; counterirritant* [zinc oxide; menthol] 20.6%●0.44%

Calm-X tablets (discontinued 2008) OTC *anticholinergic; antiemetic; antivertigo agent; motion sickness preventative* [dimenhydrinate] 50 mg

Cal-Nate film-coated tablets (discontinued 2009) ℞ *prenatal vitamin/mineral/calcium/iron supplement; stool softener* [multiple vitamins & minerals; calcium; iron (as carbonyl and ferrous gluconate); folic acid; docusate sodium; hydrogenated oil] ±●125●27●1●50 mg ⊡ kola nut

calomel NF

CaloMist nasal spray (discontinued 2010) ℞ *once-daily maintenance administration following intramuscular vitamin B_{12} therapy* [cyanocobalamin] 25 mcg/0.1 mL dose

Calphosan IV injection ℞ *calcium replacement* [calcium glycerophosphate; calcium lactate] 50●50 mg/10 mL (0.08 mEq Ca/mL) ⊡ clofezone

Calphron tablets ℞ *calcium supplement; buffering agent for hyperphosphatemia in end-stage renal failure (orphan)* [calcium (as acetate)] 169 mg (667 mg) ⊡ Claforan; Kolephrin

calteridol INN *pharmaceutic aid* [also: calteridol calcium]

calteridol calcium USAN, BAN *pharmaceutic aid* [also: calteridol]

Caltha palustris *medicinal herb* [see: cowslip]

Caltrate 600 film-coated tablets OTC *calcium supplement* [calcium (as carbonate)] 600 mg (1500 mg)

Caltrate 600 + D tablets OTC *calcium supplement* [calcium (as carbonate); vitamin D] 600 mg•400 IU

Caltrate 600 + D Plus Minerals tablets, chewable tablets OTC *calcium/mineral supplement* [calcium (as carbonate); multiple minerals; vitamin D; hydrogenated oil] 600 mg• ± • 400 IU

Caltrate 600 + Iron/Vitamin D film-coated tablets (discontinued 2008) OTC *dietary supplement* [calcium carbonate; ferrous fumarate; vitamin D] 600 mg•18 mg•125 IU

Caltrate Colon Health tablets OTC *calcium supplement* [calcium; vitamin D; hydrogenated oil] ± •200 IU

Caltrate Plus tablets (discontinued 2008) OTC *dietary supplement* [calcium carbonate; vitamin D; multiple minerals] 600 mg•200 IU• ±

Caltro tablets (discontinued 2008) OTC *calcium supplement* [calcium; vitamin D] 250 mg•125 IU ⑦ coal tar; Kaletra

calumba; calumba root; calumbo *medicinal herb* [see: colombo]

calusterone USAN, INN *antineoplastic*

Calvite P & D tablets OTC *mineral supplement* [calcium; phosphorus; vitamin D] ± • ± •120 IU

Calypte test kit for professional use ℞ *urine test for HIV-1 antibodies*

Cama Arthritis Pain Reliever tablets (discontinued 2007) OTC *analgesic; antipyretic; anti-inflammatory; antirheumatic* [aspirin (buffered with magnesium oxide and aluminum hydroxide)] 500 mg

camazepam INN

cambendazole USAN, INN, BAN *anthelmintic*

Cambia oral solution ℞ *analgesic; non-steroidal anti-inflammatory drug for osteoarthritis, rheumatoid arthritis,* ankylosing spondylitis, and dysmenorrhea [diclofenac (as potassium)] 50 mg/5 mL

camellia oil JAN

Camellia sinensis *medicinal herb* [see: green tea]

Cameo Oil OTC *bath emollient*

camiglibose USAN, INN *antidiabetic*

Camila tablets (in packs of 28) ℞ *oral contraceptive (progestin only)* [norethindrone] 0.35 mg ⑦ COMLA

camiverine INN

camomile *medicinal herb* [see: chamomile]

camonagrel INN

camostat INN [also: camostat mesilate]

camostat mesilate JAN [also: camostat]

cAMP (cyclic adenosine monophosphate) [see: adenosine phosphate]

CAMP (cyclophosphamide, Adriamycin, methotrexate, procarbazine HCl) *chemotherapy protocol for non–small cell lung cancer (NSCLC)* ⑦ COMP

Campath IV infusion ℞ *monoclonal antibody antineoplastic for B-cell chronic lymphocytic leukemia (B-CLL; orphan); investigational (Phase III) cerebral anti-inflammatory for multiple sclerosis* [alemtuzumab] 30 mg/mL

camphetamide [see: camphotamide]

Campho-Phenique topical liquid, gel OTC *mild anesthetic; anti-infective; counterirritant* [camphor; phenol; eucalyptus oil] 10.8%•4.7%• ±

Campho-Phenique Cold Sore Treatment and Scab Relief cream OTC *anesthetic for cold sores and fever blisters* [pramoxine HCl; petrolatum] 1%•30%

camphor (d-camphor; dl-camphor) USP, JAN *topical antipruritic; mild local anesthetic; counterirritant* [also: trans-π-oxocamphor] ⑦ comfrey

camphor, monobromated USP

camphorated opium tincture [now: paregoric]

camphorated parachlorophenol [see: parachlorophenol, camphorated]

camphoric acid USP

camphotamide INN

Campral enteric-coated delayed-release tablets ℞ GABA/taurine analogue for the treatment of alcoholism [acamprosate calcium] 333 mg

Camptosar IV infusion ℞ topoisomerase I inhibitor; antineoplastic for metastatic colorectal cancer [irinotecan HCl] 20 mg/mL

camptothecin-11 (CPT-11) [see: irinotecan]

camsilate INN combining name for radicals or groups [also: camsylate]

camsylate USAN, BAN combining name for radicals or groups [also: camsilate]

Camvirex investigational (orphan) pediatric HIV/AIDS infections [rubitecan]

camylofin INN

Canada fleabane medicinal herb [see: fleabane; horseweed]

Canada pitch tree medicinal herb [see: hemlock]

Canada root medicinal herb [see: pleurisy root]

Canada tea medicinal herb [see: wintergreen]

canagliflozin investigational (Phase III) sodium-glucose transporter 2 (SGLT-2) inhibitor to increase the excretion of glucose in the urine for type 2 diabetes

canaigre (Rumex hymenosepalus) medicinal herb for a variety of disease states and used as a purported substitute for ginseng; not generally regarded as safe and effective because of high tannin content and possible mutagenic effect when used internally ② ginger

canakinumab monoclonal anti-inflammatory for cryopyrin-associated periodic syndrome (CAPS) and its variants, familial cold autoinflammatory syndrome (FCAS), and Muckle-Wells syndrome (orphan); investigational for systemic juvenile idiopathic arthritis (SJIA)

Canasa rectal suppositories ℞ anti-inflammatory for active ulcerative colitis, proctosigmoiditis, and proctitis [mesalamine (5-aminosalicylic acid)] 1000 mg

canbisol INN

Cancidas powder for IV infusion ℞ antifungal for candidiasis, candidemia, invasive aspergillosis and other resistant fungal infections [caspofungin acetate] 50, 70 mg/vial

candesartan USAN, INN angiotensin receptor blocker (ARB) for hypertension

candesartan cilexetil USAN angiotensin receptor blocker (ARB) for hypertension and heart failure

candicidin USAN, USP, INN, BAN polyene antifungal

Candida albicans skin test antigen diagnostic aid for diminished cellular immunity; test for HIV patients to assess TB antigen response

CandidaSure reagent slides for professional use ℞ in vitro diagnostic aid for Candida albicans in the vagina

Candin intradermal injection ℞ diagnostic aid for diminished cellular immunity; test for HIV patients to assess TB antigen response [Candida albicans skin test antigen] 0.1 mL ② quinidine

candleberry; candleberry myrtle medicinal herb [see: bayberry; tung seed]

candocuronium iodide INN

candoxatril USAN, INN, BAN antihypertensive

candoxatrilat USAN, INN, BAN antihypertensive

Cankaid oral solution OTC anti-inflammatory; antiseptic [carbamide peroxide] 10%

cankerroot medicinal herb [see: gold thread]

canna; channa medicinal herb [see: kanna]

cannabidinol (CBD) INN, BAN a nonpsychoactive derivative of the Cannabis sativa (marijuana) plant; investigational (Phase III) in the U.S. and approved in Canada and Europe as an analgesic for pain associated with cancer and multiple sclerosis

Cannabis sativa (marijuana; marihuana; hashish) euphoric/hallucinogenic street drug made from the resin or dried leaves and flowering tops of the *cannabis plant; medicinal herb for asthma, analgesia, leprosy, and loss of appetite*

canrenoate potassium USAN *aldosterone antagonist* [also: canrenoic acid; potassium canrenoate]

canrenoic acid INN, BAN *aldosterone antagonist* [also: canrenoate potassium; potassium canrenoate]

canrenone USAN, INN *aldosterone antagonist*

cantharides JAN

cantharidin *topical keratolytic*

Cantil tablets ℞ *GI anticholinergic/antispasmodic; adjunctive treatment for peptic ulcers* [mepenzolate bromide] 25 mg

CAP (cellulose acetate phthalate) [q.v.]

CAP (cyclophosphamide, Adriamycin, Platinol) *chemotherapy protocol for non–small cell lung cancer (NSCLC) and mesothelioma*

Capacet capsules ℞ *barbiturate sedative; analgesic; antipyretic* [butalbital; acetaminophen; caffeine] 50•325•40 mg

Capastat Sulfate powder for IM injection ℞ *tuberculostatic* [capreomycin sulfate] 1 g/vial

CAPE (caffeic acid phenethyl ester) *antimicrobial substance found in bee propolis*

Cape aloe *medicinal herb* [see: aloe]

cape gum *medicinal herb* [see: acacia]

capecitabine USAN, INN, BAN *oral fluoropyrimidine (a 5-FU prodrug) antineoplastic for metastatic breast and colorectal cancer; also used for pancreatic cancer*

capers (Capparis spinosa) flower buds and leaves *medicinal herb for skin disorders and for reducing the effects of enlarged capillaries*

Capex shampoo ℞ *corticosteroidal antiinflammatory; antiseborrheic* [fluocinolone acetonide] 0.01% ☒ Copegus

Caphosol oral solution OTC *saline laxative; electrolytes* [monobasic sodium phosphate; dibasic sodium phosphate; calcium chloride; sodium chloride] 0.9•3.2•5.2•56.9 g

capimorelin tartrate [see: capromorelin tartrate]

Capital with Codeine oral suspension ℞ *narcotic antitussive; analgesic; antipyretic* [codeine phosphate; acetaminophen] 12•120 mg/5 mL

Capitrol shampoo (discontinued 2010) ℞ *antibacterial and antifungal for seborrheic dermatitis* [chloroxine] 2% ☒ Gabitril

caplet (dosage form) *capsule-shaped tablet* ☒ cobalt

Capmist DM caplets OTC *antitussive; decongestant; expectorant* [dextromethorphan hydrobromide; pseudoephedrine HCl; guaifenesin] 25•30•600 mg

capmul 8210 [see: monoctanoin]

capobenate sodium USAN *antiarrhythmic*

capobenic acid USAN, INN *antiarrhythmic*

Capoten tablets ℞ *angiotensin-converting enzyme (ACE) inhibitor for hypertension, congestive heart failure (CHF), and left ventricular dysfunction (LVD) after MI; also used for the treatment of Raynaud phenomenon* [captopril] 12.5, 25, 50, 100 mg

Capozide 25/15; Capozide 25/25; Capozide 50/15; Capozide 50/25 tablets (discontinued 2010) ℞ *combination angiotensin-converting enzyme (ACE) inhibitor and diuretic for hypertension* [captopril; hydrochlorothiazide] 25•15 mg; 25•25 mg; 50•15 mg; 50•25 mg

Capparis spinosa medicinal herb [see: capers]

capreomycin INN, BAN *bactericidal antibiotic; tuberculostatic* [also: capreomycin sulfate]

capreomycin sulfate USAN, USP, JAN *bactericidal antibiotic; tuberculostatic* [also: capreomycin]

Caprogel *investigational (orphan) topical treatment for traumatic hyphema of the eye* [aminocaproic acid]

capromab INN *monoclonal antibody; imaging adjunct for prostate cancer and* *its metastases* [also: capromab pende-tide]

capromab pendetide USAN *monoclonal antibody; after on-site radiolabeling with indium In 111, it becomes* **indium In 111 capromab**, *a radiodiagnostic imaging agent for new or recurrent prostate cancer and its metastases* [also: capromab]

capromorelin tartrate USAN *growth hormone secretagogue for anti-aging, congestive heart failure, and catabolic illness*

caproxamine INN, BAN

caprylidene *dietary supplement to induce hyperketonemia for the management of mild-to-moderate Alzheimer disease; source of medium-chain triglycerides*

capsaicin *counterirritant; topical analgesic for muscle and joint pain, and for the management of neuropathic pain due to postherpetic neuralgia (orphan); investigational (orphan) for erythromelalgia and painful HIV-related neuropathy* 0.025%, 0.075% topical

Capsella bursa-pastoris medicinal herb [see: shepherd's purse]

Capsicum frutescens; C. annuum medicinal herb [see: cayenne]

capsicum oleoresin *topical analgesic; counterirritant*

Capsin lotion OTC *counterirritant; analgesic for muscle and joint pain* [capsaicin] 0.025%, 0.075% ☒ Cubicin; kebuzone; quipazine

Capsulets (trademarked dosage form) *sustained-release caplet*

captab (dosage form) *capsule-shaped tablet*

captamine INN *depigmentor* [also: captamine HCl]

captamine HCl USAN *depigmentor* [also: captamine]

captodiame INN, BAN

captodiame HCl [see: captodiame]

captodiamine HCl [see: captodiame]

captopril USAN, USP, INN, BAN, JAN *angiotensin-converting enzyme (ACE) inhibitor for hypertension, congestive heart failure (CHF), and left ventricu-*

lar dysfunction (LVD) after MI; also used for the treatment of Raynaud phenomenon 12.5, 25, 50, 100 mg oral

captopril & hydrochlorothiazide *combination angiotensin-converting enzyme (ACE) inhibitor and diuretic for hypertension* 25•15, 25•25, 50•15, 50•25 mg oral

capuride USAN, INN *hypnotic* ☒ Key-Pred

Capzasin Quick Relief gel OTC *counterirritant; analgesic for muscle and joint pain; mild anesthetic; antipruritic* [capsaicin; menthol] 0.025%•10%

Capzasin-HP cream OTC *counterirritant; analgesic for muscle and joint pain* [capsaicin] 0.1%

Capzasin-P cream OTC *counterirritant; analgesic for muscle and joint pain* [capsaicin] 0.035%

Carac cream ℞ *antineoplastic for actinic keratoses (AK)* [fluorouracil] 0.5% ☒ Coreg; Kuric

caracemide USAN, INN *antineoplastic*

Carafate tablets, oral suspension ℞ *treatment for duodenal ulcer* [sucralfate] 1 g; 1 g/10 mL ☒ Geravite

caramel NF *coloring agent* ☒ Gerimal

caramiphen INN, BAN *antitussive*

caramiphen edisylate *antitussive*

caramiphen HCl [see: caramiphen]

caraway (*Carum carvi*) NF *seeds medicinal herb for acid indigestion, appetite stimulation, colic, gas, gastrointestinal spasms, and uterine cramps*

caraway oil NF ☒ coral; Kerol

carazolol INN, BAN ☒ Kerasal AL

Carb PSE 12 DM oral suspension ℞ *antitussive; antihistamine; decongestant* [dextromethorphan tannate; carbinoxamine tannate; pseudoephedrine tannate] 27.5•3.2•45.2 mg/5 mL

Carb Pseudo-Tan oral suspension ℞ *antitussive; decongestant* [carbetapentane tannate; pseudoephedrine tannate] 25•75 mg/5 mL

carbacephems *a class of bactericidal antibiotics similar to second-generation cephalosporins (q.v.)*

carbachol USP, INN, BAN, JAN *ophthalmic cholinergic; miotic for surgery; antiglaucoma agent* [also: carbacholine chloride]

carbacholine chloride *ophthalmic cholinergic; miotic for surgery; antiglaucoma agent* [also: carbachol]

carbacrylamine resins

carbadipimidine HCl [see: carpipramine dihydrochloride]

carbadox USAN, INN, BAN *antibacterial*

Carbaglu tablets for oral solution ℞ *treatment for acute hyperammonemia due to a deficiency of the hepatic enzyme N-acetylglutamate synthetase (NAGS) (orphan)* [carglumic acid] 200 mg

carbaldrate INN

carbamate choline chloride [see: carbachol]

carbamazepine USAN, USP, INN, BAN, JAN *iminostilbene anticonvulsant; analgesic for trigeminal neuralgia; antipsychotic for manic episodes of a bipolar disorder; also used for restless legs syndrome (RLS), alcohol withdrawal, and postherpetic neuralgia* 100, 200, 300, 400 mg oral; 100 mg/5 mL oral

carbamide [see: urea]

carbamide peroxide USP *topical dental antiseptic; cerumenolytic to emulsify and disperse ear wax*

N-carbamoylarsanilic acid [see: carbarsone]

carbamoylcholine chloride [see: carbachol]

O-carbamoylsalicylic acid lactam [see: carsalam]

carbamylcholine chloride [see: carbachol]

carbamylglutamic acid [now: carglumic acid]

carbamylmethylcholine chloride [see: bethanechol chloride]

carbantel INN *anthelmintic* [also: carbantel lauryl sulfate]

carbantel lauryl sulfate USAN *anthelmintic* [also: carbantel]

carbapenems *a class of broad-spectrum antibiotics that are effective against both gram-positive and gram-negative bacteria* [also called: "penems"]

Carbaphen 12 oral liquid ℞ *antitussive; antihistamine; decongestant* [carbetapentane tannate; chlorpheniramine tannate; phenylephrine tannate] 60•8•20 mg/5 mL

carbaril INN [also: carbaryl]

carbarsone USP, INN

carbaryl BAN [also: carbaril]

carbasalate calcium INN *analgesic* [also: carbaspirin calcium]

carbaspirin calcium USAN *analgesic* [also: carbasalate calcium]

Carbastat solution (discontinued 2010) ℞ *direct-acting miotic for ophthalmic surgery* [carbachol] 0.01%

Carbatab-12 tablets ℞ *antitussive; decongestant; expectorant* [carbetapentane citrate; phenylephrine HCl; guaifenesin] 60•15•600 mg

Carbatrol extended-release capsules ℞ *iminostilbene anticonvulsant; analgesic for trigeminal neuralgia; also used for restless legs syndrome (RLS), alcohol withdrawal, and postherpetic neuralgia* [carbamazepine] 100, 200, 300 mg

Carbatuss oral liquid ℞ *antitussive; decongestant; expectorant* [carbetapentane citrate; phenylephrine HCl; guaifenesin] 20•10•100 mg/5 mL

Carbatuss CL oral liquid (discontinued 2007) ℞ *antitussive; decongestant; expectorant* [carbetapentane citrate; phenylephrine HCl; potassium guaiacolsulfonate] 20•10•100 mg/5 mL

Carbaxefed RF oral drops (discontinued 2007) ℞ *decongestant; antihistamine* [pseudoephedrine HCl; carbinoxamine maleate] 15•1 mg/mL

carbazeran USAN, INN *cardiotonic*

carbazochrome INN, JAN

carbazochrome salicylate INN

carbazochrome sodium sulfonate INN

carbazocine INN

carbenicillin INN, BAN *extended-spectrum penicillin antibiotic* [also: carbenicillin disodium; carbenicillin sodium]

carbenicillin disodium USAN, USP *extended-spectrum penicillin antibiotic* [also: carbenicillin; carbenicillin sodium]

carbenicillin indanyl sodium USAN, USP *extended-spectrum penicillin antibiotic* (base=76.4%) [also: carindacillin]

carbenicillin phenyl sodium USAN *antibacterial* [also: carfecillin]

carbenicillin potassium USAN *antibacterial*

carbenicillin sodium JAN *antibacterial* [also: carbenicillin disodium; carbenicillin]

carbenoxolone INN, BAN *corticosteroid; anti-inflammatory* [also: carbenoxolone sodium]

carbenoxolone sodium USAN *corticosteroid; anti-inflammatory* [also: carbenoxolone]

carbenzide INN

carbesilate INN *combining name for radicals or groups*

carbetapentane citrate NF *antitussive* [also: pentoxyverine]

carbetapentane tannate *antitussive*

Carbetaplex oral liquid (discontinued 2007) ℞ *antitussive; decongestant; expectorant* [carbetapentane citrate; phenylephrine HCl; guaifenesin] 20•15•100 mg/5 mL

carbetimer USAN, INN *antineoplastic*

carbetocin INN, BAN *uterotonic agent to prevent postpartum hemorrhage following cesarean section*

Carbex tablets (discontinued 2009) ℞ *monoamine oxidase inhibitor (MAOI); dopaminergic for Parkinson disease* [selegiline HCl] 5 mg

Carbic DS pediatric syrup (discontinued 2007) ℞ *decongestant; antihistamine* [pseudoephedrine HCl; carbinoxamine maleate] 25•2 mg/5 mL

carbidopa USAN, USP, INN, BAN, JAN *decarboxylase inhibitor; potentiator of* **levodopa** *for Parkinson disease (no effect when given alone)*

carbidopa & levodopa *dopamine precursor plus potentiator for Parkinson*

disease (orphan) 10•100, 25•100, 25•250, 50•200 mg oral

carbifene INN *analgesic* [also: carbiphene HCl; carbiphene]

carbimazole INN, BAN

carbinoxamine INN, BAN *antihistamine for allergic rhinitis* [also: carbinoxamine maleate]

Carbinoxamine syrup, oral drops (discontinued 2007) ℞ *decongestant; antihistamine* [pseudoephedrine HCl; carbinoxamine maleate] 60•4 mg/5 mL; 25•2 mg/mL

carbinoxamine maleate USP *antihistamine for allergic rhinitis* [also: carbinoxamine] 4 mg oral; 4 mg/5 mL oral

carbinoxamine maleate & carbinoxamine tannate *antihistamine for allergic rhinitis* 2•6 mg/5 mL oral

carbinoxamine maleate & hydrocodone bitartrate & pseudoephedrine HCl *antihistamine; antitussive; decongestant* 2•5•30 mg/5 mL oral

carbinoxamine tannate *antihistamine for allergic rhinitis*

carbinoxamine tannate & carbinoxamine maleate *antihistamine for allergic rhinitis* 6•2 mg/5 mL oral

carbiphene BAN *analgesic* [also: carbiphene HCl; carbifene]

carbiphene HCl USAN *analgesic* [also: carbifene; carbiphene]

Carbocaine injection, dental injection ℞ *local anesthetic* [mepivacaine HCl] 1%, 1.5%, 2%; 3%

Carbocaine with Neo-Cobefrin dental injection ℞ *local anesthetic; vasoconstrictor* [mepivacaine HCl; levonordefrin] 2%•1:20 000

carbocisteine INN, BAN *mucolytic* [also: carbocysteine]

carbocloral USAN, INN, BAN *hypnotic*

carbocromen INN *coronary vasodilator* [also: chromonar HCl]

carbocysteine USAN *mucolytic* [also: carbocisteine]

Carbodex DM oral drops (discontinued 2007) ℞ *antitussive; antihistamine; decongestant; for children 1–18 months* [dextromethorphan hydrobromide; carbinoxamine maleate; pseudoephedrine HCl] 4•2•15 mg/mL

Carbodex DM syrup (discontinued 2007) ℞ *antitussive; antihistamine; decongestant* [dextromethorphan hydrobromide; brompheniramine maleate; pseudoephedrine HCl] 15•4•45 mg/5 mL

carbodimid calcium [see: calcium carbimide]

Carbofed DM oral drops (discontinued 2007) ℞ *antitussive; antihistamine; decongestant; for children 1–24 months* [dextromethorphan hydrobromide; carbinoxamine maleate; pseudoephedrine HCl] 4•1•15 mg/mL

Carbofed DM syrup (discontinued 2009) ℞ *antitussive; antihistamine; decongestant* [dextromethorphan hydrobromide; brompheniramine maleate; pseudoephedrine HCl] 15•4•45 mg/5 mL

carbofenotion INN [also: carbophenothion]

Carb-O-Lac HP cream ℞ *keratolytic and moisturizer/emollient for dry, rough, or cracked feet* [urea; ammonium lactate] 20•10%

carbol-fuchsin solution (or paint) USP *antifungal*

carbolic acid [see: phenol]

carbolin [see: carbachol]

carbolonium bromide BAN [also: hexcarbacholine bromide]

carbomer INN, BAN *emulsifying and suspending agent* [also: carbomer 910]

carbomer 1342 NF *emulsifying and suspending agent*

carbomer 910 USAN, NF *emulsifying and suspending agent* [also: carbomer]

carbomer 934 USAN, NF *emulsifying and suspending agent*

carbomer 934P USAN, NF *emulsifying and suspending agent*

carbomer 940 USAN, NF *emulsifying and suspending agent*

carbomer 941 USAN, NF *emulsifying and suspending agent*

carbomycin INN

carbon *element* (C)

carbon, activated

carbon C 13 urea *diagnostic aid for detection of* H. pylori *in the stomach*

carbon C 14 urea *diagnostic aid for* H. pylori *in the stomach* [also: ^{14}C urea]

carbon dioxide (CO_2) USP *respiratory stimulant*

carbon tetrachloride NF *solvent*

carbonic acid, calcium salt [see: calcium carbonate]

carbonic acid, dilithium salt [see: lithium carbonate]

carbonic acid, dipotassium salt [see: potassium carbonate]

carbonic acid, disodium salt [see: sodium carbonate]

carbonic acid, magnesium salt [see: magnesium carbonate]

carbonic acid, monoammonium salt [see: ammonium carbonate]

carbonic acid, monopotassium salt [see: potassium bicarbonate]

carbonic acid, monosodium salt [see: sodium bicarbonate]

carbonic anhydrase inhibitors *a class of diuretic agents that reduce the rate of aqueous humor formation, resulting in decreased intraocular pressure; available in both systemic (tablets) and topical (eye drops) forms*

carbonis detergens, liquor (LCD) [see: coal tar]

carbonyl iron *hematinic; iron supplement (100% elemental iron as microparticles)*

carbophenothion BAN [also: carbofenotion]

Carb-O-Philic cream OTC *moisturizer; emollient*

carboplatin USAN, INN, BAN *alkylating antineoplastic for ovarian and other cancers* 50, 150, 450, 600 mg injection

carboprost USAN, INN, BAN *oxytocic*

carboprost methyl USAN *oxytocic*

carboprost trometanol BAN *oxytocic; prostaglandin-type abortifacient* [also: carboprost tromethamine]

carboprost tromethamine USAN, USP *oxytocic; prostaglandin-type abortifacient* [also: carboprost trometanol]

Carboptic Drop-Tainers (eye drops) (discontinued 2009) ℞ *antiglaucoma agent; direct-acting miotic* [carbachol] 3%

carboquone INN

carbose D [see: carboxymethylcellulose sodium]

Carbo-Tax (carboplatin, Taxol) [with or without filgrastim hematopoietic] *chemotherapy protocol for ovarian cancer, breast cancer, and adenocarcinoma* [also: CaT; CT; PC]

carbovir *investigational (orphan) agent for AIDS and symptomatic HIV infections*

carboxyimamidate [see: carbetimer]

carboxymethylcellulose calcium NF *tablet disintegrant*

carboxymethylcellulose sodium USP *bulk laxative; suspending and viscosity-increasing agent; ophthalmic moisturizer; tablet excipient* [also: carmellose; carmellose sodium]

carboxymethylcellulose sodium 12 NF *suspending and viscosity-increasing agent*

carbromal NF, INN

carbubarb INN

carbubarbital [see: carbubarb]

carburazepam INN

carbutamide INN, BAN

carbuterol INN, BAN *bronchodilator* [also: carbuterol HCl]

carbuterol HCl USAN *bronchodilator* [also: carbuterol]

carcainium chloride INN

carcinoembryonic antigen (CEA)

cardamom seed NF

cardamom [see: bitter cardamom]

Cardec oral drops OTC *decongestant; antihistamine; for children 6–12 years* [phenylephrine HCl; chlorpheniramine maleate] 3.5•1 mg/mL

Cardec syrup (discontinued 2009) ℞ *decongestant; antihistamine* [phenylephrine HCl; chlorpheniramine maleate] 12.5•4 mg/5 mL

Cardec DM oral drops (discontinued 2008) ℞ *antitussive; antihistamine; decongestant; for children 6–24 months* [dextromethorphan hydrobromide;

chlorpheniramine maleate; phenylephrine HCl] 3•1•3.5 mg/mL

Cardene capsules (discontinued 2010) ℞ *vasodilator for chronic stable angina* [nicardipine HCl] 20, 30 mg

Cardene I.V. injection (discontinued 2011) ℞ *calcium channel blocker for the short-term treatment of hypertension* [nicardipine HCl] 0.1, 0.2 mg/mL

Cardene SR sustained-release capsules ℞ *calcium channel blocker for hypertension* [nicardipine HCl] 30, 45, 60 mg

Cardenz tablets OTC *vitamin/mineral supplement* [multiple vitamins & minerals]

cardiac glycosides *a class of cardiovascular drugs that increase the force of cardiac contractions* [also called: digitalis glycosides]

Cardiac T test ℞ *in vitro diagnostic aid for troponin T (indicator of cardiac damage) in whole blood*

cardiacs *a class of agents that stimulate or otherwise affect the heart (a term used in folk medicine)* ② Kerodex; Kredex

cardiamid [see: nikethamide]

cardin *medicinal herb* [see: blessed thistle]

Cardiolite injection ℞ *myocardial perfusion agent for cardiac SPECT imaging* [technetium Tc 99m sestamibi] 5 mL

Cardi-Omega 3 capsules (discontinued 2008) OTC *dietary supplement* [multiple vitamins & minerals; omega-3 fatty acids (eicosapentaenoic acid and docosahexaenoic acid)] ±•1000 mg (180 mg EPA; 120 mg DHA)

cardioplegic solution (calcium chloride, magnesium chloride, potassium chloride, sodium chloride) [q.v.]

cardioprotective agents *a class of potent intracellular chelating agents which protect the heart from the effects of doxorubicin*

Cardiotek tablets OTC *vitamin/amino acid supplement* [multiple vitamins; folic acid; L-arginine] ±•0.8•75 mg

Cardiotek Rx film-coated tablets ℞ *vitamin/amino acid supplement* [vitamins B_6 and B_{12}; folic acid; L-arginine HCl] 50•0.5•2•500 mg

Cardizem IV injection (discontinued 2008) ℞ *calcium channel blocker for atrial fibrillation or paroxysmal supraventricular tachycardia (PSVT)* [diltiazem HCl] 5 mg/mL

Cardizem Lyo-Ject (prefilled syringe) ℞ *calcium channel blocker for atrial fibrillation or paroxysmal supraventricular tachycardia (PSVT)* [diltiazem HCl] 25 mg

Cardizem tablets ℞ *antianginal; antihypertensive; antiarrhythmic; calcium channel blocker* [diltiazem HCl] 30, 60, 90, 120 mg

Cardizem CD sustained-release capsules ℞ *antihypertensive; antianginal; antiarrhythmic; calcium channel blocker* [diltiazem HCl] 120, 180, 240, 300, 360 mg

Cardizem LA extended-release caplets ℞ *antihypertensive; antianginal; calcium channel blocker* [diltiazem HCl] 120, 180, 240, 300, 360, 420 mg

cardophyllin [see: aminophylline]

Cardura tablets ℞ *alpha₁-adrenergic blocker for hypertension and benign prostatic hyperplasia (BPH)* [doxazosin mesylate] 1, 2, 4, 8 mg

Cardura XL extended-release tablets ℞ *alpha₁-adrenergic blocker for benign prostatic hyperplasia (BPH)* [doxazosin mesylate] 4, 8 mg

carebastine INN

carena [see: aminophylline]

CareNatal DHA film-coated tablets + capsules (discontinued 2009) ℞ *prenatal vitamin/mineral/calcium/iron/omega-3 supplement* [multiple vitamins & minerals; calcium (as citrate); iron (as ferrous bisglycinate); folic acid + docosahexaenoic acid (DHA)] ±•200•29•1 mg (tablets) + 250 mg (capsules)

Ca-Rezz topical wash, soap OTC *disinfectant/antiseptic; medicated cleanser for acne* [triclosan] 0.3%; 0.3%, 0.25%, 0.2%

carfecillin INN, BAN *antibacterial* [also: carbenicillin phenyl sodium]

carfenazine INN *antipsychotic* [also: carphenazine maleate; carphenazine]

carfentanil INN *narcotic analgesic* [also: carfentanil citrate]

carfentanil citrate USAN *narcotic analgesic* [also: carfentanil]

carfilzomib *investigational (Phase III) proteasome inhibitor antineoplastic for multiple myeloma*

carfimate INN ⑨ crufomate

cargentos [see: silver protein]

carglumic acid *oral treatment for acute hyperammonemia due to a deficiency of the hepatic enzyme N-acetylglutamate synthetase (NAGS) (orphan)*

cargutocin INN

cariabamate *investigational (Phase III) anticonvulsant*

Carica papaya *medicinal herb* [see: papaya]

Carimune NF powder for IV infusion ℞ *passive immunizing agent for HIV and idiopathic thrombocytopenic purpura (ITP); investigational (orphan) for Guillain-Barré syndrome; also used for myasthenia gravis and multiple sclerosis* [immune globulin (IVIG)] 3, 6, 12 g/dose

carindacillin INN, BAN *extended-spectrum penicillin antibiotic* [also: carbenicillin indanyl sodium]

carisbamate *investigational (NDA filed) anticonvulsive for adjunctive treatment of partial onset seizures*

carisoprodol USP, INN, BAN *skeletal muscle relaxant* 250, 350 mg oral

carisoprodol & aspirin *skeletal muscle relaxant; analgesic* 200•325 mg oral

carisoprodol & aspirin & codeine phosphate *skeletal muscle relaxant; narcotic analgesic* 200•325•16 mg oral

carline thistle *(Carlina acaulis)* root *medicinal herb used as a carminative, diaphoretic, digestive, diuretic, febrifuge, and, in large doses, an emetic and purgative*

carmantadine USAN, INN *antiparkinsonian*

carmellose INN *suspending agent; tablet excipient* [also: carboxymethylcellulose sodium; carmellose sodium]

carmellose sodium BAN *suspending agent; tablet excipient* [also: carboxymethylcellulose sodium; carmellose]

carmetizide INN

carminatives *a class of agents that relieve flatulence*

carminomycin HCl [now: carubicin HCl]

carmofur INN

Carmol 10 lotion OTC *moisturizer; emollient; keratolytic* [urea] 10% ⍰ Gerimal

Carmol 20 cream OTC *moisturizer; emollient; keratolytic* [urea] 20% ⍰ Gerimal

Carmol 40 cream, gel R *moisturizer; emollient; keratolytic* [urea] 40% ⍰ Gerimal

Carmol HC cream R *corticosteroidal anti-inflammatory; moisturizer; emollient* [hydrocortisone acetate; urea] 1%•10%

Carmol Scalp Treatment lotion R *antibiotic; keratolytic* [sulfacetamide sodium; urea] 10%•10%

carmoxirole INN

carmustine USAN, INN, BAN *nitrosourea-type alkylating antineoplastic for brain tumors, multiple myeloma, Hodgkin disease, and non-Hodgkin lymphomas; polymer implant for recurrent malignant glioma (orphan)*

Carnation Follow-Up oral liquid, powder for oral liquid OTC *total or supplementary infant feeding*

carnauba wax [see: wax, carnauba]

carnidazole USAN, INN, BAN *antiprotozoal*

carnitine INN *vitamin* B_t

L-carnitine [see: levocarnitine]

Carnitor tablets, oral solution, IV injection or infusion R *dietary amino acid for primary and secondary genetic carnitine deficiency (orphan) and end-stage renal disease (orphan); investigational (orphan) for pediatric cardiomyopathy* [levocarnitine] 330 mg; 100 mg/mL; 500 mg/2.5 mL, 1 g/5 mL

Carnitor SF sugar-free oral solution R *dietary amino acid for primary and secondary genetic carnitine deficiency (orphan) and end-stage renal disease (orphan); investigational (orphan) for pediatric cardiomyopathy* [levocarnitine] 100 mg/mL

carnosine *natural anti-carbonylation agent that prevents cross-linking of protein and collagen; antioxidant; dipeptide of beta-alanine and L-histidine*

carocainide INN

Caroid enteric-coated tablets OTC *stimulant laxative* [bisacodyl] 5 mg

β-carotene [see: beta carotene]

caroverine INN

caroxazone USAN, INN *antidepressant*

carpenter's herb *medicinal herb* [see: woundwort]

carpenter's square *medicinal herb* [see: figwort]

carperidine INN, BAN

carperone INN

carphenazine BAN *antipsychotic* [also: carphenazine maleate; carfenazine]

carphenazine maleate USAN, USP *antipsychotic* [also: carfenazine; carphenazine]

carpindolol INN

Carpine eye drops R *antiglaucoma agent; direct-acting miotic* [pilocarpine HCl] 1%, 2%, 4%

carpipramine INN

carpipramine dihydrochloride [see: carpipramine]

carpolene [now: carbomer 934P]

carprazidil INN

carprofen USAN, INN, BAN *nonsteroidal anti-inflammatory drug (NSAID); analgesic; antipyretic; approved for humans, but currently marketed only for veterinary use* 25, 50, 100 mg oral

carpronium chloride INN

Carpuject (trademarked delivery form) *prefilled syringe*

Carpuject Smartpak (trademarked delivery form) *prefilled cartridge-needle unit package*

CarraFoam; CarraWash topical liquid OTC *skin cleanser for incontinence* *care* [aloe vera; acemannan] 🔲 Geravim; Kerafoam

carrageenan NF *suspending and viscosity-increasing agent*

CarraKlenz topical liquid OTC *wound cleanser for intact skin* [aloe vera; acemannan]

CarraSmart gel OTC *hydrogel wound dressing* [acemannan]

Carrasyn; Carrasyn V gel OTC *hydrogel wound dressing* [acemannan] 🔲 chrysin; garcinia

carrot (*Daucus carota*) oil from the dried seed and root *medicinal herb for edema, gas, and worms; also used as a nutritional and vitamin supplement and stimulant; may possibly protect the heart and liver* 🔲 Geriot

carsalam INN, BAN

carsatrin INN *cardiotonic* [also: carsatrin succinate]

carsatrin succinate USAN *cardiotonic* [also: carsatrin]

cartazolate USAN, INN *antidepressant*

carteolol INN, BAN *topical antiglaucoma agent; beta-blocker for hypertension* [also: carteolol HCl]

carteolol HCl USAN *topical antiglaucoma agent; beta-blocker for hypertension* [also: carteolol] 1%

Carthamus tinctorius *medicinal herb* [see: safflower]

Cartia XT extended-release capsules ℞ *antihypertensive; antianginal; antiarrhythmic; calcium channel blocker* [diltiazem HCl] 120, 180, 240, 300 mg

carticaine BAN *amide local anesthetic for dentistry* [also: articaine] 🔲 Corticaine

Cartrix (delivery form) *prefilled syringe*

Cartrol Filmtabs (film-coated tablets) OTC *beta-blocker for hypertension* [carteolol HCl] 2.5, 5 mg

carubicin INN *antineoplastic* [also: carubicin HCl]

carubicin HCl USAN *antineoplastic* [also: carubicin]

Carum carvi NF *medicinal herb* [see: caraway]

carumonam INN, BAN *antibacterial* [also: carumonam sodium] 🔲 germanium

carumonam sodium USAN *antibacterial* [also: carumonam]

carvedilol USAN, INN, BAN, JAN *alpha- and beta-blocker for hypertension, congestive heart failure (CHF), and left ventricular dysfunction (LVD) following myocardial infarction (MI); also used for chronic angina pectoris and idiopathic cardiomyopathy* 3.125, 6.25, 12.5, 25 mg oral

carvedilol phosphate *alpha- and beta-blocker for hypertension, congestive heart failure (CHF), and left ventricular dysfunction (LVD) following myocardial infarction (MI); also used for chronic angina pectoris and idiopathic cardiomyopathy*

carvotroline HCl USAN *antipsychotic*

Caryophyllus aromaticus *medicinal herb* [see: cloves]

carzelesin USAN *antineoplastic*

carzenide INN

casanthranol USAN, USP *stimulant laxative*

casanthranol & docusate sodium *stimulant laxative; stool softener* 30•100 mg

Cascara Aromatic oral liquid (discontinued 2010) OTC *stimulant laxative* [cascara sagrada; alcohol 18%]

cascara fluidextract, aromatic USP *stimulant laxative; investigational (orphan) to speed the evacuation of an oral drug overdose* 2–6 mL oral

cascara sagrada USP *stimulant laxative*

cascara sagrada (*Frangula purshiana; Rhamnus purshiana*) bark *medicinal herb for constipation, cough, and gallbladder, intestinal, and liver disorders; chronic use can cause hypokalemia and melanosis coli* [see also: buckthorn]

cascarin [see: casanthranol]

Casec powder (discontinued 2009) OTC *protein supplement* [calcium caseinate]

Casodex film-coated tablets ℞ *antian-drogen antineoplastic for prostate cancer* [bicalutamide] 50 mg

casopitant *investigational (NDA filed) NK-1 receptor antagonist for the prevention of chemotherapy-induced nausea and vomiting*

caspofungin acetate USAN *systemic echinocandin antifungal for candidiasis, candidemia, invasive aspergillosis and other resistant fungal infections*

Cassia acutifolia; C. angustifolia; C. senna medicinal herb [see: senna]

cassia oil [see: cinnamon oil]

CAST (Color Allergy Screening Test) reagent sticks for professional use ℞ *in vitro diagnostic aid for immunoglobulin E in serum* ⧉ Cocet

Castaderm topical liquid OTC *antifungal; astringent; antiseptic* [resorcinol; boric acid; acetone; basic fuchsin; phenol; alcohol 9%]

Castel Minus; Castel Plus topical liquid OTC *antifungal; antiseptic* [resorcinol; acetone; basic fuchsin; alcohol 11.5%]

Castellani Paint Modified topical solution ℞ *antifungal; antibacterial; keratolytic* [basic fuchsin; phenol; resorcinol]

Castellani's paint [see: carbol-fuchsin solution]

Castile soap

castor oil USP *stimulant laxative*

CaT (carboplatin, Taxol) *chemotherapy protocol for adenocarcinoma, non–small cell lung cancer (NSCLC), small cell lung cancer (SCLC), and ovarian cancer* [also: Carbo-Tax; PC]

Cataflam tablets ℞ *analgesic; nonsteroidal anti-inflammatory drug (NSAID) for osteoarthritis, rheumatoid arthritis, ankylosing spondylitis, and dysmenorrhea* [diclofenac (as potassium)] 50 mg

Catapres tablets ℞ *antihypertensive; also used for ADHD, opioid and methadone withdrawal, and smoking cessation* [clonidine HCl] 0.1, 0.2, 0.3 mg

Catapres-TTS-1; Catapres-TTS-2; Catapres-TTS-3 7-day transdermal patch ℞ *antihypertensive; also used for ADHD and smoking cessation* [clonidine HCl] 0.1 mg/day (2.5 mg); 0.2 mg/day (5 mg); 0.3 mg/day (7.5 mg)

Catatrol *bicyclic antidepressant; investigational (orphan) for cataplexy and narcolepsy* [viloxazine HCl]

catchfly *medicinal herb* [see: dogbane]

catchweed *medicinal herb* [see: bedstraw]

catechins *a class of natural polyphenolic antioxidants found in green tea and grape seed extract, used for their anticarcinogenic, anti-inflammatory, and antiatherosclerotic properties and to promote thermogenesis* [see also: epicatechins; kunecatechins]

catechol-O-methyltransferase (COMT) [see: COMT inhibitors]

catgut suture [see: absorbable surgical suture]

Catha edulis the plant from which cathinone, a naturally occurring stimulant, is derived [see also: cathinone; methcathinone]

Catharanthus roseus medicinal herb [see: periwinkle]

cathartics *a class of agents that cause vigorous evacuation of the bowels by increasing bulk, stimulating peristaltic action, etc.* [also called: purgatives]

Cathflo Activase powder for intracatheter instillation ℞ *tissue plasminogen activator (tPA) thrombolytic to keep open (TKO) central venous access devices (CVADs) (not therapeutic)* [alteplase] 2.2 mg/vial

cathine INN ⧉ Kao-Tin; K-Tan

cathinone INN *an extract of the* Catha edulis *plant, a naturally occurring stimulant* [see also: *Catha edulis;* methcathinone] ⧉ cotinine

cathomycin sodium [see: novobiocin sodium]

catkins willow *medicinal herb* [see: willow]

catmint *medicinal herb* [see: catnip]

catnip (Nepeta cataria) plant *medicinal herb for colds, colic, convulsions, diarrhea, digestion, fever, flu, gas, hives,* *nervous conditions, and stimulating delayed menses*

Catrix Correction cream OTC *moisturizer; emollient*

catrup *medicinal herb* [see: catnip]

cat's claw *(Uncaria guianensis; U. tomentosa)* inner bark *medicinal herb for cancer, Candida infections, chronic fatigue, contraception, Crohn disease, diverticulitis, hypertension, irritable bowel, lupus, parasites, PMS, ulcers, and viral infections; also used as immune booster*

catswort *medicinal herb* [see: catnip]

Caucasian walnut *medicinal herb* [see: English walnut]

Caulophyllum thalictroides medicinal herb [see: blue cohosh]

caustics *a class of escharotic or corrosive agents that destroy living tissue* [also called: cauterants]

cauterants *a class of escharotic or corrosive agents that destroy living tissue* [also called: caustics]

CAV (cyclophosphamide, Adriamycin, vincristine) *chemotherapy protocol for small cell lung cancer (SCLC), osteosarcoma, and Merkel cell carcinoma* [also known as: VAC (for lung cancer only)]

CAVE (cyclophosphamide, Adriamycin, vincristine, etoposide) *chemotherapy protocol for small cell lung cancer (SCLC)*

CAV/EP (cyclophosphamide, Adriamycin, vincristine, etoposide, Platinol) *chemotherapy protocol for small cell lung cancer (SCLC)* ⌧ CVP

Caverject intracavernosal injection, Luer-lock single-use autoinjector ℞ *vasodilator for erectile dysfunction* [alprostadil] 5, 10, 20, 40 mcg/mL

Caverject Impulse powder for intracavernosal injection in prefilled syringe ℞ *vasodilator for erectile dysfunction* [alprostadil] 10, 20 mcg/0.5 mL dose

CA-VP16; CAVP16 (cyclophosphamide, Adriamycin, VP-16) *chemo-*

therapy protocol for small cell lung cancer (SCLC) ⌧ CVP

cayenne *(Capsicum annuum; C. frutescens)* fruit *medicinal herb for arthritis, bleeding, cold feet, diabetes, high blood pressure, kidney disorders, rheumatism, poor circulation, strokes, topical neuritis syndromes, tumors, and ulcers*

Cayston solution for inhalation ℞ *antibiotic for* Pseudomonas aeruginosa *infections in cystic fibrosis patients* (orphan) [aztreonam] 75 mg/dose ⌧ guaisteine

Caziant tablets (in packs of 28) ℞ *triphasic oral contraceptive* [desogestrel; ethinyl estradiol]
Phase 1 (7 days): 0.1 mg•25 mcg;
Phase 2 (7 days): 0.125 mg•25 mcg;
Phase 3 (7 days): 0.15 mg•25 mcg;
Counters (7 days)

CBD (cannabidinol) [q.v.]

CC (carboplatin, cyclophosphamide) *chemotherapy protocol for ovarian cancer*

CCNU (chloroethyl-cyclohexyl-nitrosourea) [see: lomustine]

CD4, recombinant soluble human (rCD4) *investigational (Phase II, orphan) antiviral for AIDS*

CD4 human truncated 369 AA polypeptide *investigational (orphan) treatment for AIDS*

CD4 immunoglobulin G, recombinant human *investigational (orphan) for AIDS*

CD5-T lymphocyte immunotoxin *investigational (orphan) for graft vs. host disease following bone marrow transplants*

CD-33 [see: ricin (blocked) conjugated murine MCA myeloid cells]

CdA (2-chloro-2′-deoxyadenosine) [see: cladribine]

CDB (cisplatin, dacarbazine, BCNU) *chemotherapy protocol for malignant melanoma*

CDDP; C-DDP (cis-diamminedichloroplatinum) [see: cisplatin]

CDDP/VP; CDDP/VP-16 (cisplatin, etoposide) *chemotherapy protocol for brain tumors*

CDE (cyclophosphamide, doxorubicin, etoposide) [with filgrastim hematopoietic] *chemotherapy protocol for HIV-related non-Hodgkin lymphoma*

CDP-571 *investigational (Phase III, orphan) anti-TNFα (tumor necrosis factor alpha) antibody CB-0010 for steroid-dependent Crohn disease*

CDP-cholin [see: citicoline]

CEA (carcinoembryonic antigen)

CEA-Cide Y-90 *investigational (orphan) antineoplastic for colorectal, pancreatic, ovarian, and small cell lung cancer (SCLC)* [yttrium Y 90 labetuzumab]

Ceanothus americanus medicinal herb [see: New Jersey tea]

CEA-Scan powder for injection *investigational (orphan) imaging agent for detection of recurrent or metastatic thyroid cancers* [arcitumomab] 1.25 mg

Ceclor Pulvules (capsules), powder for oral suspension ℞ *second-generation cephalosporin antibiotic* [cefaclor] 250 mg; 125, 187, 250, 375 mg/5 mL ⧆ Sochlor; Xclair; Zyclara

Ceclor CDpak extended-release tablets (in compliance packs of 14) ℞ *second-generation cephalosporin antibiotic* [cefaclor] 500 mg

Cecon oral drops OTC *vitamin C supplement* [ascorbic acid] 100 mg/mL

Cedax capsules, powder for oral suspension ℞ *third-generation cephalosporin antibiotic* [ceftibuten] 400 mg; 90, 180 mg/5 mL ⧆ ciadox; Cidex; Sudex; Z-Dex

cedefingol USAN *antipsoriatic; antineoplastic adjunct*

cedelizumab USAN *monoclonal antibody; prophylaxis of rejection of solid organ allograft; immunomodulator for autoimmune diseases*

CEE (conjugated equine estrogen) [see: estrogens, conjugated]

CeeNu capsules, dose pack ℞ *nitrosourea-type alkylating antineoplastic for brain tumors and Hodgkin disease* [lomustine] 10, 40, 100 mg; 2 × 100 mg + 2 × 40 mg + 2 × 10 mg

CEF (cyclophosphamide, epirubicin, fluorouracil) [with Bactrim antibiotic] *chemotherapy protocol for breast cancer* [also: FEC]

cefacetrile INN *antibacterial* [also: cephacetrile sodium]

cefacetrile sodium [see: cephacetrile sodium]

cefaclor USAN, USP, INN, BAN, JAN *second-generation cephalosporin antibiotic* 250, 375, 500 mg oral; 125, 187, 250, 375 mg/5 mL oral

cefadroxil USAN, USP, INN, BAN *first-generation cephalosporin antibiotic* 500, 1000 mg oral

cefadroxil hemihydrate *first-generation cephalosporin antibiotic* 250, 500 mg/5 mL oral

cefalexin INN, JAN *first-generation cephalosporin antibiotic* [also: cephalexin]

cefaloglycin INN *antibacterial* [also: cephaloglycin]

cefalonium INN [also: cephalonium]

cefaloram INN [also: cephaloram]

cefaloridine INN *antibacterial* [also: cephaloridine]

cefalotin INN *first-generation cephalosporin antibiotic* [also: cephalothin sodium; cephalothin]

cefalotin sodium [see: cephalothin sodium]

cefamandole USAN, INN *second-generation cephalosporin antibiotic* [also: cephamandole]

cefamandole nafate USAN, USP *second-generation cephalosporin antibiotic* [also: cephamandole nafate]

cefamandole sodium USP *second-generation cephalosporin antibiotic*

cefaparole USAN, INN *antibacterial*

cefapirin INN, BAN *first-generation cephalosporin antibiotic* [also: cephapirin sodium]

cefapirin sodium [see: cephapirin sodium]

cefatrizine USAN, INN, BAN *antibacterial*

cefazaflur INN *antibacterial* [also: cefazaflur sodium]

cefazaflur sodium USAN *antibacterial* [also: cefazaflur]

cefazedone INN, BAN

cefazolin USP, INN *first-generation cephalosporin antibiotic* [also: cephazolin]

cefazolin sodium USAN, USP *first-generation cephalosporin antibiotic* [also: cephazolin sodium] 0.5, 1, 5, 10, 20 g injection

cefbuperazone USAN, INN *antibacterial*

cefcanel INN

cefcanel daloxate INN

cefdinir USAN, INN *third-generation cephalosporin antibiotic* 300 mg oral; 125, 250 mg/5 mL oral

cefditoren pivoxil *broad-spectrum cephalosporin antibiotic* 200, 400 mg oral

cefedrolor INN

cefempidone INN, BAN

cefepime USAN, INN *fourth-generation cephalosporin antibiotic* 1, 2 g injection

cefepime HCl USAN *fourth-generation cephalosporin antibiotic* 0.5, 1, 2 g injection

cefetamet USAN, INN *veterinary antibacterial*

cefetecol USAN, INN, BAN *antibacterial*

cefetrizole INN

cefivitril INN

cefixime USAN, USP, INN, BAN *third-generation cephalosporin antibiotic* ⚗ Zyvoxam

Cefizox powder or frozen premix for IV or IM injection ℞ *third-generation cephalosporin antibiotic* [ceftizoxime sodium] 0.5, 1, 2, 10 g

cefmenoxime INN *antibacterial* [also: cefmenoxime HCl]

cefmenoxime HCl USAN, USP *antibacterial* [also: cefmenoxime]

cefmepidium chloride INN

cefmetazole USAN, INN *second-generation cephalosporin antibiotic*

cefmetazole sodium USAN, USP, JAN *second-generation cephalosporin antibiotic*

cefminox INN

Cefobid powder or frozen premix for IV or IM injection (discontinued 2007) ℞ *third-generation cephalospo-*

rin antibiotic [cefoperazone sodium] 1, 2, 10 g ⚗ Cevi-Bid

cefodizime INN *cephalosporin antibiotic*

Cefol Filmtabs (film-coated tablets) (discontinued 2009) ℞ *vitamin supplement* [multiple vitamins; folic acid] ± •0.5 mg ⚗ Savella; Zyflo

cefonicid INN, BAN *second-generation cephalosporin antibiotic* [also: cefonicid monosodium]

cefonicid monosodium USAN *second-generation cephalosporin antibiotic* [also: cefonicid]

cefonicid sodium USAN, USP *second-generation cephalosporin antibiotic*

cefoperazone INN, BAN *third-generation cephalosporin antibiotic* [also: cefoperazone sodium]

cefoperazone sodium USAN, USP *third-generation cephalosporin antibiotic* [also: cefoperazone]

ceforanide USAN, USP, INN, BAN *cephalosporin antibiotic* ⚗ Zofran ODT

Cefotan powder for IV or IM injection (discontinued 2009) ℞ *cephamycin antibiotic* [cefotetan disodium] 1, 2, 10 g

cefotaxime INN, BAN *third-generation cephalosporin antibiotic* [also: cefotaxime sodium]

cefotaxime sodium USAN, USP *third-generation cephalosporin antibiotic* [also: cefotaxime] 0.5, 1, 2, 10 g injection

cefotetan USAN, INN, BAN *cephamycin antibiotic*

cefotetan disodium USAN, USP *cephamycin antibiotic* 1, 2, 10 g/vial injection

cefotiam INN, BAN *antibacterial* [also: cefotiam HCl]

cefotiam HCl USAN *antibacterial* [also: cefotiam]

cefoxazole INN [also: cephoxazole]

cefoxitin USAN, INN, BAN *cephamycin antibiotic*

cefoxitin sodium USAN, USP, BAN *cephamycin antibiotic* 1, 2, 10 g/vial injection

cefpimizole USAN, INN *antibacterial*

cefpimizole sodium USAN, JAN *antibacterial*

cefpiramide USAN, USP, INN *antibacterial* ☒ sevopramide

cefpiramide sodium USAN, JAN *antibacterial*

cefpirome INN, BAN *antibacterial* [also: cefpirome sulfate]

cefpirome sulfate USAN, JAN *antibacterial* [also: cefpirome]

cefpodoxime INN, BAN *broad-spectrum third-generation cephalosporin antibiotic* [also: cefpodoxime proxetil]

cefpodoxime proxetil USAN, JAN *broad-spectrum third-generation cephalosporin antibiotic* [also: cefpodoxime] 100, 200 mg oral; 50, 100 mg/5 mL oral

cefprozil USAN, INN *second-generation cephalosporin antibiotic* 250, 500 mg oral; 125, 250 mg/5 mL oral

cefquinome INN, BAN *veterinary antibacterial*

cefquinome sulfate USAN *veterinary antibacterial*

cefradine INN *first-generation cephalosporin antibiotic* [also: cephradine]

cefrotil INN

cefroxadine USAN, INN *antibacterial*

cefsulodin INN, BAN *antibacterial* [also: cefsulodin sodium]

cefsulodin sodium USAN *antibacterial* [also: cefsulodin]

cefsumide INN

ceftaroline fosamil *broad-spectrum cephalosporin antibiotic for complicated skin and skin structure infections (cSSSI), methicillin-resistant* S. aureus *(MRSA), and multidrug-resistant* Streptococcus pneumoniae *(MDRSP)*

ceftazidime USAN, USP, INN, BAN, JAN *third-generation cephalosporin antibiotic* 0.5, 1, 2, 6 g injection

cefteram INN

ceftezole INN

ceftibuten USAN, INN, BAN *third-generation cephalosporin antibiotic*

Ceftin film-coated tablets, oral suspension ℞ *second-generation cephalospo-* rin *antibiotic* [cefuroxime axetil] 125, 250, 500 mg; 125, 250 mg/5 mL

ceftiofur INN, BAN *veterinary antibacterial* [also: ceftiofur HCl]

ceftiofur HCl USAN *veterinary antibacterial* [also: ceftiofur]

ceftiofur sodium USAN *veterinary antibacterial*

ceftiolene INN

ceftioxide INN

ceftizoxime INN, BAN *third-generation cephalosporin antibiotic* [also: ceftizoxime sodium]

ceftizoxime sodium USAN, USP *third-generation cephalosporin antibiotic* [also: ceftizoxime]

ceftobiprole *investigational (NDA filed) broad-spectrum cephalosporin antibiotic for complicated skin and skin structure infections (SSSIs) and community-acquired pneumonia (CAP)*

ceftriaxone INN, BAN *third-generation cephalosporin antibiotic* [also: ceftriaxone sodium]

ceftriaxone sodium USAN, USP *third-generation cephalosporin antibiotic* [also: ceftriaxone] 0.25, 0.5, 1, 2, 10 g injection

cefuracetime INN, BAN

cefuroxime USAN, INN, BAN *second-generation cephalosporin antibiotic*

cefuroxime axetil USAN, USP, BAN *second-generation cephalosporin antibiotic* 125, 250, 500 mg oral; 125, 250 mg/5 mL oral

cefuroxime pivoxetil USAN *second-generation cephalosporin antibiotic*

cefuroxime sodium USP, BAN *second-generation cephalosporin antibiotic* 0.75, 1.5, 7.5 g injection

cefuzonam INN

Cefzil film-coated tablets, powder for oral suspension (discontinued 2008) ℞ *second-generation cephalosporin antibiotic* [cefprozil] 250, 500 mg; 125, 250 mg/5 mL

Cefzon (foreign name for U.S. product **Omnicef**) ☒ Zefazone

celandine *(Chelidonium majus)* root and plant *medicinal herb used as an* *analgesic, antispasmodic, caustic, diaphoretic, diuretic, narcotic, and purgative*

Celebrex capsules ℞ *COX-2 inhibitor; nonsteroidal anti-inflammatory drug (NSAID) for osteoarthritis, rheumatoid arthritis, ankylosing spondylitis, and primary dysmenorrhea; reduces polyp growth in familial adenomatous polyposis* [celecoxib] 50, 100, 200, 400 mg

celecoxib USAN *COX-2 inhibitor; nonsteroidal anti-inflammatory drug (NSAID) for osteoarthritis, rheumatoid arthritis, ankylosing spondylitis, and primary dysmenorrhea; reduces polyp growth in familial adenomatous polyposis*

celery (Apium graveolens) root, stem, and seeds *medicinal herb for aiding digestion, arthritis, cancer, diuresis, gas, headache, hysteria, inducing menstruation, lumbago, nervousness, rheumatism, and terminating lactation* ⊘ Sular; Xolair

Celestone syrup ℞ *corticosteroidal anti-inflammatory* [betamethasone] 0.6 mg/5 mL ⊘ sulisatin

Celestone Soluspan intrabursal, intra-articular, intralesional injection ℞ *corticosteroidal anti-inflammatory* [betamethasone sodium phosphate; betamethasone acetate] 3•3 mg/mL

Celexa film-coated tablets, oral solution ℞ *selective serotonin reuptake inhibitor (SSRI) for major depression; also used for obsessive-compulsive disorder (OCD), post-traumatic stress disorder (PTSD), generalized anxiety disorder (GAD), and premenstrual dysphoric disorder (PMDD)* [citalopram hydrobromide] 10, 20, 40 mg; 10 mg/5 mL ⊘ Cylex; Salex; Xolox

celgosivir HCl USAN *antiviral; alpha-glucosidase I inhibitor for HIV*

celiprolol INN, BAN *antihypertensive; antianginal; beta-blocker* [also: celiprolol HCl]

celiprolol HCl USAN *antihypertensive; antianginal; beta-blocker* [also: celiprolol]

cellacefate INN *tablet-coating agent* [also: cellulose acetate phthalate; cellacephate]

cellacephate BAN *tablet-coating agent* [also: cellulose acetate phthalate; cellacefate]

CellCept capsules, film-coated caplets, powder for oral suspension ℞ *immunosuppressant for allogenic renal, hepatic, or cardiac transplants (orphan); investigational (orphan) for pemphigus vulgaris* [mycophenolate mofetil] 250 mg; 500 mg; 200 mg/mL

CellCept powder for IV infusion ℞ *immunosuppressant for allogenic renal, hepatic, or cardiac transplants* [mycophenolate mofetil HCl] 500 mg

cellulase USAN *digestive enzyme*

cellulolytic enzyme [see: cellulase]

cellulose *bulk laxative*

cellulose, absorbable [see: cellulose, oxidized]

cellulose, ethyl ester [see: ethylcellulose]

cellulose, hydroxypropyl methyl ether [see: hydroxypropyl methylcellulose]

cellulose, microcrystalline NF *tablet and capsule diluent* [also: dispersible cellulose]

cellulose, oxidized USP *topical hemostat*

cellulose, oxidized regenerated USP *local hemostatic*

cellulose, sodium carboxymethyl [see: carboxymethylcellulose sodium]

cellulose acetate NF *tablet-coating agent; insoluble polymer membrane*

cellulose acetate butyrate [see: cabufocon A; cabufocon B]

cellulose acetate dibutyrate [see: porofocon A; porofocon B]

cellulose acetate phthalate (CAP) NF *tablet-coating agent* [also: cellacefate; cellacephate]

cellulose carboxymethyl ether, sodium salt [see: carboxymethylcellulose sodium]

cellulose diacetate [see: cellulose acetate]

cellulose dihydrogen phosphate, disodium salt [see: cellulose sodium phosphate]

cellulose disodium phosphate [see: cellulose sodium phosphate]

cellulose ethyl ether [see: ethylcellulose]

cellulose gum, modified [now: croscarmellose sodium]

cellulose methyl ether [see: methylcellulose]

cellulose nitrate [see: pyroxylin]

cellulose sodium phosphate (CSP) USAN, USP *antiurolithic to prevent stone formation in absorptive hypercalciuria Type I*

cellulosic acid [see: cellulose, oxidized]

Celluvisc solution OTC *ophthalmic moisturizer/lubricant* [carboxymethylcellulose] 1%

celmoleukin INN *immunostimulant*

Celontin Kapseals (capsules) ℞ *succinimide anticonvulsant for petit mal (absence) seizures* [methsuximide] 300 mg

celucloral INN, BAN

Cenafed tablets, syrup (discontinued 2009) OTC *nasal decongestant* [pseudoephedrine HCl] 60 mg; 30 mg/5 mL

Cenafed Plus tablets (discontinued 2007) OTC *decongestant; antihistamine* [pseudoephedrine HCl; triprolidine HCl] 60•2.5 mg

Cena-K oral liquid ℞ *electrolyte replenisher* [potassium (as chloride)] 20, 40 mEq/15 mL ② senega; zinc

Cenestin film-coated tablets ℞ *synthetic estrogen for the treatment of postmenopausal symptoms* [synthetic conjugated estrogens, A] 0.3, 0.45, 0.625, 0.9, 1.25 mg

Cenhist chewable tablets OTC *decongestant; antihistamine* [phenylephrine HCl; brompheniramine maleate] 15•6 mg

Cenogen Ultra capsules (discontinued 2010) ℞ *vitamin/mineral/iron supplement* [multiple vitamins & minerals; iron (as ferrous fumarate); folic acid] ≐•106•1 mg

Cenolate IV, IM, or subcu injection ℞ *vitamin therapy; antiscorbutic* [vitamin C (as sodium ascorbate)] 500 mg/mL (562.5 mg/mL)

Centany ointment, kit (ointment + gauze pads) ℞ *antibiotic for impetigo due to* S. aureus *or* S. pyogenes [mupirocin] 2%

Centaurea cyanus medicinal herb [see: cornflower]

centaury *(Erythraea centaurium)* plant *medicinal herb for aiding digestion, blood cleansing, fever, and promoting menstruation*

Centella asiatica medicinal herb [see: gotu kola]

Center-Al subcu or IM injection ℞ *allergenic sensitivity testing (subcu); allergenic desensitization therapy (IM)* [allergenic extracts, alum-precipitated] ② zinterol

Centergy DM oral drops ℞ *antitussive; antihistamine; decongestant* [dextromethorphan hydrobromide; chlorpheniramine maleate; phenylephrine HCl] 3•1•2 mg/mL

Centovir *investigational (orphan) treatment and prophylaxis of CMV infections in allogenic bone marrow transplants* [monoclonal antibody IgM (C-58) to cytomegalovirus (CMV)]

Centoxin *investigational (orphan) for gram-negative bacteremia in endotoxin shock* [nebacumab]

centrazene [see: simtrazene]

centrophenoxine [see: meclofenoxate]

Centrum chewable tablets OTC *vitamin/mineral/calcium/iron supplement* [multiple vitamins & minerals; calcium (as carbonate); iron (as carbonyl iron); folic acid] ≐•108•18•0.4 mg

Centrum tablets OTC *vitamin/mineral/calcium/iron supplement* [multiple vitamins & minerals; calcium (as carbonate and dibasic calcium phosphate); iron (as ferrous fumarate); folic acid; hydrogenated oil] ≐• 200•18•0.5 mg

Centrum, Advanced Formula tablets (discontinued 2008) OTC *vita-*

min/mineral/iron supplement [multiple vitamins & minerals; iron (as ferrous fumarate); folic acid; biotin] ≜•18• 0.4•0.03 mg

Centrum Cardio tablets OTC *vitamin/ mineral/calcium/iron supplement* [multiple vitamins & minerals; calcium (as dibasic calcium phosphate); iron (as ferrous fumarate); folic acid] ≜• 54•3•0.2 mg

Centrum High Potency oral liquid OTC *vitamin/mineral/iron supplement* [multiple vitamins & minerals; iron (as ferrous gluconate); biotin; alcohol] ≜•3•0.1 mg/5 mL

Centrum Jr. + Extra C; Centrum Jr. + Extra Calcium chewable tablets (discontinued 2008) OTC *vitamin/ mineral/calcium/iron supplement* [multiple vitamins & minerals; calcium; iron; folic acid; biotin] ≜•108•18• 0.4•0.045 mg; ≜•160•18•0.4• 0.045 mg

Centrum Jr. with Iron tablets (discontinued 2008) OTC *vitamin/mineral/ iron supplement* [multiple vitamins & minerals; iron; folic acid; biotin] ≜• 18 mg•0.4 mg•45 mcg

Centrum Kids Complete; Centrum Kids Dora the Explorer; Centrum Kids SpongeBob Squarepants chewable tablets OTC *vitamin/mineral/ calcium/iron supplement* [multiple vitamins & minerals; calcium (as carbonate); iron (as carbonyl iron); folic acid] ≜•108•18•0.4 mg

Centrum Performance tablets OTC *vitamin/mineral/calcium/iron supplement* [multiple vitamins & minerals; calcium (as carbonate); iron (as ferrous fumarate); folic acid; biotin; hydrogenated oil] ≜•100•18•0.4•0.04 mg

Centrum Silver tablets, chewable tablets OTC *vitamin/mineral supplement* [multiple vitamins & minerals; folic acid; biotin; lutein; hydrogenated oil] ≜•500•30•250 mcg; ≜• 500•45•250 mcg

Centrum Silver Ultra Women's tablets OTC *vitamin/mineral supplement* [multiple vitamins & minerals; folic acid; biotin; lutein; hydrogenated oil] ≜•400•30•300 mcg

centruoides (scorpion) immune F(ab′)2, equine *treatment for venomous scorpion stings (orphan)*

Ceo-Two suppository OTC CO_2-*releasing laxative* [sodium bicarbonate; potassium bitartrate]

Cēpacol mouthwash/gargle OTC *oral antiseptic* [cetylpyridinium chloride] 0.05%

Cēpacol Anesthetic troches (discontinued 2008) OTC *mucous membrane anesthetic; antiseptic* [benzocaine; cetylpyridinium chloride] 10 mg•0.07%

Cēpacol Dual Relief Sore Throat + Coating spray OTC *mucous membrane anesthetic; emollient* [benzocaine; glycerin] 5%•33%

Cēpacol Dual Relief Sore Throat + Cough spray OTC *mucous membrane anesthetic; antitussive; emollient* [benzocaine; dextromethorphan hydrobromide; glycerin] 5%•30%•30%

Cēpacol Fizzlers oral disintegrating tablets OTC *mucous membrane anesthetic* [benzocaine] 6 mg

Cēpacol Maximum Strength lozenges (discontinued 2010) OTC *mucous membrane anesthetic* [benzocaine] 10 mg

Cēpacol Menthol Regular Strength lozenges OTC *mild anesthetic; antipruritic; counterirritant* [menthol] 3 mg

Cēpacol Sore Throat lozenges OTC *mucous membrane anesthetic; antipruritic; counterirritant* [benzocaine; menthol] 10•2, 10•2.1, 10•2.6, 10• 3.6, 10•4.5 mg

Cēpacol Sore Throat oral liquid (discontinued 2008) OTC *decongestant; analgesic; antipyretic* [pseudoephedrine HCl; acetaminophen] 60•640 mg/30 mL

Cēpacol Sore Throat spray OTC *mucous membrane anesthetic; emollient* [dyclonine HCl; glycerin] 0.1%•33%

Cēpacol Sore Throat+Coating Relief Maximum Numbing lozenges OTC *mucous membrane anesthetic; emollient* [benzocaine; pectin] 15•5 mg

Cēpacol Sore Throat Maximum Numbing lozenges OTC *mucous membrane anesthetic; antipruritic; counterirritant* [benzocaine; menthol] 15•2.1, 15•2.6, 15•3.6, 15•4 mg

Cēpacol Sore Throat Postnasal Drip lozenges OTC *mild anesthetic; antipruritic; counterirritant* [menthol] 4.5 mg

Cēpacol Throat lozenges OTC *antiseptic* [cetylpyridinium chloride] 0.07%

Cēpacol Ultra Sore Throat Plus Cough lozenges OTC *antitussive; mucous membrane anesthetic* [dextromethorphan hydrobromide; benzocaine] 5•7.5 mg

Cēpacol Viractin oral cream, oral gel (discontinued 2007) OTC *mucous membrane anesthetic for cold sores and fever blisters* [tetracaine HCl] 2%

Cēpastat Sore Throat lozenges OTC *mild anesthetic; antipruritic; counterirritant* [phenol] 14.5, 29 mg

cephacetrile sodium USAN, USP *antibacterial* [also: cefacetrile]

Cephadyn caplets ℞ *barbiturate sedative; analgesic; antipyretic* [butalbital; acetaminophen] 50•650 mg

cephalexin USAN, USP, BAN *first-generation cephalosporin antibiotic* [also: cefalexin] 250, 500 mg oral; 125, 250 mg/5 mL oral

cephalexin HCl USAN, USP *first-generation cephalosporin antibiotic*

cephaloglycin USAN, USP, BAN *antibacterial* [also: cefaloglycin]

cephalonium BAN [also: cefalonium]

cephaloram BAN [also: cefaloram]

cephaloridine USAN, USP, BAN *antibacterial* [also: cefaloridine]

cephalosporin N [see: adicillin]

cephalosporins *a class of bactericidal antibiotics, divided into first-, second-, and third-generation; higher generations have increasing efficacy against gram-negative and decreasing efficacy against gram-positive bacteria*

cephalothin BAN *first-generation cephalosporin antibiotic* [also: cephalothin sodium; cefalotin]

cephalothin sodium USAN, USP *first-generation cephalosporin antibiotic* [also: cefalotin; cephalothin]

cephamandole BAN *second-generation cephalosporin antibiotic* [also: cefamandole]

cephamandole nafate BAN *second-generation cephalosporin antibiotic* [also: cefamandole nafate]

cephamycins *a class of bactericidal antibiotics similar to second-generation cephalosporins (q.v.)*

cephapirin sodium USAN, USP *first-generation cephalosporin antibiotic* [also: cefapirin]

cephazolin BAN *first-generation cephalosporin antibiotic* [also: cefazolin]

cephazolin sodium BAN *first-generation cephalosporin antibiotic* [also: cefazolin sodium]

cephoxazole BAN [also: cefoxazole]

cephradine USAN, USP, BAN *first-generation cephalosporin antibiotic* [also: cefradine]

Cephulac oral/rectal solution ℞ *synthetic disaccharide used to prevent and treat portal-systemic encephalopathy* [lactulose] 10 g/15 mL

Ceplene *investigational (Phase III) histamine H_2 receptor agonist for malignant melanoma and acute myeloid leukemia (AML)* [histamine dihydrochloride]

CEPP (cyclophosphamide, etoposide, prednisone, procarbazine) *chemotherapy protocol for non-Hodgkin lymphoma*

CEPPB (cyclophosphamide, etoposide, prednisone, procarbazine, bleomycin) *chemotherapy protocol for non-Hodgkin lymphoma* ⍰ SE BPO

Ceprotin powder for IV injection ℞ *replacement therapy for severe congenital protein C deficiency in children and adults to prevent or treat thrombosis, pulmonary emboli, and purpura fulmi-*

nans (orphan) [protein C concentrate (human)] 500, 1000 U ☑ sparteine

Ceptaz powder for IV or IM injection ℞ *third-generation cephalosporin antibiotic* [ceftazidime pentahydrate] 1, 2 g

CERA (continuous erythropoietin receptor activator) [q.v.]

CeraLyte powder for oral liquid, ready-to-use oral liquid OTC *supplementary feeding to maintain hydration and electrolyte balance in infants with diarrhea or vomiting* [rice-based formula]

ceramide trihexosidase (CTH) & agalsidase beta *investigational (orphan) enzyme replacement therapy for Fabry disease*

CeraVe; CeraVe AM; CeraVe PM; CeraVe Moisturizing lotion OTC *moisturizer/emollient*

Cerebyx IV or IM injection ℞ *hydantoin anticonvulsant for grand mal status epilepticus (orphan)* [fosphenytoin sodium (phenytoin sodium equivalent)] 75 (50) mg/mL ☑ Surbex

Ceredase IV infusion ℞ *glucocerebrosidase enzyme replacement for Gaucher disease type I (orphan)* [alglucerase] 80 U/mL

Cerefolin tablets ℞ *vitamin B supplement for homocystinemia* [multiple B vitamins; folic acid (as L-methylfolate)] ± • 5.635 mg

Cerefolin NAC caplets ℞ *vitamin B supplement for homocystinemia* [multiple B vitamins; folic acid; N-acetylcysteine] ± • 5.6 • 600 mg

cerelose [see: glucose]

Ceresine *investigational (orphan) for severe head trauma* [sodium dichloroacetate]

Cerezyme powder for IV infusion ℞ *glucocerebrosidase enzyme replacement for type 1 Gaucher disease (orphan)* [imiglucerase] 40 U/mL

Cerisa wash ℞ *antibiotic and keratolytic for acne* [sulfacetamide sodium; sulfur] 10% • 1% ☑ Xerese

cerium *element (Ce)*

cerium nitrate & silver sulfadiazine *investigational (orphan) for life-threatening burns*

cerium oxalate USP

cerivastatin sodium USAN *HMG-CoA reductase inhibitor for hyperlipidemia and hypertriglyceridemia (discontinued 2001 due to safety concerns)*

Cernevit-12 powder for IV injection ℞ *parenteral vitamin therapy* [multiple vitamins; folic acid; biotin] ± • 414 • 60 mcg

Ceron oral drops (discontinued 2011) ℞ *decongestant; antihistamine; drops for children 6–24 months* [phenylephrine HCl; chlorpheniramine maleate] 3.5 • 1 mg/mL ☑ Sereine

Ceron syrup ℞ *decongestant; antihistamine; drops for children 6–24 months* [phenylephrine HCl; chlorpheniramine maleate] 12.5 • 4 mg/5 mL ☑ Sereine

ceronapril USAN, INN *antihypertensive*

Ceron-DM oral drops (discontinued 2010) ℞ *antitussive; antihistamine; decongestant; for children 6–24 months* [dextromethorphan hydrobromide; chlorpheniramine maleate; phenylephrine HCl] 3 • 1 • 3.5 mg/mL

Ceron-DM syrup ℞ *antitussive; antihistamine; decongestant* [dextromethorphan hydrobromide; chlorpheniramine maleate; phenylephrine HCl] 15 • 4 • 12.5 mg/5 mL

Cerovite Advanced Formula tablets OTC *vitamin/mineral/calcium/iron supplement* [multiple vitamins & minerals; calcium (as ascorbate and carbonate); iron (as ferrous fumarate); folic acid; biotin] ± • 162 • 18 • 0.4 • 0.03 mg

Cerovite Jr. chewable tablets OTC *vitamin/mineral/calcium/iron supplement* [multiple vitamins & minerals; calcium; iron; folic acid; biotin] ± • 108 • 18 • 0.4 • 0.045 mg

Cerovite Senior tablets (discontinued 2008) OTC *geriatric vitamin/mineral supplement* [multiple vitamins & minerals; folic acid; biotin] ± • 200 • 30 mcg

Certagen film-coated tablets OTC *vitamin/mineral/calcium/iron supplement* [multiple vitamins & minerals; calcium (as carbonate and dicalcium phosphate); iron (as ferrous fumarate); folic acid; biotin] ≟•162•18•0.4•0.03 mg

Certagen oral liquid OTC *vitamin/mineral/iron supplement* [multiple vitamins & minerals; iron (as ferrous gluconate); biotin] ≟•3•0.1 mg/5 mL

Certagen Senior tablets (discontinued 2008) OTC *geriatric vitamin/mineral supplement* [multiple vitamins & minerals; folic acid; biotin] ≟•200•30 mcg

CertaVite oral liquid OTC *vitamin/mineral/iron supplement* [multiple vitamins & minerals; iron (as ferrous gluconate); alcohol] ≟•3 mg

CertaVite Golden tablets (discontinued 2008) OTC *geriatric vitamin/mineral supplement* [multiple vitamins & minerals; biotin] ≟•30 mcg

CertaVite with Lutein tablets OTC *vitamin/mineral/calcium/iron supplement* [multiple vitamins & minerals; calcium (as carbonate or dibasic calcium phosphate); iron (as ferrous fumarate); folic acid; biotin] ≟•18•162•0.4•0.03 mg

certolizumab pegol *immunomodulator; pegylated Fab fragment anti-TNF (tumor necrosis factor) anti-inflammatory for moderate to severe Crohn disease and rheumatoid arthritis*

Certriad *investigational (NDA filed) antihyperlipidemic drug combination; a statin drug to lower LDL cholesterol and triglycerides plus a fibrate drug to raise HDL cholesterol* [rosuvastatin calcium; fenofibrate]

Cerubidine powder for IV injection ℞ *antineoplastic for various lymphocytic and nonlymphocytic leukemias* [daunorubicin (as HCl)] 20 mg

ceruletide USAN, INN, BAN *gastric secretory stimulant*

ceruletide diethylamine USAN *gastric secretory stimulant*

Cervarix IM injection ℞ *vaccine for cervical cancer and precancerous lesions in women 10–25 years* [human papillomavirus (HPV) recombinant vaccine, bivalent (HPV types 16 and 18)] 20•20 mcg/0.5 mL dose

Cervidil vaginal insert ℞ *prostaglandin for cervical ripening at term* [dinoprostone] 10 mg

Cesamet capsules ℞ *antiemetic for nausea and vomiting associated with cancer chemotherapy; restricted use due to the high possibility of disturbing psychomimetic reactions and psychological dependence* [nabilone] 1 mg

Cesia tablets (in packs of 28) ℞ *triphasic oral contraceptive* [desogestrel; ethinyl estradiol]
Phase 1 (7 days): 0.1 mg•25 mcg;
Phase 2 (7 days): 0.125 mg•25 mcg;
Phase 3 (7 days): 0.15 mg•25 mcg;
Counters (7 days)

cesium *element (Cs)*

cesium (¹³¹Cs) chloride INN *radioactive agent* [also: cesium chloride Cs 131]

cesium chloride Cs 131 USAN *radioactive agent* [also: cesium (¹³¹Cs) chloride]

Ceta topical liquid OTC *soap-free therapeutic skin cleanser*

Ceta Plus capsules (discontinued 2010) ℞ *narcotic analgesic; antipyretic* [hydrocodone bitartrate; acetaminophen] 5•500 mg

cetaben INN *antihyperlipoproteinemic* [also: cetaben sodium] ⊡ zotepine

cetaben sodium USAN *antihyperlipoproteinemic* [also: cetaben]

Cetacaine topical liquid, gel, ointment, aerosol ℞ *anesthetic; antiseptic* [benzocaine; tetracaine HCl; butamben; benzalkonium chloride] 14%•2%•2%•0.5%

Cetacort lotion ℞ *corticosteroidal anti-inflammatory* [hydrocortisone] 0.25%, 0.5% ⊡ S-T Cort

Cetafen; Cetafen Extra film-coated tablets OTC *analgesic; antipyretic* [acetaminophen] 325 mg; 500 mg ⊡ Cytovene

Cetaklenz topical liquid OTC *soap-free skin cleanser* [cetyl alcohol; propylene glycol; sodium lauryl sulfate; stearyl alcohol]

cetalkonium *antiseptic*

cetalkonium chloride USAN, INN, BAN *topical anti-infective*

Cetamide ophthalmic ointment (discontinued 2008) ℞ *antibiotic* [sulfacetamide sodium] 10%

cetamolol INN *antiadrenergic (beta-blocker)* [also: cetamolol HCl]

cetamolol HCl USAN *antiadrenergic (beta-blocker)* [also: cetamolol]

Cetaphil cream, lotion, cleansing bar, cleansing solution OTC *soap-free therapeutic skin cleanser*

Cetaphil Daily Advance lotion OTC *moisturizer/emollient*

cethexonium chloride INN

cetiedil INN *peripheral vasodilator* [also: cetiedil citrate] ☒ Stadol

cetiedil citrate USAN *peripheral vasodilator; investigational (orphan) for sickle cell disease crisis* [also: cetiedil]

cetirizine INN, BAN *second-generation peripherally selective piperazine antihistamine for allergic rhinitis and chronic idiopathic urticaria* [also: cetirizine HCl]

cetirizine HCl USAN *second-generation peripherally selective piperazine antihistamine for allergic rhinitis and chronic idiopathic urticaria; also used for bronchial asthma* [also: cetirizine] 5, 10 mg oral; 5 mg/5 mL oral

Cetirizine Hydrochloride Allergy, Children's; Children's Cetirizine Chloride Hives Relief syrup OTC *nonsedating antihistamine for allergy and hives* [cetirizine HCl] 5 mg/5 mL

cetobemidone [see: ketobemidone]

cetocycline INN *antibacterial* [also: cetocycline HCl]

cetocycline HCl USAN *antibacterial* [also: cetocycline]

cetofenicol INN *antibacterial* [also: cetophenicol]

cetohexazine INN

cetomacrogol 1000 INN, BAN

cetophenicol USAN *antibacterial* [also: cetofenicol]

cetophenylbutazone [see: kebuzone]

cetostearyl alcohol NF *emulsifying agent*

cetotetrine HCl [now: cetocycline HCl]

cetotiamine INN

cetoxime INN, BAN

cetoxime HCl [see: cetoxime]

CETP (cholesterol ester transfer protein) [q.v.]

Cetraria islandica medicinal herb [see: Iceland moss]

Cetraxal ear drops ℞ *broad-spectrum fluoroquinolone antibiotic* [ciprofloxacin (as HCl)] 0.2%

cetraxate INN *GI antiulcerative* [also: cetraxate HCl]

cetraxate HCl USAN *GI antiulcerative* [also: cetraxate]

cetrimide INN, BAN *topical antiseptic* ☒ sweet wormwood

cetrimonium bromide INN *topical antiseptic* [also: cetrimonium chloride]

cetrimonium chloride BAN *topical antiseptic* [also: cetrimonium bromide]

cetrorelix acetate USAN *gonadotropin-releasing hormone (GnRH) antagonist for infertility*

Cetrotide subcu injection ℞ *gonadotropin-releasing hormone (GnRH) antagonist for infertility* [cetrorelix acetate] 0.25, 3 mg

cetuximab USAN *monoclonal antibody to epidermal growth factor receptor (EGFR); antineoplastic for metastatic colorectal cancer and squamous cell carcinoma (SCC) of the head and neck (orphan); investigational (Phase III) for numerous other cancers*

cetyl alcohol NF *emulsifying and stiffening agent*

cetyl esters wax NF *stiffening agent*

cetyldimethylbenzyl ammonium chloride [see: cetalkonium chloride]

cetylpyridinium chloride USP, INN, BAN *topical antiseptic; preservative*

cetyltrimethyl ammonium bromide

CEV (cyclophosphamide, etoposide, vincristine) *chemotherapy protocol for small cell lung cancer (SCLC)*

Cevi-Bid tablets OTC *vitamin C supplement* [ascorbic acid] 500 mg ⑨ Cefobid

cevimeline HCl USAN *cholinergic and muscarinic receptor agonist for dry mouth due to Sjögren syndrome* 30 mg oral

cevitamic acid [see: ascorbic acid]

cevitan [see: ascorbic acid]

ceylon gelatin [see: agar]

Cezin-S capsules (discontinued 2008) ℞ *geriatric vitamin/mineral supplement* [multiple vitamins & minerals; folic acid] ± •0.5 mg

CF (carboplatin, fluorouracil) *chemotherapy protocol for head and neck cancer*

CF (cisplatin, fluorouracil) *chemotherapy protocol for adenocarcinoma, gastric cancer, and anal cancer* [also: cisplatin + fluorourail; FUP]

CFC (chlorofluorocarbons) *the type of propellant used in older aerosol and pressurized metered-dose inhaler (pMDI) delivery systems; these are being replaced with products that use HFA-134a propellant (q.v.)*

CFM (cyclophosphamide, fluorouracil, mitoxantrone) *chemotherapy protocol for breast cancer* [also known as: CNF; FNC]

CFTR (cystic fibrosis transmembrane conductance regulator) [q.v.]

CG (chorionic gonadotropin) [see: gonadotropin, chorionic]

CGF (*Chlorella* growth factor) [q.v.]

CGF (Control Gel Formula) dressing [see: DuoDERM CGF]

CGRP (calcitonin gene-related peptide) antagonists *investigational (Phase III) class of agents for migraine headaches*

CGU WC oral liquid ℞ *narcotic antitussive; expectorant* [codeine phosphate; guaifenesin] 6.3•100 mg/5 mL

chalk, precipitated [see: calcium carbonate, precipitated]

Chamaelirium luteum *medicinal herb* [see: false unicorn]

CHAMOCA (cyclophosphamide, hydroxyurea, actinomycin D, methotrexate, Oncovin, calcium folinate, Adriamycin) *chemotherapy protocol for gestational trophoblastic neoplasm* [also known as: modified Bagshawe protocol]

chamomile (*Anthemis nobilis*; *Matricaria chamomilla*) *flowers medicinal herb for appetite stimulation, bronchitis, excessive menstruation with cramps, fever, gastrointestinal cramps, hysteria, inflammation, insomnia, nervousness, rheumatic disorders, and parasites*

channa; canna *medicinal herb* [see: kanna]

Chantel Vitamin E cream OTC *emollient* [vitamin E]

Chantix film-coated caplets ℞ *nicotine receptor agonist/antagonist; a non-nicotine smoking cessation aid; also used to reduce alcohol cravings* [varenicline (as tartrate)] 0.5, 1 mg

CHAP (cyclophosphamide, Hexalen, Adriamycin, Platinol) *chemotherapy protocol for ovarian cancer*

Chap Stick Medicated Lip Balm stick, jar, squeezable tube OTC *mild anesthetic; antipruritic; counterirritant; moisturizer; protectant; emollient* [camphor; menthol; phenol] 1%• 0.6%•0.5%

chaparral (*Larrea divaricata*; *L. glutinosa*; *L. tridentata*) *leaves and stems medicinal herb for arthritis, blood cleansing, bronchitis, cancer, chickenpox, colds, leukemia, rheumatic pain, stomach pain, and tumors; not generally regarded as safe and effective due to liver toxicity and the stimulation of some tumors*

CharcoAid oral suspension OTC *adsorbent antidote for poisoning* [activated charcoal] 15 g/120 mL, 30 g/150 mL

CharcoAid 2000 oral liquid, granules OTC *adsorbent antidote for poisoning*

[activated charcoal] 15 g/120 mL, 50 g/240 mL; 15 g

charcoal *gastric adsorbent/detoxicant; antiflatulent* 260 mg oral

charcoal, activated USP *general purpose antidote/adsorbent* 15, 30, 40, 120, 240 g, 208 mg/mL oral

Charcoal Plus enteric-coated tablets OTC *adsorbent; detoxicant* [activated charcoal] 250 mg

CharcoCaps capsules OTC *adsorbent; detoxicant; antiflatulent* [charcoal] 260 mg

Chardonna-2 tablets (discontinued 2008) ℞ *GI/GU anticholinergic/antispasmodic; sedative* [belladonna extract; phenobarbital] 15•15 mg

chaste tree *(Vitex agnus-castus)* dried ripe fruit *medicinal herb for acne, balancing progesterone and estrogen production, increasing lactation, ovarian insufficiency, premenstrual breast pain, regulating menstrual cycle, and uterine bleeding*

chaulmosulfone INN

checkerberry *medicinal herb* [see: squaw vine; wintergreen]

cheese plant; cheeseflower *medicinal herb* [see: mallow]

cheese rennet *medicinal herb* [see: bedstraw]

Cheetah oral suspension ℞ *radiopaque contrast medium for gastrointestinal imaging* [barium sulfate] 2.2%

chelafrin [see: epinephrine]

Chelated Manganese tablets OTC *manganese supplement* [manganese] 20, 50 mg

chelating agents *a class of agents that prevent bodily absorption of and cause the excretion of substances such as heavy metals*

chelen [see: ethyl chloride]

Chelidonium majus *medicinal herb* [see: celandine]

Chelone glabra *medicinal herb* [see: turtlebloom]

Chemet capsules ℞ *heavy metal chelating agent for lead poisoning (orphan); investigational (orphan) for mercury*

poisoning and cysteine kidney stones [succimer] 100 mg

Chemo-Pin (trademarked delivery form) *chemical-dispensing pin*

Chemstrip 2 GP; Chemstrip 2 LN; Chemstrip 7; Chemstrip 9; Chemstrip 10 with SG; Chemstrip uGK reagent strips OTC *in vitro diagnostic aid for multiple urine products*

Chemstrip 4 the OB; Chemstrip 6; Chemstrip 8 reagent strips (discontinued 2008) OTC *in vitro diagnostic aid for multiple urine products*

Chemstrip bG reagent strips for home use (discontinued 2008) OTC *in vitro diagnostic aid for blood glucose*

Chemstrip K reagent strips for professional use ℞ *in vitro diagnostic aid for acetone (ketones) in the urine*

Chemstrip Micral reagent strips for professional use ℞ *in vitro diagnostic aid for albumin (protein) in the urine*

Chemstrip uG reagent strips for home use (discontinued 2008) OTC *in vitro diagnostic aid for urine glucose*

chenic acid [now: chenodiol]

Chenix tablets (name changed to **Chenodal** in 2010)

Chenodal film-coated tablets ℞ *anticholelithogenic for radiolucent gallstones* [chenodiol] 250 mg

chenodeoxycholic acid INN, BAN *anticholelithogenic* [also: chenodiol]

chenodiol USAN *anticholelithogenic for radiolucent gallstones (orphan); investigational (orphan) for cerebrotendinous xanthomatosis* [also: chenodeoxycholic acid]

Chenofalk *investigational (orphan) agent for cerebrotendinous xanthomatosis* [chenodiol]

Cheracol Cough syrup (discontinued 2007) ℞ *narcotic antitussive; expectorant* [codeine phosphate; guaifenesin; alcohol 4.75%] 20•200 mg/10 mL

Cheracol D Cough Formula; Cheracol Plus syrup OTC *antitussive; expectorant* [dextromethorphan hydrobromide; guaifenesin; alcohol 4.75%] 10•100 mg/5 mL

Cheracol Sore Throat spray OTC *mild mucous membrane anesthetic; antipruritic; counterirritant* [phenol] 1.4%

Cheratussin AC syrup ℞ *narcotic antitussive; expectorant* [codeine phosphate; guaifenesin; alcohol 3.5%] 10•100 mg/5 mL

Cheratussin DAC oral liquid ℞ *narcotic antitussive; decongestant; expectorant* [codeine phosphate; pseudoephedrine HCl; guaifenesin; alcohol 2.1%] 10•30•100 mg/5 mL

cherry, black; choke cherry; rum cherry *medicinal herb* [see: wild black cherry]

cherry, black; poison black cherry *medicinal herb* [see: belladonna]

cherry birch *medicinal herb* [see: birch]

cherry juice NF

chervil (*Anthriscus cerefolium*) flowering plant *medicinal herb used as a digestive, diuretic, expectorant, and stimulant*

chervil, sweet *medicinal herb* [see: sweet cicely]

chestnut *medicinal herb* [see: horse chestnut]

Chewable Multivitamins with Fluoride pediatric tablets (discontinued 2008) ℞ *vitamin supplement; dental caries preventative* [multiple vitamins; fluoride; folic acid] ≛•1•0.3 mg

Chewable Triple Vitamins with Fluoride pediatric tablets (discontinued 2008) ℞ *vitamin supplement; dental caries preventative* [vitamins A, C, and D; fluoride] 2500 IU•60 mg•400 IU•1 mg

Chewable Vitamin C chewable tablets OTC *vitamin C supplement* [ascorbic acid and sodium ascorbate] 250, 500 mg

Chew-C chewable tablets OTC *vitamin C supplement* [ascorbic acid and sodium ascorbate] 500 mg

chicken's toes *medicinal herb* [see: coral root]

chickweed (*Stellaria media*) plant *medicinal herb for appetite suppression, bleeding, blood cleansing, convulsions,* *obesity, skin rashes, and ulcers; also used as a homeopathic remedy for psoriasis and rheumatic pain*

chicory (*Chicorium intybus*) plant and root *medicinal herb for blood cleansing, cardiac disease, jaundice, liver disorders, promoting expectoration, and removal of calcium deposits*

Chigg Away lotion OTC *antibacterial; antiseptic; anesthetic* [sulfur; benzocaine] 10%•5%

Chiggerex ointment (discontinued 2011) OTC *anesthetic; antipruritic; counterirritant* [benzocaine; camphor; menthol]

Chigger-Tox topical liquid (discontinued 2011) OTC *anesthetic* [benzocaine]

Chikusetsu ginseng (*Panax pseudo-ginseng*) *medicinal herb* [see: ginseng]

Children's Chewable Vitamins OTC *vitamin supplements* [multiple vitamins; folic acid] ≛•300 mcg

Children's Chewable Vitamins + Iron tablets OTC *vitamin/iron supplements* [multiple vitamins; iron (as ferrous fumarate); folic acid] ≛•12•0.3 mg

Children's Elixir DM Cough & Cold (discontinued 2007) OTC *antitussive; antihistamine; decongestant* [dextromethorphan hydrobromide; brompheniramine maleate; pseudoephedrine HCl] 5•1•15 mg/5 mL

Children's Ibuprofen Cold oral suspension (discontinued 2007) OTC *analgesic; antipyretic; nonsteroidal anti-inflammatory drug; nasal decongestant* [ibuprofen; pseudoephedrine] 100•15 mg/5 mL

Children's Loratadine syrup OTC *nonsedating antihistamine for allergic rhinitis* [loratadine] 5 mg/5 mL

chili pepper; chilies *medicinal herb* [see: cayenne]

chillifolinum [see: quillifoline]

Chimaphila umbellata *medicinal herb* [see: pipsissewa]

chimeric monoclonal antibodies *antibodies cloned from a single cell genetically engineered to combine the* antigen-binding part of a murine (mouse/rat) antibody with the effector part of a human antibody, to prevent rejection by the human immune system [see: monoclonal antibodies]

chinchona *medicinal herb* [see: quinine]

Chinese cucumber *(Trichosanthes kirilowii)* gourd and root *medicinal herb for abscesses, amenorrhea, cough, diabetes, edema, fever, inducing abortion, invasive moles, jaundice, polyuria, and tumors*

Chinese gelatin [see: agar]

Chinese isinglass [see: chiniofon]

Chinese rhubarb *medicinal herb* [see: rhubarb]

chinethazone [see: quinethazone]

chiniofon NF, INN

Chionanthus virginica medicinal herb [see: fringe tree]

ChiRhoStim powder for IV injection ℞ *diagnostic aid for pancreatic function* [secretin, human] 16, 40 mcg/vial

chitosamine [see: glucosamine]

chitosan *natural cellulose-like biopolymer extracted from marine animal exoskeletons and used as a treatment for hypercholesterolemia, hyperlipidemia, and obesity; also used topically as an antimicrobial and vulnerary*

chittem bark *medicinal herb* [see: buckthorn; cascara sagrada]

Chlamydiazyme reagent kit for professional use ℞ *in vitro diagnostic aid for Chlamydia trachomatis* [solid phase enzyme immunoassay]

Chlo-Amine chewable tablets OTC *antihistamine* [chlorpheniramine maleate] 2 mg ⧆ calamine; gallamine

chlophedianol BAN *antitussive* [also: chlophedianol HCl; clofedanol]

chlophedianol HCl USAN *antitussive* [also: clofedanol; chlophedianol]

chlophenadione [see: clorindione]

chloquinate [see: cloquinate]

chloracyzine INN

chloral betaine USAN, NF, BAN *sedative* [also: cloral betaine]

chloral hydrate USP, BAN *nonbarbiturate sedative and hypnotic; also abused*

as a street drug 500 mg oral; 250, 500 mg/5 mL oral

chloral hydrate betaine [see: chloral betaine]

chloralformamide USP

chloralodol INN [also: chlorhexadol]

chloralose (α-chloralose) INN

chloralurethane [see: carbocloral]

chlorambucil USP, INN, BAN *nitrogen mustard–type alkylating antineoplastic for multiple leukemias and lymphomas; also used for other malignancies*

chloramidobenzol [see: clofenamide]

chloramine [now: chloramine-T]

chloramine-T NF [also: tosylchloramide sodium]

chloramiphene [see: clomiphene citrate]

chloramphenicol USP, INN, BAN, JAN *bacteriostatic antibiotic; antirickettsial* ⧆ cloramfenicol

chloramphenicol palmitate USP, JAN *antibacterial; antirickettsial* 150 mg/5 mL oral ⧆ cloramfenicol pantotenate

chloramphenicol pantothenate complex USAN *antibacterial; antirickettsial* [also: cloramfenicol pantotenate complex]

chloramphenicol sodium succinate USP, JAN *antibacterial; antirickettsial* 100 mg/mL injection ⧆ cloramfenicol

chloranautine [see: dimenhydrinate]

ChloraPrep One-Step swabs OTC *antiseptic* [chlorhexidine gluconate; isopropyl alcohol] 2%•70%

chlorarsen [see: dichlorophenarsine HCl]

Chlorascrub Swab; Chlorascrub Swabstick; Chlorascrub Maxi swabs OTC *antiseptic* [chlorhexidine gluconate; isopropyl alcohol] 3.15%•70% (1 mL; 1.6 mL; 5.1 mL)

Chloraseptic mouthwash/gargle OTC *oral antiseptic; antipruritic/counterirritant; mild local anesthetic* [phenol] 1.4%

Chloraseptic, Children's lozenges OTC *mucous membrane anesthetic* [benzocaine] 5 mg

Chloraseptic Defense Daily Health Strips orally disintegrating film OTC *vitamin/mineral supplement* [vitamin C; zinc]

Chloraseptic Kids' Sore Throat orally disintegrating film OTC *mucous membrane anesthetic; antipruritic; counterirritant* [benzocaine; menthol] 2•2 mg

Chloraseptic Sore Throat lozenges, orally disintegrating film OTC *mucous membrane anesthetic; antipruritic; counterirritant* [benzocaine; menthol] 6•10 mg; 3•3 mg

Chloraseptic Sore Throat oral liquid (discontinued 2008) OTC *analgesic; antipyretic* [acetaminophen] 166.6 mg/5 mL

Chloraseptic Sore Throat; Chloraseptic Kids' Sore Throat spray OTC *antipruritic/counterirritant; mild local anesthetic* [phenol] 1.4%; 0.5%

Chloraseptic Sugar Free Sore Throat lozenges OTC *mucous membrane anesthetic; antipruritic; counterirritant; (some flavors contain an antitussive)* [benzocaine; menthol; (dextromethorphan)]

chlorazanil INN

chlorazanil HCl [see: chlorazanil]

chlorazodin INN [also: chloroazodin]

chlorazone [see: chloramine-T]

chlorbenzoxamine INN

chlorbenzoxamine HCl [see: chlorbenzoxamine]

chlorbetamide INN, BAN

chlorbutanol [see: chlorobutanol]

chlorbutin [see: chlorambucil]

chlorbutol BAN *antimicrobial agent* [also: chlorobutanol]

chlorcinnazine [see: clocinizine]

chlorcyclizine INN, BAN *antihistamine* [also: chlorcyclizine HCl]

chlorcyclizine HCl USP *antihistamine* [also: chlorcyclizine]

chlordantoin USAN, BAN *antifungal* [also: clodantoin]

Chlordex GP syrup ℞ *antitussive; decongestant; antihistamine; expectorant* [dextromethorphan hydrobromide; phenylephrine HCl; chlorpheniramine maleate; guaifenesin] 7.5•10•2•100 mg/5 mL

chlordiazepoxide USP, INN, BAN, JAN *benzodiazepine anxiolytic; sedative; alcohol withdrawal aid*

chlordiazepoxide HCl USAN, USP, BAN, JAN *benzodiazepine anxiolytic; sedative; alcohol withdrawal aid; sometimes abused as a street drug* 5, 10, 25 mg oral

chlordiazepoxide HCl & clidinium bromide *anxiolytic; GI anticholinergic* 5•2.5 mg

chlordimorine INN

Chlorella a genus of single-cell algae used as a source of multiple vitamins and minerals, protein, chlorellin, chlorophyll and Chlorella growth factor (q.v.); immune enhancer and chelator of heavy metals

Chlorella **growth factor (CGF)** *natural extract of the nucleus of Chlorella algae (q.v.) that is widely used in wound healing and skin disorders*

Chloresium ointment, solution (discontinued 2010) OTC *vulnerary and deodorant for wounds, burns, and ulcers* [chlorophyllin copper complex] 0.5%; 0.2%

Chloresium tablets (discontinued 2010) OTC *systemic deodorant for ostomy, breath, and body odors* [chlorophyllin copper complex] 14 mg

chlorethate [see: clorethate]

chlorethyl [see: ethyl chloride]

Chlorex-A caplets (discontinued 2008) ℞ *decongestant; antihistamine; sleep aid* [phenylephrine HCl; chlorpheniramine maleate; phenyltoloxamine citrate] 20•4•40 mg

Chlorex-A 12 oral suspension (discontinued 2009) ℞ *decongestant; antihistamine; sleep aid* [phenylephrine tannate; chlorpheniramine tannate; pyrilamine tannate] 5•2•12.5 mg/5 mL

chlorfenisate [see: clofibrate]

chlorfenvinphos BAN [also: clofenvinfos]

chlorguanide HCl [see: chloroguanide HCl]

chlorhexadol BAN [also: chloralodol]

chlorhexidine INN, BAN *broad-spectrum antimicrobial* [also: chlorhexidine gluconate]

chlorhexidine gluconate USAN *broad-spectrum antimicrobial; investigational (orphan) for oral mucositis in bone marrow transplant patients* [also: chlorhexidine] 0.12% oral rinse; 2% topical wipes

chlorhexidine HCl USAN, BAN *broad-spectrum antimicrobial*

chlorhexidine phosphanilate USAN *broad-spectrum antimicrobial*

chlorimiphenin [see: imiclopazine]

chlorimpiphenine [see: imiclopazine]

chlorinated & iodized peanut oil [see: chloriodized oil]

chlorindanol USAN *spermaticide* [also: clorindanol]

chlorine *element (Cl)* ⧈ Klaron

chloriodized oil USP

chlorisondamine chloride INN, BAN

chlorisondamone chloride [see: chlorisondamine chloride]

chlormadinone INN, BAN *progestin* [also: chlormadinone acetate]

chlormadinone acetate USAN, NF *progestin* [also: chlormadinone]

chlormerodrin NF, INN, BAN

chlormerodrin (^{197}Hg) INN *renal function test; radioactive agent* [also: chlormerodrin Hg 197]

chlormerodrin Hg 197 USAN, USP *renal function test; radioactive agent* [also: chlormerodrin (^{197}Hg)]

chlormerodrin Hg 203 USAN, USP *renal function test; radioactive agent*

chlormeroprin [see: chlormerodrin]

chlormethazanone [see: chlormezanone]

chlormethiazole BAN [also: clomethiazole]

chlormethine INN *nitrogen mustard-type alkylating antineoplastic* [also: mechlorethamine HCl; mustine; nitrogen mustard N-oxide HCl]

chlormethylencycline [see: clomocycline]

chlormezanone INN, BAN *mild anxiolytic*

chlormidazole INN, BAN

chlornaphazine INN

chloroacetic acid [see: monochloroacetic, dichloroacetic, or trichloroacetic acid]

8-chloroadenosine monophosphate, cyclic (8-Cl cAMP) [see: tocladesine]

chloroazodin USP [also: chlorazodin]

5-chlorobenzoxazolinone [see: chlorzoxazone]

chlorobutanol NF, INN *antimicrobial agent; preservative* [also: chlorbutol]

chlorochine [see: chloroquine]

chlorocresol USAN, NF, INN *antiseptic; disinfectant*

2-chloro-2′-deoxyadenosine (CdA) [now: cladribine]

chlorodeoxylincomycin [see: clindamycin]

chloroethane [see: ethyl chloride]

2-chloroethyl-3-sarcosinamide-1-nitrosourea *investigational (orphan) for malignant glioma*

chloroform NF *solvent*

chloroguanide HCl USP *antimalarial; dihydrofolate reductase inhibitor* [also: proguanil]

chloroguanide HCl & atovaquone *combination dihydrofolate reductase inhibitor and antiprotozoal for malaria* 100•250 mg oral

chloroguanide triazine pamoate [see: cycloguanil pamoate]

chloro-iodohydroxyquinoline [see: clioquinol]

chlorolincomycin [see: clindamycin]

Chloromag *injection* ℞ *magnesium replacement therapy* [magnesium chloride hexahydrate] 200 mg/mL

chloromethapyrilene citrate [see: chlorothen citrate]

Chloromycetin *powder for eye drops (discontinued 2009)* ℞ *antibiotic* [chloramphenicol] 25 mg/15 mL

Chloromycetin Sodium Succinate *powder for IV injection* ℞ *broad-spectrum bacteriostatic antibiotic* [chloramphenicol sodium succinate] 100 mg/mL

p-chlorophenol [see: parachlorophenol]

chlorophenothane NF [also: clofenotane; dicophane]

chlorophenoxamide [see: clefamide]

chlorophenylmercury [see: phenylmercuric chloride]

chlorophyll, water soluble [see: chlorophyllin]

chlorophyllin *vulnerary; oral deodorant for ostomy, breath, and body odors; topical deodorant for wounds and ulcers* 20 mg oral

chlorophyllin copper complex USAN *oral deodorant for ostomy, breath, and body odors; topical deodorant for wounds and ulcers*

chloroprednisone INN

chloroprednisone acetate [see: chloroprednisone]

chloroprocaine INN *injectable local anesthetic* [also: chloroprocaine HCl]

chloroprocaine HCl USP *injectable local anesthetic; central or peripheral nerve block, including lumbar and epidural block* [also: chloroprocaine] 2%, 3% injection

chloropyramine INN [also: halopyramine]

chloropyrilene INN, BAN [also: chlorothen citrate]

chloroquine USP, INN, BAN *amebicide; antimalarial* ▣ Klor-Con

chloroquine diphosphate [see: chloroquine phosphate]

chloroquine HCl USP *amebicide; antimalarial* [also: chloroquine]

chloroquine phosphate USP, BAN *amebicide; antimalarial; lupus erythematosus suppressant* (base=60%) 150, 250, 300, 500 mg oral

chloroserpidine INN

N-chlorosuccinimide [see: succinchlorimide]

chlorothen citrate NF [also: chloropyrilene]

chlorothenium citrate [see: chlorothen citrate]

chlorothenylpyramine [see: chlorothen]

chlorothiazide USP, INN, BAN *diuretic; antihypertensive* 250, 500 mg oral

chlorothiazide sodium USAN, USP *diuretic; antihypertensive* 500 mg injection

chlorothymol NF

chlorotoxin *investigational (orphan) antineoplastic for malignant glioma*

chlorotrianisene USP, INN, BAN *estrogen for hormone replacement therapy or inoperable prostatic cancer*

chloroxine USAN *antibacterial and antifungal for seborrheic dermatitis of the scalp*

chloroxylenol USP, INN, BAN *antiseptic*

chlorozone [see: chloramine-T]

chlorpenthixol [see: clopenthixol]

chlorphenamine INN *antihistamine* [also: chlorpheniramine maleate; chlorpheniramine]

chlorphenamine maleate [see: chlorpheniramine maleate]

chlorphenecyclane [see: clofenciclan]

chlorphenesin INN, BAN *skeletal muscle relaxant* [also: chlorphenesin carbamate]

chlorphenesin carbamate USAN, JAN *skeletal muscle relaxant* [also: chlorphenesin]

chlorphenindione [see: clorindione]

chlorpheniramine BAN *alkylamine antihistamine* [also: chlorpheniramine maleate; chlorphenamine]

chlorpheniramine maleate USP *alkylamine antihistamine* [also: chlorphenamine; chlorpheniramine] 4, 8, 12 mg oral

chlorpheniramine maleate & codeine phosphate *antihistamine; narcotic antitussive* 2•10 mg/5 mL oral

chlorpheniramine maleate & dextromethorphan hydrobromide & pseudoephedrine HCl *antihistamine; antitussive; decongestant* 4•30•30 mg oral

chlorpheniramine maleate & phenylephrine HCl *antihistamine; decongestant* 4•20 mg oral; 4•12.5 mg/5 mL oral; 1•3.5 mg/mL oral

chlorpheniramine maleate & pseu-doephedrine HCl *antihistamine; decongestant* 8•120, 12•100, 12•120 mg oral

chlorpheniramine polistirex USAN *alkylamine antihistamine*

chlorpheniramine polistirex & hydrocodone polistirex *antihistamine; narcotic antitussive* 8•10 mg/5 mL oral

chlorpheniramine tannate *alkylamine antihistamine*

chlorpheniramine tannate & pseu-doephedrine tannate *antihistamine; decongestant*

chlorpheniramine tannate & pyril-amine tannate & phenylephrine tannate *antihistamine; decongestant* 2•12.5•5 mg/5 mL oral

chlorphenoctium amsonate INN, BAN

chlorphenotane [see: chlorophenothane]

chlorphenoxamine INN, BAN [also: chlorphenoxamine HCl]

chlorphenoxamine HCl USP [also: chlorphenoxamine]

chlorphentermine INN, BAN *anorectic* [also: chlorphentermine HCl]

chlorphentermine HCl USAN *anorectic* [also: chlorphentermine]

chlorphenylindandione [see: clorindione]

chlorphthalidone [see: chlorthalidone]

chlorprocaine chloride [see: chloroprocaine HCl]

chlorproethazine INN [also: chlorproethazine HCl]

chlorproethazine HCl [also: chlorproethazine]

chlorproguanil INN, BAN

chlorproguanil HCl [see: chlorproguanil]

chlorpromazine USP, INN, BAN *conventional (typical) phenothiazine antipsychotic for schizophrenia and manic episodes of a bipolar disorder; antiemetic for nausea and vomiting*

chlorpromazine HCl USP, BAN, JAN *phenothiazine antipsychotic for schizophrenia, manic episodes of a bipolar*

disorder, pediatric hyperactivity, and severe pediatric behavioral problems; treatment for acute intermittent porphyria, nausea/vomiting, and intractable hiccoughs 10, 25, 50, 100, 200 mg oral; 25 mg/mL injection

chlorpromazine hibenzate JAN *conventional (typical) phenothiazine antipsychotic for schizophrenia and manic episodes of a bipolar disorder; antiemetic for nausea and vomiting*

chlorpromazine phenolphthalinate JAN *conventional (typical) phenothiazine antipsychotic for schizophrenia and manic episodes of a bipolar disorder; antiemetic for nausea and vomiting*

chlorpromazine tannate USP, INN, BAN *conventional (typical) phenothiazine antipsychotic for schizophrenia and manic episodes of a bipolar disorder; antiemetic for nausea and vomiting*

chlorpropamide USP, INN, BAN, JAN *sulfonylurea antidiabetic that stimulates insulin secretion in the pancreas* 100, 250 mg oral

chlorprophenpyridamine maleate [see: chlorpheniramine maleate]

chlorprothixene USAN, USP, INN, BAN *thioxanthene antipsychotic*

chlorpyrifos BAN

chlorquinaldol INN, BAN

chlortalidone INN *antihypertensive; diuretic* [also: chlorthalidone]

chlortetracycline INN, BAN *antibiotic; antiprotozoal* [also: chlortetracycline bisulfate]

chlortetracycline bisulfate USP *antibiotic; antiprotozoal* [also: chlortetracycline]

chlortetracycline calcium *antibiotic; antiprotozoal*

chlortetracycline HCl USP, BAN *antibiotic; antiprotozoal*

chlorthalidone USAN, USP, BAN *antihypertensive; diuretic for congestive heart failure, hepatic cirrhosis, and corticosteroid therapy* [also: chlortalidone] 25, 50, 100 mg oral

chlorthalidone & atenolol *combination diuretic and beta-blocker for hypertension* 25•50, 25•100 mg oral

chlorthenoxazin BAN [also: chlorthenoxazine]

chlorthenoxazine INN [also: chlorthenoxazin]

chlorthiazide [see: chlorothiazide]

chlortrianisestrol [see: chlorotrianisene]

Chlor-Trimeton Allergy 8 Hour; Chlor-Trimeton Allergy 12 Hour timed-release tablets OTC *antihistamine* [chlorpheniramine maleate] 8 mg; 12 mg

Chlor-Trimeton Allergy-D 4 Hour tablets (discontinued 2007) OTC *decongestant; antihistamine* [pseudoephedrine sulfate; chlorpheniramine maleate] 60•4 mg

Chlor-Trimeton Allergy-D 12 Hour sustained-release tablets (discontinued 2007) OTC *decongestant; antihistamine* [pseudoephedrine sulfate; chlorpheniramine maleate] 120•8 mg

chlorzoxazone USP, INN, BAN, JAN *skeletal muscle relaxant* 250, 375, 500, 750 mg oral

chlosudimeprimylum [see: clopamide]

ChlVPP (chlorambucil, vinblastine, procarbazine, prednisone/prednisolone) *chemotherapy protocol for Hodgkin lymphoma* (note: prednisone is preferred in the U.S.; prednisolone is preferred in the U.K.)

ChlVPP/EVA (chlorambucil, vinblastine, procarbazine, prednisone/prednisolone; etoposide, vincristine, Adriamycin) *chemotherapy protocol for Hodgkin lymphoma* (note: prednisone is preferred in the U.S.; prednisolone is preferred in the U.K.)

CHO cells, recombinant [see: CD4, human truncated]

choice dielytra *medicinal herb* [see: turkey corn]

Choice DM fingerstick test kit for home use OTC *in vitro diagnostic aid for glycosylated hemoglobin levels*

Choice DM; Choice DM Sugar-Free oral liquid OTC *enteral nutritional therapy for abnormal glucose tolerance* [lactose-free formula] 237 mL; 325 mL

Choice DM Daily Moisurizing lotion OTC *moisturizer; emollient*

Choice DM Gentle Care mouthwash OTC

choke cherry; black choke *medicinal herb* [see: wild black cherry]

Cholac oral/rectal solution (discontinued 2007) ℞ *synthetic disaccharide used to prevent and treat portal-systemic encephalopathy* [lactulose] 10 g/15 mL ⓦ shellac

cholagogues *a class of agents that stimulate the flow of bile into the duodenum*

cholalic acid [see: dehydrocholic acid]

cholecalciferol (vitamin D₃) USP, BAN, JAN *fat-soluble vitamin* (1 mcg= 400 IU) [also: colecalciferol] 1000, 50 000 IU oral

cholera vaccine USP *active bacterin for cholera* (Vibrio cholerae)

cholesterin [see: cholesterol]

cholesterol NF *emulsifying agent*

cholesterol ester transfer protein (CETP) inhibitor *a class of investigational antihyperlipidemics that raise HDL cholesterol levels and decrease plaque formation in the arteries*

cholestrin [see: cholesterol]

cholestyramine BAN *bile salts ion-exchange resin; cholesterol-lowering antihyperlipidemic* [also: cholestyramine resin; colestyramine]

Cholestyramine Light powder for oral suspension ℞ *cholesterol-lowering antihyperlipidemic; treatment for pruritus due to partial biliary obstruction; also used for diarrhea and as an antidote to* Clostridium difficile *and digitalis toxicity* [cholestyramine resin] 4 g/dose

cholestyramine resin USP *bile salts ion-exchange resin; cholesterol-lowering antihyperlipidemic; treatment for pruritus due to partial biliary obstruction; also used for diarrhea and as an antidote to* Clostridium difficile *and digitalis toxicity* [also: colestyramine;

cholestyramine] 4 g powder for oral solution

Choletec IV injection ℞ *radioactive hepatobiliary imaging agent for chole-scintigraphy* [technetium Tc 99m mebrofenin] 100 mCi in 45 mg

cholic acid [see: dehydrocholic acid]

Cholidase tablets (discontinued 2008) OTC *dietary lipotropic; vitamin supplement* [choline; inositol; vitamins B_6, B_{12}, and E] 185•150•2.5•0.005•7.5 mg

choline *lipotropic supplement* 375, 650 mg oral

choline alfoscerate INN

choline bitartrate NF *lipotropic supplement* 250 mg oral

choline bromide hexamethylenedicarbamate [see: hexacarbacholine bromide]

choline chloride INN *lipotropic supplement; investigational (orphan) for choline deficiency of long-term parenteral nutrition*

choline chloride acetate [see: acetylcholine chloride]

choline chloride carbamate [see: carbachol]

choline chloride succinate [see: succinylcholine chloride]

choline dihydrogen citrate NF *lipotropic supplement* 650 mg oral

choline fenofibrate *PPARα agonist for primary hypercholesterolemia, hypertriglyceridemia, and mixed dyslipidemia*

choline gluconate INN

choline glycerophosphate [see: choline alfoscerate]

choline perchlorate, nitrate ester [see: nitricholine perchlorate]

choline salicylate USAN, INN, BAN *analgesic; antipyretic; anti-inflammatory; antirheumatic*

choline theophyllinate INN, BAN *bronchodilator* [also: oxtriphylline]

cholinergic agonists *a class of agents that produce effects similar to those of the parasympathetic nervous system* [also called: parasympathomimetics]

cholinesterase inhibitors *a class of drugs which increase acetylcholine neurotransmitters, used as a cognition adjuvant in Alzheimer dementia* [also called: acetylcholinesterase (AChE) inhibitors]

Cholinoid capsules OTC *dietary lipotropic; vitamin supplement* [choline (as bitartrate); inositol; multiple B vitamins; vitamin C; lemon bioflavonoids] 334•334•±•300•300 mg

Cholografin Meglumine injection ℞ *radiopaque contrast medium for cholecystography and cholangiography* [iodipamide meglumine (49.2% iodine)] 520 mg/mL (257 mg/mL)

chondodendron tomentosum [see: tubocurarine chloride]

chondrocyte-alginate *investigational (orphan) gel suspension for vesicoureteral reflux in children*

chondroitin 4-sulfate [see: danaparoid sodium]

chondroitin 6-sulfate [see: danaparoid sodium]

chondroitin sulfate *natural remedy for arthritis, blood clots, and extravasation from needle sticks after certain chemotherapy treatments*

chondroitin sulfate sodium JAN

chondroitin sulfuric acid *natural remedy* [see: chondroitin sulfate]

chondroitinase *investigational (orphan) agent for vitrectomy*

Chondrox capsules OTC *dietary supplement for osteoarthritis; protects and rebuilds cartilage in joints* [N-acetyl-D-glucosamine; glucosamine sulfate; chondroitin sulfate; manganese (as aspartate)] 500•500•800•0.17 mg

Chondrus crispus medicinal herb [see: Irish moss]

chonsurid *natural remedy* [see: chondroitin sulfate]

Chooz chewing gum OTC *antacid; calcium supplement* [calcium (as carbonate)] 500 mg (1250 mg)

CHOP (cyclophosphamide, hydroxydaunomycin, Oncovin,

prednisone) *chemotherapy protocol for non-Hodgkin lymphoma*

CHOP-Bleo (cyclophosphamide, hydroxydaunomycin, Oncovin, prednisone, bleomycin) *chemotherapy protocol for non-Hodgkin lymphoma*

choriogonadotropin alfa USAN, INN *recombinant human chorionic gonadotropin (rhCG); fertility stimulant for anovulatory women; adjuvant therapy for cryptorchidism*

chorionic gonadotrophin [see: gonadotropin, chorionic]

chorionic gonadotropin (CG) [see: gonadotropin, chorionic]

Choron-10 powder for IM injection (discontinued 2011) ℞ *a human-derived hormone used for prepubertal cryptorchidism or hypogonadism and to induce ovulation in anovulatory women* [chorionic gonadotropin] 1000 U/mL ⚗ Creon; guarana

CHP (chlorhexidine phosphanilate) [q.v.]

Christmas factor [see: factor IX complex]

Chromagen capsules (discontinued 2008) ℞ *hematinic* [iron (as ferrous fumarate); vitamin B_{12}; vitamin C; intrinsic factor concentrate] 70•0.01•150•100 mg

Chromagen film-coated caplets (discontinued 2011) ℞ *hematinic* [iron (as ferrous aspartoglycinate); vitamin B_{12}; vitamin C; intrinsic factor concentrate; succinic acid] 70•0.01•152•50•75 mg

Chromagen FA film-coated caplets ℞ *hematinic* [iron (as ferric pyrophosphate and ferrous aspartoglycinate); vitamin B_{12}; vitamin C; folic acid] 70•0.01•150•1 mg

Chromagen FA; Chromagen Forte capsules ℞ *hematinic* [iron (as ferrous fumarate); vitamin B_{12}; vitamin C; folic acid] 150•0.01•150•1 mg; 151•0.01•60•1 mg

Chromagen Forte film-coated caplets ℞ *hematinic* [iron (as ferrous fumarate, ferrous aspartoglycinate, and

elemental iron); vitamin B_{12}; vitamin C; folic acid] 151•0.01•60.8•1 mg

Chroma-Pak IV injection (discontinued 2011) ℞ *chromium supplement* [chromic chloride hexahydrate (20% elemental chromium)] 20.5, 102.5 mcg/mL (4, 20 mcg Cr/mL)

chromargyre [see: merbromin]

chromated albumin [see: albumin, chromated Cr 51 serum]

Chromelin Complexion Blender topical suspension OTC *skin darkening agent for vitiligo and hypopigmented areas* [dihydroxyacetone] 5%

chromic acid, disodium salt [see: sodium chromate Cr 51]

chromic chloride USP *dietary chromium supplement; additive to IV solutions for total parenteral nutrition* (20% elemental chromium) 20.5 mcg/mL (4 mcg/mL Cr) injection

chromic chloride Cr 51 USAN *radioactive agent*

chromic chloride hexahydrate [see: chromic chloride]

chromic phosphate Cr 51 USAN *radioactive agent*

chromic phosphate P 32 USAN, USP *antineoplastic; radioactive agent*

chromium *element (Cr); trace mineral important in glucose metabolism*

Chromium Chloride IV injection ℞ *intravenous nutritional therapy* [chromic chloride hexahydrate] 4 mcg/mL

chromium chloride [see: chromic chloride Cr 51]

chromium chloride hexahydrate [see: chromic chloride]

chromium picolinate *dietary chromium supplement*

chromium polynicotinate *dietary chromium supplement*

chromocarb INN

chromonar HCl USAN *coronary vasodilator* [also: carbocromen]

Chronoforte capsules OTC *anti-aging supplement; glycation inhibitor; antioxidant* [acetyl-L-carnitine; alpha lipoic acid; carnosine; nettle leaf;

quercetin; biotin] 333.3•50•166.7•
166.7•12.5•0.5 mg

Chronosule (trademarked dosage form) *sustained-action capsule* ℞ Granisol

Chronotab (trademarked dosage form) *sustained-action tablet*

Chronulac oral/rectal solution ℞ *hyperosmotic laxative* [lactulose] 10 g/15 mL

Chrysanthemum parthenium *medicinal herb* [see: feverfew]

Chrysanthemum vulgare *medicinal herb* [see: tansy]

chrysazin (*withdrawn from the market by the FDA*) [see: danthron]

chrysin *natural aromatase inhibitor used to block the conversion of testosterone to estrogen* ℞ Carrasyn; garcinia

chymopapain USAN, INN, BAN *proteolytic enzyme for herniated lumbar discs*

chymotrypsin USP, INN, BAN *proteolytic enzyme; zonulolytic for intracapsular lens extraction*

chymotrypsin & papain & trypsin *investigational (orphan) enzyme combination adjunct to chemotherapy for multiple myeloma*

C.I. acid orange 24 monosodium salt (color index) [see: resorcin brown]

C.I. basic violet 3 (color index) [see: gentian violet]

C.I. basic violet 14 monohydrochloride (color index) [see: fuchsin, basic]

C.I. direct blue 53 tetrasodium salt (color index) [see: Evans blue]

C.I. mordant yellow 5, disodium salt (color index) [see: olsalazine sodium]

ciadox INN ℞ Cedax; Cidex; Sudex; Z-Dex

Cialis film-coated tablets ℞ *selective vasodilator for erectile dysfunction (ED); approved for p.r.n. or q.d. dosing* [tadalafil] 2.5, 5, 10, 20 mg ℞ Salese; Silace; xylose

ciamexon INN, BAN ℞ Sumaxin

cianergoline INN

cianidanol INN

cianidol [see: cianidanol]

cianopramine INN

ciapilome INN

Ciba Vision Cleaner for Sensitive Eyes solution (discontinued 2010) OTC *surfactant cleaning solution for soft contact lenses*

Ciba Vision Saline aerosol solution OTC *rinsing/storage solution for soft contact lenses* [sodium chloride (saline solution)]

Cibacalcin subcu or IM injection ℞ *calcium regulator for Paget disease (osteitis deformans) (orphan)* [calcitonin (human)] 0.5 mg/vial

cibenzoline INN, BAN *antiarrhythmic* [also: cifenline]

cibenzoline succinate JAN *antiarrhythmic* [also: cifenline succinate]

cicaprost INN *prostacyclin analogue*

cicarperone INN

cicely, sweet *medicinal herb* [see: sweet cicely]

Cichorium intybus *medicinal herb* [see: chicory]

ciclacillin INN, BAN *antibacterial* [also: cyclacillin]

ciclactate INN

ciclafrine INN *antihypotensive* [also: ciclafrine HCl]

ciclafrine HCl USAN *antihypotensive* [also: ciclafrine]

ciclazindol USAN, INN, BAN *antidepressant*

ciclesonide *corticosteroidal anti-inflammatory; once-daily nasal aerosol for seasonal or perennial allergic rhinitis; once-daily inhalation aerosol for persistent asthma*

cicletanine USAN, INN, BAN *antihypertensive*

ciclindole INN *antidepressant* [also: cyclindole]

cicliomenol INN ℞ cyclomenol

ciclobendazole INN, BAN *anthelmintic* [also: cyclobendazole]

Ciclodan topical liquid ℞ *antifungal for tinea pedis, tinea cruris, tinea corporis, tinea versicolor, candidiasis, and seborrheic dermatitis* [ciclopirox] 8%

ciclofenazine INN *antipsychotic* [also: cyclophenazine HCl]

ciclofenazine HCl [see: cyclophenazine HCl]

cicloheximide INN *antipsoriatic* [also: cycloheximide]

ciclonicate INN

ciclonium bromide INN

ciclopirox USAN, INN, BAN *topical antifungal for tinea pedis, tinea cruris, tinea corporis, tinea versicolor, candidiasis, seborrheic dermatitis, and onychomycosis 0.77%, 8% topical; 1% shampoo; 8% nail lacquer*

ciclopirox olamine USAN, USP, JAN *topical antifungal for tinea pedis, tinea cruris, tinea corporis, tinea versicolor, candidiasis, seborrheic dermatitis, and onychomycosis 1% topical*

ciclopramine INN

cicloprofen USAN, INN, BAN *anti-inflammatory*

cicloprolol INN *antiadrenergic (beta-blocker)* [also: cicloprolol HCl; cycloprolol]

cicloprolol HCl USAN *antiadrenergic (beta-blocker)* [also: cicloprolol; cycloprolol]

ciclosidomine INN, BAN

ciclosporin INN *immunosuppressive* [also: cyclosporine; cyclosporin]

ciclotate INN *combining name for radicals or groups*

ciclotizolam INN, BAN

ciclotropium bromide INN

cicloxilic acid INN

cicloxolone INN, BAN

cicortonide INN

cicrotoic acid INN

cideferron INN ⊘ Pseudofrin

Cidex-7; Cidex Plus 28 solution OTC *broad-spectrum antimicrobial* [glutaral] 2%; 3.2% ⊘ Cedax; ciadox; Sudex; Z-Dex

cidofovir USAN, INN *nucleoside antiviral for AIDS-related cytomegalovirus (CMV) retinitis*

cidoxepin INN *antidepressant* [also: cidoxepin HCl]

cidoxepin HCl USAN *antidepressant* [also: cidoxepin]

cifenline USAN *antiarrhythmic* [also: cibenzoline]

cifenline succinate USAN *antiarrhythmic* [also: cibenzoline succinate]

cifostodine INN

ciglitazone USAN, INN *antidiabetic*

cignolin [see: anthralin]

ciheptolane INN

ciladopa INN, BAN *antiparkinsonian; dopaminergic agent* [also: ciladopa HCl]

ciladopa HCl USAN *antiparkinsonian; dopaminergic agent* [also: ciladopa]

cilansetron INN *treatment for irritable bowel syndrome*

cilastatin INN, BAN *enzyme inhibitor* [also: cilastatin sodium]

cilastatin sodium USAN, JAN *enzyme inhibitor* [also: cilastatin]

cilazapril USAN, INN, BAN, JAN *antihypertensive; ACE inhibitor*

cilazaprilat INN, BAN

cilexetil USAN *combining name for radicals or groups*

ciliary neurotrophic factor *investigational (orphan) agent for amyotrophic lateral sclerosis*

ciliary neurotrophic factor, recombinant human *investigational (orphan) agent for amyotrophic lateral sclerosis and other muscular atrophies*

"cillins" *brief term for a class of antibiotics derived from various strains of the fungus Penicillium, or their semi-synthetic analogues, whose generic names end in "cillin," such as ampicillin* [properly called: penicillins] ⊘ Selenos; Zolinza

cilmostim USAN *hematopoietic; macrophage colony-stimulating factor*

cilobamine INN *antidepressant* [also: cilobamine mesylate]

cilobamine mesylate USAN *antidepressant* [also: cilobamine]

cilofungin USAN, INN *antifungal*

ciloprost [see: iloprost]

cilostamide INN ⊘ salacetamide

cilostazol USAN, INN *antithrombotic; phosphodiesterase (PDE) III platelet aggregation inhibitor and vasodilator for* *intermittent claudication* 50, 100 mg oral

Ciloxan Drop-Tainers (eye drops), ointment ℞ *broad-spectrum fluoroquinolone antibiotic* [ciprofloxacin (as HCl)] 3 mg/mL

ciltoprazine INN

cilutazoline INN

cimaterol USAN, INN *repartitioning agent* ② Symmetrel; xamoterol

cimemoxin INN

cimepanol INN

cimetidine USAN, USP, INN, BAN, JAN *histamine H₂ antagonist for gastric and duodenal ulcers and gastric hypersecretory conditions* 200, 300, 400, 800 mg oral

cimetidine HCl USAN *histamine H₂ antagonist for gastric and duodenal ulcers and gastric hypersecretory conditions* 300 mg/5 mL oral; 300 mg/2 mL injection

Cimetidine in 0.9% Sodium Chloride IV infusion ℞ *histamine H₂ antagonist for gastric and duodenal ulcers and gastric hypersecretory conditions* [cimetidine HCl] 300 mg/50 mL bag

cimetropium bromide INN

Cimicifuga racemosa medicinal herb [see: black cohosh]

cimoxatone INN

Cimzia powder for subcu injection, subcu injection in prefilled syringes ℞ *anti-inflammatory for moderate to severe Crohn disease and rheumatoid arthritis* [certolizumab pegol] 200 mg

cinacalcet HCl *oral calcimimetic agent for hypercalcemia due to parathyroid carcinoma (orphan), primary hyperparathyroidism, or secondary hyperparathyroidism (SHPT) due to chronic kidney disease* (base=91%) 30, 60, 90 mg oral

cinalukast USAN, INN *antiasthmatic*

cinametic acid INN

cinamolol INN

cinanserin INN *serotonin inhibitor* [also: cinanserin HCl]

cinanserin HCl USAN *serotonin inhibitor* [also: cinanserin]

cinaproxen INN

cincaine chloride [see: dibucaine HCl]

cinchocaine INN, BAN *local anesthetic* [also: dibucaine]

cinchocaine HCl BAN *local anesthetic* [also: dibucaine HCl]

Cinchona succirubra; C. ledgeriana; C. calisaya medicinal herb [see: quinine]

cinchonidine sulfate NF

cinchonine sulfate NF

cinchophen NF, INN, BAN

cinecromen INN

cinepaxadil INN

cinepazet INN, BAN *antianginal* [also: cinepazet maleate]

cinepazet maleate USAN *antianginal* [also: cinepazet]

cinepazic acid INN

cinepazide INN, BAN

cinfenine INN

cinfenoac INN, BAN

cinflumide USAN, INN *muscle relaxant*

cingestol USAN, INN *progestin*

cinitapride INN

cinmetacin INN

cinnamaldehyde NF

cinnamaverine INN

cinnamedrine USAN, INN *smooth muscle relaxant*

cinnamedrine HCl *smooth muscle relaxant*

cinnamic aldehyde [now: cinnamaldehyde]

cinnamon NF

cinnamon oil NF

cinnamon (Cinnamonum zeylanicum) bark and oil *medicinal herb for diarrhea, dysmenorrhea, gastrointestinal upset, microbial and fungal infections, and gas pain; also used as an aromatic, astringent, and stimulant*

cinnamon wood *medicinal herb* [see: sassafras]

cinnarizine USAN, INN, BAN *antihistamine*

cinnarizine clofibrate INN

cinnofuradione INN

cinnofuron [see: cinnofuradione]

cinnopentazone INN *anti-inflammatory* [also: cintazone]

cinnopropazone [see: apazone]

Cinobac capsules (discontinued 2009) ℞ *urinary antibacterial* [cinoxacin] 250 mg ⊘ Sani-Pak

cinoctramide INN

cinodine HCl USAN *veterinary antibacterial*

cinolazepam INN

cinoquidox INN

cinoxacin USAN, USP, INN, BAN *urinary antibacterial*

cinoxate USAN, USP, INN *ultraviolet screen*

cinoxolone INN, BAN

cinoxopazide INN

cinperene USAN, INN *antipsychotic*

cinprazole INN

cinpropazide INN

cinquefoil *(Potentilla anserina; P. canadensis; P. reptans)* plant *medicinal herb used as an antispasmodic and astringent*

cinromide USAN, INN *anticonvulsant*

Cinryze powder for IV infusion ℞ *agent to prevent acute attacks of angioedema in adolescents or adults with hereditary angioedema (HAE)* [C1-inhibitor, human] 500 units/vial

cintazone USAN *anti-inflammatory* [also: cinnopentazone]

cintramide INN *antipsychotic* [also: cintriamide]

cintriamide USAN *antipsychotic* [also: cintramide]

cinuperone INN

cioteronel USAN, INN *antiandrogen* ⊘ citronella; soterenol; SteriNail

cipamfylline USAN *antiviral agent; tumor necrosis factor alpha inhibitor*

cipemastat USAN, INN *matrix metalloproteinase inhibitor*

cipionate INN *combining name for radicals or groups* [also: cypionate]

ciprafamide INN

ciprazafone INN

ciprefadol INN *analgesic* [also: ciprefadol succinate]

ciprefadol succinate USAN *analgesic* [also: ciprefadol]

Cipro Cystitis Pack (6 film-coated tablets) (discontinued 2008) ℞ *broad-spectrum fluoroquinolone antibiotic* [ciprofloxacin] 100 mg

Cipro film-coated tablets ℞ *broad-spectrum fluoroquinolone antibiotic* [ciprofloxacin (as HCl)] 250, 500, 750 mg

Cipro powder for oral suspension ℞ *broad-spectrum fluoroquinolone antibiotic* [ciprofloxacin] 250, 500 mg/5 mL

Cipro HC Otic ear drop suspension ℞ *broad-spectrum fluoroquinolone antibiotic; corticosteroidal anti-inflammatory* [ciprofloxacin; hydrocortisone] 0.2%•1% (2•10 mg/mL)

Cipro I.V. ℞ *broad-spectrum fluoroquinolone antibiotic* [ciprofloxacin] 200, 400 mg/vial ⊘ Spiriva

Cipro XR film-coated extended-release tablets ℞ *broad-spectrum fluoroquinolone antibiotic* [ciprofloxacin (as the base and HCl)] 500, 1000 mg

ciprocinonide USAN, INN *adrenocortical steroid*

Ciprodex ear drop suspension ℞ *broad-spectrum fluoroquinolone antibiotic; corticosteroidal anti-inflammatory* [ciprofloxacin HCl; dexamethasone] 0.3%•0.1%

ciprofibrate USAN, INN, BAN *antihyperlipoproteinemic*

ciprofloxacin USAN, INN, BAN *broad-spectrum fluoroquinolone antibiotic* 200, 400 mg injection; 212.6, 425.2 mg oral ⊘ sparfloxacin

ciprofloxacin HCl USAN, USP, JAN *broad-spectrum fluoroquinolone antibiotic* (base=74%) [3.5 mg/mL] 100, 250, 500, 750, 1000 mg oral; 287.5, 574.9 mg oral; 3.5 mg/mL eye drops ⊘ sparfloxacin

Ciprofloxacin in 5% Dextrose injection ℞ *broad-spectrum fluoroquinolone antibiotic* [ciprofloxacin] 200, 400 mg ⊘ sparfloxacin

ciprofloxacin liposomal *broad-spectrum bactericidal antibiotic; investigational (orphan) aerosolized formulation for the treatment of cystic fibrosis*

cipropride INN

ciproquazone INN

ciproquinate INN *coccidiostat for poultry* [also: cyproquinate]

ciprostene INN *platelet antiaggregatory agent* [also: ciprostene calcium]

ciprostene calcium USAN *platelet antiaggregatory agent* [also: ciprostene]

ciproximide INN *antipsychotic; antidepressant* [also: cyproximide]

ciramadol USAN, INN *analgesic*

ciramadol HCl USAN *analgesic*

cirazoline INN

Circadin *natural sleep aid; investigational (orphan) for circadian rhythm sleep disorders in blind people with no light perception* [melatonin]

Circavite-T tablets (discontinued 2008) OTC *vitamin/mineral/iron supplement* [multiple vitamins & minerals; iron] ± •12 mg

Circulase *investigational (orphan) for advanced chronic critical limb ischemia* [prostaglandin E_1 enol ester]

cirolemycin USAN, INN *antineoplastic; antibacterial*

cisapride USAN, INN, BAN, JAN *peristaltic stimulant; treatment for nocturnal heartburn due to gastroesophageal reflux disease; (withdrawn from the U.S. market in 2000 due to increased cardiac arrhythmias)*

cisatracurium besylate USAN *nondepolarizing neuromuscular blocker*

CISCA; CisCA (cisplatin, cyclophosphamide, Adriamycin) *chemotherapy protocol for bladder cancer*

CISCA$_{II}$/VB$_{IV}$ (cisplatin, cyclophosphamide, Adriamycin; vinblastine, bleomycin) *chemotherapy protocol for germ cell tumors*

cisclomiphene [now: enclomiphene]

cisconazole USAN, INN *antifungal*

cis-DDP (diamminedichloroplatinum) [see: cisplatin]

cis-diamminedichloroplatinum (DDP) [see: cisplatin]

cismadinone INN

cisplatin USAN, USP, INN, BAN *alkylating antineoplastic for metastatic testicular tumors, metastatic ovarian tumors, and advanced bladder cancer* 1 mg/mL injection

cisplatin + docetaxel *chemotherapy protocol for bladder, head, and neck cancer* [also: docetaxel + cisplatin; TC]

cisplatin & epinephrine *investigational (NDA filed, orphan) injectable gel for squamous cell carcinoma of the head and neck; investigational (orphan) for metastatic malignant melanoma*

cisplatin + fluorouracil *chemotherapy protocol for head, neck, esophageal, bladder, anal, and cervical cancer* [also: CF; FUP]

cisplatin + vinorelbine *chemotherapy protocol for head, neck, cervical and non–small cell lung cancer* [also: VC; vinorelbine + cisplatin]

cis-**platinum** [now: cisplatin]

cis-**platinum II** [now: cisplatin]

9-*cis*-retinoic acid [see: alitretinoin]

13-*cis*-retinoic acid [see: isotretinoin]

cistinexine INN

citalopram INN, BAN *selective serotonin reuptake inhibitor (SSRI) for major depression*

citalopram hydrobromide USAN *selective serotonin reuptake inhibitor (SSRI) for major depression; also used for obsessive-compulsive disorder (OCD), post-traumatic stress disorder (PTSD), generalized anxiety disorder (GAD), and premenstrual dysphoric disorder (PMDD)* 10, 20, 40 mg oral; 10 mg/5 mL oral

Citanest Forte injection ℞ *local anesthetic and vasoconstrictor for dental procedures* [prilocaine HCl; epinephrine] 4%•1:200 000

Citanest Plain injection ℞ *local anesthetic for dental procedures* [prilocaine HC] 4%

citatepine INN

citenamide USAN, INN *anticonvulsant*

citenazone INN

citicoline INN, JAN *neuroprotectant* [also: citicoline sodium]

citicoline sodium USAN *neuroprotectant* [also: citicoline]

citiolone INN

Citra pH oral solution OTC *antacid* [sodium citrate] 450 mg/5 mL

Citracal tablets OTC *calcium supplement* [calcium (as citrate)] 200 mg (950 mg)

Citracal Creamy Bites chewable tablets (discontinued 2008) OTC *calcium supplement* [calcium (as citrate); vitamin D] 500 mg•200 IU

Citracal + D3 caplets OTC *vitamin/calcium supplement* [calcium (as citrate); vitamin D] 315 mg•250 IU

Citracal Liquitab effervescent tablets OTC *calcium supplement* [calcium (as citrate)] 500 mg (2380 mg)

Citracal Plus film-coated tablets OTC *calcium/mineral supplement* [calcium (as citrate); vitamin D; multiple minerals] 250 mg•125 IU• ±

Citracal Prenatal 90 + DHA tablets + capsules ℞ *prenatal vitamin/mineral/calcium/iron/omega-3 supplement; stool softener* [multiple vitamins & minerals; calcium (as citrate); iron (as carbonyl); folic acid; docusate sodium + docosahexaenoic acid (DHA)] ±•200•90•1•50 mg (tablets) + 250 mg (capsules)

Citracal Prenatal + DHA tablets + capsules ℞ *prenatal vitamin/mineral/calcium/iron/omega-3 supplement; stool softener* [multiple vitamins & minerals; calcium (as citrate); iron (as carbonyl and ferrous gluconate); folic acid; docusate sodium + docosahexaenoic acid (DHA)] ±•125•27•1•50 mg (tablets) + 250 mg (capsules)

Citracal Prenatal Rx tablets ℞ *prenatal vitamin/mineral/calcium/iron supplement* [multiple vitamins & minerals; calcium (as citrate); iron; folic acid; docusate sodium] ±•125•27•1•50 mg

Citralax effervescent granules OTC *saline laxative* [magnesium citrate; magnesium sulfate] ② Starlix

CitraNatal DHA; CitraNatal 90 DHA tablets + capsules ℞ *prenatal vitamin/mineral/calcium/iron/omega-3 supplement; stool softener* [multiple vitamins & minerals; calcium (as citrate); iron (as carbonyl); folic acid; docusate sodium + docosahexaenoic acid (DHA)] ±•125•27•1•50 mg (tablets) + 250 mg (capsules); ±• 200•90•1•50 mg (tablets) + 250 mg (capsules)

CitraNatal Rx tablets ℞ *prenatal vitamin/mineral/calcium/iron supplement; stool softener* [multiple vitamins & minerals; calcium (as citrate); iron (as carbonyl); folic acid; docusate sodium] ±•125•27•1•50 mg

citrate dextrose [see: ACD solution]

citrate of magnesia [see: magnesium citrate]

citrate phosphate dextrose [see: anticoagulant citrate phosphate dextrose solution]

citrate phosphate dextrose adenine [see: anticoagulant citrate phosphate dextrose adenine solution]

citrated caffeine NF [see: caffeine citrate]

citric acid USP *pH adjusting agent; urinary acidifier* ② stearic acid

citric acid, magnesium oxide & sodium carbonate [see: Suby G solution]

citric acid & potassium citrate *investigational (orphan) agent for the dissolution and control of uric acid and cysteine calculi in the urinary tract*

citric acid & sodium citrate *urinary alkalinizing agent* 334•500 mg/5 mL oral

citrin [see: bioflavonoids]

Citrocarbonate effervescent granules OTC *antacid* [sodium bicarbonate; sodium citrate] 780•1820 mg/dose

Citrolith tablets ℞ *urinary alkalinizing agent* [potassium citrate; sodium citrate] 50•950 mg

citronella (Cymbopogon nardus; C. winterianus) oil *medicinal herb for gastrointestinal spasms, promoting diuresis, and worms; also used as an antibacterial; not generally regarded as safe and effective for internal use as it* *is highly toxic* ☒ cioteronel; soterenol; SteriNail

Citrotein oral liquid, powder for oral liquid OTC *enteral nutritional therapy* [lactose-free formula]

citrovorum factor [see: leucovorin calcium]

Citrucel powder, tablets OTC *bulk laxative* [methylcellulose] 2 g/tbsp. or scoop; 500 mg

Citrucel Fiber Shake; Citrucel Sugar Free powder for oral solution OTC *bulk laxative* [methylcellulose] 2 g/tbsp.

Citrus bergamia; C. aurantium *medicinal herb* [see: bergamot oil]

citrus bioflavonoids [see: bioflavonoids]

Citrus Calcium coated tablets OTC *calcium supplement* [calcium (as citrate)] 200 mg (950 mg)

Citrus Calcium + D caplets OTC *calcium supplement* [calcium (as citrate); vitamin D] 200 mg•200 IU, 315 mg•200 IU

Citrus limon *medicinal herb* [see: lemon]

Citrus paradisi *medicinal herb* [see: grapefruit]

civamide *investigational (orphan) agent for postherpetic neuralgia of the trigeminal nerve*

8-Cl cAMP (8-chloroadenosine monophosphate, cyclic) [see: tocladesine]

CLA (conjugated linoleic acid) [q.v.]

cladribine *antimetabolite antineoplastic for hairy-cell leukemia (orphan); investigational (Phase III, orphan) disease-modifying agent for relapsing multiple sclerosis; investigational (orphan) for chronic lymphocytic leukemia, myeloid leukemia, and non-Hodgkin lymphoma* 1 mg/mL injection

Claforan powder or frozen premix for IV or IM injection ℞ *third-generation cephalosporin antibiotic* [cefotaxime sodium] 0.5, 1, 2, 10 g ☒ Calphron; Kolephrin

clamidoxic acid INN, BAN

clamoxyquin BAN *antiamebic* [also: clamoxyquin HCl; clamoxyquine]

clamoxyquin HCl USAN *antiamebic* [also: clamoxyquine; clamoxyquin]

clamoxyquine INN *antiamebic* [also: clamoxyquin HCl; clamoxyquin]

clanfenur INN

clanobutin INN

clantifen INN

clara cell 10kDa protein, recombinant human *investigational (orphan) for prevention of bronchopulmonary dysplasia in neonates with respiratory distress syndrome (RDS)*

Claravis capsules ℞ *keratolytic for severe recalcitrant cystic acne* [isotretinoin] 10, 20, 30, 40 mg ☒ Klorvess

claretin-12 [see: cyanocobalamin]

Clarifoam EF topical foam ℞ *antibiotic and keratolytic for acne* [sulfacetamide sodium; sulfur] 10%•5%

Clarinex film-coated tablets, syrup ℞ *nonsedating antihistamine for allergic rhinitis and chronic idiopathic urticaria* [desloratadine] 5 mg; 2.5 mg/5 mL

Clarinex RediTabs (rapidly disintegrating tablets) ℞ *nonsedating antihistamine for allergic rhinitis and chronic idiopathic urticaria* [desloratadine] 2.5, 5 mg

Clarinex-D 12 Hour extended-release tablets ℞ *nonsedating antihistamine and decongestant for allergic rhinitis* [desloratadine; pseudoephedrine sulfate] 2.5•120 mg

Clarinex-D 24 Hour extended-release tablets ℞ *nonsedating antihistamine and decongestant for allergic rhinitis* [desloratadine; pseudoephedrine sulfate] 5•240 mg

Claripel cream (discontinued 2010) ℞ *hyperpigmentation bleaching agent* [hydroquinone] 4%

Claris soap ℞ *antibiotic and keratolytic for acne* [sulfacetamide sodium; sulfur] 10%•1% ☒ Clerz

clarithromycin USAN, INN, BAN, JAN *macrolide antibiotic* 250, 500 mg oral; 125, 250 mg/5 mL oral

clarithromycin & amoxicillin & omeprazole *combination macrolide and aminopenicillin antibiotic plus a gastric antisecretory* 500•500•20 mg oral

Claritin capsules, syrup OTC *nonsedating antihistamine for allergic rhinitis* [loratadine] 10 mg; 5 mg/5 mL

Claritin 24-Hour Allergy tablets OTC *nonsedating antihistamine for allergic rhinitis; also used for chronic idiopathic urticaria* [loratadine] 10 mg

Claritin Children's Allergy chewable tablets, oral solution OTC *nonsedating antihistamine for allergic rhinitis* [loratadine] 5 mg; 5 mg/5 mL

Claritin Eye eye drops OTC *antihistamine and mast cell stabilizer for allergic conjunctivitis* [ketotifen (as fumarate)] 0.025%

Claritin Hives Relief tablets OTC *nonsedating antihistamine for hives* [loratadine] 10 mg

Claritin Non-Drowsy Liqui-Gels (liquid-filled softgels) OTC *nonsedating antihistamine for allergic rhinitis* [loratadine] 10 mg

Claritin RediTabs (orally disintegrating tablets) OTC *nonsedating antihistamine for allergic rhinitis* [loratadine] 5, 10 mg

Claritin-D 12 Hour; Claritin-D 24 Hour extended-release tablets OTC *nonsedating antihistamine; decongestant* [loratadine; pseudoephedrine sulfate] 5•120 mg; 10•240 mg

Claviceps purpurea medicinal herb [see: ergot]

clavulanate potassium USAN, USP *beta-lactamase inhibitor; penicillin synergist*

clavulanic acid INN, BAN *beta-lactamase inhibitor; penicillin synergist*

claw, scaly dragon's; turkey claw *medicinal herb* [see: coral root]

clay, kaolin *natural material* [see: kaolin]

clazolam USAN, INN *minor tranquilizer*

clazolimine USAN, INN *diuretic*

clazuril USAN, INN, BAN *coccidiostat for pigeons* ⍰ Clozaril; glycerol

CLD-BOMP *chemotherapy protocol for cervical cancer* [see: BOMP]

Clean and Clear Foaming Facial Cleanser soap OTC *disinfectant/antiseptic; medicated cleanser for acne* [triclosan] 0.25%

Clear Eyes Contact Lens Relief eye drops OTC *antiseptic; emollient* [sorbic acid] 0.25%

Clear Eyes for Dry Eyes eye drops OTC *moisturizer; emollient* [carboxymethylcellulose sodium; glycerin] 1%•0.25%

Clear Eyes for Dry Eyes Plus Redness Relief eye drops OTC *decongestant; vasoconstrictor; moisturizer/lubricant* [naphazoline HCl; hypromellose; glycerin] 0.012%•0.8%•0.25%

Clear Eyes for Redness Relief eye drops OTC *decongestant; vasoconstrictor; moisturizer/lubricant* [naphazoline HCl; glycerin] 0.012%•0.2%

Clear Eyes Seasonal Relief eye drops OTC *decongestant; astringent* [naphazoline HCl; zinc sulfate] 0.012%•0.2%

Clearasil Acne Treatment cream OTC *keratolytic for acne* [benzoyl peroxide] 10%

Clearasil Acne-Fighting Pads OTC *keratolytic for acne* [salicylic acid; alcohol] 2%• ⍰

Clearasil Adult Care cream OTC *antiseptic, antifungal, and keratolytic for acne* [sulfur; resorcinol; alcohol 10%]

Clearasil Antibacterial Soap bar OTC *disinfectant/antiseptic; medicated cleanser for acne* [triclosan]

Clearasil Clearstick topical liquid OTC *keratolytic for acne* [salicylic acid; alcohol] 1.25%•39%, 2%•39%

Clearasil Daily Face Wash topical liquid OTC *disinfectant/antiseptic; medicated cleanser for acne* [triclosan] 0.3%

Clearasil Double Clear; Clearasil Double Textured medicated pads OTC *keratolytic for acne* [salicylic acid; alcohol] 1.25%•40%, 2%•40%; 2%•40%

Clearasil Medicated Deep Cleanser topical liquid OTC *keratolytic cleanser for acne* [salicylic acid; alcohol 42%] 0.5%

Clear-Atadine tablets OTC *nonsedating antihistamine for allergic rhinitis; also used for chronic idiopathic urticaria* [loratadine] 10 mg

Clear-Atadine Children's oral liquid OTC *nonsedating antihistamine for allergic rhinitis* [loratadine] 5 mg/5 mL

Clear-Atadine D extended-release tablets OTC *nonsedating antihistamine; decongestant* [loratadine; pseudo-ephedrine sulfate] 10•240 mg

Clearblue Easy Digital Pregnancy Test test stick plus digital readout for home use OTC *in vitro diagnostic aid; urine pregnancy test*

Clearblue Easy Ovulation Test test sticks for home use (7 sticks per package) OTC *in vitro diagnostic aid; urine ovulation test*

Clearblue Easy Pregnancy Test test stick for home use OTC *in vitro diagnostic aid; urine pregnancy test*

Clearly Cala-gel OTC *topical antihistamine* [diphenhydramine HCl]

Clearview Chlamydia test for professional use ℞ *in vitro diagnostic aid for* Chlamydia trachomatis [color-label immunoassay]

cleavers; cleaverwort *medicinal herb* [see: bedstraw]

clebopride USAN, INN *antiemetic*

Cleervue-M film-coated tablets ℞ *tetracycline antibiotic for gram-negative and gram-positive bacteria; antirickett-sial* [minocycline (as HCl)] 50 mg

clefamide INN, BAN

clemastine USAN, BAN *ethanolamine antihistamine* ⑨ galamustine

clemastine fumarate USAN, USP, BAN *ethanolamine antihistamine;* (base= 75%) 1.34, 2.68 mg oral; 0.67 mg/5 mL oral

Clematis cirrhosa; C. virginiana medicinal herb [see: woodbine]

clemeprol INN, BAN

clemizole INN, BAN

clemizole penicillin INN, BAN

clenbuterol INN, BAN

Clenia cream, foaming wash ℞ *antibiotic and keratolytic for acne, rosacea,*

and seborrheic dermatitis [sulfaceta-mide sodium; sulfur] 10%•5% ⑨ Calan; Gilenya; kaolin; khellin

clenoliximab *investigational (Phase I/II) anti-CD4 antibody for the treatment of rheumatoid arthritis*

clenpirin INN [also: clenpyrin]

clenpyrin BAN [also: clenpirin]

clentiazem INN *calcium channel antag-onist* [also: clentiazem maleate]

clentiazem maleate USAN *calcium channel antagonist* [also: clentiazem]

Clenz-Lyte powder for oral solution ℞ *pre-procedure bowel evacuant* [poly-ethylene glycol–electrolyte solution (PEG 3350, potassium chloride, sodium bicarbonate, sodium chlo-ride, sodium sulfate)]

Cleocin capsules ℞ *antibiotic; investiga-tional (orphan) for* AIDS-related Pneu-mocystis pneumonia (PCP) and sar-coidosis [clindamycin (as HCl)] 75, 150, 300 mg

Cleocin vaginal cream in prefilled applicator, vaginal ovules (supposi-tories) ℞ *antibiotic for bacterial vagi-nosis* [clindamycin phosphate] 2%; 100 mg ⑨ Galzin; glycine; Quelicin

Cleocin Pediatric granules for oral solution ℞ *antibiotic* [clindamycin (as palmitate HCl)] 75 mg/5 mL

Cleocin Phosphate IM injection ℞ *antibiotic; investigational (orphan) for* AIDS-related Pneumocystis pneumo-nia (PCP) [clindamycin (as phos-phate)] 150 mg/mL

Cleocin Phosphate IV infusion ℞ *antibiotic; investigational (orphan) for* AIDS-related Pneumocystis pneumo-nia (PCP) [clindamycin (as phos-phate)] 300, 600, 900 mg

Cleocin T gel, lotion, topical solution, pledgets ℞ *antibiotic for acne; also used for rosacea* [clindamycin phos-phate] 1%

Clerz 2 solution (discontinued 2010) OTC *rewetting solution for hard or soft contact lenses* ⑨ Claris

Clerz Plus solution OTC *rewetting solu-tion for hard or soft contact lenses*

cletoquine INN, BAN

clevidipine butyrate *calcium channel blocker for the rapid control of hypertension*

Cleviprex emulsion for IV injection ℞ *calcium channel blocker for the rapid control of hypertension* [clevidipine butyrate] 25, 50 mg

clibucaine INN

click.easy (trademarked device) *reconstitution cartridge for* **Serostim**, *used with a* **cool.click** *or* **one.click** *autoinjector*

clidafidine INN

clidanac INN

clidinium bromide USAN, USP, INN, BAN *GI/GU anticholinergic/antispasmodic; peptic ulcer adjunct*

clidinium bromide & chlordiazepoxide HCl *GI/GU anticholinergic/antispasmodic; anxiolytic* 2.5•5 mg

Climara transdermal patch ℞ *estrogen replacement therapy for the treatment of postmenopausal symptoms and prevention of postmenopausal osteoporosis* [estradiol] 25, 37.5, 50, 60, 75, 100 mcg/day

ClimaraPro transdermal patch ℞ *hormone replacement therapy for the treatment of postmenopausal symptoms and prevention of postmenopausal osteoporosis* [levonorgestrel; estradiol] 15• 45 mcg/day

climazolam INN

climbazole INN, BAN

climiqualine INN

Clinac BPO gel ℞ *keratolytic for acne* [benzoyl peroxide] 7%

clinafloxacin HCl USAN *quinolone antibacterial*

Clindagel gel ℞ *antibiotic for acne; also used for rosacea* [clindamycin phosphate] 1%

ClindaMax gel, lotion ℞ *antibiotic for acne; also used for rosacea* [clindamycin phosphate] 1%

ClindaMax vaginal cream in prefilled applicators (discontinued 2009) ℞ *antibiotic for bacterial vaginosis* [clindamycin phosphate] 2%

clindamycin USAN, INN, BAN *lincosamide antibiotic; investigational (orphan) for AIDS-related Pneumocystis pneumonia (PCP) and sarcoidosis*

clindamycin HCl USP, BAN *lincosamide antibiotic; investigational (orphan) for AIDS-related Pneumocystis pneumonia (PCP) and sarcoidosis* 75, 150, 300 mg oral

clindamycin HCl & primaquine phosphate *investigational (orphan) for AIDS-related Pneumocystis pneumonia (PCP)*

clindamycin palmitate HCl USAN, USP *lincosamide antibiotic* 75 mg/5 mL oral

clindamycin phosphate USAN, USP *lincosamide antibiotic* 1%, 2% topical; 150 mg/mL injection

clindamycin phosphate & benzoyl peroxide *lincosamide antibiotic and keratolytic for acne* 1%•5% topical

Clindesse vaginal cream in prefilled applicators ℞ *antibiotic for bacterial vaginosis* [clindamycin phosphate] 2%

Clindets pledgets ℞ *antibiotic for acne; also used for rosacea* [clindamycin; alcohol 52%] 1%

Clindets topical solution (discontinued 2010) ℞ *antibiotic for acne; also used for rosacea* [clindamycin; alcohol 52%] 1%

Clinipak (trademarked packaging form) *unit dose package*

Clinistix reagent strips for home use (discontinued 2008) OTC *in vitro diagnostic aid for urine glucose*

Clinitest reagent tablets for home use (discontinued 2008) OTC *in vitro diagnostic aid for urine glucose*

clinocaine HCl [see: procaine HCl]

clinofibrate INN

clinolamide INN

Clinoril tablets ℞ *nonsteroidal anti-inflammatory drug (NSAID) for osteoarthritis, rheumatoid arthritis, ankylosing spondylitis, acute bursitis/tendinitis, and other inflammatory conditions* [sulindac] 200 mg

clioquinol USP, INN, BAN *topical anti-bacterial/antifungal* 3% topical

clioxanide USAN, INN, BAN *anthelmintic*

clipoxamine [see: cliropamine]

cliprofen USAN, INN *anti-inflammatory*

cliropamine INN

Clivarine *investigational (orphan) for deep vein thrombosis (DVT) in pediatric or pregnant patients* [reviparin sodium]

clobamine mesylate [now: cilobamine mesylate]

clobazam USAN, INN, BAN *minor benzodiazepine tranquilizer; anxiolytic; investigational (NDA filed) anticonvulsant for seizures associated with Lennox-Gastaut syndrome (LGS)*

clobedolum [see: clonitazene]

clobenoside INN

clobenzepam INN

clobenzorex INN

clobenztropine INN

clobetasol INN, BAN *topical corticosteroidal anti-inflammatory* [also: clobetasol propionate]

clobetasol propionate USAN *topical corticosteroidal anti-inflammatory for scalp dermatoses and plaque psoriasis* [also: clobetasol] 0.05% topical

clobetasone INN, BAN *topical corticosteroidal anti-inflammatory* [also: clobetasone butyrate]

clobetasone butyrate USAN *topical corticosteroidal anti-inflammatory* [also: clobetasone]

Clobex topical spray, lotion, shampoo ℞ *corticosteroidal anti-inflammatory* [clobetasol propionate] 0.05%

clobutinol INN

clobuzarit INN, BAN

clocanfamide INN

clocapramine INN

clociguanil INN, BAN

clocinizine INN

clocortolone INN *topical corticosteroid* [also: clocortolone acetate]

clocortolone acetate USAN *topical corticosteroid* [also: clocortolone]

clocortolone pivalate USAN, USP *topical corticosteroid*

clocoumarol INN

Clocream cream OTC *moisturizer; emollient* [cod liver oil (vitamins A and E); cholecalciferol; vitamin A palmitate]

clodacaine INN

clodanolene USAN, INN *skeletal muscle relaxant*

clodantoin INN *antifungal* [also: chlordantoin]

clodazon INN *antidepressant* [also: clodazon HCl] ⑨ Caldesene

clodazon HCl USAN *antidepressant* [also: clodazon]

Cloderm cream ℞ *corticosteroidal anti-inflammatory* [clocortolone pivalate] 0.1%

clodoxopone INN

clodronate disodium *bisphosphonate bone resorption inhibitor for hypercalcemia of malignancy* [also: disodium clodronate]

clodronic acid USAN, INN, BAN *calcium regulator*

clofarabine *purine nucleoside antimetabolite antineoplastic for patients 1–21 years with acute lymphoblastic leukemia (orphan); investigational (Phase III, orphan) for acute myelogenous leukemia*

clofazimine USAN, INN, BAN *bactericidal; tuberculostatic; leprostatic (orphan); available only to physicians enrolled in the National Hansen Disease Program through the FDA*

clofedanol INN *antitussive* [also: chlophedianol HCl; chlophedianol]

clofedanol HCl [see: chlophedianol HCl]

clofenamic acid INN

clofenamide INN

clofenciclan INN

clofenetamine INN

clofenetamine HCl [see: clofenetamine]

clofenotane INN [also: chlorophenothane; dicophane]

clofenoxyde INN

clofenpyride [see: nicofibrate]

clofenvinfos INN [also: chlorfenvinphos]

Clofera oral liquid OTC *antitussive; decongestant* [chlophedianol HCl;

pseudoephedrine HCl] 12.5•30 mg/
5 mL

clofeverine INN

clofexamide INN

clofezone INN ② Calphosan

clofibrate USAN, USP, INN, BAN *triglyceride-lowering antihyperlipidemic for
primary dysbetalipoproteinemia (type
III hyperlipidemia) and hypertriglyceridemia (types IV and V hyperlipidemia)*

clofibric acid INN

clofibride INN

clofilium phosphate USAN, INN *antiarrhythmic*

clofinol [see: nicofibrate]

cloflucarban USAN *disinfectant* [also:
halocarban]

clofluperol INN, BAN *antipsychotic*
[also: seperidol HCl]

clofluperol HCl [see: seperidol HCl]

clofoctol INN

cloforex INN

clofurac INN

clogestone INN, BAN *progestin* [also:
clogestone acetate]

clogestone acetate USAN *progestin*
[also: clogestone]

cloguanamil INN, BAN [also: clogua-
namile]

cloguanamile BAN [also: cloguanamil]

Clolar IV infusion ℞ *antineoplastic for
patients 1−21 years with acute lymphoblastic leukemia (orphan); investigational
(Phase III, orphan) for acute myelogenous leukemia* [clofarabine] 1 mg/mL

clomacran INN, BAN *antipsychotic*
[also: clomacran phosphate]

clomacran phosphate USAN *antipsychotic* [also: clomacran]

clomegestone INN *progestin* [also: clomegestone acetate]

clomegestone acetate USAN *progestin*
[also: clomegestone]

clometacin INN

clometerone INN *antiestrogen* [also:
clometherone]

clometherone USAN *antiestrogen* [also:
clometerone]

clomethiazole INN [also: chlormethia-
zole]

clomethiazole edisylate USAN *GABA
(A) receptor modulator for acute
ischemic stroke*

clometocillin INN

Clomid tablets ℞ *ovulation stimulant*
[clomiphene citrate] 50 mg

clomide [see: aklomide]

clomifene INN *gonad-stimulating principle; ovulation stimulant* [also: clomiphene citrate; clomiphene]

clomifenoxide INN

clominorex USAN, INN *anorectic*

clomiphene BAN *gonad-stimulating
principle; ovulation stimulant* [also:
clomiphene citrate; clomifene]

clomiphene citrate USAN, USP *gonad-
stimulating principle; ovulation stimulant* [also: clomifene; clomiphene] 50
mg oral

clomipramine INN, BAN *tricyclic antidepressant for obsessive-compulsive disorders* [also: clomipramine HCl]

clomipramine HCl USAN *tricyclic
antidepressant for obsessive-compulsive
disorders* [also: clomipramine] 25, 50,
75 mg oral

clomocycline INN, BAN ② colimecycline

clomoxir INN

clonazepam USAN, USP, INN, BAN
*anticonvulsant; anxiolytic for panic dis-
order; also used for parkinsonian dysarthria, neuralgias, multifocal tics, and
manic episodes of a bipolar disorder;
investigational (orphan) for hyperexplexia (startle disease)* 0.125, 0.25,
0.5, 1, 2 mg oral

clonazoline INN

CloniBID sustained release *investigational (NDA filed) antihypertensive*
[clonidine HCl]

Clonicel *investigational (Phase III)
treatment for attention-deficit/hyperac-
tivity disorder (ADHD) in children*
[clonidine]

clonidine USAN, INN, BAN *centrally
acting antiadrenergic antihypertensive;
adjunct to epidural opioid analgesics for
severe cancer pain (orphan); investigational (Phase III) treatment for attention-*

deficit/hyperactivity disorder in children 0.1, 0.2, 0.3 mg/day transdermal; 0.17, 0.26 mg oral; 0.09 mg/mL oral

clonidine HCl USAN, USP, BAN *centrally acting antiadrenergic antihypertensive; central analgesic; adjunct to epidural opioid analgesics for severe cancer pain (orphan); stimulant adjunct for ADHD; also used for opioid and methadone withdrawal and smoking cessation* 0.1, 0.2, 0.3 mg oral; 0.1, 0.5 mg/mL injection; 0.1, 0.2, 0.3 mg/day transdermal

clonitazene INN, BAN

clonitrate USAN, INN *coronary vasodilator*

clonixeril USAN, INN *analgesic*

clonixin USAN, INN *analgesic*

clopamide USAN, INN, BAN *antihypertensive; diuretic*

clopenthixol USAN, INN, BAN *antipsychotic*

cloperastine INN

cloperidone INN *sedative* [also: cloperidone HCl]

cloperidone HCl USAN *sedative* [also: cloperidone]

clophenoxate [see: meclofenoxate]

clopidogrel INN, BAN *platelet aggregation inhibitor for stroke, myocardial infarction, peripheral artery disease, and acute coronary syndrome*

clopidogrel bisulfate USAN *platelet aggregation inhibitor for stroke, myocardial infarction, peripheral artery disease, and acute coronary syndrome; also used before coronary stent implantation surgery* (base=76.6%) 75 mg oral available in Europe

clopidol USAN, INN, BAN *coccidiostat for poultry*

clopimozide USAN, INN *antipsychotic*

clopipazan INN *antipsychotic* [also: clopipazan mesylate]

clopipazan mesylate USAN *antipsychotic* [also: clopipazan]

clopirac USAN, INN, BAN *anti-inflammatory*

cloponone INN, BAN

clopoxide [see: chlordiazepoxide]

clopoxide chloride [see: chlordiazepoxide HCl]

cloprednol USAN, INN, BAN *corticosteroid; anti-inflammatory*

cloprostenol INN, BAN *prostaglandin* [also: cloprostenol sodium]

cloprostenol sodium USAN *prostaglandin* [also: cloprostenol]

cloprothiazole INN ? glyprothiazol

cloquinate INN, BAN

cloquinozine INN

cloracetadol INN

cloral betaine INN *sedative* [also: chloral betaine]

cloramfenicol pantotenate complex INN *antibacterial; antirickettsial* [also: chloramphenicol pantothenate complex] ? chloramphenicol palmitate

cloranolol INN

clorarsen [see: dichlorophenarsine HCl]

clorazepate dipotassium USAN, USP *benzodiazepine anxiolytic; minor tranquilizer; alcohol withdrawal aid; anticonvulsant adjunct* [also: dipotassium clorazepate] 3.75, 7.5, 15 mg oral

clorazepate monopotassium USAN *minor tranquilizer*

clorazepic acid BAN

cloretate INN *sedative; hypnotic* [also: clorethate]

Cloretazine *investigational (orphan) for acute myelogenous leukemia*

clorethate USAN *sedative; hypnotic* [also: cloretate]

clorexolone USAN, INN, BAN *diuretic*

clorgiline INN [also: clorgyline]

clorgyline BAN [also: clorgiline]

cloricromen INN

cloridarol INN

clorindanic acid INN

clorindanol INN *spermaticide* [also: chlorindanol]

clorindione INN, BAN

clormecaine INN

clorofene INN *disinfectant* [also: clorophene]

cloroperone INN *antipsychotic* [also: cloroperone HCl]

cloroperone HCl USAN *antipsychotic* [also: cloroperone]

clorophene USAN *disinfectant* [also: clorofene]

cloroqualone INN

clorotepine INN

Clorpactin WCS-90 powder for topical solution OTC *antimicrobial* [oxychlorosene sodium] 2 g

clorprenaline INN, BAN *adrenergic; bronchodilator* [also: clorprenaline HCl]

clorprenaline HCl USAN *adrenergic; bronchodilator* [also: clorprenaline]

Clorpres tablets R *combination central antiadrenergic and diuretic for hypertension* [clonidine HCl; chlorthalidone] 0.1•15 mg; 0.2•15 mg; 0.3•15 mg

clorquinaldol [see: chlorquinaldol]

clorsulon USAN, INN *antiparasitic; fasciolicide*

clortermine INN *anorectic* [also: clortermine HCl]

clortermine HCl USAN *anorectic* [also: clortermine]

closantel USAN, INN, BAN *anthelmintic*

closilate INN *combining name for radicals or groups* [also: closylate]

closiramine INN *antihistamine* [also: closiramine aceturate]

closiramine aceturate USAN *antihistamine* [also: closiramine]

clostebol INN [also: clostebol acetate] ⑨ colestipol

clostebol acetate BAN [also: clostebol]

clostridial collagenase [see: collagenase *Clostridium histolyticum*]

Clostridium botulinum **toxin** [see: botulinum toxin]

closylate USAN, BAN *combining name for radicals or groups* [also: closilate]

clotbur *medicinal herb* [see: burdock]

clothiapine USAN, BAN *antipsychotic* [also: clotiapine]

clothixamide maleate USAN *antipsychotic* [also: clotixamide]

clotiapine INN *antipsychotic* [also: clothiapine]

clotiazepam INN

cloticasone INN, BAN *anti-inflammatory* [also: cloticasone propionate]

cloticasone propionate USAN *anti-inflammatory* [also: cloticasone]

clotioxone INN

clotixamide INN *antipsychotic* [also: clothixamide maleate]

clotixamide maleate [see: clothixamide maleate]

clotrimazole (CLT) USAN, USP, INN, BAN, JAN *broad-spectrum antifungal; investigational (orphan) for sickle cell disease and Huntington disease* 1% topical; 100 mg vaginal; 10 mg troches

clotrimazole & betamethasone dipropionate *broad-spectrum antifungal; corticosteroidal anti-inflammatory* 1%•0.05% topical

cloudberry *medicinal herb* [see: blackberry]

clove oil NF ⑨ Calafol

clover, king's; sweet clover *medicinal herb* [see: melilot]

clover, marsh *medicinal herb* [see: buckbean]

clover, purple; wild clover *medicinal herb* [see: red clover]

clover, winter *medicinal herb* [see: squaw vine]

cloves (*Caryophyllus aromaticus; Eugenia caryophyllata; Syzygium aromaticum*) seed and oil *medicinal herb for bad breath, bronchial secretions, dizziness, earache, fever, nausea, platelet aggregation inhibition, poor circulation, and thrombosis; also used topically as an analgesic and antiseptic*

clovoxamine INN

cloxacepride INN

cloxacillin INN, BAN *penicillinase-resistant penicillin antibiotic* [also: cloxacillin benzathine]

cloxacillin benzathine USP *penicillinase-resistant penicillin antibiotic* [also: cloxacillin]

cloxacillin sodium USAN, USP *penicillinase-resistant penicillin antibiotic*

cloxazolam INN

cloxestradiol INN

cloxifenol [see: triclosan]

cloximate INN

cloxiquine INN *antibacterial* [also: cloxyquin]

cloxotestosterone INN

cloxphendyl [see: cloxypendyl]

cloxypendyl INN

cloxyquin USAN *antibacterial* [also: cloxiquine]

clozapine USAN, INN, BAN *novel (atypical) dibenzapine antipsychotic for severe schizophrenia and recurrent suicidal behavior; sedative* 12.5, 25, 50, 100, 200 mg oral ⊉ Calcibon

Clozaril tablets ℞ *novel (atypical) dibenzapine antipsychotic for severe schizophrenia and recurrent suicidal behavior; sedative* [clozapine] 25, 100 mg ⊉ clazuril; glycerol

CLT (clotrimazole) [q.v.]

club, shepherd's *medicinal herb* [see: mullein]

club moss (*Lycopodium clavatum*) spores *medicinal herb used as a hemostatic and vulnerary*

cluster, wax *medicinal herb* [see: wintergreen]

C-Max gradual-release tablets (discontinued 2007) OTC *vitamin/mineral supplement* [vitamin C; multiple minerals] 1•≛ g

CMC (carboxymethylcellulose) gum [see: carboxymethylcellulose sodium]

CMF; CMF-IV (cyclophosphamide, methotrexate, fluorouracil) *chemotherapy protocol for breast cancer*

CMF/AV (cyclophosphamide, methotrexate, fluorouracil, Adriamycin, Oncovin) *chemotherapy protocol*

CMFP; CMF-P (cyclophosphamide, methotrexate, fluorouracil, prednisone) *chemotherapy protocol for breast cancer*

CMFVP (cyclophosphamide, methotrexate, fluorouracil, vincristine, prednisone) *chemotherapy protocol for breast cancer* [also known as: Cooper regimen]

C-MOPP *chemotherapy protocol for Hodgkin or non-Hodgkin lymphoma* [see: COPP]

CMV (cisplatin, methotrexate, vinblastine) *chemotherapy protocol for bladder cancer*

CMV-IGIV (cytomegalovirus immune globulin intravenous) [see: cytomegalovirus immune globulin, human]

CN2 HCl [see: mechlorethamine HCl]

CNF (cyclophosphamide, Novantrone, fluorouracil) *chemotherapy protocol for breast cancer* [also known as: CFM; FNC]

Cnicus benedictus *medicinal herb* [see: blessed thistle]

CNL8 Nail Kit topical solution ℞ *antifungal for onychomycosis* [ciclopirox; tocopherol (vitamin E)] 8%•5%

CNOP (cyclophosphamide, Novantrone, Oncovin, prednisone) *chemotherapy protocol for non-Hodgkin lymphoma*

CNTO 148 *investigational (Phase III) injectable anti-inflammatory for rheumatoid and psoriatic arthritis and ankylosing spondylitis*

CNTO 1275 *investigational (Phase III) injectable anti-inflammatory for psoriasis*

Co I (coenzyme I) [see: nadide]

CO_2 (carbon dioxide) [q.v.]

^{57}Co [see: cobaltous chloride Co 57]

^{57}Co [see: cyanocobalamin Co 57]

^{58}Co [see: cyanocobalamin (^{58}Co)]

^{60}Co [see: cobaltous chloride Co 60]

^{60}Co [see: cyanocobalamin Co 60]

coachweed *medicinal herb* [see: bedstraw]

CoaguChek PT test strips for home use OTC *in vitro diagnostic aid for the management of anticoagulation therapy*

coagulants *a class of agents that promote or accelerate clotting of the blood*

coagulation factor VIIa [see: factor VIIa, recombinant]

coagulation factor IX (human) [see: factor IX complex; nonacog alfa]

Coagulin-B *investigational (orphan) agent for moderate to severe hemophilia* [adeno-associated viral vector containing the gene for human coagulation Factor IX]

coakum *medicinal herb* [see: pokeweed]

coal tar USP *topical antieczematic; anti-seborrheic* ☒ Caltro; Kaletra

co-amoxiclav (amoxicillin & potassium clavulanate) [q.v.]

Coartem tablets ℞ *artemisinin-based combination therapy (ACT) for malaria* [artemether; lumefantrine] 20•120 mg ☒ Cort-Dome

COB (cisplatin, Oncovin, bleomycin) *chemotherapy protocol for head and neck cancer*

cobalamin concentrate USP *vitamin B₁₂; hematopoietic*

cobalt *element (Co)* ☒ caplet

cobalt-labeled vitamin B₁₂ [see: cyanocobalamin Co 57 & Co 60]

cobaltous chloride Co 57 USAN *radioactive agent*

cobaltous chloride Co 60 USAN *radioactive agent*

cobamamide INN

COBARTin *investigational (orphan) for steatorrhea in short bowel syndrome* [conjugated bile acids]

cobicistat *investigational (Phase III) anti-retroviral potentiator HIV-1 infection*

cocaine USP, BAN *topical anesthetic for mucous membranes; often abused as a street drug, derived from coca leaves* 4%, 10% topical

cocaine, crack *street drug made by converting cocaine HCl into a form that can be smoked, which causes a faster, more intense effect*

cocaine HCl USP *topical anesthetic for mucous membranes; often abused as a street drug, derived from coca leaves* 135 mg oral; 4%, 10% topical

Cocaine Viscous *topical solution* ℞ *mucous membrane anesthetic* [cocaine] 4%, 10%

cocarboxylase INN [also: co-carboxylase]

co-carboxylase BAN [also: cocarboxylase]

cocashweed *medicinal herb* [see: life root]

coccidioidin USP *dermal coccidioidomycosis test*

cocculin [see: picrotoxin]

Cocculus lacunosus; C. suberosus medicinal herb [see: levant berry]

Cocculus palmatus medicinal herb [see: colombo]

Cocet caplets ℞ *narcotic analgesic; antitussive; antipyretic* [codeine phosphate; acetaminophen] 30•650 mg ☒ CAST

Cochlearia armoracia medicinal herb [see: horseradish]

cocklebur *medicinal herb* [see: agrimony; burdock]

cockspur pepper *medicinal herb* [see: cayenne]

cockspur rye *medicinal herb* [see: ergot]

cocoa (Theobromo cacao) NF *bean medicinal herb used as a cardiac stimulant, diuretic, and vasodilator*

cocoa butter (Theobromo cacao) NF *suppository base; emollient/protectant* [also: cacao butter]

cocowort *medicinal herb* [see: shepherd's purse]

Cod Liver Oil *softgels* OTC *vitamin supplement* [vitamins A and D] 1250•130, 2500•260 IU

cod liver oil USP, BAN *vitamins A and D source; emollient/protectant*

cod liver oil, nondestearinated NF

codactide INN, BAN

Codal-DH *syrup* (discontinued 2009) ℞ *narcotic antitussive; antihistamine; sleep aid; decongestant* [hydrocodone bitartrate; pyrilamine maleate; phenylephrine HCl] 1.66•8.33•5 mg/5 mL

Codal-DM *syrup* OTC *antitussive; antihistamine; sleep aid; decongestant* [dextromethorphan hydrobromide; pyrilamine maleate; phenylephrine HCl] 10•8.33•5 mg/5 mL

CODE (cisplatin, Oncovin, doxorubicin, etoposide) [with prednisone, Bactrim, and ketoconazole] *chemotherapy protocol for small cell lung cancer (SCLC)*

codehydrogenase I [see: nadide]

codeine USP, BAN *narcotic analgesic used as an antitussive; sometimes abused as a street drug* ☒ Kadian; Quad Tann

codeine & acetaminophen *narcotic analgesic* 15•300, 30•300, 60•300 mg oral; 12•30 mg/5 mL oral

codeine phosphate USP, BAN *narcotic analgesic used as an antitussive* 15 mg/ 5 mL oral; 15, 30 mg/mL injection

codeine phosphate & aspirin *narcotic antitussive; analgesic; antipyretic* 325•15 mg oral

codeine phosphate & aspirin & carisoprodol *narcotic analgesic; skeletal muscle relaxant* 16•325•200 mg oral

codeine phosphate & butalbital & acetaminophen & caffeine *narcotic antitussive; barbiturate sedative; analgesic* 30•50•325•40 mg oral

codeine phosphate & butalbital & aspirin & caffeine *narcotic antitussive; barbiturate sedative; analgesic* 30•50•325•40 mg oral

codeine phosphate & chlorpheniramine maleate *narcotic antitussive; antihistamine* 10•2 mg/5 mL oral

codeine phosphate & guaifenesin *antitussive; narcotic analgesic; expectorant* 10•300 mg oral

codeine phosphate & promethazine HCl *narcotic antitussive; antihistamine* 10•6.25 mg/5 mL oral

codeine phosphate & promethazine HCl & phenylephrine HCl *narcotic antitussive; antihistamine; decongestant* 10•6.25•5 mg/5 mL oral

codeine polistirex USAN *narcotic analgesic used as an antitussive*

codeine sulfate USP *narcotic analgesic used as an antitussive* 15, 30, 60 mg oral; 30 mg/5 mL oral

codelcortone [see: prednisolone]

Codeprex extended-release oral suspension (discontinued 2007) ℞ *narcotic antitussive; antihistamine* [codeine polistirex; chlorpheniramine polistirex] 40•8 mg/10 mL

co-dergocrine mesylate BAN *cognition adjuvant* [also: ergoloid mesylates]

Codiclear DH syrup (discontinued 2011) ℞ *narcotic antitussive; expectorant* [hydrocodone bitartrate; guaifenesin] 3.5•300 mg/5 mL

Codimal DH syrup (discontinued 2009) ℞ *narcotic antitussive; antihistamine; decongestant* [hydrocodone bitartrate; dexchlorpheniramine maleate; phenylephrine HCl] 2•1•5 mg/5 mL

Codimal DM syrup OTC *antitussive; antihistamine; sleep aid; decongestant* [dextromethorphan hydrobromide; pyrilamine maleate; phenylephrine HCl] 10•8.33•5 mg/5 mL

Codimal PH syrup (discontinued 2009) ℞ *narcotic antitussive; antihistamine; sleep aid; decongestant* [codeine phosphate; pyrilamine maleate; phenylephrine HCl] 20•16.7•10 mg/10 mL

codorphone [now: conorphone HCl]

codoxime USAN, INN *antitussive*

Coease intraocular injection ℞ *viscoelastic agent for ophthalmic surgery* [hyaluronate sodium] 12 mg/mL

coenzyme Q10 *natural enzyme cofactor used as a cardiac protectant, free radical scavenger, and membrane stabilizer; investigational (orphan) for Huntington disease, pediatric CHF, and mitochondrial cytopathies* [also: ubiquinol; ubiquinone]

CoFactor *investigational (Phase III) chemotherapy rescue agent for fluorouracil toxicity*

coffeine [see: caffeine]

cofisatin INN

cofisatine [see: cofisatin]

cogazocine INN

Cogentin tablets, IV or IM injection ℞ *anticholinergic; antiparkinsonian* [benztropine mesylate] 0.5, 1, 2 mg; 1 mg/mL

Co-Gesic tablets ℞ *narcotic analgesic; antipyretic* [hydrocodone bitartrate; acetaminophen] 5•500 mg

Cognex capsules ℞ *cognition adjuvant for mild-to-moderate Alzheimer dementia* [tacrine HCl] 10, 20, 30, 40 mg ⑨ Kionex

Cognitex; Cognitex with Pregnenolone softgels OTC *anti-aging supplement for improving mental function*

[glyceryl phosphorylcholine; choline dihydrogen citrate; choline bitartrate; phosphatidylserine; vinpocetine; pantothenic acid; RNA/DNA; (pregnenolone)] 100•250•200•16.7•2.5•83.3•70.8(•8.3) mg

cohosh *medicinal herb* [see: black cohosh; blue cohosh; white cohosh]

Cola acuminata medicinal herb [see: kola nut]

Colace capsules, syrup, oral liquid OTC *laxative; stool softener* [docusate sodium] 50, 100 mg; 60 mg/15 mL; 150 mg/15 mL 🄪 Cal-Cee

Colace; Colace Infant/Child suppositories OTC *hyperosmolar laxative* [glycerin] 🄪 Cal-Cee

colaspase BAN *antineoplastic for acute lymphocytic leukemia (ALL)* [also: asparaginase]

Colazal capsules ℞ *gastrointestinal antiinflammatory for ulcerative colitis* [balsalazide disodium] 750 mg 🄪 Gelseal

colchamine [see: demecolcine]

colchicine USP, JAN *gout suppressant; also used for pericarditis and Behçet syndrome; investigational (orphan) to stop the progression of multiple sclerosis* 0.6 mg (1/100 gr.) oral

colchicine & probenecid *treatment for frequent, recurrent attacks of gouty arthritis* 0.5•500 mg oral

Colchicum autumnale; C. speciosum; C. vernum medicinal herb [see: autumn crocus]

Colcrys film-coated caplets ℞ *gout suppressant; also used for pericarditis and Behçet syndrome* [colchicine] 0.6 mg (1/100 gr.)

Cold & Cough Tussin softgels (discontinued 2007) OTC *antitussive; decongestant; expectorant* [dextromethorphan hydrobromide; pseudoephedrine HCl; guaifenesin] 10•30•200 mg

cold cream USP

Cold & Hot Pain Relief Therapy transdermal patch OTC *mild anesthetic; antipruritic; counterirritant* [menthol] 5%

Cold Symptoms Relief tablets (discontinued 2007) OTC *antitussive; antihistamine; decongestant; analgesic; antipyretic* [dextromethorphan hydrobromide; chlorpheniramine maleate; pseudoephedrine HCl; acetaminophen] 10•2•30•325 mg

Coldec D extended-release caplets (discontinued 2007) ℞ *decongestant; antihistamine* [pseudoephedrine HCl; carbinoxamine maleate] 80•8 mg

Coldec DM oral liquid (discontinued 2007) ℞ *antitussive; antihistamine; decongestant* [dextromethorphan hydrobromide; brompheniramine maleate; pseudoephedrine HCl] 15•4•60 mg/5 mL

Coldmist JR sustained-release tablets ℞ *decongestant; expectorant* [pseudoephedrine HCl; guaifenesin] 48•595 mg

Coldmist LA extended-release caplets ℞ *decongestant; expectorant* [pseudoephedrine HCl; guaifenesin] 85•795 mg

Coldonyl tablets OTC *decongestant; expectorant; analgesic; antipyretic* [phenylephrine HCl; guaifenesin; acetaminophen] 5•100•325 mg

colecalciferol (vitamin D₃) INN *fat-soluble vitamin* [also: cholecalciferol]

colesevelam HCl USAN *bile acid sequestrant; nonabsorbable cholesterol-lowering polymer for hyperlipidemia and to improve glycemic control in type 2 diabetes*

Colestid tablets, granules for oral suspension ℞ *cholesterol-lowering antihyperlipidemic* [colestipol HCl] 1 g; 5 g/dose

colestipol INN, BAN *bile acid sequestrant; cholesterol-lowering antihyperlipidemic* [also: colestipol HCl] 🄪 clostebol

colestipol HCl USAN, USP *bile acid sequestrant; cholesterol-lowering antihyperlipidemic* [also: colestipol] 1, 5 g oral

colestolone USAN, INN *hypolipidemic*

colestyramine INN *bile salt ion-exchange resin; antihyperlipoprotein-*

emic [also: cholestyramine resin; cholestyramine]

colestyramine resin [see: cholestyramine]

colextran INN

Colfed-A sustained-release capsules ℞ *decongestant; antihistamine* [pseudoephedrine HCl; chlorpheniramine maleate] 120•8 mg

colfenamate INN

colforsin USAN, INN *antiglaucoma agent*

colfosceril palmitate USAN, INN, BAN *pulmonary surfactant for hyaline membrane disease and neonatal respiratory distress syndrome (orphan); investigational (orphan) for adult respiratory distress syndrome (ARDS)*

colic root *medicinal herb* [see: blazing star; star grass; wild yam]

Colic Tablets OTC *natural product to relieve colic, stomach cramps, hiccups, and gas in infants* [wild yam; chamomile; bitter apple]

Colic-Ease Gripe Water oral liquid OTC *natural product to relieve colic, stomach cramps, hiccups, and gas in infants* [dill weed seed oil; caraway seed oil; cinnamon bark oil; clove bud oil; cardamom seed oil]

colimecycline INN ☒ clomocycline

colistimethate sodium USAN, USP, INN *bactericidal antibiotic* [also: colistin sulphomethate] 150 mg/vial injection

colistin INN, BAN *bactericidal antibiotic* [also: colistin sulfate] ☒ glycitein

colistin methanesulfonate [see: colistimethate sodium]

colistin sulfate USP *bactericidal antibiotic* [also: colistin]

colistin sulphomethate BAN *bactericidal antibiotic* [also: colistimethate sodium]

collagen *ophthalmic implant to block the puncta and retain moisture; urethral injection for stress urinary incontinence; dermal filler for moderate to deep facial wrinkles and folds* ☒ Glyquin; Qualaquin

collagen, purified bovine *injectable dermal filler for scars, wrinkles, and facial folds*

collagen, purified human *injectable dermal filler for scars, wrinkles, and facial folds*

collagen, purified type II *investigational (Phase III, orphan) oral treatment for juvenile rheumatoid arthritis*

collagen sponge, absorbable *topical hemostat for surgery*

collagenase *topical proteolytic enzymes for necrotic tissue debridement; investigational (orphan) for Peyronie disease*

collagenase Clostridium histolyticum *enzyme therapy for Dupuytren contracture and Peyronie disease; investigational to reduce the appearance of cellulite*

Collagenase Santyl ointment ℞ *proteolytic enzymes for debriding dermal ulcers and severely burned areas* [collagenase] 250 U/g

collard *medicinal herb* [see: skunk cabbage]

Collinsonia canadensis *medicinal herb* [see: stone root]

collodion USP *topical protectant*

colloidal aluminum hydroxide [see: aluminum hydroxide gel]

colloidal oatmeal *demulcent*

colloidal silicon dioxide [see: silicon dioxide, colloidal]

Colloral *investigational (Phase III, orphan) treatment of juvenile rheumatoid arthritis* [purified type II collagen]

Collyrium for Fresh Eyes ophthalmic solution OTC *extraocular irrigating solution* [sterile isotonic solution]

ColoCare test kit for home use OTC *in vitro diagnostic aid for fecal occult blood*

Colocort rectal suspension ℞ *corticosteroidal anti-inflammatory* [hydrocortisone] 100 mg/60 mL

colombo (Cocculus palmatus) root *medicinal herb used as an antiemetic and febrifuge*

Colomed enema *investigational (orphan) for left-sided ulcerative colitis and chronic radiation proctitis* [short chain fatty acids]

colony-stimulating factors *a class of glycoproteins that stimulate the production of granulocytes and macrophages*

Color Allergy Screening Test (CAST) reagent assay tubes ℞ *in vitro diagnostic aid for immunoglobulin E in serum*

ColoScreen slide test for professional use ℞ *in vitro diagnostic aid for fecal occult blood*

colterol INN *bronchodilator* [also: colterol mesylate] ☒ glutaral

colterol mesylate USAN *bronchodilator* [also: colterol]

colt's tail *medicinal herb* [see: fleabane; horseweed]

coltsfoot (Tussilago farfara) buds, flowers, and leaves *medicinal herb for asthma, bronchitis, dry cough, hay fever, lung disorders, excess mucus, and throat irritation*

Columbia Antiseptic powder OTC *emollient; astringent; antiseptic* [zinc oxide; talc; carbolic acid; boric acid]

columbine (Aquilegia vulgaris) plant *medicinal herb used as an astringent, diaphoretic, and diuretic*

Coly-Mycin M powder for IV or IM injection ℞ *bactericidal antibiotic* [colistimethate sodium] 150 mg

Coly-Mycin S Otic suspension ℞ *corticosteroidal anti-inflammatory; antibiotic* [hydrocortisone acetate; neomycin sulfate; colistin sulfate] 1%•4.71 mg•3 mg per mL

CoLyte powder for oral solution ℞ *pre-procedure bowel evacuant* [polyethylene glycol–electrolyte solution (PEG 3350)] 60 g/L ☒ Klout; K-Lyte

ComBgen film-coated tablets (discontinued 2009) ℞ *vitamin B supplement* [vitamins B₆ and B₁₂; folic acid] 25•0.5•2.2 mg

Combidex *investigational (NDA filed) diagnostic aid for magnetic resonance lymphangiography (MRL) to detect lymph node metastases* [ferumoxtran-10]

Combiflex capsules (discontinued 2009) ℞ *antihistamine; sleep aid; analgesic; antipyretic* [phenyltoloxamine citrate; acetaminophen; salicylamide; caffeine] 20•325•250•50 mg

Combiflex ES caplets (discontinued 2008) ℞ *antihistamine; sleep aid; analgesic; antipyretic* [phenyltoloxamine citrate; acetaminophen; magnesium salicylate; caffeine] 20•500•500•50 mg

Combigan eye drops ℞ *combination alpha₂ agonist and beta-blocker for glaucoma and ocular hypertension* [brimonidine tartrate; timolol maleate] 0.2%•0.5%

CombiPatch transdermal patch ℞ *hormone replacement therapy for postmenopausal symptoms, hypogonadism, castration, and primary ovarian failure* [estradiol; norethindrone acetate] 5•14, 5•25 mcg/day

Combipres 0.1; Combipres 0.2; Combipres 0.3 tablets (discontinued 2007) ℞ *antihypertensive; diuretic* [clonidine HCl; chlorthalidone] 0.1•15 mg; 0.2•15 mg; 0.3•15 mg

Combistix reagent strips OTC *in vitro diagnostic aid for multiple urine products*

Combivent oral inhalation aerosol ℞ *anticholinergic bronchodilator for chronic bronchospasm with COPD* [ipratropium bromide; albuterol sulfate] 18•103 mcg/dose

Combivir film-coated caplets ℞ *antiviral combination for HIV infections* [lamivudine; zidovudine] 150•300 mg

combretastatin A4 phosphate *investigational (orphan) agent for anaplastic, medullary, papillary, or follicular thyroid cancer*

Combunox film-coated caplets (discontinued 2011) ℞ *narcotic analgesic; antipyretic* [oxycodone HCl; ibuprofen] 5•400 mg

Comfort Tears eye drops OTC *moisturizer/lubricant* [hydroxyethylcellulose]

ComfortCare GP Wetting & Soaking solution OTC *disinfecting/wetting/soaking solution for rigid gas permeable contact lenses*

comfrey *(Symphytum officinale; S. tuberosum)* leaves and roots *medicinal herb for anemia, arthritis, blood cleansing, boils and sores, bruises, burns, edema, emphysema, fractures, gastric ulcers, hemorrhoids, and sprains; not generally regarded as safe and effective as it may be carcinogenic and hepatotoxic* ② camphor

comfrey, spotted *medicinal herb* [see: lungwort]

Comfyde *investigational (NDA filed) anticonvulsive for adjunctive treatment of partial onset seizures* [carisbamate]

COMLA (cyclophosphamide, Oncovin, methotrexate, leucovorin [rescue], ara-C) *chemotherapy protocol for non-Hodgkin lymphoma* ② Camila

Commiphora abssynica; C. molmol; C. myrrha medicinal herb [see: myrrh]

Commiphora mukul medicinal herb [see: guggul]

Commit lozenges (name changed to **Nicorette** in 2010)

common bugloss *medicinal herb* [see: borage]

common elder *medicinal herb* [see: elderberry]

common flax *medicinal herb* [see: flaxseed]

comosain *investigational (orphan) proteolytic enzymes for debridement of severe burns*

COMP (cyclophosphamide, Oncovin, methotrexate, prednisone) *chemotherapy protocol for non-Hodgkin lymphoma*

Compack (trademarked packaging form) *patient compliance package for oral contraceptives*

Compazine suppositories (discontinued 2009) ℞ *conventional (typical) phenothiazine antipsychotic for schizophrenia; anxiolytic; antiemetic for nausea and vomiting; also used for acute treatment of migraine headaches* [prochlorperazine] 2.5, 5, 25 mg

Compazine syrup, IV or IM injection (discontinued 2009) ℞ *conventional*

(typical) phenothiazine antipsychotic for schizophrenia; anxiolytic; antiemetic for nausea and vomiting; also used for acute treatment of migraine headaches [prochlorperazine edisylate] 5 mg/5 mL; 5 mg/mL

Compazine tablets, Spansules (sustained-release capsules) (discontinued 2009) ℞ *conventional (typical) phenothiazine antipsychotic for schizophrenia; anxiolytic; antiemetic for nausea and vomiting; also used for acute treatment of migraine headaches* [prochlorperazine maleate] 5, 10, 25 mg; 30 mg

Compete tablets OTC *vitamin/iron supplement* [multiple vitamins; iron (as ferrous gluconate); folic acid] ± • 27•0.4 mg

Compleat ready-to-use oral liquid OTC *enteral nutritional therapy* [lactose-free formula] 1000, 1500 mL

Compleat Modified Formula closed system containers OTC *enteral nutritional therapy*

Compleat Modified Formula ready-to-use oral liquid OTC *enteral nutritional therapy* [lactose-free formula]

Compleat Regular Formula ready-to-use oral liquid OTC *enteral nutritional therapy* [milk-based formula]

complement receptor type I, myristoylated recombinant *investigational (orphan) to prevent delayed graft function following solid organ transplant*

complement receptor type I, soluble recombinant human *investigational (orphan) for adult respiratory distress syndrome and to prevent postcardiopulmonary bypass syndrome in children undergoing cardiopulmonary bypass*

Complera caplets ℞ *once-daily antiretroviral combination for HIV-1 infections* [emtricitabine; tenofovir disoproxil fumarate; rilpivirine] 200• 300•25 mg

Complere tablets OTC *vitamin/mineral/calcium/iron/amino acid supplement* [multiple vitamins & minerals; calcium (as dicalcium phosphate); iron (as amino acid rice chelate); folic acid; multiple amino acids] ± • 150 • 5 • 0.03 • ± mg

Complete solution (discontinued 2010) OTC *rewetting solution for soft contact lenses*

Complete tablets OTC *vitamin/mineral/calcium/iron supplement* [multiple vitamins & minerals; calcium; iron; folic acid] ± • 162 • 18 • 0.4 mg

Complete All-in-One solution (discontinued 2010) OTC *cleaning/disinfecting/rinsing/storage solution for soft contact lenses* [polyhexamethylene biguanide] 0.0001%

Complete Daily with Lutein tablets OTC *vitamin/mineral/calcium/iron supplement* [multiple vitamins & minerals; calcium (as carbonate and dicalcium phosphate); iron (as carbonyl iron); folic acid] ± • 162 • 18 • 0.04 mg

Complete Energy caplets OTC *vitamin/mineral/calcium/iron/herbal supplement* [multiple vitamins & minerals; calcium (as carbonate and dicalcium phosphate); iron (as carbonyl iron); folic acid; herbal blend] ± • 100 • 18 • 0.4 • ± mg

Complete Senior tablets OTC *vitamin/mineral supplement* [multiple vitamins & minerals; folic acid; biotin; lutein] ± • 400 • 30 • 250 mcg

Complete Weekly Enzymatic Cleaner effervescent tablets OTC *enzymatic cleaner for soft contact lenses* [subtilisin A]

Complete Winnie the Pooh chewable tablets OTC *vitamin/mineral/calcium/iron supplement* [multiple vitamins & minerals; calcium (as carbonate and dicalcium phosphate); iron (as ferrous sulfate); folic acid] ± • 100 • 18 • 0.4 mg

Complex 15 Face cream OTC *moisturizer; emollient*

Complex 15 Hand & Body cream, lotion OTC *moisturizer; emollient*

Comply oral liquid OTC *enteral nutritional therapy* [lactose-free formula]

component pertussis vaccine (alternate name for acellular pertussis vaccine) [see: diphtheria & tetanus toxoids & acellular pertussis (DTaP) vaccine, adsorbed]

Compound 347 liquid for vaporization ℞ *inhalation general anesthetic* [enflurane]

compound 42 [see: warfarin]

compound CB3025 [see: melphalan]

compound E [see: cortisone acetate]

compound F [see: hydrocortisone]

compound orange spirit [see: orange spirit, compound]

compound S [see: zidovudine]

compound solution of sodium chloride INN *fluid and electrolyte replenisher* [also: Ringer injection]

compound solution of sodium lactate INN *electrolyte and fluid replenisher; systemic alkalizer* [also: Ringer injection, lactated]

Compound W topical liquid, gel OTC *keratolytic* [salicylic acid in collodion] 17%

Compound W Freeze Off aerosol spray OTC *cryoablation of common and plantar warts* [dimethyl ether; propane; isobutane]

Compound W One Step Wart Remover for Kids pad OTC *keratolytic* [salicylic acid] 40%

Compoz gelcaps OTC *antihistamine; sleep aid* [diphenhydramine HCl] 25 mg

Compoz Nighttime Sleep Aid tablets OTC *antihistamine; sleep aid* [diphenhydramine HCl] 50 mg

compressible sugar [see: sugar, compressible]

Compro suppositories ℞ *conventional (typical) phenothiazine antipsychotic for schizophrenia; anxiolytic; antiemetic for nausea and vomiting; also used for acute treatment of migraine headaches* [prochlorperazine] 25 mg

Computer Eye Drops (discontinued 2008) OTC *ophthalmic moisturizer and emollient* [glycerin] 1%

COMT (catechol-O-methyltransferase) inhibitors *a class of antipar-*

kinson agents that stabilize serum levo-dopa levels by inhibiting an enzyme that breaks down the levodopa before it reaches the brain

Comtan film-coated tablets ℞ COMT (catechol-O-methyltransferase) inhibitor for Parkinson disease [entacapone] 200 mg

Comtrex Day and Night Flu Therapy; Comtrex Day and Night Severe Cold and Sinus caplets OTC decongestant; analgesic; antipyretic; antihistamine added PM [phenylephrine HCl; acetaminophen; chlorpheniramine maleate added PM] 5•325 mg AM; 5•325•2 mg PM

Comtrex Day & Night Cold & Cough caplets OTC antitussive; decongestant; analgesic; antipyretic; antihistamine added PM [dextromethorphan hydrobromide; phenylephrine HCl; acetaminophen; chlorpheniramine maleate added PM] 10•5•325 mg AM; 10•5•325•2 mg PM

Comtrex Multi-Symptom Deep Chest Cold caplets OTC expectorant; analgesic; antipyretic [guaifenesin; acetaminophen] 200•325 mg

Comtrex Nighttime Cold & Cough caplets OTC antitussive; antihistamine; decongestant; analgesic; antipyretic [dextromethorphan hydrobromide; chlorpheniramine maleate; phenylephrine HCl; acetaminophen] 10•2•5•325 mg

Comtrex Non-Drowsy Cold & Cough caplets OTC antitussive; decongestant; analgesic; antipyretic [dextromethorphan hydrobromide; phenylephrine HCl; acetaminophen] 10•5•325 mg

Comvax IM injection ℞ vaccine for H. influenzae type b (HIB) and hepatitis B infections in children 1½–15 months [Haemophilus influenzae b purified capsular polysaccharide; Neisseria meningitidis OMPC; hepatitis B virus vaccine] 7.5•125•5 mcg/0.5 mL

Conal oral suspension ℞ decongestant; antihistamine; sleep aid [phenyleph-

rine tannate; chlorpheniramine tannate; pyrilamine tannate] 15•8•12.5 mg/5 mL

Conceive Pregnancy test kit for home use OTC in vitro diagnostic aid; urine pregnancy test

Concentrated Cleaner solution OTC cleaning solution for rigid gas permeable contact lenses

Conceptrol Disposable Contraceptive vaginal gel OTC spermicidal contraceptive [nonoxynol 9] 4%

Concerta OROS dual-release tablets (22% immediate release, 78% extended release) ℞ CNS stimulant; once-daily treatment for attention-deficit/hyperactivity disorder (ADHD) [methylphenidate HCl] 18, 27, 36, 54, 72 mg

Condylox solution, gel ℞ antimitotic for external genital and perianal warts [podofilox] 0.5%

cone flower, purple medicinal herb [see: echinacea]

conessine INN

conessine hydrobromide [see: conessine]

Conex Cold & Allergy tablets, oral solution OTC decongestant; antihistamine [pseudoephedrine sulfate; dexbrompheniramine maleate] 60•2 mg; 30•1 mg/5 mL

confectioner's sugar [see: sugar, confectioner's]

Confide test kit for home use (discontinued 2008) OTC in vitro diagnostic aid for HIV in the blood

congazone sodium [see: Congo red]

Congesta DM tablets OTC antitussive; expectorant [dextromethorphan hydrobromide; guaifenesin] 20•400 mg

Congestac caplets OTC decongestant; expectorant [pseudoephedrine HCl; guaifenesin] 60•400 mg

Congestaid tablets OTC nasal decongestant [pseudoephedrine HCl] 30 mg

Congo red USP

conivaptan HCl arginine vasopressin antagonist; diuretic for euvolemic and hypervolemic hyponatremia in hospitalized patients; treatment for syndrome of inappropriate antidiuretic hormone (SIADH)

conjugated bile acids [see: bile acids, conjugated]

conjugated equine estrogen (CEE) [see: estrogens, conjugated]

conjugated estrogens [see: estrogens, conjugated]

conjugated linoleic acid (CLA) *natural omega-6 essential fatty acid shown to be effective in weight management and cancer prevention*

conorfone INN *analgesic* [also: conorphone HCl]

conorfone HCl [see: conorphone HCl]

conorphone HCl USAN *analgesic* [also: conorfone]

Conray; Conray 30; Conray 43 injection ℞ *radiopaque contrast medium* [iothalamate meglumine (47% iodine)] 600 mg/mL (282 mg/mL); 300 mg/mL (141 mg/mL); 430 mg/mL (202 mg/mL)

Constilac oral/rectal solution ℞ *hyperosmotic laxative* [lactulose] 10 g/15 mL

Constulose oral/rectal solution ℞ *hyperosmotic laxative* [lactulose] 10 g/15 mL

consumptive's weed *medicinal herb* [see: yerba santa]

Contac Cold + Flu caplets OTC *decongestant; antihistamine; analgesic; antipyretic* [phenylephrine HCl; chlorpheniramine maleate; acetaminophen] 5•7•500 mg

Contac Cold + Flu Day & Night caplets OTC *decongestant; analgesic; antipyretic; antihistamine added* PM [phenylephrine HCl; acetaminophen; chlorpheniramine maleate added PM] 5•500 mg AM; 5•500•2 mg PM

conteben [see: thioacetazone; thiacetazone]

continuous erythropoietin receptor activator (CERA) *investigational (Phase III) hematopoietic for anemia in patients with chronic kidney disease*

Contrave sustained release *investigational (NDA filed) combination opiate*

blocker and antidepressant to treat obesity and reduce cardiac risk factors* [naltrexone HCl; bupropion HCl] 32•360 mg

Contrin capsules (discontinued 2008) ℞ *hematinic* [iron (as ferrous fumarate); vitamin B₁₂; vitamin C; intrinsic factor concentrate; folic acid] 110•0.015•75•240•0.5 mg

ControlPak (trademarked packaging form) *tamper-resistant unit-dose package*

ControlRx toothpaste ℞ *dental caries preventative* [fluoride (as sodium fluoride)] 0.5% (1.1%)

conval lily *medicinal herb* [see: lily of the valley]

Convallaria majalis *medicinal herb* [see: lily of the valley]

conventional (typical) antipsychotics *a class of dopamine receptor antagonists with a higher affinity to the D_2 than D_1 receptors and little affinity to the nondopaminergic receptors; high incidence of extrapyramidal side effects (EPS)* [compare to: novel (atypical) antipsychotics]

Convolvulus sepium *medicinal herb* [see: hedge bindweed]

convulsion root; convulsion weed *medicinal herb* [see: fit root]

Conyza canadensis *medicinal herb* [see: horseweed]

cool.click (trademarked delivery device) *needle-free subcutaneous injector*

Cooper regimen (cyclophosphamide, methotrexate, fluorouracil, vincristine, prednisone) *chemotherapy protocol for breast cancer* [also known as: CMFVP]

COP [see: creatinolfosfate]

COP (cyclophosphamide, Oncovin, prednisone) *chemotherapy protocol for non-Hodgkin lymphoma*

COP 1 (copolymer 1) [see: glatiramer acetate]

Copaxone subcu injection in **Autoject2** (prefilled glass syringe) ℞ *immunomodulator for relapsing-remitting multiple sclerosis (orphan)* [glatiramer acetate] 20 mg/mL

Cope tablets OTC *analgesic; antipyretic; anti-inflammatory; antacid* [aspirin; caffeine; magnesium hydroxide; aluminum hydroxide] 421•32•50•25 mg

COPE (cyclophosphamide, Oncovin, Platinol, etoposide) *chemotherapy protocol for small cell lung cancer (SCLC) and pediatric brain tumors* [also known as: baby brain I protocol]

Copegus film-coated tablets ℞ *antiviral for chronic hepatitis C infections (orphan) and clinically stable HIV disease; also used for viral hemorrhagic fevers* [ribavirin] 200 mg ② Capex

copolymer 1 (COP 1) [see: glatiramer acetate]

copovithane BAN

COPP (cyclophosphamide, Oncovin, procarbazine, prednisone) *chemotherapy protocol for Hodgkin or non-Hodgkin lymphoma*

copper *element (Cu)* ② Keppra

copper chloride dihydrate [see: cupric chloride]

copper gluconate (copper D-gluconate) USP *dietary copper supplement*

copper sulfate pentahydrate [see: cupric sulfate]

copper 10-undecenoate [see: copper undecylenate]

copper undecylenate USAN

copperhead snake antivenin [see: antivenin (Crotalidae) polyvalent]

Coprexa *investigational (orphan) for Wilson disease* [ammonium tetrathiomolybdate]

Coptis trifolia *medicinal herb* [see: gold thread]

CoQ10 [see: coenzyme Q10]

coral (Goniopora spp.; Porite spp.) *natural material used as a substrate for bone grafts and fractures and in reconstructive surgery* ② caraway oil; Kerol

Coral Calcium Plus Vitamin D & Magnesium capsules OTC *vitamin/calcium/magnesium supplement* [vitamin D; calcium (as carbonate); magnesium]

coral root (Corallorhiza odontorhiza) *medicinal herb for diaphoresis, fever, insomnia, and sedation*

coral snake antivenin [see: antivenin (Micrurus fulvius)]

corbadrine INN *adrenergic; vasoconstrictor* [also: levonordefrin]

Cordaptive extended-release tablets (available in the European Union as **Tredaptive**) *investigational (Phase III) antihyperlipidemic for hypertriglyceridemia plus prostaglandin inhibitor to prevent flushing* [niacin; laropiprant] 1000•20 mg

Cordarone tablets, IV infusion ℞ *antiarrhythmic for acute ventricular tachycardia and fibrillation (orphan)* [amiodarone HCl] 200 mg; 50 mg/mL

Cordox *investigational (Phase III, orphan) cytoprotective agent for vasoocclusive episodes of sickle cell disease* [fructose-1,6-diphosphate]

Cordran cream, ointment, lotion, tape ℞ *corticosteroidal anti-inflammatory* [flurandrenolide] 0.05%; 0.05%; 0.05%; 4 mcg/cm^2

Cordran SP cream ℞ *corticosteroidal anti-inflammatory* [flurandrenolide] 0.05%

Cordron-D; Cordron-D NR oral liquid ℞ *decongestant; antihistamine* [pseudoephedrine HCl; carbinoxamine maleate] 17.5•2 mg/5 mL; 12.5•2 mg/5 mL

Cordron-DM NR oral liquid ℞ *antitussive; antihistamine; decongestant* [dextromethorphan hydrobromide; carbinoxamine maleate; pseudoephedrine HCl] 15•3•12.5 mg/5 mL

Cordron-HC oral liquid (discontinued 2009) ℞ *narcotic antitussive; antihistamine; decongestant* [hydrocodone bitartrate; chlorpheniramine maleate; phenylephrine HCl] 1.67•2.5•20 mg/5 mL

Cordron-HC NR syrup (discontinued 2009) ℞ *narcotic antitussive; antihistamine; decongestant* [hydrocodone bitartrate; chlorpheniramine maleate;

pseudoephedrine HCl] 1.67•2.5•
17.5 mg/5 mL

Coreg Tiltab (film-coated tablets) ℞
alpha- and beta-blocker for hypertension, congestive heart failure (CHF), and left ventricular dysfunction (LVD) following myocardial infarction (MI); also used for chronic angina pectoris and idiopathic cardiomyopathy [carvedilol]
3.125, 6.25, 12.5, 25 mg ⊡ Carac;
Kuric

Coreg CR extended-release capsules ℞
alpha- and beta-blocker for hypertension, congestive heart failure (CHF), and left ventricular dysfunction (LVD) following myocardial infarction (MI) [carvedilol phosphate] 10, 20, 40, 80 mg

Corfen DM oral liquid ℞ *decongestant; antihistamine; antitussive* [phenylephrine HCl; chlorpheniramine maleate; dextromethorphan hydrobromide] 10•4•15 mg/5 mL

Corgard tablets ℞ *beta-blocker; antianginal; antihypertensive; also used for migraine prophylaxis* [nadolol] 20, 120, 160 mg

coriander *(Coriandrum sativum)* seed *medicinal herb used as antispasmodic, appetizer, carminative, and stomachic*

coriander oil NF

Coricidin D Cold, Flu, & Sinus tablets OTC *decongestant; antihistamine; analgesic; antipyretic* [phenylephrine HCl; chlorpheniramine maleate; acetaminophen] 5•2•325 mg

Coricidin HBP Chest Congestion & Cough softgels OTC *antitussive; expectorant* [dextromethorphan hydrobromide; guaifenesin] 10•200 mg

Coricidin HBP Cold & Flu tablets OTC *antihistamine; analgesic; antipyretic* [chlorpheniramine maleate; acetaminophen] 2•325 mg

Coricidin HBP Cough & Cold tablets OTC *antitussive; antihistamine* [dextromethorphan hydrobromide; chlorpheniramine maleate] 30•4 mg

Coricidin HBP Flu tablets OTC *antitussive; antihistamine; analgesic; antipyretic* [dextromethorphan hydrobro-

mide; chlorpheniramine maleate; acetaminophen] 15•2•500 mg

Corifact powder for IV infusion ℞ *systemic hemostatic/antihemophilic for congenital factor XIII deficiency (orphan)* [factor XIII concentrate, human] 1000–1600 IU/vial (actual potency is stated on each vial)

corifollitropin alfa *investigational (Phase III) follicle-stimulating hormone (FSH) for the induction of ovulation in assisted reproductive technologies (ART)*

corkwood tree *(Duboisia myoporoides)* leaves *medicinal herb used as a central nervous system stimulant and in homeopathic therapy for eye disorders; not generally regarded as safe and effective as it contains scopolamine and related alkaloids, which may be fatal in high doses*

Corlopam IV infusion ℞ *rapid-acting vasodilator for in-hospital management of hypertensive emergencies* [fenoldopam mesylate] 10 mg/mL

Corlux *GR-II antagonist; investigational (orphan) for Cushing syndrome* [mifepristone]

Cormax cream, ointment, topical liquid ℞ *corticosteroidal anti-inflammatory* [clobetasol propionate] 0.05%

cormed [see: nikethamide]

cormetasone INN *topical anti-inflammatory* [also: cormethasone acetate]

cormetasone acetate [see: cormethasone acetate]

cormethasone acetate USAN *topical anti-inflammatory* [also: cormetasone]

corn, turkey *medicinal herb* [see: turkey corn]

corn cockle *(Agrostemma githago)* seeds and root *medicinal herb for cancer, edema, exanthema, hemorrhoids, jaundice, and worms; also used as an emmenagogue and expectorant, and in homeopathic remedies for gastritis and paralysis; not generally regarded as safe and effective as it is extremely poisonous*

Corn Huskers lotion OTC *moisturizer; emollient*

corn oil NF *solvent; caloric replacement*

corn silk (stigmata maidis) *medicinal herb* [see: Indian corn]

cornflower (Centaurea cyanus) *plant medicinal herb for conjunctivitis, corneal ulcers and other eye disorders and for nervous disorders and poisonous bites and stings*

Coromega packets OTC *dietary supplement* [omega-3 fatty acids (eicosapentaenoic acid and docosahexaenoic acid); vitamin C] 650•12 mg (350 mg EPA; 230 mg DHA)

Coromega Child Brain & Body Squeezer packets OTC *dietary supplement* [omega-3 fatty acids (eicosapentaenoic acid and docosahexaenoic acid); vitamin C] 284•11.6 mg (36 mg EPA; 200 mg DHA)

corpse plant *medicinal herb* [see: fit root]

corpus luteum extract [see: progesterone]

Corque cream ℞ *corticosteroidal anti-inflammatory; antifungal; antibacterial* [hydrocortisone; clioquinol] 1%•3% ☑ Carac; Kuric

Correctol enteric-coated tablets OTC *stimulant laxative* [bisacodyl] 5 mg

CortaGel OTC *corticosteroidal anti-inflammatory* [hydrocortisone] 1%

Cortaid cream, ointment OTC *corticosteroidal anti-inflammatory* [hydrocortisone acetate] 1%

Cortaid pump spray OTC *corticosteroidal anti-inflammatory* [hydrocortisone] 1%

Cortaid Faststick roll-on stick OTC *corticosteroidal anti-inflammatory* [hydrocortisone; alcohol 55%] 1%

Cortaid with Aloe cream, ointment OTC *corticosteroidal anti-inflammatory* [hydrocortisone acetate] 0.5%

Cortamox lotion (discontinued 2011) ℞ *corticosteroidal anti-inflammatory; local anesthetic; antiseptic* [hydrocortisone acetate; pramoxine HCl; chloroxylenol] 1%•1%•0.1%

Cortane-B lotion ℞ *corticosteroidal anti-inflammatory; local anesthetic; antiseptic* [hydrocortisone acetate; pramoxine HCl; chloroxylenol] 1%•1%•0.1%

Cortane-B Aqueous; Cortane-B Otic ear drops ℞ *corticosteroidal anti-inflammatory; local anesthetic; antiseptic* [hydrocortisone; pramoxine HCl; chloroxylenol] 1%•1%•0.1%

Cort-Dome cream ℞ *corticosteroidal anti-inflammatory* [hydrocortisone] 0.5%, 1% ☑ Coartem

Cort-Dome High Potency rectal suppositories ℞ *corticosteroidal anti-inflammatory* [hydrocortisone acetate] 25 mg

Cortef tablets, oral suspension (discontinued 2009) ℞ *corticosteroid; anti-inflammatory* [hydrocortisone] 5, 10, 20 mg; 10 mg/5 mL

Cortef Feminine Itch cream OTC *corticosteroidal anti-inflammatory* [hydrocortisone acetate] 0.5%

cortenil [see: desoxycorticosterone acetate]

cortexolone [see: cortodoxone]

Cortic; Cortic-ND ear drops ℞ *corticosteroidal anti-inflammatory; local anesthetic; antiseptic* [hydrocortisone; pramoxine HCl; chloroxylenol] 1%•1%•0.1%

Corticaine cream (discontinued 2010) OTC *corticosteroidal anti-inflammatory* [hydrocortisone acetate] 0.5% ☑ carticaine

corticorelin ovine triflutate USAN, INN *corticotropin-releasing hormone; diagnostic aid for Cushing syndrome and adrenocortical insufficiency (orphan)*

corticosteroids *a class of anti-inflammatory drugs*

corticotrophin INN, BAN *adrenocorticotropic hormone; corticosteroidal anti-inflammatory; diagnostic aid* [also: corticotropin]

corticotrophin-zinc hydroxide INN *adrenocorticotropic hormone; corticosteroidal anti-inflammatory; diagnostic aid* [also: corticotropin zinc hydroxide]

corticotropin USP *adrenocorticotropic hormone; corticosteroidal anti-inflammatory; diagnostic aid* [also: corticotrophin]

corticotropin, repository USP *adreno-corticotropic hormone; corticosteroidal anti-inflammatory for infantile spasms (orphan); diagnostic aid for testing adrenocortical function*

corticotropin tetracosapeptide [see: cosyntropin]

corticotropin zinc hydroxide USP *adrenocorticotropic hormone; corticosteroidal anti-inflammatory; diagnostic aid* [also: corticotrophin-zinc hydroxide]

corticotropin-releasing factor *investigational (Phase I/II, orphan) for peritumoral brain edema*

cortisol [see: hydrocortisone]

cortisol 21-acetate [see: hydrocortisone acetate]

cortisol 21-butyrate [see: hydrocortisone butyrate]

cortisol 21-cyclopentanepropionate [see: hydrocortisone cypionate]

cortisol cyclopentylpropionate [see: hydrocortisone cypionate]

cortisol 21-valerate [see: hydrocortisone valerate]

cortisone INN, BAN *corticosteroidal anti-inflammatory* [also: cortisone acetate]

cortisone acetate USP *corticosteroidal anti-inflammatory* [also: cortisone] 25 mg oral

Cortisporin cream ℞ *corticosteroidal anti-inflammatory; antibiotic* [hydrocortisone acetate; neomycin sulfate; polymyxin B sulfate] 0.5%•3.5 mg•10 000 U per g

Cortisporin eye drop suspension (discontinued 2008) ℞ *corticosteroidal anti-inflammatory; antibiotic* [hydrocortisone; neomycin sulfate; polymyxin B sulfate] 1%•0.35%•10 000 U per mL

Cortisporin Otic ear drops ℞ *corticosteroidal anti-inflammatory; antibiotic* [hydrocortisone; neomycin sulfate; polymyxin B sulfate] 1%•5 mg•10 000 U per mL

Cortisporin-TC Otic ear drop suspension ℞ *corticosteroidal anti-inflamma-tory; antibiotic; surface-active synergist* [hydrocortisone acetate; neomycin sulfate; colistin sulfate; thonzonium bromide] 10•3.3•3•0.5 mg/mL

cortisuzol INN

cortivazol USAN, INN *corticosteroidal anti-inflammatory*

Cortizone for Kids cream OTC *corticosteroidal anti-inflammatory* [hydrocortisone] 0.5%

Cortizone-5 ointment OTC *corticosteroidal anti-inflammatory* [hydrocortisone] 0.5%

Cortizone-10 cream, ointment, topical liquid OTC *corticosteroidal anti-inflammatory* [hydrocortisone] 1%

Cortizone-10 External Anal Itch cream OTC *corticosteroidal anti-inflammatory* [hydrocortisone] 1%

Cortizone-10 Plus cream OTC *corticosteroidal anti-inflammatory* [hydrocortisone] 1%

Cortizone-10 Quickshot spray OTC *corticosteroidal anti-inflammatory* [hydrocortisone] 1%

cortodoxone USAN, INN, BAN *anti-inflammatory*

Cortone Acetate intra-articular or intralesional injection (discontinued 2007) ℞ *corticosteroidal anti-inflammatory* [cortisone acetate] 50 mg/mL

Cortrosyn powder for IM or IV injection ℞ *diagnostic aid for testing adrenocortical function* [cosyntropin] 0.25 mg

Corvert IV infusion ℞ *antiarrhythmic for atrial fibrillation/flutter* [ibutilide fumarate] 0.1 mg/mL

Corvite Free tablets ℞ *vitamin/mineral supplement* [multiple vitamins & minerals; coenzyme Q10; folic acid; biotin] ±•35•1.25•0.075 mg

corydalis (*Corydalis cava*) root *medicinal herb used as an antispasmodic, hypnotic, and antiparkinsonian*

Corydalis formosa *medicinal herb* [see: turkey corn]

Corynanthe johimbe *medicinal herb* [see: yohimbe]

Corzall oral liquid ℞ *antitussive; decongestant* [carbetapentane citrate;

pseudoephedrine HCl] 20•30 mg/5 mL ☒ cresol; Cryselle; Kerasal

Corzall Plus oral liquid ℞ *antitussive; decongestant; antihistamine; sleep aid* [carbetapentane citrate; pseudoephedrine HCl; pyrilamine maleate] 20•30•7.5 mg/5 mL

Corzall-PE oral liquid ℞ *antitussive; antihistamine; decongestant* [carbetapentane citrate; dexchlorpheniramine maleate; phenylephrine HCl] 20•1•10 mg/5 mL

Corzide 40/5; Corzide 80/5 tablets ℞ *combination beta-blocker and diuretic for hypertension* [nadolol; bendroflumethiazide] 40•5 mg; 80•5 mg

Cosmegen powder for IV injection ℞ *antibiotic antineoplastic for various tumors, carcinomas, and sarcomas; potentiator for radiation therapy* [dactinomycin] 0.5 mg/vial

CosmoDerm gel for subcu injection ℞ *dermal filler for shallow scars and fine wrinkles* [collagen, purified human] 35 mg/mL

cosmoline [see: petrolatum]

CosmoPlast gel for subcu injection ℞ *dermal filler for scars, deep wrinkles, and facial folds* [collagen, purified human, cross-linked] 35 mg/mL

Cosopt eye drops ℞ *combination carbonic anhydrase inhibitor and beta-blocker for glaucoma* [dorzolamide HCl; timolol maleate] 2%•0.5%

cosyntropin USAN *adrenocorticotropic hormone; diagnostic aid for testing adrenocortical function* [also: tetracosactide; tetracosactrin] 0.25 mg/mL injection

Cotab A; Cotab AX caplets ℞ *narcotic antitussive; antihistamine* [codeine phosphate; chlorpheniramine maleate] 10•4 mg; 20•4 mg ☒ CTAB; K-Tab; Q-Tapp

Cotabflu caplets ℞ *narcotic antitussive; antihistamine; analgesic; antipyretic* [codeine phosphate; chlorpheniramine maleate; acetaminophen] 20•4•500 mg

cotarnine chloride NF

cotarnine HCl [see: cotarnine chloride]

cotinine INN *antidepressant* [also: cotinine fumarate]

cotinine fumarate USAN *antidepressant* [also: cotinine]

Cotrim; Cotrim D.S. tablets (discontinued 2010) ℞ *broad-spectrum sulfonamide antibiotic* [sulfamethoxazole; trimethoprim] 400•80 mg; 800•160 mg

Cotrim Pediatric oral suspension (discontinued 2010) ℞ *broad-spectrum sulfonamide antibiotic* [sulfamethoxazole; trimethoprim] 200•40 mg/5 mL

co-trimoxazole BAN [also: trimethoprim + sulfamethoxazole]

cotriptyline INN

cotton, purified USP *surgical aid*

cottonseed oil NF *solvent*

cottonweed *medicinal herb* [see: milkweed]

Cotuss EX syrup (discontinued 2007) ℞ *narcotic antitussive; expectorant* [hydrocodone bitartrate; potassium guaiacolsulfonate] 2.5•120 mg/5 mL

Cotuss HD; Cotuss MS syrup (discontinued 2007) ℞ *narcotic antitussive; antihistamine; decongestant* [hydrocodone bitartrate; chlorpheniramine maleate; phenylephrine HCl] 5•8•20 mg/10 mL; 10•4•20 mg/10 mL

couch grass (*Agropyron repens*) rhizomes, roots, and stems *medicinal herb for blood cleansing, cystitis, diabetes, jaundice, kidney problems, upper respiratory tract inflammation with mucous discharge, rheumatism, and urinary infections*

coughroot *medicinal herb* [see: birthroot]

Coughtuss oral liquid (discontinued 2009) ℞ *narcotic antitussive; antihistamine; decongestant* [hydrocodone bitartrate; chlorpheniramine maleate; phenylephrine HCl] 5•2•5 mg/5 mL

coughweed *medicinal herb* [see: life root]

coughwort *medicinal herb* [see: coltsfoot]

Cough-X lozenges OTC *antitussive; mucous membrane anesthetic* [dextromethorphan hydrobromide; benzocaine] 5•2 mg

Coumadin tablets, powder for IV injection ℞ *coumarin-derivative anticoagulant* [warfarin sodium] 1, 2, 2.5, 3, 4, 5, 6, 7.5, 10 mg; 2 mg/mL

coumafos INN [also: coumaphos]

coumamycin INN *antibacterial* [also: coumermycin]

coumaphos BAN [also: coumafos]

coumarin NF *anticoagulant; investigational (orphan) for renal cell carcinoma*

coumarins *a class of anticoagulants that interfere with vitamin K-dependent clotting factors*

coumazoline INN

coumermycin USAN *antibacterial* [also: coumamycin]

coumermycin sodium USAN *antibacterial*

coumetarol INN [also: cumetharol]

counterirritants *a class of agents that produce superficial irritation in one part of the body to relieve irritation in another part*

Covaryx; Covaryx H.S. film-coated caplets ℞ *combination equine estrogen and synthetic androgen; hormone replacement therapy for postmenopausal symptoms* [esterified estrogens; methyltestosterone] 1.25•2.5 mg; 0.625•1.25 mg

covatin HCl [see: captodiame HCl]

Covera-HS extended-release film-coated tablets ℞ *antihypertensive; antianginal; antiarrhythmic; calcium channel blocker* [verapamil HCl] 180, 240 mg

cow cabbage *medicinal herb* [see: masterwort; white pond lily]

cow parsnip *medicinal herb* [see: masterwort]

cowslip (Caltha palustris) plant *medicinal herb used as an analgesic, antispasmodic, diaphoretic, diuretic, expectorant, and rubefacient*

cowslip, Jerusalem *medicinal herb* [see: lungwort]

COX-2 (cyclooxygenase-2) inhibitors *a class of nonsteroidal anti-inflammatory drugs (NSAIDs) for osteoarthritis, rheumatoid arthritis, acute pain,* *and primary dysmenorrhea; these agents also have antipyretic activity*

Cozaar film-coated tablets ℞ *angiotensin receptor blocker (ARB) for hypertension; treatment to delay the progression of diabetic nephropathy* [losartan potassium] 25, 50, 100 mg

CP (chlorambucil, prednisone) *chemotherapy protocol for chronic lymphocytic leukemia (CLL) and ovarian cancer*

CP (cyclophosphamide, Platinol) *chemotherapy protocol for ovarian cancer*

CP DEC oral drops (discontinued 2009) ℞ *decongestant; antihistamine; drops for children 6–24 months* [phenylephrine HCl; chlorpheniramine maleate] 3.5•1 mg/mL

CP DEC syrup (discontinued 2011) ℞ *decongestant; antihistamine; drops for children 6–24 months* [phenylephrine HCl; chlorpheniramine maleate] 12.5•4 mg/5 mL

CP DEC-DM oral drops (discontinued 2009) ℞ *antitussive; antihistamine; decongestant; for children 6–24 months* [dextromethorphan hydrobromide; chlorpheniramine maleate; phenylephrine HCl] 3•1•3.5 mg/mL

CP DEC-DM syrup ℞ *antitussive; antihistamine; decongestant* [dextromethorphan hydrobromide; chlorpheniramine maleate; phenylephrine HCl] 15•4•12.5 mg/5 mL

CPB WC oral liquid ℞ *narcotic antitussive; antihistamine; decongestant* [codeine phosphate; brompheniramine maleate; pseudoephedrine HCl] 6.3•1.3•10 mg/5 mL

C.P.-DM oral drops (discontinued 2007) ℞ *antitussive; antihistamine; decongestant; for children 1–24 months* [dextromethorphan hydrobromide; carbinoxamine maleate; pseudoephedrine HCl] 4•1•15 mg/mL

C-Phed Tannate oral suspension (discontinued 2007) ℞ *decongestant; antihistamine* [pseudoephedrine tannate; chlorpheniramine tannate] 150•9 mg/10 mL

C-Phen syrup, oral drops ℞ *deconges-tant; antihistamine; drops for children 6–24 months* [phenylephrine HCl; chlorpheniramine maleate] 12.5•4 mg/5 mL; 3.5•1 mg/mL ⑤ caffeine; Kuvan

C-Phen DM oral drops ℞ *antitussive; antihistamine; decongestant; for children 6–24 months* [dextromethorphan hydrobromide; chlorpheniramine maleate; phenylephrine HCl] 3•1•3.5 mg/mL ⑤ G Phen DM; Guaifen DM

C-Phen DM syrup ℞ *antitussive; antihistamine; decongestant* [dextromethorphan hydrobromide; chlorpheniramine maleate; phenylephrine HCl] 15•4•12.5 mg/5 mL ⑤ G Phen DM; Guaifen DM

CPM 8/PE 20/MSC 1.25 caplets ℞ *antihistamine; decongestant; anticholinergic to dry mucosal secretions* [chlorpheniramine maleate; phenylephrine HCl; methscopolamine nitrate] 8•20•1.25 mg

CPM 8/PSE 90/MSC 2.5 sustained-release tablets ℞ *antihistamine; decongestant; anticholinergic to dry mucosal secretions* [chorpheniramine maleate; pseudoephedrine HCl; methscopolamine nitrate] 8•90•2.5 mg

CPM PSE syrup ℞ *antihistamine; decongestant* [chlorpheniramine maleate; pseudoephedrine HCl] 2•30 mg/5 mL

CPM/PSE DM oral drops ℞ *antihistamine; decongestant; antitussive; for children 6–11 years* [chlorpheniramine maleate; pseudoephedrine HCl; dextromethorphan hydrobromide] 0.8•9•3 mg/mL

CPT-11 (camptothecin-11) [see: irinotecan]

CP-Tannic oral suspension (discontinued 2007) ℞ *decongestant; antihistamine* [pseudoephedrine tannate; chlorpheniramine tannate] 150•9 mg/10 mL

CR1 (complement receptor 1) [see: complement receptor type I]

⁵¹Cr [see: albumin, chromated Cr 51 serum]

⁵¹Cr [see: chromic chloride Cr 51]

⁵¹Cr [see: chromic phosphate Cr 51]

⁵¹Cr [see: sodium chromate Cr 51]

cramp bark *(Viburnum opulus)* bark and berries *medicinal herb for asthma, convulsions, cramps, heart palpitations, hypertension, hysteria, leg cramps, nervousness, spasm, and urinary disorders*

crampweed *medicinal herb* [see: cinquefoil]

cranberry *(Vaccinium edule; V. erythrocarpum; V. macrocarpon; V. oxycoccos; V. vitis)* fruit *medicinal herb for bladder, kidney, and urinary tract infections; also used to decrease the rate of urine degradation and odor formation in incontinent patients*

cranesbill; spotted cranesbill *medicinal herb* [see: alum root]

Crantex oral liquid ℞ *decongestant; expectorant* [phenylephrine HCl; guaifenesin] 7.5•100 mg/5 mL

Crantex ER extended-release capsules (discontinued 2007) ℞ *decongestant; expectorant* [phenylephrine HCl; guaifenesin] 10•300 mg

Crataegus laevigata; C. monogyna; C. oxyacantha medicinal herb [see: hawthorn]

crawley; crawley root *medicinal herb* [see: coral root]

Creamy Tar shampoo (discontinued 2008) OTC *antiseborrheic; antipsoriatic; antipruritic; antibacterial* [coal tar] 8.65%

Creapure *investigational (orphan) agent for amyotrophic lateral sclerosis (ALS) and Huntington disease* [creatine]

creatine *investigational (orphan) agent for amyotrophic lateral sclerosis (ALS) and Huntington disease*

creatinolfosfate INN

Creomulsion Adult Formula syrup OTC *antitussive* [dextromethorphan hydrobromide] 20 mg/15 mL

Creomulsion for Children syrup OTC *antitussive* [dextromethorphan hydrobromide] 5 mg/5 mL

Creon 5; Creon 6; Creon 10; Creon 12; Creon 20; Creon 24

(name changed to **Creon Delayed Release** in 2009) ② Choron

Creon Delayed Release capsules containing enteric-coated microspheres ℞ *porcine-derived digestive enzymes* [pancrelipase (lipase; protease; amylase)] 6•19•30, 12•38•60, 24•76•120 thousand USP units

creosote carbonate USP

Creo-Terpin oral liquid OTC *antitussive* [dextromethorphan hydrobromide; alcohol 25%] 10 mg/15 mL

cresol NF *disinfectant* ② Corzall; Cryselle; Kerasal

cresotamide INN

cresoxydiol [see: mephenesin]

crestomycin sulfate [see: paromomycin sulfate]

Crestor film-coated tablets ℞ *HMG-CoA reductase inhibitor for hypercholesterolemia, mixed dyslipidemia, and hypertriglyceridemia; reduces atheroma (plaque build-up) in arteries and serum C-reactive protein (CRP) levels to prevent stroke and myocardial infarction* [rosuvastatin (as calcium)] 5, 10, 20, 40 mg

Cresylate ear drops ℞ *antiseptic; antibacterial; antifungal* [m-cresyl acetate; chlorobutanol; alcohol] 25%•25%•1%

cresylic acid [see: cresol]

crilanomer INN

crilvastatin USAN, INN *antihyperlipidemic*

Crinone vaginal gel in prefilled applicators ℞ *natural progestin; hormone replacement or supplementation for assisted reproductive technology (ART) treatments* [progesterone] 8% (90 mg)

crisnatol INN *antineoplastic* [also: crisnatol mesylate]

crisnatol mesylate USAN *antineoplastic* [also: crisnatol]

Criticare HN ready-to-use oral liquid OTC *enteral nutritional therapy* [lactose-free formula]

Crixivan capsules ℞ *antiretroviral protease inhibitor for HIV infection* [indinavir (as sulfate)] 100, 200, 400 mg

crizotinib *anaplastic lymphoma kinase (ALK) inhibitor for non–small cell lung cancer in nonsmokers caused by a defective ALK gene*

CRNatal tablets + capsules ℞ *prenatal vitamin/mineral/calcium/iron/omega-3 supplement; stool softener* [multiple vitamins & minerals; calcium; iron (as carbonyl and ferrous gluconate); folic acid; docusate sodium + docosahexaenoic acid (DHA)] ±•100•30•1•75 mg (tablets) + 275 mg (capsules)

crobefate INN *combining name for radicals or groups*

croconazole INN

crocus, autumn *medicinal herb* [see: autumn crocus]

Crocus sativus *medicinal herb* [see: saffron]

CroFab injection ℞ *treatment of pit viper (rattlesnake, copperhead, and cottonmouth moccasin) snake bites (orphan)* [antivenin (Crotalidae) polyvalent immune Fab (ovine)]

crofelemer USAN *investigational (Phase III) treatment for AIDS-related diarrhea; investigational (Phase II) antiviral for AIDS-related genital herpes*

crofilcon A USAN *hydrophilic contact lens material*

Crolom eye drops (discontinued 2011) ℞ *mast cell stabilizer; antiallergic and antiviral for vernal keratoconjunctivitis* [cromolyn sodium] 4%

cromacate INN *combining name for radicals or groups*

cromakalim INN, BAN

cromesilate INN *combining name for radicals or groups*

cromitrile INN *antiasthmatic* [also: cromitrile sodium]

cromitrile sodium USAN *antiasthmatic* [also: cromitrile]

cromoglicic acid INN *prophylactic antiasthmatic* [also: cromolyn sodium; cromoglycic acid]

cromoglycic acid BAN *prophylactic antiasthmatic* [also: cromolyn sodium; cromoglicic acid]

cromolyn sodium USAN, USP *anti-inflammatory; mast cell stabilizer; oral inhalation treatment of allergy, asthma, and bronchospasm; intranasal treatment of allergic rhinitis; oral treatment of mastocytosis; topical treatment of vernal keratoconjunctivitis (orphan)* [also: cromoglicic acid; cromoglycic acid] 10 mg/mL inhalation; 40 mg/mL spray; 100 mg/5 mL oral; 4% eye drops

Cronassial *investigational (orphan) agent for retinitis pigmentosa* [gangliosides, sodium salts]

cronetal [see: disulfiram]

cronidipine INN

cropropamide INN, BAN

croscarmellose INN *tablet disintegrant* [also: croscarmellose sodium]

croscarmellose sodium USAN, NF *tablet disintegrant* [also: croscarmellose]

crosfumaril [see: hemoglobin crosfumaril]

crospovidone NF *tablet excipient*

cross-linked carboxymethylcellulose sodium [now: croscarmellose sodium]

cross-linked carmellose sodium [see: croscarmellose sodium]

crotaline antivenin [see: antivenin (Crotalidae) polyvalent]

crotamiton USP, INN, BAN *scabicide; antipruritic*

crotetamide INN [also: crotethamide]

crotethamide BAN [also: crotetamide]

crotoniazide INN

crotonylidenisoniazid [see: crotoniazide]

crotoxyfos BAN

crowfoot *medicinal herb* [see: alum root; buttercup]

crowfoot buttercup; acrid crowfoot; cursed crowfoot; marsh crowfoot; meadow crowfoot; tall crowfoot; water crowfoot *medicinal herb* [see: buttercup]

crown, priest's *medicinal herb* [see: dandelion]

crude tuberculin [see: tuberculin, old]

Cruex aerosol powder OTC *antifungal* [miconazole nitrate] 2%

Cruex cream OTC *antifungal* [clotrimazole] 1%

Cruex topical powder OTC *antifungal* [calcium undecylenate] 10%

crufomate USAN, INN, BAN *veterinary anthelmintic* ⍰ carfimate

cryofluorane INN *aerosol propellant* [also: dichlorotetrafluoroethane]

Cryptaz *antiprotozoal; investigational (orphan) for intestinal amebiasis* [nitazoxanide]

cryptenamine acetates

Crypto-LA slide test for professional use ℞ *in vitro diagnostic aid for* Cryptococcus neoformans *antigens*

Cryptosporidium parvum bovine colostrum IgG concentrate *investigational (orphan) treatment of cryptosporidiosis-induced diarrhea in immunocompromised patients*

Cryselle tablets (in packs of 21 and 28) ℞ *monophasic oral contraceptive; emergency postcoital contraceptive* [norgestrel; ethinyl estradiol] 0.3 mg• 30 mcg ⍰ Corzall; cresol; Kerasal

crystal violet [see: gentian violet]

crystallized trypsin [see: trypsin, crystallized]

Crystamine IM or subcu injection (discontinued 2009) ℞ *hematinic; vitamin B_{12} supplement* [cyanocobalamin] 1000 mcg/mL

Crysti 1000 IM or subcu injection (discontinued 2008) ℞ *hematinic; vitamin B_{12} supplement* [cyanocobalamin] 1000 mcg/mL

crystografin [see: meglumine diatriazole]

^{131}Cs [see: cesium chloride Cs 131]

C-Solve lotion OTC *nontherapeutic base for compounding various dermatological preparations*

CSP (cellulose sodium phosphate) [q.v.]

CT (cisplatin, Taxol) *chemotherapy protocol for ovarian, cervical, esophageal, gastric, and non–small cell lung cancer* [also: PC]

CTAB (cetyltrimethyl ammonium bromide) ⍰ Cotab; K-Tab; Q-Tapp

C-Tan D oral suspension (discontinued 2011) ℞ *decongestant; antihistamine* [phenylephrine tannate; brompheniramine tannate] 5•4 mg/5 mL

C-Tan D Plus oral suspension ℞ *decongestant; antihistamine* [phenylephrine tannate; brompheniramine tannate] 5•5 mg/5 mL

C-Tanna 12D oral suspension ℞ *antitussive; antihistamine; sleep aid; decongestant* [carbetapentane tannate; pyrilamine tannate; phenylephrine tannate] 30•30•5 mg/5 mL

CTX (cyclophosphamide) [q.v.]

⁶⁴Cu [see: cupric acetate Cu 64]

cubeb (Piper cubeba) unripe berries *medicinal herb used as an antiseptic, antisyphilitic, carminative, diuretic, expectorant, stimulant, and stomachic* ⓘ Q-Pap

Cubicin powder for IV infusion ℞ *cyclic lipopeptide antibiotic for skin and skin structure infections (SSSIs), Staphylococcus aureus bloodstream infections, and right-sided endocarditis* [daptomycin] 500 mg/vial ⓘ Capsin; kebuzone; quipazine

cucurbita (Cucurbita maxima; C. moschata; C. pepa) seeds *medicinal herb for prophylaxis, immobilization, and aiding in the expulsion of intestinal worms and parasites; also used in prostate gland disorders*

Culturelle with Lactobacillus GG; Culturelle for Kids capsules OTC *natural intestinal bacteria; probiotic; dietary supplement* [Lactobacillus GG] 10 billion live cells; 1 billion live cells

Culturette 10 Minute Group A Strep ID slide test for professional use ℞ *in vitro diagnostic test for Group A streptococcal antigens in throat swabs* [latex agglutination test]

Culver physic *medicinal herb* [see: Culver root]

Culver root (Varonicastrum virginicum) *medicinal herb for blood cleansing, diarrhea, and liver and stomach disorders*

cumetharol BAN [also: coumetarol]

cumin (Cuminum cyminum; C. odorum) seeds and oil *medicinal herb for gastric cancer; also used as an antioxidant*

cupric acetate Cu 64 USAN *radioactive agent*

cupric chloride USP *dietary copper supplement; additive to IV solutions for total parenteral nutrition (37% elemental copper)* 1.07 mg/mL (0.4 mg/mL Cu) injection

cupric sulfate USP *antidote to phosphorus overload; dietary copper supplement; additive to IV solutions for total parenteral nutrition (25% elemental copper)* 1.57 mg/mL (0.4 mg/mL Cu) injection

Cuprimine capsules ℞ *metal chelating agent for rheumatoid arthritis, Wilson disease, and cystinuria* [penicillamine] 250 mg

cuprimyxin USAN, INN *veterinary antibacterial; antifungal*

cuproxoline INN, BAN

Curaçao aloe *medicinal herb* [see: aloe]

curare [see: metocurine iodide; tubocurarine chloride]

Curcuma domestica; C. longa *medicinal herb* [see: turmeric]

cure-all *medicinal herb* [see: lemon balm]

CureLight BroadBand Model 01 (device) *red-light illuminator; used with* **Metvixia** (methyl aminolevulinate HCl) *for photodynamic therapy of precancerous actinic keratoses of the face and scalp*

Curity Sponge Sticks OTC *broad-spectrum antimicrobial* [iodine] 1%

Curity Wet Skin Scrub Pack kit (sponges + sponge sticks) OTC *broad-spectrum antimicrobial* [iodine] 1%

curium *element (Cm)*

curled dock; curly dock *medicinal herb* [see: yellow dock]

curled mint *medicinal herb* [see: peppermint]

curls, blue *medicinal herb* [see: woundwort]

Curosurf intratracheal suspension ℞ *porcine lung extract for respiratory dis-*

tress syndrome (RDS) in premature infants (orphan); also used for severe meconium aspiration in term infants [poractant alfa] 1.5, 3 mL (120, 240 mg phospholipids)

curral [see: diallybarbituric acid]

currant (Ribes nigrum; R. rubrum) leaves and fruit medicinal herb used as a diaphoretic and diuretic

custard apple medicinal herb [see: pawpaw]

custirsen sodium investigational antineoplastic for progressive metastatic prostate cancer

Cūtar Bath Oil Emulsion OTC antipsoriatic; antiseborrheic; antipruritic; emollient [coal tar (as liquor carbonis detergens)] 1.5% (7.5%)

Cūtemol cream OTC moisturizer; emollient [allantoin]

Cuticura Medicated Soap bar (discontinued 2010) OTC therapeutic skin cleanser; antiseptic [triclocarban] 1%

Cutivate cream, lotion, ointment ℞ corticosteroidal anti-inflammatory [fluticasone propionate] 0.05%; 0.05%; 0.005%

Cuvposa oral liquid ℞ GI antisecretory to prevent chronic, severe drooling [glycopyrrolate] 1 mg/5 mL

CVAD; C-VAD (cyclophosphamide, vincristine, Adriamycin, dexamethasone) [with mesna rescue and filgrastim hematopoietic] chemotherapy protocol for acute lymphocytic leukemia (ALL) and mantle cell lymphoma [note: rarely given alone; see: hyper-CVAD/HD MTX ara-C]

CVD (cisplatin, vinblastine, dacarbazine) chemotherapy protocol for malignant melanoma

CVD (cisplatin, vinblastine, dacarbazine) + IL-2I (interleukin-2 [aldesleukin], interferon [alfa]) chemotherapy protocol for malignant melanoma

CVI (carboplatin, VePesid, ifosfamide) [with mesna rescue] chemotherapy protocol for non–small cell lung cancer (NSCLC) [also known as: VIC]

CVP (cyclophosphamide, vincristine, prednisone) chemotherapy protocol for non-Hodgkin lymphoma and chronic lymphocytic leukemia (CLL)

CVPP (CCNU, vinblastine, procarbazine, prednisone) chemotherapy protocol for Hodgkin lymphoma ⑦ CAV/EP

CY-1503 investigational (Phase III, orphan) adjunct to surgery for congenital heart defects in newborns; investigational (orphan) for postischemic pulmonary reperfusion edema

CY-1899 investigational (orphan) agent for chronic active hepatitis B

cyacetacide INN [also: cyacetazide]

cyacetazide BAN [also: cyacetacide]

cyamemazine INN

cyamepromazine [see: cyamemazine]

cyanamide JAN [also: calcium carbimide]

cyani medicinal herb [see: cornflower]

Cyanide Antidote Package ℞ emergency treatment of cyanide poisoning (orphan) [sodium nitrite; sodium thiosulfate; amyl nitrite inhalant] 300 mg•12.5 g•0.3 mL

cyanoacetohydrazide [see: cyacetazide]

cyanoacrylate topical skin adhesive for closing surgical incisions and traumatic lacerations; topical mucous membrane sealant and protectant for canker and mouth sores

cyanocobalamin (vitamin B_{12}) USP, INN, BAN, JAN water-soluble vitamin; hematopoietic 50, 100, 250, 500, 1000, 2500, 5000 mcg oral; 100, 1000 mcg/mL injection

cyanocobalamin (^{57}Co) INN pernicious anemia test; radioactive agent [also: cyanocobalamin Co 57]

cyanocobalamin (^{58}Co) INN

cyanocobalamin (^{60}Co) INN pernicious anemia test; radioactive agent [also: cyanocobalamin Co 60]

cyanocobalamin Co 57 USAN, USP pernicious anemia test; radioactive agent [also: cyanocobalamin (^{57}Co)]

cyanocobalamin Co 60 USAN, USP *pernicious anemia test; radioactive agent* [also: cyanocobalamin (^{60}Co)]

Cyanoject IM or subcu injection (discontinued 2009) ℞ *hematinic; vitamin B$_{12}$ supplement* [cyanocobalamin] 1000 mcg/mL

Cyanokit powder for IV infusion ℞ *antidote to acute cyanide poisoning (orphan)* [hydroxocobalamin] 25 mg/mL (5 g/dose) ⊠ Senokot; Zincate

cyclacillin USAN, USP *antibacterial* [also: ciclacillin]

Cyclafem 1/35 tablets (in packs of 28) ℞ *monophasic oral contraceptive* [norethindrone; ethinyl estradiol] 1 mg• 35 mcg × 21 days; counters × 7 days

Cyclafem 7/7/7 tablets (in packs of 28) ℞ *triphasic oral contraceptive* [norethindrone; ethinyl estradiol] Phase 1 (7 days): 0.5 mg•35 mcg; Phase 2 (7 days): 0.75 mg•35 mcg; Phase 3 (7 days): 1 mg•35 mcg; Counters (7 days)

cyclamate calcium NF

cyclamic acid USAN, BAN *non-nutritive sweetener (banned in the U.S.)*

cyclamide [see: glycyclamide]

cyclandelate INN, BAN, JAN *peripheral vasodilator; vascular smooth muscle relaxant*

cyclarbamate INN, BAN

cyclazocine USAN, INN *analgesic*

cyclazodone INN

Cyclessa tablets (in packs of 28) ℞ *triphasic oral contraceptive; emergency postcoital contraceptive* [desogestrel; ethinyl estradiol] ⊠ Sequels Phase 1 (7 days): 0.1 mg•25 mcg; Phase 2 (7 days): 0.125 mg•25 mcg; Phase 3 (7 days): 0.15 mg•25 mcg; Counters (7 days)

cyclexanone INN

cyclic adenosine monophosphate (cAMP) [see: adenosine phosphate]

cyclic lipopeptides *a class of antibiotics that binds to bacterial membranes and causes a rapid depolarization of membrane potential, which inhibits RNA/DNA synthesis, leading to bacterial cell death*

cyclic propylene carbonate [see: propylene carbonate]

cyclindole USAN *antidepressant* [also: ciclindole]

Cyclinex-1 powder OTC *formula for infants with urea cycle disorders or gyrate atrophy*

Cyclinex-2 powder for oral liquid OTC *enteral nutritional therapy for urea cycle disorders or gyrate atrophy* [multiple essential amino acids]

cycliramine INN *antihistamine* [also: cycliramine maleate]

cycliramine maleate USAN *antihistamine* [also: cycliramine]

cyclizine USP, INN, BAN *anticholinergic; antihistamine; antiemetic; motion sickness relief* ⊠ seclazone

cyclizine HCl USP, BAN *anticholinergic; antihistamine; antiemetic; motion sickness relief*

cyclizine lactate USP, BAN *antinauseant*

cyclobarbital NF, INN [also: cyclobarbitone]

cyclobarbital calcium NF

cyclobarbitone BAN [also: cyclobarbital]

cyclobendazole USAN *anthelmintic* [also: ciclobendazole]

cyclobenzaprine INN *skeletal muscle relaxant* [also: cyclobenzaprine HCl]

cyclobenzaprine HCl USAN, USP *skeletal muscle relaxant* [also: cyclobenzaprine] 5, 7.5, 10, 15, 30 mg oral

cyclobutoic acid INN

cyclobutyrol INN

cyclocarbothiamine [see: cycotiamine]

cyclocoumarol BAN

cyclocumarol [see: cyclocoumarol]

α-cyclodextrin [see: alfadex]

cyclofenil INN, BAN

cyclofilcon A USAN *hydrophilic contact lens material*

cycloguanil embonate INN, BAN *antimalarial* [also: cycloguanil pamoate]

cycloguanil pamoate USAN *antimalarial* [also: cycloguanil embonate]

Cyclogyl Drop-Tainers (eye drops) ℞ *cycloplegic; mydriatic* [cyclopentolate HCl] 0.5%, 1%, 2%

cyclohexanehexol [see: inositol]

cyclohexanesulfamate dihydrate [see: sodium cyclamate]

cyclohexanesulfamic acid *(banned in the U.S.)* [see: cyclamic acid]

cycloheximide USAN *antipsoriatic* [also: cicloheximide]

***p*-cyclohexylhydratropic acid** [see: hexaprofen]

N-cyclohexyllinoleamide [see: clinolamide]

4-cyclohexyloxybenzoate [see: cyclomethycaine]

1-cyclohexylpropyl carbamate [see: procymate]

N-cyclohexylsulfamic acid *(banned in the U.S.)* [see: cyclamic acid]

cyclomenol INN Ⓢ cicliomenol

cyclomethicone NF *wetting agent*

cyclomethycaine INN, BAN *local anesthetic* [also: cyclomethycaine sulfate]

cyclomethycaine sulfate USP *local anesthetic* [also: cyclomethycaine]

Cyclomydril Drop-Tainers (eye drops) ℞ *cycloplegic; mydriatic* [cyclopentolate HCl; phenylephrine HCl] 0.2% •1%

cyclonium iodide [see: oxapium iodide]

cyclooxygenase-2 (COX-2) inhibitors *a class of nonsteroidal anti-inflammatory drugs (NSAIDs) for osteoarthritis, rheumatoid arthritis, acute pain, and primary dysmenorrhea; these agents also have antipyretic activity*

cyclopentamine INN, BAN [also: cyclopentamine HCl]

cyclopentamine HCl USP [also: cyclopentamine]

cyclopentaphene [see: cyclarbamate]

cyclopenthiazide USAN, INN, BAN *antihypertensive*

cyclopentolate INN, BAN *ophthalmic anticholinergic* [also: cyclopentolate HCl]

cyclopentolate HCl USP *ophthalmic anticholinergic; mydriatic; cycloplegic* [also: cyclopentolate] 1% eye drops

8-cyclopentyl 1,3-dipropylxanthine *investigational (orphan) for cystic fibrosis*

cyclophenazine HCl USAN *antipsychotic* [also: ciclofenazine]

cyclophilin inhibitors *a class of agents that treat hepatitis C virus infections*

cyclophosphamide USP, INN, BAN, JAN *nitrogen mustard–type alkylating antineoplastic for a wide variety of malignancies* 25, 50 mg oral; 0.5, 1, 2 g injection

cycloplegics *a class of drugs that paralyze the ciliary muscles of the eye*

cyclopolydimethylsiloxane [see: cyclomethicone]

cyclopregnol INN

cycloprolol BAN *antiadrenergic (beta-blocker)* [also: cicloprolol HCl; cicloprolol]

cyclopropane USP, INN *inhalation general anesthetic*

Cycloprostin *investigational (orphan) heparin replacement for hemodialysis* [epoprostenol]

cyclopyrronium bromide INN

cycloserine (L-cycloserine) USP, INN, BAN, JAN *bacteriostatic; tuberculosis retreatment; investigational (orphan) for Gaucher disease*

Cycloset tablets ℞ *dopamine agonist to suppress increased postprandial blood sugar in type 2 diabetes* [bromocriptine (as mesylate)] 0.8 mg

Cyclospire oral aerosol *investigational (orphan) to prevent and treat lung allograft and other pulmonary rejection associated with bone marrow transplantation* [cyclosporine, liposomal]

cyclosporin BAN *immunosuppressant* [also: cyclosporine; ciclosporin]

cyclosporin A [now: cyclosporine]

cyclosporine USAN, USP *immunosuppressant for transplants (orphan), rheumatoid arthritis, and psoriasis; tear stimulant for Sjögren keratoconjunctivitis sicca (orphan); investigational (orphan) for corneal melting syndrome* [also:

ciclosporin; cyclosporin] 25, 50, 100 mg oral; 100 mg/mL oral; 50 mg/mL injection

cyclosporine, liposomal *investigational (orphan) oral aerosol to prevent and treat lung allograft and other pulmonary rejection associated with bone marrow transplantation*

cyclosporine & ketoconazole *investigational (orphan) to diminish nephrotoxicity from organ transplantation*

CycloTech (trademarked delivery device) *provides premeasured doses of oral liquids and records dosing times*

cyclothiazide USAN, USP, INN, BAN *diuretic; antihypertensive*

cyclovalone INN

cycobemin [see: cyanocobalamin]

Cycofed syrup (discontinued 2007) ℞ *narcotic antitussive; decongestant* [codeine phosphate; pseudoephedrine HCl] 20•60 mg/5 mL

cycotiamine INN

cycrimine INN, BAN [also: cycrimine HCl]

cycrimine HCl USP [also: cycrimine]

Cydec oral drops (discontinued 2007) ℞ *decongestant; antihistamine* [pseudoephedrine HCl; carbinoxamine maleate] 25•2 mg/mL ⍰ Xedec; Zodeac

Cydec-DM syrup, pediatric oral drops (discontinued 2007) ℞ *antitussive; antihistamine; decongestant* [dextromethorphan hydrobromide; carbinoxamine maleate; pseudoephedrine HCl] 15•4•60 mg/5 mL; 4•2•25 mg/mL

cyfluthrin BAN

cyhalothrin BAN

cyheptamide USAN, INN *anticonvulsant*

cyheptropine INN

Cyklokapron IV infusion ℞ *systemic hemostatic for menorrhagia; also used as a surgical adjunct for patients with congenital coagulopathies (orphan); investigational (orphan) for hereditary angioneurotic edema* [tranexamic acid] 100 mg/mL

Cyklokapron tablets (discontinued 2009) ℞ *systemic hemostatic; surgical*

adjunct for patients with congenital coagulopathies (orphan) [tranexamic acid] 500 mg

Cylex; Cylex Sugar-Free lozenges OTC *mucous membrane anesthetic; antiseptic* [benzocaine; cetylpyridinium chloride] 15•5 mg ⍰ Celexa; Salex; Xolox

Cylexin *investigational (Phase III, orphan) adjunct to surgery for congenital heart defects in newborns; investigational (orphan) for postischemic pulmonary reperfusion edema* [CY-1503 (code name—generic name not yet assigned)]

Cymbalta enteric-coated delayed-release pellets in capsules ℞ *selective serotonin and norepinephrine reuptake inhibitor (SSNRI) for major depressive disorder (MDD) and generalized anxiety disorder (GAD); analgesic for diabetic peripheral neuropathy (DPN), fibromyalgia, and chronic musculoskeletal pain* [duloxetine (as HCl)] 20, 30, 60 mg ⍰ Simplet

Cymbopogon citratus medicinal herb [see: lemongrass]

Cymbopogon nardus; C. winterianus medicinal herb [see: citronella]

cymemoxine [see: cimemoxin]

Cymevene (foreign name for the U.S. product **Cytovene**)

Cynara scolymus medicinal herb [see: artichoke]

cynarine INN

Cyomin IM or subcu injection (discontinued 2009) ℞ *hematinic; vitamin B_{12} supplement* [cyanocobalamin] 1000 mcg/mL ⍰ Xeomin; Zymine

cypenamine INN, BAN *antidepressant* [also: cypenamine HCl]

cypenamine HCl USAN *antidepressant* [also: cypenamine]

cypionate USAN, BAN *combining name for radicals or groups* [also: cipionate]

cypothrin USAN *veterinary insecticide*

cyprazepam USAN, INN *sedative*

cyprenorphine INN, BAN

cyprenorphine HCl [see: cyprenorphine]

Cypripedium pubescens medicinal herb [see: lady's slipper]

cyprodemanol [see: cyprodenate]

cyprodenate INN

cyproheptadine INN, BAN *nonselective piperidine antihistamine for hypersensitivity reactions; antipruritic* [also: cyproheptadine HCl]

cyproheptadine HCl USP, JAN *nonselective piperidine antihistamine for allergic rhinitis and type I hypersensitivity reactions; antipruritic; adjunctive anaphylactic therapy; also used for post-traumatic stress disorder (PTSD)* [also: cyproheptadine] 4 mg oral; 2 mg/5 mL oral

cyprolidol INN *antidepressant* [also: cyprolidol HCl]

cyprolidol HCl USAN *antidepressant* [also: cyprolidol]

cyproquinate USAN *coccidiostat for poultry* [also: ciproquinate]

cyproterone INN, BAN *antiandrogen* [also: cyproterone acetate]

cyproterone acetate USAN *antiandrogen; investigational (orphan) for severe hirsutism* [also: cyproterone]

cyproximide USAN *antipsychotic; antidepressant* [also: ciproximide]

cyren A [see: diethylstilbestrol]

cyren B [see: diethylstilbestrol dipropionate]

cyromazine INN, BAN ☒ Seromycin

Cystadane powder for oral solution ℞ *electrolyte replenisher for homocystinuria* (orphan) [betaine HCl] 1 g

Cystagon capsules ℞ *antiurolithic for nephropathic cystinosis* (orphan) [cysteamine bitartrate] 50, 150 mg

cystamin [see: methenamine]

cysteamine USAN, BAN *antiurolithic for nephropathic cystinosis* (orphan) [also: mercaptamine]

cysteamine bitartrate *antiurolithic for nephropathic cystinosis* (orphan)

cysteamine HCl USAN *antiurolithic; investigational (orphan) for corneal cysteine accumulation in cystinosis patients*

cysteine (L-cysteine) INN *nonessential amino acid; symbols: Cys, C; investigational (orphan) for erythropoietic protoporphyria photosensitivity* [also: cysteine HCl]

cysteine HCl (L-cysteine HCl) USP *nonessential amino acid* [also: cysteine] 50 mg/mL injection

L-cysteine HCl monohydrate [see: cysteine HCl]

Cystex tablets ℞ *urinary antibiotic; analgesic; acidifier* [methenamine; sodium salicylate; benzoic acid] 162•162.5•32 mg

cystic fibrosis gene therapy *investigational (orphan) for cystic fibrosis*

cystic fibrosis transmembrane conductance regulator (CFTR) *investigational (orphan) for cystic fibrosis*

cystic fibrosis transmembrane conductance regulator, recombinant adenovirus (AdGV-CFTR) *investigational (orphan) for cystic fibrosis*

cystine (L-cystine) USAN *amino acid* ☒ Sustain; Systane

cystogen [see: methenamine]

Cystografin; Cystografin Dilute intracavitary instillation ℞ *radiopaque contrast medium for urological imaging* [diatrizoate meglumine (46.67% iodine)] 300 mg/mL (141 mg/mL); 180 mg/mL (85 mg/mL)

Cystospaz tablets ℞ *GI/GU antispasmodic; antiparkinsonian; anticholinergic "drying agent" for allergic rhinitis and hyperhidrosis* [hyoscyamine sulfate] 0.15 mg

Cysview intravesical injection ℞ *photosensitizer for fluorescence cystoscopy* [hexaminolevulinate HCl] 100 mg

Cytadren tablets (discontinued 2008) ℞ *adrenal steroid inhibitor; antisteroidal t-2.2>antineoplastic for corticotropin-producing tumors* [aminoglutethimide] 250 mg

cytarabine USAN, USP, INN, BAN, JAN *antimetabolite antineoplastic for various leukemias* 100, 500, 1000, 2000 mg injection

cytarabine, liposomal *antimetabolite antineoplastic for lymphomatous neoplastic meningitis (NM) arising from solid tumors or non-Hodgkin lymphoma (orphan)*

cytarabine HCl USAN *antiviral*

Cytisus scoparius medicinal herb [see: broom]

Cyto B2 powder for oral solution OTC *vitamin supplement* [riboflavin (vitamin B₂)] 343 mg/g

CytoGam IV infusion ℞ *prevention of primary cytomegalovirus in bone marrow and organ transplants from a CMV seropositive donor to an immunocompromised CMV seronegative recipient (orphan)* [cytomegalovirus immune globulin, solvent/detergent treated] 50 mg/mL

CytoImplant *investigational (orphan) agent for pancreatic cancer* [blood mononuclear cells, allogenic peripheral]

cytomegalovirus immune globulin (CMV-IG), human *prevention of primary cytomegalovirus in bone marrow and organ transplants from a CMV seropositive donor to an immunocompromised CMV seronegative recipient (orphan)*

cytomegalovirus immune globulin intravenous (CMV-IGIV) & ganciclovir sodium *investigational (orphan) for cytomegalovirus pneumonia in bone marrow transplant patients*

Cytomel tablets ℞ *synthetic thyroid hormone (T₃ fraction only)* [liothyronine sodium] 5, 25, 50 mcg

cytoprotective agents *a class of drugs that provide prophylaxis against the side effects of antineoplastic agents*

cytosine arabinoside (ara-C) [see: cytarabine]

cytosine arabinoside HCl [now: cytarabine HCl]

Cytosol topical liquid ℞ *for general irrigating, washing, and rinsing* [physiological irrigating solution]

Cytotec tablets ℞ *prevents NSAID-induced gastric ulcers; has been used for cervical ripening and induction of labor; use by pregnant women can cause abortion, premature birth, or birth defects* [misoprostol] 100, 200 mcg

cytotoxic lymphocyte maturation factor [see: edodekin alfa]

Cytovene capsules (discontinued 2010) ℞ *antiviral for AIDS-related cytomegalovirus (CMV) infections (orphan) and CMV retinitis (orphan)* [ganciclovir] 250, 500 mg ⊡ Cetafen

Cytovene powder for IV infusion ℞ *antiviral for AIDS-related cytomegalovirus (CMV) infections (orphan)* [ganciclovir sodium] 500 mg/vial ⊡ Cetafen

Cytoxan tablets, powder for IV injection (discontinued 2008) ℞ *antineoplastic for a wide variety of malignancies* [cyclophosphamide] 25, 50 mg; 100 mg ⊡ Staxyn

Cytra-2 solution ℞ *urinary alkalizing agent* [sodium citrate; citric acid] 500•334 mg/5 mL ⊡ Scytera; Zetar

Cytra-3 syrup ℞ *urinary alkalinizing agent* [potassium citrate; sodium citrate; citric acid] 550•500•334 mg/5 mL ⊡ Scytera; Zetar

Cytra-K oral solution ℞ *urinary alkalizing agent* [potassium citrate; citric acid] 1100•334 mg/5 mL

Cytra-LC solution ℞ *urinary alkalizer* [potassium citrate; sodium citrate; citric acid] 550•500•334 mg/5 mL

Cytuss HC; Cytuss HC NR oral liquid (discontinued 2009) ℞ *narcotic antitussive; antihistamine; decongestant* [hydrocodone bitartrate; chlorpheniramine maleate; phenylephrine HCl] 2.5•2•5 mg/5 mL; 2.5•1•5 mg/5 mL ⊡ Z-Tuss AC

CYVADIC; CY-VA-DIC; CyVADIC (cyclophosphamide, vincristine, Adriamycin, DIC) *chemotherapy protocol for bone and soft tissue sarcomas*

D (vitamin D) [q.v.]

D-2.5-W; D-5-W; D-10-W; D-20-W; D-25-W; D-30-W; D-40-W; D-50-W; D-60-W; D-70-W ℞ *intravenous nutritional therapy* [dextrose]

D3-50 capsules OTC *vitamin D supplement* [cholecalciferol (vitamin D₃)] 50 000 IU

D 400 chewable tablets OTC *vitamin D supplement* [cholecalciferol (vitamin D₃)] 400 IU

D 1000 chewable tablets OTC *vitamin supplement* [cholecalciferol (vitamin D₃)] 1000 IU

D 1000 Plus tablets OTC *vitamin/calcium supplement* [vitamins B₆, B₁₂, and D; calcium; folic acid] 10 mg•200 mcg•1000 IU•120 mg•400 mcg

D₂ (vitamin D₂) [see: ergocalciferol]

D-2000 Maximum Strength tablets OTC *vitamin/calcium supplement* [cholecalciferol (vitamin D₃); calcium] 2000 IU•180 mg

D₃ (vitamin D₃) [see: cholecalciferol]

d4T [see: stavudine]

D-5000 Super Strength tablets OTC *vitamin/calcium supplement* [cholecalciferol (vitamin D₃); calcium] 5000 IU•180 mg

D Drops oral drops OTC *vitamin D supplement* [cholecalciferol (vitamin D₃)] 1000, 2000 IU/0.03 mL

D.A. chewable tablets ℞ *decongestant; antihistamine; anticholinergic to dry mucosal secretions* [phenylephrine HCl; chlorpheniramine maleate; methscopolamine nitrate] 10•2•1.25 mg

DA (daunorubicin, ara-C) *chemotherapy protocol for acute myelocytic leukemia (AML)* [also known as: ara-C + DNR]

DAA (dihydroxyaluminum aminoacetate) [q.v.]

dabigatran etexilate *direct thrombin inhibitor; oral anticoagulant for the prevention of stroke, deep vein thrombosis (DVT), or other venous thromboembolism (VTE) following total hip or total knee replacement surgery*

dacarbazine USAN, USP, INN, BAN *alkylating antineoplastic for metastatic malignant melanoma and Hodgkin disease* 100, 200 mg injection

dacemazine INN ⑦ duazomycin

Dacex-A oral drops (discontinued 2007) ℞ *antitussive; antihistamine; decongestant; for children 3–24 months* [dextromethorphan hydrobromide; carbinoxamine maleate; phenylephrine HCl] 4•1•2 mg/mL ⑦ Desoxi; Diskus

Dacex-DM syrup ℞ *antitussive; decongestant; expectorant* [dextromethorphan hydrobromide; phenylephrine HCl; guaifenesin] 25•12.5•175 mg/5 mL

Dacex-PE extended-release caplets ℞ *antitussive; decongestant; expectorant* [dextromethorphan hydrobromide; phenylephrine HCl; guaifenesin] 30•10•600 mg

dacisteine INN

dacliximab [now: daclizumab]

daclizumab USAN, INN, BAN *immunosuppressant; monoclonal antibody (MAb) to prevent acute rejection of kidney and bone marrow transplants (orphan); investigational (Phase II) adjunct to interferon treatment of multiple sclerosis*

Dacogen IV infusion ℞ *antineoplastic for myelodysplastic syndromes (MDS); orphan); investigational (NDA filed, orphan) for chronic myelogenous leukemia and sickle cell anemia* [decitabine] 50 mg

Dacriose ophthalmic solution (discontinued 2010) OTC *extraocular irrigating solution* [sterile isotonic solution]

dactinomycin USAN, USP, BAN *antibiotic antineoplastic for various tumors, carcinomas, and sarcomas; potentiator for radiation therapy* [also: actinomycin D] 0.5 mg/vial injection

dacuronium bromide INN, BAN

DADDS (diacetyl diaminodiphenyl-sulfone) [see: acedapsone]

dagapamil INN

daidzein one of several soy isoflavones that provide cell-protective effects

daidzin isoform precursor to daidzein [q.v.]

Daily Betic tablets OTC *vitamin/mineral/calcium supplement* [multiple vitamins & minerals; calcium; folic acid; biotin] ±•100•0.2•0.075 mg

Daily Multi caplets OTC *vitamin/mineral/calcium/iron supplement* [multiple vitamins & minerals; calcium (as carbonate and dicalcium phosphate); iron (as ferrous fumarate); folic acid] ±•162•18•0.4 mg

Daily Multi 50+ caplets OTC *vitamin/mineral supplement* [multiple vitamins & minerals; folic acid; biotin; lutein] ±•400•30•300 mcg

Daily Multiple Vitamins with Iron tablets OTC *vitamin/iron supplement* [multiple vitamins; iron (as ferrous fumarate); folic acid] ±•18•0.4 mg

Daily Vitamins oral liquid, syrup OTC *vitamin supplement* [multiple vitamins; HFCS]

Daily-Vite tablets OTC *vitamin/iron supplement* [multiple vitamins; iron; folic acid] ±•18•0.4 mg ⊡ Dialyvite

Daily-Vite with Iron & Minerals tablets (discontinued 2008) OTC *vitamin/mineral/iron supplement* [multiple vitamins & minerals; iron; folic acid; biotin] ±•18•0.4•⅔ mg

Dairy Ease chewable tablets OTC *digestive aid for lactose intolerance* [lactase enzyme] 3300 U ⊡ Dry Eyes; DUROS

DairyCare delayed-release capsules OTC *digestive aid for lactose intolerance* [lactase enzyme; Lactobacillus acidophilus] 15•190 mg ⊡ DURAcare

daisy, wild medicinal herb [see: wild daisy]

Dakin solution [see: sodium hypochlorite]

Dalalone intra-articular, intralesional, soft tissue, or IM injection R corticosteroidal anti-inflammatory [dexamethasone sodium phosphate] 4 mg/mL

Dalalone D.P. intra-articular, soft tissue, or IM injection (discontinued 2009) R corticosteroidal anti-inflammatory [dexamethasone acetate] 16 mg/mL

Dalalone L.A. intralesional, intra-articular, soft tissue, or IM injection (discontinued 2009) R corticosteroidal anti-inflammatory [dexamethasone acetate] 8 mg/mL

dalanated insulin [see: insulin, dalanated]

dalbavancin glycopeptide antibiotic for anaerobic and gram-positive aerobic bacteria; investigational (NDA filed) once-weekly treatment for methicillin-resistant Staphylococcus aureus (MRSA) and methicillin-resistant S. epidermidis (MRSE)

dalbraminol INN

dalcetrapib investigational (Phase III) antihyperlipidemic; cholesterol ester transfer protein (CETP) inhibitor that raises HDL cholesterol and decreases plaque formation in the arteries

daledalin INN antidepressant [also: daledalin tosylate]

daledalin tosylate USAN antidepressant [also: daledalin]

dalfampridine potassium-channel blocker to improve walking with multiple sclerosis

dalfopristin USAN, INN streptogramin antibacterial antibiotic for life-threatening infections

dalfopristin & quinupristin two streptogramin antibiotics that are synergistically bactericidal to gram-positive infections; investigational (NDA filed) for pneumonia

Daliresp tablets R once-daily treatment for chronic obstructive pulmonary disease (COPD) [roflumilast] 500 mcg

Dallergy oral drops R decongestant; antihistamine; for children 2–12 years [phenylephrine HCl; chlorpheniramine maleate] 2•1 mg/mL

Dallergy sustained-release caplets (discontinued 2007) R decongestant; antihistamine; anticholinergic to dry muco-

sal secretions [phenylephrine HCl; chlorpheniramine maleate; methscopolamine nitrate] 20•12•2.5 mg

Dallergy tablets, chewable caplets, syrup Ŗ *decongestant; antihistamine; anticholinergic to dry mucosal secretions* [phenylephrine HCl; chlorpheniramine maleate; methscopolamine nitrate] 10•4•1.25 mg; 10•2•1.25 mg; 8•2•0.75 mg/5 mL

Dallergy DM syrup Ŗ *antitussive; decongestant; antihistamine* [dextromethorphan hydrobromide; pseudoephedrine HCl; brompheniramine maleate] 15•30•3 mg/5 mL

Dallergy PE extended-release caplets Ŗ *decongestant; antihistamine; anticholinergic to dry mucosal secretions* [phenylephrine HCl; chlorpheniramine maleate; methscopolamine nitrate] 20•8•2.5 mg

Dallergy-JR extended-release capsules, oral suspension Ŗ *decongestant; antihistamine* [phenylephrine HCl; chlorpheniramine maleate] 20•4 mg; 20•4 mg/5 mL

Dalmane capsules (discontinued 2008) Ŗ *benzodiazepine sedative and hypnotic; anticonvulsant; muscle relaxant; also abused as a street drug* [flurazepam HCl] 15, 30 mg ⧉ Dilomine; diolamine

d'Alpha E 1000 softgels OTC *vitamin supplement* [vitamin E (as *d*-alpha tocopherol)] 1000 IU

dalteparin sodium USAN, INN, BAN *a low molecular weight heparin–type anticoagulant and antithrombotic for prevention of deep vein thrombosis (DVT), venous thromboembolism (VTE), unstable angina, and myocardial infarction*

daltroban USAN, INN *immunosuppressive*

Damason-P tablets Ŗ *narcotic analgesic; antipyretic* [hydrocodone bitartrate; aspirin] 5•500 mg

dambose [see: inositol]

dametralast INN

damiana (Turnera aphrodisiaca; T. diffusa; T. microphylla) leaves *medicinal herb for bed-wetting, bron-* *chitis, emphysema, headache, hormonal imbalance, hot flashes, menopause, and Parkinson disease; also used as an aphrodisiac*

damotepine INN

danaparoid sodium USAN, BAN *glycosaminoglycan anticoagulant and antithrombotic for prevention of deep vein thrombosis (DVT)*

danazol USAN, USP, INN, BAN *anterior pituitary suppressant; gonadotropin inhibitor for endometriosis, fibrocystic breast disease, and hereditary angioedema* 50, 100, 200 mg oral

dandelion (Leontodon taraxacum; Taraxacum officinale) leaves and root *medicinal herb for anemia, analgesia, blisters, blood cleansing, blood glucose regulation, constipation, diaphoresis, dyspepsia, edema, endurance, gallbladder disease, hypertension, and liver disorders*

daniplestim USAN *treatment for chemotherapy-induced bone marrow suppression*

daniquidone BAN

danitamon [see: menadione]

danitracen INN

danofloxacin INN *veterinary antibacterial* [also: danofloxacin mesylate]

danofloxacin mesylate USAN *veterinary antibacterial* [also: danofloxacin]

danosteine INN

danshen (Salvia miltiorrhiza) *medicinal herb for abdominal pain, bruises, circulatory problems, insomnia, menstrual irregularity, and stroke; also used as an aid in granulation of wounds*

danthron USP, BAN (withdrawn from the market by the FDA) [also: dantron]

Dantrium capsules, powder for IV injection Ŗ *skeletal muscle relaxant; investigational (orphan) for neuroleptic malignant syndrome* [dantrolene sodium] 25, 50, 100 mg; 20 mg/vial (0.32 mg/mL)

dantrolene USAN, INN, BAN *skeletal muscle relaxant*

dantrolene sodium USAN, BAN *skeletal muscle relaxant; investigational* (orphan) for neuroleptic malignant syndrome 25, 50, 100 mg oral; 20 mg injection

dantron INN (withdrawn from market by FDA) [also: danthron]

dapagliflozin investigational (NDA filed) sodium-glucose transporter 2 (SGLT-2) inhibitor to increase the excretion of glucose in the urine for type 2 diabetes

Daphne mezereum medicinal herb [see: mezereon]

dapiprazole INN alpha-adrenergic blocker; miotic; neuroleptic [also: dapiprazole HCl]

dapiprazole HCl USAN alpha-adrenergic blocker; miotic; neuroleptic [also: dapiprazole]

dapoxetine investigational (NDA filed) short-acting selective serotonin reuptake inhibitor (SSRI) for various urogenital indications, including moderate to severe premature ejaculation (PE)

dapsone USAN, USP, BAN antibacterial for acne vulgaris; leprostatic; herpetiform dermatitis suppressant; investigational (Phase III, orphan) for Pneumocystis pneumonia (PCP) and toxoplasmosis 25, 100 mg oral

Daptacel IM injection ℞ active immunizing agent for diphtheria, tetanus, and pertussis; Dtap (diphtheria predominant) vaccine used in the initial immunization series of infants and children 6 weeks to 6 years [diphtheria toxoid; tetanus toxoid; acellular pertussis toxoid (DTaP vaccine)] 15 Lf•5 Lf• 10 mcg per 0.5 mL dose

daptazole [see: amiphenazole]

daptomycin USAN, INN, BAN cyclic lipopeptide antibiotic for complicated skin and skin structure infections (cSSSIs), Staphylococcus aureus bloodstream infections, and right-sided endocarditis

darapladib investigational (Phase III) lipoprotein PLA$_2$ inhibitor for atherosclerosis and acute coronary syndrome (ACS)

Daraprim tablets ℞ antimalarial; toxoplasmosis treatment adjunct [pyrimethamine] 25 mg

darbepoetin alfa USAN erythropoiesis-stimulating agent (ESA); recombinant human erythropoietin for anemia associated with chronic renal failure or chemotherapy for nonmyeloid malignancies

darbufelone mesylate USAN anti-inflammatory; antiarthritic; cyclooxygenase inhibitor; 5-lipoxygenase inhibitor

darenzepine INN

darglitazone sodium USAN oral hypoglycemic

darifenacin hydrobromide selective muscarinic M$_3$ receptor antagonist for urinary frequency, urgency, and incontinence

darodipine USAN, INN antihypertensive; bronchodilator; vasodilator

Darpaz tablets (discontinued 2010) ℞ urinary antibiotic; antiseptic; analgesic; antispasmodic [methenamine; sodium phosphate; phenyl salicylate; methylene blue; hyoscyamine sulfate] 81.6•40.8•36.2•10.8•0.12 mg

darunavir ethanolate protease inhibitor; oral antiretroviral for HIV-1 infections

darusentan investigational (Phase III) endothelin receptor antagonist (ERA) vasodilator for resistant hypertension

Darvocet A500 film-coated tablets (discontinued 2010) ℞ narcotic analgesic; antipyretic; all products containing propoxyphene were withdrawn from the market in 2010 due to safety concerns [propoxyphene napsylate; acetaminophen] 100•500 mg

Darvocet-N 50; Darvocet-N 100 tablets (discontinued 2010) ℞ narcotic analgesic; antipyretic; all products containing propoxyphene were withdrawn from the market in 2010 due to safety concerns [propoxyphene napsylate; acetaminophen] 50•325 mg; 100•650 mg

Darvon Pulvules (capsules) (discontinued 2010) ℞ narcotic analgesic for mild to moderate pain; all products containing propoxyphene were withdrawn from the market in 2010 due to safety concerns [propoxyphene HCl] 65 mg ⑨ Duraphen

Darvon Compound 32 Pulvules (capsules) (discontinued 2007) ℞ *narcotic analgesic; antipyretic* [propoxyphene HCl; aspirin; caffeine] 32•389•32.4 mg

Darvon Compound 65 Pulvules (capsules) (discontinued 2010) ℞ *narcotic analgesic; antipyretic; all products containing propoxyphene were withdrawn from the market in 2010 due to safety concerns* [propoxyphene HCl; aspirin; caffeine] 65•389•32.4 mg

Darvon-N film-coated tablets (discontinued 2010) ℞ *narcotic analgesic for mild to moderate pain; all products containing propoxyphene were withdrawn from the market in 2010 due to safety concerns* [propoxyphene napsylate] 100 mg ⦾ Duraphen

dasatinib *multiple tyrosine kinase inhibitor; antineoplastic for chronic myeloid leukemia (CML) and acute lymphoblastic leukemia in patients expressing the Philadelphia chromosome (Ph+ ALL)*

DAT (daunorubicin, ara-C, thioguanine) *chemotherapy protocol for acute myelocytic leukemia (AML)* [also known as: DCT; TAD]

datelliptium chloride INN

DaTscan IV injection ℞ *radiodiagnostic imaging agent for single photon emission computed tomography (SPECT) scans of the brain for the evaluation of parkinsonian syndromes* [ioflupane I 123] 2 mCi/mL (74 MBq/mL)

Datura stramonium medicinal herb [see: jimsonweed]

daturine hydrobromide [see: hyoscyamine hydrobromide]

Daucus carota medicinal herb [see: carrot]

daunomycin [see: daunorubicin HCl]

daunorubicin (DNR) INN, BAN *anthracycline antibiotic antineoplastic for various leukemias* [also: daunorubicin HCl]

daunorubicin citrate, liposomal *anthracycline antibiotic antineoplastic for advanced HIV-related Kaposi sarcoma (orphan)*

daunorubicin HCl USAN, USP, JAN *anthracycline antibiotic antineoplastic for various lymphocytic and nonlymphocytic leukemias* [also: daunorubicin] 20, 50 mg injection

DaunoXome IV infusion ℞ *antibiotic antineoplastic for advanced AIDS-related Kaposi sarcoma (orphan)* [daunorubicin citrate, liposomal] 2 mg/mL (50 mg/dose)

DAV (daunorubicin, ara-C, VePesid) *chemotherapy protocol for acute myelocytic leukemia (AML)*

davitamon [see: menadione]

Daxas ⓔ (available in Europe) *investigational (NDA filed) once-daily oral phosphodiesterase 4 (PDE-4) inhibitor for chronic obstructive pulmonary disease (COPD)* [roflumilast]

Dayalets Filmtabs (film-coated tablets) (discontinued 2008) OTC *vitamin supplement* [multiple vitamins; folic acid] ±•0.4 mg

Dayalets + Iron Filmtabs (film-coated tablets) (discontinued 2008) OTC *vitamin/iron supplement* [multiple vitamins; ferrous sulfate; folic acid] ±•18•0.4 mg

Dayhist-1 tablets OTC *antihistamine for allergic rhinitis and urticaria* [clemastine fumarate] 1.34 mg ⦾ Duohist

Daypro film-coated caplets ℞ *analgesic; nonsteroidal anti-inflammatory drug (NSAID) for osteoarthritis and rheumatoid arthritis* [oxaprozin] 600 mg ⦾ Dopar

Daypro Alta film-coated caplets ℞ *analgesic; nonsteroidal anti-inflammatory drug (NSAID) for osteoarthritis and rheumatoid arthritis* [oxaprozin (as potassium)] 600 mg

DayQuil Mucus Control oral liquid OTC *expectorant* [guaifenesin] 66.7 mg/5 mL

DayQuil Multi-Symptom Cold/Flu Relief LiquiCaps (liquid-filled gelcaps), oral liquid OTC *antitussive; decongestant; analgesic; antipyretic* [dextromethorphan hydrobromide;

phenylephrine HCl; acetaminophen] 10•5•325 mg; 10•5•325 mg/15 mL

DayQuil Sinex Liqui-caps (liquid-filled gelcaps) OTC *decongestant; analgesic; antipyretic* [phenylephrine HCl; acetaminophen] 5•325 mg

Daytime Sinus Relief Non-Drowsy caplets (discontinued 2007) OTC *decongestant; analgesic; antipyretic* [pseudoephedrine HCl; acetaminophen] 30•500 mg

Daytrana transdermal patch R *CNS stimulant for attention-deficit/hyperactivity disorder (ADHD)* [methylphenidate] 10, 15, 20, 30 mg/day

dazadrol INN *antidepressant* [also: dazadrol maleate]

dazadrol maleate USAN *antidepressant* [also: dazadrol]

dazepinil INN *antidepressant* [also: dazepinil HCl]

dazepinil HCl USAN *antidepressant* [also: dazepinil]

dazidamine INN

dazmegrel USAN, INN, BAN *thromboxane synthetase inhibitor*

dazolicine INN

dazopride INN *peristaltic stimulant* [also: dazopride fumarate]

dazopride fumarate USAN *peristaltic stimulant* [also: dazopride]

dazoquinast INN

dazoxiben INN, BAN *antithrombotic* [also: dazoxiben HCl]

dazoxiben HCl USAN *antithrombotic* [also: dazoxiben]

DBED (dibenzylethylenediamine dipenicillin G) [see: penicillin G benzathine]

DBM (dibromomannitol) [see: mitobronitol]

DC softgels OTC *laxative; stool softener* [docusate calcium] 240 mg

D&C Brown No. 1 (drugs & cosmetics) [see: resorcin brown]

DCA (desoxycorticosterone acetate) [q.v.]

DCA (dichloroacetate) [see: sodium dichloroacetate]

DCF (2'-deoxycoformycin) [see: pentostatin]

DCL (descarboethoxyloratadine) [q.v.]

DCT (daunorubicin, cytarabine, thioguanine) *chemotherapy protocol for acute myelocytic leukemia (AML)* [also known as: DAT; TAD]

DDAVP tablets, nasal spray, rhinal tube, subcu or IV injection R *posterior pituitary hormone for hemophilia A (orphan), von Willebrand disease (orphan), central diabetes insipidus, and nocturnal enuresis* [desmopressin acetate] 0.1, 0.2 mg; 10 mcg/dose; 0.1 mg/mL; 4 mcg/mL ⊡ DVP

DDAVP (1-deamino-8-D-arginine-vasopressin) [see: desmopressin acetate]

DDC; ddC (dideoxycytidine) [see: zalcitabine]

o,p'-DDD [now: mitotane]

DDI; ddI (dideoxyinosine) [see: didanosine]

DDP; cis-DDP (diamminedichloroplatinum) [see: cisplatin]

DDS (diaminodiphenylsulfone) [now: dapsone]

DDT (dichlorodiphenyltrichloroethane) [see: chlorophenothane]

DDVP (dichlorovinyl dimethyl phosphate) [see: dichlorvos]

DEA (diethanolamine) [q.v.]

deacetyllanatoside C [see: deslanoside]

17-deacylnorgestimate [see: norelgestromin]

deadly nightshade *medicinal herb* [see: belladonna]

deadly nightshade leaf [see: belladonna extract]

DEAE-rebeccamycin *investigational (orphan) for bile duct tumors*

deal pine *medicinal herb* [see: white pine]

1-deamino-8-D-arginine-vasopressin (DDAVP) [see: desmopressin acetate]

deanil INN *combining name for radicals or groups*

deanol BAN [also: deanol aceglumate]

deanol aceglumate INN [also: deanol]

deanol acetamidobenzoate

deba [see: barbital]

Debacterol oral solution with swab applicator ℞ *antiseptic and analgesic for ulcerating mouth and gum lesions such as aphthous ulcers (canker sores) and necrotizing ulcerative gingivitis (pyorrhea)* [sulfuric acid; sulfonated phenolics] 30%•50%

deboxamet INN

debrase *investigational (orphan) agent for debridement of acute, deep dermal burns*

Debridase *investigational (orphan) agent for débridement of acute, deep dermal burns* [debrase]

Debrisan beads, paste (discontinued 2010) ℞ *débrider and cleanser for wet wounds* [dextranomer] ⃞ Diprosone

debrisoquin sulfate USAN *antihypertensive* [also: debrisoquine]

debrisoquine INN, BAN *antihypertensive* [also: debrisoquin sulfate]

Debrox ear drops OTC *cerumenolytic to emulsify and disperse ear wax* [carbamide peroxide] 6.5%

Decadron tablets (discontinued 2010) ℞ *corticosteroidal anti-inflammatory* [dexamethasone] 0.5, 0.75 mg

Decadron Phosphate intra-articular, intralesional, soft tissue or IM injection ℞ *corticosteroidal anti-inflammatory* [dexamethasone sodium phosphate] 4 mg/mL

Decadron Phosphate IV injection ℞ *corticosteroidal anti-inflammatory* [dexamethasone sodium phosphate] 24 mg/mL

Decadron with Xylocaine soft tissue injection (discontinued 2009) ℞ *corticosteroidal anti-inflammatory; anesthetic* [dexamethasone sodium phosphate; lidocaine HCl] 4•10 mg/mL

Decagen tablets (discontinued 2008) OTC *vitamin/mineral/iron supplement* [multiple vitamins & minerals; iron; folic acid; biotin] ±•18 mg•0.4 mg•30 mcg

Decaject intra-articular, intralesional, soft tissue, or IM injection ℞ *cortico-*

steroidal anti-inflammatory [dexamethasone sodium phosphate] 4 mg/mL

Decaject-L.A. intralesional, intra-articular, soft tissue, or IM injection (discontinued 2009) ℞ *corticosteroidal anti-inflammatory* [dexamethasone acetate] 8 mg/mL

decamethonium bromide USP, INN [also: decamethonium iodide]

decamethonium iodide BAN [also: decamethonium bromide]

Decapinol oral rinse ℞ *gingivitis treatment*

decapinol [see: delmopinol]

Decavac IM injection ℞ *active immunizing agent for diphtheria and tetanus* [diphtheria & tetanus toxoids, adsorbed] 2•5 LfU per 0.5 mL dose

decavitamin USP

De-Chlor HC oral liquid (discontinued 2009) ℞ *narcotic antitussive; antihistamine; decongestant* [hydrocodone bitartrate; chlorpheniramine maleate; phenylephrine HCl] 2.5•2•10 mg/5 mL

De-Chlor HD oral liquid (discontinued 2008) ℞ *narcotic antitussive; antihistamine; decongestant* [hydrocodone bitartrate; chlorpheniramine maleate; phenylephrine HCl] 2.5•4•10 mg/5 mL

De-Chlor MR oral liquid (discontinued 2009) ℞ *narcotic antitussive; antihistamine; sleep aid; decongestant* [hydrocodone bitartrate; pyrilamine maleate; phenylephrine HCl] 10•10•10 mg/10 mL

De-Chlor NX oral liquid (discontinued 2011) ℞ *narcotic antitussive; expectorant* [hydrocodone bitartrate; potassium guaiacolsulfonate] 3•150 mg/5 mL

Decholin tablets OTC *laxative; hydrocholeretic* [dehydrocholic acid] 250 mg

decicain [see: tetracaine HCl]

decil INN *combining name for radicals or groups* ⃞ Dicel

decimemide INN

decitabine USAN, INN, BAN *DNA synthesis inhibitor; antineoplastic for myelo-*

dysplastic syndromes (MDS; orphan); investigational (NDA filed, orphan) for chronic myelogenous leukemia and sickle cell anemia

decitropine INN

declaben [now: lodelaben]

declenperone USAN, INN *veterinary sedative*

Declomycin film-coated tablets ℞ *broad-spectrum antibiotic* [demeclocycline HCl] 150, 300 mg

decloxizine INN

Decodult tablets (discontinued 2007) OTC *decongestant; antihistamine; analgesic; antipyretic* [phenylephrine HCl; chlorpheniramine maleate; acetaminophen] 5•2•300 mg

Decofed syrup (discontinued 2009) OTC *nasal decongestant* [pseudoephedrine HCl] 30 mg/5 mL

Decohistine DH oral liquid (discontinued 2007) ℞ *narcotic antitussive; antihistamine; decongestant* [codeine phosphate; chlorpheniramine maleate; pseudoephedrine HCl; alcohol 5.8%] 10•2•30 mg/5 mL

Decolate tablets (discontinued 2007) ℞ *decongestant; antihistamine; expectorant* [phenylephrine HCl; chlorpheniramine maleate; guaifenesin] 5•4•100 mg

decominol INN

Deconamine tablets (discontinued 2007) ℞ *decongestant; antihistamine* [pseudoephedrine HCl; chlorpheniramine maleate] 60•4 mg

Deconamine syrup ℞ *decongestant; antihistamine* [pseudoephedrine HCl; chlorpheniramine maleate] 30•2 mg/5 mL

Deconamine SR sustained-release capsules (discontinued 2009) ℞ *decongestant; antihistamine* [pseudoephedrine HCl; chlorpheniramine maleate] 120•8 mg

Deconex capsules ℞ *decongestant; expectorant* [phenylephrine HCl; guaifenesin] 10•390 mg

Deconex DM extended-release tablets ℞ *antitussive; decongestant;*

expectorant [dextromethorphan hydrobromide; phenylephrine HCl; guaifenesin] 30•30•900 mg

Deconex DMX caplets OTC *antitussive; decongestant; expectorant* [dextromethorphan hydrobromide; phenylephrine HCl; guaifenesin] 15•10•380 mg

Deconomed SR sustained-release capsules ℞ *decongestant; antihistamine* [pseudoephedrine HCl; chlorpheniramine maleate] 120•8 mg

Deconsal II extended-release capsules (discontinued 2007) ℞ *decongestant; expectorant* [phenylephrine HCl; guaifenesin] 20•375 mg ② doconazole

Deconsal II extended-release tablets ℞ *decongestant; expectorant* [phenylephrine HCl; guaifenesin] 25•275 mg ② doconazole

Deconsal CT chewable tablets ℞ *decongestant; antihistamine* [phenylephrine HCl; pyrilamine maleate] 10•16 mg

decoquinate USAN, INN, BAN *coccidiostat for poultry*

dectaflur USAN, INN *dental caries preventative*

Decylenes ointment OTC *antifungal* [undecylenic acid; zinc undecylenate]

deditonium bromide INN

Deep-Down Rub OTC *analgesic; mild anesthetic; antipruritic; counterirritant* [methyl salicylate; menthol; camphor] 15%•5%•0.5%

deer musk *(Moschus moschiferus) natural remedy in ancient Chinese medicine; reported to have antianginal, antibacterial, antihistaminic, anti-inflammatory, CNS-depressant, and stimulant activity in clinical studies*

deerberry *medicinal herb* [see: holly; squaw vine; wintergreen]

DEET (diethyltoluamide) [q.v.]

deferasirox *oral iron chelating agent for chronic iron overload due to blood transfusions (orphan)*

deferiprone *investigational (orphan) agent for chronic iron overload due to transfusion-dependent anemias*

deferoxamine USAN, INN *chelating agent for acute or chronic iron poisoning* [also: desferrioxamine] 500, 2000 mg/vial

deferoxamine & dextran *investigational (orphan) for acute iron poisoning*

deferoxamine HCl USAN *chelating agent for acute or chronic iron poisoning*

deferoxamine mesylate USAN, USP *chelating agent for acute or chronic iron poisoning* [also: desferrioxamine mesylate] 500, 2000 mg injection

defibrotide BAN *investigational (NDA filed, orphan) agent for thrombotic thrombocytopenic purpura and hepatic veno-occlusive disease*

Definity injection ℞ *radiopaque contrast medium to enhance echocardiography* [perflutren] 6.52 mg/mL

deflazacort USAN, INN, BAN *anti-inflammatory*

defosfamide INN

defungit sodium salt [see: bensuldazic acid]

Defy eye drops (discontinued 2010) ℞ *aminoglycoside antibiotic* [tobramycin] 0.3%

degarelix acetate *gonadotropin-releasing hormone (GnRH) blocker to reduce testosterone levels in patients with advanced prostate cancer*

Degas chewable tablets (discontinued 2008) OTC *antiflatulent* [simethicone] 80 mg ☑ Duac CS

degludec *investigational (Phase III) long-acting insulin for once-weekly injections*

Dehistine syrup ℞ *decongestant; antihistamine; anticholinergic to dry mucosal secretions* [phenylephrine HCl; chlorpheniramine maleate; methscopolamine nitrate] 10•2•1.25 mg/5 mL

dehydrated alcohol [see: alcohol, dehydrated]

Dehydrex drops *investigational (orphan) treatment for recurrent corneal erosion* [dextran 70]

dehydroacetic acid NF *preservative*

dehydroandrosterone [see: prasterone]

dehydrocholate sodium USP [also: sodium dehydrocholate]

7-dehydrocholesterol, activated [now: cholecalciferol]

dehydrocholic acid USP, INN, BAN, JAN *choleretic; laxative* 250 mg oral

dehydrocholin [see: dehydrocholic acid]

dehydroemetine INN, BAN *anti-infective for amebiasis and amebic dysentery*

dehydroepiandrosterone (DHEA) *natural hormone precursor; investigational (NDA filed, orphan) for systemic lupus erythematosus (SLE); investigational (orphan) replacement therapy for adrenal insufficiency*

dehydroepiandrosterone sulfate (DHEAS)

dehydroepiandrosterone sulfate sodium *investigational (orphan) agent for re-epithelialization of serious burns and skin graft donor sites*

Deka oral liquid (discontinued 2007) ℞ *antitussive; antihistamine; decongestant; expectorant* [dextromethorphan hydrobromide; dexbrompheniramine maleate; pseudoephrine HCl; guaifenesin] 30•1•30•200 mg/10 mL

Deka Pediatric oral drops (discontinued 2007) ℞ *antitussive; decongestant; antihistamine; expectorant; for children 1–24 months* [dextromethorphan hydrobromide; pseudoephedrine HCl; dexbrompheniramine maleate; guaifenesin] 4•12.5•0.5•40 mg/mL

delanterone INN

delapril INN *antihypertensive; angiotensin-converting enzyme (ACE) inhibitor* [also: delapril HCl]

delapril HCl USAN *antihypertensive; angiotensin-converting enzyme (ACE) inhibitor* [also: delapril]

Delatestryl IM injection ℞ *androgen replacement for hypogonadism or testosterone deficiency in men, delayed puberty in boys, and metastatic breast cancer in women; hormone replacement therapy (HRT) for postandropausal symptoms; also abused as a* *street drug* [testosterone enanthate (in oil)] 200 mg/mL

delavirdine INN *antiviral; non-nucleoside reverse transcriptase inhibitor (NNRTI) for HIV and AIDS* [also: delavirdine mesylate]

delavirdine mesylate USAN *non-nucleoside reverse transcriptase inhibitor (NNRTI); oral antiretroviral for HIV-1 infection* [also: delavirdine]

delayed-release aspirin [see: aspirin]

Delazinc ointment OTC *astringent* [zinc oxide] 25% ⧉ Dalacin C

Delcap (trademarked device) *unit dispensing cap*

Delcort cream (discontinued 2008) OTC *corticosteroidal anti-inflammatory* [hydrocortisone] 0.5%, 1%

delequamine INN *alpha₂ adrenoreceptor antagonist for sexual dysfunction* [also: delequamine HCl]

delequamine HCl USAN *alpha₂ adrenoreceptor antagonist for sexual dysfunction* [also: delequamine]

delergotrile INN

Delestrogen IM injection ℞ *synthetic estrogen for the treatment of postmenopausal symptoms and prevention of postmenopausal osteoporosis; hormonal antineoplastic for prostate and metastatic breast cancers* [estradiol valerate in oil] 10, 20, 40 mg/mL

delfantrine INN

delfaprazine INN

Delfen Contraceptive vaginal foam OTC *spermicidal contraceptive* [nonoxynol 9] 12.5%

delmadinone INN, BAN *progestin; antiandrogen; antiestrogen* [also: delmadinone acetate]

delmadinone acetate USAN *progestin; antiandrogen; antiestrogen* [also: delmadinone]

delmetacin INN

delmopinol INN

delnav [see: dioxathion]

delorazepam INN

Delos lotion ℞ *keratolytic for acne* [benzoyl peroxide] 3.5%

deloxolone INN

m-delphene [see: diethyltoluamide]

delprostenate INN, BAN

Delsym extended-release oral suspension OTC *antitussive* [dextromethorphan polistirex] 30 mg/5 mL

deltacortone [see: prednisone]

Delta-D tablets OTC *vitamin supplement* [cholecalciferol (vitamin D₃)] 400 IU

deltafilcon A USAN *hydrophilic contact lens material*

deltafilcon B USAN *hydrophilic contact lens material*

delta-1-hydrocortisone [see: prednisolone]

Deltasone tablets (discontinued 2008) ℞ *corticosteroid; anti-inflammatory* [prednisone] 2.5, 5, 10, 20 mg

delta-9-tetrahydrocannabinol (THC) [see: dronabinol]

delta-9-THC (tetrahydrocannabinol) [see: dronabinol]

Delta-Tritex cream, ointment (discontinued 2007) ℞ *corticosteroidal anti-inflammatory* [triamcinolone acetonide] 0.1%

Deltavac vaginal cream ℞ *broad-spectrum antibiotic; antiseptic; moisturizer/lubricant* [sulfanilamide; aminacrine HCl; allantoin] 15%•0.2%•2%

deltibant USAN *bradykinin antagonist for treatment of systemic inflammatory response syndrome*

deltra-stab [see: prednisolone]

delucemine HCl USAN *NMDA receptor antagonist; neuroprotectant*

Demadex IV injection (discontinued 2008) ℞ *antihypertensive; loop diuretic for congestive heart failure, hepatic cirrhosis, and renal disease* [torsemide] 10 mg/mL

Demadex tablets ℞ *antihypertensive; loop diuretic for congestive heart failure, hepatic cirrhosis, and renal disease* [torsemide] 5, 10, 20, 100 mg

dembrexine INN, BAN

dembroxol [see: dembrexine]

demecarium bromide USP, INN, BAN *antiglaucoma agent; reversible cholinesterase inhibitor miotic*

demeclocycline USP, BAN *tetracycline antibiotic*

demeclocycline HCl USP, BAN *tetracycline antibiotic; antirickettsial* 150, 300 mg oral

demecolcine INN, BAN

demecycline USAN, INN *antibacterial*

demegestone INN

demekastigmine bromide [see: demecarium bromide]

demelverine INN

Demerol tablets, syrup, IV or IM injection ℞ *narcotic analgesic; also abused as a street drug* [meperidine HCl] 50, 100 mg; 50 mg/5 mL; 25, 50, 75, 100 mg/mL

demetacin [see: delmetacin]

11-demethoxyreserpine [see: deserpidine]

demethylchlortetracycline (DMCT) [now: demeclocycline]

demethylchlortetracycline HCl [see: demeclocycline HCl]

N-demethylcodeine [see: norcodeine]

demexiptiline INN

Demi-Regroton tablets (discontinued 2007) ℞ *antihypertensive; diuretic* [chlorthalidone; reserpine] 25•0.125 mg

democonazole INN

demoxepam USAN, INN *minor tranquilizer*

demoxytocin INN

Demser capsules ℞ *antihypertensive for pheochromocytoma* [metyrosine] 250 mg

demulcents *a class of agents that soothe irritated or abraded tissues, particularly mucous membranes*

Demulen 1/35; Demulen 1/50 tablets (in Compacks of 21 or 28) (discontinued 2008) ℞ *monophasic oral contraceptive* [ethynodiol diacetate; ethinyl estradiol] 1 mg•35 mcg; 1 mg•50 mcg

denatonium benzoate USAN, NF, INN, BAN *alcohol denaturant; flavoring agent*

denaverine INN

Denavir cream ℞ *antiviral for recurrent herpes labialis* [penciclovir] 1%

Denaze oral liquid ℞ *decongestant; antihistamine; anticholinergic to dry mucosal secretions* [phenylephrine HCl; chlorpheniramine maleate; methscopolamine nitrate] 10•4•1.25 mg/5 mL ② Doan's

denbufylline INN, BAN

Dendracin Neurodendtraxcin lotion OTC *anesthetic; analgesic; antipruritic; counterirritant* [capsaicin; methyl salicylate; menthol] 0.0375%•30%•10%

denileukin diftitox USAN, INN *antineoplastic for cutaneous T-cell lymphoma (orphan)*

denipride INN

denofungin USAN *antifungal; antibacterial*

denopamine INN

Denorex Everyday Dandruff shampoo OTC *antiseborrheic; antibacterial; antifungal* [pyrithione zinc] 2%

denosumab *human monoclonal antibody to receptor activator for nuclear factor k; osteoclast regulator; subcu injection to increase bone density, treat postmenopausal osteoporosis, and prevent bone metastasis; investigational (Phase II) for rheumatoid arthritis*

denpidazone INN

Denquel toothpaste OTC *tooth desensitizer* [potassium nitrate] 5%

Denta 5000 Plus dental cream ℞ *caries preventative* [fluoride (as sodium fluoride)] 0.5% (1.1%)

DentaGel ℞ *dental caries preventative* [fluoride (as sodium fluoride)] 0.5% (1.1%)

dental antiformin [see: antiformin, dental]

dental-type silica [see: silica, dental-type]

Dentipatch transmucosal patch (discontinued 2010) ℞ *mucous membrane anesthetic* [lidocaine HCl] 46.1 mg

Dentiva lozenges OTC *mucous membrane moisturizer for dry mouth* [eucalyptus oil; menthol; peppermint oil; wintergreen oil; zinc]

Dent-O-Kain/20 topical liquid OTC *mucous membrane anesthetic* [benzocaine] 20%

Dent's Lotion-Jel OTC *mucous membrane anesthetic* [benzocaine]

Dent's Toothache Gum; Dent's Toothache Drops OTC *mucous membrane anesthetic* [benzocaine] 20%

denufosol tetrasodium *P2Y$_2$ uridine 5'-triphosphate (UTP) agonist to increase mucosal hydration and enhance mucus clearance from the lungs; investigational (Phase III, orphan) inhalation solution for cystic fibrosis*

denyl sodium [see: phenytoin sodium]

denzimol INN

deodorants *a class of agents that mask undesirable or offensive odors* [also called: antibromics]

2'-deoxycoformycin (DCF) [see: pentostatin]

deoxycorticosterone acetate [see: desoxycorticosterone acetate]

deoxycorticosterone pivalate [see: desoxycorticosterone pivalate]

deoxycortolone pivalate BAN *salt-regulating adrenocortical steroid* [also: desoxycorticosterone pivalate]

deoxycortone BAN *salt-regulating adrenocortical steroid* [also: desoxycorticosterone acetate; desoxycortone]

2'-deoxycytidine *investigational (orphan) host-protective agent in acute myelogenous leukemia*

deoxyephedrine HCl [see: methamphetamine HCl]

12-deoxyerythromycin [see: berythromycin]

1-deoxygalactonojirimycin *investigational (orphan) for Fabry disease*

deoxyribonuclease, recombinant human (rhDNase) [see: dornase alfa]

deoxyribonucleic acid (DNA)

15-deoxyspergualin trihydrochloride [now: gusperimus trihydrochloride]

Depacin capsules (discontinued 2008) OTC *analgesic; antipyretic* [acetaminophen] 325 mg

Depacon IV infusion ℞ *anticonvulsant for complex partial seizures and simple or complex absence seizures* [valproate sodium] 500 mg/vial ⑦ dibucaine

Depakene capsules ℞ *anticonvulsant for complex partial seizures and simple or complex absence seizures* [valproic acid] 250 mg ⑦ dibucaine

Depakene syrup ℞ *anticonvulsant for complex partial seizures and simple or complex absence seizures* [valproic acid] 250 mg/5 mL ⑦ dibucaine

Depakote delayed-release enteric-coated tablets ℞ *anticonvulsant for complex partial seizures and simple or complex absence seizures; treatment for manic episodes of a bipolar disorder; migraine headache prophylaxis* [divalproex sodium] 125, 250, 500 mg

Depakote sprinkle capsules ℞ *anticonvulsant for complex partial seizures and simple or complex absence seizures* [divalproex sodium] 125 mg

Depakote ER extended-release tablets ℞ *anticonvulsant for complex partial seizures and simple or complex absence seizures; treatment for manic episodes of a bipolar disorder; migraine headache prophylaxis* [divalproex sodium] 250, 500 mg

Depen titratable tablets ℞ *metal chelating agent for rheumatoid arthritis, Wilson disease, and cystinuria* [penicillamine] 250 mg

depepsen [see: sodium amylosulfate]

Deplin tablets ℞ *hematinic* [folic acid (as L-methylfolate)] 7.5, 15 mg

depMedalone 40; depMedalone 80 intralesional, soft tissue, and IM injection (discontinued 2008) ℞ *corticosteroid; anti-inflammatory; immunosuppressant* [methylprednisolone acetate] 40 mg/mL; 80 mg/mL

DepoCyt sustained-release intrathecal injection ℞ *antineoplastic for lymphomatous neoplastic meningitis (NM) arising from solid tumors or non-Hodgkin lymphoma (orphan)* [cytarabine, liposomal] 10 mg/mL

DepoDur extended-release liposomal suspension for epidural injection ℞ *narcotic analgesic* [morphine sulfate] 10 mg/mL

Depo-Estradiol IM injection ℞ *synthetic estrogen; hormone replacement therapy for the treatment of postmenopausal symptoms* [estradiol cypionate in oil] 5 mg/mL

Depoject intralesional, soft tissue, and IM injection (discontinued 2008) ℞ *corticosteroid; anti-inflammatory; immunosuppressant* [methylprednisolone acetate] 40, 80 mg/mL

Depo-Medrol intralesional, soft tissue, and IM injection ℞ *corticosteroid; anti-inflammatory; immunosuppressant* [methylprednisolone acetate] 20, 40, 80 mg/mL

Depo-Provera IM injection ℞ *long-term (3 month) injectable contraceptive (150 mg only); hormonal antineoplastic adjunct for metastatic endometrial and renal carcinoma (400 mg only)* [medroxyprogesterone acetate] 150, 400 mg/mL

Depo-Sub Q Provera 104 subcu injection in prefilled syringes ℞ *long-term (3 month) injectable contraceptive* [medroxyprogesterone acetate] 104 mg

Depo-Testosterone IM injection ℞ *androgen for hypogonadism or testosterone deficiency in men; hormone replacement therapy for postandropausal symptoms; also abused as a street drug* [testosterone cypionate (in oil)] 100, 200 mg/mL

depramine INN [also: balipramine]

deprenyl (L-deprenyl) [see: selegiline HCl]

depreotide USAN *radiopharmaceutical imaging agent*

depressants *a class of agents that reduce functional activity and vital energy in general by producing muscular relaxation and diaphoresis*

deprodone INN, BAN ☒ diperodon

deprostil USAN, INN *gastric antisecretory* ☒ dipyrocetyl

deptropine INN, BAN

deptropine citrate [see: deptropine]

depurants; depuratives *a class of agents that purify or cleanse the system, particularly the blood* [also called: pellants]

dequalinium chloride INN, BAN

Dequasine tablets OTC *dietary supplement* [multiple minerals & amino acids; vitamin C] ± • 200 mg

deracoxib USAN *COX-2 inhibitor anti-inflammatory and analgesic for osteoarthritis and rheumatoid arthritis*

deramciclane *serotonin 5-HT$_2$ receptor antagonist; antidepressant; anxiolytic*

Derifil tablets OTC *systemic deodorant for ostomy, breath, and body odors* [chlorophyllin] 100 mg ☒ Duraflu

Dermabase cream OTC *nontherapeutic base for compounding various dermatological preparations*

Dermabond topical liquid OTC *skin adhesive for closing surgical incisions and traumatic lacerations*

Dermacoat aerosol (discontinued 2007) OTC *anesthetic* [benzocaine] 4.5%

Dermacort cream, lotion ℞ *corticosteroidal anti-inflammatory* [hydrocortisone] 1%

Dermadrox ointment OTC *astringent; skin protectant; emollient* [aluminum hydroxide gel; zinc chloride; lanolin]

DermaFlex gel (discontinued 2009) OTC *anesthetic* [lidocaine; alcohol 79%] 2.5%

Dermal Therapy lotion ℞ *moisturizer; emollient; keratolytic* [urea] 20%

Dermal-Rub balm (discontinued 2010) OTC *analgesic; counterirritant* [methyl salicylate; camphor; racemic menthol; cajuput oil]

Dermamycin cream, spray OTC *antihistamine* [diphenhydramine HCl] 2%

Derma-Pax lotion OTC *antihistamine* [diphenhydramine HCl] 0.5%

DermaPhor ointment OTC *emollient* [petrolatum] 44%

Dermarest gel OTC *antihistamine; antifungal* [diphenhydramine HCl; resorcinol] 2% • 2%

Dermarest Plus gel, spray OTC *antihis-tamine; mild anesthetic; antipruritic; counterirritant* [diphenhydramine HCl; menthol] 2%•1%

Dermasept Antifungal spray liquid OTC *antifungal; antiseptic; anesthetic; astringent* [tolnaftate; tannic acid; zinc chloride; benzocaine; methylben-zethonium HCl; undecylenic acid; alcohol 58.54%] 1.017%•6.098%•5.081%•2.032%•3.049%•5.081%

Dermasil lotion OTC *bath emollient*

Derma-Smoothe/FS oil ℞ *corticoster-oidal anti-inflammatory; emollient* [flu-ocinolone acetonide] 0.01%

dermatan sulfate [see: danaparoid sodium]

dermatol [see: bismuth subgallate]

Dermatop E cream, ointment ℞ *corti-costeroidal anti-inflammatory* [predni-carbate] 0.1%

DermaVite tablets OTC *vitamin/mineral supplement* [multiple vitamins & minerals; folic acid; biotin] ±•400•600 mcg

Dermazinc cream, shampoo OTC *anti-seborrheic; antibacterial; antifungal* [pyrithione zinc] 0.25%

Derm-Cleanse topical liquid OTC *soap-free therapeutic skin cleanser*

Dermol HC anorectal cream, anorec-tal ointment ℞ *corticosteroidal anti-inflammatory* [hydrocortisone] 1%, 2.5%; 1%

Dermolate Anti-Itch cream OTC *cor-ticosteroidal anti-inflammatory* [hydro-cortisone] 0.5%

Dermolin liniment OTC *analgesic; mild anesthetic; antipruritic; counterirritant; antiseptic* [methyl salicylate; camphor; racemic menthol; mustard oil; alco-hol 8%] ⓘ Dramilin

Dermoplast aerosol spray, lotion OTC *anesthetic; antipruritic; counterirritant* [benzocaine; menthol] 20%•0.5%; 8%•0.5%

Dermoplast Antibacterial aerosol spray OTC *anesthetic; antiseptic* [ben-zocaine; benzethonium chloride] 20%•0.2%

DermOtic Oil ear drops ℞ *corticoster-oidal anti-inflammatory* [fluocinolone acetonide in oil] 0.01%

Dermovan cream OTC *nontherapeutic base for compounding various dermato-logical preparations*

Dermprotective Factor (DPF) (trade-marked ingredient) *aromatic syrup* [eriodictyon]

Dermtex HC with Aloe cream OTC *corticosteroidal anti-inflammatory* [hydrocortisone] 0.5%

Dermuspray aerosol spray ℞ *proteo-lytic enzyme for débridement of necrotic tissue; vulnerary* [trypsin; Peruvian balsam] 0.1•72.5 mg/0.82 mL

derpanicate INN

DES (diethylstilbestrol) [q.v.]

desacetyl vinblastine amide (DAVA) [see: vindesine]

desacetyl-lanatoside C [see: deslano-side]

desaglybuzole [see: glybuzole]

desamino-oxytocin [see: demoxytocin]

desaspidin INN

desciclovir USAN, INN *antiviral*

descinolone INN *corticosteroid; anti-inflammatory* [also: descinolone ace-tonide]

descinolone acetonide USAN *cortico-steroid; anti-inflammatory* [also: desci-nolone]

Desenex cream OTC *antifungal* [clo-trimazole] 1%

Desenex foam, soap OTC *antifungal* [undecylenic acid] 10%

Desenex powder (discontinued 2008) OTC *antifungal* [miconazole nitrate] 2%

Desenex powder, aerosol powder, oint-ment, cream OTC *antifungal* [undec-ylenic acid; zinc undecylenate] 25% total

Desenex, Prescription Strength spray liquid, spray powder (discon-tinued 2008) OTC *antifungal for tinea pedis, tinea cruris, and tinea corporis* [miconazole nitrate] 2%

Desenex Antifungal cream (discon-tinued 2007) OTC *antifungal for tinea*

pedis, tinea cruris, and tinea corporis [miconazole nitrate] 2%

Desenex Liquid Spray OTC *antifungal* [miconazole nitrate] 2%

DesenexMax cream (discontinued 2010) OTC *allylamine antifungal* [terbinafine HCl] 1%

deserpidine INN, BAN *antihypertensive; peripheral antiadrenergic; rauwolfia derivative*

desert herb; desert tea *medicinal herb* [see: ephedra]

desferrioxamine BAN *chelating agent for acute or chronic iron poisoning* [also: deferoxamine]

desferrioxamine mesylate BAN *chelating agent for acute or chronic iron poisoning* [also: deferoxamine mesylate]

desflurane USAN, INN *inhalation general anesthetic*

desglugastrin INN

desipramine INN, BAN *tricyclic antidepressant* [also: desipramine HCl] ⊡ diisopromine

desipramine HCl USAN, USP *tricyclic antidepressant* [also: desipramine] 10, 25, 50, 75, 100, 150 mg oral

desirudin USAN *anticoagulant; thrombin inhibitor for the prevention of deep vein thrombosis (DVT) in elective hip replacement surgery*

Desitin ointment OTC *moisturizer; emollient; astringent* [cod liver oil; zinc oxide]

Desitin Clear ointment OTC *diaper rash treatment* [white petrolatum] 60%

Desitin Creamy ointment OTC *diaper rash treatment* [zinc oxide] 10%

Desitin with Zinc Oxide powder OTC *diaper rash treatment* [zinc oxide; cornstarch] 10%•88.2%

deslanoside USP, INN, BAN *cardiotonic; cardiac glycoside*

desloratadine USAN *second-generation peripherally selective piperidine antihistamine for allergic rhinitis and chronic idiopathic urticaria; active metabolite of loratadine* 2.5, 5 mg oral

desloratadine & pseudoephedrine sulfate *antihistamine; decongestant* 5•240 mg oral

deslorelin USAN, INN *LHRH agonist*

desmethylmoramide INN

desmoglein 3 synthetic peptide *investigational (orphan) for pemphigus vulgaris*

desmophosphamide [see: defosfamide]

desmopressin INN, BAN *posterior pituitary antidiuretic hormone (ADH)* [also: desmopressin acetate]

desmopressin acetate USAN *antidiuretic; posterior pituitary antidiuretic hormone for central diabetes insipidus, hemophilia A (orphan), von Willebrand disease (orphan), and nocturnal enuresis* [also: desmopressin] 0.1, 0.2 mg oral; 4 mcg/mL injection; 10 mcg nasal spray

desocriptine INN

Desogen tablets (in packs of 28) ℞ *monophasic oral contraceptive* [desogestrel; ethinyl estradiol] 0.15 mg•30 mcg × 21 days; counters × 7 days ⊡ Diascan

desogestrel USAN, INN, BAN *progestin*

desolone [see: deprodone]

desomorphine INN, BAN

Desonate gel ℞ *corticosteroidal anti-inflammatory* [desonide] 0.05%

desonide USAN, INN, BAN *topical corticosteroidal anti-inflammatory* 0.05% topical

DesOwen ointment, cream, lotion ℞ *corticosteroidal anti-inflammatory* [desonide] 0.05%

desoximetasone USAN, USP, INN *topical corticosteroidal anti-inflammatory* [also: desoxymethasone] 0.05%, 0.25% topical

desoxycholic acid *increases secretion of bile acids*

desoxycorticosterone acetate (DCA; DOCA) USP *salt-regulating adrenocortical steroid* [also: desoxycortone; deoxycortone]

desoxycorticosterone pivalate USP *salt-regulating adrenocortical steroid* [also: deoxycortolone pivalate]

**desoxycorticosterone trimethylace-
tate** USP
desoxycortone INN *salt-regulating
adrenocortical steroid* [also: desoxycorticosterone acetate; deoxycortone]
l-**desoxyephedrine** [see: levmetamfet-
amine]
desoxyephedrine HCl [see: methamphetamine HCl]
desoxymethasone BAN *topical corticosteroidal anti-inflammatory* [also: des-
oximetasone]
Desoxyn tablets R̂ *CNS stimulant;
also abused as a street drug* [metham-
phetamine HCl] 5 mg
desoxyribonuclease [see: fibrinolysin
& desoxyribonuclease]
Despec oral drops (discontinued 2008)
R̂ *antitussive; decongestant; expectorant; for children 1–24 months* [dex-
tromethorphan hydrobromide; pseudoephedrine HCl; guaifenesin] 4•
20•10 mg/mL ⊠ Dosepak
Despec oral liquid OTC *decongestant;
expectorant* [phenylephrine HCl;
guaifenesin] 10•200 mg/10 mL ⊠
Dosepak
Despec DM extended-release tablets
(discontinued 2007) R̂ *antitussive;
decongestant; expectorant* [dextro-
methorphan hydrobromide; pseudoephedrine HCl; guaifenesin] 60•
120•800 mg
Despec DM oral liquid (discontinued
2007) R̂ *antitussive; decongestant;
expectorant* [dextromethorphan
hydrobromide; phenylephrine HCl;
guaifenesin] 30•10•200 mg/10 mL
Despec EXP syrup R̂ *narcotic antitussive; decongestant; expectorant* [dihy-
drocodeine bitartrate; pseudoephedrine HCl; guaifenesin] 7.5•15•100
mg/5 mL
Despec NR oral drops (discontinued
2010) R̂ *antitussive; decongestant;
expectorant; for children 1–24 months*
[dextromethorphan hydrobromide;
phenylephrine HCl; guaifenesin] 4•
1.5•20 mg/mL

DespecTab tablets R̂ *decongestant;
expectorant* [pseudoephedrine HCl;
guaifenesin] 40•400 mg
Desquam-E 5 gel (discontinued 2009)
R̂ *keratolytic for acne* [benzoyl perox-
ide] 5%
Desquam-E 10 gel R̂ *keratolytic for
acne* [benzoyl peroxide] 10%
Desquam-X cleansing bar R̂ *keratolytic for acne* [benzoyl peroxide] 10%
Desquam-X 5; Desquam-X 10 gel
(discontinued 2009) R̂ *keratolytic for
acne* [benzoyl peroxide] 5%; 10%
Desquam-X Wash topical liquid R̂
keratolytic for acne [benzoyl peroxide]
5%, 10%
de-Stat 3; de-Stat 4 solution (discontinued 2010) OTC *cleaning/disinfect-
ing/soaking solution for rigid gas permeable contact lenses*
destradiol [see: estradiol]
desulfated heparin [see: heparin, 2-0-
desulfated]
63-desulfohirudin [see: desirudin]
desvenlafaxine succinate *selective
serotonin and norepinephrine reuptake
inhibitor (SSNRI) for major depressive
disorder (MDD); investigational (NDA
filed) for postmenopausal vasomotor
symptoms; investigational (Phase III)
for fibromyalgia and diabetic peripheral
neuropathy; single isomer of venlafaxine*
Desyrel film-coated tablets, Dividose
(multiple-scored tablets) (discontinued 2010) R̂ *antidepressant; also used
for aggressive behavior, alcoholism,
panic disorder, agoraphobia, and cocaine
withdrawal* [trazodone HCl] 50, 100
mg; 150, 300 mg
DET (diethyltryptamine) [q.v.]
Detachol topical liquid OTC *adhesive
remover for the skin*
detajmium bitartrate INN
Detane gel (discontinued 2010) OTC
anesthetic [benzocaine] 7.5% ⊠ Dytan
detanosal INN
Detect-A-Strep slide tests for professional use R̂ *in vitro diagnostic aid for
streptococcal antigens in throat swabs*

Detecto-Seal (trademarked packaging form) *tamper-resistant parenteral package*

deterenol INN *ophthalmic adrenergic* [also: deterenol HCl]

deterenol HCl USAN *ophthalmic adrenergic* [also: deterenol]

detergents *a class of agents that cleanse wounds and sores*

detigon HCl [see: chlophedianol HCl]

detirelix INN *luteinizing hormone-releasing hormone (LHRH) antagonist* [also: detirelix acetate]

detirelix acetate USAN *luteinizing hormone-releasing hormone (LHRH) antagonist* [also: detirelix]

detomidine INN, BAN *veterinary analgesic; sedative* [also: detomidine HCl]

detomidine HCl USAN *veterinary analgesic; sedative* [also: detomidine]

detorubicin INN

detralfate INN

Detrol film-coated tablets ℞ *muscarinic receptor antagonist for urinary frequency, urgency, and incontinence* [tolterodine tartrate] 1, 2 mg

Detrol LA extended-release capsules ℞ *muscarinic receptor antagonist for urinary frequency, urgency, and incontinence* [tolterodine tartrate] 2, 4 mg

detrothyronine INN

Detussin oral liquid (discontinued 2007) ℞ *narcotic antitussive; decongestant* [hydrocodone bitartrate; pseudoephedrine HCl; alcohol 5%] 5•60 mg/5 mL

deuterium oxide USAN *radioactive agent*

devapamil INN

devazepide USAN *cholecystokinin antagonist*

devil's bones *medicinal herb* [see: wild yam]

devil's claw *(Harpagophytum procumbens)* root *medicinal herb for arrhythmias, arteriosclerosis, arthritis, blood cleansing, diabetes, hypertension, liver disease, lowering cholesterol, rheumatism, stomach disorders, and strengthening bladder and kidneys*

devil's club *(Echinopanax horridum; Fatsia horrida; Oplopanax horridus; Panax horridum)* cambium and stem *medicinal herb for arthritis, burns and cuts, colds, cough, fever, inducing vomiting and bowel evacuation, pneumonia, and tuberculosis*

devil's dung *medicinal herb* [see: asafetida]

devil's eye *medicinal herb* [see: henbane]

devil's fuge *medicinal herb* [see: mistletoe]

devil's shrub *medicinal herb* [see: eleuthero]

Devrom chewable tablets OTC *systemic deodorizer for ostomy and incontinence odors* [bismuth subgallate] 200 mg

dewberry *medicinal herb* [see: blackberry]

Dex GG TR timed-release tablets (discontinued 2007) ℞ *antitussive; expectorant* [dextromethorphan hydrobromide; guaifenesin] 60•1000 mg

Dex4 Glucose chewable tablets OTC *blood glucose elevating agent for hypoglycemia* [glucose]

dexa [see: dexamethasone]

DexAlone liquid-filled gelcaps OTC *antitussive* [dextromethorphan hydrobromide] 30 mg

dexamethasone USP, INN, BAN *corticosteroidal anti-inflammatory; investigational (orphan) for idiopathic intermediate uveitis* 0.25, 0.5, 0.75, 1, 1.5, 2, 4, 6 mg oral; 0.5 mg/5 mL oral

dexamethasone acefurate USAN, INN *corticosteroidal anti-inflammatory*

dexamethasone acetate USAN, USP, BAN *corticosteroidal anti-inflammatory*

dexamethasone dipropionate USAN *corticosteroidal anti-inflammatory*

Dexamethasone Intensol oral drops ℞ *corticosteroidal anti-inflammatory* [dexamethasone] 1 mg/mL

dexamethasone & neomycin sulfate & polymyxin B sulfate *topical ophthalmic corticosteroidal anti-inflammatory and antibiotic* 0.1%•0.35%•10 000 U/mL eye drops

dexamethasone sodium phosphate USP, BAN *corticosteroid; anti-inflammatory* 0.1% eye drops; 4, 10 mg/mL injection

dexamethasone & tobramycin *corticosteroidal anti-inflammatory; antibiotic* 0.1%•0.3% eye drops

dexamfetamine INN *CNS stimulant* [also: dextroamphetamine; dexamphetamine]

dexamisole USAN, INN *antidepressant*

dexamphetamine BAN *CNS stimulant* [also: dextroamphetamine; dexamfetamine]

dexanabinol *nonpsychotropic synthetic analogue of marijuana; investigational (Phase II, orphan) for the attenuation or amelioration of long-term neurological sequelae of severe head trauma*

Dexasol eye drops/ear drops (discontinued 2009) ℞ *corticosteroidal anti-inflammatory for corneal injury, ophthalmic inflammation, and otic inflammation* [dexamethasone (as sodium phosphate)] 0.1%

Dexasone intra-articular, intralesional, soft tissue, or IM injection ℞ *corticosteroidal anti-inflammatory* [dexamethasone sodium phosphate] 4 mg/mL

Dexasone L.A. intralesional, intra-articular, soft tissue, or IM injection (discontinued 2009) ℞ *corticosteroidal anti-inflammatory* [dexamethasone acetate] 8 mg/mL

Dexasporin ophthalmic ointment ℞ *corticosteroidal anti-inflammatory; antibiotic* [dexamethasone; neomycin sulfate; polymyxin B sulfate] 0.1%•0.35%•10 000 U/g

Dexatrim Max Daytime Appetite Control film-coated extended-release caplets OTC *vitamin/mineral/ herbal supplement* [multiple B vitamins; multiple minerals; Asian ginseng; caffeine] ±•±•250•200 mg

dexbrompheniramine INN, BAN *alkylamine antihistamine* [also: dexbrompheniramine maleate]

dexbrompheniramine maleate USP *alkylamine antihistamine* [also: dexbrompheniramine]

dexchlorpheniramine INN *alkylamine antihistamine* [also: dexchlorpheniramine maleate]

dexchlorpheniramine maleate USP *alkylamine antihistamine* [also: dexchlorpheniramine] 4, 6 mg oral; 2 mg/5 mL oral

dexchlorpheniramine tannate *alkylamine antihistamine*

dexchlorpheniramine tannate & dextromethorphan tannate & phenylephrine tannate *antihistamine; antitussive; decongestant* 2•30•20 mg/5 mL oral

dexclamol INN *sedative* [also: dexclamol HCl]

dexclamol HCl USAN *sedative* [also: dexclamol]

Dexcon-DM syrup (discontinued 2007) ℞ *antitussive; decongestant; expectorant* [dextromethorphan hydrobromide; phenylephrine HCl; guaifenesin] 20•10•100 mg/5 mL

Dexedrine Spansules (sustained-release capsules) ℞ *amphetamine; CNS stimulant; often abused as a street drug* [dextroamphetamine sulfate] 5, 10, 15 mg

Dexedrine tablets (discontinued 2008) ℞ *amphetamine; CNS stimulant; often abused as a street drug* [dextroamphetamine sulfate] 5 mg

dexetimide USAN, INN, BAN *anticholinergic*

dexetozoline INN

dexfenfluramine INN, BAN *anorexiant; appetite suppressant; serotonin reuptake inhibitor* [also: dexfenfluramine HCl]

dexfenfluramine HCl USAN *anorexiant; appetite suppressant; serotonin reuptake inhibitor* [also: dexfenfluramine]

DexFerrum IV or IM injection ℞ *hematinic* [iron dextran] 50, 100 mg/dose

DexFol tablets ℞ *vitamin supplement* [multiple B vitamins; vitamin C; folic acid; biotin] ±•60•5•0.3 mg

dexibuprofen USAN, INN *analgesic; cyclooxygenase inhibitor; anti-inflammatory*

dexibuprofen lysine USAN *analgesic; cyclooxygenase inhibitor; anti-inflammatory* [also: dexibuprofen]

Dexilant dual delayed-release capsules ℞ *proton pump inhibitor for gastric and duodenal ulcers, erosive esophagitis, gastroesophageal reflux disease (GERD), and other gastroesophageal disorders* [dexlansoprazole] 30, 60 mg

deximafen USAN, INN *antidepressant*

dexindoprofen INN

dexivacaine USAN, INN *anesthetic*

dexlansoprazole *proton pump inhibitor for gastric and duodenal ulcers, erosive esophagitis, GERD, and other gastroesophageal disorders; enantiomer of* **lansoprazole**

dexlofexidine INN

dexmedetomidine USAN, INN, BAN *sedative*

dexmedetomidine HCl *sedative for intubated and ventilated patients in an intensive care setting; premedication to anesthesia; also used for postanesthetic shivering* (base=84.75%)

dexmethylphenidate HCl CNS *stimulant for attention-deficit/hyperactivity disorder (ADHD) and narcolepsy; active isomer of methylphenidate HCl* 2.5, 5, 10 mg oral

dexnorgestrel acetime [now: norgestimate]

Dexodryl chewable caplets, oral suspension ℞ *antihistamine; anticholinergic to dry mucosal secretions* [chlorpheniramine maleate; methscopolamine nitrate] 2•1.5 mg; 2•1.5 mg/5 mL ⑫ dioxadrol

Dexone LA intralesional, intra-articular, soft tissue, or IM injection (discontinued 2009) ℞ *corticosteroidal anti-inflammatory* [dexamethasone acetate] 8 mg/mL

dexormaplatin USAN, INN *antineoplastic*

dexoxadrol INN CNS *stimulant; analgesic* [also: dexoxadrol HCl]

dexoxadrol HCl USAN CNS *stimulant; analgesic* [also: dexoxadrol]

DexPak; DexPak 6 Day; DexPak 13 Day; DexPak Jr. 10 Day TaperPak (tablets) ℞ *corticosteroidal anti-inflammatory* [dexamethasone] 1.5 mg

dexpanthenol USAN, USP, INN, BAN GI *stimulant for the prevention and treatment of postoperative paralytic ileus, intestinal atony, and decreased intestinal motility* 250 mg/mL injection

dexpemedolac USAN *analgesic*

Dexphen M oral solution ℞ *antihistamine; decongestant; anticholinergic to dry mucosal secretions* [dexchlorpheniramine maleate; phenylephrine HCl; methscopolamine nitrate] 1•10•1.25 mg/5 mL

Dexphen w/C oral liquid ℞ *narcotic antitussive; antihistamine; decongestant* [codeine phosphate; dexchlorpheniramine maleate; phenylephrine HCl] 10•1•5 mg/5 mL

dexpropranolol HCl USAN *antiarrhythmic; antiadrenergic (beta-blocker)* [also: dexpropranolol]

dexproxibutene INN

dexrazoxane USAN, INN, BAN *cardioprotectant for doxorubicin-induced cardiomyopathy (orphan) and anthracycline extravasation (orphan); chelates intracellular iron*

dexrazoxane HCl *cardioprotectant for doxorubicin-induced cardiomyopathy (orphan) and anthracycline extravasation; chelates intracellular iron* (base= 85%) 294, 589 mg injection (250, 500 mg base)

dexsecoverine INN

dexsotalol HCl USAN *class III antiarrhythmic*

dextilidine INN

dextran INN, BAN *blood flow adjuvant; plasma volume extender* [also: dextran 40]

dextran, high molecular weight [see: dextran 70]

dextran, low molecular weight [see: dextran 40]

dextran 1 *monovalent hapten for prevention of dextran-induced anaphylactic reactions; investigational (orphan) for cystic fibrosis*

dextran 40 USAN *blood flow adjuvant; plasma volume extender* [also: dextran] 10% injection

dextran 70 USAN *plasma volume extender; viscosity-increasing agent; investigational (orphan) for recurrent corneal erosion* 6% injection

dextran 75 USAN *plasma volume extender; viscosity-increasing agent* 6% injection

dextran & deferoxamine *investigational (orphan) for acute iron poisoning*

dextran sulfate *investigational (orphan) inhalant for cystic fibrosis*

dextran sulfate, sodium salt, aluminum complex [see: detralfate]

dextran sulfate sodium *investigational (orphan) for AIDS*

dextranomer INN, BAN *debrider and cleanser for wet wounds*

dextrates USAN, NF *tablet binder and diluent*

dextriferron NF, INN, BAN

dextrin NF, BAN *suspending agent; tablet binder and diluent*

dextroamphetamine USAN *CNS stimulant; often abused as a street drug, which causes strong psychic dependence* [also: dexamfetamine; dexamphetamine]

dextroamphetamine combinations [see: amphetamines, mixed]

dextroamphetamine phosphate USP *CNS stimulant*

dextroamphetamine saccharate *CNS stimulant*

dextroamphetamine sulfate USP *CNS stimulant; often abused as a street drug, which causes psychic dependence* 5, 10, 15 mg oral; 5 mg/5 mL oral

dextrobrompheniramine maleate [see: dexbrompheniramine maleate]

dextrochlorpheniramine maleate [see: dexchlorpheniramine maleate]

dextrofemine INN

dextromethorphan USP, INN, BAN *antitussive*

dextromethorphan hydrobromide USP, BAN *NMDA inhibitor and sigma-1 agonist; antitussive; treatment for involuntary emotional expression disorder (pseudobulbar affect)*

dextromethorphan hydrobromide & guaifenesin *antitussive; expectorant* 30•500 mg oral

dextromethorphan hydrobromide & promethazine HCl *antitussive; antihistamine* 15•6.25 mg/5 mL oral

dextromethorphan hydrobromide & pseudoephedrine HCl & chlorpheniramine maleate *antitussive; decongestant; antihistamine* 30•30•4 mg oral

dextromethorphan hydrobromide & pseudoephedrine HCl & guaifenesin *antitussive; decongestant; expectorant* 60•90•800 mg oral

dextromethorphan polistirex USAN *antitussive*

dextromethorphan tannate *antitussive*

dextromethorphan tannate & phenylephrine tannate & dexchlorpheniramine tannate *antitussive; decongestant; antihistamine* 30•20•2 mg/5 mL oral

dextromethorphan tannate & phenylephrine tannate & pyrilamine tannate *antitussive; decongestant; antihistamine; sleep aid* 25•15.5•15.5 mg/5 mL oral

dextromoramide INN, BAN

dextromoramide tartrate [see: dextromoramide]

dextro-pantothenyl alcohol [see: dexpanthenol]

dextropropoxiphene chloride [see: propoxyphene HCl]

dextropropoxyphene INN, BAN *narcotic analgesic* [also: propoxyphene HCl]

dextropropoxyphene HCl BAN [also: propoxyphene HCl]

dextrorphan INN, BAN *adjunct to vasospastic therapy* [also: dextrorphan HCl]

dextrorphan HCl USAN *adjunct to vasospastic therapy* [also: dextrorphan]

dextrose USP *fluid and nutrient replenisher; parenteral antihypoglycemic*

5% Dextrose and Electrolyte #48;
  5% Dextrose and Electrolyte #75;
  10% Dextrose and Electrolyte #48
  IV infusion ℞ *intravenous nutritional/electrolyte therapy* [combined electrolyte solution; dextrose]

dextrose excipient NF *tablet excipient*

Dextrose Thermoject System IV injection ℞ *diagnostic aid for the measurement of cardiac output by the thermodilution method* [dextrose] 0.9%, 5%

DextroStat tablets ℞ *amphetamine; CNS stimulant* [dextroamphetamine sulfate] 5, 10 mg

dextrothyronine [see: detrothyronine]

dextrothyroxine BAN *antihyperlipidemic* [also: dextrothyroxine sodium]

dextrothyroxine sodium USAN, USP, INN *antihyperlipidemic* [also: dextrothyroxine]

Dex-Tuss oral liquid ℞ *narcotic antitussive; expectorant* [codeine phosphate; guaifenesin] 10•300 mg/5 mL

Dex-Tuss DM oral liquid ℞ *antitussive; expectorant* [dextromethorphan hydrobromide; guaifenesin] 10•100 mg/5 mL ② docusate sodium

dexverapamil INN *adjunct to chemotherapy*

Dey-Dose (delivery device) *nebulizer*

Dey-Lute (trademarked delivery device) *nebulizer*

dezaguanine USAN, INN *antineoplastic*

dezaguanine mesylate USAN *antineoplastic*

dezinamide USAN, INN *anticonvulsant*

dezocine USAN, INN *narcotic analgesic*

DFMO (difluoromethylornithine) [see: eflornithine]

DFMO (difluoromethylornithine) HCl [see: eflornithine HCl]

DFP (diisopropyl flurophosphate) [see: isoflurophate]

DHA (docosahexaenoic acid) [q.v.; also: doconexent]

DHAD (dihydroxyanthracenedione) [see: mitoxantrone]

DHAP (dexamethasone, high-dose ara-C, Platinol) *chemotherapy protocol for non-Hodgkin lymphoma*

DHC Plus capsules ℞ *narcotic analgesic; antipyretic* [dihydrocodeine bitartrate; acetaminophen; caffeine] 16•356.4•30 mg ② DOK-Plus

DHE (dihydroergotamine) [see: dihydroergotamine mesylate]

D.H.E. 45 IV or IM injection ℞ *ergot alkaloid for the rapid control of migraine and cluster headaches* [dihydroergotamine mesylate] 1 mg/mL

DHEA (dehydroepiandrosterone) [q.v.]

D-Hist D extended-release caplets ℞ *decongestant; antihistamine; anticholinergic to dry mucosal secretions* [pseudoephedrine HCl; dexchlorpheniramine maleate; methscopolamine bromide] 45•3.5•1 mg ② Dosette; Duocet

DHPG (dihydroxy propoxymethyl guanine) [see: ganciclovir]

DHS Tar liquid shampoo, gel shampoo OTC *antiseborrheic; antipsoriatic; antipruritic; antibacterial* [coal tar] 0.5%

DHS Zinc shampoo OTC *antiseborrheic; antibacterial; antifungal* [pyrithione zinc] 2%

DHT tablets, Intensol (concentrated oral solution) (discontinued 2009) ℞ *vitamin D therapy for tetany and hypoparathyroidism* [dihydrotachysterol] 0.125, 0.2, 0.4 mg; 0.2 mg/mL

DHT (dihydrotachysterol) [q.v.]

DHT (dihydrotestosterone) [see: androstanolone; stanolone]

DI (doxorubicin, ifosfamide) [with mesna rescue; with or without filgrastim hematopoietic] *chemotherapy protocol for soft tissue sarcoma* [also known as: AI]

Diaβeta (or DiaBeta) tablets ℞ *sulfonylurea antidiabetic that stimulates insulin secretion in the pancreas* [glyburide] 1.25, 2.5, 5 mg

Diabetic Tussin oral liquid OTC *expectorant* [guaifenesin] 100 mg/5 mL

Diabetic Tussin Cold & Flu oral liquid OTC *antitussive; antihistamine;*

sleep aid; analgesic; antipyretic [dextromethorphan hydrobromide; diphenhydramine HCl; acetaminophen] 10•12.5•325 mg/5 mL

Diabetic Tussin DM oral liquid OTC *antitussive; expectorant* [dextromethorphan hydrobromide; guaifenesin] 10•100, 10•200 mg/5 mL

DiabetiDerm cream OTC *antifungal* [undecylenic acid] 10%

Diabetiks tablets OTC *vitamin/mineral/ amino acid supplement* [multiple vitamins, minerals, and amino acids; folic acid; biotin] ±•75•62.5 mcg

Diabinese tablets (discontinued 2008) ℞ *sulfonylurea antidiabetic that stimulates insulin secretion in the pancreas* [chlorpropamide] 100, 250 mg

diacerein INN

diacetamate INN, BAN

diacetolol INN, BAN *antiadrenergic (beta-blocker)* [also: diacetolol HCl]

diacetolol HCl USAN *antiadrenergic (beta-blocker)* [also: diacetolol]

diacetoxyphenylisatin [see: oxyphenisatin acetate]

diacetoxyphenyloxindol [see: oxyphenisatin acetate]

diacetrizoate sodium [see: diatrizoate sodium]

diacetyl diaminodiphenylsulfone (DADDS) [see: acedapsone]

diacetylated monoglycerides NF *plasticizer*

diacetylcholine chloride [see: succinylcholine chloride]

diacetyl-dihydroxydiphenylisatin [see: oxyphenisatin acetate]

diacetyldioxphenylisatin [see: oxyphenisatin acetate]

diacetylmorphine HCl USP *(heroin; banned in USA)* [also: diamorphine]

diacetylmorphine salts *(heroin; banned in USA)*

diacetylsalicylic acid [see: dipyrocetyl]

diacetyltannic acid [see: acetyltannic acid]

diacetylthiamine [see: acetiamine]

diagniol [see: sodium acetrizoate]

diallybarbituric acid [see: allobarbital]

diallylbarbituric acid [now: allobarbital]

diallylnortoxiferene dichloride [see: alcuronium chloride]

diallymal [see: allobarbital]

Dialpak (trademarked packaging form) *reusable patient compliance package for oral contraceptives*

Dialume capsules (discontinued 2010) ℞ *antacid* [aluminum hydroxide gel] 500 mg

Dialyte Pattern LM solution ℞ *peritoneal dialysis solution* [multiple electrolytes; dextrose] 1.5%•±, 2.5%•± , 4.5%•±

Dialyvite 800 with Zinc 15 tablets OTC *vitamin/mineral supplement* [multiple B vitamins; vitamin C; folic acid; biotin; zinc] ±•60•0.8•0.3•15 mg

Dialyvite 3000 tablets OTC *vitamin/ mineral supplement* [multiple vitamins & minerals; folic acid; biotin] ±•3•0.3 mg ⑫ Daily-Vite

Dialyvite Multi-Vitamins for Dialysis Patients tablets ℞ *vitamin/mineral supplement* [multiple vitamins; folic acid; biotin] ±•1•0.3 mg

Dialyvite with Zinc tablets ℞ *vitamin/mineral supplement* [multiple B vitamins; vitamin C; folic acid; biotin; zinc] ±•100•1•0.3•? mg

dia-mer-sulfonamides (sulfadiazine & sulfamerazine) [q.v.]

diamethine [see: dimethyltubocurarinium chloride; dimethyltubocurarine]

diamfenetide INN [also: diamphenethide]

diaminedipenicillin G [see: penicillin G benzathine]

diaminodiphenylsulfone (DDS) [now: dapsone]

3,4-diaminopyridine *investigational (orphan) for Lambert-Eaton myasthenic syndrome*

cis-diamminedichloroplatinum (DDP) [see: cisplatin]

diammonium phosphate [see: ammonium phosphate]

diamocaine INN, BAN *local anesthetic* [also: diamocaine cyclamate]

diamocaine cyclamate USAN *local anesthetic* [also: diamocaine]

diamorphine BAN *(heroin; banned in the U.S.)* [also: diacetylmorphine HCl]

Diamox Sequels (sustained-release capsules) ℞ *diuretic for edema and glaucoma; treatment for acute mountain sickness* [acetazolamide] 500 mg ⑨ DMax

Diamox tablets (discontinued 2010) ℞ *diuretic for edema and glaucoma; anticonvulsant for centrencephalic epilepsies; treatment for acute mountain sickness* [acetazolamide] 125, 250 mg ⑨ DMax

diamphenethide BAN [also: diamfenetide]

diampromide INN, BAN

diampron [see: amicarbalide]

diamthazole BAN [also: dimazole]

diamthazole dihydrochloride [see: diamthazole]

Dianabol tablets (discontinued 1982) ℞ *anabolic steroid; discontinued for human use, but the veterinary product is still available and sometimes abused as a street drug* [methandrostenolone] 2.5, 5 mg

Dianeal Low Calcium with Dextrose 1.5% (2.5%; 4.25%); Dianeal PD-2 with Dextrose 1.5% (2.5%; 3.5%; 4.25%); UltraBag Dianeal PD-2 with Dextrose 1.5% (2.5%; 4.25%) IV infusion ℞ *nutritional supplement for continuous ambulatory peritoneal dialysis patients (orphan)* [peritoneal dialysis solution; dextrose] 100 mL

diapamide USAN *diuretic; antihypertensive* [also: tiamizide]

Diaparene Baby cream OTC *diaper rash treatment*

Diaparene Cornstarch Baby powder OTC *diaper rash treatment* [cornstarch; aloe]

Diaparene Diaper Rash ointment OTC *diaper rash treatment* [zinc oxide]

Diaper Guard ointment OTC *diaper rash treatment* [dimethicone; vitamins A, D, and E; zinc oxide] 1%•±•±

Diaper Rash ointment OTC *diaper rash treatment* [zinc oxide]

diaphene [see: dibromsalan]

diaphenylsulfone [see: dapsone]

diaphoretics *a class of agents that promote profuse perspiration* [also called: sudorifics]

Diar-Aid tablets OTC *antidiarrheal; GI adsorbent* [loperamide HCl] 2 mg

diarbarone INN

Diascan reagent strips for home use OTC *in vitro diagnostic aid for blood glucose*

DiaScreen reagent strips for professional use ℞ *in vitro diagnostic aid for multiple disease markers in the urine*

Diasorb tablets, oral liquid OTC *antidiarrheal; GI adsorbent* [activated attapulgite] 750 mg; 750 mg/5 mL

Diastat AcuDial rectal gel in prefilled disposable applicators ℞ *benzodiazepine anticonvulsant for acute repetitive seizures (orphan)* [diazepam; alcohol 10%] 2.5, 5, 7.5, 10, 12.5, 15, 17.5, 20 mg/dose (2.5, 10, 20 mg/applicator)

Diastix reagent strips for home use (discontinued 2008) OTC *in vitro diagnostic aid for urine glucose*

diathymosulfone INN

diatrizoate meglumine USP *oral/parenteral radiopaque contrast medium (46.67% iodine)* [also: meglumine diatrizoate]

diatrizoate methylglucamine [see: diatrizoate meglumine]

diatrizoate sodium USP *oral/rectal/parenteral radiopaque contrast medium (59.87% iodine)* [also: sodium amidotrizoate; sodium diatrizoate]

diatrizoate sodium I 125 USAN *radioactive agent*

diatrizoate sodium I 131 USAN *radioactive agent*

diatrizoic acid USAN, USP, BAN *radiopaque contrast medium* [also: amidotrizoic acid]

Diatx tablets ℞ *hematinic* [multiple B vitamins; folic acid; biotin] ±•5•0.3 mg

Diatx Fe tablets ℞ *vitamin/iron supplement for anemia* [multiple B vitamins; folic acid; biotin; iron (as ferrous fumarate)] ± • 5 • 0.3 • 100 mg

Diatx Zn film-coated tablets ℞ *vitamin/mineral supplement* [multiple B vitamins and minerals; vitamin C; folic acid; biotin] ± • 60 • 5 • 0.3 mg

diaveridine USAN, INN, BAN *antibacterial*

diazacholesterol dihydrochloride [see: azacosterol HCl]

diazepam USAN, USP, INN, BAN, JAN *benzodiazepine anxiolytic; sedative; skeletal muscle relaxant; anticonvulsant for acute repetitive seizures (orphan); alcohol withdrawal aid; also abused as a street drug* 2, 5, 10 mg oral; 5 mg/5 mL oral; 5 mg/mL injection

Diazepam rectal gel in a prefilled applicator ℞ *benzodiazepine sedative; anxiolytic; anticonvulsant; skeletal muscle relaxant* [diazepam; alcohol 10%] 2.5, 10, 20 mg

Diazepam Intensol oral drops ℞ *benzodiazepine sedative; anxiolytic; skeletal muscle relaxant; anticonvulsant; also abused as a street drug* [diazepam; alcohol 19%] 5 mg/mL

diazinon BAN [also: dimpylate]

diaziquone USAN, INN *antineoplastic; investigational (orphan) for primary brain malignancies (astrocytomas)*

diazoxide USAN, USP, INN, BAN *emergency antihypertensive; vasodilator; glucose-elevating agent for hyperinsulinemia due to pancreatic cancer*

dibasic calcium phosphate [see: calcium phosphate, dibasic]

dibasic potassium phosphate [see: potassium phosphate, dibasic]

dibasic sodium phosphate [see: sodium phosphate, dibasic]

dibasol [see: bendazol]

dibazol [see: bendazol]

dibekacin INN, BAN

dibemethine INN

dibencil [see: penicillin G benzathine]

dibencozide [see: cobamamide]

Dibent IM injection (discontinued 2010) ℞ *gastrointestinal anticholinergic/antispasmodic for irritable bowel*

syndrome (IBS) [dicyclomine HCl] 10 mg/mL

dibenthiamine [see: bentiamine]

dibenzathione [see: sulbentine]

dibenzepin INN, BAN *antidepressant* [also: dibenzepin HCl]

dibenzepin HCl USAN *antidepressant* [also: dibenzepin]

dibenzodiazepines *a class of novel (atypical) antipsychotic agents*

dibenzothiazepines *a class of novel (atypical) antipsychotic agents*

dibenzothiazine [see: phenothiazine]

dibenzothiophene USAN *keratolytic*

dibenzoxazepines *a class of dopamine receptor antagonists with antipsychotic, hypotensive, antiemetic, antispasmodic, and antihistaminic activity*

dibenzoyl peroxide [see: benzoyl peroxide]

dibenzoylthiamin [see: bentiamine]

dibenzthion [see: sulbentine]

dibenzylethylenediamine dipenicillin G (DBED) [see: penicillin G benzathine]

Dibenzyline capsules ℞ *antihypertensive for pheochromocytoma* [phenoxybenzamine HCl] 10 mg

N,N-dibenzylmethylamine [see: dibemethine]

dibromodulcitol [see: mitolactol]

dibromohydroxyquinoline [see: broxyquinoline]

dibromomannitol (DBM) [see: mitobronitol]

dibromopropamidine BAN [also: dibrompropamidine]

4,5-dibromorhodamine 123 *investigational (orphan) for chronic myelogenous leukemia*

dibrompropamidine INN [also: dibromopropamidine]

dibromsalan USAN, INN *disinfectant*

dibrospidium chloride INN

dibucaine USP *topical anesthetic* [also: cinchocaine] 1% topical ☒ Depacon

dibucaine HCl USP *local anesthetic* [also: cinchocaine HCl]

dibudinate INN *combining name for radicals or groups*

dibunate INN *combining name for radicals or groups*

dibuprol INN

dibupyrone INN, BAN

dibusadol INN

dibutoline sulfate

DIC (dimethyl imidazole carboxamide) [see: dacarbazine]

Dical CapTabs (caplets) (discontinued 2008) OTC *calcium supplement* [calcium (as dibasic calcium phosphate); vitamin D] 117 mg•133 IU

dicalcium phosphate [see: calcium phosphate, dibasic]

Dical-D tablets (discontinued 2010) OTC *calcium supplement* [calcium (as dibasic calcium phosphate); vitamin D] 105 mg•120 IU

dicarbine INN

Dicarbosil chewable tablets OTC *antacid; calcium supplement* [calcium (as carbonate)] 200 mg (500 mg)

dicarfen INN

Dicel oral suspension ℞ *decongestant; antihistamine* [pseudoephedrine tannate; chlorpheniramine tannate] 75•5 mg/5 mL 🔟 decil

Dicel CD oral liquid OTC *decongestant; antihistamine; antitussive* [pseudoephedrine HCl; brompheniramine maleate; chlophedianol HCl] 30•2•12.5 mg/5 mL

Dicel DM chewable tablets OTC *antitussive; antihistamine; decongestant* [dextromethorphan hydrobromide; chlorpheniramine maleate; pseudoephedrine HCl] 10•2•30 mg

Dicel DM oral suspension ℞ *antitussive; antihistamine; decongestant* [dextromethorphan tannate; chlorpheniramine tannate; pseudoephedrine tannate] 25•5•75 mg/5 mL

dichlofenthion BAN

dichloralantipyrine [see: dichloralphenazone]

dichloralphenazone (chloral hydrate & phenazone) BAN *mild sedative*

dichloralphenazone & acetaminophen & isometheptane mucate *cerebral vasoconstrictor and analgesic*

for *vascular and tension headaches; "possibly effective" for migraine headaches* 100•325•65 mg oral

dichloralpyrine [see: dichloralphenazone]

dichloramine-T NF

dichloranilino imidazolin [see: clonidine HCl]

dichloren [see: mechlorethamine HCl]

dichlorisone INN

dichlorisone acetate [see: dichlorisone]

dichlormethazanone [see: dichlormezanone]

dichlormezanone INN

dichloroacetic acid *strong keratolytic/ cauterant*

dichlorodifluoromethane NF *aerosol propellant; topical refrigerant anesthetic*

dichlorodiphenyl trichloroethane (DDT) [see: chlorophenothane]

dichlorometaxylenol [see: dichloroxylenol]

dichloromethane [see: methylene chloride]

dichlorophen INN, BAN

dichlorophenarsine INN, BAN [also: dichlorophenarsine HCl]

dichlorophenarsine HCl USP [also: dichlorophenarsine]

dichlorotetrafluoroethane NF *aerosol propellant; topical refrigerant anesthetic* [also: cryofluorane]

dichlorovinyl dimethyl phosphate (DDVP) [see: dichlorvos]

dichloroxylenol INN, BAN

dichlorphenamide USP, BAN *carbonic anhydrase inhibitor; diuretic* [also: diclofenamide]

dichlorvos USAN, INN, BAN *anthelmintic*

dichysterol [see: dihydrotachysterol]

diciferron INN

dicirenone USAN, INN *hypotensive; aldosterone antagonist*

Dick test (scarlet fever streptococcus toxin)

diclazuril USAN, INN, BAN *coccidiostat for poultry*

diclofenac INN, BAN *analgesic; antiarthritic; nonsteroidal anti-inflammatory* *drug (NSAID) for ankylosing spondylitis* [also: diclofenac potassium]

diclofenac epolamine *transdermal analgesic; nonsteroidal anti-inflammatory drug (NSAID) for acute pain due to strains, sprains, and contusions*

diclofenac potassium USAN *analgesic; nonsteroidal anti-inflammatory drug (NSAID) for osteoarthritis, rheumatoid arthritis, ankylosing spondylitis, and dysmenorrhea; topical treatment for actinic keratoses* [also: diclofenac] 50 mg oral

diclofenac sodium USAN, JAN *analgesic; nonsteroidal anti-inflammatory drug (NSAID) for osteoarthritis, rheumatoid arthritis, and ankylosing spondylitis; ocular treatment for cataract extraction and corneal refractive surgery; topical treatment for actinic keratoses* 25, 50, 75, 100 mg oral; 0.1% eye drops

diclofenamide INN *carbonic anhydrase inhibitor* [also: dichlorphenamide]

diclofensine INN

diclofibrate [see: simfibrate]

diclofurime INN

diclometide INN

diclonixin INN

dicloralurea USAN, INN *veterinary food additive*

dicloxacillin USAN, INN, BAN *penicillinase-resistant penicillin antibiotic*

dicloxacillin sodium USAN, USP, BAN *penicillinase-resistant penicillin antibiotic* 250, 500 mg oral

dicobalt edetate INN, BAN

dicolinium iodide INN

Dicomal-DH syrup (discontinued 2007) ℞ *narcotic antitussive; antihistamine; sleep aid; decongestant* [hydrocodone bitartrate; pyrilamine maleate; phenylephrine HCl] 1.66•8.33•5 mg/5 mL

Dicomal-DM syrup (discontinued 2007) OTC *antitussive; antihistamine; sleep aid; decongestant* [dextromethorphan hydrobromide; pyrilamine maleate; phenylephrine HCl] 20•16.7•10 mg/10 mL

dicophane BAN [also: chlorophenothane; clofenotane]

dicoumarin [see: dicumarol]

dicoumarol INN *coumarin-derivative anticoagulant* [also: dicumarol]

dicresulene INN

Dictamnus albus *medicinal herb* [see: fraxinella]

dicumarol USAN, USP *coumarin-derivative anticoagulant* [also: dicoumarol]

dicyclomine BAN *gastrointestinal anticholinergic/antispasmodic* [also: dicyclomine HCl; dicycloverine]

dicyclomine HCl USP *gastrointestinal anticholinergic/antispasmodic for irritable bowel syndrome (IBS)* [also: dicycloverine; dicyclomine] 10, 20 mg oral; 10 mg/5 mL oral; 10 mg/mL injection

dicycloverine INN *anticholinergic* [also: dicyclomine HCl; dicyclomine]

dicycloverine HCl [see: dicyclomine HCl]

dicysteine [see: cystine]

didanosine USAN, INN, BAN *nucleoside reverse transcriptase inhibitor (NRTI); antiviral for advanced HIV-1 infection (orphan)* 125, 200, 250, 400 mg oral

didehydrodideoxythymidine [see: stavudine]

Di-Delamine gel, spray OTC *antihistamine* [diphenhydramine HCl; tripelennamine HCl] 1%•0.5%

2′,3′-dideoxyadenosine (ddA) *investigational (orphan) treatment for AIDS*

dideoxycytidine (DDC; ddC) [see: zalcitabine]

dideoxyinosine (DDI; ddI) [see: didanosine]

Didrex tablets ℞ *CNS stimulant; anorexiant* [benzphetamine HCl] 50 mg

Didronel caplets ℞ *bisphosphonate bone resorption inhibitor for Paget disease, heterotopic ossification, and hypercalcemia of malignancy (orphan); also used for corticosteroid-induced osteoporosis* [etidronate disodium] 200, 400 mg

didrovaltrate INN

didroxane [see: dichlorophen]

dieldrin INN, BAN

dielytra; choice dielytra *medicinal herb* [see: turkey corn]

diemal [see: barbital]

dienestrol USP, INN *estrogen* [also: dienoestrol]

dienoestrol BAN *estrogen* [also: dienestrol]

dienogest INN

dietamiphylline [see: etamiphyllin]

dietamiverine HCl [see: bietamiverine HCl]

diethadione INN, BAN

diethanolamine NF *alkalizing agent*

diethazine INN, BAN ⑨ Detussin

diethazine HCl [see: diethazine]

diethyl phthalate NF *plasticizer*

diethylamine p-aminobenzenestibonate [see: stibosamine]

3-diethylaminobutyranilide [see: octacaine]

diethylbarbiturate monosodium [see: barbital sodium]

diethylbarbituric acid [see: barbital]

diethylcarbamazine INN, BAN *anthelmintic for Bancroft filariasis, onchocerciasis, tropical eosinophilia, and loiasis* [also: diethylcarbamazine citrate]

diethylcarbamazine citrate (DEC) USP *anthelmintic for Bancroft filariasis, onchocerciasis, tropical eosinophilia, and loiasis* [also: diethylcarbamazine]

diethylcarbamazine dihydrogen citrate [see: diethylcarbamazine citrate]

diethyldithiocarbamate *investigational (Phase II/III, orphan) immunomodulator for HIV and AIDS*

diethyldixanthogen [see: dixanthogen]

diethylenediamine citrate [see: piperazine citrate]

diethylenetriaminepentaacetic acid (DTPA) [see: pentetic acid]

N,N-diethyllysergamide [see: lysergide]

diethylmalonylurea [see: barbital]

diethylmalonylurea sodium [see: barbital sodium]

N,N-diethylnicotinamide [see: nikethamide]

diethylnorspermine *investigational (orphan) for hepatocellular carcinoma*

diethylpropion BAN *CNS stimulant; anorexiant* [also: diethylpropion HCl; amfepramone] 75 mg oral

diethylpropion HCl USP *CNS stimulant; anorexiant* [also: amfepramone; diethylpropion] 25, 75 mg oral

diethylstilbestrol (DES) USP, INN *hormonal antineoplastic for inoperable prostatic and breast cancer* [also: stilboestrol]

diethylstilbestrol diphosphate USP *hormonal antineoplastic* [also: fosfestrol]

diethylstilbestrol dipropionate NF

p-diethylsulfamoylbenzoic acid [see: etebenecid; ethebenecid]

diethylthiambutene INN, BAN

diethyltoluamide (DEET) USP, BAN *arthropod repellent*

diethyltryptamine (DET) *a hallucinogenic street drug closely related to dimethyltryptamine (DMT), but prepared synthetically*

N,N-diethylvanillamide [see: ethamivan]

dietifen INN

dietroxine [see: diethadione]

diexanthogen [see: dixanthogen]

difebarbamate INN

difemerine INN [also: difemerine HCl]

difemerine HCl [also: difemerine]

difemetorex INN

difenamizole INN

difencloxazine INN

difencloxazine HCl [see: difencloxazine]

difenidol INN *antiemetic; antivertigo* [also: diphenidol]

difenoximide INN *antiperistaltic* [also: difenoximide HCl]

difenoximide HCl USAN *antiperistaltic* [also: difenoximide]

difenoxin USAN, INN, BAN *antiperistaltic*

difenoxin HCl *antiperistaltic*

diferuloylmethane *investigational (orphan) agent for cystic fibrosis*

difetarsone INN, BAN

difeterol INN

Differin gel, lotion ℞ *synthetic retinoid analogue for acne* [adapalene] 0.1%, 0.3%; 0.1%

Differin solution, cream, single-use pledgets ℞ *synthetic retinoid analogue for acne* [adapalene] 0.1%

Dificid film-coated tablets ℞ *macrolide antibiotic for* Clostridium difficile *infections* [fidaxomicin] 200 mg

Difil-G 400 caplets ℞ *antiasthmatic; bronchodilator; expectorant* [dyphylline; guaifenesin] 200•400 mg ⑨ Duphalac

Difil-G Forte oral liquid (discontinued 2010) ℞ *antiasthmatic; bronchodilator; expectorant* [dyphylline; guaifenesin] 100•100 mg/5 mL

diflorasone INN, BAN *topical corticosteroidal anti-inflammatory* [also: diflorasone diacetate]

diflorasone diacetate USAN, USP *topical corticosteroidal anti-inflammatory* [also: diflorasone] 0.05% topical

difloxacin INN *anti-infective; DNA gyrase inhibitor* [also: difloxacin HCl]

difloxacin HCl USAN *anti-infective; DNA gyrase inhibitor* [also: difloxacin]

difluanazine INN *CNS stimulant* [also: difluanine HCl]

difluanazine HCl [see: difluanine HCl]

difluanine HCl USAN *CNS stimulant* [also: difluanazine]

Diflucan IV infusion (discontinued 2011) ℞ *systemic triazole antifungal* [fluconazole] 2 mg/mL

Diflucan tablets, powder for oral suspension ℞ *systemic triazole antifungal* [fluconazole] 50, 100, 150, 200 mg; 10, 40 mg/mL

diflucortolone USAN, INN, BAN *corticosteroid; anti-inflammatory*

diflucortolone pivalate USAN *corticosteroid; anti-inflammatory*

diflumidone INN, BAN *anti-inflammatory* [also: diflumidone sodium]

diflumidone sodium USAN *anti-inflammatory* [also: diflumidone]

diflunisal USAN, USP, INN, BAN *anti-inflammatory; analgesic; antipyretic; antiarthritic; antirheumatic* 500 mg oral

difluoromethylornithine (DFMO) [see: eflornithine]

difluoromethylornithine HCl [see: eflornithine HCl]

difluprednate USAN, INN *topical corticosteroidal anti-inflammatory for ocular surgery*

difolliculin [see: estradiol benzoate]

diftalone USAN, INN *anti-inflammatory*

digalloyl trioleate USAN

Di-Gel oral liquid OTC *antacid; antiflatulent* [aluminum hydroxide; magnesium hydroxide; simethicone] 200•200•20 mg/5 mL ⑨ Dical

Di-Gel, Advanced Formula chewable tablets OTC *antacid; antiflatulent* [magnesium hydroxide; calcium carbonate; simethicone] 128•280•20 mg

digestants; digestives *a class of agents that promote or aid in digestion*

digestive enzymes (amylase; lipase; protease) [q.v.]

Digex capsules OTC *digestive enzymes; GI antispasmodic; antihistamine; sleep aid* [pancrelipase (amylase; protease; lipase); cellulase; hyoscyamine sulfate; phenyltoloxamine citrate] 30 mg•6 mg•1200 IU•2 mg•0.0625 mg•15 mg

Digex NF capsules ℞ *GI antispasmodic; antihistamine; sleep aid* [hyoscyamine sulfate; phenyltoloxamine citrate] 0.0625•15 mg

Digibind powder for IV injection ℞ *antidote to digoxin/digitoxin overdose (orphan)* [digoxin immune Fab (ovine)] 38 mg/vial

Digidote *investigational (orphan) antidote to cardiac glycoside intoxication* [digoxin immune Fab (ovine)]

DigiFab powder for IV injection ℞ *antidote to digoxin/digitoxin overdose (orphan)* [digoxin immune Fab (ovine)] 40 mg/vial

digitalis USP *cardiotonic*

Digitalis ambigua; D. ferriginea; D. grandiflora; D. lanata; D. lutea; D. purpurea medicinal herb [see: foxglove]

digitalis glycosides *a class of cardiovascular drugs that increase the force of cardiac contractions* [also called: cardiac glycosides]

Digitek tablets (discontinued 2008) ℞ *cardiac glycoside to increase cardiac output; antiarrhythmic* [digoxin] 0.125, 0.25 mg

digitoxin USP, INN, BAN *cardiotonic; cardiac glycoside; investigational (orphan) for soft tissue sarcomas and ovarian cancer*

digitoxin, acetyl [see: acetyldigitoxin]

α-digitoxin monoacetate [see: acetyldigitoxin]

digitoxoside [see: digitoxin]

digolil INN *combining name for radicals or groups*

digoxin USP, INN, BAN *cardiotonic; cardiac glycoside antiarrhythmic* 0.125, 0.25 mg oral, 0.05 mg/mL oral, 0.1, 0.25 mg/mL injection

digoxin antibody [see: digoxin immune Fab]

digoxin immune Fab (ovine) *antidote to digoxin/digitoxin intoxication (orphan); investigational (orphan) for other cardiac glycoside intoxication*

dihexyverine INN *anticholinergic* [also: dihexyverine HCl]

dihexyverine HCl USAN *anticholinergic* [also: dihexyverine]

Dihistine Expectorant oral liquid (discontinued 2007) ℞ *narcotic antitussive; decongestant; expectorant* [codeine phosphate; pseudoephedrine HCl; guaifenesin; alcohol 7.5%] 10•30•100 mg/5 mL

dihydan soluble [see: phenytoin sodium]

dihydralazine INN, BAN

dihydralazine sulfate [see: dihydralazine]

5,6-dihydro-5-azacytidine *investigational (orphan) for malignant mesothelioma*

dihydrobenzthiazide [see: hydrobentizide]

dihydrocodeine INN, BAN *narcotic analgesic and antitussive* [also: dihydrocodeine bitartrate]

dihydrocodeine bitartrate USP *narcotic analgesic and antitussive* [also: dihydrocodeine]

dihydrocodeine bitartrate & acetaminophen & caffeine *narcotic analgesic and antitussive* 32•712.8•60 mg

dihydrocodeine bitartrate & brompheniramine maleate & phenylephrine HCl *narcotic analgesic and antitussive; antihistamine; decongestant* 3•4•7.5 mg oral

dihydrocodeinone bitartrate [see: hydrocodone bitartrate]

DiHydro-CP syrup ℞ *narcotic antitussive; antihistamine; decongestant* [dihydrocodeine bitartrate; chlorpheniramine maleate; pseudoephedrine HCl] 7.5•2•15 mg/5 mL

dihydroergocornine [see: ergoloid mesylates]

dihydroergocristine [see: ergoloid mesylates]

dihydroergocryptine [see: ergoloid mesylates]

dihydroergotamine (DHE) INN, BAN *antiadrenergic; anticoagulant; ergot alkaloid for rapid control of migraines* [also: dihydroergotamine mesylate; dihydroergotamine mesilate]

dihydroergotamine mesilate JAN *antiadrenergic; anticoagulant; ergot alkaloid for rapid control of migraines* [also: dihydroergotamine mesylate; dihydroergotamine]

dihydroergotamine mesylate USAN, USP *antiadrenergic; anticoagulant; ergot alkaloid for the rapid control of migraine and cluster headaches* [also: dihydroergotamine; dihydroergotamine mesilate] 1 mg/mL injection

dihydroergotamine methanesulfonate [see: dihydroergotamine mesylate]

dihydroergotoxine mesylate [now: ergoloid mesylates]

dihydroergotoxine methanesulfonate [now: ergoloid mesylates]

dihydroethaverine [see: drotaverine]

dihydrofollicular hormone [see: estradiol]

dihydrofolliculine [see: estradiol]

dihydrogenated ergot alkaloids [now: ergoloid mesylates]

dihydrohydroxycodeinone [see: oxycodone]

dihydrohydroxycodeinone HCl [see: oxycodone HCl]

6-dihydro-6-iminopurine [see: adenine]

dihydroindolones *a class of dopamine receptor antagonists with conventional (typical) antipsychotic activity* [also called: indolones]

dihydroisoperparine [see: drotaverine]

dihydromorphinone HCl [now: hydromorphone HCl]

dihydroneopine [see: dihydrocodeine bitartrate]

DiHydro-PE syrup ℞ *narcotic antitussive; antihistamine; decongestant* [dihydrocodeine bitartrate; chlorpheniramine maleate; phenylephrine HCl] 3•2•7.5 mg/5 mL

dihydropyridines *a class of calcium channel blockers*

dihydrostreptomycin (DST) INN *antibacterial* [also: dihydrostreptomycin sulfate]

dihydrostreptomycin sulfate USP *antibacterial* [also: dihydrostreptomycin]

dihydrostreptomycin-streptomycin [see: streptoduocin]

dihydrotachysterol (DHT) USP, INN, BAN, JAN *fat-soluble vitamin; synthetic reduction product of tachysterol, a vitamin D isomer; calcium regulator for tetany and hypoparathyroidism*

dihydrotestosterone (DHT) *anabolic steroid; investigational (Phase II, orphan) for AIDS-wasting syndrome* [also: androstanolone; stanolone]

dihydrotheelin [see: estradiol]

dihydroxy(stearato)aluminum [see: aluminum monostearate]

dihydroxy propoxymethyl guanine (DHPG) [see: gancyclovir]

dihydroxyacetone *skin darkener for vitiligo and hypopigmented areas*

dihydroxyaluminum aminoacetate (DAA) USP *antacid*

dihydroxyaluminum sodium carbonate USP *antacid*

dihydroxyanthranol [see: anthralin]

dihydroxyanthraquinone *(withdrawn from market)* [see: danthron]

1α,25-dihydroxycholecalciferol [see: calcitriol]

24,25-dihydroxycholecalciferol *investigational (orphan) for uremic osteodystrophy*

dihydroxyestrin [see: estradiol]

5,7-dihydroxyflavone [see: chrysin]

dihydroxyfluorane [see: fluorescein]

dihydroxyphenylalanine (DOPA) [see: levodopa]

dihydroxyphenylisatin [see: oxyphenisatin acetate]

dihydroxyphenyloxindol [see: oxyphenisatin acetate]

dihydroxyprogesterone acetophenide [see: algestone acetophenide]

dihydroxypropyl theophylline [see: dyphylline]

diiodobuphenine [see: bufeniode]

diiodohydroxyquin [now: iodoquinol]

diiodohydroxyquinoline INN, BAN *antiamebic* [also: iodoquinol]

diisopromine INN ② desipramine

diisopromine HCl [see: diisopromine]

diisopropanolamine NF *alkalizing agent*

diisopropyl flurophosphate (DFP) [see: isoflurophate]

diisopropyl flurophosphonate [see: isoflurophate]

diisopropyl phosphorofluoridate [see: isoflurophate]

2,6-diisopropylphenol [see: propofol]

Dilacor XR sustained-release capsules *(discontinued 2010)* ℞ *antihypertensive; antianginal; antiarrhythmic; calcium channel blocker* [diltiazem HCl] 120, 180, 240 mg

Dilantin extended-release capsules ℞ *hydantoin anticonvulsant* [phenytoin sodium] 30, 100 mg

Dilantin Infatabs (chewable tablets) ℞ *hydantoin anticonvulsant* [phenytoin] 50 mg

Dilantin-125 oral suspension ℞ *hydantoin anticonvulsant* [phenytoin] 125 mg/5 mL

Dilatrate-SR sustained-release capsules ℞ *coronary vasodilator; antianginal* [isosorbide dinitrate] 40 mg

Dilaudid tablets, oral liquid, subcu or IM injection, suppositories ℞ *narcotic analgesic; often abused as a street drug* [hydromorphone HCl] 2, 4, 8 mg; 1 mg/mL; 1, 2, 4 mg/mL; 3 mg

Dilaudid Cough syrup (discontinued 2007) ℞ *narcotic antitussive; expectorant* [hydromorphone HCl; guaifenesin; alcohol 5%] 1•100 mg/5 mL

Dilaudid-HP subcu or IM injection; powder for subcu or IM injection ℞ *narcotic analgesic* [hydromorphone HCl] 10 mg/mL; 250 mg

dilazep INN

dilevalol INN, BAN *antihypertensive; antiadrenergic (beta-blocker)* [also: dilevalol HCl]

dilevalol HCl USAN, JAN *antihypertensive; antiadrenergic (beta-blocker)* [also: dilevalol]

Dilex-G; Dilex-G 200 syrup ℞ *antiasthmatic; bronchodilator; expectorant* [dyphylline; guaifenesin] 100•100 mg/5 mL; 100•200 mg/5 mL

Dilex-G 400 tablets ℞ *antiasthmatic; bronchodilator; expectorant* [dyphylline; guaifenesin] 200•400 mg

dilithium carbonate [see: lithium carbonate]

dill *(Anethum graveolens)* fruit and seed *medicinal herb used as an aromatic, carminative, diaphoretic, stimulant, and stomachic*

dilmefone INN

Dilomine IM injection (discontinued 2011) ℞ *gastrointestinal anticholinergic/antispasmodic for irritable bowel syndrome (IBS)* [dicyclomine HCl] 10 mg/mL ▣ Dalmane; diolamine

Dilotab tablets (discontinued 2007) OTC *decongestant; analgesic; antipyretic* [pseudoephedrine HCl; acetaminophen] 30•500 mg

Dilotab II tablets OTC *decongestant; analgesic; antipyretic* [phenylephrine HCl; acetaminophen] 5•325 mg

diloxanide INN, BAN

diloxanide furoate *investigational anti-infective for amebiasis* (available only from the Centers for Disease Control and Prevention)

Dilt-CD extended-release capsules ℞ *antihypertensive; calcium channel blocker* [diltiazem HCl] 120, 180, 240, 300 mg

Diltia XT sustained-release capsules ℞ *antihypertensive; calcium channel blocker* [diltiazem HCl] 120, 180, 240 mg

diltiazem INN, BAN *coronary vasodilator; calcium channel blocker; antianginal; antihypertensive* [also: diltiazem HCl]

diltiazem HCl USAN, USP, JAN *coronary vasodilator; calcium channel blocker; antianginal; antihypertensive; antiarrhythmic* [also: diltiazem] 30, 60, 90, 120, 180, 240, 300, 360, 420 mg oral; 5 mg/mL injection

diltiazem malate USAN *coronary vasodilator; calcium channel blocker; antianginal; antihypertensive; antiarrhythmic*

Dilt-XR extended-release capsules ℞ *antihypertensive; calcium channel blocker* [diltiazem HCl] 120, 180, 240 mg

Diltzac extended-release tablets ℞ *antihypertensive; calcium channel blocker* [diltiazem HCl] 120, 180, 240, 300, 360 mg

diluted acetic acid [see: acetic acid, diluted]

diluted alcohol [see: alcohol, diluted]

diluted hydrochloric acid [see: hydrochloric acid, diluted]

diluted sodium hypochlorite [see: sodium hypochlorite, diluted]

dimabefylline INN

dimantine INN *anthelmintic* [also: dymanthine HCl]

dimantine HCl INN [also: dymanthine HCl]

Dimaphen elixir (discontinued 2011) OTC *decongestant; antihistamine* [pseudoephedrine HCl; brompheniramine maleate] 30•2 mg/10 mL

Dimaphen DM Cold & Cough elixir OTC *antitussive; antihistamine;*

decongestant [dextromethorphan hydrobromide; brompheniramine maleate; pseudoephedrine HCl] 10•2•30 mg/10 mL

Dimaphen DM Cold & Cough, Children's oral liquid Ŗ *antitussive; antihistamine; decongestant* [dextromethorphan hydrobromide; brompheniramine maleate; phenylephrine HCl] 10•2•5 mg/10 mL

dimazole INN [also: diamthazole]

dimazole dihydrochloride [see: dimazole; diamthazole]

Dime capsules OTC *vitamin/mineral/amino acid supplement* [multiple vitamins, minerals, and amino acids; folic acid; biotin] ±•400•25 mcg

dimebolin HCl *investigational (Phase III) treatment for Alzheimer and Huntington diseases*

Dimebon *investigational (Phase III) treatment for Alzheimer and Huntington diseases* [dimebolin HCl]

dimecamine INN

dimecolonium iodide INN

dimecrotic acid INN

dimedrol [see: diphenhydramine HCl]

dimefadane USAN, INN *analgesic*

dimefilcon A USAN *hydrophilic contact lens material*

dimefline INN, BAN *respiratory stimulant* [also: dimefline HCl]

dimefline HCl USAN *respiratory stimulant* [also: dimefline]

dimefocon A USAN *hydrophobic contact lens material*

dimekolin [see: dimecolonium iodide]

dimelazine INN

dimelin [see: dimecolonium iodide]

dimemorfan INN

dimenhydrinate USP, INN, BAN *antiemetic; anticholinergic; antivertigo; motion sickness prophylaxis* 50 mg oral; 12.5 mg/4 mL oral; 50 mg/mL injection

dimenoxadol INN [also: dimenoxadole]

dimenoxadole BAN [also: dimenoxadol]

dimepheptanol INN, BAN

dimepranol INN *immunomodulator* [also: dimepranol acedoben]

dimepranol acedoben USAN *immunomodulator* [also: dimepranol]

dimepregnen INN, BAN

dimepropion BAN [also: metamfepramone]

dimeprozan INN

dimeprozinum [see: dimeprozan]

dimercaprol USP, INN *chelating agent for arsenic, gold, and mercury poisoning; adjunct to lead poisoning*

dimercaptopropanol [see: dimercaprol]

2,3-dimercaptosuccinic acid (DMSA) [see: succimer]

dimesna INN

dimesone INN, BAN

Dimetabs tablets Ŗ *anticholinergic; antiemetic; antivertigo agent; motion sickness preventative* [dimenhydrinate] 50 mg

dimetacrine INN

dimetamfetamine INN

Dimetane DX oral liquid Ŗ *antitussive; decongestant; antihistamine* [dextromethorphan hydrobromide; pseudoephedrine HCl; brompheniramine maleate] 10•30•2 mg/5 mL

Dimetapp 12-Hour Non-Drowsy Extentabs (extended-release tablets) OTC *decongestant* [pseudoephedrine HCl] 120 mg

Dimetapp Children's Cold & Allergy elixir OTC *decongestant; antihistamine* [phenylephrine HCl; brompheniramine maleate] 2.5•1 mg/10 mL

Dimetapp Children's ND Non-Drowsy Allergy orally disintegrating tablets, syrup OTC *nonsedating antihistamine for allergic rhinitis* [loratadine] 10 mg; 5 mg/5 mL

Dimetapp Decongestant Pediatric oral drops (discontinued 2009) OTC *nasal decongestant* [pseudoephedrine HCl] 7.5 mg/0.8 mL

Dimetapp Long Acting Cough Plus Cold syrup OTC *antitussive; antihistamine* [dextromethorphan hydrobromide; chlorpheniramine maleate] 15•2 mg/10 mL

Dimetapp Non-Drowsy Liqui-Gels (liquid-filled softgels) (discontinued

2009) OTC *decongestant* [pseudo-ephedrine HCl] 30 mg

Dimetapp Sinus caplets OTC *decongestant; analgesic; antipyretic* [pseudoephedrine HCl; ibuprofen] 30•200 mg

Dimetapp Toddler's Decongestant Plus Cough oral drops OTC *antitussive; decongestant; for children 2–5 years* [dextromethorphan hydrobromide; pseudoephedrine HCl] 5•2.5 mg/1.6 mL

dimethadione USAN, INN *anticonvulsant*

dimethazan 🔢 duometacin

dimethazine [see: mebolazine]

dimethicone USAN, NF, BAN *lubricant and hydrophobing agent; soft tissue prosthetic aid* [also: dimeticone]

dimethicone 350 USAN *soft tissue prosthetic aid*

dimethindene BAN *antihistamine* [also: dimethindene maleate; dimetindene]

dimethindene maleate USP *antihistamine* [also: dimetindene; dimethindene]

dimethiodal sodium INN

dimethisoquin BAN [also: dimethisoquin HCl; quinisocaine]

dimethisoquin HCl USAN [also: quinisocaine; dimethisoquin]

dimethisterone USAN, NF, INN, BAN *progestin*

dimetholizine INN

dimethothiazine BAN *serotonin inhibitor* [also: fonazine mesylate; dimetotiazine]

dimethoxanate INN, BAN

dimethoxanate HCl [see: dimethoxanate]

2,5-dimethoxy-4-methylamphetamine (DOM) *a hallucinogenic street drug derived from amphetamine, popularly called STP*

dimethoxyphenyl penicillin sodium [see: methicillin sodium]

dimethpyridene maleate [see: dimethindene maleate]

dimethyl ketone [see: acetone]

dimethyl phthalate USP

dimethyl polysiloxane [see: dimethicone]

dimethyl sulfoxide (DMSO) USAN, USP, INN *solvent; anti-inflammatory for symptomatic relief of interstitial cystitis; investigational (orphan) for traumatic brain coma; investigational (orphan) topical treatment for scleroderma and extravasation of cytotoxic drugs* [also: dimethyl sulphoxide] *50% solution*

dimethyl sulphoxide BAN *topical anti-inflammatory; solvent* [also: dimethyl sulfoxide]

dimethyl triazeno imidazole carboxamide (DIC; DTIC) [see: dacarbazine]

3-(3,5-dimethyl-1H-methylene)-1,3-dihydro-indole-2-one *investigational (orphan) for Kaposi sarcoma and von Hippel-Lindau disease*

dimethylaminoethanol (DMAE) *natural precursor to the neurotransmitter acetylcholine; readily crosses the blood-brain barrier to enhance memory and cognitive function*

dimethylaminoethanol bitartrate *natural precursor to the neurotransmitter acetylcholine; readily crosses the blood-brain barrier to enhance memory and cognitive function (base=37%)*

dimethylaminophenazone [see: aminopyrine]

dimethylcysteine [see: penicillamine]

dimethylglycine HCl (DMG) *amino acid; natural immune system booster*

dimethylhexestrol [see: methestrol]

1,5-dimethylhexylamine [see: octodrine]

5,5-dimethyl-2,4-oxazolidinedione (DMO) [see: dimethadione]

dimethyloxyquinazine [see: antipyrine]

o,α-dimethylphenethylamine [see: ortetamine]

dimethylsiloxane polymers [see: dimethicone]

dimethylthiambutene INN, BAN

dimethyltryptamine (DMT) *hallucinogenic street drug derived from a plant* *native to South America and the West Indies*

dimethyltubocurarine BAN [also: dimethyltubocurarinium chloride]

dimethyltubocurarine iodide [see: metocurine iodide]

dimethyltubocurarinium chloride INN [also: dimethyltubocurarine]

dimethylxanthine [see: theophylline]

dimeticone INN *lubricant and hydrophobing agent; soft tissue prosthetic aid* [also: dimethicone]

dimetindene INN *antihistamine* [also: dimethindene maleate; dimethindene]

dimetindene maleate [see: dimethindene maleate]

dimetipirium bromide INN

dimetofrine INN

dimetotiazine INN *serotonin inhibitor* [also: fonazine mesylate; dimethothiazine]

dimetridazole INN, BAN

dimevamide INN

dimevamide sulfate [see: dimevamide]

diminazene INN, BAN

dimoxamine HCl USAN *memory adjuvant*

dimoxaprost INN

dimoxyline INN

dimpylate INN [also: diazinon]

dinaline INN

Dinate IV or IM injection (discontinued 2010) ℞ *anticholinergic; antiemetic; antivertigo agent; motion sickness preventative* [dimenhydrinate] 50 mg/mL ⊠ D-Tann AT; Duonate

dinazafone INN

diniprofylline INN

dinitolmide INN, BAN

dinitrotoluamide [see: dinitolmide]

dinoprost USAN, INN, BAN *oxytocic for induction of labor; prostaglandin-type abortifacient; cervical ripening agent*

dinoprost trometamol BAN *oxytocic for induction of labor; prostaglandin-type abortifacient; cervical ripening agent* [also: dinoprost tromethamine]

dinoprost tromethamine USAN *oxytocic for induction of labor; prostaglan-*

din-type abortifacient; treatment for postpartum uterine bleeding [also: dinoprost trometamol]

dinoprostone USAN, INN, BAN *oxytocic for induction of labor; prostaglandin-type abortifacient; cervical ripening agent*

dinsed USAN, INN *coccidiostat for poultry* ⊠ Donna-Sed

dioctyl calcium sulfosuccinate [now: docusate calcium]

dioctyl potassium sulfosuccinate [now: docusate potassium]

dioctyl sodium sulfosuccinate (DSS) [now: docusate sodium]

Dioctyn softgels OTC *laxative; stool softener* [docusate sodium] 100 mg

diodone INN [also: iodopyracet]

diohippuric acid I 125 USAN *radioactive agent*

diohippuric acid I 131 USAN *radioactive agent*

diolamine USAN, INN *combining name for radicals or groups* ⊠ Dalmane; Dilomine

diolostene [see: methandriol]

dionin [see: ethylmorphine HCl]

diophyllin [see: aminophylline]

Dioscorea villosa *medicinal herb* [see: wild yam]

diosmin INN

Diostate D tablets (discontinued 2008) OTC *calcium supplement* [calcium (as dibasic calcium phosphate); vitamin D] 114 mg•133 IU

diotyrosine I 125 USAN *radioactive agent* ⊠ dotarizine

diotyrosine I 131 USAN *radioactive agent* ⊠ dotarizine

Diovan tablets ℞ *angiotensin receptor blocker (ARB) for hypertension, heart failure, and myocardial infarction* [valsartan] 40, 80, 160, 320 mg ⊠ D-Phen

Diovan HCT tablets ℞ *combination angiotensin receptor blocker (ARB) and diuretic for hypertension* [valsartan; hydrochlorothiazide] 80•12.5, 160•12.5, 160•25, 320•12.5, 320•25 mg

dioxadilol INN

dioxadrol INN *antidepressant* [also: dioxadrol HCl] ⊠ Dexodryl

dioxadrol HCl USAN *antidepressant* [also: dioxadrol]

d-**dioxadrol HCl** [see: dexoxadrol HCl]

dioxamate INN, BAN

dioxaphetyl butyrate INN, BAN

dioxathion BAN [also: dioxation]

dioxation INN [also: dioxathion]

dioxethedrin INN

dioxethedrin HCl [see: dioxethedrin]

dioxifedrine INN

dioxindol [see: oxyphenisatin acetate]

dioxyanthranol [see: anthralin]

dioxyanthraquinone (*withdrawn from market*) [see: danthron]

dioxybenzone USAN, USP, INN *ultraviolet screen*

dipalmitoylphosphatidylcholine (DPPC) [see: colfosceril palmitate]

diparcol HCl [see: diethazine HCl]

dipegyl [see: niacinamide]

dipenicillin G [see: penicillin G benzathine]

dipenine bromide BAN [also: diponium bromide]

Dipentum capsules ℞ *anti-inflammatory for ulcerative colitis* [olsalazine sodium] 250 mg

dipeptidyl peptidase-4 (DPP-4) inhibitors *a class of oral antidiabetic agents that enhance the function of the body's incretin system to increase insulin production in the pancreas and reduce glucose production in the liver*

diperodon USP, INN, BAN *topical anesthetic* Ⓓ deprodone

diperodon HCl *topical anesthetic*

diphemanil methylsulfate USP *anticholinergic* [also: diphemanil metilsulfate; diphemanil methylsulphate]

diphemanil methylsulphate BAN *anticholinergic* [also: diphemanil methylsulfate; diphemanil metilsulfate]

diphemanil metilsulfate INN *anticholinergic* [also: diphemanil methylsulfate; diphemanil methylsulphate]

Diphen AF oral liquid OTC *antihistamine; sleep aid* [diphenhydramine HCl] 12.5 mg/5 mL

Diphen Tann 25 mg/PE Tann 10 mg/CT Tann 30 mg chewable tab-

lets ℞ *antihistamine; sleep aid; decongestant; antitussive* [diphenhydramine tannate; phenylephrine tannate; carbetapentane tannate] 25•10•30 mg

diphenadione USP, INN, BAN

diphenan INN

diphenatil [see: diphemanil methylsulfate]

diphenchloxazine HCl [see: difencloxazine HCl]

diphenesenic acid [see: xenyhexenic acid]

Diphenhist caplets, capsules, oral liquid OTC *antihistamine; sleep aid* [diphenhydramine HCl] 25 mg; 25 mg; 12.5 mg/5 mL

diphenhydramine INN, BAN *ethanolamine antihistamine; antitussive; motion sickness preventative; sleep aid* [also: diphenhydramine citrate]

diphenhydramine citrate USP *ethanolamine antihistamine; antitussive; motion sickness preventative; sleep aid* [also: diphenhydramine]

diphenhydramine citrate & ibuprofen *antipyretic; antihistaminic sleep aid; analgesic* 38•200 mg oral

diphenhydramine HCl USP, BAN *ethanolamine antihistamine; antitussive; motion sickness preventative; sleep aid* 25, 50 mg oral; 50 mg/mL injection

diphenhydramine tannate *ethanolamine antihistamine; antitussive; motion sickness preventative; sleep aid*

diphenhydramine theoclate [see: dimenhydrinate]

diphenidol USAN, BAN *antiemetic; antivertigo* [also: difenidol]

diphenidol HCl USAN *antiemetic*

diphenidol pamoate USAN *antiemetic*

DiphenMax D chewable tablets (discontinued 2010) ℞ *decongestant; antihistamine; sleep aid* [phenylephrine tannate; diphenhydramine tannate] 10•25 mg

diphenmethanil methylsulfate [see: diphemanil methylsulfate]

diphenoxylate INN, BAN *antiperistaltic* [also: diphenoxylate HCl]

diphenoxylate HCl USP *antiperistaltic* [also: diphenoxylate]

diphenylacetylindandione [see: diphenadione]

diphenylalkylamines *a class of calcium channel blockers*

Diphenylan Sodium capsules ℞ *anticonvulsant* [phenytoin sodium] 30, 100 mg

diphenylbutazone [see: phenylbutazone]

diphenylbutylpiperidines [see: phenylbutylpiperidines]

diphenylcyclopenone *investigational (orphan) agent for severe alopecia areata, alopecia totalis, and alopecia universalis*

diphenylhydantoin [now: phenytoin]

diphenylhydantoin sodium [now: phenytoin sodium]

diphenylisatin [see: oxyphenisatin]

diphenylpyraline INN, BAN *antihistamine* [also: diphenylpyraline HCl]

diphenylpyraline HCl USP *antihistamine* [also: diphenylpyraline]

diphetarsone [see: difetarsone]

diphexamide iodomethylate [see: buzepide metiodide]

diphosphonic acid [see: etidronic acid]

diphosphopyridine nucleotide (DPN) [now: nadide]

diphosphoric acid, tetrasodium salt [see: sodium pyrophosphate]

diphosphothiamin [see: co-carboxylase]

diphoxazide INN

diphtheria antitoxin USP *passive immunizing agent for diphtheria* [also: diphtheria toxoid] 500 U/mL injection

diphtheria CRM$_{197}$ conjugate *carrier protein for hemophilus b and pneumococcal vaccines*

diphtheria equine antitoxin *investigational passive immunizing agent* (available only from the Centers for Disease Control and Prevention)

diphtheria & tetanus toxoids, adsorbed (DT; Td) USP *active immunizing agent for diphtheria and tetanus* 2•2, 2•5, 2•10, 6.6•5, 7.5•

7.5, 10•5, 12.5•5, 15•10 LfU/0.5 mL injection

diphtheria & tetanus toxoids & acellular pertussis (DTaP; Dtap; Tdap) vaccine *active immunizing agent for diphtheria, tetanus, and pertussis* [compare variants: Tdap; Dtap]

diphtheria & tetanus toxoids & pertussis vaccine (DTP) USP *active immunizing agent for diphtheria, tetanus, and pertussis*

diphtheria & tetanus toxoids & whole-cell pertussis vaccine (DTwP) *active immunizing agent for diphtheria, tetanus, and pertussis* 6.5•5•4, 10•5.5•4 LfU/0.5 mL injection

diphtheria toxin, diagnostic [now: diphtheria toxin for Schick test]

diphtheria toxin, inactivated diagnostic [now: Schick test control]

diphtheria toxin for Schick test USP *dermal diphtheria immunity test*

diphtheria toxoid USP *active immunizing agent for diphtheria* [also: diphtheria antitoxin]

diphtheria toxoid, adsorbed USP *active immunizing agent for diphtheria* 15 LfU/0.5 mL injection

dipipanone INN, BAN

dipipanone HCl [see: dipipanone]

dipiproverine INN

dipiproverine HCl [see: dipiproverine]

dipivalyl epinephrine (DPE) [now: dipivefrin]

dipivefrin USAN *ophthalmic adrenergic* [also: dipivefrine]

dipivefrin HCl USP *topical antiglaucoma agent* 0.1% eye drops

dipivefrine INN, BAN *ophthalmic adrenergic* [also: dipivefrin]

diponium bromide INN [also: dipenine bromide]

dipotassium carbonate [see: potassium carbonate]

dipotassium clorazepate INN *benzodiazepine anxiolytic; minor tranquilizer; anticonvulsant adjunct; alcohol withdrawal aid* [also: clorazepate dipotassium]

dipotassium hydrogen phosphate [see: potassium phosphate, dibasic]

dipotassium phosphate [see: potassium phosphate, dibasic]

dipotassium pyrosulfite [see: potassium metabisulfite]

diprafenone INN

diprenorphine INN, BAN

Diprivan emulsion for IV R *general anesthetic* [propofol] 10 mg/mL

diprobutine INN, BAN

diprofene INN

diprogulic acid INN

diproleandomycin INN

Diprolene ointment, gel, lotion R *corticosteroidal anti-inflammatory* [betamethasone dipropionate, augmented] 0.05%

Diprolene AF cream R *corticosteroidal anti-inflammatory* [betamethasone dipropionate, augmented] 0.05%

diprophylline INN, BAN *bronchodilator* [also: dyphylline]

dipropylacetic acid [see: valproic acid]

2-dipropylaminoethyl diphenylthioacetate [see: diprofene]

1,1-dipropylbutylamine [see: diprobutine]

diproqualone INN

Diprosone ointment, cream, lotion, aerosol (discontinued 2010) R *corticosteroidal anti-inflammatory* [betamethasone dipropionate] 0.05%; 0.05%; 0.05%; 0.1% ② Debrisan

diproteverine INN, BAN

diprothazine [see: dimelazine]

diprotrizoate sodium USP [also: sodium diprotrizoate]

diproxadol INN

Dipteryx odorata; D. oppositifolia medicinal herb [see: tonka bean]

dipyridamole USAN, USP, INN, BAN *coronary vasodilator; platelet aggregation inhibitor to prevent postoperative thromboembolic complications of cardiac valve replacement; diagnostic aid for coronary artery function* 25, 50, 75 mg oral; 5 mg/mL injection

dipyridamole & aspirin *coronary vasodilator; platelet aggregation inhibitor* 200•25 mg

dipyrithione USAN, INN *antibacterial; antifungal*

dipyrocetyl INN ② deprostil

dipyrone USAN, BAN *analgesic; antipyretic* [also: metamizole sodium] ② duoperone

dirithromycin USAN, INN, BAN *macrolide antibiotic*

Dirucotide *investigational (Phase III) synthetic peptide for secondary progressive multiple sclerosis*

disaccharide tripeptide glycerol dipalmitoyl *investigational (orphan) immunostimulant for pulmonary and hepatic metastases of colorectal adenocarcinoma, Ewing sarcoma, and osteosarcoma*

Disalcid film-coated tablets, capsules R *analgesic; antipyretic; anti-inflammatory; antirheumatic* [salsalate] 500, 750 mg; 500 mg

disalicylic acid [see: salsalate]

Dis-Co Pack (trademarked packaging form) *unit-dose package*

DisCoVisc prefilled syringes R *viscoelastic agent for ophthalmic surgery* [hyaluronate sodium; chondroitin sulfate sodium] 17•40 mg/mL

discutients *a class of agents that cause a dispersal or disappearance of a pathological condition, such as a tumor*

disease-modifying antirheumatic drugs (DMARDs) *a class of agents that slow the progression of rheumatic arthritis (RA) by modifying immune system response; this is in contrast to NSAIDs, which treat only the symptoms of the disease*

disinfectants *a class of agents that inhibit the growth and development of microorganisms, usually on an inanimate surface, without necessarily killing them* [see also: antiseptics; germicides]

Disinfecting Solution OTC *chemical disinfecting solution for soft contact lenses* [chlorhexidine; EDTA; thimerosal] 0.005%•0.1%•0.00%

disiquonium chloride USAN, INN *antiseptic*

Diskets (trademarked dosage form) *dispersible tablets*

Diskets dispersible tablets ℞ *narcotic analgesic; narcotic addiction detoxicant; often abused as a street drug* [methadone HCl] 40 mg

Diskhaler (trademarked delivery device) *inhalation powder dispenser for use with a* Rotadisk

Diskus (trademarked delivery device) *breath-activated inhalation powder dispenser* ☐ Dacex; Desoxi

Disney Pixar Cars Gummies; Disney Pixar Finding Nemo Gummies; Disney Winnie the Pooh Gummies OTC *vitamin/mineral supplement* [multiple vitamins and minerals; folic acid; biotin] ±•100•22.5 mcg

Disney Princess Complete Children's MultiVitamin chewable tablets OTC *vitamin/mineral/iron supplement* [multiple vitamins & minerals; iron (as ferrous sulfate); folic acid; biotin] ±•18•0.4•0.04 mg

disobutamide USAN, INN *antiarrhythmic*

disodium carbenicillin [see: carbenicillin disodium]

disodium carbonate [see: sodium carbonate]

disodium cefotetan [see: cefotetan disodium]

disodium chromate [see: sodium chromate]

disodium clodronate tetrahydrate [available in Canada; investigational (orphan) in the U.S.] *bisphosphonate bone resorption inhibitor for hypercalcemia and osteolysis of malignancy*

disodium cromoglycate (DSC; DSCG) [see: cromolyn sodium]

disodium dihydrogen methylenediphosphonate [see: medronate disodium]

disodium edathamil [see: edathamil disodium]

disodium edetate BAN *metal-chelating agent* [also: edetate disodium]

disodium ethylenediamine tetraacetate [see: edetate disodium]

disodium hydrogen phosphate [see: sodium phosphate]

disodium hydrogen phosphate heptahydrate [see: sodium phosphate, dibasic]

disodium hydrogen phosphate hydrate [see: sodium phosphate, dibasic]

(disodium) methylene diphosphonate (MDP) [now: medronate disodium]

disodium phosphate [see: sodium phosphate, dibasic]

disodium phosphate heptahydrate [see: sodium phosphate]

disodium phosphonoacetate monohydrate [see: fosfonet sodium]

disodium phosphorofluoridate [see: sodium monofluorophosphate]

disodium pyrosulfite [see: sodium metabisulfite]

disodium silibinin dihemisuccinate *investigational (orphan) antitoxin for* Amanita phalloides (*mushroom*) *intoxication*

disodium sulfate decahydrate [see: sodium sulfate]

disodium thiosulfate pentahydrate [see: sodium thiosulfate]

disofenin USAN, INN, BAN *carrier agent in diagnostic tests*

disogluside INN

disoprofol [see: propofol]

disopromine HCl [see: diisopromine HCl]

disoproxil *combining name for radicals or groups* [also: soproxil]

disopyramide USAN, INN, BAN *antiarrhythmic for severe ventricular arrhythmias*

disopyramide phosphate USAN, USP, BAN *antiarrhythmic for severe ventricular arrhythmias* 100, 150 mg oral

disoxaril USAN, INN *antiviral*

Di-Spaz capsules, IM injection (discontinued 2011) ℞ *gastrointestinal anticholinergic/antispasmodic for irrita-*

ble bowel syndrome (IBS) [dicyclomine HCl] 10 mg; 10 mg/mL

Dispenserpak (trademarked packaging form) *unit-of-use package*

DisperMox tablets for oral suspension ℞ *aminopenicillin antibiotic* [amoxicillin] 200, 400 mg

dispersible cellulose BAN *tablet and capsule diluent* [also: cellulose, microcrystalline]

Dispertab (trademarked dosage form) *delayed-release tablet*

Dispette (trademarked delivery device) *disposable pipette*

Dispos-a-Med (trademarked dosage form) *solution for inhalation*

distaquaine [see: penicillin V]

distigmine bromide INN, BAN

disulergine INN

disulfamide INN [also: disulphamide]

disulfiram USP, INN, BAN *deterrent to alcohol consumption* 250, 500 mg oral

disulfurous acid, dipotassium salt [see: potassium metabisulfite]

disulfurous acid, disodium salt [see: sodium metabisulfite]

disulphamide BAN [also: disulfamide]

disuprazole INN

ditazole INN

ditekiren USAN *antihypertensive; renin inhibitor*

ditercalinium chloride INN

dithiazanine BAN [also: dithiazanine iodide]

dithiazanine iodide USP, INN [also: dithiazanine]

dithranol INN, BAN *topical antipsoriatic* [also: anthralin] ⊡ deterenol

D.I.T.I.-2 vaginal cream ℞ *broad-spectrum antibiotic; antiseptic; moisturizer/lubricant* [sulfanilamide; aminacrine HCl; allantoin] 15%•0.2%•2%

ditiocarb sodium INN

ditiomustine INN

ditolamide INN

ditophal INN, BAN

Ditropan tablets, syrup (discontinued 2009) ℞ *urinary antispasmodic for urge urinary incontinence and frequency* [oxybutynin chloride] 5 mg; 5 mg/5 mL

Ditropan XL extended-release tablets ℞ *urinary antispasmodic for urge urinary incontinence and frequency* [oxybutynin chloride] 5, 10, 15 mg

diuretics *a class of agents that stimulate increased excretion of urine* ⊡ Drytex

Diurigen tablets (discontinued 2008) ℞ *diuretic* [chlorothiazide] 500 mg ⊡ DuraGen

Diuril oral suspension ℞ *diuretic* [chlorothiazide] 250 mg/5 mL ⊡ Doral

Diuril powder for IV injection ℞ *diuretic* [chlorothiazide sodium] 500 mg ⊡ Doral

Diuril tablets (discontinued 2008) ℞ *diuretic* [chlorothiazide] 250, 500 mg ⊡ Doral

Diutensen-R tablets (discontinued 2007) ℞ *antihypertensive* [methyclothiazide; reserpine] 2.5•0.1 mg

divabuterol INN

divalproex sodium USAN *anticonvulsant for complex partial seizures and simple or complex absence seizures; treatment for manic episodes of a bipolar disorder; migraine headache prophylaxis; valproic acid derivative* [also: valproate semisodium; semisodium valproate] 125, 250, 500 mg oral

divanilliden cyclohexanone [see: cyclovalone]

divaplon INN

Divide-Tab (trademarked dosage form) *scored tablet*

Dividose (trademarked dosage form) *multiple-scored tablets*

Divigel transdermal gel ℞ *estrogen-replacement therapy for moderate-to-severe hot flashes associated with menopause* [estradiol] 0.1% (0.25, 0.5, 1.0 g/pkt.)

diviminol [see: viminol]

divinyl ether [see: vinyl ether]

divinyl oxide [see: vinyl ether]

dixamone bromide [see: methantheline bromide]

dixanthogen INN

dixarit [see: clonidine]

dizatrifone INN

dizocilpine INN *neuroprotective; NMDA (N-methyl-D-aspartate) antagonist* [also: dizocilpine maleate]

dizocilpine maleate USAN *neuroprotective; NMDA (N-methyl-D-aspartate) antagonist* [also: dizocilpine]

D-Lay (trademarked dosage form) *timed-release tablet*

D-mab *a slang term for* **denosumab** [q.v.]

DMAE (dimethylaminoethanol) [q.v.]

DMARDs (disease-modifying antirheumatic drugs) *a class of agents that slow the progression of rheumatic arthritis (RA) by modifying immune system response; this is in contrast to NSAIDs, which treat only the symptoms of the disease*

DMax syrup (discontinued 2007) ℞ *antitussive; antihistamine; decongestant* [dextromethorphan hydrobromide; carbinoxamine maleate; phenylephrine HCl] 30•8•16 mg/10 mL ⚠ Diamox

DMax Pediatric oral drops (discontinued 2007) ℞ *antitussive; antihistamine; decongestant; for children 1–24 months* [dextromethorphan hydrobromide; carbinoxamine maleate; phenylephrine HCl] 4•2•2 mg/mL

DM/CPM/PE/GG syrup ℞ *antitussive; antihistamine; decongestant; expectorant* [dextromethorphan hydrobromide; chlorpheniramine maleate; phenylephrine HCl; guaifenesin] 15•2•10•100 mg/5 mL

DMCT (demethylchlortetracycline) [see: demeclocycline]

DMG (dimethylglycine) [q.v.]

DML lotion OTC *moisturizer; emollient*

DML Forte cream OTC *moisturizer; emollient*

DMO (dimethyl oxazolidinedione) [see: dimethadione]

DMP 777 *investigational (orphan) for the management of cystic fibrosis lung disease*

DM/PE/CPM oral liquid ℞ *antitussive; decongestant; antihistamine* [dextro-

methorphan hydrobromide; phenylephrine HCl; chlorpheniramine maleate] 3•1.5•1 mg/5 mL

DM/PSE/BPM syrup ℞ *antitussive; decongestant; antihistamine* [dextromethorphan hydrobromide; pseudoephedrine HCl; brompheniramine maleate] 30•50•3 mg/5 mL

DMSA (dimercaptosuccinic acid) [see: succimer]

DMSO (dimethyl sulfoxide) [q.v.]

DMT (dimethyltryptamine) *street drug* [q.v.]

DNA (deoxyribonucleic acid)

DNA polymerase [see: reverse transcriptase inhibitors; non-nucleoside reverse transcriptase inhibitors]

DNase (recombinant human deoxyribonuclease I) [see: dornase alfa]

DNR (daunorubicin) [q.v.]

Doak Tar shampoo (discontinued 2011) OTC *antiseborrheic; antipsoriatic; antipruritic; antibacterial* [coal tar] 1.2%

Doak Tar Oil bath oil, topical liquid (discontinued 2011) OTC *antiseborrheic; antipsoriatic; antipruritic; antibacterial* [coal tar (as tar distillate)] 0.8% (2%)

Doan's caplets OTC *analgesic; antirheumatic* [magnesium salicylate] 325, 377, 500 mg ⚠ Denaze

Doan's P.M. caplets OTC *analgesic; antirheumatic; antihistamine; sleep aid* [magnesium salicylate; diphenhydramine HCl] 580•25 mg

dobupride INN

dobutamine USAN, INN, BAN *vasopressor for cardiac shock*

dobutamine HCl USAN, USP, BAN *vasopressor for cardiac shock* 12.5 mg/mL injection

Dobutamine HCl in 5% Dextrose IV injection ℞ *vasopressor for cardiac shock* [dobutamine HCl] 250, 100, 1000 mg

dobutamine lactobionate USAN *cardiotonic*

dobutamine tartrate USAN *cardiotonic*

DOCA (desoxycorticosterone acetate) [q.v.]

docarpamine INN

docebenone USAN, INN *5-lipoxygenase inhibitor*

Docefrez injection ℞ *antineoplastic for advanced or metastatic breast, prostate, stomach, head, neck, and non–small cell lung cancer (NSCLC); also used for ovarian, esophageal, and other cancers* [docetaxel] 20, 80 mg/vial

docetaxel USAN, INN *antineoplastic for advanced or metastatic breast, prostate, stomach, head, neck, and non–small cell lung cancer (NSCLC); also used for ovarian, esophageal, and other cancers; analogue to paclitaxel* 10, 20, 40 mg/mL injection

docetaxel + cisplatin *chemotherapy protocol for non–small cell lung cancer (NSCLC)* [also: cisplatin + docetaxel; TC]

dock, curled; curly dock; narrow dock; sour dock *medicinal herb* [see: yellow dock]

dock, patience; sweet dock *medicinal herb* [see: bistort]

doconazole USAN, INN *antifungal* ☑ Deconsal

doconexent INN *omega-3 marine triglyceride* [also: docosahexaenoic acid (DHA)]

docosahexaenoic acid (DHA) *natural omega-3 fatty acid used to prevent a wide range of degenerative diseases; high concentrations are found in the brain, where supplementation may increase brain function; effective in treating depression and other brain disorders* [also: doconexent]

docosahexaenoic acid & paclitaxel *investigational (orphan) taxane for hormone-refractory prostate cancer*

docosanol (n-docosanol) USAN *antiviral for herpes simplex labialis; topical treatment of oral herpes simplex type 1*

docosil INN *combining name for radicals or groups*

DocQlace softgels OTC *laxative; stool softener* [docusate sodium] 100 mg

Docu oral liquid; syrup OTC *laxative; stool softener* [docusate sodium] 150 mg/15 mL; 20 mg/5 mL

docusate calcium USAN, USP *laxative; stool softener* 240 mg oral

docusate potassium USAN, USP *laxative; stool softener*

docusate sodium USAN, USP, BAN *stool softener; surfactant/wetting agent* [also: sodium dioctyl sulfosuccinate] 50, 100, 250 mg oral; 50 mg/15 mL oral ☑ Dex-Tuss DM

docusate sodium & casanthranol *stool softener; stimulant laxative* 100•30 mg

Docusate with Casanthranol capsules OTC *stool softener; stimulant laxative* [docusate sodium; casanthranol] 100•30 mg

Docusoft-S capsules OTC *laxative; stool softener* [docusate sodium] 100 mg

Docusol Mini-Enema disposable enema OTC *laxative; stool softener* [docusate sodium] 283 mg

dodecafluoropentane [see: perflenapent]

dodeclonium bromide INN

2-dodecylisoquinolinium bromide [see: lauryl isoquinolinium bromide]

dofamium chloride INN, BAN

dofetilide USAN, INN, BAN *potassium channel blocker; antiarrhythmic for the conversion of atrial fibrillation/atrial flutter*

dofosfate INN *combining name for radicals or groups*

dog grass *medicinal herb* [see: couch grass]

dog poison (Aethusa cynapium) plant *medicinal herb used as an antispasmodic and emetic in homeopathic remedies; not generally regarded as safe and effective as ingestion may be fatal*

dogbane (Apocynum androsaemifolium) root *medicinal herb used as a cathartic, diuretic, emetic, expectorant, stimulant, and sudorific*

dogwood, black; black alder dogwood *medicinal herb* [see: buckthorn; cascara sagrada]

244   DOK-Plus

DOK-Plus syrup OTC *stimulant laxative; stool softener* [casanthranol; docusate sodium; alcohol 10%] 30•60 mg/15 mL ☑ DHC Plus

DOK-Plus tablets OTC *stimulant laxative; stool softener* [sennosides; docusate sodium] 8.6•50 mg ☑ DHC Plus

Dolacet capsules ℞ *narcotic analgesic; antipyretic* [hydrocodone bitartrate; acetaminophen] 5•500 mg ☑ Dulcet

dolantal [see: meperidine HCl]

dolantin [see: meperidine HCl]

dolasetron INN *serotonin 5-HT₃ receptor antagonist; antiemetic to prevent nausea and vomiting following chemotherapy or surgery; also used to prevent radiation-induced nausea and vomiting* [also: dolasetron mesylate]

dolasetron mesylate USAN *serotonin 5-HT₃ receptor antagonist; antiemetic to prevent nausea and vomiting following chemotherapy or surgery; also used to prevent radiation-induced nausea and vomiting* [also: dolasetron]

Dolgic caplets ℞ *barbiturate sedative; analgesic; antipyretic* [butalbital; acetaminophen] 50•650 mg

Dolgic LQ oral solution ℞ *barbiturate sedative; analgesic; antipyretic* [butalbital; acetaminophen; caffeine; alcohol 7.4%] 50•325•40 mg/15 mL

Dolgic Plus oral liquid ℞ *barbiturate sedative; analgesic; antipyretic* [butalbital; acetaminophen; caffeine] 50•750•40 mg

doliracetam INN

Dolobid film-coated tablets (discontinued 2007) ℞ *analgesic; antiarthritic; antirheumatic; anti-inflammatory; antipyretic* [diflunisal] 250, 500 mg

dolomite *nutritional supplement; source of calcium and magnesium*

Dolomite tablets (discontinued 2008) OTC *mineral supplement* [calcium; magnesium] 130•78 mg

Dolono elixir (discontinued 2008) OTC *analgesic; antipyretic* [acetaminophen] 160 mg/5 mL

Dolophine HCl tablets ℞ *narcotic analgesic; narcotic addiction detoxi-*

cant; often abused as a street drug [methadone HCl] 5, 10 mg

Dolorac cream (discontinued 2008) OTC *analgesic; counterirritant* [capsaicin] 0.025%

dolosal [see: meperidine HCl]

Dolsed sugar-coated tablets (discontinued 2008) ℞ *urinary antibiotic; analgesic; antispasmodic; acidifier* [methenamine; phenyl salicylate; atropine sulfate; methylene blue; hyoscyamine sulfate; benzoic acid] 40.8•18.1•0.03•5.4•0.03•4.5 mg

dolutegravir *investigational (Phase III) antiviral for HIV infections*

dolvanol [see: meperidine HCl]

DOM (2,5-dimethoxy-4-methylamphetamine) *a hallucinogenic street drug derived from amphetamine, popularly called STP*

domazoline INN *anticholinergic* [also: domazoline fumarate]

domazoline fumarate USAN *anticholinergic* [also: domazoline]

Domeboro powder packets, effervescent tablets OTC *astringent wet dressing (modified Burow solution)* [aluminum sulfate; calcium acetate]

Domeboro Otic [see: Otic Domeboro]

Dome-Paste medicated gauze bandage OTC *protection and support of extremities* [zinc oxide; calamine; gelatin]

domestrol [see: diethylstilbestrol]

domibrom [see: domiphen bromide]

domiodol USAN, INN *mucolytic*

domiphen bromide USAN, BAN *topical anti-infective*

domipizone INN

Domol Bath and Shower Oil OTC *bath emollient*

domoprednate INN

domoxin INN

domperidone USAN, INN, BAN, JAN *antiemetic for diabetic gastroparesis and chronic gastritis*

domperidone maleate INN, BAN *antiemetic for diabetic gastroparesis and chronic gastritis* (base=78.6%)

Donatuss DC oral liquid ℞ *narcotic antitussive; decongestant; expectorant* [dihydrocodone bitartrate; phenylephrine HCl; guaifenesin] 7.5•7.5•50 mg/5 mL

Donatussin oral drops ℞ *decongestant; expectorant; for children 1–24 months* [phenylephrine HCl; guaifenesin] 1.5•20 mg/mL

Donatussin syrup ℞ *antitussive; decongestant; antihistamine; expectorant* [dextromethorphan hydrobromide; phenylephrine HCl; chlorpheniramine maleate; guaifenesin] 15•10•2•100 mg/5 mL

Donatussin DC syrup ℞ *narcotic antitussive; decongestant; expectorant* [hydrocodone bitartrate; phenylephrine HCl; guaifenesin] 2.5•6•120 mg/5 mL

Donatussin DM oral drops ℞ *antitussive; antihistamine; decongestant; for children 3–24 months* [dextromethorphan hydrobromide; chlorpheniramine maleate; phenylephrine HCl] 3•1•1.5 mg/mL

Donatussin DM syrup OTC *antitussive; decongestant; expectorant* [dextromethorphan hydrobromide; pseudoephedrine HCl; guaifenesin] 15•30•150 mg/5 mL

donepezil HCl USAN *reversible acetylcholinesterase (AChE) inhibitor; cognition adjuvant for Alzheimer dementia; also used for vascular dementia, post-stroke aphasia, and memory improvement in multiple sclerosis patients* 5, 10 mg oral

donetidine USAN, INN, BAN *antagonist to histamine H_2 receptors*

dong quai (*Angelica polymorpha; A. sinensis; A. dahurica*) root *medicinal herb for allergies, anemia, blood cleansing, constipation, female hormonal problems, hypertension, internal bleeding, menopausal symptoms, nourishing brain, and ulcers; not generally regarded as safe and effective as it contains coumarins and safrole*

Donna-Sed elixir ℞ *GI antispasmodic; anticholinergic; sedative* [atropine sulfate; scopolamine hydrobromide;

hyoscyamine hydrobromide; phenobarbital] 0.0194•0.0065•0.1037•16.2 mg/5 mL ☒ dinsed

Donnatal Extentabs (extended-release tablets), tablets, elixir ℞ *GI/GU anticholinergic/antispasmodic; sedative* [atropine sulfate; scopolamine hydrobromide; hyoscyamine sulfate; phenobarbital] 0.0582•0.0195•0.3111•48.6 mg; 0.0194•0.0065•0.1037•16.2 mg; 0.0194•0.0065•0.1037•16.2 mg/5 mL

DOPA (dihydroxyphenylalanine) [see: levodopa]

L-dopa [see: levodopa]

dopamantine USAN, INN *antiparkinsonian*

dopamine INN, BAN *vasopressor for cardiac, pulmonary, traumatic, septic, or renal shock* [also: dopamine HCl]

dopamine HCl USAN, USP *vasopressor for cardiac, pulmonary, traumatic, septic, or renal shock; also used for chronic obstructive pulmonary disease (COPD), congestive heart failure (CHF), and respiratory distress syndrome (RDS) in infants* [also: dopamine] 40, 80, 160 mg/mL injection

Dopamine HCl in 5% Dextrose IV injection ℞ *vasopressor for cardiac, pulmonary, traumatic, septic, or renal shock; also used for chronic obstructive pulmonary disease (COPD), congestive heart failure (CHF), and respiratory distress syndrome (RDS) in infants* [dopamine HCl; dextrose] 200, 400, 800 mg

dopaminergics *a class of antiparkinsonian agents that affect the dopamine neurotransmitters in the brain*

Dopar capsules (discontinued 2010) ℞ *dopamine precursor for Parkinson disease* [levodopa] 100, 250, 500 mg ☒ Daypro

dopexamine USAN, INN, BAN *cardiovascular agent*

dopexamine HCl USAN, BAN *cardiovascular agent*

Dopram IV injection or infusion ℞ *CNS stimulant; analeptic; adjunct to* *postanesthesia "stir-up"; respiratory stimulant for chronic obstructive pulmonary disease (COPD); also used for apnea of prematurity* [doxapram HCl] 20 mg/mL

dopropidil INN

doqualast INN

Doral caplets ℞ *benzodiazepine sedative and hypnotic* [quazepam] 7.5, 15 mg ⊠ Diuril

dorastine INN *antihistamine* [also: dorastine HCl]

dorastine HCl USAN *antihistamine* [also: dorastine]

doreptide INN

doretinel USAN, INN *antikeratinizing agent*

Doribax IV infusion ℞ *broad-spectrum carbapenem antibiotic for complicated urinary tract infections (cUTI), including pyelonephritis, and complicated intra-abdominal infections (cIAI); investigational (Phase III, orphan) for nosocomial pneumonia* [doripenem] 500 mg

doripenem *broad-spectrum carbapenem antibiotic for complicated urinary tract infections (cUTI), including pyelonephritis, and complicated intra-abdominal infections (cIAI); investigational (Phase III, orphan) for nosocomial pneumonia*

Dormarex 2 tablets OTC *antihistamine; sleep aid; motion sickness preventative* [diphenhydramine HCl] 50 mg

dormethan [see: dextromethorphan hydrobromide]

Dormin caplets, capsules OTC *antihistamine; sleep aid* [diphenhydramine HCl] 25 mg

dormiral [see: phenobarbital]

dormonal [see: barbital]

dornase alfa USAN, INN *mucolytic to reduce viscoelasticity of sputum in cystic fibrosis patients (orphan)*

Doryx coated pellets in capsules, delayed-release tablets ℞ *tetracycline antibiotic* [doxycycline hyclate] 75, 100, 150 mg ⊠ Droxia

dorzolamide HCl USAN *topical carbonic anhydrase inhibitor for glaucoma* 2% eye drops

dorzolamide HCl & timolol maleate *combination carbonic anhydrase inhibitor and beta-blocker for glaucoma* 2%• 0.5% eye drops

D.O.S. softgels OTC *laxative; stool softener* [docusate sodium] 100, 250 mg

Dosa-Trol Pack (trademarked packaging form) *unit-of-use package*

dose dense CAF (cyclophosphamide, Adriamycin, fluorouracil) *chemotherapy protocol for breast cancer*

dose dense epirubicin + paclitaxel + cyclophosphamide, sequential [with filgrastim hematopoietic and mesna rescue] *chemotherapy protocol for breast cancer*

Dosepak (trademarked packaging form) *unit-of-use package* ⊠ Despec

dosergoside INN

Dosette (trademarked packaging form) *injectable unit-of-use system (vials, ampules, syringes, etc.)* ⊠ Duocet

Dospan (trademarked dosage form) *controlled-release tablets*

Dostinex tablets (discontinued 2008) ℞ *dopamine agonist for hyperprolactinemia* [cabergoline] 0.5 mg

dosulepin INN *antidepressant* [also: dothiepin HCl; dothiepin; dosulepin HCl]

dosulepin HCl JAN *antidepressant* [also: dothiepin HCl; dosulepin; dothiepin]

dotarizine INN ⊠ diotyrosine

dotefonium bromide INN

dothiepin BAN *antidepressant* [also: dothiepin HCl; dosulepin; dosulepin HCl]

dothiepin HCl USAN *antidepressant* [also: dosulepin; dothiepin; dosulepin HCl]

Double Antibiotic ointment OTC *antibiotic* [polymyxin B sulfate; bacitracin zinc] 10 000•500 U/g

Double Ice ArthriCare [see: ArthriCare, Double Ice]

Double-Action Toothache Kit tablets + topical liquid OTC *analgesic; antipyretic + mucous membrane anes-*

thetic [acetaminophen + benzocaine; alcohol 74%] 325 mg + ≗

Dovonex cream, ointment, scalp solution ℞ *antipsoriatic* [calcipotriene] 0.005%

DOX (doxorubicin) → CMF (cyclophosphamide, methotrexate, fluorouracil), sequential *chemotherapy protocol for breast cancer*

doxacurium chloride USAN, INN, BAN *nondepolarizing neuromuscular blocker; muscle relaxant; adjunct to anesthesia*

doxaminol INN

doxapram INN, BAN *respiratory stimulant; analeptic* [also: doxapram HCl]

doxapram HCl USAN, USP *CNS stimulant; analeptic; adjunct to postanesthesia "stir-up"; respiratory stimulant for chronic obstructive pulmonary disease (COPD); also used for apnea of prematurity* [also: doxapram] 20 mg/mL injection

doxaprost USAN, INN *bronchodilator*

doxate [see: docusate sodium]

doxazosin INN, BAN *alpha₁-adrenergic blocker for hypertension and benign prostatic hyperplasia (BPH)* [also: doxazosin mesylate]

doxazosin mesylate USAN *alpha₁-adrenergic blocker for hypertension and benign prostatic hyperplasia (BPH)* [also: doxazosin] 1, 2, 4, 8 mg oral

doxefazepam INN

doxenitoin INN

doxepin INN, BAN *tricyclic antidepressant; anxiolytic; topical antihistamine* [also: doxepin HCl]

doxepin HCl USAN, USP *tricyclic antidepressant; anxiolytic; low-dose treatment for chronic insomnia; anxiolytic; topical antihistamine* [also: doxepin] 10, 25, 50, 75, 100, 150 mg oral; 10 mg/mL oral

doxercalciferol USAN *synthetic vitamin D analogue; serum calcium regulator for hyperparathyroidism due to chronic kidney disease*

doxibetasol INN [also: doxybetasol]

Doxidan delayed-release tablets OTC *stimulant laxative* [bisacodyl] 5 mg

doxifluridine INN, JAN *antineoplastic*

Doxil IV injection suspension ℞ *antineoplastic for Kaposi sarcoma, ovarian cancer (orphan), and multiple myeloma (orphan); investigational (Phase III) for breast cancer* [doxorubicin HCl, liposome-encapsulated] 20, 60 mg/vial

doxofylline USAN, INN *bronchodilator*

doxorubicin USAN, INN, BAN *anthracycline antibiotic antineoplastic*

doxorubicin HCl USP *anthracycline antibiotic antineoplastic* 10, 20, 50 mg, 2 mg/mL injection

doxorubicin HCl, liposome-encapsulated (LED) *anthracycline antibiotic antineoplastic for Kaposi sarcoma, ovarian cancer (orphan), and multiple myeloma (orphan); investigational (Phase III) for breast cancer*

doxorubicin + streptozocin *chemotherapy protocol for islet-cell carcinoma*

doxpicodin HCl [now: doxpicomine HCl]

doxpicomine INN *analgesic* [also: doxpicomine HCl]

doxpicomine HCl USAN *analgesic* [also: doxpicomine]

Doxy 100; Doxy 200 powder for IV infusion ℞ *tetracycline antibiotic* [doxycycline hyclate] 100 mg/vial; 200 mg/vial

doxybetasol BAN [also: doxibetasol]

doxycycline USAN, USP, INN, BAN *tetracycline antibiotic for the treatment of rosacea; antirickettsial; malaria prophylaxis* 40, 150 mg oral; 25 mg/5 mL oral

doxycycline calcium USP *tetracycline antibiotic; antiprotozoal*

doxycycline fosfatex USAN, BAN *tetracycline antibiotic*

doxycycline hyclate USP *tetracycline antibiotic; periodontitis treatment* 20, 50, 75, 100, 500 mg oral; 100 mg/vial injection

doxycycline monohydrate *tetracycline antibiotic* 50, 75, 100, 150 mg oral

doxylamine INN, BAN *antihistamine; sleep aid* [also: doxylamine succinate]

doxylamine succinate USP *antihistamine; sleep aid* [also: doxylamine]

Doxytex oral liquid ℞ *antihistamine; sleep aid; for children 2–6 years* [doxylamine succinate] 2.5 mg/2.5 mL

DPE (dipivalyl epinephrine) [now: dipivefrin]

DPF [see: Dermprotective Factor]

D-Phen 1000 extended-release caplets ℞ *decongestant; expectorant* [phenylephrine HCl; guaifenesin] 30•1000 mg ⑨ Diovan

DPN (diphosphopyridine nucleotide) [now: nadide]

DPP-4 (dipeptidyl peptidase-4) inhibitors *a class of oral antidiabetic agents that enhance the function of the body's incretin system to increase insulin production in the pancreas and reduce glucose production in the liver*

DPPC (dipalmitoylphosphatidylcholine) [see: colfosceril palmitate]

DPPE (diethyl-phenylmethyl-phenoxy ethenamine) HCl [see: tesmilifene HCl]

Dr. Brown's Home Drug Testing System OTC *in vitro diagnostic aid for detection of multiple illicit drugs in the urine*

Dr. Dermi-Heal ointment OTC *vulnerary; antipruritic; astringent* [allantoin; zinc oxide; Peruvian balsam] 1%• 2 • 2

Dr. Edwards' Olive tablets OTC *stimulant laxative* [sennosides] 8.6 mg

Dr. Scholl's Advanced Pain Relief Corn Removers; Dr. Scholl's Callus Removers; Dr Scholl's Clear Away; Dr. Scholl's Corn Removers medicated discs OTC *keratolytic* [salicylic acid in a rubber-based vehicle] 40%

Dr. Scholl's Clear Away OneStep; Dr. Scholl's OneStep Corn Removers medicated strips OTC *keratolytic* [salicylic acid in a rubber-based vehicle] 40%

Dr. Scholl's Corn/Callus Remover topical liquid OTC *keratolytic* [salicylic acid in flexible collodion] 17%

Dr. Scholl's Cracked Heel Relief cream OTC *anesthetic; antiseptic* [lidocaine HCl; benzalkonium chloride] 2%•0.13%

Dr. Scholl's Moisturizing Corn Remover Kit medicated discs + cushions + moisturizing cream OTC *keratolytic* [salicylic acid in a rubber-based vehicle] 40%

Dr. Scholl's Wart Remover Kit topical liquid + adhesive pads OTC *keratolytic* [salicylic acid in flexible collodion] 17%

Dr. Smith's Adult Care; Dr. Smith's Diaper ointment OTC *astringent; moisturizer; emollient* [zinc oxide] 10%

draflazine USAN *cardioprotectant*

dragée (French for "sugar plum") *a sugar-coated pill or medicated confection* [pronounced "drah zhá"]

dragon's claw, scaly *medicinal herb* [see: coral root]

dragonwort *medicinal herb* [see: bistort]

Dramamine oral liquid (discontinued 2011) ℞ *antinauseant; antiemetic; antivertigo agent; motion sickness preventative* [dimenhydrinate] 15.62 mg/5 mL

Dramamine tablets, chewable tablets OTC *antinauseant; antiemetic; antivertigo agent; motion sickness preventative* [dimenhydrinate] 50 mg; 50 mg

Dramamine, Children's oral liquid (discontinued 2011) OTC *antinauseant; antiemetic; antivertigo agent; motion sickness preventative* [dimenhydrinate; alcohol 5%] 12.5 mg/5 mL

Dramamine Less Drowsy Formula tablets OTC *anticholinergic; antihistamine; antivertigo agent; motion sickness preventative* [meclizine HCl] 25 mg

Dramanate IV or IM injection ℞ *antinauseant; antiemetic; antivertigo agent; motion sickness preventative* [dimenhydrinate] 50 mg/mL

dramarin [see: dimenhydrate]

dramedilol INN

Dramilin IV or IM injection ℞ *antinauseant; antiemetic; antivertigo agent; motion sickness preventative* [dimenhydrinate] 50 mg/mL ⑨ Dermolin

dramyl [see: dimenhydrate]

draquinolol INN

drazidox INN

Drepanol *investigational (orphan) for prophylactic treatment of sickle cell disease* [OM 401 (code name—generic name not yet assigned)]

dribendazole USAN, INN *anthelmintic*

dricol [see: amidephrine]

Dri/Ear ear drops OTC *antiseptic; emollient* [isopropyl alcohol; glycerin] 95%•5%

dried aluminum hydroxide gel [see: aluminum hydroxide gel, dried]

dried basic aluminum carbonate [see: aluminum carbonate, basic]

dried ferrous sulfate [see: ferrous sulfate, dried]

dried yeast [see: yeast, dried]

DriHist SR sustained-release caplets ℞ *decongestant; antihistamine; anticholinergic to dry mucosal secretions* [phenylephrine HCl; chlorpheniramine maleate; methscopolamine nitrate] 20•8•2.5 mg

drinidene USAN, INN *analgesic*

Drisdol capsules ℞ *vitamin deficiency therapy for refractory rickets, familial hypophosphatemia, and hypoparathyroidism* [ergocalciferol (vitamin D₂)] 50 000 IU

Drisdol Drops for oral or IM administration OTC *vitamin supplement; vitamin deficiency therapy for refractory rickets, familial hypophosphatemia, and hypoparathyroidism* [ergocalciferol (vitamin D₂)] 8000 IU/mL

Dristan 12-Hr. nasal spray OTC *nasal decongestant* [oxymetazoline HCl] 0.05%

Dristan Cold, Maximum Strength caplets OTC *decongestant; antihistamine; analgesic; antipyretic* [pseudoephedrine HCl; brompheniramine maleate; acetaminophen] 30•2•500 mg

Dristan Cold Multi-Symptom Formula tablets OTC *decongestant; antihistamine; analgesic; antipyretic* [phenylephrine HCl; chlorpheniramine maleate; acetaminophen] 5•2•325 mg

Dristan Fast Acting Formula nasal spray (discontinued 2009) OTC *nasal decongestant; antihistamine* [phenylephrine HCl; pheniramine maleate] 0.5%•0.2%

Dritho-Scalp cream ℞ *antipsoriatic for the scalp* [anthralin] 0.5%

Drixomed sustained-release tablets (discontinued 2008) ℞ *decongestant; antihistamine* [pseudoephedrine sulfate; dexbrompheniramine maleate] 120•6 mg

Drixoral 12-Hour Non-Drowsy Formula extended-release tablets (discontinued 2009) OTC *nasal decongestant* [pseudoephedrine sulfate] 120 mg

Drixoral Cold & Allergy extended-release tablets OTC *decongestant; antihistamine* [pseudoephedrine sulfate; dexbrompheniramine maleate] 120•6 mg

drobuline USAN, INN *antiarrhythmic*

drocarbil NF

drocinonide USAN, INN *anti-inflammatory*

droclidinium bromide INN

drocode [see: dihydrocodeine]

drofenine INN

droloxifene INN *antiestrogen antineoplastic*

droloxifene citrate USAN *antineoplastic; antiestrogen*

drometrizole USAN, INN *ultraviolet screen*

dromostanolone propionate USAN, USP *antineoplastic* [also: drostanolone]

dronabinol USAN, USP, INN *cannabinoid; antiemetic for chemotherapy; appetite stimulant for AIDS patients (orphan); investigational (Phase III) analgesic for pain associated with cancer and multiple sclerosis* 2.5, 5, 10 mg oral

dronedarone HCl *multi-channel antiarrhythmic that affects the calcium, potassium, and sodium channels; used to treat atrial fibrillation and atrial flutter*

drop chalk [see: calcium carbonate]

dropberry *medicinal herb* [see: Solomon's seal]

Drop-Dose (trademarked delivery form) *prefilled eye drop dispenser*

dropempine INN

droperidol USAN, USP, INN, BAN *general anesthetic; antiemetic; antipsychotic*

Dropperettes (delivery form) *prefilled droppers*

droprenilamine USAN, INN *coronary vasodilator*

dropropizine INN, BAN

Drop-Tainers (trademarked delivery form) *prefilled eye drop dispenser*

drospirenone USAN *progestin; spirono-lactone analogue; aldosterone antagonist; androgen and mineralocorticoid blocker*

drospirenone & ethinyl estradiol *monophasic oral contraceptive* 3•0.02, 3•0.03 mg

drostanolone INN, BAN *antineoplastic* [also: dromostanolone propionate]

drotaverine INN

drotebanol INN, BAN

drotrecogin alfa *recombinant human activated protein C (rhAPC); thrombo-lytic/fibrinolytic for severe sepsis*

DroTuss oral liquid ℞ *narcotic antitus-sive; decongestant; antihistamine; expectorant* [hydrocodone bitartrate; pseudoephedrine HCl; chlorphenir-amine maleate; guaifenesin] 2.5•15•2•100 mg/5 mL 🔾 Duratuss

droxacin INN *antibacterial* [also: drox-acin sodium]

droxacin sodium USAN *antibacterial* [also: droxacin]

Droxia capsules ℞ *sickle cell anemia treatment (orphan); also used for throm-bocythemia and as adjunctive therapy for HIV* [hydroxyurea] 200, 300, 400 mg 🔾 Doryx

droxicainide INN

droxicam INN

droxidopa INN *synthetic precursor of norepinephrine; investigational (NDA filed, orphan) for neurogenic orthostatic hypotension*

droxifilcon A USAN *hydrophilic contact lens material*

droxinavir HCl USAN *antiviral; HIV-1 protease inhibitor*

droxypropine INN, BAN

Dry Eyes eye drops OTC *moisturizer/lubricant* [polyvinyl alcohol] 1.4% 🔾 Dairy Ease; DUROS

Dry Eyes ophthalmic ointment OTC *moisturizer/lubricant* [white petrolatum; mineral oil] 🔾 Dairy Ease; DUROS

DryMax syrup ℞ *antihistamine; decon-gestant; anticholinergic to dry mucosal secretions* [chorpheniramine maleate; pseudoephedrine HCl; methscopol-amine nitrate] 4•30•1.25 mg/5 mL

Dryopteris filix-mas *medicinal herb* [see: aspidium]

Dryphen Multi-Symptom Formula tablets OTC *decongestant; antihista-mine; analgesic; antipyretic* [phenyl-ephrine HCl; chlorpheniramine mal-eate; acetaminophen] 5•2•325 mg

Drysec sustained-release tablets ℞ *decongestant; antihistamine; anticholin-ergic to dry mucosal secretions* [phen-ylephrine HCl; chlorpheniramine maleate; methscopolamine nitrate] 20•8•2.5 mg

Drysol solution ℞ *astringent for hyper-hidrosis* [aluminum chloride (hexahy-drate)] 20% 🔾 Durasal

Drytergent topical liquid OTC *soap-free therapeutic skin cleanser*

Drytex lotion OTC *keratolytic cleanser for acne* [salicylic acid; acetone; iso-propyl alcohol] ?•10%•40% 🔾 diuretics

Dryvax powder for reconstitution (dis-continued 2009) ℞ *active immuniza-tion against smallpox using the multi-ple-puncture technique (scarification); licensed for restricted use and available only from the CDC* [smallpox vac-cine] 100 million infectious vaccinia viruses/mL

DSC; DSCG (disodium cromogly-cate) [see: cromolyn sodium]

D-S-S capsules OTC *laxative; stool sof-tener* [docusate sodium] 100 mg

DSS (dioctyl sodium sulfosucci-nate) [now: docusate sodium]

DST (dihydrostreptomycin) [q.v.]

DT; Td (diphtheria & tetanus [tox-oids]) *the designation DT (or TD) denotes the pediatric vaccine; Td denotes the adult vaccine* [see: diphtheria & tetanus toxoids, adsorbed]

D-Tab film-coated extended-release caplets ℞ *decongestant; expectorant* [phenylephrine HCl; guaifenesin] 40•1200 mg

D-Tann chewable tablets, oral suspension ℞ *decongestant; antihistamine; sleep aid* [phenylephrine tannate; diphenhydramine tannate] 10•25 mg; 7.5•25 mg/5 mL

D-Tann AT oral suspension ℞ *antitussive; antihistamine; sleep aid* [carbetapentane tannate; diphenhydramine tannate] 30•25 mg/5 mL ⊞ Dinate; Duonate

D-Tann CD oral suspension ℞ *antitussive; antihistamine; sleep aid; decongestant* [carbetapentane tannate; diphenhydramine tannate; phenylephrine tannate] 30•25•15 mg/5 mL

D-Tann CT tablets, oral suspension ℞ *antitussive; antihistamine; sleep aid; decongestant* [carbetapentane tannate; diphenhydramine tannate; phenylephrine tannate] 30•25•10 mg; 30•25•7.5 mg/5 mL

D-Tann DM oral suspension ℞ *antitussive; antihistamine; sleep aid; decongestant* [dextromethorphan tannate; diphenhydramine tannate; phenylephrine tannate] 75•25•7.5 mg/5 mL

Dtap (diphtheria, tetanus, & acellular pertussis) vaccine Dtap (diphtheria predominant) is the vaccine used in the initial immunization series of infants and children 6 weeks to 6 years; compare to Tdap [see: diphtheria & tetanus toxoids & acellular pertussis (DTaP; Dtap; Tdap) vaccine]

DTaP (diphtheria & tetanus [tox-oids] & acellular pertussis [vaccine]) [q.v.]

DTIC (dimethyl triazeno imidazole carboxamide) [see: dacarbazine]

DTIC + tamoxifen *chemotherapy protocol for malignant melanoma*

DTIC-ACTD; DTIC-ACT-D (DTIC, actinomycin D) *chemotherapy protocol*

DTIC-Dome IV injection ℞ *antineoplastic for metastatic malignant melanoma and Hodgkin disease* [dacarbazine] 100, 200 mg

DTP (diphtheria & tetanus [tox-oids] & pertussis [vaccine]) [q.v.]

DTPA (diethylenetriaminepenta-acetic acid) [see: pentetic acid]

DTPA (diethylenetriaminepenta-acetic acid) technetium (^{99m}Tc), human serum albumin [see: technetium Tc 99m pentetate]

DTwP (diphtheria & tetanus [tox-oids] & whole-cell pertussis [vaccine]) [q.v.]

Duac CS gel ℞ *antibiotic and keratolytic for acne* [clindamycin; benzoyl peroxide] 1%•5% ⊞ Degas

Dual Action Complete chewable tablets OTC *combination antacid and histamine H_2 antagonist for acid indigestion and heartburn* [calcium carbonate; magnesium hydroxide; famotidine] 800•165•10 mg

duazomycin USAN, INN *antineoplastic* ⊞ dacemazine

duazomycin A [see: duazomycin]
duazomycin B [see: azotomycin]
duazomycin C [see: ambomycin]
Duboisia myoporoides *medicinal herb* [see: corkwood]

duck's foot *medicinal herb* [see: mandrake]

ducodal [see: oxycodone]

Duet chewable tablets (discontinued 2011) ℞ *prenatal vitamin/mineral/calcium/iron supplement* [multiple vitamins & minerals; calcium; iron (as ferrous fumarate and ferrous bisglycinate); folic acid] ≛•100•29•1 mg ⊞ Caduet

Duet tablets (discontinued 2011) ℞ *vitamin/mineral/calcium/iron supplement* [multiple vitamins & minerals; calcium; iron] ≛•200•29 mg ⊞ Caduet

Duet DHA tablets + capsules (discontinued 2011) ℞ *prenatal vitamin/mineral/calcium/iron/omega-3 supplement* [multiple vitamins & minerals; calcium; iron (as ferrous bisglycinate HCl); folic acid + docosahexaenoic acid (DHA)] ±•200•29•1 mg (tablets) + 200 mg (capsules)

Duet DHA^{EC} Duet DHA^EC enteric-coated tablets + capsules (discontinued 2011) ℞ *prenatal vitamin/mineral/calcium/iron/omega-3 supplement* [multiple vitamins & minerals; calcium; iron; folic acid + docosahexaenoic acid (DHA)] ±•200•29•1 mg (tablets) + 200 mg (capsules)

Duetact tablets ℞ *antidiabetic combination for type 2 diabetes that increases cellular response to insulin and stimulates insulin secretion in the pancreas* [pioglitazone HCl; glimepiride] 30•2, 30•4 mg

Duexis tablets ℞ *analgesic; antipyretic; nonsteroidal anti-inflammatory drug (NSAID) for minor aches and pains; gastric antisecretory* [ibuprofen; famotidine] 800•26.6 mg

Dulcet (trademarked dosage form) *chewable tablet* ☒ Dolacet

Dulcolax enteric-coated tablets OTC *stimulant laxative* [bisacodyl] 5 mg

Dulcolax oral liquid OTC *saline laxative; antacid* [magnesium hydroxide] 400 mg/5 mL

Dulcolax suppositories (discontinued 2007) OTC *stimulant laxative* [bisacodyl] 10 mg

Dulcolax Balance powder for oral solution OTC *laxative; bowel evacuant* [polyethylene glycol 3350] 17 g/dose

Dulcolax Bowel Prep Kit 4 enteric-coated tablets + 1 suppository OTC *pre-procedure bowel evacuant* [bisacodyl] 5 mg; 10 mg

Dulcolax Stool Softener softgels OTC *laxative; stool softener* [docusate sodium] 100 mg

DuLeek-Dp tablets ℞ *hematinic* [folic acid (as L-methylfolate)] 7.5, 15 mg

Dulera oral inhalation aerosol ℞ *combination corticosteroidal anti-inflammatory and beta agonist bronchodilator for chronic asthma* [mometasone furoate; formoterol fumarate] 100•5, 200•5 mcg

Dull-C powder for oral liquid OTC *vitamin C supplement* [ascorbic acid] 4.24 g/tsp.

dulofibrate INN

duloxetine INN *selective serotonin and norepinephrine reuptake inhibitor (SSNRI) for depression* [also: duloxetine HCl]

duloxetine HCl USAN *selective serotonin and norepinephrine reuptake inhibitor for major depressive disorder and generalized anxiety disorder; analgesic for diabetic peripheral neuropathy, fibromyalgia, and chronic musculoskeletal pain* (base=89%) [also: duloxetine] 20, 30, 60 mg oral

dulozafone INN

dumorelin INN

duneryl [see: phenobarbital]

Duocaine injection ℞ *local anesthetic; peripheral nerve block for ophthalmic surgery* [bupivacaine HCl; lidocaine HCl] 3.75•10 mg/mL

Duocet tablets ℞ *narcotic analgesic; antipyretic* [hydrocodone bitartrate; acetaminophen] 5•500 mg ☒ Dosette

DuoDerm CGF; DuoDerm Extra Thin; DuoDerm Hydroactive adhesive dressings OTC *occlusive wound dressing* [hydrocolloid gel]

DuoDerm Hydroactive paste, granules OTC *wound dressing* [hydrocolloid gel] 30 g; 5 g

Duodopa investigational (orphan) *dopamine precursor plus potentiator for late-stage Parkinson disease* [levodopa; carbidopa]

DuoDote prefilled IM auto-injectors ℞ *antidote to organophosphate nerve agents and organophosphate insecticide poisoning* [atropine; pralidoxime chloride] 2.1•600 mg

DuoFilm patch OTC *keratolytic* [salicylic acid in a rubber-based vehicle] 40%

DuoFilm topical liquid OTC *keratolytic* [salicylic acid in flexible collodion] 17%

Duohist DH oral liquid ℞ *narcotic antitussive; antihistamine; decongestant* [dihydrocodeine bitartrate; chlorpheniramine maleate; phenylephrine HCl] 7.25•2•5 mg/5 mL ⊡ Dayhist

duometacin INN

duomycin [see: chlortetracycline HCl]

Duonate-12 oral suspension (discontinued 2007) ℞ *decongestant; antihistamine; sleep aid* [phenylephrine tannate; pyrilamine tannate] 5•30 mg/5 mL ⊡ Dinate; D-Tann AT

DuoNeb oral inhalation aerosol ℞ *anticholinergic bronchodilator for chronic obstructive pulmonary disease (COPD)* [ipratropium bromide; albuterol sulfate] 0.5•3 mg/dose

duoperone INN *neuroleptic* [also: duoperone fumarate] ⊡ dipyrone

duoperone fumarate USAN *neuroleptic* [also: duoperone]

DuoPlant gel ℞ *keratolytic* [salicylic acid in flexible collodion] 17%

DuoPlavin ⊕ *investigational (NDA filed) platelet aggregation inhibitor combination* [clopidogrel; aspirin]

duotal [see: guaiacol carbonate]

Duotan PD pediatric oral suspension (discontinued 2007) ℞ *decongestant; antihistamine* [pseudoephedrine tannate; dexchlorpheniramine tannate] 75•2.5 mg/5 mL

DuoVisc prefilled syringes ℞ *dispersive/cohesive viscoelastic agent for ophthalmic surgery* [Viscoat (q.v.); ProVisc (q.v.)] 0.35•0.4, 0.5•0.55 mL

Duphalac oral/rectal solution ℞ *hyperosmotic laxative* [lactulose] 10 g/15 mL

duponol [see: sodium lauryl sulfate]

dupracetam INN

Durabac capsules ℞ *analgesic; antipyretic; antihistamine* [acetaminophen; salicylamide; phenyltoloxamine citrate] 325•250•20 mg

Durabac Forte tablets ℞ *analgesic; antipyretic; antihistamine* [acetaminophen; magnesium salicylate; phenyl-

toloxamine citrate; caffeine] 500•500•20•50 mg

Duracaps (dosage form) *sustained-release capsules*

DURAcare II solution (discontinued 2010) OTC *surfactant cleaning solution for soft contact lenses* ⊡ DairyCare

Duraclon continuous epidural infusion ℞ *central analgesic; adjunct to opioid analgesics for severe cancer pain (orphan)* [clonidine HCl] 100, 500 mcg/mL

DuraDEX extended-release tablets (discontinued 2007) ℞ *antitussive; expectorant* [dextromethorphan hydrobromide; guaifenesin] 20•1200 mg

Duradrin capsules (discontinued 2008) ℞ *cerebral vasoconstrictor and analgesic for vascular and tension headaches; "possibly effective" for migraine headaches* [isometheptene mucate; dichloralphenazone; acetaminophen] 65•100•325 mg

Duradryl syrup ℞ *decongestant; antihistamine; anticholinergic to dry mucosal secretions* [phenylephrine HCl; chlorpheniramine maleate; methscopolamine nitrate] 10•2•1.25 mg/5 mL

Duraflex Comfort gel OTC *analgesic; mild anesthetic; antipruritic; counterirritant* [aloe; methyl salicylate; menthol; camphor; capsicum; urea]

Duraflu tablets ℞ *antitussive; decongestant; expectorant; analgesic; antipyretic* [dextromethorphan hydrobromide; pseudoephedrine HCl; guaifenesin; acetaminophen] 20•60•200•500 mg ⊡ Derifil

DuraGen ℞ *resorbable graft matrix to repair the dura mater following brain surgery or traumatic injury* ⊡ Diurigen

Duragesic-12; Duragesic-25; Duragesic-50; Duragesic-75; Duragesic-100 transdermal patch ℞ *narcotic analgesic* [fentanyl] 12.5 mcg/hr.; 25 mcg/hr.; 50 mcg/hr.; 75 mcg/hr.; 100 mcg/hr.

Durahist sustained-release tablets (discontinued 2009) ℞ *decongestant; antihistamine; anticholinergic to dry muco-*

sal secretions [pseudoephedrine HCl; chlorpheniramine maleate; methscopolamine bromide] 60•8•1.25 mg

Durahist D extended-release caplets (discontinued 2009) ℞ *decongestant; antihistamine; anticholinergic to dry mucosal secretions* [pseudoephedrine HCl; dexchlorpheniramine maleate; methscopolamine bromide] 45•3.5• 1 mg

Duramist Plus 12-Hour Decongestant nasal spray OTC *nasal decongestant* [oxymetazoline HCl] 0.05%

Duramorph IV, IM, or subcu injection ℞ *narcotic analgesic* [morphine sulfate] 0.5, 1 mg/mL

duramycin *investigational (orphan) agent for cystic fibrosis*

durapatite USAN *prosthetic aid* [also: calcium phosphate, tribasic; hydroxyapatite]

Duraphen II; Duraphen 1000 extended-release tablets (discontinued 2008) ℞ *decongestant; expectorant* [phenylephrine HCl; guaifenesin] 25•800 mg; 30•1000 mg ℞ Darvon

Duraphen II DM extended-release tablets (discontinued 2007) ℞ *antitussive; decongestant; expectorant* [dextromethorphan hydrobromide; phenylephrine HCl; guaifenesin] 20•20•800 mg

Duraphen Forte extended-release tablets (discontinued 2007) ℞ *antitussive; decongestant; expectorant* [dextromethorphan hydrobromide; phenylephrine HCl; guaifenesin] 30•30•1200 mg

DuraPrep Surgical Solution self-contained applicator OTC *broad-spectrum antimicrobial prep for surgical procedures* [iodine; isopropyl alcohol] 0.7%•74%

DuraProxin; DuraProxin ES transdermal patch OTC *analgesic; mild anesthetic; antipruritic; counterirritant* [methyl salicylate; camphor; menthol] 10%•3%•1.25%

Durasal II sustained-release tablets (discontinued 2007) ℞ *decongestant;*

expectorant [pseudoephedrine HCl; guaifenesin] 60•600 mg ℞ Drysol

DuraSite (trademarked dosage form) *polymer-based eye drops*

DuraSolv (trademarked dosage form) *orally disintegrating tablets*

Durasphere injection ℞ *tissue-bulking agent for female stress urinary incontinence* [carbon-coated beads]

Dura-Tab (trademarked dosage form) *sustained-release tablet*

DuraTan DM oral suspension (discontinued 2009) ℞ *antitussive; antihistamine; decongestant* [dextromethorphan tannate; brompheniramine tannate; phenylephrine tannate] 20•8•20 mg/5 mL

DuraTan Forte oral suspension (discontinued 2009) ℞ *antitussive; antihistamine; decongestant* [dextromethorphan tannate; dexchlorpheniramine tannate; pseudoephedrine tannate] 30•3.5•45 mg/5 mL

DuraTan PE oral suspension (discontinued 2009) ℞ *decongestant; antihistamine; anticholinergic to dry mucosal secretions* [phenylephrine HCl; chlorpheniramine maleate; methscopolamine nitrate] 10•2•1.5 mg/5 mL

Duratears Naturale ophthalmic ointment OTC *moisturizer/lubricant* [white petrolatum; mineral oil; lanolin]

Duration nasal spray OTC *nasal decongestant* [oxymetazoline HCl] 0.05%

Duratuss; Duratuss GP extended-release tablets ℞ *decongestant; expectorant* [phenylephrine HCl; guaifenesin] 25•900 mg; 25•1200 mg ℞ DroTuss

Duratuss A extended-release tablets ℞ *decongestant; expectorant; analgesic; antipyretic* [phenylephrine HCl; guaifenesin; acetaminophen] 20• 600•650 mg ℞ DroTuss

Duratuss AC 12 Tannate oral suspension (discontinued 2010) ℞ *antitussive; antihistamine; sleep aid; decongestant* [dextromethorphan tannate; diphenhydramine tannate; phenylephrine tannate] 30•25•30 mg/5 mL

Duratuss CS extended-release caplets ℞ *antitussive; expectorant* [carbetapentane citrate; guaifenesin] 60•900 mg

Duratuss DA capsules ℞ *decongestant; antihistamine* [pseudoephedrine HCl; chlorpheniramine maleate] 100•12 mg

Duratuss DM elixir (discontinued 2010) ℞ *antitussive; expectorant* [dextromethorphan hydrobromide; guaifenesin] 25•225 mg/5 mL

Duratuss HD elixir ℞ *narcotic antitussive; decongestant; expectorant* [hydrocodone bitartrate; phenylephrine HCl; guaifenesin] 2.5•10•225 mg/5 mL

Duratuss PE extended-release tablets (discontinued 2008) ℞ *decongestant; expectorant* [phenylephrine HCl; guaifenesin] 30•1050 mg

Dura-Vent/DA sustained-release tablets ℞ *decongestant; antihistamine; anticholinergic to dry mucosal secretions* [phenylephrine HCl; chlorpheniramine maleate; methscopolamine nitrate] 20•8•2.5 mg

Duraxin capsules (discontinued 2007) ℞ *antihistamine; sleep aid; analgesic; antipyretic* [phenyltoloxamine citrate; acetaminophen; salicylamide] 25•325•200 mg

Durezol eye drop emulsion ℞ *corticosteroidal anti-inflammatory for ocular surgery* [difluprednate] 0.05% ⊡ Drysol

Duricef capsules, tablets, powder for oral suspension (discontinued 2008) ℞ *first-generation cephalosporin antibiotic* [cefadroxil] 500 mg; 1000 mg; 125, 250, 500 mg/5 mL

DUROS (trademarked delivery device) *implantable drug carrier, osmotically driven to provide a daily dose of several micrograms for up to one year; it is not biodegradable and must be removed or replaced when exhausted* ⊡ Dairy Ease; Dry Eyes

Dur-Tann DM oral suspension ℞ *antitussive; antihistamine; decongestant* [dextromethorphan tannate; brom-

pheniramine tannate; phenylephrine tannate] 20•8•20 mg/5 mL

Dur-Tann Forte oral suspension ℞ *antitussive; antihistamine; decongestant* [dextromethorphan tannate; dexchlorpheniramine tannate; pseudoephedrine tannate] 30•3.5•45 mg/5 mL

dusting powder, absorbable USP *surgical glove lubricant*

dutasteride USAN *5α-reductase blocker; inhibits the conversion of testosterone to dihydrotestosterone (DHT); treatment for benign prostatic hyperplasia (BPH); also used to prevent prostate cancer* 0.5 mg oral

DVP (daunorubicin, vincristine, prednisone) *chemotherapy protocol for acute lymphocytic leukemia (ALL)*

dwarf ginseng *(Panax trifolius) medicinal herb* [see: ginseng]

dwarf palm; dwarf palmetto *medicinal herb* [see: saw palmetto]

dwarf sumach *medicinal herb* [see: sumach]

Dyazide capsules ℞ *antihypertensive; diuretic* [triamterene; hydrochlorothiazide] 37.5•25 mg

dyclocaine BAN *topical anesthetic* [also: dyclonine HCl; dyclonine]

dyclonine INN *mucous membrane anesthetic* [also: dyclonine HCl; dyclocaine]

dyclonine HCl USP *mucous membrane anesthetic* [also: dyclonine; dyclocaine]

dydrogesterone USAN, USP, INN, BAN *progestin*

dyer's broom *(Genista tinctoria) flowering twigs medicinal herb used as an aperient, diuretic, stimulant, and vasoconstrictor*

dyer's bugloss *medicinal herb* [see: henna *(Alkanna)*]

dyer's saffron *medicinal herb* [see: safflower]

dyer's weed *medicinal herb* [see: goldenrod]

Dyflex-G tablets ℞ *antiasthmatic; bronchodilator; expectorant* [dyphylline; guaifenesin] 200•200 mg

dyflos BAN *antiglaucoma agent; irreversible cholinesterase inhibitor miotic* [also: isoflurophate]

Dy-G oral liquid ℞ *antiasthmatic; bronchodilator; expectorant* [dyphylline; guaifenesin] 100•100 mg/5 mL

dylate [see: clonitrate]

Dylix elixir ℞ *antiasthmatic; bronchodilator* [dyphylline] 100 mg/15 mL

dymanthine HCl USAN *anthelmintic* [also: dimantine HCl]

Dymenate IV or IM injection ℞ *antinauseant; antiemetic; antivertigo; motion sickness preventative* [dimenhydrinate] 50 mg/mL

Dynabac enteric-coated delayed-release tablets (discontinued 2008) ℞ *once-daily macrolide antibiotic for respiratory and dermatological infections* [dirithromycin] 250 mg

Dynacin capsules, film-coated tablets ℞ *tetracycline antibiotic for gram-negative and gram-positive bacteria; antirickettsial* [minocycline (as HCl)] 50, 75, 100 mg

DynaCirc capsules (discontinued 2010) ℞ *antihypertensive; dihydropyridine calcium channel blocker* [isradipine] 2.5, 5 mg

DynaCirc CR controlled-release tablets ℞ *once-daily antihypertensive; dihydropyridine calcium channel blocker* [isradipine] 5, 10 mg

dynacoryl [see: nikethamide]

Dynafed Asthma Relief tablets OTC *bronchodilator; decongestant; expectorant* [ephedrine HCl; guaifenesin] 25•200 mg

Dynafed E.X. tablets (discontinued 2008) OTC *analgesic; antipyretic* [acetaminophen] 500 mg

Dynafed Jr., Children's chewable tablets (discontinued 2008) OTC *analgesic; antipyretic* [acetaminophen] 80 mg

Dyna-Hex Skin Cleanser; Dyna-Hex 2 Skin Cleanser topical liquid OTC *broad-spectrum antimicrobial; germicidal* [chlorhexidine gluconate; alcohol 4%] 4%; 2%

dynamine *investigational (orphan) agent for Lambert-Eaton myasthenic syndrome and Charcot-Marie-Tooth disease*

dynarsan [see: acetarsone]

Dynatuss DF syrup (discontinued 2007) ℞ *narcotic antitussive; expectorant* [hydrocodone bitartrate; guaifenesin] 5•200 mg/10 mL

Dynatuss EX syrup ℞ *antitussive; decongestant; expectorant* [dextromethorphan hydrobromide; phenylephrine HCl; guaifenesin] 30•10•200 mg/5 mL

Dynex sustained-release caplets (discontinued 2007) ℞ *decongestant; expectorant* [pseudoephedrine HCl; guaifenesin] 90•1200 mg

Dynex LA dual-release caplets ℞ *decongestant; expectorant* [phenylephrine HCl; guaifenesin (50% immediate release; 50% extended release)] 30•800 mg

Dynex VR dual-release capsules ℞ *antitussive; expectorant* [carbetapentane citrate (sustained release); guaifenesin (immediate release)] 30•400 mg

dyphylline USP *antiasthmatic; bronchodilator* [also: diprophylline]

dyphylline & guaifenesin *antiasthmatic; bronchodilator; expectorant* 200•200 mg oral

Dyphylline-GG elixir OTC *antiasthmatic; bronchodilator; expectorant* [dyphylline; guaifenesin] 100•100 mg/15 mL

Dyphylline-GG ES caplets ℞ *antiasthmatic; bronchodilator; expectorant* [dyphylline; guaifenesin] 200•300 mg

Dyprotex pads OTC *diaper rash treatment* [zinc oxide; dimethicone] 40%•2.5%

Dyrenium capsules ℞ *antihypertensive; potassium-sparing diuretic for congestive heart failure, cirrhosis of the liver, nephrotic syndrome, idiopathic edema, and steroid-induced edema* [triamterene] 50, 100 mg

Dysport injection ℞ *neurotoxin complex for cervical dystonia (orphan) and facial wrinkles; also used for achalasia,*

Frey syndrome, palmar hyperhidrosis, and Tourette syndrome [abobotulinumtoxin A] 300, 500 U/vial

dysprosium *element (Dy)*

Dytan chewable tablets, oral suspension ℞ *antihistamine; sleep aid* [diphenhydramine tannate] 25 mg; 25 mg/5 mL ⌇ Detane

Dytan-CD oral suspension (discontinued 2009) ℞ *antitussive; antihistamine; sleep aid; decongestant* [carbetapentane tannate; diphenhydramine tannate; phenylephrine tannate] 30•25•15 mg/5 mL

Dytan-CS tablets, oral suspension ℞ *antitussive; antihistamine; sleep aid; decongestant* [carbetapentane tannate; diphenhydramine tannate; phenylephrine tannate] 30•25•10 mg; 30•25•7.5 mg/5 mL

Dytan-D chewable tablets (discontinued 2009) ℞ *decongestant; antihistamine; sleep aid* [phenylephrine tannate; diphenhydramine tannate] 10•25 mg

Dytan-D oral suspension ℞ *decongestant; antihistamine; sleep aid* [phenylephrine tannate; diphenhydramine tannate] 7.5•25 mg/5 mL

E₂C (estradiol cypionate) [q.v.]

EACA (epsilon-aminocaproic acid) [see: aminocaproic acid]

EAP (etoposide, Adriamycin, Platinol) *chemotherapy protocol for gastric and small bowel cancer*

ear, lion's *medicinal herb* [see: motherwort]

Ear-Dry ear drops OTC *antiseptic; astringent* [boric acid] 2.75% ⌇ Auro-Dri

Ear-Eze ear drops (discontinued 2010) ℞ *corticosteroidal anti-inflammatory; antibiotic* [hydrocortisone; neomycin sulfate; polymyxin B sulfate] 1%•5 mg•10 000 U per mL ⌇ Aerius; Iressa; Oracea; OROS; Urso

Ear-Gesic ear drops ℞ *anesthetic; analgesic; vasoconstrictor* [benzocaine; antipyrine; phenylephrine HCl] 5%•5%•0.25% ⌇ Urogesic

EarSol-HC ear drops OTC *corticosteroidal anti-inflammatory; antiseptic* [hydrocortisone; alcohol 44%] 1%

earthnut oil [see: peanut oil]

Easprin delayed-release enteric-coated tablets ℞ *analgesic; antipyretic; anti-inflammatory; antirheumatic* [aspirin] 975 mg ⌇ aceperone; azaperone; esuprone

Easter giant *medicinal herb* [see: bistort]

Easy A1C fingerstick test kit for home use OTC *in vitro diagnostic aid for glycosylated hemoglobin levels*

EasyInjector (trademarked delivery device) *self-injector*

ebastine USAN, INN *antihistamine* ⌇ epostane

ebiratide INN

ebrotidine INN

ebselen INN ⌇ epicillin

EC (epicatechin); ECG, ECg (epicatechin gallate) [q.v.]

EC (etoposide, carboplatin) *chemotherapy protocol for lung and prostate cancer and Merkel cell carcinoma*

ecadotril USAN, INN *antihypertensive*

ecalcidene USAN *antipsoriatic*

ecallantide *kallikrein inhibitor for acute attacks of hereditary angioedema (HAE) (orphan)*

ecamsule USAN *UVA sunscreen*

ecarazine [see: todralazine]

EC-ASA (enteric-coated aspirin) [see: aspirin]

ecastolol INN

Ecee Plus tablets OTC *vitamin/mineral supplement* [vitamins C and E; zinc

sulfate; magnesium sulfate] 100•
165•80•70 mg

**echinacea (*Echinacea angustifolia;
E. purpurea; E. pallida*)** root
*medicinal herb for anemia, blood dis-
eases, blood poisoning, boils, dizziness,
immune system stimulation, lymph disorders, promoting wound healing, prostate disorders, skin infections, and
snake bites*

echinocandins *a class of antifungals*
[also: glucan synthesis inhibitors]

Echinopanax horridum *medicinal herb*
[see: devil's club]

echothiophate iodide USP *antiglaucoma
agent; irreversible cholinesterase inhibitor
miotic* [also: ecothiopate iodide]

ecipramidil INN

eclanamine INN *antidepressant* [also:
eclanamine maleate]

eclanamine maleate USAN *antidepressant* [also: eclanamine]

eclazolast USAN, INN *antiallergic; mediator release inhibitor*

EC-Naprosyn enteric-coated delayed-
release caplets ℞ *analgesic; nonsteroidal anti-inflammatory drug (NSAID)
for osteoarthritis, rheumatoid arthritis,
juvenile arthritis, ankylosing spondylitis, primary dysmenorrhea, bursitis/ten-
dinitis, and other mild to moderate pain*
[naproxen] 375, 500 mg

ecogramostim BAN

ecomustine INN

econazole USAN, INN, BAN *topical antifungal*

econazole nitrate USAN, USP, BAN
topical antifungal 1% topical

Econo B & C caplets (discontinued
2008) OTC *vitamin supplement* [multi-
ple B vitamins; vitamin C] ±•300
mg

Econopred Plus Drop-Tainers (eye
drop suspension) (discontinued 2010)
℞ *corticosteroidal anti-inflammatory*
[prednisolone acetate] 1%

ecopipam HCl USAN *selective dopamine receptor antagonist for addiction*

ecostigmine iodide [see: echothiophate iodide]

ecothiopate iodide INN, BAN *antiglaucoma agent; irreversible cholinesterase
inhibitor miotic* [also: echothiophate
iodide]

Ecotrin enteric-coated tablets, enteric-
coated caplets OTC *analgesic; antipyretic; anti-inflammatory; antiarthritic*
[aspirin] 325, 500 mg

Ecotrin Low Strength enteric-coated
tablets OTC *analgesic; antipyretic;
anti-inflammatory; antiarthritic* [aspi-
rin] 81 mg

Ecovia *investigational (orphan) for
Huntington disease* [remacemide HCl]

ecraprost USAN *treatment of peripheral
occlusive disease*

ecteinascidin [see: trabectedin]

ectylurea BAN

eculizumab *monoclonal antibody; antihemolytic for paroxysmal nocturnal
hemoglobinuria (PNH; orphan); investigational (orphan) for idiopathic membranous glomerular nephropathy*

Ed-A-Hist sustained-release tablets,
oral liquid ℞ *decongestant; antihistamine* [phenylephrine HCl; chlorpheniramine maleate] 20•8 mg; 10•
4 mg/5 mL

Ed-A-Hist DM oral liquid ℞ *antitussive; antihistamine; decongestant* [dex-
tromethorphan hydrobromide;
chlorpheniramine maleate; phenylephrine HCl] 15•4•10 mg/5 mL

Ed-Apap, Children's oral liquid OTC
analgesic; antipyretic [acetaminophen]
160 mg/5 mL

Ed-Bron G oral liquid ℞ *antiasthmatic;
bronchodilator; expectorant* [dyphyl-
line; guaifenesin] 150•100 mg/15 mL

Ed-Bron GP oral liquid OTC *decongestant; expectorant* [phenylephrine
HCl; guaifenesin] 5•100 mg/5 mL

Ed-ChlorPed D oral drops ℞ *decongestant; antihistamine; for children 2–
12 years* [phenylephrine HCl; chlorpheniramine maleate] 5•2 mg/mL

Ed-Chlorped Jr. oral liquid OTC *antihistamine* [chlorpheniramine male-
ate] 2 mg/5 mL

Ed-Chlor-Tan caplets ℞ *antihistamine* [chlorpheniramine tannate] 8 mg

Ed-Flex capsules (discontinued 2007) ℞ *antihistamine; sleep aid; analgesic; antipyretic* [phenyltoloxamine citrate; acetaminophen; salicylamide] 20•300•200 mg (note: one of two products with the same name)

Ed-Flex capsules (discontinued 2007) ℞ *antihistamine; sleep aid; analgesic; antipyretic* [phenyltoloxamine citrate; acetaminophen; magnesium salicylate] 20•500•500 mg (note: one of two products with the same name)

Ed-Spaz tablets, orally disintegrating tablets ℞ *GI/GU antispasmodic; antiparkinsonian; anticholinergic "drying agent" for allergic rhinitis and hyperhidrosis* [hyoscyamine sulfate] 0.125 mg

ED-TLC; ED-Tuss HC oral liquid (discontinued 2009) ℞ *narcotic antitussive; antihistamine; decongestant* [hydrocodone bitartrate; chlorpheniramine maleate; phenylephrine HCl] 1.67•2•5 mg/5 mL; 3.5•4•10 mg/5 mL

Ed-Tuss HC syrup (discontinued 2007) ℞ *narcotic antitussive; antihistamine; decongestant* [hydrocodone bitartrate; chlorpheniramine maleate; phenylephrine HCl] 2.5•4•10 mg/5 mL

edamine [see: ethylenediamine]

Edarbi tablets ℞ *angiotensin receptor blocker (ARB) for hypertension* [azilsartan medoxomil] 40, 80 mg

edathamil [now: edetate calcium disodium]

edathamil calcium disodium [now: edetate calcium disodium]

edathamil disodium [now: edetate disodium]

edatrexate USAN, INN *antineoplastic; methotrexate analogue*

Edecrin tablets ℞ *loop diuretic for congestive heart failure, hepatic cirrhosis, and renal disease* [ethacrynic acid] 25 mg

Edecrin Sodium powder for IV injection ℞ *loop diuretic for congestive heart failure, hepatic cirrhosis, and renal disease* [ethacrynate sodium] 50 mg

edelfosine INN

edetate calcium disodium USAN, USP *heavy metal chelating agent for acute or chronic lead poisoning and lead encephalopathy* [also: sodium calcium edetate; sodium calciumedetate; calcium disodium edetate]

edetate dipotassium USAN *chelating agent*

edetate disodium USP *chelating agent; preservative; antioxidant* [also: disodium edetate] 150 mg/mL injection

edetate magnesium disodium *chelating agent for atherosclerosis*

edetate sodium USAN *chelating agent*

edetate trisodium USAN *chelating agent*

edetic acid NF, INN, BAN *chelating agent*

edetol USAN, INN *alkalizing agent*

Edex injection, pre-filled syringes ℞ *vasodilator for erectile dysfunction* [alprostadil] 10, 20, 40 mcg/mL ☑ ADEKs; Adoxa; Iodex

edifolone INN *antiarrhythmic* [also: edifolone acetate]

edifolone acetate USAN *antiarrhythmic* [also: edifolone]

edisilate INN *combining name for radicals or groups* [also: edisylate]

edisylate USAN, BAN *combining name for radicals or groups* [also: edisilate]

edithamil [see: edetate ...]

Edluar sublingual tablets ℞ *imidazopyridine sedative and hypnotic for the short-term treatment of insomnia* [zolpidem tartrate] 5, 10 mg

edobacomab USAN *monoclonal antibody to endotoxin for gram-negative sepsis*

edodekin alfa USAN *antiasthmatic; immunomodulator*

edogestrone INN, BAN

edonentan USAN *endothelin A (ETA) inhibitor for heart failure*

edoxudine USAN, INN *antiviral*

edrecolomab USAN *investigational (orphan) antineoplastic adjunct for pancreatic cancer*

edrofuradene [see: nifurdazil]

edrophone chloride [see: edrophonium chloride]

edrophonium chloride USP, INN, BAN *short-acting anticholinesterase muscle stimulant; diagnostic aid for myasthenia gravis; antidote to curare*

EDTA (ethylenediaminetetraacetic acid) [see: edetate disodium]

EDTA calcium [see: edetate calcium disodium]

Edurant film-coated tablets R̥ *nonnucleoside reverse transcriptase inhibitor (NNRTI) for HIV-1 infection* [rilpivirine (as HCl)] 25 mg

E.E.S. granules for oral suspension R̥ *macrolide antibiotic* [erythromycin ethylsuccinate] 200 mg/5 mL

EES (erythromycin ethylsuccinate) [q.v.]

E.E.S. 200 oral suspension (discontinued 2008) R̥ *macrolide antibiotic* [erythromycin ethylsuccinate] 200 mg/5 mL

E.E.S. 400 Filmtabs (film-coated tablets), oral suspension R̥ *macrolide antibiotic* [erythromycin ethylsuccinate] 400 mg; 400 mg/5 mL

efalizumab *recombinant humanized monoclonal antibody (rhuMAb) to leukocyte function–associated antigen-1 (LFA-1); immunosuppressant for moderate to severe plaque psoriasis*

efaproxiral *investigational (NDA filed, orphan) radiosensitizer for brain tumors*

Efaproxyn *investigational (NDA filed, orphan) radiosensitizer for brain tumors* [efaproxiral]

efaroxan INN, BAN

efavirenz *non-nucleoside reverse transcriptase inhibitor (NNRTI); oral antiretroviral for HIV-1 infection*

efavirenz & emtricitabine & tenofovir disoproxil fumarate *antiviral combination therapy for HIV infection in adults* 600•200•300 mg oral

efegatran sulfate USAN *antithrombotic*

efetozole INN

effector molecules *a class of cytotoxic or radioactive drugs delivered to specific tissue—usually a cancerous tumor—*

by *targeted monoclonal antibody vehicles (T-MAVs; q.v.)*

Effer-K effervescent tablets R̥ *electrolyte replenisher* [potassium (as bicarbonate and citric acid)] 10, 20, 25 mEq

Effervescent Potassium effervescent tablets (discontinued 2007) R̥ *electrolyte replenisher* [potassium (as bicarbonate and citrate)] 25 mEq

Effervescent Potassium Chloride effervescent tablets for oral solution R̥ *electrolyte replenisher* [potassium (as chloride)] 25 mEq

Effexor tablets (discontinued 2011) R̥ *selective serotonin and norepinephrine reuptake inhibitor (SSNRI) for major depressive disorder (MDD)* [venlafaxine (as HCl)] 37.5, 75, 100 mg

Effexor XR extended-release capsules R̥ *selective serotonin and norepinephrine reuptake inhibitor (SSNRI) for major depressive disorder (MDD), generalized anxiety disorder (GAD), social anxiety disorder (SAD), and panic disorder* [venlafaxine (as HCl)] 37.5, 75, 150 mg

Effient film-coated tablets R̥ *platelet aggregation inhibitor for patients with acute coronary syndrome (ACS)* [prasugrel (as HCl)] 5, 10 mg

Efidac 24 dual-release tablets OTC *antihistamine* [chlorpheniramine maleate] 16 mg (4 mg immediate release, 12 mg extended release)

Efidac 24 Pseudoephedrine dual-release tablets (discontinued 2009) OTC *nasal decongestant* [pseudoephedrine HCl] 240 mg (60 mg immediate release, 180 mg extended release)

eflornithine INN, BAN *antineoplastic; antiprotozoal; topical hair growth inhibitor* [also: eflornithine HCl]

eflornithine HCl USAN *antiprotozoal for* Trypanosoma brucei gambiense *(sleeping sickness) infection (orphan); topical hair growth inhibitor; investigational (orphan) for AIDS-related Pneumocystis pneumonia (PCP)* [also: eflornithine]

efloxate INN

eflumast INN

Efodine ointment OTC broad-spectrum antimicrobial [povidone-iodine] 1%

eformoterol fumarate BAN long-acting beta$_2$ agonist; sympathomimetic bronchodilator for asthma [also: formoterol; formoterol fumarate]

EFP (etoposide, fluorouracil, Platinol) chemotherapy protocol for gastric and small bowel cancer

efrotomycin USAN, INN, BAN veterinary growth stimulant

Efudex cream, topical solution (discontinued 2010) ℞ antineoplastic for actinic keratoses (AK) and basal cell carcinomas (BCC) [fluorouracil] 5%; 5% ⑨ Avidoxy

Efudex Occlusion Pack cream + bandages (discontinued 2009) ℞ antineoplastic for actinic keratoses (AK) and basal cell carcinomas (BCC) [fluorouracil] 5%

efungumab investigational (Phase III, orphan) for invasive candidiasis and other severe fungal infections

EGC (epigallocatechin); EGCG, EGCg (epigallocatechin gallate) [q.v.]

EGFR (epidermal growth factor receptor) inhibitors [q.v.]

Egrifta powder for subcu injection ℞ agent for the reduction of excess abdominal fat due to HIV-associated lipodystrophy [tesamorelin (as acetate)] 1 mg

egtazic acid USAN, INN pharmaceutic aid

Egyptian privet medicinal herb [see: henna (Lawsonia)]

Egyptian thorn medicinal herb [see: acacia]

EHDP (ethane hydroxydiphosphonate) [see: etidronate disodium]

Ehrlich 594 [see: acetarsone]

Ehrlich 606 [see: arsphenamine]

eicosapentaenoic acid (EPA) natural omega-3 fatty acid used to prevent a wide range of degenerative diseases; precursor to the anti-inflammatory and anticoagulant series 3 prostaglandins; effective in treating depression and other mental disorders [also: icosapent]

8 in 1 (methylprednisolone, vincristine, lomustine, procarbazine, hydroxyurea, cisplatin, cytarabine, dacarbazine) chemotherapy protocol for pediatric brain tumors ⑨ Attain

8-MOP capsules ℞ systemic psoralens for psoriasis, repigmentation of idiopathic vitiligo, and cutaneous T-cell lymphoma (CTCL); used to increase tolerance to sunlight and enhance pigmentation [methoxsalen] 10 mg

einsteinium element (Es)

eIPV (enhanced, inactivated polio vaccine) [see: poliovirus vaccine, enhanced inactivated]

elacridar HCl USAN chemotherapy potentiator; multi-drug-resistance inhibitor

elantrine USAN, INN anticholinergic

elanzepine INN ⑨ olanzapine

Elaprase injection ℞ iduronate-2-sulfatase enzyme to improve walking capacity in patients with Hunter syndrome (mucopolysaccharidosis II; MPS II; orphan) [idursulfase] 2 mg/mL

elastofilcon A USAN hydrophilic contact lens material

elbanizine INN

elcatonin INN, JAN investigational (orphan) intrathecal treatment of intractable pain

eldacimibe USAN antihyperlipidemic; antiatherosclerotic; AcylCoA transferase (ACAT) inhibitor

Eldepryl capsules ℞ monoamine oxidase inhibitor (MAOI); dopaminergic for Parkinson disease (orphan) [selegiline HCl] 5 mg

elder flower; elderberry (Sambucus canadensis; S. ebulus; S. nigra; S. racemosa) berries and flowers medicinal herb for allergies, asthma, bronchitis, colds, constipation, edema, fever, hay fever, pneumonia, and sinus congestion; also used topically as an astringent

Eldercaps capsules (discontinued 2008) ℞ vitamin/mineral supplement [multiple vitamins & minerals; folic acid] ≛ • 1 mg

Eldertonic oral liquid OTC *vitamin/ mineral supplement* [multiple B vitamins & minerals; alcohol 13.5%]

eldexomer INN

Eldopaque; Eldopaque-Forte cream OTC *hyperpigmentation bleaching agent; sunscreen* [hydroquinone in a sunblock base] 2%; 4%

Eldoquin-Forte cream OTC *hyperpigmentation bleaching agent* [hydroquinone] 4%

elecampane *(Inula helenium)* root *medicinal herb for chronic bronchitis and cough*

electrocortin [see: aldosterone]

eledoisin INN

Elestat eye drops ℞ *antihistamine and mast cell stabilizer for allergic conjunctivitis* [epinastine HCl] 0.05% ⧄ AlaSTAT

Elestrin transdermal gel in a metered-dose pump ℞ *estrogen replacement therapy for postmenopausal symptoms* [estradiol] 0.06% (0.52 mg/dose) ⧄ alosetron

eletriptan hydrobromide USAN *vascular serotonin 5-HT$_{1B/1D/1F}$-receptor agonist for the acute treatment of migraine* (base=82.5%)

eleuthero *(Eleutherococcus senticosus)* root *medicinal herb for age spots, blood diseases, depression, hemorrhage, immune system stimulation, increasing endurance and longevity, normalizing blood pressure, platelet aggregation inhibition, sexual stimulation, and stress* [previously called: Siberian ginseng]

Elevess subcu injection ℞ *dermal filler for facial wrinkles and scar remediation* [cross-linked hyaluronic acid; lidocaine] ⧄ Eliphos; Ulefsa

ELF (etoposide, leucovorin/levoleucovorin [rescue], fluorouracil) *chemotherapy protocol for gastric cancer*

elfazepam USAN, INN *veterinary appetite stimulant*

elfdock; elfwort *medicinal herb* [see: elecampane]

elgodipine INN

Elidel cream ℞ *immunomodulator for atopic dermatitis* [pimecrolimus] 1%

Eligard sustained-release subcu injection ℞ *antihormonal antineoplastic for advanced prostate cancer* [leuprolide acetate] 7.5 mg (1-month depot), 22.5 mg (3-month depot), 30 mg (4-month depot), 45 mg (6-month depot) ⧄ Allegra

Elimite cream ℞ (available OTC in Canada as **Kwellada-P** lotion) *parasiticide for scabies and lice; also used for papulopustular rosacea* [permethrin] 5% ⧄ Alimta

Eliphos tablets ℞ *calcium supplement; buffering agent for hyperphosphatemia in end-stage renal disease* [calcium (as acetate)] 169 mg (667 mg) ⧄ Elevess; Ulefsa

eliprodil INN *treatment for ischemic stroke*

Eliquis ⓔ tablets *investigational (Phase III) antithrombotic for deep vein thrombosis (DVT), venous thromboembolism (VTE), and stroke prevention* [apixaban]

Elite OB with DHA caplets ℞ *prenatal vitamin/mineral/iron/omega-3 supplement* [multiple vitamins & minerals; iron (as ferrous fumarate); folic acid; omega-3 fatty acids (DHA and EPA)] ≟•28•1.25•200 mg

Elitek powder for IV infusion ℞ *antineoplastic for leukemia, lymphoma, and solid tumor malignancies (orphan)* [rasburicase] 1.5, 7.5 mg

Elixomin elixir (discontinued 2008) ℞ *antiasthmatic; bronchodilator* [theophylline] 80 mg/15 mL

Elixophyllin capsules (discontinued 2008) ℞ *antiasthmatic; bronchodilator* [theophylline] 100, 200 mg

Elixophyllin elixir ℞ *antiasthmatic; bronchodilator* [theophylline] 80 mg/ 15 mL

Elixophyllin GG oral liquid (discontinued 2007) ℞ *antiasthmatic; bronchodilator; expectorant* [theophylline; guaifenesin] 100•100 mg/15 mL

Elixophyllin-KI elixir (discontinued 2007) ℞ *antiasthmatic; bronchodila-*

tor; expectorant [theophylline; potassium iodide] 80•130 mg/15 mL

ElixSure Children's Congestion syrup OTC *decongestant* [pseudoephedrine HCl] 15 mg/5 mL

ElixSure Children's Cough syrup OTC *antitussive* [dextromethorphan hydrobromide] 7.5 mg/5 mL

ElixSure Fever Reducer/Pain Reliever oral solution OTC *analgesic; antipyretic* [acetaminophen] 160 mg/ 5 mL

ElixSure IB oral suspension OTC *analgesic; antipyretic; nonsteroidal anti-inflammatory drug (NSAID) for minor aches and pains* [ibuprofen] 100 mg/5 mL

ella tablets R̶ *emergency postcoital contraceptive that is effective when taken up to 5 days after unprotected sex* [ulipristal acetate] 30 mg

ellagic acid INN

ellaOne Ⓔ (European name for U.S. product ella) Ⓓ aloin

Ellence IV infusion R̶ *anthracycline antibiotic antineoplastic for breast cancer (orphan)* [epirubicin HCl] 50, 200 mg/vial

elliptinium acetate INN, BAN

elm, American; Indian elm; moose elm; red elm; rock elm; sweet elm; winged elm *medicinal herb* [see: slippery elm]

Elmiron capsules R̶ *urinary tract anti-inflammatory and analgesic for interstitial cystitis (orphan)* [pentosan polysulfate sodium] 100 mg

elmustine INN

elnadipine INN

Elocon ointment, cream, lotion R̶ *corticosteroidal anti-inflammatory* [mometasone furoate] 0.1% Ⓓ Ala-Quin; Alcaine; Aloquin; elucaine

Elon Barrier Protectant liquid OTC *skin protectant*

Elon Dual Defense Antifungal Formula topical liquid OTC *antifungal* [undecylenic acid] 25%

Eloxatin IV infusion R̶ *alkylating antineoplastic for advanced or metastatic colorectal cancers; also used for non-*

Hodgkin lymphoma and advanced ovarian cancer (orphan) [oxaliplatin] 50, 100, 200 mg

elsamitrucin USAN, INN *antineoplastic*

Elspar powder for IV or IM injection R̶ *antineoplastic adjunct for acute lymphocytic leukemia* [asparaginase] 10 000 IU

Elta SilverGel 2" × 2", 4" × 4" dressings OTC *broad-spectrum antimicrobial; premedicated dressings for adjunctive burn treatment* [silver (elemental)] 55 ppm (parts per million)

Elta SilverGel gel OTC *broad-spectrum antimicrobial for minor burns and superficial cuts, lacerations, and abrasions; may be used under a doctor's supervision for serious burns, skin ulcers, skin grafts, and surgical wounds* [silver (elemental)] 55 ppm

eltanolone INN *IV anesthetic*

eltenac INN

eltoprazine INN

eltrombopag *hematopoietic; oral thrombopoietin (TPO) receptor agonist to increase platelet production in idiopathic thrombocytopenic purpura (ITP)*

elucaine USAN, INN *gastric anticholinergic* Ⓓ Ala-Quin; Alcaine; Aloquin; Elocon

elvitegravir *investigational (Phase III) integrase inhibitor antiretroviral for drug-resistant HIV-1 infection*

Elymus repens medicinal herb [see: couch grass]

elziverine INN

EMA (estramustine L-alanine) [q.v.]

EMA 86 (etoposide, mitoxantrone, ara-C) *chemotherapy protocol for acute myelocytic leukemia (AML)*

Emadine eye drops R̶ *antihistamine for allergic conjunctivitis* [emedastine difumarate] 0.05%

Embeda extended-release capsules R̶ *abuse-resistant opioid for moderate to severe pain; the sequestered opioid antagonist is released only if crushed, chewed, or dissolved in alcohol for abuse* [morphine sulfate; naltrexone

HCl (sequestered)] 20•0.8, 30•1.2, 50•2, 60•2.4, 80•3.2, 100•4 mg

embinal [see: barbital sodium]

embonate INN, BAN *combining name for radicals or groups* [also: pamoate]

embramine INN, BAN ⍰ ampyrimine; imipramine

embramine HCl [see: embramine]

Embrex 600 chewable tablets ℞ *vitamin/mineral/calcium/iron supplement* [multiple vitamins & minerals; calcium; iron (as carbonyl); folic acid] ±•240•90•1 mg

embutramide USAN, INN, BAN *veterinary anesthetic; veterinary euthanasia*

Emcyt capsules ℞ *nitrogen mustard-type alkylating antineoplastic for metastatic or progressive prostatic carcinoma* [estramustine phosphate sodium] 140 mg

emedastine INN *ophthalmic antihistamine* [also: emedastine difumarate]

emedastine difumarate USAN, JAN *ophthalmic antihistamine for allergic conjunctivitis* [also: emedastine]

Emend capsules ℞ *antiemetic for chemotherapy-induced and postoperative nausea and vomiting* [aprepitant] 40, 80, 125 mg ⍰ Immun-Aid

Emend IV infusion ℞ *antiemetic for chemotherapy-induced nausea and vomiting* [fosaprepitant (as dimeglumine)] 115, 150 mg (188, 245 mg) ⍰ Immun-Aid

emepronium bromide INN, BAN

emepronium carrageenate BAN

emetic herb; emetic weed *medicinal herb* [see: lobelia]

emetics *a class of agents that induce vomiting*

emetine BAN *antiamebic* [also: emetine HCl] ⍰ iometin

emetine bismuth iodide [see: emetine HCl]

emetine HCl USP *amebicide* [also: emetine]

Emetrol oral solution OTC *antiemetic for nausea associated with influenza, morning sickness, motion sickness, inhalation anesthesia, or food and drink indiscretions* [phosphorated carbohy-

drate solution (fructose, dextrose, and phosphoric acid)] 1.87 g•1.87 g•21.5 mg ⍰ amiterol

EMF oral liquid OTC *protein supplement* [multiple amino acids] 15 g protein

Emgel gel ℞ *antibiotic for acne* [erythromycin; alcohol 77%] 2%

emiglitate INN, BAN

emilium tosilate INN *antiarrhythmic* [also: emilium tosylate]

emilium tosylate USAN *antiarrhythmic* [also: emilium tosilate]

emitefur USAN *antineoplastic for stomach, colorectal, breast, pancreatic, and non–small cell lung cancers (NSCLC)* ⍰ amitivir

EMLA (eutectic mixture of local anesthetics) cream, adhesive disc ℞ *anesthetic* [lidocaine; prilocaine] 2.5%•2.5% ⍰ Emollia; emu oil

emmenagogues *a class of agents that induce or increase menstruation*

Emollia lotion OTC *moisturizer; emollient* ⍰ EMLA; emu oil

emollient laxatives *a subclass of laxatives that work by retarding colonic absorption of fecal water to soften the stool and ease its movement through the intestines* [see also: laxatives]

emollients *a class of dermatological agents that soften and soothe the skin*

emonapride INN ⍰ Omnipred

emopamil INN

Emoquette tablets (in packs of 28) ℞ *monophasic oral contraceptive* [desogestrel; ethinyl estradiol] 0.15 mg•30 mcg × 21 days; counters × 7 days ⍰ Umecta

emorfazone INN

Empirin tablets OTC *analgesic; antipyretic; anti-inflammatory; antirheumatic* [aspirin] 325 mg ⍰ amiperone

Empirin with Codeine No. 3 & No. 4 tablets ℞ *narcotic antitussive; analgesic; antipyretic; also abused as a street drug* [codeine phosphate; aspirin] 30•325 mg; 60•325 mg

Emsam transdermal patch ℞ *monoamine oxidase inhibitor (MAOI); once-daily treatment for major depressive dis-

order (MDD) [selegiline] 6, 9, 12 mg/day

emtricitabine USAN *synthetic cytosine analogue; antiviral nucleoside analogue reverse transcriptase inhibitor for HIV-1 infection; also used for hepatitis B virus (HBV) infection*

emtricitabine & tenofovir disoproxil fumarate & efavirenz *antiviral combination therapy for HIV infection in adults* 200•300•600 mg oral

Emtriva capsules, oral solution ℞ *antiviral nucleoside analogue reverse transcriptase inhibitor for HIV-1 infection; also used for hepatitis B virus (HBV) infection* [emtricitabine] 200 mg; 10 mg/mL

emtryl [see: dimetridazole]

emu oil *natural remedy for arthritis pain, hair loss prevention, and chronic skin disorders* ⊠ EMLA; Emollia

emulsifying wax [see: wax, emulsifying]

Emulsoil oral emulsion OTC *stimulant laxative* [castor oil] 95%

EM·V (estramustine, vinblastine) *chemotherapy protocol for prostate cancer* [also known as: estramustine + vinblastine] ⊠ EMF

emylcamate INN, BAN

Enablex extended-release tablets ℞ *selective muscarinic receptor antagonist for urinary frequency, urgency, and incontinence* [darifenacin hydrobromide] 7.5, 15 mg

enadoline INN *analgesic* [also: enadoline HCl]

enadoline HCl USAN *analgesic; investigational (orphan) for severe head injury* [also: enadoline]

enalapril INN, BAN *antihypertensive; angiotensin-converting enzyme (ACE) inhibitor; treatment for congestive heart failure (CHF)* [also: enalapril maleate]

enalapril maleate USAN, USP *antihypertensive; angiotensin-converting enzyme (ACE) inhibitor; treatment for congestive heart failure (CHF)* [also: enalapril] 2.5, 5, 10, 20 mg oral

enalapril maleate & hydrochlorothiazide *combination angiotensin-converting enzyme (ACE) inhibitor and diuretic for hypertension* 5•12.5, 10•25 mg oral

enalaprilat USAN, USP, INN, BAN *antihypertensive; angiotensin-converting enzyme (ACE) inhibitor* 1.25 mg/mL injection

enalkiren USAN, INN *antihypertensive; renin inhibitor*

enallynymal sodium [see: methohexital sodium]

enantate INN *combining name for radicals or groups* [also: enanthate]

enanthate USAN, USP, BAN *combining name for radicals or groups* [also: enantate]

enantiomer [def.] *One of a pair of chemical compounds having the same molecular formula, but with the atoms arranged in mirror image. Subdivided into* (+) *(formerly d- or dextro-) and* (−) *(formerly l- or levo-).* [see also: isomer; racemic]

Enbrel powder for subcu injection, prefilled syringes ℞ *soluble tumor necrosis factor receptor (sTNFR) inhibitor for rheumatoid arthritis, juvenile rheumatoid arthritis (orphan), psoriatic arthritis, and ankylosing spondylitis; investigational (orphan) for Wegener granulomatosis* [etanercept] 25 mg/vial; 25, 50 mg

enbucrilate INN, BAN

encainide INN, BAN *antiarrhythmic* [also: encainide HCl]

encainide HCl USAN *antiarrhythmic* [also: encainide]

Encare vaginal suppositories OTC *spermicidal contraceptive* [nonoxynol 9] 2.27%

enciprazine INN, BAN *minor tranquilizer* [also: enciprazine HCl]

enciprazine HCl USAN *minor tranquilizer* [also: enciprazine]

enclomifene INN [also: enclomiphene]

enclomiphene USAN [also: enclomifene]

encyprate USAN, INN *antidepressant*

EndaCod-C oral liquid ℞ *narcotic antitussive; antihistamine* [codeine phosphate; chlorpheniramine maleate] 10•2 mg/5 mL

EndaCod-DC oral liquid ℞ *narcotic antitussive; decongestant* [codeine phosphate; pseudoephedrine HCl] 10•30 mg/5 mL

EndaCof caplets (discontinued 2007) ℞ *narcotic antitussive; expectorant* [hydrocodone bitartrate; guaifenesin] 2.5•300 mg

EndaCof-AC syrup ℞ *narcotic antitussive; antihistamine* [codeine phosphate; brompheniramine maleate] 10•2 mg/5 mL

EndaCof-C oral liquid ℞ *narcotic antitussive; antihistamine* [codeine phosphate; chlorpheniramine maleate] 10•2 mg/5 mL

EndaCof-DC oral liquid ℞ *narcotic antitussive; decongestant* [codeine phosphate; pseudoephedrine HCl] 10•30 mg/5 mL

EndaCof-DH oral liquid (discontinued 2010) ℞ *narcotic antitussive; antihistamine; decongestant* [dihydrocodeine bitartrate; brompheniramine maleate; phenylephrine HCl] 3•4•7.5 mg/5 mL

EndaCof-DM syrup (discontinued 2009) ℞ *antitussive; antihistamine; decongestant* [dextromethorphan hydrobromide; brompheniramine maleate; pseudoephedrine HCl] 30•4•60 mg/5 mL

EndaCof-PD oral drops (discontinued 2010) OTC *antitussive; antihistamine; decongestant; for children 1–24 months* [dextromethorphan hydrobromide; brompheniramine maleate; pseudoephedrine HCl] 3•1•12.5 mg/mL

EndaCof-XP oral liquid (discontinued 2007) ℞ *narcotic antitussive; expectorant* [hydrocodone bitartrate; guaifenesin] 5•400 mg/10 mL

Endacon oral liquid ℞ *antitussive; decongestant; expectorant* [dextromethorphan hydrobromide; phenylephrine HCl; guaifenesin] 20•10•100 mg/5 mL

Endagen-HD oral liquid (discontinued 2007) ℞ *narcotic antitussive; antihistamine; decongestant* [hydrocodone bitartrate; chlorpheniramine maleate; phenylephrine HCl] 3.4•4•10 mg/10 mL ⑨ indecainide

Endal CD syrup ℞ *narcotic antitussive; antihistamine; decongestant* [codeine phosphate; chlorpheniramine maleate; phenylephrine HCl] 7.5•2•5 mg/5 mL

Endal HD syrup (discontinued 2007) ℞ *narcotic antitussive; antihistamine; sleep aid; decongestant* [hydrocodone bitartrate; diphenhydramine HCl; phenylephrine HCl] 4•25•15 mg/10 mL

Endal HD Plus syrup (discontinued 2009) ℞ *narcotic antitussive; antihistamine; decongestant* [hydrocodone bitartrate; chlorpheniramine maleate; phenylephrine HCl] 3.5•2•7.5 mg/5 mL

EndaRoid cream ℞ *corticosteroidal anti-inflammatory; local anesthetic* [hydrocortisone acetate; pramoxine] 1%•1% ⑨ Android; Inderide

endiemal [see: metharbital]

endive *medicinal herb* [see: chicory]

endive, white; wild endive *medicinal herb* [see: dandelion]

endixaprine INN

endobenzyline bromide

endocaine [see: pyrrocaine]

Endocet tablets ℞ *narcotic analgesic; antipyretic* [oxycodone HCl; acetaminophen] 5•325, 7.5•325, 7.5•500, 10•325, 10•650 mg

endolate [see: meperidine HCl]

Endometrin vaginal inserts ℞ *natural progestin; hormone replacement or supplementation for assisted reproductive technology (ART) treatments* [progesterone, micronized] 100 mg

endomide INN

endomycin

endostatin protein, recombinant human *investigational (orphan) for* neuroendocrine tumors and metastatic melanoma

endothelin-1 receptor antagonists *a class of vasodilator antihypertensives that block the action of endothelin-1 (ET-1), a vascular vasoconstrictor more potent than angiotensin II*

endothelin-A (EtA; ETA; ET$_A$) receptor antagonists *a class of anti-neoplastic agents that mediate the action of endothelin-1 (ET-1) to retard the proliferation of cancerous cells*

endralazine INN, BAN *antihypertensive* [also: endralazine mesylate]

endralazine mesylate USAN *antihypertensive* [also: endralazine]

Endrate IV infusion (discontinued 2008) ℞ *chelating agent for hypercalcemia and ventricular arrhythmias due to digitalis toxicity* [edetate disodium] 150 mg/mL

endrisone INN *topical ophthalmic anti-inflammatory* [also: endrysone]

endrysone USAN *topical ophthalmic anti-inflammatory* [also: endrisone]

Enduret (trademarked dosage form) *prolonged-action tablet* ▣ woundwort

Enduron tablets ℞ *antihypertensive; diuretic* [methyclothiazide] 5 mg

Enecat CT concentrated rectal suspension ℞ *radiopaque contrast medium for gastrointestinal imaging* [barium sulfate] 5%

enefexine INN

Enerjets lozenges OTC *CNS stimulant; analeptic* [caffeine] 75 mg

enestebol INN

EnfaCare [see: Enfamil EnfaCare]

Enfalyte ready-to-use oral liquid OTC *supplementary feeding to maintain hydration and electrolyte balance in infants with diarrhea or vomiting* 33.8 oz bottles ▣ Infalyte

Enfamil oral liquid, powder for oral liquid OTC *total or supplementary infant feeding*

Enfamil EnfaCare oral liquid, powder for oral liquid OTC *enriched formula for premature infants* [milk-based formula] 3 oz. bottles; 14 oz. cans

Enfamil Fer-In-Sol drops OTC *iron supplement* [iron (as ferrous sulfate)] 15 mg/mL

Enfamil Human Milk Fortifier powder OTC *supplement to breast milk*

Enfamil LactoFree oral liquid, concentrate for oral liquid, powder for oral liquid OTC *hypoallergenic infant formula* [milk-based formula, lactose free] 946 mL; 384 mL; 397 g

Enfamil LIPIL with Iron Nursette bottles, ready-to-use oral liquid, concentrate for oral liquid, powder for oral liquid OTC *infant formula fortified with omega-3 fatty acids* 3, 6 oz. bottles; 32 oz. cans; 13 oz. cans; 12.9, 25.9 oz. cans

Enfamil Next Step oral liquid, powder for oral liquid OTC *total or supplementary infant feeding*

Enfamil Premature Formula oral liquid OTC *total or supplementary infant feeding*

Enfamil with Iron oral liquid, powder for oral liquid OTC *total or supplementary infant feeding*

enfenamic acid INN

enflurane USAN, USP, INN, BAN *inhalation general anesthetic* 125, 250 mL

enfuvirtide *fusion inhibitor that prevents HIV from binding to T-cells, thus preventing viral entry into healthy cells*

Engerix-B IM injection ℞ *active immunizing agent for hepatitis B and D in adults* [hepatitis B virus vaccine, inactivated, recombinant] 20 mcg/mL

English elm *(Ulmus campestris) medicinal herb* [see: slippery elm]

English hawthorn *medicinal herb* [see: hawthorn]

English ivy *(Hedera helix) leaves medicinal herb used as an antispasmodic and antiexanthematous agent*

English oak *(Quercus robur) medicinal herb* [see: white oak]

English valerian *medicinal herb* [see: valerian]

English walnut *(Juglans regia) leaves medicinal herb used as an astringent*

englitazone INN *antidiabetic* [also: englitazone sodium]

englitazone sodium USAN *antidiabetic* [also: englitazone]

enhanced, inactivated polio vaccine (eIPV) [see: poliovirus vaccine, enhanced inactivated]

Enhancer powder for oral suspension ℞ *radiopaque contrast medium for gastrointestinal imaging* [barium sulfate] 98%

enhexymal [see: hexobarbital]

eniclobrate INN

enilconazole USAN, INN, BAN *antifungal*

enilospirone INN

eniluracil USAN *antineoplastic potentiator for fluorouracil; uracil reductase inhibitor*

enisoprost USAN, INN *antiulcerative; investigational (orphan) to reduce cyclosporine nephrotoxicity and acute rejection following organ transplants*

Enisyl tablets OTC *dietary amino acid supplement* [L-lysine] 334, 500 mg ⚗ anise oil; Anusol; Enseal; Unisol

Enjuvia film-coated tablets ℞ *hormone replacement therapy for severe postmenopausal vasomotor symptoms* [synthetic conjugated estrogens, B] 0.3, 0.45, 0.625, 0.9, 1.25 mg

Enlive! ready-to-use oral liquid OTC *enteral nutritional therapy* [whey protein–based formula] 240 mL ⚗ One-Alpha

Enlon IV or IM injection ℞ *short-acting muscle stimulant; diagnostic aid for myasthenia gravis; antidote to curare* [edrophonium chloride] 10 mg/mL ⚗ inulin

Enlon Plus IV or IM injection ℞ *muscle stimulant; adjunctive treatment for an overdose of curare or neuromuscular blockers* [edrophonium chloride; atropine sulfate] 10•0.14 mg

enloplatin USAN, INN *antineoplastic*

Ennds tablets OTC *systemic deodorant for ostomy, breath, and body odors* [chlorophyllin copper complex] 10 mg

enocitabine INN ⚗ ancitabine

enofelast USAN, INN *antiasthmatic*

enolicam INN *anti-inflammatory; antirheumatic* [also: enolicam sodium]

enolicam sodium USAN *anti-inflammatory; antirheumatic* [also: enolicam]

enoxacin USAN, INN, BAN, JAN *broadspectrum fluoroquinolone antibiotic*

enoxamast INN

enoxaparin BAN *a low molecular weight heparin–type anticoagulant and antithrombotic for the prevention of deep vein thrombosis (DVT), unstable angina, and myocardial infarction* [also: enoxaparin sodium]

enoxaparin sodium USAN, INN *a low molecular weight heparin–type anticoagulant and antithrombotic for the prevention of deep vein thrombosis (DVT), unstable angina, and myocardial infarction* [also: enoxaparin] 100, 150 mg/mL injection

enoximone USAN, INN, BAN *cardiotonic*

enoxolone INN, BAN

enphenemal [see: mephobarbital]

enpiprazole INN, BAN

enpiroline INN *antimalarial* [also: enpiroline phosphate]

enpiroline phosphate USAN *antimalarial* [also: enpiroline]

enprazepine INN

Enpresse tablets (in packs of 28) ℞ *triphasic oral contraceptive; emergency postcoital contraceptive* [levonorgestrel; ethinyl estradiol]
Phase 1 (6 days): 0.5 mg•30 mcg;
Phase 2 (5 days): 0.75 mg•40 mcg;
Phase 3 (10 days): 0.125 mg•30 mcg;
Counters (7 days)

enprofen [now: furaprofen]

enprofylline USAN, INN *bronchodilator*

enpromate USAN, INN *antineoplastic*

enprostil USAN, INN, BAN *antisecretory; antiulcerative*

enramycin INN

enrofloxacin USAN, INN, BAN *veterinary antibacterial*

Enseal (trademarked dosage form) *enteric-coated tablet* ⚗ anise oil; Anusol; Enisyl; Unisol

Ensure oral liquid, powder for oral liquid OTC *enteral nutritional therapy* [lactose-free formula]

Ensure pudding OTC *enteral nutritional therapy* [milk-based formula] 150 g

Ensure Glucerna beverage, bars OTC *diabetic nutritional supplements/snacks*

Ensure High Calcium ready-to-use oral liquid OTC *enteral nutritional therapy for postmenopausal women*

Ensure High Protein ready-to-use oral liquid OTC *enteral nutritional therapy* [lactose-free formula] 237 mL

Ensure HN; Ensure with Fiber ready-to-use oral liquid OTC *enteral nutritional therapy* [lactose-free formula]

Ensure Plus; Ensure Plus HN oral liquid OTC *enteral nutritional therapy* [lactose-free formula]

EN-tab (trademarked dosage form) *enteric-coated tablet*

entacapone USAN COMT *(catechol-O-methyltransferase) inhibitor for Parkinson disease*

entecavir USAN *nucleoside reverse transcriptase inhibitor (NRTI); antiviral for chronic hepatitis B virus (HBV) infection*

enteramine [see: serotonin]

Entereg capsules ℞ *peripherally acting opioid receptor antagonist for postoperative ileus (POI); restores normal bowel function after surgery* [alvimopan] 12 mg

Entero Vu oral suspension (discontinued 2009) ℞ *radiopaque contrast agent for small bowel imaging* [barium sulfate] 13%, 24% in 600 mL

Entero Vu powder for oral liquid ℞ *radiopaque contrast agent for small bowel imaging* [barium sulfate] 100 g packets

Entero-Test; Entero-Test Pediatric string capsules for professional use ℞ *in vitro diagnostic aid for GI disorders*

Entertainer's Secret throat spray OTC *saliva substitute*

Entex oral liquid ℞ *decongestant; expectorant* [phenylephrine HCl; guaifenesin] 7.5•100 mg/5 mL

Entex ER extended-release capsules (discontinued 2007) ℞ *decongestant; expectorant* [phenylephrine HCl; guaifenesin] 10•300 mg

Entex HC oral liquid ℞ *narcotic antitussive; decongestant; expectorant* [hydrocodone bitartrate; pseudoephedrine HCl; guaifenesin] 3.75•22.5•50 mg/5 mL

Entex LA dual-release capsules ℞ *decongestant; expectorant* [phenylephrine HCl (extended release); guaifenesin (immediate release)] 30•400 mg

Entex LA dual-release tablets ℞ *decongestant; expectorant (50% immediate release; 50% extended release)* [phenylephrine HCl; guaifenesin] 30•800 mg

Entex LQ oral liquid OTC *decongestant; expectorant* [phenylephrine HCl; guaifenesin] 10•100 mg/5 mL

Entex PSE dual-release capsules ℞ *decongestant; expectorant* [pseudoephedrine HCl (extended release); guaifenesin (immediate release)] 120•400 mg

Entex PSE sustained-release caplets ℞ *decongestant; expectorant* [pseudoephedrine HCl; guaifenesin] 50•525 mg

Entocort EC oral capsules for ileal release ℞ *corticosteroidal anti-inflammatory for Crohn disease* [budesonide (micronized)] 3 mg

Entri-Pak (delivery form) *liquid-filled pouch*

Entrition 0.5 oral liquid (discontinued 2008) OTC *enteral nutritional therapy* [lactose-free formula]

Entrition HN Entri-Pak (liquid-filled pouch) OTC *enteral nutritional therapy* [lactose-free formula]

Entrobar oral suspension ℞ *radiopaque contrast medium for gastrointestinal imaging* [barium sulfate] 50%

EntroEase oral suspension (discontinued 2008) ℞ *radiopaque contrast medium for gastrointestinal imaging* [barium sulfate] 13%

EntroEase Dry powder for oral suspension (discontinued 2008) ℞ *radiopaque contrast medium for gastrointestinal imaging* [barium sulfate] 92%

Entsol nasal spray, intranasal gel OTC *nasal moisturizer* [sodium chloride (saline solution)] 🄰 Antizol

Entsol Nasal Wash solution OTC *nasal irrigant and moisturizer* [sodium chloride (saline solution)]

entsufon INN *detergent* [also: entsufon sodium]

entsufon sodium USAN *detergent* [also: entsufon]

Entuss oral liquid (discontinued 2007) ℞ *narcotic antitussive; expectorant* [hydrocodone bitartrate; potassium guaiacolsulfonate] 5•300 mg/5 mL

Enuclene eye drops OTC *cleaning, wetting and lubricating agent for artificial eyes* [tyloxapol] 0.25%

Enulose oral/rectal solution ℞ *synthetic disaccharide used to prevent and treat portal-systemic encephalopathy* [lactulose] 10 g/15 mL

enviomycin INN

enviradene USAN, INN *antiviral*

Enviro-Stress slow-release tablets (discontinued 2008) OTC *vitamin/mineral supplement* [multiple vitamins & minerals; folic acid] ±•0.4 mg

enviroxime USAN, INN *antiviral*

enzacamene USAN *ultraviolet sunscreen*

Enzone cream ℞ *corticosteroidal anti-inflammatory; anesthetic* [hydrocortisone acetate; pramoxine HCl] 1%•1% 🄰 Anacin; inosine; Unasyn

Enzymatic Cleaner for Extended Wear tablets (discontinued 2010) OTC *enzymatic cleaner for soft contact lenses* [pork pancreatin]

E-Oil oral concentrate, topical liquid OTC *vitamin supplement* [vitamin E] 100 IU/0.25 mL

Eovist IV injection ℞ *paramagnetic contrast agent for MRIs of the liver* [gadoxetate disodium] 181.43 mg/mL in 10 mL vials 🄰 Evista

EP (etoposide, Platinol) [with or without filgrastim hematopoietic]

chemotherapy protocol for adenocarcinoma, lung cancer, testicular cancer, neuroendocrine tumors, and thymoma

EPA capsules (discontinued 2008) OTC *dietary supplement* [omega-3 fatty acids (eicosapentaenoic acid and docosahexaenoic acid)] 1000 mg (180 mg EPA; 120 mg DHA)

EPA (eicosapentaenoic acid) [q.v.; also: icosapent]

epalrestat INN *treatment for diabetic neuropathy*

epanolol USAN, INN, BAN

eperezolid USAN *antibacterial*

eperisone INN 🄰 euprocin

epervudine INN

ephedra (*Ephedra* spp.) plant *medicinal herb for asthma, blood cleansing, bronchitis, bursitis, chills, colds, edema, fever, flu, headache, kidney disorders, nasal congestion, and venereal disease* 🄰 Ivy-Dry

ephedrine USP, BAN *sympathomimetic bronchodilator; nasal decongestant; vasopressor for shock*

ephedrine HCl USP, BAN *sympathomimetic bronchodilator; nasal decongestant; vasopressor for shock*

ephedrine sulfate USP *sympathomimetic bronchodilator; nasal decongestant; vasopressor for acute hypotensive shock* [also: ephedrine sulphate] 25 mg oral; 50 mg/mL injection

ephedrine sulphate BAN *sympathomimetic bronchodilator; nasal decongestant* [also: ephedrine sulfate]

ephedrine tannate *sympathomimetic bronchodilator; nasal decongestant*

Epi-C concentrated oral suspension ℞ *radiopaque contrast medium for gastrointestinal imaging* [barium sulfate] 150% 🄰 APC; Apo-K; EPOCH

epicainide INN

epicatechin (EC); epicatechin gallate (ECG; ECg) *natural polyphenolic antioxidants found in green tea, believed to be primarily responsible for its anticarcinogenic property* [see also: epicatechins; epigallocatechin]

epicatechins *a class of natural polyphenolic antioxidants found in green tea and grape seed extract, used for their anticarcinogenic, anti-inflammatory, and antiatherosclerotic properties and to promote thermogenesis* [see also: catechins; kunecatechins]

epicillin USAN, INN, BAN *antibacterial* ⊉ ebselen

EpiCream ℞ *moisturizer; emollient*

epicriptine INN

epidermal growth factor (EGF), human *investigational (orphan) for acceleration of corneal regeneration and the healing of severe burns*

epidermal growth factor receptor (EGFR) inhibitors *a class of antineoplastics, predominantly monoclonal antibodies, that suppress the growth of breast, colorectal, head, and neck cancers; includes HER1 (q.v.), HER2 (q.v.), HER3, and HER4* [also known as: human epidermal growth factor receptor (HER) inhibitors]

Epidrin capsules ℞ *cerebral vasoconstrictor and analgesic for vascular and tension headaches; "possibly effective" for migraine headaches* [isometheptene mucate; dichloralphenazone; acetaminophen] 65•100•325 mg

Epiduo gel ℞ *synthetic retinoid analogue; keratolytic* [adapalene; benzoyl peroxide] 0.1%•2.5%

epiestriol INN [also: epioestriol] ⊉ Abstral

Epifoam aerosol foam ℞ *corticosteroidal anti-inflammatory; anesthetic* [hydrocortisone acetate; pramoxine] 1%•1%

epigallocatechin (EGC); epigallocatechin gallate (EGCG; EGCg) *natural polyphenolic antioxidants found in green tea, believed to be primarily responsible for its anticarcinogenic property* [see also: epicatechins]

epilin [see: dietifen]

Epilyt lotion concentrate OTC *moisturizer; emollient*

epimestrol USAN, INN, BAN *anterior pituitary activator*

Epinal eye drops (discontinued 2009) ℞ *antiglaucoma agent* [epinephryl borate] 0.5%, 1% ⊉ Abenol

epinastine INN *antihistamine and mast cell stabilizer* [also: epinastine HCl]

epinastine HCl *antihistamine and mast cell stabilizer for allergic conjunctivitis* [also: epinastine] 0.05% eye drops

epinephran [see: epinephrine]

epinephrine USP, INN *vasoconstrictor; sympathomimetic bronchodilator; topical antiglaucoma agent; vasopressor for shock; emergency treatment of anaphylaxis* [also: adrenaline] 1:1000 (0.1 mg/mL) injection

epinephrine bitartrate USP *sympathomimetic bronchodilator; ophthalmic adrenergic; topical antiglaucoma agent*

epinephrine bitartrate & articaine HCl *vasoconstrictor; local anesthetic* ⊉•4% injection

epinephrine bitartrate & prilocaine HCl *vasoconstrictor; local anesthetic* 0.005 mg/mL•4% injection

epinephrine borate *topical antiglaucoma agent*

epinephrine & cisplatin *investigational (NDA filed, orphan) injectable gel for squamous cell carcinoma of the head and neck; investigational (orphan) for metastatic malignant melanoma*

epinephrine HCl *sympathomimetic bronchodilator; nasal decongestant; topical antiglaucoma agent; vasopressor for shock; emergency treatment of anaphylaxis* 0.1% eye drops; 1:1000, 1:10 000 (1, 0.1 mg/mL) injection

Epinephrine Mist inhalation aerosol OTC *sympathomimetic bronchodilator and vasopressor for bronchial asthma* [epinephrine] 0.22 mg/spray

epinephryl borate USAN, USP *adrenergic; topical antiglaucoma agent*

epioestriol BAN [also: epiestriol] ⊉ Abstral

EpiPen; EpiPen Jr. auto-injector (automatic IM injection device) ℞ *vasopressor for shock; emergency treatment of anaphylaxis* [epinephrine] 1:1000 (1 mg/mL); 1:2000 (0.5 mg/mL)

epipropidine USAN, INN *antineoplastic*

EpiQuin Micro cream ℞ *hyperpigmentation bleaching agent* [hydroquinone (in a base containing vitamins A, C, and E)] 4%

epirizole USAN, INN *analgesic; antiinflammatory*

epiroprim INN

epirubicin INN, BAN *anthracycline antibiotic antineoplastic* [also: epirubicin HCl]

epirubicin HCl USAN, JAN *anthracycline antibiotic antineoplastic for breast cancer (orphan)* [also: epirubicin] 10, 50, 200 mg/vial injection

epirubicin + paclitaxel + cyclophosphamide, sequential, dose dense [with filgrastim hematopoietic and mesna rescue] *chemotherapy protocol for breast cancer*

epitetracycline HCl USP *antibacterial*

epithiazide USAN, BAN *antihypertensive; diuretic* [also: epitizide]

epithioandrostanol [see: epitiostanol]

epitiostanol INN

epitizide INN *antihypertensive; diuretic* [also: epithiazide]

Epitol tablets ℞ *iminostilbene anticonvulsant; analgesic for trigeminal neuralgia; also used for restless legs syndrome (RLS), alcohol withdrawal, and postherpetic neuralgia* [carbamazepine] 200 mg ⊘ Apetil

Epivir film-coated tablets, oral solution ℞ *antiviral for HIV infection* [lamivudine] 150, 300 mg; 10 mg/mL

Epivir-HBV film-coated caplets, oral solution ℞ *antiviral for hepatitis B virus (HBV) infection* [lamivudine] 100 mg; 5 mg/mL

eplerenone USAN *aldosterone receptor antagonist for hypertension and congestive heart failure (CHF); improves survival after a cardiovascular event* 25, 50 mg oral

EPO (epoetin alfa) [q.v.]

EPO (evening primrose oil) [see: evening primrose]

EPOCH (etoposide, prednisone, Oncovin, cyclophosphamide, hydroxydaunomycin) [with Bactrim antibiotic] *chemotherapy protocol for non-Hodgkin lymphoma* ⊘ APC; Apo-K; Epi-C

EPOCH, dose-adjusted [with filgrastim hematopoietic and Bactrim plus azithromycin or clarithromycin antibiotic] *chemotherapy protocol for B-cell lymphoma and non-Hodgkin lymphoma associated with HIV infections* [see: EPOCH]

epoetin alfa (EPO) USAN, INN, BAN, JAN *hematopoietic to stimulate RBC production for anemia of chronic renal failure, HIV, and chemotherapy (orphan) and to reduce the need for blood transfusions in surgery; investigational (orphan) for myelodysplastic syndrome*

epoetin beta USAN, INN, BAN, JAN *erythropoiesis-stimulating agent (ESA) for the treatment of anemia due to chronic renal failure (orphan)*

Epogen IV or subcu injection ℞ *hematopoietic to stimulate RBC production for anemia of chronic renal failure, HIV, and chemotherapy (orphan) and to reduce the need for blood transfusions in surgery* [epoetin alfa] 2000, 3000, 4000, 10 000, 20 000 U/mL ⊘ Apokyn; Opcon-A

epoprostenol USAN, INN *platelet aggregation inhibitor and vasodilator for pulmonary hypertension (orphan); investigational (orphan) heparin replacement for hemodialysis*

epoprostenol sodium USAN, BAN *platelet aggregation inhibitor and vasodilator for pulmonary hypertension (orphan); investigational (orphan) heparin replacement for hemodialysis* 0.5, 1.5 mg injection

epostane USAN, INN, BAN *interceptive* ⊘ ebastine

epoxytropine tropate methylbromide [see: methscopolamine bromide]

epratuzumab *investigational (Phase III, orphan) monoclonal antibody to CD22, radiolabeled with yttrium Y 90 for AIDS-related non-Hodgkin lymphoma;*

investigational (Phase III) for systemic
lupus erythematosus (SLE)

eprazinone INN

eprinomectin USAN veterinary antiparasitic

epristeride USAN, INN, BAN alpha reductase inhibitor

eprosartan USAN angiotensin receptor blocker (ARB) for hypertension

eprosartan mesylate USAN angiotensin receptor blocker (ARB) for hypertension

eprovafen INN

eproxindine INN

eprozinol INN

epsikapron [see: aminocaproic acid]

epsilon-aminocaproic acid (EACA) [see: aminocaproic acid]

epsiprantel INN, BAN

Epsom salt granules OTC saline laxative [magnesium sulfate]

Epsom salt [see: magnesium sulfate]

e.p.t. Quick Stick test stick for home use OTC in vitro diagnostic aid; urine pregnancy test

eptacog alfa (activated) activated recombinant human blood coagulation Factor VII (rFVIIa) for hemophilia A and B

eptaloprost INN

eptamestrol [see: etamestrol]

eptaprost [see: eptaloprost]

eptastatin sodium [see: pravastatin sodium]

eptastigmine INN treatment for Alzheimer disease

eptazocine INN

eptifibatide glycoprotein (GP) IIb/IIIa receptor antagonist; platelet aggregation inhibitor for acute coronary syndrome, unstable angina, myocardial infarction, and cardiac surgery

Epulor oral liquid OTC enteral nutritional therapy [milk-based formula] 1.5 oz./pouch

Epzicom film-coated caplets ℞ once-daily antiretroviral nucleoside reverse transcriptase inhibitor (NRTI) for HIV infection [abacavir (as sulfate); lamivudine] 600•300 mg

Equagesic tablets ℞ analgesic; antipyretic; anti-inflammatory; anxiolytic; sedative [aspirin; meprobamate] 325•200 mg

Equalactin chewable tablets OTC bulk laxative; antidiarrheal [calcium polycarbophil] 625 mg

Equetro extended-release capsules ℞ iminostilbene antipsychotic for manic episodes of a bipolar disorder; also used for restless legs syndrome (RLS), alcohol withdrawal, and postherpetic neuralgia [carbamazepine] 100, 200, 300 mg

Equilet chewable tablets OTC antacid; calcium supplement [calcium (as carbonate)] 200 mg (500 mg) ⊡ Accolate

equilin USP estrogen

Equipoise brand name for boldenone undecylenate, a veterinary anabolic steroid abused as a street drug ⊡ Aquabase

Equisetum arvens medicinal herb [see: horsetail]

Eraxis powder for IV infusion ℞ antifungal for candidemia of the internal organs, esophageal candidiasis, and other serious fungal infections [anidulafungin] 50, 100 mg/vial

Erbitux IV infusion ℞ antineoplastic for metastatic colorectal cancer and squamous cell carcinoma (SCC) of the head and neck (orphan); investigational (Phase III) for brain, breast, bladder, gastric, lung, prostate, and pancreatic cancers [cetuximab] 100, 200 mg/vial

erbium element (Er) ⊡ europium

erbulozole USAN, INN antineoplastic adjunct

erbumine USAN, INN, BAN combining name for radicals or groups

Ercaf tablets ℞ migraine-specific vasoconstrictor [ergotamine tartrate; caffeine] 1•100 mg ⊡ Airacof

erdosteine INN

Erechtites hieracfolia medicinal herb [see: pilewort]

ergocalciferol (vitamin D₂) USP, INN, BAN, JAN fat-soluble vitamin for refractory rickets, familial hypophosphatemia, *and hypoparathyroidism* (1 mg=40 000 IU) 50 000 U oral; 8000 U/mL oral

ergoloid mesylates USAN, USP *cognition adjuvant for age-related mental capacity decline* [also: co-dergocrine mesylate] 0.5, 1 mg oral

Ergomar sublingual tablets ℞ *prophylaxis or treatment of migraine and other vascular headaches* [ergotamine tartrate] 2 mg

ergometrine INN, BAN *oxytocic for induction of labor* [also: ergonovine maleate]

ergonovine maleate USP *oxytocic for the induction of labor and prevention of postpartum and postabortal hemorrhage* [also: ergometrine]

ergosterol, activated [see: ergocalciferol]

ergot (*Claviceps purpurea*) dried sclerotia *medicinal herb used as an abortifacient, emmenagogue, hemostatic, oxytocic, and vasoconstrictor; source of ergotamine and LSD* ☒ Irrigate

ergot alkaloids [see: ergoloid mesylates]

ergotamine INN, BAN *migraine-specific analgesic* [also: ergotamine tartrate]

ergotamine tartrate USP *prophylaxis or treatment of migraine and other vascular headaches* [also: ergotamine]

ergotamine tartrate & caffeine *prophylaxis or treatment of migraine and other vascular headaches* 1•100 mg oral

Ergotrate Maleate tablets ℞ *oxytocic for the induction of labor and prevention of postpartum and postabortal hemorrhage* [ergonovine maleate] 0.2 mg

eribulin mesylate *microtubulin inhibitor antineoplastic for metastatic breast cancer; derived from the Japanese black sponge*

ericolol INN

Erigeron canadensis medicinal herb [see: fleabane; horseweed]

eriodictyon NF

Eriodictyon californicum medicinal herb [see: yerba santa]

eritrityl tetranitrate INN *coronary vasodilator* [also: erythrityl tetranitrate]

erizepine INN ☒ AeroSpan

erlizumab USAN *monoclonal antibody to treat reperfusion injury following acute myocardial infarction*

erlotinib HCl *human epidermal growth factor receptor type 1 (HER1) inhibitor; tyrosine kinase inhibitor; antineoplastic for advanced or metastatic non–small cell lung and pancreatic cancer; investigational (orphan) for malignant gliomas* (base=91.5%)

E-R-O Ear Drops OTC *cerumenolytic to emulsify and disperse ear wax* [carbamide peroxide] 6.5% ☒ Auro Ear Drops

erocainide INN

errhines *a class of agents that promote nasal discharge or secretion* ☒ Orencia; Orinase

Errin tablets (in packs of 28) ℞ *oral contraceptive (progestin only)* [norethindrone] 0.35 mg ☒ iron

ersofermin USAN, INN *wound healing agent; transglutaminase inhibitor for the treatment of scar tissue*

Ertaczo cream ℞ *antifungal* [sertaconazole nitrate] 2%

ertapenem sodium USAN *broad-spectrum carbapenem antibiotic*

Erwinase *investigational (orphan) antineoplastic for acute lymphocytic leukemia* [erwinia L-asparaginase]

erwinia L-asparaginase *investigational (orphan) antineoplastic for acute lymphocytic leukemia*

Ery Pads pledgets ℞ *antibiotic for acne* [erythromycin; alcohol 60.5%] 2%

Eryc delayed-release capsules containing enteric-coated pellets ℞ *macrolide antibiotic* [erythromycin] 250 mg ☒ ara-G; ARC

EryDerm 2% topical solution ℞ *antibiotic for acne* [erythromycin; alcohol 77%] 2%

Erygel gel ℞ *antibiotic for acne* [erythromycin; alcohol 92%] 2% ☒ Orajel

Eryngium aquaticum medicinal herb [see: water eryngo]

EryPed oral drops ℞ *macrolide antibiotic* [erythromycin ethylsuccinate] 100 mg/2.5 mL ☒ AeroBid

EryPed 200; EryPed 400 oral suspension ℞ *macrolide antibiotic* [erythromycin ethylsuccinate] 200 mg/5 mL; 400 mg/5 mL ⍰ AeroBid

Ery-Tab enteric-coated delayed-release tablets ℞ *macrolide antibiotic* [erythromycin] 250, 333, 500 mg

erythorbic acid

Erythraea centaurium medicinal herb [see: centaury]

erythrityl tetranitrate USAN, USP *coronary vasodilator; antianginal* [also: eritrityl tetranitrate]

Erythrocin Lactobionate powder for IV injection ℞ *macrolide antibiotic* [erythromycin lactobionate] 500, 1000 mg/vial

Erythrocin Stearate Filmtabs (film-coated tablets) ℞ *macrolide antibiotic* [erythromycin stearate] 250, 500 mg

erythrol tetranitrate [now: erythrityl tetranitrate]

erythromycin USP, INN, BAN *macrolide antibiotic* 250, 500 mg oral; 2% topical; 0.5% ophthalmic

erythromycin 2′-acetate octadecanoate [see: erythromycin acistrate]

erythromycin 2′-acetate stearate [see: erythromycin acistrate]

erythromycin acistrate USAN, INN *macrolide antibiotic*

erythromycin B [see: berythromycin]

erythromycin & benzoyl peroxide *antibiotic and keratolytic for acne* 3%•5% topical

erythromycin estolate USAN, USP, BAN *macrolide antibiotic*

erythromycin ethyl succinate BAN *macrolide antibiotic* [also: erythromycin ethylsuccinate]

erythromycin ethylcarbonate USP *macrolide antibiotic*

erythromycin ethylsuccinate (EES) USP *macrolide antibiotic* [also: erythromycin ethyl succinate] 400 mg oral; 200, 400 mg/5 mL oral

erythromycin ethylsuccinate & sulfisoxizole *antibiotic combination for acute otitis media in children* 200•600 mg oral

erythromycin gluceptate USP *macrolide antibiotic*

erythromycin glucoheptonate [see: erythromycin gluceptate]

erythromycin lactobionate USP *macrolide antibiotic*

erythromycin lauryl sulfate, propionyl [now: erythromycin estolate]

erythromycin monoglucoheptonate [see: erythromycin gluceptate]

erythromycin octadecanoate [see: erythromycin stearate]

erythromycin 2′-propanoate [see: erythromycin propionate]

erythromycin propionate USAN *macrolide antibiotic*

erythromycin 2′-propionate dodecyl sulfate [see: erythromycin estolate]

erythromycin propionate lauryl sulfate [now: erythromycin estolate]

erythromycin salnacedin USAN *macrolide antibiotic for acne vulgaris*

erythromycin stearate USP, BAN *macrolide antibiotic* 250, 500 mg oral

erythromycin stinoprate INN *macrolide antibiotic*

Erythronium americanum medicinal herb [see: adder's tongue]

erythropoietin, recombinant human (rEPO) [see: epoetin alfa; epoetin beta]

erythrosine sodium USP *dental disclosing agent*

Eryzole granules for oral suspension (discontinued 2010) ℞ *antibiotic* [erythromycin ethylsuccinate; sulfisoxazole acetyl] 200•600 mg/5 mL ⍰ Orasol; uracil

esafloxacin INN

esaprazole INN

Esbriet ⍤ (available in the European union) *investigational (NDA filed, orphan) TGF-beta inhibitor for idiopathic pulmonary fibrosis (IPF)* [pirfenidone]

escalated BEACOPP (bleomycin, etoposide, Adriamycin, cyclophosphamide, Oncovin, procarbazine, prednisone) [with filgrastim hematopoietic] *chemotherapy protocol for Hodgkin lymphoma*

escitalopram oxalate USAN *selective serotonin reuptake inhibitor (SSRI) for major depressive disorder (MDD) and generalized anxiety disorder (GAD); also used for post-traumatic stress disorder (PTSD); isomer of citalopram*

Esclim transdermal patch (discontinued 2009) ℞ *estrogen replacement therapy for the treatment of postmenopausal symptoms* [estradiol] 25, 37.5 mcg/day ☒ Oesclim

esculamine INN

eseridine INN

eserine [see: physostigmine]

esflurbiprofen INN, BAN

Esgic caplets, capsules ℞ *barbiturate sedative; analgesic; antipyretic* [butalbital; acetaminophen; caffeine] 50•325•40 mg

Esgic-Plus caplets, capsules ℞ *barbiturate sedative; analgesic; antipyretic* [butalbital; acetaminophen; caffeine] 50•500•40 mg

ESHAP (etoposide, Solu-Medrol, high-dose ara-C, Platinol) *chemotherapy protocol for non-Hodgkin lymphoma*

esilate INN *combining name for radicals or groups* [also: esylate] ☒ Isolyte

Esimil tablets (discontinued 2007) ℞ *antihypertensive; diuretic* [hydrochlorothiazide; guanethidine monosulfate] 25•10 mg ☒ Isomil

Eskalith CR controlled-release tablets (discontinued 2007) ℞ *antipsychotic for manic episodes* [lithium carbonate] 450 mg

Eskimo Kids oral liquid OTC *dietary supplement* [omega-3 fatty acids (eicosapentaenoic acid and docosahexaenoic acid); vitamin D] 800 mg•100 IU (270 mg EPA; 180 mg DHA)

eslicarbazepine acetate *investigational (NDA filed) once-daily adjunctive therapy for partial-onset seizures in adults*

esmolol INN, BAN *antihypertensive; beta-blocker* [also: esmolol HCl]

esmolol HCl USAN *antiarrhythmic; antihypertensive; beta-blocker; treatment for supraventricular tachycardia and intraoperative/postoperative tachycardia or hypertension; also used for unstable angina* [also: esmolol] 10 mg/mL injection

Esmya *investigational (Phase III) selective progesterone receptor modulator for uterine fibroids (myoma)* [ulipristal acetate]

Esocor P oral suspension ℞ *antitussive; antihistamine; decongestant* [dextromethorphan hydrobromide; chlorpheniramine maleate; pseudoephedrine HCl] 30•4•30 mg/5 mL

E-Solve lotion OTC *nontherapeutic base for compounding various dermatological preparations*

esomeprazole magnesium USAN *oral proton pump inhibitor for gastric and duodenal ulcers, erosive esophagitis, gastroesophageal reflux disease (GERD), and other gastroesophageal disorders; isomer of omeprazole*

esomeprazole sodium *injectable proton pump inhibitor for the short-term treatment of GERD in patients who cannot take the drug orally; isomer of omeprazole*

esorubicin INN *antineoplastic* [also: esorubicin HCl]

esorubicin HCl USAN *antineoplastic* [also: esorubicin]

Esotérica Dry Skin Treatment lotion OTC *moisturizer; emollient*

Esotérica Facial; Esotérica Regular cream OTC *hyperpigmentation bleaching agent* [hydroquinone] 2%

Esotérica Soap OTC *bath emollient*

Esotérica Sunscreen cream OTC *hyperpigmentation bleaching agent; sunscreen* [hydroquinone; padimate O; oxybenzone] 2%•3.3%•2.5%

esproquin HCl USAN *adrenergic* [also: esproquine]

esproquine INN *adrenergic* [also: esproquin HCl]

Essential ProPlus powder for oral solution OTC *oral protein supplement* with vitamins and minerals [soy protein; multiple vitamins and minerals]

estazolam USAN, INN *benzodiazepine sedative and hypnotic* 1, 2 mg oral

Ester-C Plus Multi-Mineral capsules OTC *vitamin C/mineral supplement with multiple bioflavonoids* [vitamin C; multiple minerals; citrus bioflavonoids; acerola; rose hips; rutin] 425•±•50•12.5•12.5•5 mg

Ester-C Plus Vitamin C capsules OTC *vitamin C/calcium supplement with multiple bioflavonoids* [vitamin C; calcium; citrus bioflavonoids; acerola; rose hips; rutin] 500•62•25•10•10•5 mg; 1000•125•200•25•25•25 mg

esterified estrogens [see: estrogens, esterified]

esterifilcon A USAN *hydrophilic contact lens material*

estilben [see: diethylstilbestrol dipropionate]

estolate INN *combining name for radicals or groups*

estomycin sulfate [see: paromomycin sulfate]

Estrace tablets ℞ *estrogen replacement therapy for the treatment of postmenopausal symptoms and prevention of postmenopausal osteoporosis; palliative therapy for prostate and metastatic breast cancers* [estradiol, soy-derived] 0.5, 1, 2 mg

Estrace Vaginal cream ℞ *estrogen replacement for postmenopausal atrophic vaginitis* [estradiol] 0.1 mg/g

Estraderm transdermal patch ℞ *estrogen replacement therapy for the treatment of postmenopausal symptoms and prevention of postmenopausal osteoporosis* [estradiol] 50, 100 mcg/day

estradiol USP, INN *estrogen replacement therapy for the treatment of postmenopausal disorders and the prevention of postmenopausal osteoporosis; palliative therapy for breast and prostate cancers; may be naturally derived or a synthetic analogue* [also: oestradiol] 0.5, 1, 2 mg oral

estradiol acetate *synthetic estrogen; hormone replacement therapy for the treatment of postmenopausal symptoms*

estradiol-17β *estrogen replacement therapy for postmenopausal disorders*

estradiol benzoate USP, INN, JAN [also: oestradiol benzoate]

estradiol 17-cyclopentanepropionate [see: estradiol cypionate]

estradiol cypionate USP *synthetic estrogen; hormone replacement therapy for the treatment of postmenopausal symptoms*

estradiol dipropionate NF, JAN

estradiol enanthate USAN *estrogen*

estradiol hemihydrate *synthetic estrogen; topical hormone therapy for atrophic vaginitis* (base=97%)

estradiol 17-heptanoate [see: estradiol enanthate]

estradiol monobenzoate [see: estradiol benzoate]

estradiol 17-nicotinate 3-propionate [see: estrapronicate]

estradiol & norethindrone acetate *a mixture of natural and synthetic hormones; hormone replacement therapy for postmenopausal symptoms* 1•0.5 mg oral

estradiol phosphate polymer [see: polyestradiol phosphate]

Estradiol Transdermal System patch ℞ *estrogen replacement therapy for the treatment of postmenopausal symptoms and prevention of postmenopausal osteoporosis* [estradiol] 25, 37.5, 50, 60, 75, 100 mcg/day

estradiol 17-undecanoate [see: estradiol undecylate]

estradiol undecylate USAN, INN *estrogen*

estradiol valerate USP, INN, JAN *synthetic estrogen; hormone replacement therapy for the treatment of postmenopausal symptoms and the prevention of postmenopausal osteoporosis; hormonal antineoplastic for breast and prostate cancers* [also: oestradiol valerate] 10, 20, 40 mg/mL injection

Estra-L 40 IM injection ℞ *estrogen replacement therapy for postmenopausal symptoms; antineoplastic for prostatic cancer* [estradiol valerate in oil] 40 mg/mL ☒ Ezetrol

estramustine USAN, INN, BAN *nitrogen mustard-type alkylating antineoplastic*

estramustine phosphate sodium USAN, BAN, JAN *nitrogen mustard-type alkylating antineoplastic for prostate cancer*

estramustine + vinblastine *chemotherapy protocol for prostate cancer* [also known as: EM-V]

estrapronicate INN

Estrasorb topical emulsion ℞ *estrogen replacement therapy for postmenopausal symptoms* [estradiol (as hemihydrate)] 25 mcg/pouch

Estratest; Estratest H.S. sugar-coated tablets ℞ *combination equine estrogen and synthetic androgen; hormone replacement therapy for postmenopausal symptoms* [esterified estrogens; methyltestosterone] 1.25•2.5 mg; 0.625•1.25 mg

estrazinol INN *estrogen* [also: estrazinol hydrobromide]

estrazinol hydrobromide USAN *estrogen* [also: estrazinol]

Estring vaginal ring ℞ *three-month estrogen replacement for postmenopausal atrophic vaginitis* [estradiol] 2 mg (7.5 mcg/day) ☒ Oestring

estriol USP *estrogen* [also: estriol succinate; oestriol succinate] ☒ Ezetrol

estriol succinate INN *estrogen* [also: estriol; oestriol succinate]

estrobene [see: diethylstilbestrol]

estrobene DP [see: diethylstilbestrol dipropionate]

estrofurate USAN, INN *estrogen*

Estrogel transdermal gel ℞ *estrogen replacement therapy for postmenopausal symptoms* [estradiol] 0.06% (0.75 mg/dose)

estrogenic substances, conjugated [see: estrogens, conjugated]

estrogenine [see: diethylstilbestrol]

estrogens *a class of sex hormones that includes estradiol, estrone, and estriol; also used as an antineoplastic*

estrogens, conjugated USP, JAN *a mixture of equine estrogens; hormone replacement therapy for the treatment of postmenopausal symptoms and prevention of postmenopausal osteoporosis; palliative therapy for breast and prostate cancers*

estrogens, esterified USP *a mixture of equine estrogens; hormone replacement therapy for the treatment of postmenopausal disorders; palliative therapy for breast and prostate cancers*

estrogens, esterified & methyltestosterone *combination equine estrogen and synthetic androgen; hormone replacement therapy for postmenopausal symptoms* 0.625•1.25, 1.25•2.5 mg oral

estrogens A, synthetic conjugated (SCE-A) *a mixture of 9 synthetic estrogenic substances; hormone replacement therapy for postmenopausal symptoms* 0.625 mg/g vaginal cream

estrogens B, synthetic conjugated (SCE-B) *a mixture of 10 synthetic estrogenic substances; hormone replacement therapy for severe postmenopausal vasomotor symptoms*

estromenin [see: diethylstilbestrol]

estrone USP, INN *bioidentical human estrogen; natural hormone replacement therapy for postmenopausal disorders; palliative therapy for breast and prostate cancers* [also: oestrone] ☒ isoetarine

estrone hydrogen sulfate [see: estrone sodium sulfate]

estrone sodium sulfate *synthetic estrogen*

Estrophasic (trademarked/patented dosing regimen) *gradual estrogen intake with steady progestin intake*

estropipate USP *natural estrogen replacement therapy for the treatment of postmenopausal symptoms and prevention of postmenopausal osteoporosis; a stabilized form of estrone, the bioidentical human estrogen* 0.75, 1.5, 3, 6 mg oral

Estrostep 21 tablets (in packs of 21) (discontinued 2008) ℞ *triphasic oral contraceptive; treatment for acne vulgaris in females* [norethindrone acetate; ethinyl estradiol]
Phase 1 (5 days): 1 mg•20 mcg;
Phase 2 (7 days): 1 mg•30 mcg;
Phase 3 (9 days): 1 mg•35 mcg

Estrostep Fe tablets (in packs of 28) ℞ *triphasic oral contraceptive; iron supplement* [norethindrone acetate; ethinyl estradiol; ferrous fumarate]
Phase 1 (5 days): 1•0.02•75 mg;
Phase 2 (7 days): 1•0.03•75 mg;
Phase 3 (9 days): 1•0.035•75 mg;
Counters (7 days): 0•0•75 mg

esuprone INN ⑦ aceperone; aspirin; azaperone; Easprin

esylate USAN, BAN *combining name for radicals or groups* [also: esilate] ⑦

Isolyte E

eszopiclone *nonbarbiturate sedative and hypnotic for chronic insomnia; isomer of* zopiclone 1, 2, 3 mg oral

etabenzarone INN

etabonate USAN, INN *combining name for radicals or groups*

etacepride INN

etacrynic acid INN, JAN *antihypertensive; loop diuretic* [also: ethacrynic acid]

etafedrine INN, BAN *adrenergic* [also: etafedrine HCl]

etafedrine HCl USAN *adrenergic* [also: etafedrine]

etafenone INN ⑦ etifenin

etafilcon A USAN *hydrophilic contact lens material*

etamestrol INN

etaminile INN

etamiphyllin INN [also: etamiphylline]

etamiphyllin methesculetol [see: metescufylline]

etamiphylline BAN [also: etamiphyllin]

etamivan INN *central and respiratory stimulant* [also: ethamivan]

etamocycline INN

etamsylate INN *hemostatic* [also: ethamsylate]

etanercept USAN *soluble tumor necrosis factor receptor (sTNFR) inhibitor for rheumatoid arthritis, juvenile rheumatoid arthritis (orphan), psoriatic arthritis, and ankylosing spondylitis; investigational (orphan) for Wegener granulomatosis*

etanidazole USAN, INN *antineoplastic; hypoxic cell radiosensitizer*

etanterol INN

etaperazine [see: perphenazine]

etaqualone INN

etarotene USAN, INN *keratolytic*

etasuline INN ⑦ etozolin

etazepine INN ⑦ atosiban

etazolate INN *antipsychotic* [also: etazolate HCl]

etazolate HCl USAN *antipsychotic* [also: etazolate]

etebenecid INN [also: ethebenecid]

etenzamide BAN [also: ethenzamide]

eterobarb USAN, INN, BAN *anticonvulsant*

etersalate INN

ethacridine INN [also: ethacridine lactate; acrinol]

ethacridine lactate [also: ethacridine; acrinol]

ethacrynate sodium USAN, USP *loop diuretic for congestive heart failure, hepatic cirrhosis, and renal disease*

ethacrynic acid USAN, USP, BAN *loop diuretic for congestive heart failure, hepatic cirrhosis, and renal disease* [also: etacrynic acid]

ethambutol INN, BAN *bacteriostatic; primary tuberculostatic* [also: ethambutol HCl]

ethambutol HCl USAN, USP *bacteriostatic; primary tuberculostatic* [also: ethambutol] 100, 400 mg oral

ethamivan USAN, USP, BAN *central and respiratory stimulant* [also: etamivan]

Ethamolin IV injection ℞ *sclerosing agent for bleeding esophageal varices (orphan)* [ethanolamine oleate] 5%

ethamsylate USAN, BAN *hemostatic* [also: etamsylate]

ethanol JAN *topical anti-infective/antiseptic; astringent; solvent; a widely* *abused "legal street drug" used to produce euphoria* [also: alcohol]

ethanol, dehydrated JAN *antidote* [also: alcohol, dehydrated]

ethanolamine oleate USAN *sclerosing agent for bleeding esophageal varices (orphan)* [also: monoethanolamine oleate]

ethanolamines *a class of antihistamines that includes diphenhydramine HCl and clemastine fumarate*

ethaverine INN *peripheral vasodilator*

ethaverine HCl *peripheral vasodilator for peripheral and vascular insufficiency due to arterial spasm* [also: ethaverine]

ethchlorvynol USP, INN, BAN *sedative; hypnotic*

ethebenecid BAN [also: etebenecid]

EtheDent chewable tablets ℞ *dental caries preventative* [sodium fluoride] 0.25, 0.5, 1 mg

EtheDent dental cream (discontinued 2009) ℞ *caries preventative* [fluoride (as sodium fluoride)] 0.5% (1.1%)

ethenzamide INN, JAN [also: etenzamide]

ether USP *inhalation anesthetic*

Ethezyme; Ethezyme 830 ointment (discontinued 2010) ℞ *proteolytic enzyme for débridement of necrotic tissue; vulnerary* [papain; urea] 1 100 000 U•100 mg per gram; 830 000 IU•100 mg per gram

ethiazide INN, BAN

ethidium bromide [see: homidium bromide]

ethinamate USP, INN, BAN *sedative; hypnotic*

ethinyl estradiol USP *estrogen replacement therapy for the treatment of postmenopausal disorders; palliative therapy for prostate and breast cancers; investigational (orphan) for Turner syndrome* [also: ethinylestradiol; ethinyloestradiol]

ethinyl estradiol & drospirenone *monophasic oral contraceptive* 0.02•3, 0.3•3 mg

ethinyl estradiol & levonorgestrel *monophasic oral contraceptive; extended-cycle (3 months) biphasic oral contraceptive* 20•90, 30•50, 30•125, 40•75 mcg; Phase 1: 30•150 mcg, Phase 2: 10•0 mcg

ethinyl estradiol & norethindrone acetate *monophasic oral contraceptive* 0.005•1, 0.02•1, 0.03•1, 0.035•0.4, 0.035•0.5, 0.035•0.75, 0.035•1, 0.25•0.8 mg

ethinyl estradiol & norgestimate *monophasic oral contraceptive* 25•180, 25•215, 25•250, 35•215, 35•250 mcg

ethinylestradiol INN *estrogen replacement therapy for the treatment of postmenopausal disorders; palliative therapy for prostate and breast cancers* [also: ethinyl estradiol; ethinyloestradiol]

ethinyloestradiol BAN *estrogen replacement therapy for the treatment of postmenopausal disorders; palliative therapy for prostate and breast cancers* [also: ethinyl estradiol; ethinylestradiol]

ethiodized oil USP *parenteral radiopaque contrast medium (37% iodine)*

ethiodized oil (^{131}I) INN *antineoplastic; radioactive agent* [also: ethiodized oil I 131]

ethiodized oil I 131 USAN *antineoplastic; radioactive agent* [also: ethiodized oil (^{131}I)]

Ethiodol intracavitary instillation (discontinued 2010) ℞ *radiopaque contrast medium for lymphography and gynecological imaging* [ethiodized oil (37% iodine)] 1284 mg/mL (475 mg/mL)

ethiofos [now: amifostine]

ethionamide USAN, USP, INN, BAN *bacteriostatic; tuberculosis retreatment*

ethisterone NF, INN, BAN ② itasetron

Ethmozine film-coated tablets (discontinued 2008) ℞ *antiarrhythmic for severe ventricular arrhythmias* [moricizine HCl] 200, 250, 300 mg

ethodryl [see: diethylcarbamazine citrate]

ethoglucid BAN [also: etoglucid]

ethoheptazine BAN [also: ethoheptazine citrate]

ethoheptazine citrate NF, INN [also: ethoheptazine]

ethohexadiol USP

ethomoxane INN, BAN

ethomoxane HCl [see: ethomoxane]

ethonam nitrate USAN antifungal [also: etonam]

ethopabate BAN

ethopropazine BAN anticholinergic; antiparkinsonian [also: ethopropazine HCl; profenamine]

ethopropazine HCl USP anticholinergic; antiparkinsonian [also: profenamine; ethopropazine]

ethosalamide BAN [also: etosalamide]

ethosuximide USAN, USP, INN, BAN succinimide anticonvulsant 250 mg oral; 250 mg/5 mL oral

ethotoin USP, INN, BAN hydantoin anticonvulsant

ethoxarutine [see: ethoxazorutoside]

ethoxazene HCl USAN analgesic [also: etoxazene]

ethoxazorutoside INN

ethoxyacetanilide (withdrawn from market) [see: phenacetin]

o-ethoxybenzamide [see: ethenzamide; etenzamide]

ETH-Oxydose oral drops (discontinued 2009) ℞ narcotic analgesic [oxycodone HCl] 20 mg/mL

ethoxzolamide USP

Ethrane liquid for vaporization ℞ inhalation general anesthetic [enflurane] ⍰ ATryn

ethybenztropine USAN, BAN anticholinergic [also: etybenzatropine]

ethyl acetate NF solvent

ethyl alcohol (EtOH; ETOH) [now: alcohol; ethanol]

ethyl aminobenzoate (ethyl p-aminobenzoate) JAN topical anesthetic; nonprescription diet aid [also: benzocaine]

ethyl 2-benzimidazolecarbamate [see: lobendazole]

ethyl N-benzylcyclopropanecarbamate [see: encyprate]

ethyl biscoumacetate NF, INN, BAN

ethyl biscumacetate [see: ethyl biscoumacetate]

ethyl carbamate [now: urethane]

ethyl carfluzepate INN

ethyl cartrizoate INN

ethyl chloride USP topical refrigerant anesthetic

ethyl dibunate USAN, INN, BAN antitussive

ethyl dirazepate INN

ethyl eicosapentaenoate investigational (orphan) agent for Huntington disease

ethyl ether [see: ether]

ethyl p-fluorophenyl sulfone [see: fluoresone]

ethyl p-hydroxybenzoate [see: ethylparaben]

ethyl loflazepate INN

ethyl nitrite NF

ethyl oleate NF vehicle

ethyl oxide [see: ether]

ethyl vanillin NF flavoring agent

ethylcellulose NF tablet binder

ethylchlordiphene [see: etofamide]

ethyldicoumarol [see: ethyl biscoumacetate]

ethylene NF inhalation general anesthesia ⍰ Atolone

ethylene disterate [see: glycol distearate]

ethylenediamine USP, JAN

ethylenediaminetetraacetate [see: edetate disodium]

ethylenediaminetetraacetic acid (EDTA) [see: edetate disodium]

N,N-ethylenediarsanilic acid [see: difetarsone]

ethylenedinitrilotetraacetate disodium [see: edetate disodium]

ethylestrenol USAN, INN anabolic steroid; also abused as a street drug [also: ethyloestrenol; ethylnandrol]

ethylhexanediol [see: ethohexadiol]

2-ethylhexyl diphenyl phosphate [see: octicizer]

2-ethylhexyl p-methoxycinnamate [see: octinoxate]

2-ethylhexyl salicylate [see: octisalate]

ethylhydrocupreine HCl NF

ethylmethylthiambutene INN, BAN

ethylmorphine BAN [also: ethylmorphine HCl]

ethylmorphine HCl NF [also: ethylmorphine]

ethylnandrol JAN *anabolic steroid; also abused as a street drug* [also: ethylestrenol; ethyloestrenol]

ethylnorepinephrine HCl USP *sympathomimetic bronchodilator*

ethyloestradiol BAN *estrogen* [also: ethinyl estradiol]

ethyloestrenol BAN *anabolic steroid; also abused as a street drug* [also: ethylestrenol; ethylnandrol]

ethylpapaverine HCl [see: ethaverine HCl]

ethylparaben NF *antifungal agent*

ethylphenacemide [see: pheneturide]

ethylstibamine [see: stibosamine]

2-ethylthioisonicotinamide [see: ethionamide]

ethynerone USAN, INN *progestin*

ethynodiol BAN *progestin* [also: ethynodiol diacetate; etynodiol]

ethynodiol diacetate USAN, USP *progestin* [also: etynodiol; ethynodiol]

(−)-5-ethynylnicotine [see: altinicline]

5-ethynyluracil [see: eniluracil]

Ethyol powder for IV infusion ℞ *chemoprotective agent for cisplatin and paclitaxel chemotherapy (orphan); treatment for moderate to severe xerostomia following postoperative radiation therapy (orphan); investigational (orphan) for cyclophosphamide-induced granulocytopenia* [amifostine] 500 mg/vial

ethypicone INN

ethypropymal sodium [see: probarbital sodium]

etibendazole USAN, INN *anthelmintic*

eticlopride INN

eticyclidine INN

etidocaine USAN, INN, BAN *injectable local anesthetic*

etidocaine HCl *injectable local anesthetic*

etidronate disodium USAN, USP *bisphosphonate bone resorption inhibitor for Paget disease, heterotopic ossification, and hypercalcemia of malignancy (orphan); also used for corticosteroid-induced osteoporosis; investigational (orphan) for metabolic bone disease* 200, 400 mg oral

etidronate monosodium

etidronate sodium (*this term is used only when the form of sodium cannot be more accurately identified*)

etidronate tetrasodium

etidronate trisodium

etidronic acid USAN, INN, BAN *calcium regulator*

etifelmine INN

etifenin USAN, INN, BAN *diagnostic aid* ⑨ etafenone

etifoxin BAN [also: etifoxine]

etifoxine INN [also: etifoxin]

etilamfetamine INN

etilefrine INN

etilefrine pivalate INN

etintidine INN *antagonist to histamine H_2 receptors* [also: etintidine HCl]

etintidine HCl USAN *antagonist to histamine H_2 receptors* [also: etintidine]

etiocholanedione *investigational (orphan) for aplastic anemia and Prader-Willi syndrome*

etipirium iodide INN

etiproston INN

etiracetam INN

etiroxate INN

etisazole INN, BAN

etisomicin INN, BAN

etisulergine INN

etizolam INN

etobedolum [see: etonitazene]

etocarlide INN

etocrilene INN *ultraviolet screen* [also: etocrylene]

etocrylene USAN *ultraviolet screen* [also: etocrilene]

etodolac USAN, INN, BAN *analgesic; nonsteroidal anti-inflammatory drug (NSAID) for osteoarthritis, rheumatoid arthritis, juvenile rheumatoid arthritis, and other chronic pain* [also: etodolic acid] 200, 300, 400, 500, 600 mg oral

R-etodolac *investigational (orphan) treatment for chronic lymphocytic leukemia*

etodolic acid INN *analgesic; antiarthritic; nonsteroidal anti-inflammatory drug (NSAID)* [also: etodolac]

etodroxizine INN

etofamide INN

etofenamate USAN, INN, BAN *analgesic; anti-inflammatory*

etofenprox INN

etofibrate INN

etoformin INN *antidiabetic* [also: etoformin HCl]

etoformin HCl USAN *antidiabetic* [also: etoformin]

etofuradine INN ⊉ atevirdine

etofylline INN

etofylline clofibrate INN *antihyperlipoproteinemic* [also: theofibrate]

etoglucid INN [also: ethoglucid]

EtOH; ETOH (ethyl alcohol) [now: alcohol]

etolorex INN

etolotifen INN

etoloxamine INN

etomidate USAN, INN, BAN *rapid-acting nonbarbiturate general anesthetic; hypnotic* 2 mg/mL injection

etomidoline INN

etomoxir INN

etonam INN *antifungal* [also: ethonam nitrate]

etonam nitrate [see: ethonam nitrate]

etonitazene INN, BAN

etonogestrel USAN, INN *progestin for vaginal (1 month) and parenteral (3 years) contraception; also used as a male contraceptive (parenteral)*

etoperidone INN *antidepressant* [also: etoperidone HCl]

etoperidone HCl USAN *antidepressant* [also: etoperidone]

etophylate [see: acepifylline]

Etopophos powder for IV injection ℞ *antineoplastic for testicular and small cell lung cancers (SCLC)* [etoposide (as phosphate)] 100 mg/vial

etoposide USAN, INN, BAN *antineoplastic* 50 mg oral; 20 mg/mL injection

etoposide phosphate USAN *antineoplastic for testicular and small cell lung cancers (SCLC)*

etoprindole INN

etoprine USAN *antineoplastic*

etoricoxib USAN *antiarthritic; antipyretic; COX-2 inhibitor; nonsteroidal anti-inflammatory drug (NSAID)*

etorphine INN, BAN ⊉ Etrafon; Otrivin

etosalamide INN [also: ethosalamide]

etoxadrol INN *anesthetic* [also: etoxadrol HCl]

etoxadrol HCl USAN *anesthetic* [also: etoxadrol]

etoxazene INN *analgesic* [also: ethoxazene HCl]

etoxazene HCl [see: ethoxazene HCl]

etoxeridine INN, BAN

etozolin USAN, INN *diuretic* ⊉ etasuline

etrabamine INN

Etrafon; Etrafon-A; Etrafon-Forte tablets ℞ *conventional (typical) phenothiazine antipsychotic for schizophrenia and psychotic disorders; antidepressant* [perphenazine; amitriptyline HCl] 2•25 mg; 4•10 mg; 4•25 mg ⊉ etorphine; Otrivin

Etrafon 2−10 tablets (discontinued 2009) ℞ *conventional (typical) phenothiazine antipsychotic for schizophrenia and psychotic disorders; antidepressant* [perphenazine; amitriptyline HCl] 2•10 mg ⊉ etorphine; Otrivin

etravirine *non-nucleoside reverse transcriptase inhibitor (NNRTI) for drug-resistant HIV-1 infections*

etretin [see: acitretin]

etretinate USAN, INN, BAN, JAN *systemic antipsoriatic; retinoic acid analogue*

etryptamine INN, BAN *CNS stimulant* [also: etryptamine acetate]

etryptamine acetate USAN *CNS stimulant* [also: etryptamine]

etybenzatropine INN *anticholinergic* [also: ethybenztropine]

etymemazine INN

etymemazine HCl [see: etymemazine]

etynodiol INN *progestin* [also: ethynodiol diacetate; ethynodiol]

etyprenaline [see: isoetharine]

eucaine HCl NF

Eucalyptamint ointment, gel OTC *mild anesthetic; antipruritic; counterir-*

ritant; antiseptic [menthol; eucalyptus oil] 16%• ♀; 8%• ♀

eucalyptol USAN *antiseptic/germicide*

eucalyptus (Eucalyptus globulus) oil *medicinal herb for bronchitis, lung disorders, neuralgia, and skin sores; source of bioflavonoids*

eucalyptus oil NF *topical antiseptic*

eucatropine INN, BAN *ophthalmic anticholinergic* [also: eucatropine HCl]

eucatropine HCl USP *ophthalmic anticholinergic* [also: eucatropine]

Eucerin cream OTC *nontherapeutic base for compounding various dermatological preparations*

Eucerin cream, lotion OTC *moisturizer; emollient*

Eucerin Itch-Relief Moisturizing spray OTC *mild anesthetic; antipruritic; counterirritant* [menthol] 0.15%

Eucerin Plus lotion OTC *moisturizer; emollient* [sodium lactate; urea] 5%• 5%

eucodal [see: oxycodone]

Eucrease ⓔ *combination DPP-4 inhibitor for type 2 diabetes that increases insulin production in the pancreas, reduces glucose production in the liver, and increases cellular response to insulin* [vildagliptin; metformin] ⊉ ocrase

euflavine [see: acriflavine]

Euflexxa intra-articular injection in prefilled syringes ℞ *viscoelastic lubricant and "shock absorber" for osteoarthritis and temporomandibular joint syndrome* [hyaluronate sodium] 20 mg/2 mL ⊉ Avelox; I-Valex

Eugenia caryophyllata medicinal herb [see: cloves]

Eugenia pimenta medicinal herb [see: allspice]

eugenol USP *dental analgesic*

eukadol [see: oxycodone]

Eulexin capsules (discontinued 2009) ℞ *antineoplastic for prostate cancer* [flutamide] 125 mg

Euonymus atropurpureus medicinal herb [see: wahoo]

Eupatorium cannabinum medicinal herb [see: hemp agrimony]

Eupatorium perfoliatum medicinal herb [see: boneset]

Eupatorium purpureum medicinal herb [see: queen of the meadow]

Euphorbia poinsettia; E. pulcherrima medicinal herb [see: poinsettia]

euphoretics; euphoriants; euphoragens *a class of agents that produce euphoria*

Euphrasia officinalis; E. rostkoviana; E. strica medicinal herb [see: eyebright]

euprocin INN *topical anesthetic* [also: euprocin HCl] ⊉ eperisone

euprocin HCl USAN *topical anesthetic* [also: euprocin]

euquinine [see: quinine ethylcarbonate]

Eurax cream, lotion ℞ *scabicide; antipruritic* [crotamiton] 10% ⊉ Urex

European alder; European black alder; European buckthorn *medicinal herb* [see: buckthorn]

European aspen *medicinal herb* [see: black poplar]

europium *element (Eu)* ⊉ erbium

EVA (etoposide, vinblastine, Adriamycin) *chemotherapy protocol for Hodgkin lymphoma*

Evac-Q-Mag carbonated oral liquid OTC *saline laxative* [magnesium citrate; citric acid; potassium citrate]

Evac-Q-Tabs tablets OTC *stimulant laxative* [bisacodyl] 5 mg

Evac-U-Gen chewable tablets OTC *stimulant laxative* [sennosides] 10 mg

EvaMist metered-dose transdermal spray ℞ *hormone replacement for postmenopausal vasomotor symptoms* [estradiol] 1.53 mg/spray

evandamine INN

evening primrose (Oenothera biennis) bark, leaves, oil *medicinal herb for cardiovascular health, hypertension, mastalgia, multiple sclerosis, nerves, obesity, premenstrual syndrome, prostate disorders, rheumatoid arthritis, and skin disorders*

everlasting (Anaphalis margaritacea; Gnaphalium polycephalum; G. uliginosum) plant *medicinal herb used* as an astringent, diaphoretic, febrifuge, pectoral, vermifuge, and vulnerary

evernimicin USAN antibiotic

everolimus mTOR kinase inhibitor; oral antineoplastic for advanced renal cell carcinoma and subependymal giant cell astrocytoma (SGCA) secondary to tuberous sclerosis complex (TSC); immunosuppressant for the prevention of transplant rejection

Evista film-coated tablets ℞ selective estrogen receptor modulator (SERM) for the prevention and treatment of postmenopausal osteoporosis; hormone antagonist for breast cancer (orphan); also used for uterine leiomyomas, pubertal gynecomastia, and prostate cancer [raloxifene HCl] 60 mg ☑ Eovist

E-Vitamin ointment OTC emollient [vitamin E] 30 mg/g ☑ iofetamine

Evithrom topical solution ℞ hemostatic to minimize blood loss during surgery [thrombin, human] 800–1200 U/mL

Evoclin topical foam ℞ antibiotic for acne; also used for rosacea [clindamycin phosphate] 1% ☑ ivoqualine

Evolence subcu injection in prefilled syringes ℞ dermal filler for moderate to deep facial wrinkles and folds [collagen, purified porcine] 3.5%

Evoxac capsules ℞ cholinergic and muscarinic receptor agonist for treatment of dry mouth due to Sjögren syndrome [cevimeline HCl] 30 mg

Evra [see: Ortho Evra]

Exact vanishing cream OTC keratolytic for acne [benzoyl peroxide] 5% ☑ Oxecta

Exactacain aerosol spray ℞ topical anesthetic for surgical or endoscopic procedures [benzocaine; butamben; tetracaine HCl] 14%•2%•2%

exalamide INN 5

Exalgo extended-release tablets ℞ narcotic analgesic [hydromorphone HCl] 8, 12, 16 mg

Exall-D oral liquid ℞ antitussive; decongestant; expectorant [carbetapentane citrate; pseudoephedrine HCl; guaifenesin] 10•30•100 mg/5 mL

exametazime USAN, INN, BAN regional cerebral perfusion imaging aid

exaprolol INN antiadrenergic (beta-blocker) [also: exaprolol HCl]

exaprolol HCl USAN antiadrenergic (beta-blocker) [also: exaprolol]

exatecan mesylate USAN antineoplastic; topoisomerase I inhibitor

Excedrin Aspirin Free caplets, geltabs OTC analgesic; antipyretic; anti-inflammatory [acetaminophen; caffeine] 500•65 mg

Excedrin Back & Body caplets OTC analgesic; antipyretic; anti-inflammatory [acetaminophen; buffered aspirin] 250•250 mg

Excedrin Extra Strength caplets, tablets, geltabs OTC analgesic; antipyretic; anti-inflammatory [acetaminophen; aspirin; caffeine] 250•250•65 mg

Excedrin Migraine tablets OTC analgesic for relief of migraine headache syndrome, including prodrome, pain, and associated symptoms [acetaminophen; aspirin; caffeine] 250•250•65 mg

Excedrin P.M. oral liquid, liquigels OTC analgesic; antipyretic; antihistamine; sleep aid [acetaminophen; diphenhydramine HCl] 1000•50 mg/30 mL; 500•25 mg

Excedrin P.M. tablets, caplets, geltabs OTC analgesic; antipyretic; antihistamine; sleep aid [acetaminophen; diphenhydramine HCl] 500•38 mg

Excedrin QuickTabs (orally dissolving tablets) (discontinued 2008) OTC analgesic; antipyretic; anti-inflammatory [acetaminophen; caffeine] 500•65 mg

Excedrin Sinus Headache film-coated tablets OTC analgesic; antipyretic; decongestant [acetaminophen; phenylephrine HCl] 325•5 mg

Excedrin Tension Headache caplets, geltabs OTC analgesic; antipyretic; anti-inflammatory [acetaminophen; caffeine] 500•65 mg

Excita Extra premedicated condom OTC spermicidal/barrier contraceptive [nonoxynol 9] 8%

ExeClear-C syrup ℞ *narcotic antitussive; expectorant* [codeine phosphate; guaifenesin] 10•200 mg/5 mL

ExeClear-DM syrup (discontinued 2010) ℞ *antitussive; decongestant; expectorant* [dextromethorphan hydrobromide; pseudoephedrine HCl; guaifenesin] 15•30•150 mg/5 mL

ExeCof extended-release tablets ℞ *antitussive; decongestant; expectorant* [dextromethorphan hydrobromide; phenylephrine HCl; guaifenesin] 60•40•1000 mg

ExeFen DMX extended-release tablets ℞ *antitussive; decongestant; expectorant* [dextromethorphan hydrobromide; pseudoephedrine HCl; guaifenesin] 40•80•780 mg

ExeFen DMX tablets OTC *antitussive; decongestant; expectorant* [dextromethorphan hydrobromide; pseudoephedrine HCl; guaifenesin] 20•60•400 mg

ExeFen-PD extended-release caplets ℞ *decongestant; expectorant* [phenylephrine HCl; guaifenesin] 10•600 mg

Exelbine injectable emulsion *investigational (NDA filed) antineoplastic for non–small cell lung cancer* [vinorelbine]

Exelderm solution ℞ *antifungal* [sulconazole nitrate] 1%

Exelon capsules, oral solution ℞ *acetylcholinesterase inhibitor to increase cognition in Alzheimer and Parkinson disease* [rivastigmine tartrate] 1.5, 3, 4.5, 6 mg; 2 mg/mL ▣ ioxilan

Exelon Patch ℞ *acetylcholinesterase inhibitor to increase cognition in Alzheimer and Parkinson disease* [rivastigmine] 4.6, 9.5 mg/day

exemestane INN *aromatase inhibitor; antihormonal antineoplastic for advanced breast cancer in postmenopausal women (orphan)* 25 mg oral

exenatide *synthetic exendin-4 analogue; incretin mimetic antidiabetic for type 2 diabetes that improves the body's normal glucose-sensing mechanisms and slows gastric emptying; synthetic analogue of Gila monster saliva*

exepanol INN

ExeTuss; ExeTuss GP extended-release caplets ℞ *decongestant; expectorant* [phenylephrine HCl; guaifenesin] 25•900 mg; 25•1200 mg

ExeTuss DM extended-release tablets ℞ *antitussive; decongestant; expectorant* [dextromethorphan hydrobromide; phenylephrine HCl; guaifenesin] 25•20•600 mg

Exforge film-coated tablets ℞ *combination calcium channel blocker and angiotensin receptor blocker (ARB) for hypertension* [amlodipine besylate; valsartan] 5•160, 5•320, 10•160, 10•320 mg

Exforge HCT film-coated tablets ℞ *combination calcium channel blocker, angiotensin receptor blocker (ARB), and diuretic for hypertension* [amlodipine besylate; valsartan; hydrochlorothiazide] 5•160•12.5, 5•160•25, 10•160•12.5, 10•160•25, 10•320•25 mg

Ex-Histine syrup (discontinued 2007) ℞ *decongestant; antihistamine; anticholinergic to dry mucosal secretions* [phenylephrine HCl; chlorpheniramine maleate; methscopolamine bromide] 20•4•2.5 mg/10 mL

Exidine Skin Cleanser; Exidine-2 Scrub; Exidine-4 Scrub topical liquid OTC *broad-spectrum antimicrobial; germicidal* [chlorhexidine gluconate; alcohol 4%] 4%; 2%; 4%

exifone INN

exiproben INN

exisulind *investigational (NDA filed, orphan) antineoplastic for familial adenomatous polyposis (FAP; also known as adenomatous polyposis coli, or APC)*

Exjade tablets ℞ *once-daily iron chelating agent for chronic iron overload due to blood transfusions (orphan)* [deferasirox] 125, 250, 500 mg

Ex-Lax tablets, chocolated chewable tablets OTC *stimulant laxative* [sennosides] 15 mg

Ex-Lax Gentle Strength caplets OTC *stimulant laxative; stool softener* [sennosides; docusate sodium] 10•65 mg

Ex-Lax Maximum Relief tablets OTC *stimulant laxative* [sennosides] 25 mg

Ex-Lax Stool Softener caplets OTC *laxative; stool softener* [docusate sodium] 100 mg

Ex-Lax Ultra enteric-coated tablets OTC *stimulant laxative* [bisacodyl] 5 mg

Exocaine Medicated Rub; Exocaine Plus Rub (discontinued 2008) OTC *analgesic; counterirritant* [methyl salicylate] 25%; 30%

Exoderm soap OTC *antiseptic and keratolytic cleanser for acne* [salicylic acid; sulfur] 3%•10%

Exosurf *investigational (orphan) pulmonary surfactant for adult respiratory distress syndrome (ARDS)* [colfosceril palmitate]

Exosurf Neonatal intratracheal suspension ℞ *pulmonary surfactant for hyaline membrane disease and respiratory distress syndrome (orphan)* [colfosceril palmitate] 108 mg

Exparel *local anesthetic; investigational (NDA filed) long-acting formulation for postsurgical pain management* [bupivacaine HCl]

expectorants *a class of drugs that promote the ejection of mucus from the respiratory tract*

Expidet (trademarked dosage form) *fast-dissolving dose*

Exratuss oral suspension (discontinued 2007) ℞ *antitussive; antihistamine; decongestant* [carbetapentane tannate; chlorpheniramine tannate; phenylephrine tannate] 30•4•12.5 mg

exsiccated sodium arsenate [see: sodium arsenate, exsiccated]

Extavia powder for subcu injection ℞ *immunomodulator for relapsing-remitting multiple sclerosis (orphan)* [interferon beta-1b] 0.3 mg (8 MIU)/dose

Extencap (trademarked dosage form) *extended-release capsule*

extended insulin zinc [see: insulin zinc, extended]

Extendryl chewable tablets ℞ *decongestant; antihistamine; anticholinergic to dry mucosal secretions* [phenylephrine HCl; chlorpheniramine maleate; methscopolamine nitrate] 10•2•1.25 mg

Extendryl syrup ℞ *decongestant; antihistamine; anticholinergic to dry mucosal secretions* [phenylephrine HCl; dexchlorpheniramine maleate; methscopolamine nitrate] 10•1•1.25 mg/5 mL

Extendryl DM extended-release tablets ℞ *antitussive; antihistamine; anticholinergic to dry mucosal secretions* [dextromethorphan hydrobromide; chlorpheniramine maleate; methscopolamine nitrate] 30•8•2.5 mg

Extendryl G extended-release tablets ℞ *decongestant; expectorant* [phenylephrine HCl; guaifenesin] 30•1000 mg

Extendryl GCP oral solution ℞ *antitussive; decongestant; expectorant* [carbetapentane citrate; phenylephrine HCl; guaifenesin] 15•5•100 mg/5 mL

Extendryl JR sustained-release pediatric capsules (discontinued 2007) ℞ *decongestant; antihistamine; anticholinergic to dry mucosal secretions* [phenylephrine HCl; chlorpheniramine maleate; methscopolamine nitrate] 10•4•1.25 mg

Extendryl PEM extended-release tablets ℞ *decongestant; anticholinergic to dry mucosal secretions* [phenylephrine HCl; methscopolamine nitrate] 30•1.25 mg

Extendryl SR sustained-release capsules (discontinued 2007) ℞ *decongestant; antihistamine; anticholinergic to dry mucosal secretions* [phenylephrine HCl; chlorpheniramine maleate; methscopolamine nitrate] 20•8•2.5 mg

Extentab (trademarked dosage form) *extended-release tablet*

Extina topical foam ℞ *antifungal for seborrheic dermatitis* [ketoconazole] 2%

Extra Action Cough syrup OTC *antitussive; expectorant* [dextromethorphan hydrobromide; guaifenesin] 10•100 mg/5 mL

"Extra Strength" products [see under product name]

Extra Strength Pain Reliever PM caplets OTC *analgesic; antipyretic; antihistamine; sleep aid* [acetaminophen; diphenhydramine HCl] 500•25 mg

Extraneal IV infusion (supplied in **Ultrabag** and **Ambu-Flex**) ℞ *peritoneal dialysis solution for end-stage renal disease (orphan)* [icodextrin] 75 g

Extratuss oral suspension (discontinued 2007) ℞ *antitussive; antihistamine; decongestant* [carbetapentane tannate; brompheniramine tannate; phenylephrine tannate] 30•4•12.5 mg/5 mL

Exubera powder for oral inhalation in unit dose blisters, for use with an **Exubera Release Unit** (inhalation device) (discontinued 2007) ℞ *antidiabetic; each milligram of inhaled powder is approximately equivalent to 3 units of injected insulin* [insulin, human (rDNA)] 1, 3 mg/blister

Exubera Release Unit (trademarked delivery device) (discontinued 2007) *inhalation powder dispenser for use with* **Exubera**

eye balm; eye root *medicinal herb* [see: goldenseal]

Eye Drops (discontinued 2011) OTC *decongestant; vasoconstrictor* [tetrahydrozoline HCl] 0.05%

Eye Health & Vitality tablets OTC *vitamin/mineral supplement* [vitamins A, C, and E; multiple minerals; lutein/zeaxanthin blend] 2500 IU•175 mg•200 IU•±•3 mg

Eye Irrigating Solution OTC *extraocular irrigating solution* [sterile isotonic solution]

Eye Scrub solution OTC *eyelid cleanser for blepharitis or contact lenses*

Eye Stream ophthalmic solution OTC *extraocular irrigating solution* [sterile isotonic solution]

Eye Wash ophthalmic solution OTC *extraocular irrigating solution* [sterile isotonic solution]

eyebright *(Euphrasia officinalis; E. rostkoviana; E. strica)* plant *medicinal herb for blood cleansing, cataracts, colds, conjunctivitis, eye disorders and infections, and stimulating liver function; not generally regarded as safe and effective for topical ophthalmic use* ⊡ Iberet

Eye-Lube-A eye drops OTC *moisturizer/lubricant* [glycerin] 0.25% ⊡ Albay

Eyetamins caplets OTC *vitamin/mineral supplement* [vitamins A, C, and E; multiple minerals; lutein; zeaxanthin] 5000 IU•60 mg•30 IU•±•2 mg•95 mcg

Eylea injection *investigational (NDA filed) angiogenesis inhibitor for wet age-related macular degeneration (AMD), central retinal vein occlusion (CRVO), and diabetic macular edema (DME)* [aflibercept]

EZ Detect test kit for home use OTC *in vitro diagnostic aid for fecal occult blood*

ezetimibe USAN *antihyperlipidemic for primary hypercholesterolemia and mixed hyperlipidemia; intestinal cholesterol absorption inhibitor*

EZFE 200 capsules OTC *iron supplement* [iron] 200 mg

E-Z-Gas II effervescent granules OTC *antacid; antiflatulent; aid in endoscopic examination* [sodium bicarbonate; citric acid; simethicone] 2.21•1.53•0.04 g/dose

E-Z-HD oral suspension ℞ *radiopaque contrast medium for gastrointestinal imaging* [barium sulfate] 98%

Ezide tablets ℞ *antihypertensive; diuretic* [hydrochlorothiazide] 50 mg

ezlopitant USAN *substance P receptor antagonist for emesis, pain, and inflammation*

ezogabine USAN *potassium channel opener for adjunctive treatment of partial-onset epilepsy in adults* [also: retigabine]

E-Z-Paque; E-Z-Paque Liquid oral suspension ℞ *radiopaque contrast agent* [barium sulfate] 96%; 60%

E-Z-Paste oral cream ℞ *radiopaque contrast agent* [barium sulfate] 60%

1+1-F Creme ℞ *corticosteroidal anti-inflammatory; antifungal; antibacterial; anesthetic* [hydrocortisone; clioquinol; pramoxine] 1%•3%•1%

¹⁸F [see: fludeoxyglucose F 18]

¹⁸F [see: sodium fluoride F 18]

Fab (fragment, antigen-binding) [def.] *one side of an immunoglobulin that contains an antigen binding site*

FAB (French-American-British) [def.] *a classification system for acute leukemia*

Fablyn (available in Europe) *second-generation selective estrogen receptor modulator (SERM); investigational (NDA filed) for osteoporosis; investigational for breast cancer* [lasofoxifene tartrate]

Fabrazyme powder for IV infusion ℞ *enzyme replacement therapy for Fabry disease (orphan)* [agalsidase beta] 5.5, 37 mg/dose

FAC (fluorouracil, Adriamycin, cyclophosphamide) *chemotherapy protocol for breast cancer*

Fact Plus test kit for home use OTC *in vitro diagnostic aid; urine pregnancy test*

Factive film-coated tablets ℞ *broad-spectrum fluoroquinolone antibiotic for respiratory tract infections* [gemifloxacin (as mesylate)] 320 mg ② Viactiv

factor II (prothrombin)

factor III [see: thromboplastin]

factor VIIa, recombinant *coagulant for hemophilia A and B (orphan); investigational (orphan) for Glanzmann thrombasthenia*

factor VIII [see: antihemophilic factor]

factor VIII (rDNA) BAN *blood coagulating factor*

factor VIII fraction BAN *blood coagulating factor*

factor IX USP *systemic hemostatic; antihemophilic for factor IX deficiency (hemophilia B; Christmas disease) (orphan)* [also: factor IX complex; factor IX fraction; nonacog alfa]

factor IX complex USP *systemic hemostatic/antihemophilic for factor IX deficiency (hemophilia B; Christmas disease) (orphan)* [also: factor IX fraction; nonacog alfa]

factor IX fraction BAN *systemic hemostatic; antihemophilic* [also: factor IX complex; nonacog alfa]

factor XIII concentrate, human *systemic hemostatic/antihemophilic for congenital factor XIII deficiency (orphan)*

Factrel powder for subcu or IV injection ℞ *gonadotropin releasing hormone; diagnostic aid for anterior pituitary function* [gonadorelin HCl] 100, 500 mcg

fadrozole INN *antineoplastic; aromatase inhibitor* [also: fadrozole HCl]

fadrozole HCl USAN *antineoplastic; aromatase inhibitor* [also: fadrozole]

falintolol INN

falipamil INN

false foxglove *medicinal herb* [see: feverweed]

false unicorn (Chamaelirium luteum) root *medicinal herb used for amenorrhea, morning sickness, and preventing miscarriages; also used for colic, cough, and digestive, kidney, and prostate problems; emetic in high doses*

false valerian *medicinal herb* [see: life root]

false vervain *medicinal herb* [see: blue vervain]

FAM (fluorouracil, Adriamycin, mitomycin) *chemotherapy protocol for adenocarcinoma, gastric cancer, and pancreatic cancer*

famciclovir USAN, INN, BAN *oral antiviral for herpes labialis (cold sores), herpes simplex type 2 (genital herpes), and herpes zoster (shingles) infections; suppressive therapy for recurrent outbreaks* 125, 250, 500 mg oral

famiraprinium chloride INN

famotidine USAN, USP, INN, BAN *histamine H₂ antagonist for gastric and duodenal ulcers, gastroesophageal reflux disease (GERD), and gastric hyper-*

secretory conditions 10, 20, 40 mg oral; 40 mg/5 mL oral; 10 mg/mL injection; 20 mg/50 mL infusion

famotine INN *antiviral* [also: famotine HCl]

famotine HCl USAN *antiviral* [also: famotine]

fampridine USAN, INN *investigational (Phase III, orphan) agent for multiple sclerosis and spinal cord injury*

famprofazone INN, BAN

FAMTX (fluorouracil, Adriamycin, methotrexate) [with leucovorin rescue] *chemotherapy protocol for gastric cancer*

Famvir film-coated tablets ℞ *antiviral for herpes labialis (cold sores), herpes simplex type 2 (HSV-2, genital herpes) and herpes zoster (shingles) infections; suppressive therapy for recurrent outbreaks* [famciclovir] 125, 250, 500, 1000 mg

fananserin USAN *antipsychotic; antischizophrenic; dopamine D$_2$ and serotonin 5-HT$_2$ receptor antagonist*

Fanapt tablets ℞ *selective serotonin and dopamine antagonist; atypical antipsychotic for schizophrenia* [iloperidone] 1, 2, 4, 6, 8, 10, 12 mg

fanetizole INN, BAN *immunoregulator* [also: fanetizole mesylate]

fanetizole mesylate USAN *immunoregulator* [also: fanetizole]

Fansidar tablets (discontinued 2010) ℞ *antimalarial* [sulfadoxine; pyrimethamine] 500•25 mg

fanthridone BAN *antidepressant* [also: fantridone HCl; fantridone]

fantridone INN *antidepressant* [also: fantridone HCl; fanthridone]

fantridone HCl USAN *antidepressant* [also: fantridone; fanthridone]

FAP (fluorouracil, Adriamycin, Platinol) *chemotherapy protocol for gastric cancer*

Farbee with Vitamin C caplets (discontinued 2008) OTC *vitamin supplement* [multiple B vitamins; vitamin C] ≚•300 mg

Fareston tablets ℞ *antiestrogen antineoplastic for metastatic breast cancer in postmenopausal women (orphan); investigational (orphan) for desmoid tumors* [toremifene (as citrate)] 60 mg

farglitazar USAN *thiazolidinedione (TZD) antidiabetic that increases cellular response to insulin without increasing insulin secretion*

farnesil INN *combining name for radicals or groups* ⍰ Fer-In-Sol

faropenem [see: fropenem]

fasiplon INN

Faslodex prefilled syringe for IM injection ℞ *once monthly antiestrogen antineoplastic for metastatic breast cancer in postmenopausal women* [fulvestrant] 50 mg/mL

Faspak (trademarked packaging form) *flexible plastic bag* ⍰ Visipak

Fastic (Japanese name for U.S. product **Starlix**) ⍰ Vasotec

Fast-Trak (trademarked delivery device) *quick-loading syringe*

fat, hard NF *suppository base*

fat emulsion, intravenous *parenteral essential fatty acid replacement*

Father John's Medicine Plus oral liquid (discontinued 2007) OTC *antitussive; antihistamine; decongestant* [dextromethorphan hydrobromide; chlorpheniramine maleate; phenylephrine HCl] 10•4•10 mg/30 mL

Fatsia horrida medicinal herb [see: devil's club]

FazaClo orally disintegrating tablets ℞ *novel (atypical) dibenzapine antipsychotic for severe schizophrenia and recurrent suicidal behavior; sedative* [clozapine] 12.5, 25, 100, 150, 200 mg ⍰ Visicol

fazadinium bromide INN, BAN

fazarabine USAN, INN *antineoplastic*

5-FC (5-fluorocytosine) [see: flucytosine]

FC2 Female Condom OTC *barrier contraceptive*

F-CL (fluorouracil, leucovorin calcium [rescue]) *chemotherapy protocol for colorectal, gastric, hepatocellu-*

lar, ovarian, and pancreatic cancers; dosing regimens include: biweekly, de Gramont, Douillard, German, Mayo Clinic, post-gastrectomy, Roswell Park, and weekly [also known as: FU/LV]

FD&C Red No. 2 (Food, Drug & Cosmetic [Act]) [see: amaranth]

FD&C Red No. 3 (Food, Drug & Cosmetic [Act]) [see: erythrosine sodium]

F-ddA (fluorodideoxyadenosine) [see: lodenosine]

FDDNP ([18F] fluoroethyl [methyl] amino-2-naphthyl ethylidene malononitrile) PET scan contrast medium for detection of beta-amyloid senile plaques and neurofibrillary tangles for early detection of Alzheimer disease

18FDG (fludeoxyglucose) [see: fludeoxyglucose F 18]

FDh (2(3H) furanone di-hydro) a precursor to gamma hydroxybutyrate (GHB); a formerly legal alternative to GHB, now also illegal (Schedule I); also known as gamma butyrolactone (GBL) [see: gamma hydroxybutyrate (GHB)]

FDP (fructose-1,6-diphosphate) [q.v.]

FE Aspartate tablets OTC iron supplement [iron (as ferrous aspartate)] 18 mg (112 mg)

59Fe [see: ferric chloride Fe 59]

59Fe [see: ferric citrate (59Fe)]

59Fe [see: ferrous citrate Fe 59]

59Fe [see: ferrous sulfate Fe 59]

febantel USAN, INN, BAN veterinary anthelmintic

febarbamate INN

febricides a class of agents that relieve or reduce fever [also called: antifebriles; antipyretics; antithermics; febrifuges]

febrifuges a class of agents that relieve or reduce fever [also called: antifebriles; antipyretics; antithermics; febricides]

febuprol INN

febuverine INN

febuxostat selective xanthine oxidase inhibitor for gout-associated hyperuricemia

FEC (fluorouracil, epirubicin, cyclophosphamide) chemotherapy protocol for breast cancer [also: CEF]

feclemine INN

feclobuzone INN

FED (fluorouracil, etoposide, DDP) chemotherapy protocol for non–small cell lung cancer (NSCLC)

fedotozine INN kappa selective opioid agonist for irritable bowel syndrome

fedrilate INN

Feen-A-Mint enteric-coated tablets OTC stimulant laxative [bisacodyl] 5 mg

Feiba NF (nanofiltered) powder for IV injection or drip ℞ antihemophilic to correct factor VIII deficiency and coagulation deficiency [anti-inhibitor coagulant complex, vapor heated] 500, 1000, 2500 U/vial

Feiba VH Immuno powder for IV injection or drip (discontinued 2011) ℞ antihemophilic to correct factor VIII deficiency and coagulation deficiency [anti-inhibitor coagulant complex, vapor heated] (each bottle is labeled with dosage)

felbamate USAN, INN anticonvulsant; adjunctive therapy for Lennox-Gastaut syndrome (orphan)

Felbatol tablets, oral suspension (the FDA and the manufacturer strongly caution against its use due to adverse side effects) ℞ anticonvulsant; adjunctive therapy for Lennox-Gastaut syndrome (orphan) [felbamate] 400, 600 mg; 600 mg/5 mL

felbinac USAN, INN, BAN anti-inflammatory

Feldene capsules ℞ analgesic; nonsteroidal anti-inflammatory drug (NSAID) for osteoarthritis and rheumatoid arthritis [piroxicam] 10, 20 mg

felipyrine INN

felodipine USAN, INN, BAN vasodilator; antihypertensive; calcium channel blocker 2.5, 5, 10 mg oral

felonwood; felonwort medicinal herb [see: bittersweet nightshade]

felvizumab USAN *monoclonal antibody for prophylaxis and treatment of respiratory syncytial virus (RSV)*

felypressin USAN, INN, BAN *vasoconstrictor* ⑨ fluprazine

Fem pH vaginal jelly OTC *acidity modifier; antiseptic* [acetic acid, glacial; oxyquinoline sulfate] 0.9%•0.025%

Fem-1 tablets (discontinued 2007) OTC *analgesic; antipyretic; diuretic* [acetaminophen; pamabrom] 500•25 mg

female fern *(Polypodium vulgare)* root *medicinal herb used as an anthelmintic, cholagogue, demulcent, and purgative*

female regulator *medicinal herb* [see: life root]

Femara film-coated tablets ℞ *aromatase inhibitor; estrogen antagonist; antineoplastic for early, advanced, or metastatic breast cancer in postmenopausal women* [letrozole] 2.5 mg

FemBack caplets (discontinued 2008) OTC *analgesic; antipyretic; antihistamine; sleep aid* [acetaminophen; salicylamide; phenyltoloxamine citrate] 150•150•44 mg

Fem-Cal; Fem-Cal Plus tablets OTC *calcium/mineral supplement* [calcium (as carbonate); multiple minerals; vitamin D] 250 mg•±•100 IU

Fem-Cal Citrate tablets OTC *mineral supplement* [calcium (as citrate); vitamin D; multiple minerals] ±•100 IU•±

Femcon Fe chewable tablets (in packs of 28) ℞ *monophasic oral contraceptive; iron supplement* [norethindrone; ethinyl estradiol; ferrous fumarate] 0.4 mg•35 mcg•75 mg × 21 days; 0•0•75 mg × 7 days

femhrt 1/5 tablets (in packs of 28) ℞ *a mixture of synthetic and equine hormones; hormone replacement therapy for postmenopausal symptoms* [norethindrone acetate; ethinyl estradiol] 1 mg•5 mcg

femhrtLo tablets (in packs of 28) ℞ *a mixture of synthetic and equine hormones; hormone replacement therapy*

for postmenopausal symptoms [norethindrone acetate; ethinyl estradiol] 0.5 mg•2.5 mcg

Feminique Disposable Douche vaginal solution OTC *acidity modifier; cleanser and deodorizer* [vinegar (acetic acid)]

Femizol-M vaginal cream (discontinued 2009) OTC *antifungal* [miconazole nitrate] 2%

femoxetine INN

Femring vaginal ring ℞ *synthetic estrogen; three-month hormone replacement for postmenopausal atrophic vaginitis* [estradiol acetate] 12.4 mg (50 mcg/day), 24.8 mg (100 mcg day)

FemSoft urethral insert ℞ *treatment for stress urinary incontinence* [silicone plug]

Femtrace tablets ℞ *synthetic estrogen; hormone replacement for postmenopausal symptoms* [estradiol acetate] 0.45, 0.9, 1.8 mg

Fem-V kit for home use OTC *in vitro diagnostic aid for vaginal infections*

fenabutene INN

fenacetinol INN

fenaclon INN

fenadiazole INN ⑨ Vandazole

fenaftic acid INN

fenalamide USAN, INN *smooth muscle relaxant*

fenalcomine INN

fenamifuril INN

fenamisal INN *antibacterial; tuberculostatic* [also: phenyl aminosalicylate]

fenamole USAN, INN *anti-inflammatory* ⑨ Venomil

fenaperone INN

fenarsone [see: carbarsone]

fenasprate [see: benorilate]

fenbendazole USAN, INN, BAN *anthelmintic*

fenbenicillin INN [also: phenbenicillin]

fenbufen USAN, INN, BAN *anti-inflammatory*

fenbutrazate INN [also: phenbutrazate]

fencamfamin INN, BAN

fencamfamin HCl [see: fencamfamin]

fencarbamide INN *anticholinergic* [also: phencarbamide]

fenchlorphos BAN *systemic insecticide* [also: ronnel; fenclofos]

fencilbutirol USAN, INN *choleretic*

fenclexonium metilsulfate INN

fenclofenac USAN, INN, BAN *anti-inflammatory*

fenclofos INN *systemic insecticide* [also: ronnel; fenchlorphos]

fenclonine USAN, INN *serotonin inhibitor*

fenclorac USAN, INN *anti-inflammatory*

fenclozic acid INN, BAN

fendiline INN

fendizoate INN *combining name for radicals or groups*

fendosal USAN, INN, BAN *anti-inflammatory* ⊗ Vandazole

feneritrol INN

Fenesin DM IR tablets OTC *antitussive; expectorant* [dextromethorphan hydrobromide; guaifenesin] 15•400 mg

fenestrel USAN, INN *estrogen*

fenethazine INN ⊗ phenothiazine

fenethylline BAN *CNS stimulant* [also: fenethylline HCl; fenetylline] ⊗ phenythilone; Ventolin

fenethylline HCl USAN *CNS stimulant* [also: fenetylline; fenethylline]

fenetradil INN

fenetylline INN *CNS stimulant* [also: fenethylline HCl; fenethylline] ⊗ Ventolin

fenflumizole INN

fenfluramine INN, BAN *anorexiant; CNS depressant* [also: fenfluramine HCl]

fenfluramine HCl USAN *anorexiant; CNS depressant* [also: fenfluramine]

fenfluthrin INN, BAN

fengabine USAN, INN, BAN *mood regulator*

fenharmane INN ⊗ pheniramine

fenimide USAN, INN, BAN *antipsychotic* ⊗ Vanamide

feniodium chloride INN

fenipentol INN

fenirofibrate INN

fenisorex USAN, INN, BAN *anorectic*

fenleuton USAN *5-lipoxygenase inhibitor for asthma*

fenmetozole INN *antidepressant; narcotic antagonist* [also: fenmetozole HCl]

fenmetozole HCl USAN *antidepressant; narcotic antagonist* [also: fenmetozole]

fenmetramide USAN, INN, BAN *antidepressant*

fennel *(Anethum foeniculum; Foeniculum officinale; F. vulgare)* seeds *medicinal herb for colic, gas, intestinal problems, promoting expectoration, stimulating lactation and menses, and sedation in children* ⊗ phenol; vanilla

fennel oil NF

fenobam USAN, INN *sedative*

fenocinol INN

fenoctimine INN *gastric antisecretory* [also: fenoctimine sulfate]

fenoctimine sulfate USAN *gastric antisecretory* [also: fenoctimine]

fenofibrate INN, BAN *fibric acid derivative; PPARα agonist for primary hypercholesterolemia, hypertriglyceridemia, and mixed dyslipidemia; also used for hyperuricemia* 54, 67, 107, 134, 160, 200 mg oral

Fenoglide tablets ℞ *antihyperlipidemic for primary hypercholesterolemia, hypertriglyceridemia, and mixed dyslipidemia; also used for hyperuricemia* [fenofibrate] 40, 120 mg ⊗ Vancoled

fenoldopam INN, BAN *dopamine agonist; vasodilator for hypertensive emergencies* [also: fenoldopam mesylate]

fenoldopam mesylate USAN *dopamine agonist; rapid-acting vasodilator for in-hospital management of hypertensive emergencies* [also: fenoldopam] 10 mg/mL injection

fenoprofen USAN, INN, BAN *analgesic; nonsteroidal anti-inflammatory drug (NSAID)*

fenoprofen calcium USAN, USP, BAN *analgesic; nonsteroidal anti-inflammatory drug (NSAID) for osteoarthritis, rheumatoid arthritis, and other mild to moderate pain; also used for juvenile rheumatoid arthritis, migraine head-*

aches, and sunburn pain 200, 300, 600 mg oral

fenoterol USAN, INN, BAN *bronchodilator; beta-blocker* [also: fenoterol hydrobromide] 🔟 Phentrol

fenoterol hydrobromide JAN *bronchodilator; antiasthmatic; beta-blocker* [also: fenoterol]

fenoverine INN

fenoxazol [see: pemoline]

fenoxazoline INN

fenoxazoline HCl [see: fenoxazoline]

fenoxedil INN

fenoxypropazine INN [also: phenoxypropazine]

fenozolone INN

fenpentadiol INN

fenperate INN

fenpipalone USAN, INN *anti-inflammatory*

fenpipramide INN, BAN

fenpiprane INN, BAN

fenpiprane HCl [see: fenpiprane]

fenpiverinium bromide INN

fenprinast INN *bronchodilator; antiallergic* [also: fenprinast HCl]

fenprinast HCl USAN *bronchodilator; antiallergic* [also: fenprinast]

fenproporex INN

fenprostalene USAN, INN, BAN *luteolysin*

fenquizone USAN, INN *diuretic* 🔟 Vancocin

fenretinide USAN, INN *investigational (Phase II) synthetic retinoid to slow the progression of macular degeneration*

fenspiride INN *bronchodilator; antiadrenergic (alpha-blocker)* [also: fenspiride HCl]

fenspiride HCl USAN *bronchodilator; antiadrenergic (alpha-blocker)* [also: fenspiride]

fentanyl INN, BAN *narcotic analgesic; also abused as a street drug* [also: fentanyl citrate] 12.5, 25, 50, 75, 100 mcg/hr. transdermal; 0.1, 0.2, 0.4, 0.6, 0.8 mg oral transmucosal

fentanyl citrate USAN, USP, JAN *narcotic analgesic for breakthrough pain in cancer patients; adjunct to anesthesia; also abused as a street drug* [also: fen-

tanyl] 200, 400, 600, 800, 1200, 1600 mcg oral transmucosal

Fentanyl Citrate Transmucosal lozenge on a stick ℞ *narcotic analgesic for anesthesia premedication* [fentanyl citrate] 200, 400, 600, 800, 1200, 1600 mcg

fentanyl HCl *transdermal narcotic analgesic for short-term management of postoperative pain* (base=90%)

fenthion BAN 🔟 phenytoin

fentiazac USAN, INN, BAN *anti-inflammatory*

fenticlor USAN, INN, BAN *topical anti-infective*

fenticonazole INN, BAN *antifungal* [also: fenticonazole nitrate]

fenticonazole nitrate USAN *antifungal* [also: fenticonazole]

fentonium bromide INN

Fentora buccal tablets ℞ *transmucosal narcotic analgesic for chronic pain in opioid-tolerant cancer patients* [fentanyl (as citrate)] 100, 200, 400, 600, 800 mcg

fenugreek (Trigonella foenum-grae-cum) seeds *medicinal herb for boils, bronchial secretions, cellulitis, diabetes, hypercholesterolemia, kidney stones, lung infections, promoting expectoration, stomach irritation, and tuberculosis*

fenyramidol INN *analgesic; skeletal muscle relaxant* [also: phenyramidol HCl]

fenyripol INN *skeletal muscle relaxant* [also: fenyripol HCl]

fenyripol HCl USAN *skeletal muscle relaxant* [also: fenyripol]

Feocyte prolonged-action tablets (discontinued 2008) ℞ *hematinic* [iron (as ferrous fumarate, ferrous gluconate, and ferrous sulfate); desiccated liver; vitamins B_6, B_{12}, and C; folic acid] 110•15•2•0.05•100•0.8 mg

FeoGen capsules ℞ *hematinic* [iron (as ferrous fumarate); vitamin B_{12}; vitamin C; intrinsic factor concentrate] 66•0.01•250•100 mg

FeoGen FA; FeoGen Forte gelcaps ℞ *hematinic* [iron; vitamins B_{12} & C;

folic acid] 66•0.01•250•1 mg; 151•
0.01•60•1 mg

Feosol tablets OTC *iron supplement* [carbonyl iron] 45 mg (note: multiple products with the same name) ☑ PhosLo; VaZol; VSL

Feosol tablets OTC *iron supplement* [iron (as ferrous sulfate)] 65 mg (325 mg) (note: multiple products with the same name) ☑ PhosLo; VaZol; VSL

Feosol tablets OTC *iron supplement* [iron (as ferrous sulfate, dried)] 65 mg (200 mg) (note: multiple products with the same name) ☑ PhosLo; VaZol; VSL

fepentolic acid INN

fepitrizol INN

fepradinol INN

feprazone INN, BAN

fepromide INN

feprosidnine INN

Feraheme IV injection OTC *iron replacement for iron deficiency in patients with chronic kidney disease* [iron (as ferumoxytol)] 30 mg/mL

Feratab tablets OTC *iron supplement* [iron (as ferrous sulfate, dried)] 60 mg

Fer-Gen-Sol drops (discontinued 2011) OTC *iron supplement* [iron (as ferrous sulfate)] 15 mg/0.6 mL ☑ voriconazole

Fergon tablets OTC *iron supplement* [iron (as ferrous gluconate)] 27 mg

Feridex I.V. injection R *radiopaque contrast medium to enhance MRIs of the liver* [ferumoxides] 11.2 mg iron

Fer-In-Sol drops (name changed to **Enfamil Fer-In-Sol** in 2009) ☑ farnesil

Fer-Iron drops OTC *iron supplement* [iron (as ferrous sulfate)] 15 mg/mL

fermium *element (Fm)*

fern; fern brake *medicinal herb* [see: buckhorn brake; female fern]

fern, flowering; king's fern; water fern *medicinal herb* [see: buckhorn brake]

FernBlock capsules OTC *herbal remedy that protects skin from sun damage by absorbing ultraviolet rays and quench-* *ing free radicals* [*Polypodium leucotomos*] 240 mg

fern-leaved foxglove *medicinal herb* [see: feverweed]

Fero-Folic-500 controlled-release Filmtabs (film-coated tablets) (discontinued 2008) R *hematinic* [iron (as ferrous sulfate); vitamin C; folic acid] 105•500•0.8 mg

Fero-Grad-500 controlled-release tablets OTC *vitamin/iron supplement* [iron (as ferrous sulfate); sodium ascorbate] 105•500 mg

FeroSul tablets OTC *iron supplement* [iron (as ferrous sulfate)] 65 mg ☑ Virasal; vorozole

Ferotrinsic capsules (discontinued 2008) R *hematinic* [iron (as ferrous fumarate); vitamin B$_{12}$; vitamin C; intrinsic factor concentrate; folic acid] 110•0.015•75•240•0.5 mg

Ferralet 90 film-coated tablets R *hematinic* [carbonyl iron; vitamins B$_{12}$ and C; folic acid; docusate sodium] 90•0.012•120•1•50 mg

Ferralet Plus tablets (discontinued 2008) OTC *vitamin/iron supplement* [iron (as ferrous gluconate); vitamin B$_{12}$; vitamin C; folic acid] 46•0.025•400•0.8 mg

Ferretts film-coated caplets OTC *iron supplement* [iron (as ferrous fumarate)] 106 mg ☑ Fortaz

Ferrex 150 capsules OTC *iron supplement* [iron (as polysaccharide-iron complex)] 150 mg

Ferrex 150 Forte capsules R *hematinic* [iron (as elemental iron and polysaccharide iron); vitamin B$_{12}$; folic acid] 150•0.025•1 mg

Ferrex 150 Forte Plus capsules R *hematinic* [iron (as polysaccharide-iron complex); vitamins B$_{12}$ and C; folic acid] 150•0.025•60•1 mg

Ferrex 150 Plus capsules OTC *vitamin/iron supplement* [iron (as polysaccharide-iron complex); vitamin C] 150 mg•50 mg

Ferrex PC; Ferrex PC Forte film-coated tablets R *vitamin/mineral/iron*

supplement for pregnancy and lactation [multiple vitamins & minerals; iron (as polysaccharide-iron complex); folic acid] ± • 60 • 1 mg

ferric ammonium citrate NF

ferric ammonium sulfate

ferric cacodylate NF

ferric chloride (FeCl₃)

ferric chloride Fe 59 (⁵⁹FeCl₃) USAN *radioactive agent*

ferric citrate (⁵⁹Fe) INN

ferric citrochloride NF

ferric fructose USAN, INN *hematinic*

ferric glycerophosphate NF

ferric hexacyanoferrate (insoluble Prussian blue) *chelating agent for internal contamination with radioactive or nonradioactive cesium and/or thallium (orphan)*

ferric hyaluronate *adhesion barrier for open gynecological and lower GI surgery*

ferric hydroxide sucrose complex [see: iron sucrose; saccharated ferric oxide]

ferric hypophosphite NF

ferric oxide NF *coloring agent*

ferric oxide, red NF

ferric oxide, yellow NF

ferric pyrophosphate, soluble NF

ferric subsulfate NF *hemostatic used in a solution or paste to control superficial bleeding from skin biopsies, cervical biopsies, colposcopy, etc.*

ferricholinate [see: ferrocholinate]

ferriclate calcium sodium USAN *hematinic* [also: calcium sodium ferriclate]

Ferriprox *investigational (orphan) agent for chronic iron overload due to transfusion-dependent anemias* [deferiprone]

ferristene USAN *paramagnetic imaging agent for MRI*

Ferrlecit IV infusion ℞ *hematinic for iron deficiency due to chronic hemodialysis with erythropoietin therapy* [iron (as sodium ferric gluconate)] 62.5 mg/5 mL

ferrocholate [see: ferrocholinate]

ferrocholinate INN

Ferrocyte Plus film-coated caplets ℞ *hematinic* [iron (as ferrous fumarate);

multiple vitamins & minerals; folic acid] 106 • ± • 1 mg

Ferrogel Forte softgels ℞ *hematinic* [iron (as ferrous fumarate); vitamin B₁₂; vitamin C; folic acid] 151 • 0.01 • 60 • 1 mg

ferropolimaler INN

Ferro-Sequels timed-release tablets OTC *iron supplement* [iron (as ferrous fumarate); docusate sodium] 50 • 100 mg

ferrotrenine INN

ferrous aspartate *hematinic; iron supplement (16% elemental iron)*

ferrous citrate Fe 59 USAN, USP *radioactive agent*

ferrous fumarate USP *hematinic; iron supplement (33% elemental iron)* 90, 324 mg oral

ferrous gluconate USP *hematinic; iron supplement (11.6% elemental iron)* 225, 300, 324, 325 mg oral

ferrous lactate NF

ferrous orotate JAN

ferrous sulfate (FeSO₄ · 7H₂O) USP, JAN *hematinic; iron supplement (20% elemental iron)* 135, 140, 325 mg (27, 45, 65 mg Fe) oral; 220, 300 mg (44, 60 mg Fe)/5 mL oral; 75 mg (15 mg Fe)/mL oral

ferrous sulfate, dried (FeSO₄ · xH₂O) USP *hematinic; iron supplement (30% elemental iron)* 160 mg (50 mg Fe) oral

ferrous sulfate, exsiccated [see: ferrous sulfate, dried]

ferrous sulfate Fe 59 (⁵⁹FeSO₄) USAN *radioactive agent*

fertirelin INN, BAN *veterinary gonadotropin-releasing hormone* [also: fertirelin acetate]

fertirelin acetate USAN *veterinary gonadotropin-releasing hormone* [also: fertirelin]

ferucarbotran USAN *superparamagnetic diagnostic aid*

Ferula assafoetida; F. foetida; F. rubricaulis *medicinal herb* [see: asafetida; asafoetida]

ferumoxides USAN *parenteral radi-opaque contrast medium to enhance MRIs of the liver*

ferumoxsil USAN *oral MRI contrast medium for upper GI tract imaging*

ferumoxtran-10 USAN *superparamagnetic diagnostic aid; investigational (NDA filed) for magnetic resonance lymphangiography (MRL) to detect lymph node metastases*

ferumoxytol *iron replacement for iron deficiency in patients with chronic kidney disease*

FeSO₄ (ferrous sulfate) [q.v.]

fesoterodine fumarate *muscarinic receptor antagonist for overactive bladder*

Fetal Fibronectin Test kit for professional use ℞ *in vitro diagnostic aid for fetal fibronectin in vaginal secretions at 24–34 weeks, a predictor of preterm delivery*

fetal neural cells [see: neural cells, porcine fetal]

fetid hellebore (Helleborus foetidus) [see: hellebore]

Fe-Tinic 150 capsules (discontinued 2009) ℞ *hematinic* [iron (as polysaccharide-iron complex)] 150 mg

Fe-Tinic 150 Forte capsules ℞ *hematinic* [iron (as polysaccharide-iron complex); vitamin B₁₂; folic acid] 150•0.025•1 mg

fetoxilate INN *smooth muscle relaxant* [also: fetoxylate HCl; fetoxylate]

fetoxylate BAN *smooth muscle relaxant* [also: fetoxylate HCl; fetoxilate]

fetoxylate HCl USAN *smooth muscle relaxant* [also: fetoxilate; fetoxylate]

fever root *medicinal herb* [see: coral root]

fever twig *medicinal herb* [see: bittersweet nightshade]

FeverAll; Children's FeverAll; Infant's FeverAll; Junior FeverAll suppositories OTC *analgesic; antipyretic* [acetaminophen] 650 mg; 120 mg; 80 mg; 325 mg

FeverAll, Children's; Junior FeverAll Sprinkle Caps (powder) (discontinued 2008) OTC *analgesic; antipyretic* [acetaminophen] 80 mg; 160 mg

feverbush *medicinal herb* [see: winterberry]

feverfew (Chrysanthemum parthenium; Leucanthemum parthenium; Pyrethrum parthenium; Tanacetum parthenium) leaves and flowers *medicinal herb used as an aspirin substitute for chills, colds, fever, inflammation, and migraine and sinus headache*

feverweed (Gerardia pedicularia) plant *medicinal herb used as an antiseptic, diaphoretic, febrifuge, and sedative*

fexicaine INN

fexinidazole INN

Fexmid film-coated tablets ℞ *skeletal muscle relaxant* [cyclobenzaprine HCl] 7.5 mg

fexofenadine HCl USAN *second-generation peripherally selective piperidine antihistamine for allergic rhinitis and chronic idiopathic urticaria* 30, 60, 180 mg oral

fexofenadine HCl & pseudoephedrine HCl *antihistamine and decongestant combination for allergic rhinitis* 60•120, 180•240 mg oral

fezatione INN

fezolamine INN *antidepressant* [also: fezolamine fumarate]

fezolamine fumarate USAN *antidepressant* [also: fezolamine]

FGF-20 (fibroblast growth factor-20) [q.v.]

fiacitabine (FIAC) USAN, INN *antiviral*

fialuridine (FIAU) USAN, INN *investigational (orphan) antiviral for chronic active hepatitis B5*

Fiber Choice chewable tablets OTC *vitamin/mineral supplement* [multiple vitamins and minerals; folic acid] ≜ •200 mcg

Fiber Therapy Original Texture powder for oral solution OTC *bulk laxative* [psyllium hydrophilic mucilloid] 3.4 g/tsp.

Fiberall powder OTC *bulk laxative* [psyllium hydrophilic mucilloid] 3.5 g/tsp.

FiberCon tablets OTC *bulk laxative; antidiarrheal* [calcium polycarbophil] 500 mg

Fiberlan oral liquid OTC *enteral nutritional therapy* [lactose-free formula]

Fiber-Lax tablets OTC *bulk laxative; antidiarrheal* [calcium polycarbophil] 625 mg

FiberNorm tablets OTC *bulk laxative; antidiarrheal* [calcium polycarbophil] 625 mg

Fibersure powder for oral solution OTC *bulk laxative; antidiarrheal; dietary fiber supplement* [inulin]

fibracillin INN

Fibricor tablets ℞ *antihyperlipidemic for primary hypercholesterolemia, hypertriglyceridemia, and mixed dyslipidemia; also used for hyperuricemia* [fenofibric acid] 35, 105 mg

fibrin INN

fibrin sealant, human *topical agent to adhere autologous skin grafts to wounds due to burns; dressing treatment to control bleeding during cardiovascular surgery*

fibrinase [see: factor XIII]

fibrinogen (^{125}I) INN [also: fibrinogen I 125]

fibrinogen, human USP *systemic hemostatic to control bleeding in fibrinogen-deficient patients* (orphan)

fibrinogen I 125 USAN *vascular patency test; radioactive agent* [also: fibrinogen (^{125}I)]

fibrinoligase [see: factor XIII]

fibrinolysin, human INN [also: plasmin]

fibrin-stabilizing factor (FSF) [see: factor XIII]

fibroblast growth factor, basic (bFGF) [see: ersofermin]

fibroblast growth factor-20, recombinant human (rhFGF-20) *investigational (orphan) for radiation-induced oral mucositis*

fibroblast interferon [now: interferon beta]

Fibrogammin P (name changed to **Corifact** upon marketing release in 2011)

fibronectin *investigational (orphan) for nonhealing corneal ulcers or epithelial defects*

Ficus carica *medicinal herb* [see: fig]

fidaxomicin *oral macrolide antibiotic for* Clostridium difficile *infections*

Fidelin *natural hormone precursor; investigational (NDA filed, orphan) for systemic lupus erythematosus (SLE); investigational (orphan) replacement therapy for adrenal insufficiency* [dehydroepiandrosterone (DHEA)]

fiduxosin HCl USAN *alpha$_{1a}$-adrenoceptor antagonist for benign prostatic hyperplasia (BPH)*

fig (Ficus carica) *fruit medicinal herb used as a demulcent, emollient, and laxative*

figwort (Scrophularia nodosa) *leaves, stems, and roots medicinal herb for abrasions, athlete's foot, cradle cap, fever, impetigo, restlessness, skin diseases, and skin tumors*

filaminast USAN *selective phosphodiesterase IV inhibitor for asthma*

filenadol INN

filgrastim USAN, INN, BAN *hematopoietic stimulant for severe chronic neutropenia (orphan), acute myeloid leukemia (AML), and bone marrow transplants; investigational (Phase III, orphan) cytokine for AIDS-related cytomegalovirus retinitis; investigational (orphan) for myelodysplastic syndrome biosimilar (available in Europe):* 300 mcg/mL injection

Filipendula ulmaria *medicinal herb* [see: meadowsweet]

filipin USAN, INN *antifungal* ☒ Velban

Filmix *investigational (orphan) neurosonographic contrast medium for intracranial tumors* [microbubble contrast agent]

Filmlok (trademarked dosage form) *film-coated tablet*

Filmseal (trademarked dosage form) *film-coated tablet* ☒ flumizole

Filmtabs (trademarked dosage form) *film-coated tablets*

Finac lotion OTC *keratolytic for acne* [salicylic acid; isopropyl alcohol] 2%•22.5% ℞ FNC

Finacea gel ℞ *antimicrobial and keratolytic for mild to moderate rosacea* [azelaic acid] 15% ℞ Phenazo

Finajet; Finaplix *brand names for trenbolone acetate, a European veterinary anabolic steroid abused as a street drug*

finasteride USAN, INN, BAN *alphareductase inhibitor; androgen hormone inhibitor for benign prostatic hyperplasia (BPH) and androgenic alopecia in men; investigational for aggressive prostate tumors* 5 mg oral

Finevin cream ℞ *antimicrobial and keratolytic for inflammatory acne vulgaris* [azelaic acid] 20%

finger leaf *medicinal herb* [see: cinquefoil]

fingolimod *immunomodulator; oral treatment for relapsing multiple sclerosis*

Fioricet tablets ℞ *barbiturate sedative; analgesic; antipyretic* [butalbital; acetaminophen; caffeine] 50•325•40 mg

Fioricet with Codeine capsules ℞ *narcotic antitussive; barbiturate sedative; analgesic* [codeine phosphate; butalbital; acetaminophen; caffeine] 30•50•325•40 mg

Fiorinal capsules ℞ *barbiturate sedative; analgesic; antipyretic* [butalbital; aspirin; caffeine] 50•325•40 mg

Fiorinal with Codeine capsules ℞ *barbiturate sedative; narcotic antitussive; analgesic; antipyretic* [butalbital; codeine phosphate; aspirin; caffeine] 50•30•325•40 mg

fipexide INN

Firazyr subcu injection ℞ *treatment for hereditary angioedema (HAE) (orphan)* [icatibant acetate] 10 mg/mL

fireweed *medicinal herb* [see: pilewort]

Firmagon subcu injection ℞ *gonadotropin-releasing hormone (GnRH) blocker to reduce testosterone levels in patients with advanced prostate cancer* [degarelix (as acetate)] 80, 120 mg/vial

First Choice reagent strips for home use OTC *in vitro diagnostic aid for blood glucose*

First Duke's Mouthwash oral suspension ℞ *topical antihistamine; topical anti-inflammatory; topical antifungal* [diphenhydramine; hydrocortisone; nystatin] 525•60•600 mg/bottle

First Mary's Mouthwash oral suspension ℞ *topical antihistamine; topical anti-inflammatory; topical antifungal; topical antibiotic* [diphenhydramine; hydrocortisone; nystatin; tetracycline HCl] 450•60•1200•1500 mg/bottle

First Response; First Response Early Result test stick for home use OTC *in vitro diagnostic aid; urine pregnancy test*

First Response Ovulation Predictor test kit for home use OTC *in vitro diagnostic aid to predict ovulation time*

fisalamine [see: mesalamine]

fit root (Monotropa uniflora) *medicinal herb used as an antispasmodic, febrifuge, nervine, and sedative*

FIV-ASA suppositories ℞ *anti-inflammatory for active ulcerative colitis, proctosigmoiditis, and proctitis* [mesalamine (5-aminosalicylic acid)] 500 mg

5 + 2 protocol (cytarabine, daunorubicin) *chemotherapy protocol for acute myelocytic leukemia (AML)*

5 + 2 protocol (cytarabine, mitoxantrone) *chemotherapy protocol for acute myelocytic leukemia (AML)*

5-ALA HCl; ALA [see: aminolevulinic acid HCl]

5% Alcohol and 5% Dextrose in Water; 10% Alcohol and 5% Dextrose in Water IV infusion ℞ *for caloric replacement and rehydration* [dextrose; alcohol] 5%•5%; 10%•5%

5 Benzagel; 10 Benzagel gel ℞ *keratolytic for acne* [benzoyl peroxide] 5%; 10%

5% Travert and Electrolyte No. 2; 10% Travert and Electrolyte No. 2 IV infusion ℞ *intravenous nutritional/electrolyte therapy* [combined electrolyte solution; invert sugar (50% dextrose + 50% fructose)]

506U78 *investigational (orphan) for chronic lymphocytic leukemia*

5-FC (5-fluorocytosine) [see: flucytosine]

five-finger grass; five fingers *medicinal herb* [see: cinquefoil]

five-fingers root *medicinal herb* [see: ginseng]

5-HT (5-hydroxytryptamine) [see: serotonin]

5-HT₃ (hydroxytryptamine) receptor antagonists *a class of antiemetic and antinauseant agents used primarily after emetogenic cancer chemotherapy* [also called: selective serotonin 5-HT₃ blockers]

5-HTP (5-hydroxytryptophan) [see: L-5 hydroxytryptophan]

FL (flutamide, leuprolide acetate) *chemotherapy protocol for prostate cancer*

flag, sweet; myrtle flag *medicinal herb* [see: calamus]

flag lily; poison flag; water flag *medicinal herb* [see: blue flag]

Flagyl film-coated tablets, capsules ℞ *antibiotic; antiprotozoal; amebicide* [metronidazole] 250, 500 mg; 375 mg ② Ful-Glo

Flagyl topical *investigational (orphan) treatment for advanced decubitus ulcers and active perianal Crohn disease* [metronidazole]

Flagyl ER film-coated extended-release tablets ℞ *once-daily antibiotic for bacterial vaginosis* [metronidazole] 750 mg

Flagyl IV powder for injection (discontinued 2010) ℞ *antibiotic; antiprotozoal; amebicide* [metronidazole HCl] 500 mg

flamenol INN

Flammacerium *investigational (orphan) for life-threatening burns* [silver sulfadiazine; cerium nitrate]

Flanders Buttocks ointment OTC *diaper rash treatment* [zinc oxide; Peruvian balsam]

flannel flower *medicinal herb* [see: mullein]

Flarex Drop-Tainers (eye drop suspension) ℞ *corticosteroidal anti-inflammatory* [fluorometholone (as acetate)] 0.1% ② Fluarix

FlashDose (trademarked dosage form) *orally disintegrating tablets*

Flatulex drops OTC *antiflatulent* [simethicone] 40 mg/0.6 mL

Flatulex tablets (discontinued 2009) OTC *adsorbent; detoxicant; antiflatulent* [activated charcoal; simethicone] 250•80 mg

flavamine INN

flavine [see: acriflavine HCl]

flavocoxid *natural flavonoids and flavins; natural COX-2 inhibitor; analgesic and anti-inflammatory for the dietary management of osteoarthritis*

flavodic acid INN

flavodilol INN *antihypertensive* [also: flavodilol maleate]

flavodilol maleate USAN *antihypertensive* [also: flavodilol]

flavonoid [see: troxerutin]

Flavons tablets OTC *dietary supplement* [mixed bioflavonoids] 500 mg

Flavons-500 tablets OTC *dietary supplement* [citrus bioflavonoids] 500 mg

flavoxate INN, BAN *smooth muscle relaxant; urinary antispasmodic* [also: flavoxate HCl]

flavoxate HCl USAN *anticholinergic; smooth muscle relaxant; urinary antispasmodic* [also: flavoxate] 100 mg oral

flaxseed (Linum usitatissimum) *medicinal herb for arthritis, autoimmune diseases, colds, constipation, cough, heart disease, lowering cholesterol levels, skin disorders, and urinary tract infections*

flazalone USAN, INN, BAN *anti-inflammatory* ② flusalan

FLe (fluorouracil, levamisole) *chemotherapy protocol for colorectal cancer*

flea seed; fleawort *medicinal herb* [see: plantain]

fleabane; horseweed (Erigeron canadensis) plant *medicinal herb used as* *an astringent, diuretic, and hemostatic* ⑤ Velban

fleawort; flea seed *medicinal herb* [see: plantain]

Flebogamma 5%; Flebogamma 10% IV infusion ℞ *passive immunizing agent for primary (inherited) immunodeficiency disorders; also used for Guillain-Barré syndrome, myasthenia gravis, and multiple sclerosis* [immune globulin (IGIV)] 5% (0.5, 2.5, 5, 10 g/dose); 10% (5, 10, 20 g/dose)

flecainide INN, BAN *antiarrhythmic* [also: flecainide acetate]

flecainide acetate USAN *antiarrhythmic* [also: flecainide] 50, 100, 150 mg oral

Flector transdermal patch ℞ *analgesic; nonsteroidal anti-inflammatory drug (NSAID) for acute pain due to strains, sprains, and contusions* [diclofenac (as epolamine)] 180 mg

Fleet disposable enema OTC *saline laxative* [monobasic sodium phosphate; dibasic sodium phosphate] 7•19 g/ 118 mL dose

Fleet Babylax rectal liquid OTC *hyperosmolar laxative* [glycerin] 4 mL/dose

Fleet Bisacodyl disposable enema OTC *stimulant laxative* [bisacodyl] 10 mg/ 30 mL dose

Fleet Laxative enteric-coated tablets, suppositories OTC *stimulant laxative* [bisacodyl] 5 mg; 10 mg

Fleet Medicated Wipes cleansing pads OTC *moisturizer and cleanser for external rectal/vaginal areas; astringent; antiseptic; antifungal* [hamamelis water (witch hazel); glycerin; alcohol] 50%•10%•7%

Fleet Mineral Oil disposable enema OTC *emollient laxative* [mineral oil] 118 mL dose

Fleet Pain Relief anorectal wipes OTC *local anesthetic* [pramoxine HCl; glycerin] 1%•12%

Fleet Phospho-soda oral solution (discontinued 2009) OTC *saline laxative* [monobasic sodium phosphate; dibasic sodium phosphate] 7.2•2.7 g/15 mL

Fleet Phospho-soda EZ-Prep two-dose kit (discontinued 2009) OTC *pre-procedure bowel evacuant* [monobasic sodium phosphate; dibasic sodium phosphate] First dose: 21.6•5.4 g/45 mL; Second dose: 14.4•3.6 g/30 mL

Fleet Prep Kit No. 1 and No. 2 (discontinued 2009) OTC *pre-procedure bowel evacuant* [other Fleet products in combination kits]

Fleet Prep Kit No. 3 oral liquid + 4 tablets + enema OTC *pre-procedure bowel evacuant* [**Fleet Phospho-soda** (liquid); bisacodyl (tablets and enema)] 45 mL; 5 mg; 10 mg/30 mL

flerobuterol INN

fleroxacin USAN, INN *antibacterial*

flesinoxan INN *antidepressant; anxiolytic*

flestolol INN *antiadrenergic (beta-blocker)* [also: flestolol sulfate]

flestolol sulfate USAN *antiadrenergic (beta-blocker)* [also: flestolol]

fletazepam USAN, INN, BAN *skeletal muscle relaxant*

Fletcher's Castoria oral liquid OTC *stimulant laxative* [senna concentrate] 33.3 mg/mL

fleur-de-lis *medicinal herb* [see: blue flag]

Flexall gel OTC *mild anesthetic; antipruritic; counterirritant* [menthol] 7%

Flex-all 454 gel OTC *analgesic; mild anesthetic; antipruritic; counterirritant* [methyl salicylate; menthol] ≟•16%

Flexaphen capsules (discontinued 2009) ℞ *skeletal muscle relaxant; analgesic; antipyretic* [chlorzoxazone; acetaminophen] 250•300 mg

Flex-Care Especially for Sensitive Eyes solution (discontinued 2010) OTC *chemical disinfecting solution for soft contact lenses* [note: the soft contact indication is different from RGP contact indication for the same product]

Flex-Care Especially for Sensitive Eyes solution (discontinued 2010) OTC *disinfecting/wetting/soaking solution for rigid gas permeable contact lenses* [note: the RGP contact indication is different from soft contact indication for the same product]

Flexderm sheets OTC *absorbent wound dressing* [hydrogel polymer]

Flexeril film-coated tablets ℞ *skeletal muscle relaxant* [cyclobenzaprine HCl] 5, 10 mg

FlexiGel Strands wound dressing OTC *absorbent dressing*

Flexon IV or IM injection ℞ *skeletal muscle relaxant; analgesic; anticholinergic* [orphenadrine citrate] 30 mg/mL ⧉ Floxin; fluquazone

FlexPack HP test for professional use ℞ *diagnostic aid for serum IgG antibodies to* H. pylori *(for peptic ulcers)*

FlexPen (trademarked delivery form) *disposable prefilled self-injector for insulin*

Flex-Power Performance Sports cream OTC *analgesic* [trolamine salicylate] 10%

Flextra-DS tablets ℞ *analgesic; antipyretic; antihistamine; sleep aid* [acetaminophen; phenyltoloxamine citrate] 500•50 mg

Flexzan; Flexzan Extra adhesive sheets OTC *absorbent, semi-occlusive wound dressing* [polyurethane foam]

flibanserin USAN *agent to block serotonin and boost dopamine; rapid-acting antidepressant; investigational (Phase III) agent to increase sexual desire and arousal in women*

Flintstones; Flintstones with Extra C chewable tablets OTC *vitamin supplement* [multiple vitamins; folic acid] ≟•300 mcg

Flintstones Complete chewable tablets OTC *vitamin/mineral/calcium/iron supplement* [multiple vitamins & minerals; calcium; iron (as ferrous fumarate); folic acid; biotin] ≟• 100•18•0.4•0.04 mg

Flintstones Gummies; Flintstones Sour Gummies OTC *vitamin/mineral supplement* [multiple vitamins and minerals; folic acid; biotin] ≟•100• 27.5 mcg

Flintstones Plus Calcium chewable tablets OTC *vitamin/mineral supplement* [multiple vitamins and minerals; folic acid] ≟•300 mcg

Flintstones Plus Iron chewable tablets OTC *vitamin/iron supplement* [multiple vitamins; iron (as ferrous fumarate); folic acid] ≟•15•0.3 mg

Flo-Coat rectal suspension ℞ *radiopaque contrast medium for gastrointestinal imaging* [barium sulfate] 100%

Flocor investigational (Phase III, orphan) *coagulation inhibitor for treatment of sickle cell vaso-occlusive crisis; investigational (orphan) for severe burns and for vasospasm following cerebral aneurysm repair* [poloxamer 188]

floctafenine USAN, INN, BAN *analgesic*

Flolan IV infusion ℞ *platelet aggregation inhibitor and vasodilator for pulmonary hypertension (orphan); investigational (orphan) heparin replacement for hemodialysis* [epoprostenol sodium] 0.5, 1.5 mg

Flomax capsules ℞ *alpha₁-adrenergic blocker for benign prostatic hyperplasia (BPH); also used as adjunctive therapy for ureteral stones* [tamsulosin HCl] 0.4 mg

flomoxef INN

Flonase nasal spray in a metered-dose pump ℞ *once-daily corticosteroidal anti-inflammatory for seasonal or perennial allergic rhinitis* [fluticasone propionate] 50 mcg/dose

Flo-Pack (trademarked delivery form) *vial for IV drip* ⧉ Folbic

Flo-Pred oral suspension ℞ *corticosteroid; anti-inflammatory* [prednisolone acetate] 15 mg/5 mL

flopropione INN

Floranex chewable tablets OTC *natural intestinal bacteria; probiotic; dietary supplement* [Lactobacillus acidophilus; L. bulgaricus] 1 million CFU total

florantyrone INN, BAN

Flora-Q capsules ℞ *natural intestinal bacteria; probiotic; dietary supplement* [Lactobacillus acidophilus; L. paracasei; Bifidobacterium; Streptococcus thermophilus] 8 million CFU

Florastor capsules OTC *natural intestinal bacteria; probiotic; dietary supplement* [*Saccharomyces boulardii lyo*] 250 mg

Florastor Kids oral powder OTC *natural intestinal bacteria; probiotic; dietary supplement* [*Saccharomyces boulardii lyo*] 250 mg

florbetapir F 18 *investigational (NDA filed) radioactive contrast agent to visualize beta-amyloid plaques on PET scans, which is used to detect Alzheimer disease*

flordipine USAN, INN *antihypertensive*

floredil INN

Florentine iris *medicinal herb* [see: orris root]

floretione [see: fluoresone]

florfenicol USAN, INN, BAN *veterinary antibacterial*

Florical capsules, tablets OTC *calcium/fluoride supplement* [calcium (as carbonate); sodium fluoride] 146•8.3 mg

Florida Sunburn Relief lotion OTC *mild anesthetic; antipruritic; counterirritant; antiseptic* [phenol; camphor; menthol; benzyl alcohol] 0.4%• 0.2%•0.15%•3%

florifenine INN

Florinef Acetate tablets ℞ *replacement therapy for adrenocortical insufficiency in Addison disease* [fludrocortisone acetate] 0.1 mg

Florone cream, ointment ℞ *corticosteroidal anti-inflammatory* [diflorasone diacetate] 0.05% ⃞ fluorine; valerian

Florone E cream ℞ *corticosteroidal anti-inflammatory; emollient* [diflorasone diacetate] 0.05% ⃞ fluorine; valerian

floropipamide [now: pipamperone]

floropipeton [see: propyperone]

Florvite pediatric oral drops (discontinued 2008) ℞ *vitamin supplement; dental caries preventative* [multiple vitamins; sodium fluoride] ±•0.25, ±•0.5 mg/mL

Florvite; Florvite Half Strength pediatric chewable tablets (discontinued 2008) ℞ *vitamin supplement;*

dental caries preventative [multiple vitamins; sodium fluoride; folic acid] ±•1•0.3 mg; ±•0.5•0.3 mg

Florvite + Iron pediatric oral drops (discontinued 2008) ℞ *vitamin/iron supplement; dental caries preventative* [multiple vitamins & minerals; sodium fluoride; ferrous sulfate] ±• 0.25•10, ±•0.5•10 mg/mL

Florvite + Iron; Half Strength Florvite + Iron pediatric chewable tablets (discontinued 2008) ℞ *vitamin/iron supplement; dental caries preventative* [multiple vitamins & minerals; sodium fluoride; ferrous sulfate; folic acid] ±•1•12•0.3 mg; ±•0.5•12• 0.3 mg

flosequinan USAN, INN, BAN *antihypertensive; vasodilator; treatment for congestive heart failure*

flotrenizine INN

Flovent Diskus (prefilled inhalation powder device) ℞ *corticosteroidal anti-inflammatory for chronic asthma; not indicated for acute attacks* [fluticasone propionate] 50, 100, 250 mcg/dose

Flovent Rotadisk (inhalation powder) (discontinued 2007) ℞ *corticosteroidal anti-inflammatory for chronic asthma; not indicated for acute attacks* [fluticasone propionate] 50, 100, 250 mcg/dose

Flovent HFA inhalation aerosol in a metered-dose inhaler ℞ *corticosteroidal anti-inflammatory for chronic asthma; not indicated for acute attacks* [fluticasone propionate] 44, 110, 220 mcg/dose

floverine INN ⃞ Fluvirin

flower velure *medicinal herb* [see: coltsfoot]

flower-de-luce *medicinal herb* [see: blue flag]

floxacillin USAN *antibacterial* [also: flucloxacillin]

floxacrine INN

Floxin film-coated tablets ℞ *broad-spectrum fluoroquinolone antibiotic* [ofloxacin] 200, 300, 400 mg ⃞ Flexon; fluquazone

Floxin UroPak (3-day supply) (discontinued 2008) ℞ *broad-spectrum fluoroquinolone antibiotic* [ofloxacin] 6 tablets × 200 mg ⊡ Flexon; fluquazone

Floxin Otic ear drops ℞ *broad-spectrum fluoroquinolone antibiotic* [ofloxacin] 0.3%

Floxin Otic Singles (premeasured containers) ℞ *broad-spectrum fluoroquinolone antibiotic* [ofloxacin] 0.3% (0.75 mg per 0.25 mL container)

floxuridine USAN, USP, INN *antimetabolic antineoplastic for GI adenocarcinoma metastatic to the liver; investigational (orphan) for intraperitoneal treatment of gastric cancer; also used for ovarian and kidney cancer* 500 mg injection

Flu OIA (Optical ImmunoAssay) test for professional use ℞ *rapid (less than 20 minutes) diagnostic aid for influenza A and B in sputum, nasal aspirate, or nasopharyngeal swab*

fluacizine INN ⊡ volazocine

flualamide INN

fluanisone INN, BAN

Fluarix suspension for IM injection in prefilled syringes ℞ *seasonal influenza virus types A and B vaccine for patients ≥ 3 years* [influenza split-virus vaccine (preservative free)] 0.5 mL/dose ⊡ Flarex

fluazacort USAN, INN *anti-inflammatory*

flubanilate INN *CNS stimulant* [also: flubanilate HCl]

flubanilate HCl USAN *CNS stimulant* [also: flubanilate]

flubendazole USAN, INN, BAN *antiprotozoal*

flubenisolone [see: betamethasone]

flubepride INN

flubuperone [see: melperone]

Flucaine eye drops ℞ *local anesthetic; corneal disclosing agent* [proparacaine HCl; fluorescein sodium] 0.5%• 0.25%

flucarbril INN

flucetorex INN

flucindole USAN, INN *antipsychotic*

fluciprazine INN

fluclorolone acetonide INN, BAN *corticosteroid; anti-inflammatory* [also: flucloronide]

flucloronide USAN *corticosteroid; anti-inflammatory* [also: fluclorolone acetonide]

flucloxacillin INN, BAN *antibacterial* [also: floxacillin]

fluconazole USAN, INN, BAN *systemic triazole antifungal* 50, 100, 150, 200 mg oral; 50, 200 mg/5 mL oral; 2 mg/mL injection ⊡ valconazole

flucrilate INN *tissue adhesive* [also: flucrylate]

flucrylate USAN *tissue adhesive* [also: flucrilate]

flucytosine USAN, USP, INN, BAN *systemic antifungal* 250, 500 mg oral

fludalanine USAN, INN *antibacterial*

Fludara powder for IV injection ℞ *antineoplastic for chronic lymphocytic leukemia (CLL) and non-Hodgkin lymphoma (orphan)* [fludarabine phosphate] 50 mg

fludarabine INN *antimetabolite antineoplastic* [also: fludarabine phosphate]

fludarabine phosphate USAN *antimetabolite antineoplastic for chronic lymphocytic leukemia (CLL) and non-Hodgkin lymphoma (orphan)* [also: fludarabine] 25, 50 mg injection

fludazonium chloride USAN, INN *topical anti-infective*

fludeoxyglucose (^{18}F) INN *diagnostic aid; radioactive agent* [also: fludeoxyglucose F 18]

fludeoxyglucose F 18 USAN, USP *diagnostic aid; radioactive agent* [also: fludeoxyglucose (^{18}F)] 20–200 mCi/mL injection

fludiazepam INN

fludorex USAN, INN *anorectic; antiemetic*

fludoxopone INN

fludrocortisone INN, BAN *salt-regulating adrenocortical steroid; mineralocorticoid* [also: fludrocortisone acetate]

fludrocortisone acetate USP *salt-regulating adrenocortical steroid; mineralocorticoid; for adrenocortical insufficiency* *in Addison disease* [also: fludrocortisone] 0.1 mg oral

fludroxicortide [see: flurandrenolide]

fludroxycortide INN *topical corticosteroid* [also: flurandrenolide; flurandrenolone]

flufenamic acid USAN, INN, BAN *anti-inflammatory*

flufenisal USAN, INN *analgesic*

flufosal INN

flufylline INN

flugestone INN, BAN *progestin* [also: flurogestone acetate]

flugestone acetate [see: flurogestone acetate]

fluindarol INN

fluindione INN

Flumadine film-coated tablets ℞ *antiviral for the prophylaxis and treatment of influenza A infection* [rimantadine HCl] 100 mg

Flumadine syrup (discontinued 2008) ℞ *antiviral; prophylaxis and treatment for influenza A virus* [rimantadine HCl] 50 mg/5 mL

flumazenil USAN, INN, BAN *benzodiazepine antagonist to reverse anesthesia or treat overdose; also used for hepatic encephalopathy* 0.1 mg/mL injection

flumazepil [see: flumazenil]

flumecinol INN *investigational (orphan) agent for neonatal hyperbilirubinemia*

flumedroxone INN, BAN

flumequine USAN, INN, BAN *antibacterial*

flumeridone USAN, INN, BAN *antiemetic*

flumetasone INN *corticosteroid; anti-inflammatory* [also: flumethasone]

flumethasone USAN, BAN *topical corticosteroidal anti-inflammatory* [also: flumetasone]

flumethasone pivalate USAN, USP, BAN *topical corticosteroidal anti-inflammatory*

flumethiazide INN, BAN

flumethrin BAN

flumetramide USAN, INN *skeletal muscle relaxant*

flumexadol INN

flumezapine USAN, INN, BAN *antipsychotic; neuroleptic*

fluminorex USAN, INN *anorectic*

FluMist prefilled single-use intranasal sprayers ℞ *seasonal influenza types A and B vaccine for patients 2–49 years* [influenza virus vaccine, live attenuated (preservative free)] 0.5 mL/dose

flumizole USAN, INN *anti-inflammatory* Ⓡ Filmseal

flumoxonide USAN, INN *adrenocortical steroid*

flunamine INN

flunarizine INN, BAN *vasodilator* [also: flunarizine HCl]

flunarizine HCl USAN *investigational (orphan) vasodilator for alternating hemiplegia* [also: flunarizine]

flunidazole USAN, INN *antiprotozoal*

flunisolide USAN, USP, INN, BAN *corticosteroidal anti-inflammatory for chronic asthma and rhinitis* 0.025% (25 mcg/dose) nasal spray

flunisolide acetate USAN *anti-inflammatory*

flunisolide hemihydrate [see: flunisolide]

flunitrazepam USAN, INN, BAN, JAN *benzodiazepine sedative and hypnotic; also abused as a "date rape" street drug*

flunixin USAN, INN, BAN *anti-inflammatory; analgesic*

flunixin meglumine USAN *anti-inflammatory; analgesic*

flunoprost INN

flunoxaprofen INN

fluocinolide [now: fluocinonide]

fluocinolone BAN *topical corticosteroidal anti-inflammatory* [also: fluocinolone acetonide]

fluocinolone acetonide USAN, USP, INN *topical corticosteroidal anti-inflammatory; ocular implant for uveitis (orphan)* [also: fluocinolone] 0.01%, 0.025% topical

fluocinonide USAN, USP, INN, BAN *topical corticosteroidal anti-inflammatory* 0.05% topical

fluocortin INN *anti-inflammatory* [also: fluocortin butyl]

fluocortin butyl USAN, BAN *anti-inflammatory* [also: fluocortin]

fluocortolone USAN, INN, BAN *corticosteroid; anti-inflammatory*

fluocortolone caproate USAN *corticosteroid; anti-inflammatory*

Fluonex cream Ŗ *corticosteroidal anti-inflammatory* [fluocinonide] 0.05%

Fluonid topical solution Ŗ *corticosteroidal anti-inflammatory* [fluocinolone acetonide] 0.01%

fluopromazine BAN *antipsychotic* [also: triflupromazine]

Fluoracaine eye drops Ŗ *local anesthetic; corneal disclosing agent* [proparacaine HCl; fluorescein sodium] 0.5%•0.25%

fluoracizine [see: fluacizine]

Fluor-A-day chewable tablets, oral drops Ŗ *dental caries preventative* [sodium fluoride] 0.25 mg; 0.125 mg/mL

fluorescein USP, BAN, JAN *ophthalmic diagnostic agent*

fluorescein, soluble [now: fluorescein sodium]

Fluorescein Lite antecubital venous injection Ŗ *ophthalmic diagnostic agent* [fluorescein sodium] 10%

fluorescein sodium USP, BAN, JAN *ophthalmic diagnostic agent* 2% eye drops

fluorescein sodium & benoxinate HCl *corneal disclosing agent; topical ophthalmic anesthetic* 0.25%•0.4% eye drops

fluorescein sodium & proparacaine HCl *corneal disclosing agent; topical ophthalmic anesthetic* 0.25%•0.5% eye drops

Fluorescite antecubital venous injection Ŗ *ophthalmic diagnostic agent* [fluorescein sodium] 10%

Fluoresoft eye drops Ŗ *diagnostic aid in fitting contact lenses* [fluorexon] 0.35%

fluoresone INN

Fluorets ophthalmic strips OTC *corneal disclosing agent* [fluorescein sodium] 1 mg

fluorexon *diagnosis and fitting aid for contact lenses*

fluorhydrocortisone acetate [see: fludrocortisone acetate]

Fluoride tablets OTC *dental caries preventative* [sodium fluoride] 2.21 mg

Fluoride Loz lozenges Ŗ *dental caries preventative* [sodium fluoride] 2.21 mg

Fluoridex Daily Defense Sensitivity Relief toothpaste OTC *tooth desensitizer; dental caries preventative* [potassium nitrate; sodium fluoride] 5%• 1.1%

Fluorigard oral rinse OTC *dental caries preventative; antiseptic* [sodium fluoride; alcohol 6%] 0.05%

fluorine *element (F)* ⑨ Florone; valerian

fluorine F 18 fluorodeoxyglucose [see: fludeoxyglucose F 18]

Fluorinse oral rinse Ŗ *dental caries preventative* [sodium fluoride] 0.2%

Fluor-I-Strip; Fluor-I-Strip A.T. ophthalmic strips (discontinued 2008) Ŗ *corneal disclosing agent* [fluorescein sodium] 9 mg; 1 mg

Fluoritab chewable tablets, drops Ŗ *dental caries preventative* [sodium fluoride] 1.1, 2.2 mg; 0.125 mg/drop

fluormethylprednisolone [see: dexamethasone]

5-fluorocytosine (5-FC) [see: flucytosine]

fluorodeoxyglucose F 18 [see: fludeoxyglucose F 18]

fluorodideoxyadenosine (F-ddA) [see: lodenosine]

fluorometholone USP, INN, BAN *topical ophthalmic corticosteroidal anti-inflammatory* 0.1% eye drops

fluorometholone acetate USAN *topical ophthalmic corticosteroidal anti-inflammatory*

fluoromethylene deoxycytidine (FMdC) [now: tezacitabine]

Fluoroperm 32 Ŗ *hydrophobic contact lens material* [paflufocon C]

Fluoroperm 62 Ŗ *hydrophobic contact lens material* [paflufocon B]

Fluoroperm 92 Ŗ *hydrophobic contact lens material* [paflufocon A]

Fluoroperm 151 Ŗ *hydrophobic contact lens material* [paflufocon D]

Fluoroplex cream Ŗ *antineoplastic for actinic keratoses (AK)* [fluorouracil] 1%

Fluoroplex topical solution (discontinued 2008) ℞ *antineoplastic for actinic keratoses (AK)* [fluorouracil] 1%

fluoroquinolones *a class of synthetic, broad-spectrum, antimicrobial, bactericidal antibiotics*

fluorosalan USAN *disinfectant* [also: flusalan]

fluorouracil (5-FU) USAN, USP, INN, BAN *antimetabolite antineoplastic for colorectal (orphan), esophageal (orphan), breast, stomach, and pancreatic cancers; topical treatment for actinic keratoses and basal cell carcinoma; investigational (orphan) for glioblastoma multiforme* 50 mg/mL injection; 2%, 5% topical

fluorouracil + interferon alfa-2a *investigational (orphan) chemotherapy protocol for esophageal and advanced colorectal carcinoma*

fluorouracil + leucovorin (rescue) *chemotherapy protocol for metastatic colorectal cancer*

fluoruridine deoxyribose [see: floxuridine]

fluostigmine [see: isoflurophate]

Fluothane liquid for vaporization (discontinued 2010) ℞ *inhalation general anesthetic* [halothane]

fluotracen INN *antipsychotic; antidepressant* [also: fluotracen HCl]

fluotracen HCl USAN *antipsychotic; antidepressant* [also: fluotracen]

fluoxetine USAN, INN, BAN *selective serotonin reuptake inhibitor (SSRI) for depression, obsessive-compulsive disorder, bulimia nervosa, premenstrual dysphoric disorder, and panic disorder*

fluoxetine HCl USAN *selective serotonin reuptake inhibitor (SSRI) for major depressive disorder, obsessive-compulsive disorder, bulimia nervosa, premenstrual dysphoric disorder, and panic disorder; investigational (orphan) for autism and body dysmorphic disorder* 10, 20, 40, 90 mg oral; 20 mg/5 mL oral

fluoximesterone [see: fluoxymesterone]

fluoxiprednisolone [see: triamcinolone]

fluoxymesterone USP, INN, BAN *oral androgen for hypogonadism or testosterone deficiency in men, delayed puberty in boys, and metastatic breast cancer in women; hormone replacement therapy (HRT) for postandropausal symptoms* 10 mg oral

fluparoxan INN, BAN *antidepressant* [also: fluparoxan HCl]

fluparoxan HCl USAN *antidepressant* [also: fluparoxan]

flupenthixol BAN *thioxanthene antipsychotic* [also: flupentixol]

flupentixol INN *thioxanthene antipsychotic* [also: flupenthixol]

fluperamide USAN, INN *antiperistaltic*

fluperlapine INN

fluperolone INN, BAN *corticosteroid; anti-inflammatory* [also: fluperolone acetate]

fluperolone acetate USAN *corticosteroid; anti-inflammatory* [also: fluperolone]

fluphenazine INN, BAN *conventional (typical) phenothiazine antipsychotic for schizophrenia and psychotic disorders* [also: fluphenazine enanthate]

fluphenazine decanoate *conventional (typical) phenothiazine antipsychotic for schizophrenia and psychotic disorders; used for prolonged parenteral neuroleptic therapy* 25 mg/mL injection

fluphenazine enanthate USP *conventional (typical) phenothiazine antipsychotic for schizophrenia and psychotic disorders* [also: fluphenazine]

fluphenazine HCl USP, BAN *conventional (typical) phenothiazine antipsychotic for schizophrenia and psychotic disorders* 1, 2.5, 5, 10 mg oral; 2.5 mg/5 mL oral; 5 mg/mL oral; 2.5 mg/L injection

flupimazine INN

flupirtine INN, BAN *non-narcotic analgesic* [also: flupirtine maleate]

flupirtine maleate USAN *non-narcotic analgesic* [also: flupirtine]

flupranone INN

fluprazine INN ⊘ felypressin

fluprednidene INN, BAN

fluprednisolone USAN, NF, INN, BAN *corticosteroid; anti-inflammatory*

fluprednisolone valerate USAN *corticosteroid; anti-inflammatory*

fluprofen INN, BAN

fluprofylline INN

fluproquazone USAN, INN, BAN *analgesic*

fluprostenol INN, BAN *prostaglandin* [also: fluprostenol sodium]

fluprostenol sodium USAN *prostaglandin* [also: fluprostenol]

fluquazone USAN, INN *anti-inflammatory* ☑ Flexon; Floxin

Flura tablets ℞ *dental caries preventative* [sodium fluoride] 2.2 mg

fluracil [see: fluorouracil]

fluradoline INN *analgesic* [also: fluradoline HCl]

fluradoline HCl USAN *analgesic* [also: fluradoline]

Flura-Drops ℞ *dental caries preventative* [sodium fluoride] 0.55 mg/drop

Flura-Loz lozenges ℞ *dental caries preventative* [sodium fluoride] 2.2 mg

flurandrenolide USAN, USP *topical corticosteroid* [also: fludroxycortide; flurandrenolone] 0.05% topical

flurandrenolone BAN *topical corticosteroid* [also: flurandrenolide; fludroxycortide]

flurantel INN

Flurate eye drops (discontinued 2010) ℞ *topical anesthetic; corneal disclosing agent* [benoxinate HCl; fluorescein sodium] 0.4%•0.25%

flurazepam INN, BAN *benzodiazepine sedative and hypnotic; anticonvulsant; muscle relaxant; also abused as a street drug* [also: flurazepam HCl]

flurazepam HCl USAN, USP *benzodiazepine sedative and hypnotic; anticonvulsant; muscle relaxant; also abused as a street drug* [also: flurazepam] 15, 30 mg oral

flurbiprofen USAN, USP, INN, BAN *analgesic; nonsteroidal anti-inflammatory drug (NSAID) for osteoarthritis and rheumatoid arthritis* 50, 100 mg oral

flurbiprofen sodium USP *prostaglandin synthesis inhibitor; ophthalmic nonsteroidal anti-inflammatory drug (NSAID); intraoperative miosis inhibitor* 0.03% eye drops

Fluress eye drops ℞ *topical anesthetic; corneal disclosing agent* [benoxinate HCl; fluorescein sodium] 0.4%•0.25%

fluretofen USAN, INN *anti-inflammatory; antithrombotic*

flurfamide [now: flurofamide]

flurithromycin INN

flurocitabine USAN, INN *antineoplastic*

Fluro-Ethyl aerosol spray ℞ *refrigerant anesthetic* [ethyl chloride; dichlorotetrafluoroethane] 25%•75%

flurofamide USAN, INN *urease enzyme inhibitor*

flurogestone acetate USAN *progestin* [also: flugestone]

flurothyl USAN, USP, BAN *CNS stimulant* [also: flurotyl]

flurotyl INN *CNS stimulant* [also: flurothyl]

Flurox eye drops ℞ *topical anesthetic; corneal disclosing agent* [benoxinate HCl; fluorescein sodium] 0.4%•0.25% ☑ Flarex

fluroxene USAN, NF, INN *inhalation anesthetic*

fluroxyspiramine [see: spiramide]

flusalan INN *disinfectant* [also: fluorosalan] ☑ flazalone

flusoxolol INN, BAN

fluspiperone USAN, INN *antipsychotic*

fluspirilene USAN, INN, BAN *diphenylbutylpiperidine antipsychotic*

Flutabs caplets ℞ *antitussive; decongestant; expectorant; analgesic; antipyretic* [dextromethorphan hydrobromide; pseudoephedrine HCl; guaifenesin; acetaminophen] 20•60•200•500 mg

flutamide USAN, INN, BAN *antiandrogen antineoplastic for prostate cancer* 125 mg oral

flutazolam INN

flutemazepam INN

Flutex ointment, cream (discontinued 2009) ℞ *corticosteroidal anti-inflam-*

matory [triamcinolone acetonide] 0.025%, 0.1%, 0.5% ② Foltx

flutiazin USAN, INN *veterinary anti-inflammatory*

fluticasone INN, BAN *corticosteroidal anti-inflammatory for chronic asthma or allergic rhinitis* [also: fluticasone propionate]

fluticasone furoate *corticosteroidal anti-inflammatory; nasal aerosol for seasonal or perennial allergic rhinitis*

fluticasone propionate USAN *topical corticosteroidal anti-inflammatory; oral inhalation aerosol for chronic asthma; nasal aerosol for seasonal or perennial allergic rhinitis* [also: fluticasone] 0.005%, 0.05% topical; 50 mcg nasal spray

Flutiform *investigational (Phase III) combination inhaled corticosteroidal anti-inflammatory and bronchodilator for mild-to-moderate asthma* [fluticasone propionate; formoterol fumarate]

flutizenol INN

flutomidate INN

flutonidine INN

flutoprazepam INN

flutrimazole INN

flutroline USAN, INN *antipsychotic*

flutropium bromide INN

FluTuss HC oral liquid (discontinued 2009) ℞ *narcotic antitussive; antihistamine; decongestant* [hydrocodone bitartrate; brompheniramine maleate; phenylephrine HCl] 2.5•4•7.5 mg/5 mL

fluvastatin INN, BAN *HMG-CoA reductase inhibitor for hypercholesterolemia and atherosclerosis* [also: fluvastatin sodium]

fluvastatin sodium USAN *HMG-CoA reductase inhibitor for hypercholesterolemia, hypertriglyceridemia, mixed dyslipidemia, atherosclerosis, and coronary heart disease (CHD)* [also: fluvastatin]

Fluvirin suspension for IM injection in prefilled syringes ℞ *seasonal influenza virus types A and B vaccine for patients ≥ 4 years* [influenza split-

virus vaccine (preservative free)] 0.5 mL/dose ② floverine

Fluvirin suspension for IM injection in multidose vials ℞ *seasonal influenza virus types A and B vaccine for patients ≥ 4 years* [influenza split-virus vaccine (with thimerosal preservative)] 0.5 mL/dose (mercury 25 mcg/dose) ② floverine

fluvoxamine INN, BAN *selective serotonin reuptake inhibitor (SSRI) for obsessive-compulsive disorder (OCD)* [also: fluvoxamine maleate]

fluvoxamine maleate USAN *selective serotonin reuptake inhibitor (SSRI) for obsessive-compulsive disorder (OCD) and social anxiety disorder; also used for depression, bulimia nervosa, and panic disorder* [also: fluvoxamine] 25, 50, 100 mg oral

flux root *medicinal herb* [see: pleurisy root]

fluzinamide USAN, INN *anticonvulsant*

Fluzone suspension for IM injection in prefilled syringes ℞ *seasonal influenza virus types A and B vaccine for patients ≥ 6 months* [influenza split-virus vaccine (preservative free)] 0.25, 0.5 mL/dose

Fluzone suspension for IM injection in multidose vials ℞ *seasonal influenza virus types A and B vaccine for patients ≥ 6 months* [influenza split-virus vaccine (with thimerosal preservative)] 0.5 mL/dose (mercury 25 mcg/dose)

Fluzone High-Dose suspension for IM injection in prefilled syringes ℞ *seasonal influenza virus types A and B vaccine for patients ≥ 65 years* [influenza split-virus vaccine (preservative free)] 0.5 mL/dose (with 4 times the hemagglutinin activity of **Fluzone**)

fluzoperine INN

flytrap *medicinal herb* [see: dogbane]

FMdC (fluoromethylene deoxycytidine) [now: tezacitabine]

FML; FML Forte eye drop suspension ℞ *corticosteroidal anti-inflammatory* [fluorometholone] 0.1%; 0.25%

FML S.O.P. ophthalmic ointment ℞ *corticosteroidal anti-inflammatory* [fluorometholone] 0.1%

FML-S eye drop suspension (discontinued 2009) ℞ *corticosteroidal anti-inflammatory; antibiotic* [fluorometholone; sulfacetamide sodium] 0.1%•10%

FNC (fluorouracil, Novantrone, cyclophosphamide) *chemotherapy protocol for breast cancer* [also known as: CFM; CNF]

foal's foot *medicinal herb* [see: coltsfoot]

Foamicon chewable tablets (discontinued 2008) OTC *antacid* [aluminum hydroxide; magnesium trisilicate] 80•20 mg ☒ fomocaine

Focalin tablets ℞ *CNS stimulant for attention-deficit/hyperactivity disorder (ADHD)* [dexmethylphenidate HCl] 2.5, 5, 10 mg

Focalin XR dual-release capsules (50% immediate release, 50% delayed release) ℞ *CNS stimulant for attention-deficit/hyperactivity disorder (ADHD)* [dexmethylphenidate HCl] 5, 10, 15, 20, 30, 40 mg

focofilcon A USAN *hydrophilic contact lens material*

fodipir USAN *excipient*

Foeniculum officinale; F. vulgare *medicinal herb* [see: fennel]

Foille spray (discontinued 2011) OTC *anesthetic; antiseptic* [benzocaine; chloroxylenol] 5%•0.63%

Foille Medicated First Aid ointment, aerosol spray OTC *anesthetic; antiseptic* [benzocaine; chloroxylenol] 5%•0.1%; 5%•0.6%

Foille Plus aerosol spray (discontinued 2011) OTC *anesthetic; antiseptic* [benzocaine; alcohol 57.33%] 5%

folacin [see: folic acid]

folate [see: folic acid]

folate sodium USP

Folbee Plus film-coated tablets ℞ *vitamin supplement* [multiple B vitamins; vitamin C; folic acid; biotin] ≚•60•5•0.3 mg

Folbee Plus CZ film-coated tablets ℞ *vitamin/mineral supplement* [multiple B vitamins and minerals; vitamin C; folic acid; biotin] ≚•60•5•0.3 mg

Folbic tablets ℞ *vitamin B supplement* [vitamins B_6 and B_{12}; folacin] 25•0.002•2.5 mg ☒ Flo-Pack

Folergot-DF tablets (discontinued 2008) ℞ *GI/GU anticholinergic/antispasmodic; sedative; analgesic* [belladonna alkaloids; phenobarbital; ergotamine tartrate] 0.2•40•0.6 mg

folescutol INN

Folgard tablets OTC *vitamin B supplement* [vitamins B_6 and B_{12}; folic acid] 10•0.115•0.8 mg

Folgard Rx film-coated tablets ℞ *vitamin B supplement* [vitamins B_6 and B_{12}; folic acid] 25•0.001•2.2 mg

folic acid USP, INN, BAN *vitamin B_c; vitamin M; hematopoietic; birth defect preventative* 0.4, 0.8, 1 mg oral; 5 mg/mL injection

folinate-SF calcium [see: leucovorin calcium]

folinic acid [see: leucovorin calcium]

follicle-stimulating hormone (FSH) BAN [also: menotropins]

follidrin [see: estradiol benzoate]

Follistim AQ subcu or IM injection ℞ *recombinant follicle-stimulating hormone (FSH) for the induction of ovulation in women and spermatogenesis in men; adjunct to assisted reproductive technologies (ART)* [follitropin beta] 75, 150 FSH units/vial

Follistim AQ Cartridge prefilled Follistim Pen cartridges for subcu or IM injection ℞ *recombinant follicle-stimulating hormone (FSH) for the induction of ovulation in women and spermatogenesis in men; adjunct to assisted reproductive technologies (ART)* [follitropin beta] 150, 300, 600, 600 FSH units/cartridge

follitropin alfa INN *recombinant follicle-stimulating hormone (FSH) for the induction of ovulation in women and spermatogenesis in men (orphan);*

adjunct to assisted reproductive technologies (ART)

follitropin beta INN *recombinant follicle-stimulating hormone (FSH) for the induction of ovulation in women and spermatogenesis in men; adjunct to assisted reproductive technologies (ART)* [also: menotropins]

follotropin [see: menotropins]

Follow-Up [see: Carnation Follow-Up]

Folmor tablets ℞ *nutritional supplement for homocystinemia* [folic acid; vitamins B_6 and B_{12}; Primorine (q.v.)] 2.5•25•2•875 mg

Folotyn IV injection ℞ *antineoplastic for peripheral T-cell lymphoma* [pralatrexate] 20 mg/mL

Folpace tablets ℞ *vitamin/magnesium supplement* [vitamins B_6, B_{12}, and E; folic acid; magnesium] 25 mg•425 mcg•100 IU•2.05 mg•100 mg ⊡ Phillips'

Foltrin capsules ℞ *hematinic* [iron (as ferrous fumarate); vitamin B_{12}; vitamin C; intrinsic factor concentrate; folic acid] 110•0.015•75•240•0.5 mg ⊡ Voltaren

Foltx film-coated tablets ℞ *vitamin B therapy for arteriosclerosis, cardiovascular and peripheral vascular disease, and neurological disorders* [vitamins B_6 and B_{12}; folic acid] 25•0.002•2.5 mg ⊡ Flutex

Folvite IM injection ℞ *hematinic* [folic acid] 5 mg/mL ⊡ Velivet

fomepizole USAN, INN *alcohol dehydrogenase inhibitor; antidote to methanol or ethylene glycol poisoning (orphan)* 1 g/mL injection

fomidacillin INN, BAN

fominoben INN [also: fominoben HCl]

fominoben HCl JAN [also: fominoben]

fomocaine INN, BAN ⊡ Foamicon

fonatol [see: diethylstilbestrol]

fonazine mesylate USAN *serotonin inhibitor* [also: dimetotiazine; dimethothiazine]

fondaparinux sodium *selective factor Xa inhibitor; antithrombotic for prevention of deep vein thrombosis (DVT)*

and acute pulmonary embolism (PE) following abdominal or orthopedic surgery 2.5 mg/0.5 mL, 5 mg/0.4 mL, 7.5 mg/0.6 mL, 10 mg/0.8 mL injection

fontarsol [see: dichlorophenarsine HCl]

fopirtoline INN

Foradil encapsulated powder for inhalation (used with an **Aerolizer** device) ℞ *twice-daily bronchodilator for asthma, COPD, and emphysema* [formoterol fumarate] 12 mcg/dose

Forane liquid for vaporization ℞ *inhalation general anesthetic* [isoflurane] ⊡ 4-N-1

forasartan USAN *angiotensin receptor blocker (ARB) for hypertension and congestive heart failure (CHF)*

foreign colombo *medicinal herb* [see: colombo]

forfenimex INN

Formalaz topical liquid in a roll-on bottle ℞ *drying agent for pre- and postsurgical removal of warts* [formaldehyde] 10%

formaldehyde solution USP *disinfectant; anhidrotic for hyperhidrosis and bromhidrosis* 10% topical

Formalyde-10 spray ℞ *anhidrotic for hyperhidrosis and bromhidrosis* [formaldehyde] 10%

formebolone INN, BAN

formetamide [see: formetorex]

formetorex INN

formidacillin [see: fomidacillin]

forminitrazole INN, BAN

formocortal USAN, INN, BAN *corticosteroid; anti-inflammatory*

formoterol INN *long-acting beta$_2$ agonist (LABA); sympathomimetic bronchodilator for asthma and bronchospasm* [also: eformoterol; formoterol fumarate]

formoterol fumarate USAN, JAN *long-acting beta$_2$ agonist (LABA); sympathomimetic bronchodilator for asthma and bronchospasm, and for the long-term treatment of COPD* [also: formoterol; eformoterol fumarate]

Formula 44 Cough Relief oral liquid OTC *antitussive* [dextromethorphan hydrobromide; alcohol 5%] 10 mg/5 mL

Formula 44D Cough & Head Congestion Relief oral liquid OTC *antitussive; decongestant* [dextromethorphan hydrobromide; phenylephrine HCl] 20•10 mg/15 mL

Formula 44E Cough & Chest Congestion Relief; Pediatric Formula 44e Cough & Chest Congestion Relief oral liquid OTC *antitussive; expectorant* [dextromethorphan hydrobromide; guaifenesin] 20•200 mg/15 mL; 10•100 mg/15 mL

Formula 44M Cough, Cold, & Flu Relief oral liquid OTC *antitussive; antihistamine; analgesic; antipyretic* [dextromethorphan hydrobromide; chlorpheniramine maleate; acetaminophen] 30•4•650 mg/20 mL

Formula 44m Cough & Cold Relief, Pediatric oral liquid OTC *antitussive; antihistamine; for adults and children ≥ 6 years* [dextromethorphan hydrobromide; chlorpheniramine maleate] 15•2 mg/15 mL

Formula 405 cleansing bar, cream OTC *therapeutic skin cleanser*

Formula B tablets ℞ *vitamin supplement* [multiple B vitamins; vitamin C; folic acid] ±•500•0.5 mg

Formula B Plus tablets ℞ *vitamin/mineral/iron supplement* [multiple vitamins & minerals; iron (as ferrous fumarate); folic acid; biotin] ±•27•0.8•0.15 mg

Formula EM oral solution OTC *antiemetic for nausea associated with influenza, morning sickness, motion sickness, inhalation anesthesia, or food and drink indiscretions* [phosphorated carbohydrate solution (fructose; dextrose; phosphoric acid)] 118 mL (44•44•5 g)

Formula VM-2000 tablets (discontinued 2008) OTC *dietary supplement* [multiple vitamins & minerals; multiple amino acids; iron; folic acid; biotin] ±•5 mg•0.2 mg•50 mcg

Formulation R anorectal cream OTC *temporary relief of hemorrhoidal symptoms* [phenylephrine HCl; glycerin; petrolatum] 0.25%•12%•18%

Formulation R anorectal ointment OTC *temporary relief of hemorrhoidal symptoms* [phenylephrine HCl; mineral oil; petrolatum] 0.25%•14%•72%

4'-formylacetanilide thiosemicarbazone [see: thioacetazone; thiacetazone]

foropafant INN

forskolin [see: colforsin]

Forta Drink powder OTC *enteral nutritional therapy* [lactose-free formula]

Forta Shake powder OTC *enteral nutritional therapy* [milk-based formula]

Fortamet extended-release film-coated tablets ℞ *biguanide antidiabetic that decreases hepatic glucose production and increases cellular response to insulin* [metformin HCl] 500, 1000 mg

Fortavit oral liquid OTC *vitamin/mineral/iron supplement* [multiple vitamins & minerals; iron (as ferrous sulfate); folic acid] ±•10•0.9 mg/15 mL

Fortaz powder or frozen premix for IV or IM injection ℞ *third-generation cephalosporin antibiotic* [ceftazidime] 0.5, 1, 2, 6 g ⊡ Ferretts

Fortel Midstream test stick for professional use ℞ *in vitro diagnostic aid; urine pregnancy test*

Fortel Plus test kit for home use OTC *in vitro diagnostic aid; urine pregnancy test*

Fortéo subcu injection via prefilled self-injector ℞ *parathyroid hormone (PTH) for glucocorticoid-induced osteoporosis in men and women, primary or hypogonadal osteoporosis in men, and postmenopausal osteoporosis in women* [teriparatide] 20 mcg/day (600 mcg/2.4 mL injector)

Fortesta topical gel in a metered-dose pump ℞ *androgen for hypogonadism or testosterone deficiency in men; hormone replacement therapy (HRT) for postandropausal symptoms* [testosterone] 10 mg/0.5 mL pump

Fortical nasal spray in a metered-dose inhaler ℞ *calcium regulator for post-menopausal osteoporosis* [calcitonin (salmon)] 200 U/0.9 mL dose

fortimicin A [now: astromicin sulfate]

40 winks capsules OTC *antihistamine; sleep aid* [diphenhydramine HCl] 50 mg

Forzest (Indian name for U.S. product **Cialis**)

Fosamax tablets, oral solution ℞ *bis-phosphonate bone resorption inhibitor for Paget disease and corticosteroid-induced or age-related osteoporosis in men and women; investigational (orphan) for bone manifestations of Gaucher disease and pediatric osteogenesis imperfecta* [alendronate sodium] 5, 10, 35, 40, 70 mg; 70 mg/bottle

Fosamax Plus D caplets ℞ *once-weekly bisphosphonate bone resorption inhibitor and vitamin D supplement for age-related osteoporosis in men and women* [alendronate sodium; chole-calciferol] 70 mg•70mcg (2800 IU), 70•140 mcg (5600 IU)

fosamprenavir calcium USAN *anti-retroviral; HIV-1 protease inhibitor; prodrug of amprenavir* (amprenavir conversion=86%)

fosamprenavir sodium USAN *anti-retroviral; HIV-1 protease inhibitor; prodrug of amprenavir*

fosaprepitant dimeglumine *anti-emetic for chemotherapy-induced nausea and vomiting; prodrug of aprepitant* (aprepitant conversion=61%)

fosarilate USAN, INN *antiviral*

fosazepam USAN, INN, BAN *hypnotic*

Foscan *investigational* (NDA filed, orphan) *palliative treatment for head and neck cancer* [temoporfin]

foscarnet sodium USAN, INN, BAN *antiviral for cytomegalovirus (CMV) and various herpes viruses (HSV-1, HSV-2)* 24 mg/mL injection

Foscavir IV injection (discontinued 2008) ℞ *antiviral for cytomegalovirus (CMV) retinitis and herpes simplex virus (HSV) infections in immunocom-promised patients* [foscarnet sodium] 24 mg/mL

foscolic acid INN

fosenazide INN

fosenopril sodium [see: fosinopril sodium]

fosfestrol INN, BAN *antineoplastic; estrogen* [also: diethylstilbestrol diphosphate]

fosfocreatinine INN

fosfomycin USAN, INN, BAN *antibacterial* [also: fosfomycin calcium; fosfomycin sodium]

fosfomycin calcium JAN *antibacterial* [also: fosfomycin; fosfomycin sodium]

fosfomycin sodium JAN *antibacterial* [also: fosfomycin; fosfomycin calcium]

fosfomycin tromethamine USAN *broad-spectrum bactericidal antibiotic for urinary tract infections*

fosfonet sodium USAN, INN *antiviral*

fosfosal INN ⍰ Phosphasal

Fosfree tablets OTC *vitamin/calcium/iron supplement* [multiple vitamins; calcium (as gluconate, lactate, and carbonate); iron (as ferrous gluconate)] ± •175.4•14.5 mg

fosfructose trisodium USAN *cardio-protectant*

fosinopril INN, BAN *antihypertensive; angiotensin-converting enzyme (ACE) inhibitor; adjunctive treatment for congestive heart failure (CHF)* [also: fosinopril sodium]

fosinopril sodium USAN *antihypertensive; angiotensin-converting enzyme (ACE) inhibitor; adjunctive treatment for congestive heart failure (CHF)* [also: fosinopril] 10, 20, 40 mg oral

fosinopril sodium & hydrochlorothiazide *combination angiotensin-converting enzyme (ACE) inhibitor and diuretic for hypertension* 10•12.5, 20•12.5 mg

fosinoprilat USAN, INN *antihypertensive*

fosmenic acid INN

fosmidomycin INN

fosphenytoin INN *hydantoin anticonvulsant* [also: fosphenytoin sodium]

fosphenytoin sodium USAN *hydantoin anticonvulsant for grand mal status epi-*

lepticus (orphan) (phenytoin sodium equivalent=0.67%) [also: fosphenytoin] 75 mg/mL injection (equivalent to 50 mg/mL phenytoin sodium)

fospirate USAN, INN *veterinary anthelmintic*

fospropofol disodium *injectable general anesthetic; prodrug of* **propofol**

fosquidone USAN, INN, BAN *antineoplastic*

Fosrenol chewable tablets ℞ *phosphate binder for hyperphosphatemia in end-stage renal disease (ESRD)* [lanthanum (as carbonate)] 500, 750, 1000 mg

fostedil USAN, INN *vasodilator; calcium channel blocker*

Fosteum capsule ℞ *dietary supplement for the management of osteopenia and osteoporosis* [genistein; zinc chelazome; cholecalciferol (vitamin D₃)] 27 mg•20 mg•200 IU 🔲 P-Hist DM

Fostex Acne Cleansing cream OTC *keratolytic for acne* [salicylic acid] 2%

Fostex Acne Medication Cleansing bar OTC *medicated cleanser for acne* [salicylic acid] 2%

Fostex Medicated Cleansing Shampoo OTC *antiseborrheic; keratolytic* [sulfur; salicylic acid] 2%•2%

fostriecin INN *antineoplastic* [also: fostriecin sodium]

fostriecin sodium USAN *antineoplastic* [also: fostriecin]

fosveset USAN *ligant excipient*

fotemustine INN, BAN

fo-ti; ho-shou-wu *(Polygonum multiflorum)* root *medicinal herb for atherosclerosis, blood cleansing, constipation, improving liver and kidney function, insomnia, malaria, muscle aches, TB, and weak bones; also used to increase fertility, prevent aging, and promote longevity*

Fototar cream OTC *antipsoriatic; antiseborrheic* [coal tar] 2%

fotretamine INN

Fouchet reagent (solution)

4 Hair softgel capsules (discontinued 2008) OTC *vitamin/mineral/iron supplement* [multiple vitamins & miner-

als; iron; folic acid; biotin] ≛•2.5•33.3•0.25 mg

4 Nails softgel capsules (discontinued 2008) OTC *vitamin/mineral/calcium/iron supplement* [multiple vitamins & minerals; calcium; iron; folic acid; biotin] ≛•167•3•0.333•0.0083 mg

4 Trace Elements IV injection ℞ *intravenous nutritional therapy* [multiple trace elements (metals)]

4-Way Fast Acting nasal spray OTC *nasal decongestant* [phenylephrine HCl] 1%

4-Way Menthol nasal spray OTC *nasal decongestant; mild anesthetic* [phenylephrine HCl; menthol] 1%• ≛

4-Way Moisturizing Relief nasal spray OTC *nasal decongestant* [xylometazoline HCl] 0.1%

40DS02 *investigational (orphan) for chronic iron overload due to transfusional treatments*

4-N-1 cream OTC *moisturizer; emollient* [dimethicone] 1% 🔲 Forane

Fourneau 309 (available only from the Centers for Disease Control) (discontinued 2011) ℞ *antiparasitic for African trypanosomiasis and onchocerciasis* [suramin sodium]

foxglove *(Digitalis ambigua; D. ferriginea; D. grandiflora; D. lanata; D. lutea; D. purpurea)* leaves *medicinal herb for asthma, burns, congestive heart failure, edema, promoting wound healing, and sedation; not generally regarded as safe and effective for children as ingestion can be fatal*

foxglove, American; false foxglove; fern-leaved foxglove *medicinal herb* [see: feverweed]

foxtail *medicinal herb* [see: club moss]

frabuprofen INN

Fractar (trademarked ingredient) *antipsoriatic; antiseborrheic* [crude coal tar]

Fragaria vesca medicinal herb [see: strawberry]

Fragmin deep subcu injection, prefilled syringes ℞ *anticoagulant/antithrombotic for prevention of deep vein thrombosis (DVT) and venous throm-*

boembolism (VTE) after abdominal or hip replacement surgery, unstable angina, and myocardial infarction [dalteparin sodium] 10 000, 25 000 IU (64, 160 mg)/mL; 2500, 5000, 7500, 10 000, 12 500, 15 000, 18 000 IU (16, 32, 48, 64, 80, 96, 115 mg)

framycetin INN, BAN anti-infective wound dressing

francium element (Fr)

Frangula purshiana medicinal herb [see: cascara sagrada]

frankincense (Boswellia serrata) leaves and bark medicinal herb for anaphylaxis, arthritis, asthma, blood cleansing, bronchial disorders, dysentery, rheumatism, skin ailments, ulcers, and wound healing

fraxinella (Dictamnus albus) root, plant, and seed medicinal herb used as an anthelmintic, diuretic, emmenagogue, expectorant, and febrifuge

FreAmine III 3% (8.5%) with Electrolytes IV infusion ℞ total parenteral nutrition (8.5% only); peripheral parenteral nutrition (both) [multiple essential and nonessential amino acids; electrolytes] ⧋ furomine

FreAmine III 8.5%; FreAmine III 10% IV infusion ℞ total parenteral nutrition; peripheral parenteral nutrition [multiple essential and nonessential amino acids] ⧋ furomine

FreAmine HBC 6.9% IV infusion ℞ nutritional therapy for high metabolic stress [multiple branched-chain essential and nonessential amino acids; electrolytes]

Free & Clear shampoo OTC soap-free therapeutic cleanser

Freedavite tablets OTC vitamin/mineral/calcium/iron supplement [multiple vitamins & minerals; calcium (as ascorbate and carbonate); iron (as ferrous fumarate); folic acid] ≛•20•1.8•0.4 mg

FreeStyle Lite reagent strips for home use OTC in vitro diagnostic aid for blood glucose that is unaffected by non-glucose sugars such as maltose and galactose

Freezone topical liquid OTC keratolytic [salicylic acid in a collodion-like vehicle] 13.6% ⧋ Furacin

frentizole USAN, INN, BAN immunoregulator

Fresenius Propoven emulsion for IV infusion ℞ general anesthetic [propofol] 10 mg/mL

Freshkote eye drops ℞ moisturizer/lubricant for moderate to severe dry eye [polyvinyl alcohol; polyvinyl pyrrolidone] 2.7%•2%

fringe tree (Chionanthus virginica) bark medicinal herb used as an aperient, diuretic, febrifuge, and tonic

fronepidil INN

fropenem INN broad-spectrum carbapenem antibiotic

frost plant; frost weed; frostwort medicinal herb [see: rock rose]

Frova film-coated tablets ℞ vascular serotonin 5-$HT_{1B/1D}$ receptor agonist for the acute treatment of migraine [frovatriptan succinate] 2.5 mg

frovatriptan succinate USAN vascular serotonin 5-$HT_{1B/1D}$ receptor agonist for the acute treatment of migraine

froxiprost INN

β-fructofuranosidase [see: sacrosidase]

fructose (D-fructose) USP nutrient; caloric replacement [also: levulose; compare to: high fructose corn syrup]

fructose-1,6-diphosphate (FDP) investigational (Phase III, orphan) cytoprotective agent for vaso-occlusive episodes of sickle cell disease

Fruit C 100; Fruit C 200; Fruit C 500 chewable tablets OTC vitamin C supplement [ascorbic acid and calcium ascorbate] 100 mg; 200 mg; 500 mg

Fruity Chews Children's chewable tablets OTC vitamin supplement [multiple vitamins; folic acid] ≛•300 mcg

Fruity Chews with Iron chewable tablets OTC vitamin/iron supplement [multiple vitamins; iron (as ferrous fumarate); folic acid] ≛•12•0.3 mg

frusemide BAN *antihypertensive; loop diuretic* [also: furosemide]

FSF (fibrin-stabilizing factor) [see: factor XIII]

FSH (follicle-stimulating hormone) [see: menotropins]

ftalofyne INN *veterinary anthelmintic* [also: phthalofyne]

ftaxilide INN

ftivazide INN

ftormetazine INN

ftorpropazine INN

5-FU (5-fluorouracil) [see: fluorouracil]

fubrogonium iodide INN

fuchsin, basic USP *topical antibacterial/ antifungal*

Fucus versiculosus medicinal herb [see: kelp]

FUDR powder for intra-arterial infusion ℞ *antimetabolic antineoplastic for GI adenocarcinoma metastatic to the liver; investigational (orphan) for intraperitoneal treatment of gastric cancer; also used for ovarian and kidney cancer* [floxuridine] 500 mg

FUDR; FUdR (5-fluorouracil deoxyribonucleoside) [see: floxuridine]

fuge, devil's *medicinal herb* [see: mistletoe]

Ful-Glo ophthalmic strips OTC *corneal disclosing agent* [fluorescein sodium] 0.6 mg ⊉ Flagyl

Full Spectrum B with Vitamin C tablets OTC *vitamin supplement* [multiple B vitamins; vitamin C; folic acid; biotin] ±•60•0.8•0.3 mg

Full Term test kit for professional use ℞ *in vitro diagnostic aid for fetal fibronectin; an elevated level indicates an increased risk of preterm birth*

fulmicoton [see: pyroxylin]

FU/LV (fluorouracil, leucovorin [rescue]) *chemotherapy protocol for colorectal, gastric, hepatocellular, ovarian, and pancreatic cancers; dosing regimens include: biweekly, de Gramont, Douillard, German, Mayo Clinic, postgastrectomy, Roswell Park, and weekly* [also known as: F-CL]

FU/LV/CPT-11 (fluorouracil, leucovorin [rescue], irinotecan) *chemotherapy protocol for colorectal cancer; dosing regimens include: Doullard regimen, Saltz regimen, and modified Saltz regimen* [also known as: IFL; also: ILF (for gastric cancer)]

fulvestrant USAN *steroidal selective estrogen receptor down-regulator; antiestrogen antineoplastic for metastatic breast cancer in postmenopausal women*

fumagillin INN, BAN

Fumaria officinalis medicinal herb [see: fumitory]

fumaric acid NF *acidifier*

Fumatinic sustained-release capsules ℞ *hematinic* [iron (as ferrous fumarate); vitamin B_{12}; vitamin C] 66•0.005•60 mg

fumitory (*Fumaria officinalis*) plant *medicinal herb for cardiovascular disorders, constipation, eczema, edema, and hepatobiliary disorders*

fumoxicillin USAN, INN *antibacterial*

Funduscein-10; Funduscein-25 antecubital venous injection (discontinued 2008) ℞ *ophthalmic diagnostic agent* [fluorescein sodium] 10%; 25% ⊉ vindesine

Fungi Cure Intensive topical liquid spray OTC *antifungal* [clotrimazole] 1%

Fungi Cure Maximum Strength topical liquid OTC *antifungal* [undecylenic acid; alcohol 70%] 25%

fungicidin [see: nystatin]

fungimycin USAN *antifungal* ⊉ vancomycin

Fungi-Nail topical liquid OTC *antifungal; keratolytic; anesthetic; antiseptic* [resorcinol; salicylic acid; chloroxylenol; benzocaine; alcohol 50%] 1%•2%•2%•0.5% ⊉ vincanol

Fungizone powder for IV infusion (discontinued 2008) ℞ *systemic polyene antifungal* [amphotericin B deoxycholate] 50 mg/vial ⊉ fenquizone; Vancocin

Fung-O topical liquid OTC *keratolytic* [salicylic acid] 17%

Fungoid tincture OTC *antifungal for tinea pedis, tinea cruris, and tinea corporis* [miconazole nitrate] 2%

Fungoid·HC cream ℞ *corticosteroidal anti-inflammatory; antipruritic; antifungal; antibacterial* [miconazole nitrate; hydrocortisone] 2%•1%

FUP (fluorouracil, Platinol) *chemotherapy protocol for gastric and biliary tract cancer* [also: CF; cisplatin + fluorouracil]

fuprazole INN ⏚ Vaprisol

furacilin [see: nitrofurazone]

Furacin topical solution, cream (discontinued 2009) ℞ *broad-spectrum antibacterial; adjunct to burn therapy and skin grafting* [nitrofurazone] 0.2% ⏚ Freezone

Furacin Soluble Dressing ointment (discontinued 2009) ℞ *broad-spectrum antibacterial; adjunct to burn therapy and skin grafting* [nitrofurazone] 0.2%

furacrinic acid INN, BAN

Furadantin oral suspension ℞ *urinary antibiotic* [nitrofurantoin] 25 mg/5 mL

furafylline INN ⏚ verofylline

Furalan tablets ℞ *urinary antibiotic* [nitrofurantoin] 50, 100 mg ⏚ Verelan; Virilon

furalazine INN

furaltadone INN, BAN

Furamide (available only from the Centers for Disease Control and Prevention) *investigational anti-infective for amebiasis* [diloxanide furoate]

2(3H) furanone di-hydro (FDh) *a precursor to gamma hydroxybutyrate (GHB); a formerly legal alternative to GHB, now also illegal (Schedule I); also known as gamma butyrolactone (GBL)* [see: gamma hydroxybutyrate (GHB)]

furaprofen USAN, INN *anti-inflammatory*

furazabol INN

furazolidone USP, INN, BAN *bactericidal; antiprotozoal; treatment of diarrhea and enteritis due to bacterial or protozoal organisms*

furazolium chloride USAN, INN *antibacterial*

furazolium tartrate USAN *antibacterial*

furbucillin INN

furcloprofen INN

furegrelate INN *thromboxane synthetase inhibitor* [also: furegrelate sodium]

furegrelate sodium USAN *thromboxane synthetase inhibitor* [also: furegrelate]

furethidine INN, BAN

furfenorex INN

furfuryltrimethylammonium iodide [see: furtrethonium iodide]

furidarone INN

furmethoxadone INN

furobufen USAN, INN *anti-inflammatory*

furodazole USAN, INN *anthelmintic*

furofenac INN

furomazine INN

furomine USAN, INN, BAN *ligand* ⏚ FreAmine

furosemide USAN, USP, INN, JAN *antihypertensive; loop diuretic for congestive heart failure, hepatic cirrhosis, and renal disease* [also: frusemide] 20, 40, 80 mg oral; 10 mg/mL oral; 40 mg/5 mL oral; 10 mg/mL injection

furostilbestrol INN

furoxicillin [see: fumoxicillin]

Furoxone tablets (discontinued 2008) ℞ *bactericidal; antiprotozoal; treatment of diarrhea and enteritis due to bacterial or protozoal organisms* [furazolidone] 100 mg ⏚ Viroxyn

fursalan USAN, INN *disinfectant*

fursultiamine INN

furterene INN

furtrethonium iodide INN

furtrimethonium iodide [see: furtrethonium iodide]

fusafungine INN, BAN

fusidate sodium USAN *antibiotic for staphylococcal and other gram-positive infections*

fusidic acid USAN, INN, BAN *topical and systemic antibiotic for staphylococcal and other gram-positive infections*

fusidic acid, sodium salt [see: fusidate sodium]

Fusilev injection ℞ *antidote to folic acid antagonists; chemotherapy "rescue agent" for osteosarcoma and colorectal* *cancer* [levoleucovorin (as calcium)] 50 mg (64 mg)

Fuzeon powder for subcu injection ℞ *fusion inhibitor for HIV infection* [enfu-virtide] 90 mg/mL (108 mg/dose) ⊠ Visine; Vusion

fuzlocillin INN, BAN

FZ (flutamide, Zoladex) *chemotherapy protocol for prostate cancer*

G Phen DM film-coated extended-release tablets (discontinued 2007) ℞ *antitussive; decongestant; expectorant* [dextromethorphan hydrobromide; phenylephrine HCl; guaifenesin] 60•40•600 mg ⊠ C-Phen DM; Guaifen DM

G17DT immunogen *investigational (orphan) agent for gastric cancer and adenocarcinoma of the pancreas*

⁶⁷**Ga** [see: gallium citrate Ga 67]

GAA (glucosidase-alpha acid) [see: alglucosidase alfa]

GABA (gamma-aminobutyric acid) [see: γ-aminobutyric acid]

gabapentin USAN, INN *anticonvulsant; treatment for postherpetic neuralgia; investigational (orphan) for amyotrophic lateral sclerosis; investigational (Phase III) for moderate to severe postmenopausal hot flashes* 100, 300, 400, 600, 800 mg oral; 250 mg/5 mL oral

gabapentin enacarbil *treatment for moderate-to-severe restless legs syndrome (RLS); gabapentin prodrug*

Gabapentin GR *investigational (Phase III) extended-release formulation for the treatment of postherpetic neuralgia; investigational (Phase III) for moderate to severe postmenopausal hot flashes* [gabapentin]

Gabarone tablets (discontinued 2009) ℞ *anticonvulsant for partial-onset seizures; treatment for postherpetic neuralgia* [gabapentin] 100, 300, 400 mg ⊠ gepirone; Quibron

Gabbromicina *investigational (orphan) agent for tuberculosis and Mycobacte-* *rium avium complex (MAC)* [aminosidine]

gabexate INN

Gabitril tablets ℞ *anticonvulsant; adjunctive treatment for partial seizures* [tiagabine HCl] 2, 4, 12, 16 mg ⊠ Capitrol

Gablofen intrathecal injection ℞ *skeletal muscle relaxant for intractable spasticity due to multiple sclerosis, cerebral palsy, or spinal cord injury (orphan)* [baclofen] 0.05, 0.5, 2 mg/mL

gaboxadol INN GABA_A *agonist*

Gadavist IV injection ℞ *paramagnetic contrast agent to enhance MRIs of the brain and central nervous system* [gadobutrol] 1 mmol/mL (604.72 mg/mL)

gadobenate dimeglumine USAN *parenteral gadolinium-based contrast agent (GBCA) to enhance MRIs of the brain, spine, and other CNS tissue* [also: gadobenic acid]

gadobenic acid INN *parenteral gadolinium-based contrast agent (GBCA) for MRI* [also: gadobenate dimeglumine]

gadobutrol INN *parenteral gadolinium-based contrast agent (GBCA) to enhance MRIs of the brain and central nervous system*

gadodiamide USAN, INN, BAN *parenteral gadolinium-based contrast agent (GBCA) for thoracic, abdominal, pelvic, and retroperitoneal imaging and to enhance MRIs of the brain, spine, and other CNS tissue*

gadofosveset trisodium USAN *parenteral gadolinium-based contrast agent (GBCA) for vascular enhancement in magnetic resonance angiography (MRA)*

gadolinium *element* (Gd)
gadolinium texaphyrin (Gd·Tex)
[now: motexafin gadolinium]
gadopenamide INN
gadopentetate dimeglumine USAN *parenteral gadolinium-based contrast agent (GBCA) for imaging of the head and neck, and to enhance MRIs of the brain, spine, and other CNS tissue* [also: gadopentetic acid]
gadopentetic acid INN, BAN *parenteral gadolinium-based contrast agent (GBCA) for imaging of the head and neck, and to enhance MRIs of the brain, spine, and other CNS tissue* [also: gadopentetate dimeglumine]
gadoteric acid INN
gadoteridol USAN, INN, BAN *parenteral gadolinium-based contrast agent (GBCA) for head and neck imaging and to enhance MRIs of the brain, spine, and other CNS tissue*
gadoversetamide USAN, INN *parenteral gadolinium-based contrast agent (GBCA) to enhance MRIs of the brain, head, and spine and liver structure and vascularity*
gadoxanum USAN *gadolinium-xanthan gum complex; diagnostic aid*
gadoxetate disodium *parenteral gadolinium-based contrast agent (GBCA) for MRIs of the liver*
gadozelite USAN *gadolinium zeolite complex; diagnostic aid*
gaiactamine [see: guaiactamine]
gaietamine [see: guaiactamine]
galactagogues *a class of agents that promote or increase the flow of breast milk* [also called: lactagogues]
α-D-galactopyranose [see: galactose]
galactose USAN *ultrasound contrast medium*
α-galactosidase [see: agalsidase alfa]
galamustine INN ② clemastine
galangal (*Alpinia galanga; A. officinarum*) *rhizomes medicinal herb for diuresis, fungal infections, gas, hypertension, tumors, ulcers, and worms; also used as an antiplatelet agent*

galantamine USAN, INN *acetylcholinesterase inhibitor to increase cognition in Alzheimer disease*
galantamine hydrobromide USAN *acetylcholinesterase inhibitor to increase cognition in Alzheimer disease* 4, 8, 12, 16, 24 mg oral
galanthamine [see: galantamine]
Galardin *investigational (orphan) matrix metalloproteinase (MMP) inhibitor for corneal ulcers* [ilomastat]
galdansetron INN, BAN *antiemetic* [also: galdansetron HCl]
galdansetron HCl USAN *antiemetic* [also: galdansetron]
Galeopsis tetrahit *medicinal herb* [see: hemp nettle]
Galium aparine; G. verum *medicinal herb* [see: bedstraw]
Galium odoratum *medicinal herb* [see: sweet woodruff]
galiximab *investigational (Phase III) antineoplastic for leukemia*
gallamine BAN *neuromuscular blocker* [also: gallamine triethiodide] ② calamine; Chlo-Amine
gallamine triethiodide USP, INN *neuromuscular blocker; muscle relaxant* [also: gallamine]
gallamone triethiodide [see: gallamine triethiodide]
gallic acid NF ② Gly-Oxide
gallic acid, bismuth basic salt [see: bismuth subgallate]
gallium *element* (Ga) ② Kolyum
gallium (⁶⁷Ga) citrate INN *radiopaque contrast medium; radioactive agent* [also: gallium citrate Ga 67] ② Kolyum
gallium citrate Ga 67 USAN, USP *radiopaque contrast medium; radioactive agent* [also: gallium (⁶⁷Ga) citrate]
gallium nitrate USAN *bone resorption inhibitor for hypercalcemia of malignancy (orphan)*
gallium nitrate nonahydrate [see: gallium nitrate]
gallopamil INN, BAN
gallotannic acid [see: tannic acid]
gallstone solubilizing agents *a class of drugs that dissolve gallstones*

galosemide INN ② Calcium

galsulfase *recombinant human enzyme*
N-*acetylgalactosamine 4-sulfatase;*
treatment for mucopolysaccharidosis VI
(*MPS VI; Maroteaux-Lamy syndrome*)
(*orphan*)

galtifenin INN

Galvus ⓔ tablets (available in the
Europe) *investigational (NDA filed)*
DPP-4 inhibitor for type 2 diabetes that
enhances the function of the body's
incretin system to increase insulin pro-
duction in the pancreas and reduce glu-
cose production in the liver [vildaglip-
tin] 50 mg

Galzin capsules ℞ *copper blocking/com-*
plexing agent for Wilson disease
(*orphan*) [zinc acetate] 25, 50 mg ②
Cleocin; glycine; Quelicin

GamaSTAN S/D IM injection ℞
immunizing agent for hepatitis A, mea-
sles, varicella, and rubella; treatment
for immunoglobulin G deficiency and
acquired agammaglobulinemia [immune
globulin, solvent/detergent treated]
2, 10 mL

gamfexine USAN, INN *antidepressant*

gamma benzene hexachloride [now:
lindane]

gamma butyraldehyde (GHB-alde-
hyde) *a precursor to gamma hydroxy-*
butyrate (GHB) [see: gamma hydroxy-
butyrate]

gamma butyrolactone (GBL) *precur-*
sor to gamma hydroxybutyrate (GHB);
a formerly legal alternative to GHB,
now also illegal (Schedule I); also known
as 2(3H) furanone di-hydro (FDh)
[see: gamma hydroxybutyrate (GHB)]

gamma globulin [see: globulin,
immune]

gamma hydroxybutyrate (GHB) *a*
CNS depressant used as an anesthetic
in some countries; sometimes abused as
a "date rape" street drug; illegal in the
U.S. (Schedule I) as GHB, but avail-
able (Schedule III) as sodium oxybate
to treat cataplexy due to narcolepsy
[also known as: sodium oxybate]

gamma hydroxybutyric (GHB)
acid *investigational (orphan) CNS*
depressant for narcolepsy, cataplexy,
sleep paralysis, hypnagogic hallucina-
tions, and automatic behavior

gamma oryzanol; gamma-oz *medici-*
nal herb [see: rice bran oil]

gamma-aminobutyric acid (GABA)
[see: γ-aminobutyric acid]

gamma-c cDNA, retroviral vector
investigational (orphan) for X-linked
severe combined immunodeficiency dis-
ease (SCID)

Gammagard Liquid subcu or IV infusion ℞ *passive immunizing agent for*
primary (inherited) immunodeficiency
disorders; investigational (Phase III) for
Alzheimer disease; also used for Guil-
lain-Barré syndrome, myasthenia gravis,
and multiple sclerosis [immune globulin (IGIV)] 10% (1, 2.5, 5, 10, 20 g/
dose)

Gammagard S/D freeze-dried powder
for IV infusion ℞ *passive immunizing*
agent for HIV, idiopathic thrombocyto-
penic purpura (ITP), B-cell chronic
lymphocytic leukemia, and Kawasaki
syndrome [immune globulin (IGIV),
solvent/detergent treated] 50 mg/mL

gamma-hydroxybutyrate sodium
[see: sodium oxybate]

gamma-linolenic acid (GLA) *natural*
omega-6 fatty acid; investigational
(*orphan*) *for juvenile rheumatoid arthritis*

gammaphos [now: ethiofos]

Gammar-P I.V. (pasteurized) powder
for IV infusion (discontinued 2007)
℞ *passive immunizing agent and immu-*
nomodulator for HIV; pediatric treat-
ment of primary immune deficiency
(*PID*) [immune globulin, heat treated;
human albumin] 5%•3%

gamma-vinyl GABA (gamma-ami-
nobutyric acid) [see: vigabatrin]

gamolenic acid INN, BAN

Gamunex IV infusion ℞ *passive*
immunizing agent for primary humoral
immunodeficiency, idiopathic thrombo-
cytopenic purpura (ITP), and chronic
inflammatory demyelinating polyneu-

ropathy (CIDP) (orphan) [immune globulin (IGIV), chromatography purified] 10% (1, 2.5, 10, 20 g/dose)

Gamunex-C IV infusion or subcu injection ℞ *passive immunizing agent for primary humoral immunodeficiency, idiopathic thrombocytopenic purpura (ITP), and chronic inflammatory demyelinating polyneuropathy (CIDP) (orphan)* [immune globulin, human] 10% (1, 2.5, 5, 10, 20 g/dose)

ganaxolone USAN *investigational (orphan) neuroactive steroid for infantile spasms*

ganciclovir USAN, INN, BAN *antiviral for AIDS-related cytomegalovirus (CMV) infections (orphan) and CMV retinitis (orphan); investigational (NDA filed, orphan) for herpetic keratitis* [also: ganciclovir sodium] 250, 500 mg oral; 500 mg injection

ganciclovir sodium USAN *antiviral for cytomegalovirus retinitis (orphan)* [also: ganciclovir] 500 mg injection

ganciclovir sodium & cytomegalovirus immune globulin intravenous (CMV-IGIV) *investigational (orphan) for cytomegalovirus pneumonia in bone marrow transplant patients*

Ganeden Sustenex capsules OTC *natural intestinal bacteria; probiotic; dietary supplement* [BC30] 2 billion cells

ganglefene INN

gangliosides, sodium salts *investigational (orphan) agent for retinitis pigmentosa*

Ganidin NR oral liquid ℞ *expectorant* [guaifenesin] 100 mg/5 mL

ganirelix INN *gonadotropin-releasing hormone (GnRH) antagonist for infertility* [also: ganirelix acetate]

ganirelix acetate USAN *gonadotropin-releasing hormone (GnRH) antagonist for infertility* [also: ganirelix] 250 mcg/0.5 mL injection

Ganite IV infusion ℞ *bone resorption inhibitor for hypercalcemia of malignancy (orphan)* [gallium nitrate] 25 mg/mL

Gani-Tuss NR oral liquid ℞ *narcotic antitussive; expectorant* [codeine phosphate; guaifenesin] 10•100 mg/5 mL

Gani-Tuss-DM NR oral liquid ℞ *antitussive; expectorant* [dextromethorphan hydrobromide; guaifenesin] 10•100 mg/5 mL

Gantrisin Pediatric oral suspension (discontinued 2010) ℞ *broad-spectrum sulfonamide antibiotic* [sulfisoxazole (as acetyl); alcohol 0.3%] 500 mg/5 mL

gapicomine INN

gapromidine INN

Garamycin eye drops, ophthalmic ointment (discontinued 2010) ℞ *aminoglycoside antibiotic* [gentamicin sulfate] 3 mg/mL; 3 mg/g

garcinia (*Garcinia cambogia*) fruit *medicinal herb for appetite suppressant, thermogenesis, and weight control* 🄓 Carrasyn; chrysin

Gardasil IM injection ℞ *vaccine for genital warts (condylomata acuminata) and anal cancer in men and women 9–26 years; cervical cancer and precancerous or dysplastic vaginal, vulvar, or cervical intraepithelial neoplasia in women 9–26 years* [human papillomavirus (HPV) recombinant vaccine, quadrivalent (HPV types 6, 11, 16, and 18)] 20•40•40•20 mcg/0.5 mL dose

garden nightshade *medicinal herb* [see: bittersweet nightshade]

garden patience *medicinal herb* [see: yellow dock]

Garfield; Garfield Plus Extra C chewable tablets (discontinued 2008) OTC *vitamin supplement* [multiple vitamins; folic acid] ±•0.3 mg

Garfield Complete with Minerals chewable tablets (discontinued 2008) OTC *vitamin/mineral/iron supplement* [multiple vitamins & minerals; iron; folic acid; biotin] ±•18•0.4•0.04 mg

Garfield Plus Iron chewable tablets (discontinued 2008) OTC *vitamin/iron supplement* [multiple vitamins; iron; folic acid] ±•15•0.3 mg

garget *medicinal herb* [see: pokeweed]

garlic *(Allium sativum)* bulb *medicinal herb for asthma, cancer immunity, diabetes, digestive disorders, ear infections, flatulence, hypercholesterolemia, hypertension, and infectious diseases* ⑦ Keralac

Garlique enteric-coated caplets OTC *herbal supplement for cardiovascular support* [garlic bulb extract] ≥ 5000 mcg allicin ⑦ Keralac

Gas chewable tablets OTC *antiflatulent* [simethicone] 125 mg

gas gangrene antitoxin, pentavalent

gas gangrene antitoxin, polyvalent [see: gas gangrene antitoxin, pentavalent]

Gas Permeable Daily Cleaner solution (discontinued 2010) OTC *cleaning solution for rigid gas permeable contact lenses*

Gas Relief chewable tablets, drops OTC *antiflatulent* [simethicone] 80, 125 mg; 40 mg/0.6 mL

Gas-Ban tablets OTC *antacid; antiflatulent* [calcium carbonate; simethicone] 300•40 mg ⑦ Kao-Spen

Gas-Ban DS oral liquid OTC *antacid; antiflatulent* [aluminum hydroxide; magnesium hydroxide; simethicone] 400•400•40 mg/5 mL

gastric acid inhibitors [see: proton pump inhibitors]

gastric mucin BAN

Gastroccult slide test for professional use ℞ *in vitro diagnostic aid for gastric occult blood*

Gastrocrom oral solution ℞ *mastocytosis treatment (orphan)* [cromolyn sodium] 100 mg/5 mL

Gastrografin oral solution ℞ *radiopaque contrast medium for gastrointestinal imaging* [diatrizoate meglumine; diatrizoate sodium (48.29% total iodine)] 660•100 mg/mL (367 mg/mL)

Gastro-Test string capsules for professional use ℞ *in vitro diagnostic aid for GI disorders*

Gas-X chewable tablets, softgels OTC *antiflatulent* [simethicone] 80, 125 mg; 125 mg

Gas-X Infant Drops, Baby oral drops OTC *antiflatulent* [simethicone] 20 mg/0.3 mL

Gas-X Thin Strips (orally dissolving film) OTC *antiflatulent* [simethicone] 62.5 mg

Gas-X with Maalox chewable tablets OTC *antiflatulent; antacid* [simethicone; calcium carbonate] 125•500 mg

gatifloxacin USAN *broad-spectrum fluoroquinolone antibiotic* 0.3% eye drops

Gattex *investigational (Phase III) glucagon-like peptide 2 (GLP-2) analogue for short bowel syndrome* [teduglutide]

gaultheria oil [see: methyl salicylate]

Gaultheria procumbens *medicinal herb* [see: wintergreen]

gauze, absorbent USP *surgical aid*

gauze, petrolatum USP *surgical aid*

gauze bandage [see: bandage, gauze]

gavestinel USAN *N-methyl-D-aspartate (NMDA) receptor antagonist for stroke*

GaviLAX powder for oral solution OTC *laxative; bowel evacuant* [polyethylene glycol 3350] 17 g/dose ⑦ Keflex

gavilimomab *investigational (orphan) monoclonal antibody for acute graft vs. host disease*

GaviLyte-C; Gavilyte-G oral solution ℞ *pre-procedure bowel evacuant* [PEG 3350; sodium bicarbonate; sodium chloride; sodium sulfate; potassium chloride] 240•6.72•5.84•22.72•2.98 g/4 L bottle; 236•6.74•5.86•22.74•2.97 g/4 L bottle

Gaviscon chewable tablets OTC *antacid* [aluminum hydroxide; magnesium trisilicate] 80•14.2 mg

Gaviscon oral liquid OTC *antacid* [aluminum hydroxide; magnesium carbonate] 31.7•119.3 mg/5 mL

Gaviscon Antacid chewable tablets OTC *antacid* [aluminum hydroxide; magnesium carbonate] 160•105 mg

Gaviscon Relief Formula chewable tablets, oral liquid OTC *antacid* [aluminum hydroxide; magnesium carbonate] 160•105 mg; 254•237.5 mg/5 mL

GBH *a mistaken acronym for gamma hydroxybutyrate (GHB)* [see: gamma hydroxybutyrate]

G-Bid DM TR extended-release tablets (discontinued 2007) R̲ *antitussive; expectorant* [dextromethorphan hydrobromide; guaifenesin] 60•1200 mg

GBL (gamma butyrolactone) *precursor to gamma hydroxybutyrate (GHB); a formerly legal alternative to GHB, now also illegal (Schedule I); also known as 2(3H) furanone di-hydro (FDh)* [see: gamma hydroxybutyrate]

G-CSF (granulocyte colony-stimulating factor) [see: filgrastim]

Gd texaphyrin [see: motexafin gadolinum]

Gebauer's Spray and Stretch topical spray R̲ *refrigerant anesthetic* [tetrafluoroethane; pentafluoropropane]

gedocarnil INN *treatment of central nervous system disorders*

gefarnate INN, BAN

gefitinib *epidermal growth factor receptor-tyrosine kinase inhibitor (EGFR-TKI); antineoplastic for advanced or metastatic non–small cell lung cancer (NSCLC)*

gelatin NF *encapsulating, suspending, binding and coating agent*

gelatin film, absorbable USP *topical hemostat for surgery*

gelatin solution, special intravenous [see: polygeline]

gelatin sponge, absorbable USP *topical hemostat for surgery*

gelcaps (dosage form) *soft gelatin capsules*

Gelclair oral gel R̲ *"swish and spit" treatment for oral mucositis or lesions; occlusive coating for exposed nerve endings* [povidone; hyaluronic acid] 15 mL/pkt.

Gelfilm; Gelfilm Ophthalmic R̲ *topical hemostat for surgery* [absorbable gelatin film]

Gelfoam powder R̲ *topical hemostat for surgery* [absorbable gelatin powder]

Gelfoam sponge, packs, dental packs, prostatectomy cones R̲ *topical hemostat for surgery* [absorbable gelatin sponge]

Gel-Kam tooth gel OTC *dental caries preventative* [stannous fluoride] 0.4%

Gel-Kam Rinse OTC *dental caries preventative* [stannous fluoride] 0.63%

Gelnique gel R̲ *urinary antispasmodic for urge urinary incontinence and frequency* [oxybutynin chloride] 10% (100 mg/sachet)

Gelseal (trademarked dosage form) *soft gelatin capsule* ☑ Colazal

gelsemium *(Bignonia sempervirens; Gelsemium nitidum; G. sempervirens)* plant *medicinal herb for asthma, neuralgia, and respiratory disorders; not generally regarded as safe and effective as it is highly toxic*

gelsolin, recombinant human *investigational (orphan) for respiratory symptoms of cystic fibrosis and bronchiectasis*

Gel-Tin gel OTC *dental caries preventative* [stannous fluoride] 0.4%

Gelusil chewable tablets OTC *antacid; antiflatulent* [aluminum hydroxide; magnesium hydroxide; simethicone] 200•200•25 mg ☑ Colazal

gemazocine INN

gemcadiol USAN, INN *antihyperlipoproteinemic*

gemcitabine USAN, INN, BAN *antimetabolite antineoplastic*

gemcitabine + carboplatin *chemotherapy protocol for mesothelioma and bladder, ovarian, and non–small cell lung cancer (NSCLC)*

gemcitabine-cis (gemcitabine, cisplatin) *chemotherapy protocol for non–small cell lung cancer (NSCLC) and mesothelioma* [also: gemcitabine + cisplatin (for many other cancers)]

gemcitabine + cisplatin *chemotherapy protocol for bladder, cervical, ovarian, pancreatic, nasopharyngeal, and biliary tract cancer* [also: gemcitabine-cis (for lung cancer and mesothelioma)]

gemcitabine HCl USAN *antimetabolite antineoplastic for advanced or metastatic breast, ovarian, pancreatic, and non–small cell lung cancers (NSCLC); also used for biliary, bladder, and testicular cancer* 0.2, 1, 2 g/vial injection

gemcitabine + vinorelbine *chemotherapy protocol for non–small cell lung cancer (NSCLC), mesothelioma, and soft tissue sarcoma* [also: G+V; vinorelbine + gemcitabine (for lung cancer only)]

gemeprost USAN, INN, BAN *prostaglandin*

gemfibrozil USAN, USP, INN, BAN *triglyceride-lowering antihyperlipidemic for hypertriglyceridemia (types IV and V hyperlipidemia) and coronary heart disease* 600 mg oral

gemifloxacin mesylate USAN *broad-spectrum fluoroquinolone antibiotic for respiratory tract infections*

gemopatrilat USAN *antihypertensive; angiotensin-converting enzyme (ACE) inhibitor; vasopeptidase inhibitor (VPI); treatment for congestive heart failure (CHF)*

gemtuzumab ozogamicin USAN *monoclonal antibody–targeted chemotherapy agent for acute myeloid leukemia (orphan)*

Gemzar powder for IV infusion ℞ *antimetabolite antineoplastic for advanced or metastatic breast, ovarian, pancreatic, and non–small cell lung cancers (NSCLC); also used for biliary, bladder, and testicular cancer* [gemcitabine HCl] 200, 1000 mg/dose

Genac tablets OTC *decongestant; antihistamine* [pseudoephedrine HCl; triprolidine HCl] 60•2.5 mg ② Gonak; Kank-a

Genacol Cold & Flu Relief tablets (discontinued 2007) OTC *antitussive; antihistamine; decongestant; analgesic; antipyretic* [dextromethorphan hydrobromide; chlorpheniramine maleate; pseudoephedrine HCl; acetaminophen] 15•2•30•500 mg

Genahist capsules, oral liquid OTC *antihistamine; sleep aid* [diphenhydramine HCl] 25 mg; 12.5 mg/5 mL

Genahist tablets (discontinued 2010) OTC *antihistamine; sleep aid* [diphenhydramine HCl] 25 mg

Genantussidex oral liquid (discontinued 2007) ℞ *antitussive; decongestant; expectorant* [dextromethorphan hydrobromide; phenylephrine HCl; guaifenesin] 30•10•200 mg/5 mL

Genapap tablets, rapid-release gelcaps OTC *analgesic; antipyretic* [acetaminophen] 325 mg; 500 mg

Genapap, Children's chewable tablets OTC *analgesic; antipyretic* [acetaminophen] 80 mg

Genapap, Children's elixir (discontinued 2008) OTC *analgesic; antipyretic* [acetaminophen] 160 mg/5 mL

Genapap, Infants' drops (discontinued 2008) OTC *analgesic; antipyretic* [acetaminophen] 100 mg/mL

Genaphed tablets OTC *nasal decongestant* [pseudoephedrine HCl] 30 mg ② Confide

Genaphed Plus tablets ℞ *decongestant; antihistamine* [pseudoephedrine HCl; chlorpheniramine maleate] 60•4 mg

Genasal nasal spray OTC *nasal decongestant* [oxymetazoline HCl] 0.05% ② Goniosol; Gynazole; Konsyl

Genasense *antisense antineoplastic; investigational (NDA filed, orphan) for malignant melanoma; investigational (Phase III, orphan) for multiple myeloma and chronic lymphocytic leukemia (CLL)* [augmerosen; oblimersen sodium]

Genasoft softgels OTC *laxative; stool softener* [docusate sodium] 100 mg ② Goniosoft

Genaspor cream OTC *antifungal* [tolnaftate] 1%

Genaton chewable tablets OTC *antacid* [aluminum hydroxide; magnesium trisilicate] 80•20 mg

Genaton oral liquid OTC *antacid* [aluminum hydroxide; magnesium carbonate] 31.7•137.3 mg/5 mL

Genaton, Extra Strength chewable tablets OTC *antacid* [aluminum hydroxide; magnesium carbonate] 160•105 mg

Genatuss DM syrup OTC *antitussive; expectorant* [dextromethorphan hydrobromide; guaifenesin] 10•100 mg/5 mL

Gen-bee with C caplets (discontinued 2008) OTC *vitamin supplement* [multiple B vitamins; vitamin C] ± •300 mg

Gendex 75 IV infusion ℞ *plasma volume expander for shock due to hemorrhage, burns, or surgery* [dextran 75] 6%

gene plasmid hVEGF165 [see: vascular endothelial growth factor 165, human]

Genebrom-DM oral liquid (discontinued 2007) ℞ *antitussive; antihistamine; decongestant* [dextromethorphan hydrobromide; brompheniramine maleate; pseudoephedrine HCl] 20•4•60 mg/10 mL

Genebs tablets, caplets (discontinued 2010) OTC *analgesic; antipyretic* [acetaminophen] 325, 500 mg; 500 mg

Genelan-NF oral liquid (discontinued 2007) ℞ *antitussive; antihistamine; decongestant; expectorant* [dextromethorphan hydrobromide; chlorpheniramine maleate; phenylephrine HCl; guaifenesin] 30•4•20•200 mg/10 mL

Generess Fe chewable tablets (in 28-day packs) ℞ *monophasic oral contraceptive; iron supplement (as separate tablets)* [norethindrone; ethinyl estradiol; ferrous fumarate] 0.8 mg•25 mcg × 21 days; 75 mg × 28 days

Generet-500 timed-release tablets (discontinued 2008) OTC *vitamin/iron supplement* [iron (as ferrous sulfate); multiple B vitamins; vitamin C (as sodium ascorbate)] 105• ± •500 mg ⑨ Kineret

Generix-T tablets OTC *vitamin/mineral/calcium/iron supplement* [multiple vitamins & minerals; calcium (as dicalcium phosphate); iron (as ferrous sulfate)] ± •58•15 mg

Generlac oral/rectal solution ℞ *hyperosmotic laxative* [lactulose] 10 g/15 mL

GenESA computer-controlled IV infusion device ("GenESA System") (discontinued 2007) ℞ *cardiac stressor for diagnosis of coronary artery disease* [arbutamine HCl] 0.05 mg/mL ⑨ Canasa

Gene-T-Press oral liquid (discontinued 2007) ℞ *antitussive; decongestant; expectorant* [dextromethorphan hydrobromide; phenylephrine HCl; guaifenesin] 15•5•200 mg/5 mL

Geneye eye drops (discontinued 2009) OTC *decongestant; vasoconstrictor* [tetrahydrozoline HCl] 0.05%

Genfiber powder OTC *bulk laxative* [psyllium hydrophilic mucilloid] 3.4 g/tsp.

Gengraf capsules, oral drops ℞ *immunosuppressant for allogenic kidney, liver, and heart transplants (orphan), rheumatoid arthritis (RA), and psoriasis* [cyclosporine] 25, 100 mg; 100 mg/mL

Genista tinctoria *medicinal herb* [see: dyer's broom]

genistein *one of several soy isoflavones that provide cell-protective effects*

genistin *isoform precursor to genistein* [q.v.]

Gen-K powder for oral solution ℞ *electrolyte replenisher* [potassium (as chloride)] 20 mEq/pkt.

genophyllin [see: aminophylline]

Genoptic eye drops (discontinued 2010) ℞ *aminoglycoside antibiotic* [gentamicin sulfate] 3 mg/mL

Genoptic S.O.P. ophthalmic ointment (discontinued 2009) ℞ *aminoglycoside antibiotic* [gentamicin sulfate] 3 mg/g

Genotropin MiniQuick (prefilled syringes in packs of 7) ℞ *growth hormone for children and adults with congenital or endogenous growth hormone deficiency (GHD), short bowel syndrome, or AIDS-wasting syndrome; for children with Turner syndrome, Prader-Willi syndrome, or renal-induced growth failure* [somatropin] 0.2, 0.4, 0.6, 0.8, 1, 1.2, 1.4, 1.6, 1.8, 2 mg (0.6, 1.2, 1.8, 2.4, 3, 3.6, 4.2, 4.8, 5.4, 6 IU) per syringe

Genotropin powder for subcu injection ℞ *growth hormone for children and adults with congenital or endogenous growth hormone deficiency (GHD),* *short bowel syndrome, or AIDS-wasting syndrome; for children with Turner syndrome, Prader-Willi syndrome, or renal-induced growth failure* [somatropin] 5.8, 13.8 mg (17.4, 41.4 IU) per vial

Genprin tablets OTC *analgesic; antipyretic; anti-inflammatory; antirheumatic* [aspirin] 325 mg

Gentacidin eye drops (discontinued 2009) ℞ *aminoglycoside antibiotic* [gentamicin sulfate] 3 mg/mL

Gentak ophthalmic ointment ℞ *aminoglycoside antibiotic* [gentamicin sulfate] 3 mg/g

gentamicin BAN *aminoglycoside antibiotic* [also: gentamicin sulfate]

gentamicin sulfate USAN, USP *aminoglycoside antibiotic* [also: gentamicin] 3 mg/mL eye drops; 3 mg/g ophthalmic; 0.1% topical; 10, 40 mg/mL injection

gentamicin sulfate, liposomal *investigational (orphan) agent for disseminated* Mycobacterium avium-intracellulare *infection*

Gentamicin Sulfate in 0.9% Sodium Chloride injection ℞ *aminoglycoside antibiotic* [gentamicin sulfate; sodium chloride] 0.8, 0.9, 1, 1.2, 1.4, 1.6 mg/mL (60, 70, 80, 90, 100 mg/dose)

gentamicin-impregnated polymethyl methacrylate (PMMA) beads *investigational (orphan) agent for chronic osteomyelitis*

GenTeal Mild; GenTeal Mild to Moderate eye drops OTC *moisturizer/lubricant* [hypromellose] 0.2%; 0.3%

GenTeal Moderate to Severe gel OTC *ophthalmic moisturizer/lubricant* [carboxymethylcellulose sodium; hypromellose] 0.25%•0.3%

Gentex 30 oral liquid ℞ *antitussive; decongestant; expectorant* [carbetapentane citrate; phenylephrine HCl; guaifenesin] 30•8•200 mg/5 mL ☒ Cognitex

Gentex HC oral liquid ℞ *narcotic antitussive; decongestant; expectorant* [hydrocodone bitartrate; phenylephrine HCl; guaifenesin] 2.5•7.5•100 mg/5 mL

Gentex LA extended-release caplets ℞ *decongestant; expectorant* [phenylephrine HCl; guaifenesin] 23.75•650 mg

gentian (*Gentiana lutea*) root *medicinal herb for aiding digestion, appetite stimulation, arthritis, hysteria, jaundice, liver disorders, and sore throat*

gentian violet *topical anti-infective/antifungal* [also: methylrosanilinium chloride] 1%, 2%

gentisic acid ethanolamide NF *complexing agent*

Gentle Cream OTC *moisturizer; emollient*

Gentle Iron capsules OTC *vitamin/iron supplement for anemia* [iron (as ferrous bisglycinate); vitamin B_{12}; vitamin C; folic acid] 28•0.08•60•0.4 mg

Gentran 40 IV injection ℞ *plasma volume expander for shock due to hemorrhage, burns, or surgery* [dextran 40] 10% ☒ Contrin

Gentran 70 IV infusion ℞ *plasma volume expander for shock due to hemorrhage, burns, or surgery* [dextran 70] 6% ☒ Contrin

Geocillin film-coated caplets (discontinued 2008) ℞ *extended-spectrum penicillin antibiotic* [carbenicillin indanyl sodium] 500 mg (382 mg base)

Geodon capsules ℞ *antipsychotic for schizophrenia and manic episodes of a bipolar disorder* [ziprasidone HCl] 20, 40, 60, 80 mg ☒ codeine; Kadian; Quad Tann

Geodon powder for IM injection ℞ *antipsychotic for rapid control of acute agitation in schizophrenic patients* [ziprasidone mesylate] 20 mg ☒ codeine; Kadian; Quad Tann

gepefrine INN

gepirone INN *azapirone tranquilizer; anxiolytic; antidepressant* [also: gepirone HCl] ☒ Gabarone; Quibron

gepirone HCl USAN *azapirone tranquilizer; anxiolytic; antidepressant* [also: gepirone]

Geranium maculatum *medicinal herb* [see: alum root]

2-geranylhydroquinone [see: gero-quinol]

Gerardia pedicularia medicinal herb [see: feverweed]

Geravim oral liquid OTC *vitamin/mineral/iron supplement* [multiple B vitamins & minerals; iron (as ferrous gluconate); alcohol 18%] ±•2.5 mg ⑨ CarraFoam; Kerafoam

Geravite elixir (discontinued 2008) OTC *geriatric vitamin supplement* [multiple B vitamins] ⑨ Carafate

Gerber Baby Low Iron Formula oral liquid, powder for oral liquid OTC *total or supplementary infant feeding*

Gerber Soy Formula powder OTC *hypoallergenic infant formula* [soy protein formula]

Geref powder for IV injection (discontinued 2010) ℞ *diagnostic aid for pituitary function; treatment for growth hormone deficiency (orphan), anovulation (orphan), and AIDS-related weight loss (orphan)* [sermorelin acetate] 50 mcg

Geri SS lotion OTC *moisturizer; emollient*

Geridium tablets ℞ *urinary tract analgesic for relief of pain, burning, urgency, and frequency due to mucosal irritation from surgery, catheterization, endoscopic procedures, or trauma; adjunct to antibacterial agents for urinary tract infections* [phenazopyridine HCl] 100, 200 mg ⑨ Karidium

Geri-Hydrolac cream OTC *moisturizer; emollient* [ammonium lactate] 12%

Geri-Hydrolac 5%; Geri-Hydrolac 12% lotion OTC *moisturizer; emollient* [ammonium lactate] 5%; 12%

Gerimal sublingual tablets, tablets ℞ *cognition adjuvant for age-related mental capacity decline* [ergoloid mesylates] 0.5, 1 mg; 1 mg ⑨ caramel

Gerimed film-coated tablets (discontinued 2008) OTC *geriatric vitamin/mineral supplement* [multiple vitamins & minerals]

Geri-Mucil powder for oral solution OTC *bulk laxative* [psyllium husk] 3.4 g/tsp.

Geriot film-coated tablets (discontinued 2008) OTC *vitamin/mineral/iron supplement* [multiple vitamins & minerals; iron (as carbonyl iron); folic acid; biotin] ±•50•0.4•0.045 mg ⑨ carrot

Geri-Silk bath oil OTC *moisturizer; emollient* [mineral oil]

Geri-Soft lotion OTC *moisturizer; emollient*

Geritol Complete tablets OTC *vitamin/mineral/calcium/iron supplement* [multiple vitamins & minerals; calcium; iron (as ferrous fumarate); folic acid; biotin] ±•148•16•0.4•0.038 mg

Geritol Extend caplets (discontinued 2008) OTC *vitamin/mineral/iron supplement* [multiple vitamins & minerals; ferrous fumarate; folic acid] ±• 10•0.2 mg

Geritol with Ferrex 18 Tonic oral liquid OTC *vitamin/iron supplement* [multiple B vitamins; iron (as ferric pyrophosphate); choline bitartrate; methionine; alcohol 12%] ±•6• 16.7•8.33 mg/5 mL

Geritonic oral liquid OTC *vitamin/iron supplement* [multiple B vitamins & minerals; ferric ammonium citrate; liver fraction 1; alcohol 20%] ±• 105•375 mg/15 mL

Geri-Tussin DM oral liquid OTC *antitussive; expectorant* [dextromethorphan hydrobromide; guaifenesin] 10•100 mg/5 mL

Geri-Vite oral liquid OTC *vitamin/mineral/iron supplement* [multiple B vitamins & minerals; iron (as ferrous gluconate); alcohol 18%] ±•2.5 mg ⑨ Carafate

German valerian *medicinal herb* [see: valerian]

Germanin (available only from the Centers for Disease Control) (discontinued 2011) ℞ *antiparasitic for African trypanosomiasis and onchocerciasis* [suramin sodium]

germanium *element (Ge)* ⑨ carumonam

germicides *a class of agents that destroy micro-organisms* [see also: antiseptics; disinfectants]

geroquinol INN

Geroton Forte oral liquid (discontinued 2008) OTC *geriatric vitamin/mineral supplement* [multiple B vitamins & minerals; alcohol 13.5%]

gesarol [see: chlorophenothane]

gestaclone USAN, INN *progestin*

gestadienol INN

gestanin [see: allyloestrenol]

Gestiva (name changed to **Makena** upon marketing release in 2011)

gestodene USAN, INN, BAN *progestin*

gestonorone caproate USAN, INN *progestin* [also: gestronol]

gestrinone USAN, INN *progestin*

gestronol BAN *progestin* [also: gestonorone caproate]

Get Better Bear Sore Throat Pops OTC *throat emollient and protectant* [pectin] 19 mg

Gets-It topical liquid OTC *keratolytic* [salicylic acid; zinc chloride; alcohol 28%]

gevotroline INN *antipsychotic* [also: gevotroline HCl]

gevotroline HCl USAN *antipsychotic* [also: gevotroline]

Gevrabon oral liquid (discontinued 2008) OTC *vitamin/mineral supplement* [multiple B vitamins & minerals; alcohol 18%]

Gevral tablets (discontinued 2008) OTC *vitamin/mineral/iron supplement* [multiple vitamins & minerals; ferrous fumarate; folic acid] ≛•18 mg•0.4 mg

Gevral Protein powder (discontinued 2010) OTC *oral protein supplement* [calcium caseinate; sucrose]

G-F 20 [see: hylan G-F 20]

GFN (guaifenesin) [q.v.]

GFN 550/PSE 60/DM 30 sustained-release tablets (discontinued 2007) Ɽ *expectorant; decongestant; antitussive* [guaifenesin; pseudoephedrine HCl; dextromethorphan hydrobromide] 550•60•30 mg

GFN 600/Phenylephrine 20 tablets Ɽ *expectorant; decongestant* [guaifenesin; phenylephrine HCl] 600•20 mg

GFN 600/PSE 60/DM 30 sustained-release caplets Ɽ *expectorant; decongestant; antitussive* [guaifenesin; pseudoephedrine HCl; dextromethorphan hydrobromide] 600•60•30 mg

GFN 1000/DM 50 sustained-release caplets (discontinued 2007) Ɽ *expectorant; antitussive* [guaifenesin; dextromethorphan hydrobromide] 1000•50 mg ⧄ C-Phen DM; G Phen DM; Guaifen DM

GFN 1000/DM 60; GFN 1200/DM 60 sustained-release caplets Ɽ *expectorant; antitussive* [guaifenesin; dextromethorphan hydrobromide] 1000•60 mg; 1200•60 mg ⧄ C-Phen DM; G Phen DM; Guaifen DM

GFN 1200/DM 20/PE 40 extended-release tablets Ɽ *expectorant; antitussive; decongestant* [guaifenesin; dextromethorphan hydrobromide; phenylephrine HCl] 1200•20•40 mg

GFN 1200/DM 60/PSE 120 sustained-release caplets (discontinued 2007) Ɽ *expectorant; antitussive; decongestant* [guaifenesin; dextromethorphan hydrobromide; pseudoephedrine HCl] 1200•60•120 mg

GFN/PSE sustained-release tablets Ɽ *expectorant; decongestant* [guaifenesin; pseudoephedrine HCl] 1200•120 mg

GHB (gamma hydroxybutyrate) *a CNS depressant used as an anesthetic in some countries, produced and abused as a "date rape" street drug in the U.S.; illegal in the U.S. (Schedule I)* [the sodium salt is medically known as sodium oxybate]

GHB-aldehyde (gamma butyraldehyde) *a precursor to gamma hydroxybutyrate* [see: gamma hydroxybutyrate]

GHRF; GH-RF (growth hormone-releasing factor) [q.v.]

Gianvi film-coated tablets (in packs of 28) Ɽ *monophasic oral contraceptive in a novel 24-day regimen; also approved to treat premenstrual dysphoric disorder*

(PMDD) and acne vulgaris [drospire-none; ethinyl estradiol] 3 mg•20 mcg × 24 days; counters × 4 days ② Januvia

Gilead, balm of medicinal herb [see: balm of Gilead]

Gilenya capsules ℞ treatment for relapsing multiple sclerosis (MS) [fingolimod] 0.5 mg ② Calan; Clenia; Jalyn; kaolin; khellin

Gilphex TR film-coated caplets ℞ decongestant; expectorant [phenylephrine HCl; guaifenesin] 10•388 mg

Giltuss oral liquid (discontinued 2009) ℞ antitussive; decongestant; expectorant [dextromethorphan hydrobromide; phenylephrine HCl; guaifenesin] 15•10•300 mg/5 mL ② Glutose

Giltuss Ped-C oral liquid (discontinued 2009) ℞ narcotic antitussive; decongestant; expectorant; for children 2–12 years [codeine phosphate; phenylephrine HCl; guaifenesin] 3•2.5•50 mg/5 mL

Giltuss Pediatric oral liquid (discontinued 2009) ℞ antitussive; decongestant; expectorant; for children 2–12 years [dextromethorphan hydrobromide; phenylephrine HCl; guaifenesin] 3•2.5•50 mg/5 mL

Giltuss TR capsules OTC antitussive; decongestant; expectorant [dextromethorphan hydrobromide; phenylephrine HCl; guaifenesin] 14•7•288 mg

Giltuss TR tablets (discontinued 2009) OTC antitussive; decongestant; expectorant [dextromethorphan hydrobromide; phenylephrine HCl; guaifenesin] 30•20•600 mg

ginger (Zingiber officinale) root medicinal herb for childhood diseases, colds, colic, dizziness, fever, flu, gas pains, headache, indigestion, morning sickness, nausea, poor circulation, toothache, and vestibular disorders

ginger, wild medicinal herb [see: wild ginger]

ginkgo (Ginkgo biloba) leaves medicinal herb for Alzheimer disease, antioxidant, anxiety, asthma, attention-deficit disorder, chilblains, cerebral insufficiency, dementia, dizziness, memory loss, poor circulation, Raynaud disease, stroke, and tinnitus

ginseng (Panax spp.) root medicinal herb for age spots, blood diseases, depression, hemorrhage, increasing endurance and longevity, and stress; also used as an aphrodisiac

ginseng, blue; yellow ginseng medicinal herb [see: blue cohosh]

giparmen INN ② Cuprimine

giractide INN

girisopam INN

gitalin NF [also: gitalin amorphous] ② guaietolin

gitalin amorphous INN [also: gitalin]

gitaloxin INN

gitoformate INN

gitoxin 16-formate [see: gitaloxin]

gitoxin pentaacetate [see: pengitoxin]

GLA (gamma-linolenic acid) [q.v.]

glacial acetic acid [see: acetic acid, glacial]

Gladase ointment ℞ proteolytic enzyme for débridement of necrotic tissue; vulnerary [papain; urea] 830 000 U•100 mg per g

Gladase-C ointment ℞ proteolytic enzyme for débridement of necrotic tissue; vulnerary; topical wound deodorant [papain; urea; chlorophyllin copper complex] 521 700 U/g•10%•0.5%

glafenine INN, JAN

glaphenine [see: glafenine]

glatiramer acetate USAN immunomodulator for relapsing-remitting multiple sclerosis (orphan)

Glauber salt [see: sodium sulfate]

glaucarubin

glaze, pharmaceutical NF tablet-coating agent

glaziovine INN

Gleevec film-coated tablets ℞ antineoplastic for chronic myeloid leukemia (orphan), acute lymphoblastic leukemia, chronic eosinophilic leukemia, myelodysplastic disease, gastrointestinal stromal tumors (orphan), systemic mastocytosis, and dermatofibrosarcoma protuber-

ans [imatinib mesylate] 100, 400 mg
🔟 Glivec

glemanserin USAN, INN *anxiolytic*

gleptoferron USAN, INN, BAN *veterinary hematinic*

Gliadel wafers ℞ *nitrosourea-type alkylating antineoplastic cerebral implants for excised brain tumors* [carmustine] 7.7 mg

gliamilide USAN, INN *antidiabetic*

glibenclamide INN, BAN *sulfonylurea antidiabetic that stimulates insulin secretion in the pancreas* [also: glyburide]

glibornuride USAN, INN, BAN *antidiabetic*

glibutimine INN

glicaramide INN

glicetanile INN *antidiabetic* [also: glicetanile sodium]

glicetanile sodium USAN *antidiabetic* [also: glicetanile]

gliclazide INN, BAN *sulfonylurea antidiabetic that stimulates insulin secretion in the pancreas*

glicondamide INN

glidazamide INN

gliflumide USAN, INN *antidiabetic*

glimepiride USAN, INN, BAN *sulfonylurea antidiabetic that stimulates insulin secretion in the pancreas* 1, 2, 4 mg oral

glipentide [see: glisentide]

glipizide USAN, INN, BAN *sulfonylurea antidiabetic for type 2 diabetes that stimulates insulin secretion in the pancreas* 5, 10 mg oral

Glipizide ER extended-release tablets ℞ *sulfonylurea antidiabetic that stimulates insulin secretion in the pancreas* [glipizide] 2.5, 5, 10 mg

glipizide & metformin HCl *antidiabetic combination for type 2 diabetes that stimulates insulin secretion in the pancreas, decreases hepatic glucose production, and increases cellular response to insulin* 2.5•250, 2.5•500, 5•500 mg

gliquidone INN, BAN

glisamuride INN

glisentide INN

glisindamide INN

glisolamide INN

glisoxepide INN, BAN

globin zinc insulin INN [also: insulin, globin zinc]

globulin, aerosolized pooled immune *investigational (orphan) agent for respiratory syncytial virus lower respiratory tract disease*

globulin, immune USP *passive immunizing agent for HIV, ITP, CLL, PID, CIDP, and bone marrow transplantation; infection prophylaxis in pediatric HIV (orphan); investigational (orphan) for juvenile rheumatoid arthritis, GI disturbances due to autism, and idiopathic myopathies* [also see: Rh$_O$D immune globulin]

globulin, immune, with high titers of West Nile virus antibodies *investigational (orphan) passive immunizing agent for the West Nile virus*

globulin, immune human serum [now: globulin, immune]

Glossets (trademarked dosage form) *sublingual or rectal administration*

gloxazone USAN, INN, BAN *veterinary anaplasmodastat*

gloximonam USAN, INN *antibacterial*

GlucaGen Diagnostic Kit IV injection ℞ *agent to inhibit movement of the gastrointestinal tract during radiographic procedures* [glucagon, recombinant] 1 mg

GlucaGen Emergency Kit; GlucaGen HypoKit subcu, IV, or IM injection ℞ *emergency treatment of hypoglycemic crisis* [glucagon, recombinant] 1 mg

glucagon USP, INN, BAN *antidiabetic; glucose elevating agent; diagnostic aid for GI imaging*

Glucagon Diagnostic Kit IM or IV injection ℞ *to inhibit GI tract movement during radiographic procedures* [glucagon, recombinant] 1 mg (1 U)

Glucagon Emergency Kit subcu, IM, or IV injection ℞ *emergency treatment for hypoglycemic crisis* [glucagon, recombinant] 1 mg (1 U)

glucalox INN [also: glycalox] 🔟 GlycoLax

glucametacin INN

glucan synthesis inhibitors *a class of antifungals* [also: echinocandins]

D-glucaric acid, calcium salt tetrahydrate [see: calcium saccharate]

gluceptate USAN, USP, INN, BAN *combining name for radicals or groups*

gluceptate sodium USAN *pharmaceutic aid*

Glucerna; Glucerna Select; Glucerna Weight Loss Shake ready-to-use oral liquid OTC *enteral nutritional therapy for abnormal glucose tolerance* [milk- and soy-based formula] 325 mL ⊠ glycerin

D-glucitol [see: sorbitol]

D-glucitol hexanicotinate [see: sorbinicate]

β-glucocerebrosidase, macrophage-targeted [see: alglucerase]

glucocerebrosidase, recombinant retroviral vector *investigational (orphan) enzyme replacement for types I, II, or III Gaucher disease*

glucocerebrosidase-β-glucosidase [see: alglucerase]

glucocorticoids *a class of adrenal cortical steroids that modify the body's immune response*

Glucofilm reagent strips for home use OTC *in vitro diagnostic aid for blood glucose*

glucoheptonic acid, calcium salt [see: calcium glucepate]

glucomannan (*Amorphophallus konjac*) root *medicinal herb for constipation, diverticular disease, hemorrhoids, hypercholesterolemia, and obesity; it may produce altered insulin requirements or hypoglycemia in diabetics*

Glucometer Encore; Glucometer Elite reagent strips for home use OTC *in vitro diagnostic aid for blood glucose*

D-gluconic acid, calcium salt [see: calcium gluconate]

D-gluconic acid, magnesium salt [see: magnesium gluconate]

D-gluconic acid, monopotassium salt [see: potassium gluconate]

D-gluconic acid, monosodium salt [see: sodium gluconate]

Glucophage film-coated tablets ℞ *biguanide antidiabetic that decreases hepatic glucose production and increases cellular response to insulin* [metformin HCl] 500, 850, 1000 mg

Glucophage XR extended-release caplets ℞ *once-daily biguanide antidiabetic* [metformin HCl] 500, 750 mg

β-D-glucopyranuronamide [see: glucuronamide]

glucosamine USAN, INN *pharmaceutic aid; natural remedy for osteoarthritis*

glucosamine sulfate *natural remedy for osteoarthritis*

glucose NF *blood glucose elevating agent for hypoglycemia; diagnostic aid for diabetes; tablet binder and coating agent* ⊠ Caelyx

d-glucose [see: dextrose]

d-glucose monohydrate [see: dextrose]

glucose oxidase

glucose polymers *caloric replacement*

Glucostix reagent strips for home use OTC *in vitro diagnostic aid for blood glucose*

glucosulfamide INN

glucosulfone INN

glucosylceramidase [see: alglucerase]

Glucotrol tablets ℞ *sulfonylurea antidiabetic that stimulates insulin secretion in the pancreas* [glipizide] 5, 10 mg

Glucotrol XL extended-release tablets ℞ *sulfonylurea antidiabetic that stimulates insulin secretion in the pancreas* [glipizide] 2.5, 5, 10 mg

Glucovance film-coated caplets ℞ *antidiabetic combination for type 2 diabetes that stimulates insulin secretion in the pancreas, decreases hepatic glucose production, and increases cellular response to insulin* [glyburide; metformin HCl] 1.25•250, 2.5•500, 5•500 mg

glucurolactone INN

glucuronamide INN, BAN

Glumetza extended-release film-coated tablets ℞ *biguanide antidiabetic that decreases hepatic glucose production and* increases cellular response to insulin [metformin HCl] 500, 1000 mg

glunicate INN

gluside [see: saccharin]

gluside, soluble [see: saccharin sodium]

glusoferron INN

glutamic acid (L-glutamic acid) USAN, INN *nonessential amino acid; symbols: Glu, E* 340, 500 mg oral

glutamic acid HCl *gastric acidifier*

glutamine (L-glutamine) USAN, USP, JAN *nonessential amino acid that reduces fatigue, increases exercise endurance, and strengthens the GI tract; growth hormone secretagogue; investigational (orphan) for short bowel syndrome and sickle cell disease; symbol: Gln, Q*

glutamine & somatropin *investigational (orphan) for GI malabsorption due to short bowel syndrome*

L-glutamyl-L-tryptophan *investigational (orphan) agent for AIDS-related Kaposi sarcoma*

glutaral USAN, USP, INN *disinfectant* ☒ colterol

glutaraldehyde [see: glutaral]

Glutarex-1 powder OTC *formula for infants with glutaric aciduria type I* ☒ Klotrix

Glutarex-2 powder OTC *enteral nutritional therapy for glutaric aciduria type I* ☒ Klotrix

glutasin [see: glutamic acid HCl]

glutathione *endogenous antioxidant produced in the liver; unstable as an oral supplement; endogenous levels are increased by using transdermal preparations, by supplementing its precursors, MSM and NAC (q.v.), or by regenerating it with SAMe (q.v.)*

L-glutathione, reduced *investigational (orphan) for AIDS-related cachexia*

glutaurine INN

glutethimide USP, INN, BAN *sedative; sometimes abused as a street drug*

Glutofac tablets (discontinued 2008) OTC *vitamin/mineral supplement* [multiple vitamins & minerals]

Glutofac-ZX film-coated caplets ℞ *vitamin/mineral supplement* [multiple vitamins & minerals; folic acid; biotin; lutein] ± •2.8•0.2•0.5 mg

Glutose oral gel OTC *blood glucose elevating agent for hypoglycemia* [glucose] 40% ☒ Giltuss

glyburide USAN *sulfonylurea antidiabetic for type 2 diabetes that stimulates insulin secretion in the pancreas* [also: glibenclamide] 1.25, 1.5, 2.5, 3, 4.5, 5, 6 mg oral

glyburide & metformin HCl *antidiabetic combination for type 2 diabetes that stimulates insulin secretion in the pancreas, decreases hepatic glucose production, and increases cellular response to insulin* 1.25•250, 2.5•500, 5•500 mg oral

glybutamide [see: carbutamide]

glybuthiazol INN

glybuthizol [see: glybuthiazol]

glybuzole INN

glycalox BAN [also: glucalox]

glyceol *investigational (orphan) agent for decreasing intracranial hypertension or cerebral edema*

glycerides oleiques polyoxyethylenes [see: peglicol 5 oleate]

glycerin USP *humectant; solvent; osmotic diuretic; hyperosmotic laxative; emollient/protectant; ophthalmic moisturizer* [also: glycerol] ☒ Glucerna

glycerol INN *humectant; solvent; osmotic diuretic; hyperosmotic laxative; emollient/protectant; monoctanoin component D* [also: glycerin] ☒ clazuril; Clozaril

glycerol, iodinated USAN, BAN *(disapproved for use as an expectorant in 1991)*

glycerol 1-decanoate *monoctanoin component B* [see: monoctanoin]

glycerol 1,2-dioctanoate *monoctanoin component C* [see: monoctanoin]

glycerol 1-octanoate *monoctanoin component A* [see: monoctanoin]

glycerol phosphate, manganese salt [see: manganese glycerophosphate]

glyceryl behenate NF *tablet and capsule lubricant*

glyceryl borate [see: boroglycerin]

glyceryl guaiacolate [now: guaifenesin]

glyceryl monostearate NF *emulsifying agent*

glyceryl triacetate [now: triacetin]

glyceryl trierucate *investigational (orphan) agent for adrenoleukodystrophy* [also: glyceryl trioleate]

glyceryl trinitrate BAN *coronary vasodilator* [also: nitroglycerin]

glyceryl trioleate *investigational (orphan) agent for adrenoleukodystrophy* [also: glyceryl trierucate]

glycerylaminophenaquine [see: glafenine]

Glyceryl-T capsules, oral liquid (discontinued 2007) ℞ *antiasthmatic; bronchodilator; expectorant* [theophylline; guaifenesin] 150•90 mg; 150•90 mg/15 mL

glycinato dihydroxyaluminum hydrate [see: dihydroxyaluminum aminoacetate]

glycine USP, INN *nonessential amino acid; urologic irrigant; symbols: Gly, G* [also: aminoacetic acid] 1.5% ☒ Cleocin; Galzin; Quelicin

glycine aluminum-zirconium complex [see: aluminum zirconium tetrachlorohydrex gly; aluminum zirconium trichlorohydrex gly]

Glycine max medicinal herb [see: soy]

glycine2-human glucagon-like peptide-2, recombinant *investigational (orphan) for short bowel syndrome*

glycitein *one of several soy isoflavones that provide cell-protective effects* ☒ colistin

glycitin *isoform precursor to glycitein* [q.v.]

glyclopyramide INN

glycobiarsol USP, INN [also: bismuth glycollylarsanilate]

glycocholate sodium [see: sodium glycocholate]

glycocoll [see: glycine]

glycol distearate USAN *thickening agent*

GlycoLax powder for oral solution ℞ *laxative; bowel evacuant* [polyethylene glycol 3350] 17 g/dose ☒ glucalox

glycolic acid *mild exfoliant and keratolytic*

glycolipodipsipeptides *a class of broad-spectrum antibiotics that are bactericidal against gram-positive aerobic and anaerobic bacteria*

p-**glycolophenetidide** [see: fenacetinol]

glycopeptides *a class of antibiotic antineoplastics*

glycophenylate [see: mepenzolate bromide]

glycoprotein (GP) IIb/IIIa receptor antagonists *a class of platelet aggregation inhibitors for acute coronary syndrome, unstable angina, myocardial infarction, and cardiac surgery*

glycopyrrolate USAN, USP *GI anticholinergic/antispasmodic; antisecretory to prevent chronic, severe drooling; adjunctive therapy for peptic ulcers* [also: glycopyrronium bromide] 1, 2 mg oral; 0.2 mg/mL injection

glycopyrrone bromide [see: glycopyrrolate]

glycopyrronium bromide INN, BAN *GI antispasmodic; antisecretory; peptic ulcer adjunct* [also: glycopyrrolate]

glycosaminoglycans *a class of anticoagulants used for the prophylaxis of postoperative deep vein thrombosis (DVT)*

glycosides, cardiac *a class of cardiovascular drugs that increase the force of cardiac contractions* [also called: digitalis glycosides]

glycyclamide INN, BAN

glycylcyclines *a class of bacteriostatic, antimicrobial antibiotics; a derivative of tetracyclines that have greater efficacy against tetracycline-resistant infections*

glycyrrhetinic acid [see: enoxolone]

glycyrrhiza NF

Glycyrrhiza glabra; G. palidiflora; G. uralensis medicinal herb [see: licorice]

glydanile sodium [now: glicetanile sodium]

glyhexamide USAN, INN *antidiabetic*

glyhexylamide [see: metahexamide]

Glylorin *investigational (Phase III, orphan) for nonbullous congenital ichthyosiform erythroderma (a.k.a. congenital primary ichthyosis)* [monolaurin]

glymidine BAN *antidiabetic* [also: glymidine sodium]

glymidine sodium USAN, INN *antidiabetic* [also: glymidine]

glymol [see: mineral oil]

Glynase PresTabs (micronized tablets) ℞ *sulfonylurea antidiabetic that stimulates insulin secretion in the pancreas* [glyburide] 1.5, 3, 6 mg

glyoctamide USAN, INN *antidiabetic*

Gly-Oxide oral solution OTC *antiseptic* [carbamide peroxide] 10% ⑦ gallic acid

glyparamide USAN *antidiabetic*

glyphylline [see: dyphylline]

glypinamide INN

Glypressin *investigational (orphan) for bleeding esophageal varices and hepatorenal syndrome* [terlipressin]

glyprothiazol INN ⑦ cloprothiazole

glyprothizol [see: glyprothiazol]

Glyquin cream ℞ *hyperpigmentation bleaching agent* [hydroquinone (in a sunscreen base)] 4% ⑦ Qualaquin

Glyquin-XM cream ℞ *hyperpigmentation bleaching agent* [hydroquinone (in a sunscreen base with vitamin E)] 4%

Glyset tablets ℞ *antidiabetic agent for type 2 diabetes; alpha-glucosidase inhibitor that delays the digestion of dietary carbohydrates* [miglitol] 25, 50, 100 mg ⑦ Calcet

glysobuzole INN [also: isobuzole]

GM-CSF (granulocyte-macrophage colony-stimulating factor) [see: regramostim; sargramostim; molgramostim]

Gnaphalium polycephalum; G. uliginosum medicinal herb [see: everlasting]

GNP Cold Head Congestion Daytime caplets OTC *antitussive; decongestant; analgesic; antipyretic* [dextromethorphan hydrobromide; phenylephrine HCl; acetaminophen] 10•5•325 mg

Gn-RH, GnRH (gonadotropin-releasing hormone) *an endogenous hormone, produced in the hypothalamus, which stimulates the release of luteinizing hormone (LH) and follicle-stimulating hormone (FSH) from the pituitary* [also known as: luteinizing hormone–releasing hormone (LH-RH)]

goatweed *medicinal herb* [see: St. John's wort]

gold *element (Au)*

gold Au 198 USAN, USP *antineoplastic; liver imaging aid; radioactive agent*

Gold Bond Antiseptic First Aid Quick Spray OTC *antiseptic; antipruritic; counterirritant* [benzethonium chloride; menthol] 0.13%•1%

Gold Bond Intensive Healing cream OTC *moisturizer; emollient; anesthetic* [dimethicone; pramoxine HCl] 6%•1%

Gold Bond Medicated Triple Action Relief lotion OTC *moisturizer; emollient; mild anesthetic; antipruritic; counterirritant* [dimethicone; menthol] 5%•0.15%

Gold Bond Pain Relieving Foot roll-on liquid, cream OTC *mild anesthetic; antipruritic; counterirritant* [menthol; capsaicin] 16%•⑦

gold sodium thiomalate USP *antirheumatic (50% gold)* [also: sodium aurothiomalate] 50 mg/mL injection

gold sodium thiosulfate NF [also: sodium aurotiosulfate]

gold thioglucose [see: aurothioglucose]

gold thread (*Coptis trifolia*) root *medicinal herb used as an antiphlogistic, bitter tonic, and sedative*

golden senecio *medicinal herb* [see: life root]

goldenrod (*Solidago nemoralis; S. odora; S. virgaurea*) leaves and flowering tops *medicinal herb used as an astringent, carminative, diaphoretic, diuretic, and stimulant*

goldenseal (*Hydrastis canadensis*) rhizome and root *medicinal herb used as an antibiotic and antiseptic and for internal bleeding, colon inflammation, eye infections, liver disorders, menorrhagia, mouth sores, muscular pain, sciatic pain, and vaginitis*

golimumab *anti-TNF-alpha monoclonal antibody for rheumatoid arthritis, psoriatic arthritis, and ankylosing spondylitis*

GoLYTELY powder for oral solution ℞ *pre-procedure bowel evacuant* [polyethylene glycol–electrolyte solution (PEG 3350)] 60 g/L

gonacrine [see: acriflavine]

gonadorelin INN, BAN *gonad-stimulating principle* [also: gonadorelin acetate]

gonadorelin acetate USAN *gonadotropin-releasing hormone for the induction of ovulation in women with hypothalamic amenorrhea (orphan); diagnostic aid for fertility* [also: gonadorelin]

gonadorelin HCl USAN *gonad-stimulating principle; synthetic luteinizing hormone–releasing hormone (LH-RH); in vivo diagnostic aid for anterior pituitary function*

gonadotrophin, chorionic INN, BAN *a hormone produced by human placenta (chorion) and extracted from the urine of pregnant women; used for prepubertal cryptorchidism or hypogonadism and to induce ovulation in anovulatory women; also used for rapid weight loss* [also: gonadotropin, chorionic]

gonadotrophin, serum INN

gonadotropin, chorionic USP *a hormone produced by human placenta (chorion) and extracted from the urine of pregnant women; used for prepubertal cryptorchidism or hypogonadism and to induce ovulation in anovulatory women; also used for rapid weight loss* [also: gonadotrophin, chorionic] 500, 1000, 2000 IU/mL injection

gonadotropin, serum [see: gonadotrophin, serum]

gonadotropin-releasing hormone (Gn-RH) *an endogenous hormone, produced in the hypothalamus, which stimulates the release of luteinizing hormone (LH) and follicle-stimulating hormone (FSH) from the pituitary* [also known as: luteinizing hormone–releasing hormone (LH-RH)]

gonadotropin-releasing hormone analogs *a class of hormonal antineoplastics*

gonadotropins *a class of hormones that stimulate the ovaries, including follicle-stimulating hormone and luteinizing hormone*

Gonak ophthalmic solution OTC *gonioscopic examination aid* [hydroxypropyl methylcellulose] 2.5% ⊘ Kank-a

Gonal-f subcu injection ℞ *recombinant follicle-stimulating hormone (FSH) for induction of ovulation or spermatogenesis (orphan); adjunct to assisted reproductive technologies (ART)* [follitropin alfa] 75, 450, 1050 IU

Gonal-f RFF Pen (prefilled syringes) ℞ *recombinant follicle-stimulating hormone (FSH) for induction of ovulation; adjunct to assisted reproductive technologies (ART)* [follitropin alfa] 300, 450, 900 IU

Gonic powder for IM injection (discontinued 2010) ℞ *a human-derived hormone used for prepubertal cryptorchidism or hypogonadism and to induce ovulation in anovulatory women* [chorionic gonadotropin] 1000 U/mL ⊘ Kank-a

Goniopora **spp.** *natural material* [see: coral]

Gonioscopic Prism Solution Drop-Tainers (eye drops) (discontinued 2008) OTC *agent for bonding gonioscopic prisms to the eye* [hydroxyethyl cellulose]

Goniosoft eye drops OTC *ophthalmic moisturizer/lubricant* [hypromellose; benzalkonium chloride] 2.5%•0.01%

Goniosol ophthalmic solution OTC *gonioscopic examination aid* [hydroxypropyl methylcellulose] 2.5% ⊘ Gynazole; Konsyl

Gonozyme Diagnostic reagent kit for professional use ℞ *in vitro diagnostic aid for Neisseria gonorrhoeae*

Good Sense Pain Relief Allergy Sinus gelcaps (discontinued 2007) OTC *decongestant; antihistamine; analgesic; antipyretic* [pseudoephedrine

HCl; chlorpheniramine maleate; acetaminophen] 30•2•500 mg

Good Sense Sinus caplets (discontinued 2007) OTC *decongestant; antihistamine; analgesic; antipyretic* [pseudoephedrine HCl; chlorpheniramine maleate; acetaminophen] 30•2•500 mg

Good Start; Good Start Essentials; Good Start Supreme oral liquid, powder for oral liquid OTC *total or supplementary infant feeding*

Goody's Body Pain oral powder OTC *analgesic; antipyretic; anti-inflammatory* [acetaminophen; aspirin] 325•500 mg/dose

Goody's Extra Strength oral powder OTC *analgesic; antipyretic; anti-inflammatory* [acetaminophen; aspirin; caffeine] 325•500•65 mg/dose

Goody's Fast Pain Relief oral powder OTC *analgesic; antipyretic; anti-inflammatory* [acetaminophen; aspirin; caffeine] 260•520•32.5 mg/dose

Goody's PM oral powder OTC *analgesic; antipyretic; antihistamine; sleep aid* [acewtaminophen; diphenhydramine citrate] 500•38 mg/packet

goose grass *medicinal herb* [see: bedstraw; cinquefoil]

goose hair; gosling weed *medicinal herb* [see: bedstraw]

Gordobalm OTC *analgesic; mild anesthetic; antipruritic; counterirritant; antiseptic* [methyl salicylate; menthol; camphor; alcohol 16%]

Gordochom topical solution OTC *antifungal; antiseptic* [undecylenic acid; chloroxylenol] 25%•3%

Gordofilm topical liquid ℞ *keratolytic* [salicylic acid in flexible collodion] 16.7%

Gordogesic Creme OTC *analgesic; counterirritant* [methyl salicylate] 10%

Gordon's Urea 40% cream ℞ *keratolytic for the removal of dystrophic nails* [urea] 40%

Gormel Creme OTC *moisturizer; emollient; keratolytic* [urea] 20%

goserelin USAN, INN, BAN *hormonal antineoplastic for prostate and breast cancer; luteinizing hormone-releasing hormone (LHRH) agonist* [also: goserelin acetate]

goserelin acetate JAN *hormonal antineoplastic for prostatic carcinoma, breast cancer, and endometriosis; luteinizing hormone-releasing hormone (LHRH) agonist* [also: goserelin]

gosling weed; goose grass; goose hair *medicinal herb* [see: bedstraw]

gossypol (Gossypium spp.) seed oil *medicinal herb for male and female contraception; not generally regarded as safe and effective as male sterility may be irreversible; investigational (orphan) for cancer of the adrenal cortex*

gotu kola (Centella asiatica; Hydrocotyle asiatica) entire plant *medicinal herb for abscesses, hypertension, contraception, leprosy, nervous breakdown, physical and mental fatigue, promoting wound healing, and rheumatism*

goutberry *medicinal herb* [see: blackberry]

govafilcon A USAN *hydrophilic contact lens material*

GP-500 tablets (discontinued 2007) ℞ *decongestant; expectorant* [pseudoephedrine HCl; guaifenesin] 120•500 mg

G/P 1200/60 sustained-release tablets (discontinued 2007) ℞ *expectorant; decongestant* [guaifenesin; pseudoephedrine HCl] 1200•60 mg

GP IIb/IIIa inhibitors [see: glycoprotein (GP) IIb/IIIa receptor antagonists]

gp100 adenoviral gene therapy *investigational (Phase III, orphan) theraccine for metastatic melanoma*

gp160 (glycoprotein 160) antigens *investigational (orphan) antiviral (therapeutic, Phase II) and vaccine (preventative, Phase I) for HIV and AIDS*

grace, herb of *medicinal herb* [see: rue]

Gradumet (trademarked dosage form) *controlled-release tablet*

Grafco topical swab ℞ *antiseptic* [silver nitrate; potassium nitrate] 75%•25%

graftskin *a living, bilayered skin construct for diabetic foot ulcers and pressure sores (the epidermal layer is living human keratinocytes; the dermal layer is living human fibroblasts)*

Gralise tablets ℞ *anticonvulsant for partial-onset seizures; treatment for postherpetic neuralgia* [gabapentin] 300, 600 mg

gramicidin USP, INN *antibacterial antibiotic*

gramicidin & neomycin sulfate & polymyxin B sulfate *topical antibiotic* 0.025 mg•1.75 mg•10 000 U per mL eye drops

gramicidin S INN

Graminis rhizoma **medicinal herb** [see: couch grass]

Grandpa's Wonder Pine Tar conditioner OTC *antiseborrheic; antipsoriatic; antipruritic; antibacterial* [pine tar]

granisetron USAN, INN, BAN *serotonin 5-HT₃ receptor antagonist; antiemetic to prevent nausea and vomiting following chemotherapy, radiation, or surgery*

granisetron HCl USAN *serotonin 5-HT₃ receptor antagonist; antiemetic to prevent nausea and vomiting following chemotherapy, radiation, or surgery* (base=89%) 1 mg oral; 2 mg/10 mL oral; 0.1, 1, 4 mg/mL injection

Granisol oral solution ℞ *antiemetic to prevent nausea and vomiting following chemotherapy* [granisetron (as HCl)] 1 mg/5 mL ▢ Chronosule

Granul-Derm aerosol spray ℞ *proteolytic enzyme for débridement of necrotic tissue; vulnerary* [trypsin; Peruvian balsam; castor oil] 0.1•72.5•650 mg/ 0.82 mL

Granulex aerosol spray ℞ *proteolytic enzyme for débridement of necrotic tissue; vulnerary* [trypsin; Peruvian balsam; castor oil] 0.12•87•788 mg/g

granulocyte colony-stimulating factor (G-CSF), recombinant [see: filgrastim]

granulocyte-macrophage colony-stimulating factor (GM-CSF) [see: regramostim; sargramostim; molgramostim]

GranuMed aerosol spray ℞ *proteolytic enzyme for débridement of necrotic tissue; vulnerary* [trypsin; Peruvian balsam] 0.1•72.5 mg/0.82 mL

grape, bear's *medicinal herb* [see: uva ursi]

grape, Rocky Mountain; wild Oregon grape *medicinal herb* [see: Oregon grape]

grapefruit (Citrus paradisi) *medicinal herb for potassium replacement; the pectin is used to help reduce cholesterol and promote regression of atherosclerosis*

grapeseed (Vitis coigetiae; V. vinifera) *oil medicinal herb for dental caries; also used as a dietary source of essential fatty acids and tocopherols*

grapeseed extract *natural free radical scavenger for inflammatory collagen disease and peripheral vascular disease; contains 92%–95% procyanidolic oligomers (PCOs)*

grass burdock *medicinal herb* [see: burdock]

grass myrtle *medicinal herb* [see: calamus]

Gratiola officinalis **medicinal herb** [see: hedge hyssop]

gravelroot *medicinal herb* [see: queen of the meadow]

graybeard tree *medicinal herb* [see: fringe tree]

Grazax ⒠ *sublingual tablet (approved in the EU) investigational (Phase III) oral allergy immunotherapy (AIT) for seasonal allergy to timothy grass in patients 5–17 years old*

great wild valerian *medicinal herb* [see: valerian]

greater celandine *medicinal herb* [see: celandine]

green broom; greenweed *medicinal herb* [see: dyer's broom]

Green Glo ophthalmic strips ℞ *diagnostic aid for ophthalmic abnormalities* [lissamine green] 1.5 mg

green hellebore *(Veratrum viride)*
medicinal herb [see: hellebore]

green soap [see: soap, green]

green tea *(Camellia sinensis)* leaves
*medicinal herb used as an antihyperlip-
idemic, antimicrobial, antineoplastic,
and antioxidant; also used to promote
longevity by attenuating severe fatal
diseases*

**Green Throat Spray; Red Throat
Spray** OTC *mild mucous membrane
anaesthetic; antipruritic; counterirritant*
[phenol] 1.4%

greenweed; green broom *medicinal
herb* [see: dyer's broom]

grepafloxacin INN *broad-spectrum fluoroquinolone antibiotic*

grepafloxacin HCl USAN *broad-spectrum fluoroquinolone antibiotic*

Grifola frondosa medicinal herb [see:
maitake mushrooms]

Grifols [see: Human Albumin Grifols]

Grifulvin V tablets R *systemic antifungal* [griseofulvin (microsize)] 500 mg

Grindelia squarrosia medicinal herb
[see: gum weed]

Gripe Water [see: Baby's Bliss Gripe
Water; Colic-Ease Gripe Water;
Wellements Organic Gripe Water]

griseofulvin USP, INN, BAN *systemic
antifungal* 125 mg/5 mL oral

Gris-PEG film-coated tablets R *systemic antifungal* [griseofulvin (ultra-
microsize)] 125, 250 mg

ground apple *medicinal herb* [see:
chamomile]

ground berry *medicinal herb* [see: win-
tergreen]

ground holly *medicinal herb* [see: pip-
sissewa]

ground lemon *medicinal herb* [see:
mandrake]

ground lily *medicinal herb* [see: birth-
root]

ground raspberry *medicinal herb* [see:
goldenseal]

ground squirrel pea *medicinal herb*
[see: twin leaf]

ground thistle *medicinal herb* [see: carline thistle]

**group B streptococcus immune
globulin** [see: streptococcus immune
globulin, group B]

growth hormone, human (hGH)
[see: somatropin]

**growth hormone-releasing factor
(GHRF; GH-RF)** *investigational
(orphan) for inadequate endogenous
growth hormone in children*

GRX Vitamin E cream OTC *emollient*
[tocopheryl acetate (vitamin E)]
1000 U

G-strophanthin [see: ouabain]

guabenxan INN

guacetisal INN

guafecainol INN

GUAI 800/DM 30 sustained-release
tablets R *expectorant; antitussive*
[guaifenesin; dextromethorphan
hydrobromide] 800•30 mg

guaiac

guaiacol NF ② guggul

p-**guaiacol** [see: mequinol]

guaiacol carbonate NF

guaiacol glyceryl ether [see: guaifen-
esin]

guaiactamine INN

guaiapate USAN, INN *antitussive*

guaiazulene soluble [see: sodium gua-
lenate]

guaietolin INN

Guaifed sustained-release capsules R
decongestant; expectorant [phenyleph-
rine HCl; guaifenesin] 15•400 mg ②
CVD

Guaifed syrup (discontinued 2007)
OTC *decongestant; expectorant* [pseu-
doephedrine HCl; guaifenesin] 60•
400 mg/10 mL ② CVD

Guaifed-PD sustained-release capsules
R *decongestant; expectorant* [phenyl-
ephrine HCl; guaifenesin] 7.5•200 mg

Guaifen DM extended-release tablets
R *antitussive; decongestant; expectorant*
[dextromethorphan hydrobromide;
phenylephrine HCl; guaifenesin]
20•40•1200 mg ② C-Phen DM; G
Phen DM

Guaifen PE extended-release tablets ℞ *decongestant; expectorant* [phenylephrine HCl; guaifenesin] 25•800 mg

guaifenesin USAN, USP, INN *expectorant* [also: guaiphenesin] 200 mg oral; 100 mg/5 mL oral

guaifenesin & codeine phosphate *expectorant; narcotic antitussive; narcotic analgesic* 300•10 mg oral

guaifenesin & dextromethorphan hydrobromide *expectorant; antitussive* 500•30 mg oral

Guaifenesin DM extended-release caplets (discontinued 2007) ℞ *antitussive; expectorant* [dextromethorphan hydrobromide; guaifenesin] 30•600 mg

Guaifenesin DM syrup OTC *antitussive; expectorant* [dextromethorphan hydrobromide; guaifenesin] 10•100 mg/5 mL

Guaifenesin DM NR oral liquid ℞ *antitussive; expectorant* [dextromethorphan hydrobromide; guaifenesin] 10•100 mg/5 mL

guaifenesin & dyphylline *expectorant; antiasthmatic; bronchodilator* 200•200 mg oral

guaifenesin & hydrocodone bitartrate *expectorant; narcotic antitussive* 100•5 mg/5 mL oral

Guaifenesin NR oral liquid ℞ *expectorant* [guaifenesin] 100 mg/5 mL

guaifenesin & phenylephrine HCl *expectorant; decongestant* 600•15, 600•40, 900•25, 900•30, 1200•30 mg oral; 200•5 mg/5 mL oral

guaifenesin & pseudoephedrine HCl *expectorant; decongestant* 500•60, 595•48, 795•85, 800•90, 1200•50 mg oral

guaifenesin & pseudoephedrine HCl & dextromethorphan hydrobromide *expectorant; decongestant; antitussive* 800•90•60 mg oral

Guaifenesn DM 1000/60 extended-release caplets ℞ *expectorant; antitussive* [guaifenesin; dextromethorphan hydrobromide] 1000•60 mg

Guaifenex DM extended-release caplets ℞ *antitussive; expectorant* [dextromethorphan hydrobromide; guaifenesin] 30•600 mg

Guaifenex GP extended-release film-coated tablets ℞ *decongestant; expectorant* [pseudoephedrine HCl; guaifenesin] 120•1200 mg

Guaifenex PSE 60; Guaifenex PSE 85; Guaifenex PSE 120 extended-release caplets ℞ *decongestant; expectorant* [pseudoephedrine HCl; guaifenesin] 60•600 mg; 85•795 mg; 120•600 mg

guaifylline INN *bronchodilator; expectorant* [also: guaithylline]

GuaiMAX-D extended-release caplets ℞ *decongestant; expectorant* [pseudoephedrine HCl; guaifenesin] 120•600 mg

guaimesal INN ⧉ Kemsol

Guaimist DM syrup (discontinued 2007) ℞ *antitussive; decongestant; expectorant* [dextromethorphan hydrobromide; pseudoephrine HCl; guaifenesin] 15•40•100 mg/5 mL

Guaipax PSE sustained-release tablets ℞ *decongestant; expectorant* [pseudoephedrine HCl; guaifenesin] 120•600 mg

guaiphenesin BAN *expectorant* [also: guaifenesin]

guaisteine INN ⧉ Cayston

guaithylline USAN *bronchodilator; expectorant* [also: guaifylline]

guamecycline INN, BAN

guanabenz USAN, INN *centrally acting antiadrenergic antihypertensive*

guanabenz acetate USAN, USP, JAN *centrally acting antiadrenergic antihypertensive* 4, 8 mg oral

guanacline INN, BAN *antihypertensive* [also: guanacline sulfate]

guanacline sulfate USAN *antihypertensive* [also: guanacline]

guanadrel INN *antihypertensive* [also: guanadrel sulfate]

guanadrel sulfate USAN, USP *antihypertensive* [also: guanadrel]

guanatol HCl [see: chloroguanide HCl]

guanazodine INN
guancidine INN *antihypertensive* [also: guancydine]
guancydine USAN *antihypertensive* [also: guancidine]
guanethidine INN, BAN *antihypertensive* [also: guanethidine monosulfate]
guanethidine monosulfate USAN, USP *antihypertensive; investigational (orphan) for reflex sympathetic dystrophy and causalgia* [also: guanethidine]
guanethidine sulfate USAN, USP, JAN *antihypertensive*
guanfacine INN, BAN *antihypertensive; antiadrenergic* [also: guanfacine HCl]
guanfacine HCl USAN *antihypertensive; antiadrenergic; selective alpha$_{2A}$ receptor agonist; nonstimulant treatment for attention-deficit/hyperactivity disorder (ADHD); investigational (orphan) for fragile X syndrome* [also: guanfacine] 1, 2 mg oral
guanidine HCl *cholinergic muscle stimulant for Eaton-Lambert myasthenic syndrome* 125 mg oral
guanisoquin sulfate USAN *antihypertensive* [also: guanisoquine]
guanisoquine INN *antihypertensive* [also: guanisoquin sulfate] ⑨ quinisocaine
guanoclor INN, BAN *antihypertensive* [also: guanoclor sulfate]
guanoclor sulfate USAN *antihypertensive* [also: guanoclor]
guanoctine INN *antihypertensive* [also: guanoctine HCl]
guanoctine HCl USAN *antihypertensive* [also: guanoctine]
guanoxabenz USAN, INN *antihypertensive*
guanoxan INN, BAN *antihypertensive* [also: guanoxan sulfate]
guanoxan sulfate USAN *antihypertensive* [also: guanoxan]
guanoxyfen INN *antihypertensive; antidepressant* [also: guanoxyfen sulfate]
guanoxyfen sulfate USAN *antihypertensive; antidepressant* [also: guanoxyfen]
Guaphenyl II capsules ℞ *decongestant; expectorant* [phenylephrine HCl; guaifenesin] 20•375 mg

Guaphenyl LA dual-release capsules ℞ *decongestant; expectorant* [phenylephrine HCl (extended release); guaifenesin (immediate release)] 30•400 mg
guar gum NF *dietary fiber supplement; tablet binder and disintegrant* ⑨ karaya gum
guarana (*Paullinia cupana; P. sorbilis*) seed paste *medicinal herb for dysentery, malaria, and weight reduction* ⑨ Choron
guaranine [see: caffeine]
guggul (*Commiphora mukul*) plant *medicinal herb for hypercholesterolemia and for arthritis and weight reduction in Ayurvedic medicine* ⑨ guaiacol
Guiadrine DM sustained-release caplets (discontinued 2007) ℞ *antitussive; expectorant* [dextromethorphan hydrobromide; guaifenesin] 30•600 mg
Guiatuss syrup OTC *expectorant* [guaifenesin] 100 mg/5 mL
Guiatuss AC syrup ℞ *narcotic antitussive; expectorant* [codeine phosphate; guaifenesin; alcohol 3.5%] 10•100 mg/5 mL
Guiatuss DAC syrup ℞ *narcotic antitussive; decongestant; expectorant* [codeine phosphate; pseudoephedrine HCl; guaifenesin; alcohol 1.9%] 10•30•100 mg/5 mL
Guiatuss DM syrup OTC *antitussive; expectorant* [dextromethorphan hydrobromide; guaifenesin] 10•100 mg/5 mL
gum arabic *medicinal herb* [see: acacia]
gum ivy *medicinal herb* [see: English ivy]
gum myrrh tree *medicinal herb* [see: myrrh]
gum plant *medicinal herb* [see: comfrey; yerba santa]
gum senegal [see: acacia]
gum tree, hemlock *medicinal herb* [see: hemlock]
gum weed (*Grindelia squarrosia*) flowering top and leaves *medicinal herb for asthma, bronchitis, bladder infection, poison ivy and oak, and psoriasis and other skin disorders*

guncotton, soluble [see: pyroxylin]

gusperimus INN *immunosuppressant; investigational (orphan) for acute renal graft rejection* [also: gusperimus trihydrochloride; gusperimus HCl]

gusperimus HCl JAN *immunosuppressant* [also: gusperimus trihydrochloride; gusperimus]

gusperimus trihydrochloride USAN *immunosuppressant* [also: gusperimus; gusperimus HCl]

gutta percha USP *dental restoration agent*

GyMiso *investigational (orphan) for complete expulsion of the products of conception after intrauterine fetal death* [misoprostol]

gymnema (Gymnema melicida; G. sylvestre) leaves and roots *medicinal herb for diabetes, hyperactivity, and hypoglycemia*

Gynazole-1 vaginal cream in prefilled applicator ℞ *antifungal* [butoconazole nitrate] 2% ☒ Genasal; Goniosol; Konsyl

Gynecort Female Creme cream *corticosteroidal anti-inflammatory* [hydrocortisone acetate] 1%

Gyne-Lotrimin 3 vaginal inserts, vaginal cream, combination pack (cream + inserts) OTC *antifungal* [clotrimazole] 200 mg; 2%; 200 mg + 1%

Gyne-Lotrimin 7 vaginal cream OTC *antifungal* [clotrimazole] 1%

gynergon [see: estradiol]

Gynodiol tablets ℞ *estrogen replacement therapy for the treatment of postmenopausal symptoms and prevention of postmenopausal osteoporosis; palliative therapy for prostate and metastatic breast cancers* [estradiol] 0.5, 1, 1.5, 2 mg

gynoestryl [see: estradiol]

Gynol II Contraceptive vaginal gel, vaginal jelly OTC *spermicidal contraceptive (for use with a diaphragm)* [nonoxynol 9] 2%; 3%

Gynostemma pentaphyllum *medicinal herb* [see: jiaogulan]

Gynovite Plus tablets OTC *vitamin/mineral/calcium/iron supplement* [multiple vitamins & minerals; calcium (as citrate); iron (as amino acid chelate); folic acid] ±•83.3•3•0.07 mg

Gy-Pak (trademarked packaging form) *unit-of-issue package* ☒ K-Pek

gypsy weed *medicinal herb* [see: speedwell]

Gyrocap (trademarked dosage form) *timed-release capsule*

H

H 9600 SR sustained-release caplets (discontinued 2007) ℞ *decongestant; expectorant* [pseudoephedrine HCl; guaifenesin] 90•600 mg

H₁ blockers *a class of antihistamines* [also called: histamine H₁ antagonists]

H₂ blockers *a class of gastrointestinal antisecretory agents* [also called: histamine H₂ antagonists]

²H (deuterium) [see: deuterium oxide]

H₂¹⁵O [see: water O 15]

³H (tritium) [see: tritiated water]

HAART (highly active antiretroviral therapy) *multi-drug therapy given to HIV-positive patients to prevent pro-*gression to AIDS; *a generic term applied to several different anti-HIV protocols*

hachimycin INN, BAN

Haemophilus influenzae b conjugate vaccine (HbCV) (*Haemophilus influenzae* type b capsular polysaccharide vaccine [HbPV], covalently bound to tetanus toxoid) *active bacterin for H. influenzae type b*

hafnium *element (Hf)*

Hair Booster Vitamin tablets (discontinued 2008) OTC *vitamin/mineral/iron supplement* [multiple B vitamins & minerals; iron; folic acid] ±•18•0.4 mg

Hairvite tablets OTC *vitamin/mineral/ calcium/iron supplement* [multiple vitamins & minerals; calcium; iron (as amino acid chelate); folic acid; hydrogenated oil] ± • 75 • 4.5 • 0.4 mg

Halac Kit cream + lotion ℞ *corticosteroidal anti-inflammatory + antipruritic; emollient* [halobetasol propionate (cream) + ammonium lactate (lotion)] 0.05% + 12%

halarsol [see: dichlorophenarsine HCl]

Halaven IV injection ℞ *microtubulin inhibitor antineoplastic for metastatic breast cancer* [eribulin mesylate] 0.5 mg/mL (1 mg/vial)

halazepam USAN, USP, INN, BAN *benzodiazepine anxiolytic; sedative*

halazone USP, INN *disinfectant; water purifier*

halcinonide USAN, USP, INN, BAN *topical corticosteroidal anti-inflammatory*

Halcion tablets ℞ *benzodiazepine sedative and hypnotic* [triazolam] 0.25 mg

Haldol IM injection ℞ *conventional (typical) butyrophenone antipsychotic; antispasmodic/antidyskinetic for Tourette syndrome; treatment for severe pediatric behavioral disorders such as aggression, combativeness, hyperexcitability, and poor impulse control* [haloperidol (as lactate)] 5 mg/mL

Haldol Decanoate 100 long-acting IM injection ℞ *conventional (typical) butyrophenone antipsychotic; antispasmodic/antidyskinetic for Tourette syndrome; treatment for severe pediatric behavioral disorders such as aggression, combativeness, hyperexcitability, and poor impulse control* [haloperidol (as decanoate)] 100 mg/mL

Haldol Decanoate 50 long-acting IM injection (discontinued 2010) ℞ *conventional (typical) butyrophenone antipsychotic; antispasmodic/antidyskinetic for Tourette syndrome; treatment for severe pediatric behavioral disorders such as aggression, combativeness, hyperexcitability, and poor impulse control* [haloperidol (as decanoate)] 50 mg/mL

Halenol, Children's oral liquid (discontinued 2008) OTC *analgesic; antipyretic* [acetaminophen] 160 mg/5 mL

haletazole INN [also: halethazole]

halethazole BAN [also: haletazole]

Haley's M-O oral liquid OTC *saline/ emollient laxative* [magnesium hydroxide; mineral oil] 900 mg • 3.75 mL per 15 mL

HalfLytely Bowel Prep Kit powder for oral solution; 4 enteric-coated delayed-release tablets ℞ *pre-procedure bowel evacuant* [polyethylene glycol 3350 (solution); bisacodyl (tablets)] 2 L; 5 mg

Halfprin 81 enteric-coated tablets OTC *analgesic; antipyretic; anti-inflammatory; antirheumatic* [aspirin] 81 mg

Hall's Plus lozenges OTC *mild anesthetic; antipruritic; counterirritant* [menthol] 10 mg

Hall's Sugar Free Mentho-Lyptus lozenges OTC *mild anesthetic; antipruritic; counterirritant; antiseptic* [menthol; eucalyptus oil] 5 • 2.8, 6 • 2.8 mg

Halls Zinc Defense lozenges OTC *antiseptic to relieve sore throat* [zinc acetate] 5 mg

hallucinogens *a class of agents that induce hallucinations*

halobetasol propionate USAN *topical corticosteroidal anti-inflammatory* [also: ulobetasol] 0.05% topical

halocarban INN *disinfectant* [also: cloflucarban]

halocortolone INN

halocrinic acid [see: brocrinat]

halofantrine INN, BAN *antimalarial* [also: halofantrine HCl]

halofantrine HCl USAN *antimalarial (orphan)* [also: halofantrine]

Halofed tablets OTC *nasal decongestant* [pseudoephedrine HCl] 30, 60 mg

halofenate USAN, INN, BAN *antihyperlipoproteinemic; uricosuric*

halofuginone INN *antiprotozoal* [also: halofuginone hydrobromide]

halofuginone hydrobromide USAN *antiprotozoal; investigational (orphan) for scleroderma* [also: halofuginone]

Halog ointment, cream, solution ℞
corticosteroidal anti-inflammatory [halcinonide] 0.1%

Halog-E cream (discontinued 2009) ℞
corticosteroidal anti-inflammatory [halcinonide] 0.1%

halometasone INN

halonamine INN

halopemide USAN, INN *antipsychotic*

halopenium chloride INN, BAN

haloperidol USAN, USP, INN, BAN *conventional (typical) butyrophenone antipsychotic; antispasmodic/antidyskinetic for Tourette syndrome; treatment for severe pediatric behavioral disorders such as aggression, combativeness, hyperexcitability, and poor impulse control* 0.5, 1, 2, 5, 10, 20 mg oral

haloperidol decanoate USAN, BAN *conventional (typical) butyrophenone antipsychotic; antispasmodic/antidyskinetic for Tourette syndrome; treatment for severe pediatric behavioral disorders such as aggression, combativeness, hyperexcitability, and poor impulse control* 50, 100 mg/mL injection

haloperidol lactate *conventional (typical) butyrophenone antipsychotic; antispasmodic/antidyskinetic for Tourette syndrome; treatment for severe pediatric behavioral disorders such as aggression, combativeness, hyperexcitability, and poor impulse control* 2 mg/mL oral; 5 mg/mL injection

halopone chloride [see: halopenium chloride]

halopredone INN *topical anti-inflammatory* [also: halopredone acetate]

halopredone acetate USAN *topical anti-inflammatory* [also: halopredone]

haloprogesterone USAN, INN *progestin*

haloprogin USAN, USP, INN, JAN *antibacterial; antifungal*

halopyramine BAN [also: chloropyramine]

halothane USP, INN, BAN *inhalation general anesthetic*

Halotussin syrup OTC *expectorant* [guaifenesin; alcohol 3.5%] 100 mg/5 mL

haloxazolam INN

haloxon INN, BAN

halquinol BAN *topical anti-infective* [also: halquinols]

halquinols USAN *topical anti-infective* [also: halquinol]

Hamamelis virginiana *medicinal herb* [see: witch hazel]

hamamelis water *medicinal herb* [see: witch hazel]

hamycin USAN, INN *antifungal*

HandiHaler (trademarked delivery device) *inhalation powder dispenser*

hard fat [see: fat, hard]

hardock *medicinal herb* [see: burdock]

hareburr *medicinal herb* [see: burdock]

Harpagophytum procumbens *medicinal herb* [see: devil's claw]

hashish *(Cannabis sativa)* *euphoric/hallucinogenic street drug made from the resin of the flowering tops of the cannabis plant*

Havrix adult IM injection, pediatric IM injection ℞ *immunization against hepatitis A virus (HAV)* [hepatitis A vaccine, inactivated] 1440 ELISA units (EL.U.)/mL; 720 EL.U./0.5 mL

haw *medicinal herb* [see: hawthorn]

Hawaiian Tropic Cool Aloe with I.C.E. gel OTC *anesthetic; antipruritic; counterirritant* [lidocaine; menthol]

hawthorn *(Crataegus laevigata; C. monogyna; C. oxyacantha)* flowers, leaves, and berries *medicinal herb for angina pectoris, arrhythmias, arteriosclerosis, enlarged heart, high or low blood pressure, hypoglycemia, palpitations, and tachycardia; also used as an antiseptic* ② Hytrin

Hayfebrol oral liquid (discontinued 2007) OTC *decongestant; antihistamine* [pseudoephedrine HCl; chlorpheniramine maleate] 60•4 mg/10 mL

hazel, snapping; hazelnut *medicinal herb* [see: witch hazel]

HBIG (hepatitis B immune globulin) [q.v.]

hBNP (human B-type natriuretic peptide) [see: nesiritide; nesiritide citrate]

1% HC ointment ℞ *corticosteroidal anti-inflammatory* [hydrocortisone] 1%
HC (hydrocortisone) [q.v.]
4-HC (4-hydroperoxycyclophosphamide) [q.v.]
HC Derma-Pax topical liquid OTC *corticosteroidal anti-inflammatory; antihistamine; antiseptic* [hydrocortisone; pyrilamine maleate; chlorpheniramine maleate; chlorobutanol] 0.5%•0.44%•0.06%•25%
HC Pram 1%; HC Pram 2.5% anorectal cream ℞ *corticosteroidal anti-inflammatory; local anesthetic* [hydrocortisone acetate; pramoxine] 1%•1%; 2.5%•1%
HC Pramoxine anorectal cream ℞ *corticosteroidal anti-inflammatory; local anesthetic* [hydrocortisone acetate; pramoxine] 2.5%•1%
HCA (hydrocortisone acetate) [q.v.]
hCG (human chorionic gonadotropin) [see: gonadotropin, chorionic]
HCT (hydrochlorothiazide) [q.v.]
HCTZ (hydrochlorothiazide) [q.v.]
HD 85 oral/rectal suspension ℞ *radiopaque contrast medium for gastrointestinal imaging* [barium sulfate] 85%
HD 200 Plus powder for oral suspension ℞ *radiopaque contrast medium for gastrointestinal imaging* [barium sulfate] 98%
HDCV (human diploid cell vaccine) [see: rabies vaccine]
HDMTX; HD MTX (high-dose methotrexate) [with leucovorin rescue] *chemotherapy protocol for bone sarcoma*
Head & Shoulders; Head & Shoulders Dry Scalp shampoo OTC *antiseborrheic; antibacterial; antifungal* [pyrithione zinc] 1%
Head & Shoulders Intensive Treatment lotion/shampoo OTC *antiseborrheic; dandruff treatment* [selenium sulfide] 1%
heal-all *medicinal herb* [see: figwort; stone root; woundwort]
healing herb *medicinal herb* [see: comfrey]

Healon; Healon GV intraocular injection ℞ *viscoelastic agent for ophthalmic surgery* [hyaluronate sodium] 10 mg/mL; 14 mg/mL
Healon Yellow intraocular injection (discontinued 2009) ℞ *viscoelastic agent for ophthalmic surgery; diagnostic agent* [hyaluronate sodium; fluorescein sodium] 10•0.005 mg/mL
Healon5 intraocular injection in preloaded syringes ℞ *viscoelastic agent for ophthalmic surgery* [hyaluronate sodium 5000] 23 mg/mL
Healthy Kids Vitamins D₃ chewable tablets OTC *vitamin D supplement* [cholecalciferol (vitamin D₃)] 400 IU
heart, mother's; shepherd's heart *medicinal herb* [see: shepherd's purse]
Heart Vitality tablets OTC *vitamin/mineral supplement* [vitamins B₆ and B₁₂; multiple minerals; coenzyme Q10; phytosterols; folic acid] 1•0.003•±•6•1•0.2 mg
Heartline enteric-coated tablets OTC *analgesic; antipyretic; anti-inflammatory; antirheumatic* [aspirin] 81 mg
Heather tablets (in packs of 28) ℞ *oral contraceptive (progestin only)* [norethindrone] 0.35 mg
heather (Calluna vulgaris) flowering shoots *medicinal herb used as an antiseptic, cholagogue, diaphoretic, diuretic, expectorant, and vasoconstrictor*
heavy liquid petrolatum [see: mineral oil]
heavy water (D₂O) [see: deuterium oxide]
Hectorol capsules, bolus injection during dialysis ℞ *synthetic vitamin D analogue; serum calcium regulator for hyperparathyroidism due to chronic kidney disease* [doxercalciferol] 0.5, 1, 2.5 mcg; 2 mcg/mL
hedaquinium chloride INN, BAN
Hedeoma pulegeoides *medicinal herb* [see: pennyroyal]
Hedera helix *medicinal herb* [see: English ivy]
hedge bindweed (Convolvulus sepium) flowering plant and roots *medicinal*

herb used as a cholagogue, febrifuge, and purgative

hedge garlic ***(Sisymbrium alliaria)*** *medicinal herb* [see: garlic]

hedge hyssop ***(Gratiola officinalis)*** plant *medicinal herb used as a cardiac, diuretic, purgative, and vermifuge*

hedge-burs *medicinal herb* [see: bedstraw]

"hedgehog" proteins *a class of novel human proteins that induce the formation of regenerative tissue*

Heet Liniment OTC *analgesic; counterirritant; antiseptic* [methyl salicylate; camphor; capsaicin; alcohol 70%] 15%•3.6%•0.025%

hefilcon A USAN *hydrophilic contact lens material*

hefilcon B USAN *hydrophilic contact lens material*

hefilcon C USAN *hydrophilic contact lens material*

helenien [see: xantofyl palmitate]

Helianthemum canadense *medicinal herb* [see: rock rose]

helicon [see: aspirin]

Helicosol powder for oral solution ℞ *diagnostic aid for detection of* H. pylori *in the stomach* [carbon C 13 urea]

Helidac 14-day dose-pack ℞ *combination treatment for active duodenal ulcer with* H. pylori *infection* [bismuth subsalicylate (chewable tablets); metronidazole (tablets); tetracycline HCl (capsules)] 8 × 262.4 mg; 4 × 250 mg; 4 × 500 mg (per day)

heliomycin INN

heliox *helium-oxygen mixture used for respiratory distress* (usually an 80%•20% mix) ⑨ Hyalex

helium USP *diluent for gases; element (He)*

Helixate FS powder for IV injection ℞ *systemic hemostatic; antihemophilic for the prevention and control of bleeding in classical hemophilia (hemophilia A) and von Willebrand disease (orphan)* [antihemophilic factor concentrate, recombinant] 250, 500, 1000, 2000 IU/vial

hellebore (*Helleborus* spp.; *Veratrum* spp.) rhizome *medicinal herb used as an antihypertensive; not generally regarded as safe and effective for internal consumption due to toxicity*

Helleborus **spp.** *medicinal herb* [see: hellebore]

helmet flower *medicinal herb* [see: aconite; sandalwood; skullcap]

helmet pod *medicinal herb* [see: twin leaf]

HEMA (2-hydroxyethyl methacrylate) *contact lens material*

Hemabate IM injection ℞ *prostaglandin-type abortifacient; for postpartum uterine bleeding* [carboprost tromethamine] 250 mcg/mL

Hema-Check slide tests for home use OTC *in vitro diagnostic aid for fecal occult blood*

Hema-Combistix reagent strips OTC *in vitro diagnostic aid for multiple urine products*

Hemastix reagent strips for professional use ℞ *in vitro diagnostic aid for urine occult blood*

Hematest reagent tablets for professional use ℞ *in vitro diagnostic aid for fecal occult blood*

Hematide *investigational (NDA filed) synthetic peptide–based erythropoiesis-stimulating agent (ESA) to increase RBC production for anemia due to chronic renal failure* [peginesatide]

hematin [now: hemin]

Hematinic film-coated tablets ℞ *hematinic* [iron (as ferrous fumarate); folic acid] 324•1 mg

Hematinic Plus Vitamins and Minerals tablets ℞ *hematinic* [iron (as ferrous fumarate); multiple vitamins & minerals; folic acid] 106•≛•1 mg

hematinics *a class of iron-containing agents for the prevention and treatment of iron-deficiency anemia*

hematopoietics *a class of antianemic agents that promote the formation of red blood cells*

Hematrol *synthetic progestin; investigational (orphan) for immune thrombocy-*

topenic purpura (ITP) [medroxyprogesterone acetate]

heme arginate *investigational (orphan) for acute symptomatic porphyria and myelodysplastic syndrome*

HemeSelect Collection kit for home use OTC *in vitro diagnostic aid for fecal occult blood* [for use with **HemeSelect Reagent** kit]

HemeSelect Reagent kit for professional use ℞ *in vitro diagnostic aid for fecal occult blood* [for use with **HemeSelect Collection** kit]

Hemex *investigational (orphan) for acute porphyric syndromes* [hemin; zinc mesoporphyrin]

hemiacidrin [see: citric acid, glucono-delta-lactone & magnesium carbonate]

hemin *enzyme inhibitor for acute intermittent porphyria (AIP), porphyria variegata, and hereditary coproporphyria (orphan)*

hemin & zinc mesoporphyrin *investigational (orphan) for acute porphyric syndromes*

hemlock (Tsuga canadensis) bark *medicinal herb used as an astringent, diaphoretic, and diuretic* ☒ Humalog

Hemoccult slide tests for professional use, test tape for professional use ℞ *in vitro diagnostic aid for fecal occult blood*

Hemoccult II slide tests for professional use ℞ *in vitro diagnostic aid for fecal occult blood*

Hemoccult II Dispenserpak; Hemoccult II Dispenserpak Plus slide tests for home use OTC *in vitro diagnostic aid for fecal occult blood*

Hemoccult SENSA; Hemoccult II SENSA slide tests for professional use ℞ *in vitro diagnostic aid for fecal occult blood*

Hemocitrate *investigational (orphan) adjunct to leukapheresis procedures* [sodium citrate]

Hemocyte tablets OTC *iron supplement* [iron (as ferrous fumarate)] 106 mg

Hemocyte Plus elixir (discontinued 2008) ℞ *hematinic* [iron (as polysac-charide-iron complex); multiple B vitamins & minerals; folic acid] 12•≛•0.33 mg

Hemocyte Plus tablets (discontinued 2008) ℞ *hematinic* [iron (as ferrous fumarate); multiple B vitamins & minerals; vitamin C (as sodium ascorbate); folic acid] 106•≛•200•1 mg

Hemocyte-F elixir ℞ *hematinic* [iron (as polysaccharide-iron complex); cyanocobalamin; folic acid] 100•0.025•1 mg/5 mL

Hemocyte-F tablets (discontinued 2008) ℞ *hematinic* [iron (as ferrous fumarate); folic acid] 106•1 mg

Hemofil M IV injection ℞ *systemic hemostatic; antihemophilic for the prevention and control of bleeding in classical hemophilia (hemophilia A) and von Willebrand disease (orphan)* [antihemophilic factor concentrate, human] 2–20 IU/mg

hemoglobin crosfumaril USAN, INN *blood substitute*

Hemopad fibrous dressing ℞ *topical hemostat for surgery* [microfibrillar collagen hemostat] 2.5 × 5, 5 × 8, 8 × 10 cm ☒ Humibid

Hemophilus b conjugate vaccine [see: *Haemophilus* b conjugate vaccine (HbCV)]

Hemorid for Women cream OTC *anesthetic and vasoconstrictor for hemorrhoids* [pramoxine HCl; phenylephrine HCl] 1%•0.25%

Hemorid for Women lotion OTC *emollient and protectant for hemorrhoids* [mineral oil; petrolatum; glycerin]

Hemorid for Women rectal suppositories OTC *vasoconstrictor and astringent for hemorrhoids* [zinc oxide; phenylephrine HCl] 11%•0.25%

Hemorrhoidal HC rectal suppositories ℞ *corticosteroidal anti-inflammatory for hemorrhoids* [hydrocortisone acetate] 25 mg

hemostatics *a class of therapeutic blood modifiers that arrest the flow of blood* [see also: astringents; styptics]

Hemotene fibrous dressing (discontinued 2008) ℞ *topical hemostat for surgery* [microfibrillar collagen hemostat] 1 g ☑ Humatin

Hemovit film-coated tablets ℞ *hematinic* [multiple B vitamins; vitamin C; folic acid; biotin] ± • 60 • 1 • 0.3 mg

Hemoxin *investigational (orphan) for sickle cell disease* [niprisan]

hemp *medicinal herb* [see: marijuana]

hemp agrimony *(Eupatorium cannabinum)* plant *medicinal herb used as a cholagogue, diaphoretic, diuretic, emetic, expectorant, and purgative*

hemp nettle *(Galeopsis tetrahit)* plant *medicinal herb used as an astringent, diuretic, and expectorant*

Hem-Prep anorectal ointment, rectal suppositories OTC *temporary relief of hemorrhoidal symptoms; vasoconstrictor; astringent; emollient* [phenylephrine HCl; zinc oxide] 0.025% • 11%; 0.25% • 11%

Hemril Uniserts (rectal suppositories) OTC *temporary relief of hemorrhoidal symptoms* [bismuth subgallate; bismuth resorcin compound; benzyl benzoate; Peruvian balsam; zinc oxide] 2.25% • 1.75% • 1.2% • 1.8% • 11%

Hemril-HC Uniserts (suppositories) ℞ *corticosteroidal anti-inflammatory for hemorrhoids* [hydrocortisone acetate] 25 mg

henbane *(Hyoscyamus niger)* plant *medicinal herb used as an anodyne, antispasmodic, calmative, and narcotic; primarily used externally because of its high toxicity*

heneicosafluorotripropylamine [see: perfluamine]

henna *(Alkanna tinctoria)* root *medicinal herb used as an astringent, antibiotic, and cosmetic dye; not generally regarded as safe and effective*

henna *(Lawsonia inermis)* leaves *medicinal herb used as an astringent*

HEOD (hexachloro-epoxy-octahydro-dimethanonaththalene) [see: dieldrin]

Hepacid *investigational (orphan) treatment for hepatocellular carcinoma* [pegylated arginine deiminase]

HepaGam B IM injection ℞ *treatment for acute exposure to blood containing hepatitis B surface antigen (HBsAg); prophylaxis against hepatitis B infection after maternal, social, or sexual exposure to hepatitis B* [hepatitis B immune globulin, solvent/detergent treated] 5% (50 mg/mL)

Hepandrin *investigational (orphan) anabolic steroid for alcoholic hepatitis* [oxandrolone]

heparin BAN *anticoagulant; antithrombotic* [also: heparin calcium]

heparin, 2-0-desulfated *investigational (orphan) for cystic fibrosis*

heparin, unfractionated *investigational (orphan) oral treatment for sickle cell disease*

heparin calcium USP *anticoagulant; antithrombotic* [also: heparin]

Heparin I.V. Flush prefilled syringe ℞ *IV flush for catheter patency (not therapeutic)* [heparin sodium] 1 U/mL

Heparin Lock Flush solution ℞ *IV flush for catheter patency (not therapeutic)* [heparin sodium] 10, 100 U/mL

heparin sodium USP, INN, BAN *anticoagulant; antithrombotic* 1000, 2000, 2500, 5000, 7500, 10 000, 20 000, 40 000 U/mL injection

Heparin Sodium in 5% Dextrose IV injection ℞ *anticoagulant* [heparin sodium] 40, 50 U/mL

heparin sodium & sodium chloride 0.45% *anticoagulant; antithrombotic* 12 500 U • 250 mL, 25 000 U • 250 mL, 25 000 U • 500 mL injection

heparin sodium & sodium chloride 0.9% *anticoagulant; antithrombotic* 1000 U • 500 mL, 2000 U • 1000 mL injection

heparin sulfate [see: danaparoid sodium]

heparin whole blood [see: blood, whole]

HepatAmine IV infusion ℞ *nutritional therapy for hepatic failure and hepatic* *encephalopathy* [multiple branched-chain essential and nonessential amino acids; electrolytes]

HepatAssist *investigational (orphan) for severe liver failure* [xenogeneic hepatocytes]

hepatica *(Hepatica acutiloba; H. triloba)* leaves and flowers *medicinal herb used as a diuretic and pectoral*

Hepatic-Aid II Instant Drink powder (discontinued 2009) OTC *enteral nutritional treatment for chronic liver disease* [multiple branched chain amino acids]

hepatics *a class of agents that affect the liver (a term used in folk medicine)*

hepatitis A vaccine, inactivated *active immunizing agent for the hepatitis A virus (HAV)*

hepatitis B immune globulin (HBIG) USP *passive immunizing agent; treatment for acute exposure to blood containing hepatitis B surface antigen (HBsAg); prophylaxis against hepatitis B infection after transplant (orphan), maternal, social, or sexual exposure to hepatitis B*

hepatitis B surface antigen (HBsAg) [see: hepatitis B virus vaccine, inactivated]

hepatitis B virus vaccine, inactivated USP *active immunizing agent for hepatitis B and D*

hepatitis C virus immune globulin, human *investigational (orphan) prophylaxis against hepatitis C infection in liver transplant patients*

HepeX-B *investigational (orphan) prophylaxis against hepatitis B reinfection in liver transplant patients*

Hepflush-10 solution ℞ *IV flush for catheter patency (not therapeutic)* [heparin sodium] 10 U/mL

Hep-Forte capsules OTC *vitamin supplement* [multiple vitamins & food products; folic acid; biotin] ±•60•3.3 mcg

Heplisav *investigational (Phase III) active immunizing agent for hepatitis B* [hepatitis B surface antigen]

Hep-Lock; Hep-Lock U/P solution ℞ *IV flush for catheter patency (not therapeutic)* [heparin sodium] 10, 100 U/mL

HEPP (H-chain ε [IgE] pentapeptide) [see: pentigetide]

hepronicate INN

Hepsera tablets ℞ *antiviral for chronic hepatitis B virus (HBV) infection* [adefovir dipivoxil] 10 mg

heptabarb INN [also: heptabarbitone]

heptabarbital [see: heptabarb; heptabarbitone]

heptabarbitone BAN [also: heptabarb]

heptaminol INN, BAN

heptaminol HCl [see: heptaminol]

2-heptanamine [see: tuaminoheptane]

2-heptanamine sulfate [see: tuaminoheptane sulfate]

heptaverine INN

heptolamide INN

hepzidine INN

HER (human epidermal growth factor receptor) inhibitors [q.v.]

HER1 (human epidermal growth factor receptor 1) inhibitors *a class of antineoplastics that suppress the growth of lung and pancreatic cancers*

HER2 (human epidermal growth factor receptor 2) inhibitors *a class of antineoplastics, predominantly monoclonal antibodies, that suppress the growth of breast cancer*

Heracleum lanatum medicinal herb [see: masterwort]

herb of grace *medicinal herb* [see: rue]

HercepTest test kit ℞ *diagnostic aid for the HER2 protein, used to screen patients who may benefit from treatment with Herceptin*

Herceptin powder for IV infusion ℞ *monoclonal antibody antineoplastic for metastatic HER2-overexpressing breast and gastric cancers; investigational (orphan) for pancreatic cancer* [trastuzumab] 440 mg

Hercules woundwort *medicinal herb* [see: woundwort]

heroin *potent narcotic analgesic street drug which is highly addictive; banned in the*

U.S. [medically known as diamorphine and diacetylmorphine HCl]
heroin HCl *(banned in the U.S.)* [see:
diacetylmorphine HCl]
Herpecin L lip balm OTC *vulnerary;
sunblock* [dimethicone; meradimate;
octinoxate; octisalate; oxybenzone]
1%•5%•7.5%•5%•6%
**herpes simplex virus, genetically
modified (G207)** *investigational
(orphan) agent for malignant glioma*
herpes simplex virus gene *investigational (orphan) for primary and metastatic brain tumors*
Herrick Lacrimal Plug ℞ *blocks the
puncta and canaliculus to eliminate tear
loss in keratitis sicca* [silicone plug]
HES (hydroxyethyl starch) [see:
hetastarch]
Hespan IV infusion ℞ *plasma volume
expander for shock due to hemorrhage,
burns, surgery* [hetastarch] 6%
hesperidin *a bioflavonoid (q.v.)*
hesperidin methyl chalcone [see:
bioflavonoids]
hetacillin USAN, USP, INN, BAN *antibacterial*
hetacillin potassium USAN, USP *antibacterial*
hetaflur USAN, INN, BAN *dental caries
preventative*
hetastarch USAN, BAN *plasma volume
extender* [also: hydroxyethylstarch]
6% injection
heteronium bromide USAN, INN, BAN
anticholinergic
Hetrazan tablets (discontinued 2009)
℞ *anthelmintic for Bancroft filariasis,
onchocerciasis, tropical eosinophilia,
and loiasis* [diethylcarbamazine cit-
rate] 50 mg
**hexaammonium molybdate tetra-
hydrate** [see: ammonium molybdate]
Hexabrix injection ℞ *radiopaque contrast medium* [ioxaglate meglumine;
ioxaglate sodium (54.3% total
iodine)] 393•196 mg/mL (320
mg/mL)
**HexaCAF; Hexa-CAF (hexameth-
ylmelamine, cyclophosphamide,**

amethopterin, fluorouracil) *chemotherapy protocol for ovarian cancer*
hexacarbacholine bromide INN
[also: carbolonium bromide]
hexachlorane [see: lindane]
hexachlorocyclohexane [see: lindane]
hexachlorophane BAN *topical anti-
infective; detergent* [also: hexachloro-
phene]
hexachlorophene USP, INN *topical
anti-infective; detergent* [also: hexa-
chlorophane]
hexacyclonate sodium INN
hexacyprone INN
hexadecanoic acid [see: palmitic acid]
**hexadecanoic acid, methylethyl
ester** [see: isopropyl palmitate]
hexadecanol [see: cetyl alcohol]
hexadecylamine hydrofluoride [see:
hetaflur]
hexadecylpyridinium chloride [see:
cetylpyridinium chloride]
**hexadecyltrimethylammonium bro-
mide** [see: cetrimonium bromide]
**hexadecyltrimethylammonium
chloride** [see: cetrimonium chloride]
**2,4-hexadienoic acid, potassium
salt** [see: potassium sorbate]
hexadiline INN
hexadimethrine bromide INN, BAN
hexadiphane [see: prozapine]
Hexadrol Phosphate intra-articular,
intralesional, soft tissue, or IM injection (discontinued 2010) ℞ *corticosteroidal anti-inflammatory* [dexa-
methasone sodium phosphate] 4, 10,
20 mg/mL
hexadylamine [see: hexadiline]
Hexafed sustained-release film-coated
tablets (discontinued 2007) ℞ *decongestant; antihistamine* [pseudoephed-
rine HCl; dexchlorpheniramine
maleate] 60•4 mg
hexafluorenium bromide USAN, USP
*skeletal muscle relaxant; succinylcholine
synergist* [also: hexafluronium bromide]
hexafluorodiethyl ether [see: fluro-
thyl]
hexaflurone bromide [see: hexafluorenium bromide]

hexafluronium bromide INN *skeletal muscle relaxant; succinylcholine synergist* [also: hexafluorenium bromide]

Hexalen capsules ℞ *antineoplastic for advanced ovarian adenocarcinoma (orphan)* [altretamine] 50 mg

hexamarium bromide [see: distigmine bromide]

hexametazime BAN

hexamethone bromide [see: hexamethonium bromide]

hexamethonium bromide INN, BAN

hexamethylenamine [now: methenamine]

hexamethylenamine mandelate [see: methenamine mandelate]

hexamethylenetetramine [see: methenamine]

hexamethylmelamine (HMM; HXM) [see: altretamine]

hexamidine INN

hexamine hippurate BAN *urinary antibacterial* [also: methenamine hippurate]

hexamine mandelate [see: methenamine mandelate]

hexaminolevulinate (HAL) *photosensitizer for fluorescence cystoscopy; derivative of aminolevulinic acid*

hexaminolevulinate HCl *photosensitizer for fluorescence cystoscopy; derivative of aminolevulinic acid* (base=85%)

hexapradol INN

hexaprofen INN, BAN

hexapropymate INN, BAN

hexasonium iodide INN

hexavitamin USP

Hexavitamin tablets (discontinued 2008) OTC *vitamin supplement* [multiple vitamins]

hexcarbacholine bromide INN [also: carbolonium bromide]

hexedine USAN, INN *antibacterial*

hexemal [see: cyclobarbital]

hexestrol NF, INN

hexetidine BAN

hexicide [see: lindane]

hexinol [see: cyclomenol]

hexobarbital USP, INN

hexobarbital sodium NF

hexobendine USAN, INN, BAN *vasodilator*

hexocyclium methylsulphate BAN [also: hexocyclium methylsulfate; hexocyclium metilsulfate]

hexocyclium metilsulfate INN [also: hexocyclium methylsulfate; hexocyclium methylsulphate]

hexoprenaline INN, BAN *tocolytic; bronchodilator* [also: hexoprenaline sulfate]

hexoprenaline sulfate USAN, JAN *tocolytic; bronchodilator* [also: hexoprenaline]

hexopyrimidine [see: hexetidine]

hexopyrrolate [see: hexopyrronium bromide]

hexopyrronium bromide INN

hexydaline [see: methenamine mandelate]

hexylcaine INN *local anesthetic* [also: hexylcaine HCl]

hexylcaine HCl USP *local anesthetic* [also: hexylcaine]

hexylene glycol NF *humectant; solvent*

hexylresorcinol USP *anthelmintic; topical antiseptic*

1-hexyltheobromine [see: pentifylline]

H·F Gel *investigational (orphan) emergency treatment for hydrofluoric acid burns* [calcium gluconate]

HFA-134a (hydrofluoroalkane) *propellant used in CFC-free aerosol delivery systems*

HFCS (high fructose corn syrup) *nontherapeutic ingredient for sweetening oral liquids* [compare to: fructose]

hFSH (human follicle-stimulating hormone) [now: menotropins]

HFZ (homofenazine) [q.v.]

197Hg [see: chlormerodrin Hg 197]

197Hg [see: merisoprol acetate Hg 197]

197Hg [see: merisoprol Hg 197]

203Hg [see: chlormerodrin Hg 203]

203Hg [see: merisoprol acetate Hg 203]

hGH (human growth hormone) [see: somatropin]

hibenzate INN *combining name for radicals or groups* [also: hybenzate]

Hiberix powder for injection ℞ *vaccine booster for* H. influenzae *type b (HIB) infections in children 15 months to 4 years* [Haemophilus influenzae b conjugate vaccine] 10 mcg ⑫ Hiprex

Hibiclens sponge/brush (discontinued 2010) OTC *broad-spectrum antimicrobial; germicidal* [chlorhexidine gluconate; alcohol 4%] 4%

Hibiclens Antiseptic/AntiMicrobial Skin Cleanser topical liquid (discontinued 2010) OTC *broad-spectrum antimicrobial; germicidal* [chlorhexidine gluconate; alcohol 4%] 4%

hibiscus (*Hibiscus sabdariffa* and other species) flowers and leaves *medicinal herb for cancer, edema, heart problems and nervous disorders; also used topically as an emollient; not generally regarded as safe and effective*

Hibistat Germicidal Hand Rinse topical liquid OTC *broad-spectrum antimicrobial; germicidal* [chlorhexidine gluconate; alcohol 70%] 0.5%

Hibistat Towelette OTC *broad-spectrum antimicrobial; germicidal* [chlorhexidine gluconate; alcohol 70%] 0.5%

HibTITER IM injection (discontinued 2008) ℞ *vaccine for* H. influenzae *type b (HIB) infections in children 2–71 months* [Haemophilus influenzae b conjugate vaccine (with a diphtheria CRM$_{197}$ carrier)] 10•(25) mcg/0.5 mL

Hi-C DAZE (high-dose cytarabine, daunorubicin, azacitidine, etoposide) *chemotherapy protocol for acute myelogenous leukemia (AML)*

Hi-Cal VM nutrition bar OTC *enteral nutritional therapy for HIV and AIDS*

Hicon oral solution ℞ *radioactive antineoplastic for thyroid carcinoma; thyroid inhibitor for hyperthyroidism* [sodium iodide I 131] 1000 mCi/mL (250, 500, 1000 mCi/dose)

Hi-Cor 1.0; Hi-Cor 2.5 cream ℞ *corticosteroidal anti-inflammatory* [hydrocortisone] 1%; 2.5%

HIDA (hepatoiminodiacetic acid) [see: lidofenin]

HIDAC; HiDAC (high-dose ara-C) *chemotherapy protocol for various leukemias* [also known as: HDCA]

Hieracium pilosella *medicinal herb* [see: mouse ear]

high angelica *medicinal herb* [see: angelica]

high fructose corn syrup (HFCS) *nontherapeutic ingredient for sweetening oral liquids* [compare to: fructose]

high molecular weight dextran [see: dextran 70]

high osmolar contrast media (HOCM) *a class of older radiopaque agents that have a high osmolar concentration of iodine (the contrast agent), which corresponds to a higher incidence of adverse reactions* [also called: ionic contrast media]

High Potency B with C 300 caplets OTC *vitamin supplement* [multiple B vitamins; vitamin C] ≛•300 mg

High Potency Balanced B-50 tablets OTC *vitamin supplement* [multiple B vitamins; folic acid; biotin] ≛• 400•50 mcg

High Potency Balanced B-100 timed-release tablets OTC *vitamin supplement* [multiple B vitamins; folic acid; biotin] ≛•400•100 mcg

High Potency D-1000 softgels OTC *vitamin supplement* [cholecalciferol (vitamin D$_3$)] 1000 IU

High Potency N-Vites tablets (discontinued 2008) OTC *vitamin supplement* [multiple B vitamins; vitamin C] ≛•500 mg

High Potency Vitamins and Minerals tablets OTC *vitamin/mineral/calcium/iron supplement* [multiple vitamins & minerals; calcium (as dicalcium phosphate); iron (as ferrous fumarate); folic acid] ≛•60•18•0.4 mg

hilafilcon A USAN *hydrophilic contact lens material*

hilafilcon B USAN *hydrophilic contact lens material*

hillberry *medicinal herb* [see: wintergreen]

Hiltonol *investigational (orphan) agent for orthopoxvirus infections* [polyinosinic-polycytidilic acid]

Himalayan ginseng (Panax pseudoginseng) *medicinal herb* [see: ginseng]

hindheel *medicinal herb* [see: tansy]

hini *medicinal herb* [see: Culver root]

hioxifilcon A USAN *hydrophilic contact lens material*

Hipotest tablets (discontinued 2008) OTC *dietary supplement* [multiple vitamins & minerals; multiple food products; calcium; iron; biotin] ± • 53.5•50•0.001 mg

Hi-Po-Vites tablets (discontinued 2008) OTC *dietary supplement* [multiple vitamins & minerals; multiple food products; iron; folic acid; biotin] ±•6•0.4•1 mg

Hiprex tablets ℞ *urinary antibiotic* [methenamine hippurate] 1 g ②

Hiberix

Hirudo medicinalis *natural treatment* [see: leeches]

Histacol DM Pediatric oral drops (discontinued 2007) OTC *antitussive; antihistamine; decongestant; for children 1–18 months* [dextromethorphan hydrobromide; brompheniramine maleate; pseudoephedrine HCl] 4•1•15 mg/mL

Histacol DM Pediatric syrup (discontinued 2010) ℞ *antitussive; decongestant; antihistamine; expectorant* [dextromethorphan hydrobromide; pseudoephedrine HCl; brompheniramine maleate; guaifenesin] 5•30•2•50/5 mL

Histade sustained-release capsules (discontinued 2007) ℞ *decongestant; antihistamine* [pseudoephedrine HCl; chlorpheniramine maleate] 120•12 mg

Histamax D oral drops ℞ *decongestant; antihistamine; for children 1–24 months* [phenylephrine HCl; carbinoxamine maleate] 1.5•1.5 mg/mL

histamine dihydrochloride USAN *histamine H_2 receptor agonist; investigational (NDA filed, orphan) adjuvant to* interleukin-2 *for stage IV malignant melanoma and acute myeloid leukemia (AML)*

histamine H_1 antagonists *a class of antihistamines* [also called: H_1 blockers]

histamine H_2 antagonists *a class of gastrointestinal antisecretory agents* [also called: H_2 blockers]

histamine phosphate USP *gastric secretory stimulant; diagnostic aid for pheochromocytoma*

histantin [see: chlorcyclizine HCl]

histapyrrodine INN

Histatab D tablets ℞ *antihistamine; decongestant; anticholinergic to dry mucosal secretions* [dexchlorpheniramine maleate; pseudoephedrine HCl; methscopolamine nitrate] 3.5•45•1 mg

Histatab Plus tablets (discontinued 2007) OTC *decongestant; antihistamine* [phenylephrine HCl; chlorpheniramine maleate] 5•2 mg

Hista-Vent DA sustained-release caplets (discontinued 2008) ℞ *decongestant; antihistamine; anticholinergic to dry mucosal secretions* [phenylephrine HCl; chlorpheniramine maleate; methscopolamine nitrate] 20•8•2.5 mg

Histenol-Forte tablets (discontinued 2007) OTC *antitussive; decongestant; analgesic; antipyretic* [dextromethorphan hydrobromide; pseudoephedrine HCl; acetaminophen] 10•30•325 mg

Histex oral liquid ℞ *decongestant; antihistamine* [pseudoephedrine HCl; chlorpheniramine maleate] 30•2 mg/5 mL

Histex I/E extended-release capsules ℞ *antihistamine for allergic rhinitis* [carbinoxamine maleate] 10 mg

Histex CT film-coated timed-release tablets ℞ *antihistamine for allergic rhinitis* [carbinoxamine maleate] 8 mg

Histex HC oral liquid (discontinued 2009) ℞ *narcotic antitussive; antihistamine; decongestant* [hydrocodone bitartrate; carbinoxamine maleate; pseudoephedrine HCl] 5•2•30 mg/5 mL

Histex Pd oral liquid ℞ *antihistamine for allergic rhinitis* [carbinoxamine maleate] 4 mg/5 mL

Histex SR extended-release caplets, extended-release capsules ℞ *decongestant; antihistamine* [pseudoephedrine HCl; brompheniramine maleate] 120•10 mg

Histex SR film-coated, sustained-release tablets (discontinued 2007) ℞ *decongestant; antihistamine; analgesic; antipyretic* [phenylephrine HCl; chlorpheniramine maleate; acetaminophen] 40•8•500 mg

histidine (L-histidine) USAN, USP, INN *amino acid (essential in infants and in renal failure, nonessential otherwise); symbols: His, H*

histidine monohydrochloride NF

495-L-histidineglucosylceramidase [see: imiglucerase]

Histinex HC syrup ℞ *narcotic antitussive; antihistamine; decongestant* [hydrocodone bitartrate; chlorpheniramine maleate; phenylephrine HCl] 2.5•2•5 mg/5 mL

Histinex PV syrup (discontinued 2009) ℞ *narcotic antitussive; antihistamine; decongestant* [hydrocodone bitartrate; chlorpheniramine maleate; pseudoephedrine HCl] 2.5•2• 30 mg/5 mL

Histolyn-CYL intradermal injection (discontinued 2010) ℞ *diagnostic aid for histoplasmosis* [histoplasmin (mycelial derivative)] 1:100

histoplasmin USP *dermal histoplasmosis test; Histoplasma capsulatum cultures in mycelial or yeast lysate form* 1:100 injection (yeast lysate form)

histrelin USAN, INN *LHRH agonist; investigational (orphan) for acute intermittent porphyria, hereditary coproporphyria, and variegate porphyria*

histrelin acetate *LHRH agonist to suppress the release of endogenous gonadotropin; subcu implant for the palliative treatment of advanced prostate cancer and central precocious puberty (orphan)*

Histussin HC oral liquid (discontinued 2007) ℞ *narcotic antitussive; antihistamine; decongestant* [hydrocodone bitartrate; dexbrompheniramine maleate; phenylephrine HCl] 2.5•1•5 mg/5 mL

HIV immune globulin (HIVIG) *investigational (Phase III, orphan) immunomodulator for AIDS and maternal/fetal HIV transfer*

HIV protease inhibitors *a class of antivirals that block HIV replication*

HIV vaccine [see: AIDS vaccine]

HIV-1 LA test [see: Recombigen HIV-1 LA]

HIVAB HIV-1 EIA; HIVAB HIV-1/ HIV-2 EIA; HIVAB HIV-2 EIA reagent kit for professional use ℞ *in vitro diagnostic aid for HIV antibodies* [enzyme immunoassay (EIA)]

HIVAG-1 reagent kit for professional use ℞ *in vitro diagnostic aid for HIV antibodies* [enzyme immunoassay (EIA)]

hive vine *medicinal herb* [see: squaw vine]

HIV-IG *investigational (Phase III, orphan) immunomodulator for AIDS and maternal/fetal HIV transfer* [HIV immune globulin]

HIV-neutralizing antibodies *investigational (orphan) treatment for AIDS*

Hizentra self-injector ℞ *once-weekly immune replacement therapy for genetic disorders* [immune globulin] 20%

HLA-B7/beta2M DNA lipid complex *investigational (Phase III, orphan) for invasive and metastatic melanoma*

HMB (β-hydroxy-β-methylbutyrate) [q.v.]

HMB (homatropine methylbromide) [q.v.]

HMDP (hydroxymethylene diphosphonate) [see: oxidronic acid]

hMG (human menopausal gonadotropin) [see: menotropins]

HMG-CoA (3-hydroxy-3-methylglutaryl-coenzyme A) reductase inhibitors *a class of antihyperlipidemics that markedly reduce serum LDL* *and total cholesterol and, to a lesser extent, VLDL and triglycerides* [also called: "statins"]

HMM (hexamethylmelamine) [see: altretamine]

HN₂ (nitrogen mustard) [see: mechlorethamine HCl]

hoarhound *medicinal herb* [see: horehound]

hock heal *medicinal herb* [see: woundwort]

hog apple *medicinal herb* [see: mandrake; noni]

hogweed *medicinal herb* [see: broom; masterwort]

Hold DM lozenges OTC *antitussive* [dextromethorphan hydrobromide] 5 mg

holly (Ilex aquifolium; I. opaca; I. vomitoria) leaves and berries *medicinal herb used as a CNS stimulant and emetic; not generally regarded as safe and effective*

holly, ground *medicinal herb* [see: pipsissewa]

holly bay *medicinal herb* [see: magnolia]

holly-leaved barberry; holly mahonia *medicinal herb* [see: Oregon grape]

holmium *element (Ho)*

holy thistle; blessed cardus *medicinal herb* [see: blessed thistle]

homarylamine INN

homatropine BAN *ophthalmic anticholinergic* [also: homatropine hydrobromide] ℞ HumatroPen

homatropine hydrobromide USP *ophthalmic anticholinergic; cycloplegic; mydriatic* [also: homatropine] 5% eye drops

homatropine methylbromide USP, INN, BAN *anticholinergic*

homatropine methylbromide & hydrocodone bitartrate *anticholinergic; narcotic antitussive* 1.5•5 mg/5 mL oral

Home Access; Home Access Express test kit for home use OTC *in vitro diagnostic aid for HIV in the blood*

Home Access Hepatitis C Check test kit for home use OTC *in vitro diagnostic aid for hepatitis C in the blood*

homidium bromide INN, BAN

Hominex-1 powder OTC *formula for infants with homocystinuria or hypermethioninemia*

Hominex-2 powder OTC *enteral nutritional therapy for homocystinuria or hypermethioninemia*

homochlorcyclizine INN, BAN

homofenazine (HFZ) INN

homoharringtonine *investigational (orphan) agent for chronic myelogenous leukemia*

homomenthyl salicylate [see: homosalate]

homopipramol INN

homosalate USAN, INN *ultraviolet sunscreen*

4-homosulfanilamide [see: mafenide]

homprenorphine INN, BAN

honey *natural remedy used as an antibacterial and wound healing agent and as a gargle to promote expectoration; not generally regarded as safe and effective for infants because of possible* Clostridium botulinum *contamination*

honeybee venom *natural remedy* [see: bee venom]

honeybloom *medicinal herb* [see: dogbane]

hoodwart *medicinal herb* [see: skullcap]

hopantenic acid INN

hops (Humulus lupulus) flower *medicinal herb for aiding digestion, appetite stimulation, bronchitis, cystitis, delirium, edema, headache, hyperactivity, insomnia, intestinal cramps, menstrual disorders, nervousness, pain, excessive sexual desire, and tuberculosis*

hoquizil INN *bronchodilator* [also: hoquizil HCl]

hoquizil HCl USAN *bronchodilator* [also: hoquizil]

Hordeum vulgare *medicinal herb* [see: barley]

horehound (Marrubium vulgare) plant *medicinal herb for asthma, colds and cough, croup, inducing diaphoresis and diuresis, intestinal parasites, lung disorders, promoting expectoration, and respiratory disorders*

Horizant extended-release tablets ℞ *treatment for moderate-to-severe restless legs syndrome (RLS); investigational (NDA filed) for postherpetic neuralgia* [gabapentin enacarbil] 600 mg

horse chestnut (*Aesculus californica; A. glabra; A. hippocastanum*) nuts and leaves *medicinal herb for arthritis, colds and congestion, hemorrhoids, rheumatism, and varicose veins; not generally regarded as safe and effective for internal use as it is highly toxic*

horse-elder; horseheal *medicinal herb* [see: elecampane]

horsefoot; horsehoof *medicinal herb* [see: coltsfoot]

horsemint (*Monarda punctata*) leaves and flowering tops *medicinal herb used as a cardiac, carminative, diaphoretic, diuretic, emmenagogue, stimulant, and sudorific*

horseradish (*Armoracia lapathiofolia; A. rusticana*) root *medicinal herb for appetite stimulation, colic, cough, edema, expelling afterbirth, hay fever, poor circulation, sciatic pain, sinus disorders, and skin and internal tumors; also used as a vermifuge*

horsetail (*Equisetum arvens*) plant *medicinal herb for bladder disorders, brittle nails, glandular disorders, internal bleeding, nosebleeds, poor circulation, tuberculosis, and urinary disorders*

horseweed; fleabane (*Erigeron canadensis*) plant *medicinal herb used as an astringent, diuretic, and hemostatic*

ho-shou-wu; fo-ti (*Polygonum multiflorum*) root *medicinal herb for atherosclerosis, blood cleansing, constipation, improving liver and kidney function, insomnia, malaria, muscle aches, tuberculosis, and weak bones; also used to increase fertility, prevent aging, and promote longevity*

H.P. Acthar Gel IM or subcu injectable gel ℞ *corticosteroidal anti-inflammatory for infantile spasms (orphan); diagnostic aid for testing adrenocortical function* [corticotropin, repository] 80 U/mL

HPA-23 *investigational (orphan) treatment for AIDS*

HPMCP (hydroxypropyl methylcellulose phthalate) [q.v.]

HPMPC (3-hydroxy-2-phosphonomethoxypropyl cytosine [dihydrate]) [see: cidofovir]

H-R Lubricating vaginal jelly OTC *moisturizer/lubricant* [hydroxypropyl methylcellulose]

HspE7 *investigational (orphan) agent for recurrent respiratory papillomatosis*

5-HT (5-hydroxytryptamine) [see: serotonin]

HT (human thrombin) [see: thrombin]

HT; 3-HT (3-hydroxytyramine) [see: dopamine]

5-HTP (5-hydroxytryptophan) [see: L-5 hydroxytryptophan]

huckleberry *medicinal herb* [see: bilberry]

Humalog vials, prefilled syringe cartridges, and disposable pen injectors for subcu injection ℞ *rapid-acting insulin analogue for diabetes* [insulin lispro, human (rDNA)] 100 U/mL; 150 U/1.5 mL, 300 U/3 mL; 300 U/3 mL ⚠ hemlock

Humalog KwikPen disposable pen injectors for subcu injection ℞ *rapid-acting insulin analogue for diabetes* [insulin lispro, human (rDNA)] 100 U/mL

Humalog Mix 50/50 vials and disposable pen injectors for subcu injection ℞ *dual-acting insulin analogue for diabetes* [insulin lispro protamine; insulin lispro, human (rDNA)] 50%•50% (100 U/mL total)

Humalog Mix 50/50 KwikPen disposable pen injectors for subcu injection ℞ *dual-acting insulin analogue for diabetes* [insulin lispro protamine; insulin lispro, human (rDNA)] 50%•50% (100 U/mL total)

Humalog Mix 75/25 vials and disposable pen injectors for subcu injection ℞ *dual-acting insulin analogue for diabetes* [insulin lispro protamine;

insulin lispro, human (rDNA)]
75%•25% (100 U/mL total)

Humalog Mix 75/25 KwikPen disposable pen injectors for subcu injection ℞ *dual-acting insulin analogue for diabetes* [insulin lispro protamine; insulin lispro, human (rDNA)] 75%•25% (100 U/mL total)

human acid alpha-glucosidase [see: alglucosidase alfa]

Human Albumin Grifols IV infusion ℞ *blood volume expander for shock, burns, and hypoproteinemia* [human albumin] 25%

human amniotic fluid-derived surfactant [see: surfactant, human amniotic fluid derived]

human anti–transforming growth factor [see: anti–transforming growth factor; monoclonal antibody to transforming growth factor]

human B-type natriuretic peptide (hBNP) [see: nesiritide; nesiritide citrate]

human chorionic gonadotropin (hCG) [see: gonadotropin, chorionic]

human complement receptor [see: complement receptor type I, soluble recombinant human]

human diploid cell vaccine (HDCV) [see: rabies vaccine]

human epidermal growth factor receptor (HER) inhibitors *a class of antineoplastics, predominantly monoclonal antibodies, that suppress the growth of breast, colorectal, head, and neck cancers; includes HER1 (q.v.), HER2 (q.v.), HER3, and HER4* [also known as: epidermal growth factor receptor (EGFR) inhibitors]

human follicle-stimulating hormone (hFSH) [now: menotropins]

human growth hormone (hGH) JAN *growth hormone* [also: somatropin]

human growth hormone, recombinant (rhGH) [see: somatropin]

human growth hormone releasing factor (hGH-RF) [see: growth hormone-releasing factor (GH-RF)]

human immunodeficiency virus (HIV) immune globulin (HIVIG) [see: HIV immune globulin]

human insulin [see: insulin, human; insulin aspart; insulin aspart protamine]

human menopausal gonadotropin (hMG) [see: menotropins]

human monoclonal antibodies *antibodies cloned from a single human cell* [see: monoclonal antibodies]

human papillomavirus (HPV), recombinant *vaccine for genital warts (condylomata acuminata), cervical cancer, and precancerous or dysplastic vaginal, vulvar, or cervical intraepithelial neoplasia caused by HPV infections*

human papillomavirus (HPV) recombinant vaccine, bivalent (HPV types 16 and 18) *vaccine for cervical cancer and precancerous lesions in women 10–25 years*

human papillomavirus (HPV) recombinant vaccine, quadrivalent (HPV types 6, 11, 16, and 18) *vaccine for genital warts (condylomata acuminata) and anal cancer in men and women 9–26 years; cervical cancer and precancerous or dysplastic vaginal, vulvar, or cervical intraepithelial neoplasia in women 9–26 years*

human serum albumin diethylenetriaminepentaacetic acid (DTPA) technetium (⁹⁹ᵐTc) JAN *radioactive agent* [also: technetium Tc 99m pentetate]

human superoxide dismutase (SOD) [see: superoxide dismutase, human]

Human Surf *investigational (orphan) agent for the prevention and treatment of respiratory distress syndrome (RDS) in premature infants* [surfactant, human amniotic fluid derived]

human T-cell inhibitor [see: muromonab-CD3]

human T-cell lymphotrophic virus type III (HTLV-III) [now: human immunodeficiency virus (HIV)]

Human T-Lymphotropic Virus Type I EIA reagent kit for profes-

sional use ℞ *in vitro diagnostic aid for
HTLV I antibody in serum or plasma*
[enzyme immunoassay (EIA)]

humanized monoclonal antibodies
*antibodies cloned from a single murine
(mouse/rat) cell, then genetically altered
to prevent rejection by the human
immune system* [see: monoclonal
antibodies]

HumaPen Memoir (trademarked
delivery device) ℞ *digital insulin self-
injector with 16-dose memory, for use
with* **Humalog** (insulin lispro)

Humate-P powder for IV injection ℞
*antihemophilic for von Willebrand dis-
ease (orphan)* [antihemophilic factor
(AHF); von Willebrand factor
(VWF)] 250•600, 500•1200, 1000•
2400 U/vial

Humatin capsules ℞ *aminoglycoside
antibiotic; amebicide for acute and
chronic intestinal amebiasis* [paromo-
mycin sulfate] 250 mg ② Hemotene

Humatrix Microclysmic Gel OTC
*bacteriostatic humectant and emollient
for skin irritation due to radiation or
laser therapy*

Humatrope powder for subcu or IM
injection; prefilled cartridges for
HumatroPen (self-injection device)
℞ *growth hormone for adults or children with congenital or endogenous
growth hormone deficiency, children
with Turner syndrome or renal-induced
growth failure, or AIDS-wasting syndrome (orphan)* [somatropin] 5 mg
(15 IU) per vial; 6, 12, 24 mg (18,
36, 72 IU) per cartridge

HumatroPen (trademarked delivery
device) *subcu self-injector for* **Humatrope** ② homatropine

HuMax-CD4 *investigational (orphan)
for mycosis fungoides* [monoclonal
antibody to CD4, human]

Humenza injection *investigational
(NDA filed) active immunizing agent
for H1N1 influenza A (swine flu; Mexican pandemic flu)* [influenza virus vaccine, H1N1 (adjuvanted)] 3.8 mcg

Humibid extended-release tablets OTC
expectorant [guaifenesin] 1200 mg ②
Hemopad

Humibid CS tablets (discontinued
2007) OTC *antitussive; expectorant*
[dextromethorphan hydrobromide;
guaifenesin] 20•400 mg

Humibid DM extended-release capsules (discontinued 2007) ℞ *antitussive; expectorant* [dextromethorphan
hydrobromide; guaifenesin; potassium
guaiacolsulfonate] 50•400•200 mg

Humibid E tablets OTC *expectorant*
[guaifenesin] 400 mg ② Hemopad

Humira subcu injection in prefilled
syringes ℞ *DMARD for moderate to
severe rheumatoid arthritis (RA), juvenile rheumatoid arthritis (JRA; orphan),
psoriatic arthritis, and ankylosing spondylitis; immunostimulant for Crohn disease* [adalimumab] 20, 40 mg

HuMist Moisturizing nasal mist OTC
nasal moisturizer [sodium chloride
(saline solution)] 0.65%

Humulin 50/50 subcu injection (discontinued 2009) OTC *antidiabetic*
[isophane human insulin (rDNA);
human insulin (rDNA)] 100 U/mL

Humulin 70/30 vials and disposable
pen injectors for subcu injection OTC
antidiabetic [isophane human insulin
(rDNA); human insulin (rDNA)]
100 U/mL; 300 U/3 mL

Humulin N vials and disposable pen
injectors for subcu injection OTC
antidiabetic [isophane human insulin
(rDNA)] 100 U/mL; 300 U/3 mL

Humulin R vials and disposable pen
injectors for subcu injection OTC
antidiabetic [human insulin (rDNA)]
100 U/mL

**Humulin R Regular U-500 (concen-
trated)** subcu injection ℞ *antidiabetic*
[insulin, human (rDNA)] 500 U/mL

Humulus lupulus medicinal herb [see:
hops]

huperzine A *natural extract from Chinese club moss that enhances memory,
focus, and concentration; prevents the*

breakdown of the neurotransmitter acetylcholine

hurr-burr medicinal herb [see: burdock]

Hurricaine spray liquid, oral gel, dental swab OTC mucous membrane anesthetic [benzocaine] 20%

Hurricaine topical liquid (discontinued 2007) OTC mucous membrane anesthetic [benzocaine] 20%

HXM (hexamethylmelamine) [see: altretamine]

Hyalex tablets OTC vitamin/mineral supplement [multiple vitamins and minerals] ℞ heliox

Hyalgan intra-articular injection in vials and prefilled syringes ℞ viscoelastic lubricant and "shock absorber" for osteoarthritis and temporomandibular joint syndrome [hyaluronate sodium] 20 mg/2 mL

hyalosidase INN, BAN

hyaluronan viscoelastic lubricant and "shock absorber" for osteoarthritis of the knee

hyaluronate sodium USAN, JAN ophthalmic surgical aid; treatment for osteoarthritis and TMJ syndrome; topical treatment for dermal ulcers, wounds, and burns; veterinary synovitis agent [also: hyaluronic acid] 0.1%, 0.2% topical

hyaluronic acid BAN ophthalmic surgical aid; treatment for osteoarthritis and TMJ syndrome; dermal filler for deep wrinkles and facial folds; veterinary synovitis agent; investigational (orphan) for emphysema due to alpha$_1$-antitrypsin (AAT) deficiency [also: hyaluronate sodium]

hyaluronidase USP, INN, BAN adjuvant to increase the absorption and dispersion of injected drugs, hypodermoclysis, and subcutaneous urography; also used for diabetic retinopathy and to clear vitreous hemorrhage

hyaluronoglucosaminidase [see: hyalosidase]

hyamate [see: buramate]

Hyate:C (Porcine) powder for IV injection (discontinued 2008) ℞ systemic hemostatic; antihemophilic for the prevention and control of bleeding in classical hemophilia (hemophilia A) and von Willebrand disease (orphan) in patients with antibodies to human factor VIII [antihemophilic factor concentrate, porcine] (actual number of AHF units is indicated on the vial)

hybenzate USAN combining name for radicals or groups [also: hibenzate]

Hybri-CEAker radiodiagnostic monoclonal antibody to carcinoembryonic antigen (CEA); investigational (orphan) for the detection of colorectal carcinoma [indium In 111 altumomab pentetate]

Hybrid Capture II Chlamydia Test reagent kit for professional use ℞ in vitro diagnostic aid for Chlamydia trachomatis

Hycamtin capsules ℞ antineoplastic for small cell lung cancer (SCLC) [topotecan HCl] 0.25, 1 mg

Hycamtin powder for IV injection ℞ antineoplastic for ovarian, cervical, and small cell lung cancers; also used for non–small cell lung cancer [topotecan HCl] 4 mg/dose

hycanthone USAN, INN antischistosomal

hycanthone mesylate antischistosomal

Hycet oral liquid ℞ narcotic analgesic; antipyretic [hydrocodone bitartrate; acetaminophen; alcohol 7%] 2.5• 108 mg/5 mL

hyclate INN combining name for radicals or groups

Hycodan tablets, syrup (discontinued 2009) ℞ narcotic antitussive; anticholinergic [hydrocodone bitartrate; homatropine methylbromide] 5•1.5 mg; 5•1.5 mg/5 mL

Hycort cream, ointment ℞ corticosteroidal anti-inflammatory [hydrocortisone] 1%

Hycosin Expectorant syrup (discontinued 2007) ℞ narcotic antitussive; expectorant [hydrocodone bitartrate; guaifenesin; alcohol 10%] 5•100 mg/5 mL

Hycotuss Expectorant syrup (discontinued 2011) R̽ *narcotic antitussive; expectorant* [hydrocodone bitartrate; guaifenesin; alcohol 10%] 5•100 mg/5 mL

hydantoins *a class of anticonvulsants*

Hydase solution for injection (discontinued 2009) R̽ *adjuvant to increase the absorption and dispersion of injected drugs, hypodermoclysis, and subcutaneous urography; also used for diabetic retinopathy* [hyaluronidase (bovine)] 150 U/mL

Hydeltrasol IV, IM injection (discontinued 2008) R̽ *corticosteroid; antiinflammatory* [prednisolone sodium phosphate] 20 mg/mL

Hydergine sublingual tablets, tablets, oral liquid R̽ *cognition adjuvant for age-related mental capacity decline* [ergoloid mesylates] 0.5, 1 mg; 1 mg; 1 mg/mL

Hydex PD oral liquid (discontinued 2009) R̽ *narcotic antitussive; antihistamine; decongestant* [hydrocodone bitartrate; dexchlorpheniramine maleate; phenylephrine HCl] 4•2•5 mg/5 mL

hydracarbazine INN

hydragogues *a class of purgatives that produce abundant watery discharge from the bowels*

hydralazine INN, BAN *antihypertensive; peripheral vasodilator* [also: hydralazine HCl]

hydralazine HCl USP, JAN *antihypertensive; peripheral vasodilator; investigational (orphan) for severe intrapartum hypertension due to eclampsia or preeclampsia of pregnancy* [also: hydralazine] 10, 25, 50, 100 mg oral; 20 mg/mL injection

hydralazine HCl & hydrochlorothiazide *combination peripheral vasodilator and diuretic for hypertension* 25•25, 50•50 mg oral

hydralazine polistirex USAN *antihypertensive*

Hydramine syrup, elixir (discontinued 2007) R̽ *antihistamine; sleep aid; antitussive* [diphenhydramine HCl] 12.5 mg/5 mL

hydrangea *(Hydrangea arborescens)* leaves and root *medicinal herb for arthritis, bladder infections, gallstones, gonorrhea, gout, kidney stones, rheumatism, and urinary disorders*

Hydrap-ES tablets (discontinued 2007) R̽ *antihypertensive; vasodilator; diuretic* [hydrochlorothiazide; reserpine; hydralazine HCl] 15•0.1•25 mg

hydrargaphen INN, BAN

hydrastine USP

hydrastine HCl USP

hydrastinine HCl NF

Hydrastis canadensis *medicinal herb* [see: goldenseal]

hydrazinecarboximidamide monohydrochloride [see: pimagedine HCl]

hydrazinoxane [see: domoxin]

Hydrea capsules R̽ *antineoplastic for melanoma, squamous cell carcinoma, myelocytic leukemia, and ovarian cancer; also for thrombocythemia and as adjunctive therapy for HIV infections* [hydroxyurea] 500 mg

Hydrisalic gel R̽ *keratolytic* [salicylic acid] 6%

Hydrisea lotion OTC *moisturizer; emollient* [Dead Sea salts]

Hydrisinol cream, lotion OTC *moisturizer; emollient*

Hydro 35; Hydro 40 aerosol foam R̽ *moisturizer; emollient; keratolytic* [urea] 35%; 40%

Hydro Cobex IM injection (discontinued 2008) R̽ *hematinic; vitamin B_{12} supplement* [hydroxocobalamin] 1000 mcg/mL

Hydro GP oral liquid R̽ *narcotic antitussive; decongestant; expectorant* [hydrocodone bitartrate; phenylephrine HCl; guaifenesin] 2.5•7.5•50 mg/5 mL

hydrobentizide INN

hydrobutamine [see: butidrine]

Hydrocare Cleaning and Disinfecting solution OTC *chemical disinfecting* solution for soft contact lenses [thimerosal] 0.002%

Hydrocare Preserved Saline solution OTC *rinsing/storage solution for soft contact lenses* [sodium chloride (preserved saline solution)]

Hydrocerin cream, lotion OTC *nontherapeutic base for compounding various dermatological preparations*

Hydrocet capsules (discontinued 2009) ℞ *narcotic analgesic; antipyretic* [hydrocodone bitartrate; acetaminophen] 5•500 mg

hydrochloric acid NF *acidifying agent*

hydrochloric acid, diluted NF *acidifying agent*

hydrochlorothiazide (HCT; HCTZ) USP, INN, BAN *antihypertensive; diuretic* 12.5, 25, 50, 100 mg oral

hydrochlorothiazide & benazepril HCl *combination diuretic and angiotensin-converting enzyme (ACE) inhibitor for hypertension* 6.25•5, 12.5•10, 12.5•20, 25•20 mg oral

hydrochlorothiazide & bisoprolol fumarate *combination diuretic and beta-blocker for hypertension* 6.25•2.5, 6.25•5, 6.25•10 mg oral

hydrochlorothiazide & captopril *combination diuretic and angiotensin-converting enzyme (ACE) inhibitor for hypertension* 15•25, 25•25, 15•50, 25•50 mg oral

hydrochlorothiazide & enalapril maleate *combination diuretic and angiotensin-converting enzyme (ACE) inhibitor for hypertension* 12.5•5, 25• 10 mg oral

hydrochlorothiazide & fosinopril sodium *combination diuretic and angiotensin-converting enzyme (ACE) inhibitor for hypertension* 12.5•10, 12.5•20 mg

hydrochlorothiazide & hydralazine HCl *combination diuretic and peripheral vasodilator for hypertension* 25•25, 50•50 mg oral

hydrochlorothiazide & lisinopril *combination diuretic and angiotensin-converting enzyme (ACE) inhibitor for* hypertension 12.5•10, 12.5•20, 25• 20 mg oral

hydrochlorothiazide & losartan potassium *combination diuretic and angiotensin receptor blocker (ARB) for hypertension* 12.5•50, 12.5•100, 25• 100 mg

hydrochlorothiazide & methyldopa *combination diuretic and central antiadrenergic for hypertension* 15•250, 25•250, 30•500, 50•500 mg oral

hydrochlorothiazide & metoprolol tartrate *combination diuretic and beta-blocker for hypertension* 25•50, 25•100, 50•100 mg oral

hydrochlorothiazide & moexipril HCl *combination diuretic and angiotensin-converting enzyme (ACE) inhibitor for hypertension* 12.5•7.5, 12.5•15, 25•15 mg oral

hydrochlorothiazide & propranolol HCl *combination diuretic and beta-blocker for hypertension* 25•40, 25•80 mg oral

hydrochlorothiazide & quinapril HCl *combination diuretic and angiotensin-converting enzyme (ACE) inhibitor for hypertension* 12.5•10, 12.5•20, 25•20 mg oral

hydrochlorothiazide & triamterene *antihypertensive; potassium-sparing diuretic* 25•37.5 mg oral

hydrocholeretics *a class of gastrointestinal drugs that exert laxative effects and increase volume and water content of bile actions*

Hydrocil Instant powder OTC *bulk laxative* [psyllium hydrophilic mucilloid] 3.5 g/scoop

hydrocodone INN, BAN *antitussive* [also: hydrocodone bitartrate]

hydrocodone bitartrate USAN, USP *narcotic antitussive* [also: hydrocodone]

hydrocodone bitartrate & acetaminophen *narcotic antitussive; analgesic* 2.5•500, 5•325, 5•500, 7.5• 325, 7.5•650, 7.5•750, 10•325, 10• 500, 10•650, 10•750 mg oral; 7.5• 500, 10•325 mg/15 mL oral

hydrocodone bitartrate & guaifenesin *narcotic antitussive; expectorant* 5•100 mg/5 mL oral

hydrocodone bitartrate & homatropine methylbromide *narcotic antitussive; anticholinergic* 5•1.5 mg/5 mL oral

hydrocodone bitartrate & ibuprofen *narcotic antitussive; analgesic* 5•200, 7.5•200, 10•200 mg oral

hydrocodone bitartrate & pseudoephedrine HCl & brompheniramine maleate *narcotic antitussive; decongestant; antihistamine* 2.5•30•3 mg/5 mL oral

hydrocodone bitartrate & pseudoephedrine HCl & carbinoxamine maleate *narcotic antitussive; decongestant; antihistamine* 5•30•2 mg/5 mL oral

Hydrocodone CP syrup (discontinued 2007) ℞ *narcotic antitussive; antihistamine; decongestant* [hydrocodone bitartrate; chlorpheniramine maleate; phenylephrine HCl] 2.5•2•5 mg/5 mL

Hydrocodone GF syrup (discontinued 2007) ℞ *narcotic antitussive; expectorant* [hydrocodone bitartrate; guaifenesin] 5•100 mg/5 mL

Hydrocodone HD oral liquid (discontinued 2007) ℞ *narcotic antitussive; antihistamine; decongestant* [hydrocodone bitartrate; chlorpheniramine maleate; phenylephrine HCl] 3.33•4•10 mg/10 mL

hydrocodone polistirex USAN *narcotic antitussive*

hydrocodone polistirex & chlorpheniramine polistirex *narcotic antitussive; antihistamine* 10•8 mg/5 mL oral

hydrocodone tannate *narcotic antitussive*

Hydrocof-HC oral liquid (discontinued 2007) ℞ *narcotic antitussive; antihistamine; decongestant* [hydrocodone bitartrate; chlorpheniramine maleate; pseudoephedrine HCl] 3•2•15 mg/5 mL

Hydrocol adhesive dressings OTC *occlusive wound dressing* [hydrocolloid gel]

hydrocolloid gel *dressings for wet wounds*

Hydrocort cream ℞ *corticosteroidal anti-inflammatory* [hydrocortisone] 2.5%

hydrocortamate INN

hydrocortamate HCl [see: hydrocortamate]

hydrocortisone (HC) USP, INN, BAN *corticosteroid; anti-inflammatory* 5, 10, 20 mg oral; 0.5%, 1%, 2.5% topical

hydrocortisone aceponate INN *corticosteroid; anti-inflammatory*

hydrocortisone acetate (HCA) USP, BAN *corticosteroid; anti-inflammatory* 1%, 2% topical; 25 mg suppositories; 25, 50 mg/mL injection

hydrocortisone acetate & lidocaine HCl *corticosteroidal anti-inflammatory; local anesthetic* 3%•0.5%, 2.8%•0.55%, 2.5%•3% topical

hydrocortisone acetate & pramoxine HCl *corticosteroidal anti-inflammatory; local anesthetic* 2.5%•1% topical

hydrocortisone & acetic acid *corticosteroid; anti-inflammatory; acidifying agent* 1%•2% otic solution

hydrocortisone & acyclovir *corticosteroidal anti-inflammatory; antiviral for herpes simplex* 1%•5% topical

hydrocortisone buteprate USAN [now: hydrocortisone probutate]

hydrocortisone butyrate BAN *topical corticosteroidal anti-inflammatory* [also: hydrocortisone probutate] 0.1% topical

hydrocortisone cyclopentylpropionate *corticosteroid; anti-inflammatory* [see: hydrocortisone cypionate]

hydrocortisone cypionate USP *corticosteroid; anti-inflammatory*

hydrocortisone hemisuccinate USP *corticosteroid; anti-inflammatory*

hydrocortisone & iodoquinol *corticosteroidal anti-inflammatory; amebicide; antimicrobial* 1%•1% topical

hydrocortisone & neomycin sulfate & polymyxin B sulfate *topical oph-*

thalmic/otic corticosteroidal anti-inflammatory and antibiotic 1%•0.35%• 10 000 U/mL eye drops; 1%•10 000 U/mL•5 mg/mL ear drops

hydrocortisone probutate USAN, USP *topical corticosteroidal anti-inflammatory* [previously known as: hydrocortisone buteprate]

hydrocortisone sodium phosphate USP, BAN *corticosteroid; anti-inflammatory*

hydrocortisone sodium succinate USP, BAN *corticosteroid; anti-inflammatory*

hydrocortisone valerate USAN, USP *topical corticosteroidal anti-inflammatory 0.2% topical*

Hydrocortisone with Aloe ointment OTC *corticosteroidal anti-inflammatory; emollient* [hydrocortisone; aloe] 1%• <u>?</u>

Hydrocortone tablets ℞ *corticosteroid; anti-inflammatory* [hydrocortisone] 10, 20 mg

Hydrocortone Acetate intralesional, intra-articular, or soft tissue injection ℞ *corticosteroid; anti-inflammatory* [hydrocortisone acetate] 25, 50 mg/mL

Hydrocortone Phosphate IV, subcu, or IM injection (discontinued 2009) ℞ *corticosteroid; anti-inflammatory* [hydrocortisone sodium phosphate] 50 mg/mL

Hydrocotyle asiatica medicinal herb [see: gotu kola]

Hydrocream Base OTC *nontherapeutic base for compounding various dermatological preparations*

Hydro-Crysti 12 IM injection (discontinued 2008) ℞ *hematinic; vitamin B$_{12}$ supplement* [hydroxocobalamin] 1000 mcg/mL

HydroDIURIL tablets ℞ *antihypertensive; diuretic* [hydrochlorothiazide] 25 mg

Hydro-DP syrup (discontinued 2007) ℞ *narcotic antitussive; antihistamine; sleep aid; decongestant* [hydrocodone bitartrate; diphenhydramine HCl;

phenylephrine HCl] 2•12.5•7.5 mg/ 5 mL

HydroFed syrup ℞ *narcotic antitussive; decongestant; expectorant* [hydrocodone bitartrate; phenylephrine HCl; guaifenesin] 2.5•6•150 mg/5 mL

hydrofilcon A USAN *hydrophilic contact lens material*

hydroflumethiazide USP, INN, BAN *antihypertensive; diuretic*

hydrofluoric acid *dental caries preventative*

hydrofluoroalkane (HFA) *propellant used in CFC-free aerosol delivery systems* [usually HFA-134a]

hydrogen *element (H)*

hydrogen peroxide USP *topical anti-infective*

hydrogen tetrabromoaurate [see: bromauric acid]

hydrogenated ergot alkaloids [now: ergoloid mesylates]

hydrogenated vegetable oil [see: vegetable oil, hydrogenated]

Hydrogesic capsules ℞ *narcotic analgesic; antipyretic* [hydrocodone bitartrate; acetaminophen] 5•500 mg

Hydro-Iodoquinol 2-1 gel ℞ *corticosteroidal anti-inflammatory; antimicrobial* [hydrocortisone; iodoquinol; aloe polysaccharides] 2%•1%•1%

hydromadinone INN

Hydromet syrup ℞ *narcotic antitussive; anticholinergic* [hydrocodone bitartrate; homatropine methylbromide] 5•1.5 mg/5 mL

Hydromide syrup (discontinued 2007) ℞ *narcotic antitussive; anticholinergic* [hydrocodone bitartrate; homatropine methylbromide] 5•1.5 mg/5 mL

hydromorphinol INN, BAN

hydromorphone INN, BAN *narcotic analgesic; often abused as a street drug* [also: hydromorphone HCl]

hydromorphone HCl USP *narcotic analgesic; often abused as a street drug* [also: hydromorphone] 2, 4, 8 mg oral; 1 mg/mL oral; 3 mg rectal; 1, 2, 4, 10 mg/mL injection

hydromorphone sulfate

Hydron CP oral liquid (discontinued 2009) ℞ *narcotic antitussive; antihistamine; decongestant* [hydrocodone bitartrate; chlorpheniramine maleate; phenylephrine HCl] 5•2•10 mg/5 mL

Hydron EX; Hydron KGS oral liquid (discontinued 2011) ℞ *narcotic antitussive; expectorant* [hydrocodone bitartrate; potassium guaiacolsulfonate] 2.5•120 mg/5 mL; 5•300 mg/5 mL

Hydron PSC oral liquid (discontinued 2009) ℞ *narcotic antitussive; antihistamine; decongestant* [hydrocodone bitartrate; chlorpheniramine maleate; pseudoephedrine HCl] 5•2•30 mg/5 mL

Hydropane syrup (discontinued 2007) ℞ *narcotic antitussive; anticholinergic* [hydrocodone bitartrate; homatropine methylbromide] 5•1.5 mg/5 mL

Hydro-Par tablets ℞ *antihypertensive; diuretic* [hydrochlorothiazide] 25, 50 mg

Hydro-PC oral liquid (discontinued 2007) ℞ *narcotic antitussive; antihistamine; decongestant* [hydrocodone bitartrate; chlorpheniramine maleate; phenylephrine HCl] 2•2•5 mg/5 mL

Hydro-PC II oral liquid (discontinued 2009) ℞ *narcotic antitussive; antihistamine; decongestant* [hydrocodone bitartrate; chlorpheniramine maleate; phenylephrine HCl] 2•2•7.5 mg/5 mL

Hydropel ointment OTC *skin protectant* [silicone; hydrophobic starch derivative] 30%•10%

Hydrophed tablets (discontinued 2007) ℞ *antiasthmatic; bronchodilator; decongestant; antihistamine* [theophylline; ephedrine sulfate; hydroxyzine HCl] 130•25•10 mg

Hydrophilic ointment OTC *nontherapeutic base for compounding various dermatological preparations*

hydrophilic ointment [see: ointment, hydrophilic]

hydrophilic petrolatum [see: petrolatum, hydrophilic]

Hydropres-50 tablets (discontinued 2007) ℞ *antihypertensive; diuretic* [hydrochlorothiazide; reserpine] 50•0.125 mg

hydroquinone USP *hyperpigmentation bleaching agent* 3%, 4% topical

hydroquinone methyl ether [see: mequinol]

Hydro-Serp tablets (discontinued 2007) ℞ *antihypertensive; diuretic* [hydrochlorothiazide; reserpine] 50•0.125 mg

Hydroserpine #1; Hydroserpine #2 tablets (discontinued 2007) ℞ *antihypertensive; diuretic* [hydrochlorothiazide; reserpine] 25•0.125 mg; 50•0.125 mg

HydroSkin cream, lotion OTC *corticosteroidal anti-inflammatory* [hydrocortisone] 1%

HydroSkin ointment (discontinued 2007) OTC *corticosteroidal anti-inflammatory* [hydrocortisone] 1%

hydrotalcite INN, BAN

Hydro-Tussin CBX syrup (discontinued 2008) ℞ *decongestant; antihistamine* [pseudoephedrine HCl; carbinoxamine maleate] 25•2 mg/5 mL

Hydro-Tussin DM oral liquid (discontinued 2008) ℞ *antitussive; expectorant* [dextromethorphan hydrobromide; guaifenesin] 20•200 mg/5 mL

Hydro-Tussin HC syrup (discontinued 2009) ℞ *narcotic antitussive; antihistamine; decongestant* [hydrocodone bitartrate; chlorpheniramine maleate; pseudoephedrine HCl] 3•2•15 mg/5 mL

Hydro-Tussin HD oral liquid (discontinued 2008) ℞ *narcotic antitussive; decongestant; expectorant* [hydrocodone bitartrate; pseudoephedrine HCl; guaifenesin] 2.5•30•100 mg/5 mL

Hydro-Tussin HG syrup (discontinued 2011) ℞ *narcotic antitussive; expectorant* [hydrocodone bitartrate; guaifenesin] 3.5•100 mg/5 mL

Hydro-Tussin XP syrup ℞ *narcotic antitussive; decongestant; expectorant* [hydrocodone bitartrate; pseudoephedrine HCl; guaifenesin] 3•15•100 mg/5 mL

hydroxamethocaine BAN [also: hydroxytetracaine]

hydroxidione sodium succinate [see: hydroxydione sodium succinate]

hydroxindasate INN

hydroxindasol INN

hydroxizine chloride [see: hydroxyzine HCl]

hydroxocobalamin USAN, USP, INN, BAN, JAN *vitamin B₁₂; hematopoietic; antidote to acute cyanide poisoning (orphan)* [also: hydroxocobalamin acetate] 1 mg/mL injection

hydroxocobalamin acetate JAN *vitamin B₁₂; hematopoietic* [also: hydroxocobalamin]

hydroxocobalamin & sodium thiosulfate *investigational (orphan) for severe acute cyanide poisoning*

hydroxocobemine [see: hydroxocobalamin]

3-hydroxy-2-phosphonomethoxypropyl cytosine (HPMPC) dihydrate [see: cidofovir]

N-hydroxyacetamide [see: acetohydroxamic acid]

4′-hydroxyacetanilide [see: acetaminophen]

4′-hydroxyacetanilide salicylate [see: acetaminosalol]

hydroxyamfetamine INN *ophthalmic adrenergic; mydriatic* [also: hydroxyamphetamine hydrobromide; hydroxyamphetamine]

hydroxyamphetamine BAN *ophthalmic adrenergic; mydriatic* [also: hydroxyamphetamine hydrobromide; hydroxyamfetamine]

hydroxyamphetamine hydrobromide USP *ophthalmic adrenergic/vasoconstrictor; mydriatic* [also: hydroxyamfetamine; hydroxyamphetamine]

4-hydroxyanisole (4HA); *p*-**hydroxyanisole** [see: mequinol]

hydroxyapatite BAN *prosthetic aid* [also: durapatite; calcium phosphate, tribasic]

2′-hydroxybenzamide [see: salicylamide]

2′-hydroxybenzoic acid [see: salicylic acid]

o-**hydroxybenzyl alcohol** [see: salicyl alcohol]

hydroxybutanedioic acid [see: malic acid]

4-hydroxybutanoic acid [see: gamma hydroxybutyrate (GHB)]

4-hydroxybutanoic acid, sodium salt [see: sodium oxybate]

hydroxybutyrate sodium, gamma [see: sodium oxybate]

hydroxycarbamide INN *antineoplastic* [also: hydroxyurea]

hydroxychloroquine INN, BAN *antimalarial; lupus erythematosus suppressant* [also: hydroxychloroquine sulfate]

hydroxychloroquine sulfate USP *antimalarial; antirheumatic; lupus erythematosus suppressant* (base=77.5%) [also: hydroxychloroquine] 200 mg oral

25-hydroxycholecalciferol [see: calcifediol]

hydroxycincophene [see: oxycinchophen]

hydroxydaunomycin [see: doxorubicin]

14-hydroxydihydromorphine [see: hydromorphinol]

hydroxydione sodium succinate INN, BAN

1α-hydroxyergocalciferol [see: doxercalciferol]

hydroxyethyl cellulose NF *suspending and viscosity-increasing agent; ophthalmic aid*

2-hydroxyethyl methacrylate (HEMA) *contact lens material*

hydroxyethyl starch (HES) [see: hetastarch]

hydroxyethylstarch JAN *plasma volume extender* [also: hetastarch]

hydroxyhexamide

3-hydroxyisovalerate; β-hydroxyiso-valerate [see: β-hydroxy-β-methyl-butyrate (HMB)]

hydroxylapatite [see: durapatite; calcium phosphate, tribasic]

hydroxymagnesium aluminate [see: magaldrate]

hydroxymesterone [see: medrysone]

6-hydroxymethylacylfulvene *investigational (orphan) for advanced or metastatic pancreatic cancer*

β-hydroxy-β-methylbutyrate (HMB) *an endogenous metabolite of the amino acid L-leucine; a natural supplement taken to prevent exercise-induced muscle breakdown (proteolysis), resulting in larger muscle gains from resistance training; may have immunomodulatory effects*

hydroxymethylene diphosphonate (HMDP) [see: oxidronic acid]

hydroxymethylgramicidin [see: methocidin]

N-hydroxynaphthalimide diethyl phosphate [see: naftalofos]

hydroxypethidine INN, BAN

hydroxyphenamate USAN *minor tranquilizer* [also: oxyfenamate]

N-4-hydroxyphenylretinamide [see: fenretinide]

hydroxyprocaine INN, BAN

hydroxyprogesterone INN, BAN *naturally occurring progestin for amenorrhea, metrorrhagia, and dysfunctional uterine bleeding*

hydroxyprogesterone caproate USP, INN, JAN *synthetic progestin to prevent preterm birth in women with a history of spontaneous preterm delivery* [also: 17 alpha-hydroxyprogesterone caproate]

2-hydroxypropanoic acid, calcium salt, hydrate [see: calcium lactate]

hydroxypropyl cellulose NF *topical protectant; emulsifying and coating agent* [also: hydroxypropylcellulose]

hydroxypropyl methylcellulose USP *suspending and viscosity-increasing agent; ophthalmic moisturizer and surgical aid; vaginal moisturizer/lubricant* [also: hypromellose; hydroxypropylmethylcellulose]

hydroxypropyl methylcellulose 1828 USP

hydroxypropyl methylcellulose phthalate (HPMCP) NF *tablet-coating agent* [also: hydroxypropylmethylcellulose phthalate]

hydroxypropyl methylcellulose phthalate 200731 NF *tablet-coating agent*

hydroxypropyl methylcellulose phthalate 220824 NF *tablet-coating agent*

hydroxypropylcellulose JAN *topical protectant; emulsifying and coating agent* [also: hydroxypropyl cellulose]

hydroxypropylmethylcellulose JAN *suspending and viscosity-increasing agent; ophthalmic surgical aid* [also: hydroxypropyl methylcellulose; hypromellose]

hydroxypropylmethylcellulose phthalate JAN *tablet-coating agent* [also: hydroxypropyl methylcellulose phthalate]

hydroxypyridine tartrate INN

hydroxyquinoline *topical antiseptic and protectant*

4'-hydroxysalicylanilide [see: osalmid]

hydroxystearin sulfate NF

hydroxystenozole INN

hydroxystilbamidine INN, BAN *antileishmanial* [also: hydroxystilbamidine isethionate]

hydroxystilbamidine isethionate USP *antileishmanial* [also: hydroxystilbamidine]

hydroxysuccinic acid [see: malic acid]

hydroxytetracaine INN [also: hydroxamethocaine]

hydroxytoluic acid INN, BAN

5-hydroxytryptamine₁ (5-HT₁) [see: serotonin]

5-hydroxytryptamine₃ (5-HT₃) receptor antagonists *a class of antinauseant and antiemetic agents used primarily after emetogenic cancer chemotherapy*

5-hydroxytryptophan (5-HTP) [see: L-5 hydroxytryptophan]

3-hydroxytyramine (HT; 3-HT) [see: dopamine]

hydroxyurea USAN, USP, BAN *antimetabolite antineoplastic for melanoma, squamous cell carcinoma, myelocytic leukemia, and ovarian cancer; treatment for sickle cell anemia (orphan); also for thrombocythemia and as adjunctive therapy for HIV infections* [also: hydroxycarbamide] 500 mg oral

1α-hydroxyvitamin D₂ [see: doxercalciferol]

hydroxyzine INN, BAN *anxiolytic; minor tranquilizer; antiemetic; piperazine antihistamine; antipruritic* [also: hydroxyzine HCl]

hydroxyzine HCl USP *anxiolytic; minor tranquilizer; antiemetic; piperazine antihistamine; antipruritic* [also: hydroxyzine] 10, 25, 50 mg oral; 10 mg/5 mL oral; 25, 50 mg/mL injection

hydroxyzine pamoate USP *anxiolytic; minor tranquilizer; antiemetic; piperazine antihistamine; antipruritic* 25, 50, 100 mg oral

Hyflex-650 tablets (discontinued 2009) ℞ *analgesic; antipyretic; antihistamine; sleep aid* [acetaminophen; phenyltoloxamine citrate] 650•60 mg

HyGel gel ℞ *wound healing agent for skin irritations, dermal ulcers, wounds, and burns* [hyaluronate sodium] 0.2%

Hygenic Cleansing anorectal pads OTC *moisturizer and cleanser for external rectal/vaginal areas; astringent* [witch hazel] 50%

Hygroton tablets (discontinued 2010) ℞ *antihypertensive; diuretic* [chlorthalidone] 100 mg

Hy-KXP oral liquid (discontinued 2011) ℞ *narcotic antitussive; expectorant* [hydrocodone bitartrate; potassium guaiacolsulfonate] 4.5•300 mg/5 mL

Hylaform gel for subcu injection in prefilled syringes (discontinued 2010) ℞ *dermal filler for wrinkles and facial folds* [hylan B] 5.5 mg/mL

hylan B *hyaluronic acid gel-based dermal filler*

hylan G-F 20 *hyaluronic acid gel-fluid (G-F) polymer mixture for osteoarthritis and TMJ syndrome*

Hylenex solution for injection ℞ *adjuvant to increase the absorption and dispersion of injected drugs, hypodermoclysis, and subcutaneous urography; also used for diabetic retinopathy* [hyaluronidase (recombinant human)] 150 U/mL

Hylira gel ℞ *wound healing agent for skin irritations, dermal ulcers, wounds, and burns* [hyaluronate sodium] 0.2%

Hylorel tablets (discontinued 2008) ℞ *antihypertensive* [guanadrel sulfate] 10, 25 mg

hymecromone USAN, INN *choleretic*

HyoMax tablets ℞ *GI/GU antispasmodic; anticholinergic* [hyoscyamine sulfate] 0.125 mg

HyoMax-FT chewable tablets ℞ *GI/GU antispasmodic; anticholinergic* [hyoscyamine sulfate] 0.125 mg

Hyophen tablets ℞ *urinary antibiotic; antiseptic; analgesic; antispasmodic* [methenamine; phenyl salicylate; methylene blue; benzoic acid; hyoscyamine sulfate] 81.6•36.2•10.8•9•0.12 mg ② Hy-Phen

hyoscine hydrobromide BAN *anticholinergic CNS depressant for postencephalitic parkinsonism and other spasticities, delirium tremens and other maniacal states, and general sedation; motion sickness preventative; GI antispasmodic/antiemetic; cycloplegic; mydriatic* [also: scopolamine hydrobromide]

hyoscine methobromide BAN *anticholinergic* [also: methscopolamine bromide]

hyoscyamine (L-hyoscyamine) USP, BAN *anticholinergic; urinary antispasmodic*

hyoscyamine hydrobromide USP *GI antispasmodic; anticholinergic*

hyoscyamine sulfate USP *GI/GU antispasmodic; antiparkinsonian; anticholinergic "drying agent" for allergic rhinitis and hyperhidrosis* [also: hyoscyamine sulphate] 0.125, 0.25, 0.375 mg oral; 0.125 mg/mL oral

hyoscyamine sulphate BAN GI/GU *antispasmodic; antiparkinsonian; anticholinergic "drying agent" for allergic rhinitis and hyperhidrosis* [also: hyoscyamine sulfate]

Hyoscyamus niger medicinal herb [see: henbane]

Hyosophen tablets, elixir (discontinued 2008) ℞ *GI/GU anticholinergic/ antispasmodic; sedative* [atropine sulfate; scopolamine hydrobromide; hyoscyamine hydrobromide; phenobarbital] 0.0194•0.0065•0.1037• 16.2 mg; 0.0194•0.0065•0.1037• 16.2 mg/5 mL

Hypaque-76 injection ℞ *radiopaque contrast medium* [diatrizoate meglumine; diatrizoate sodium (48.7% total iodine)] 660•100 mg/mL (370 mg/mL)

Hypaque-Cysto intracavitary instillation (discontinued 2010) ℞ *radiopaque contrast medium for urological imaging* [diatrizoate meglumine (46.67% iodine)] 300 mg/mL (141 mg/mL)

Hypaque Meglumine 60% injection (discontinued 2010) ℞ *radiopaque contrast medium* [diatrizoate meglumine (46.67% iodine)] 600 mg/mL (282 mg/mL)

Hypaque Sodium powder for oral/ rectal solution ℞ *radiopaque contrast medium for gastrointestinal imaging* [diatrizoate sodium (59.87% iodine)] 1002 mg/g (600 mg/g)

Hypaque Sodium 50% injection (discontinued 2010) ℞ *radiopaque contrast medium* [diatrizoate sodium (46.67% iodine)] 500 mg/mL (300 mg/mL)

HyperHEP B S/D IM injection ℞ *hepatitis B immunizing agent* [hepatitis B immune globulin, solvent/detergent treated] 0.5, 1, 5 mL

hypericin *investigational (Phase III, orphan) antineoplastic for glioblastoma multiforme and cutaneous T-cell lymphoma*

Hypericum perforatum medicinal herb [see: St. John's wort]

Hyperlyte CR IV admixture ℞ *intravenous electrolyte therapy* [combined electrolyte solution]

Hypermune RSV *investigational (orphan) treatment for respiratory syncytial virus (RSV) infections* [respiratory syncytial virus immune globulin (RSV-IG)]

hyperosmotic laxatives *a subclass of laxatives that use the osmotic effect to retain water in the intestines, lowering colonic pH and increasing peristalsis* [see also: laxatives]

HyperRab S/D IM injection ℞ *passive immunizing agent for use after rabies exposure* [rabies immune globulin, solvent/detergent treated] 150 IU/mL (300, 1500 IU/dose)

HyperRHO S/D Full Dose IM injection in prefilled syringes ℞ *immunizing agent for antenatal or postpartum prophylaxis of Rh hemolytic disease of the newborn* [Rh$_O$(D) immune globulin, solvent/detergent treated] 300 mcg (≥ 1500 IU)

HyperRHO S/D Mini-Dose IM injection in prefilled syringes ℞ *obstetric Rh factor immunity suppressant* [Rh$_O$(D) immune globulin, solvent/ detergent treated] 50 mcg (≥ 250 IU)

Hyperstat IV injection (discontinued 2009) ℞ *vasodilator for hypertensive emergency* [diazoxide] 15 mg/mL

Hyphed syrup (discontinued 2009) ℞ *narcotic antitussive; antihistamine; decongestant* [hydrocodone bitartrate; chlorpheniramine maleate; pseudoephedrine HCl; alcohol 5%] 2.5•2• 30 mg/5 mL

Hy-Phen tablets (discontinued 2009) ℞ *narcotic analgesic; antipyretic* [hydrocodone bitartrate; acetaminophen] 5•500 mg ⌦ Hyophen

hyphylline [see: dyphylline]

hypnogene [see: barbital]

hypnotics *a class of agents that induce sleep*

hypochlorous acid, sodium salt [see: sodium hypochlorite]

β-hypophamine [see: vasopressin]

α-hypophamine [see: oxytocin]

hypophosphorous acid NF *antioxidant*

Hyporet (trademarked delivery form) *prefilled disposable syringe*

HypoTears eye drops OTC *moisturizer/lubricant* [polyvinyl alcohol] 1%

HypoTears ophthalmic ointment OTC *moisturizer/lubricant* [white petrolatum; mineral oil]

HypoTears PF eye drops (discontinued 2010) OTC *moisturizer/lubricant* [polyvinyl alcohol] 1%

hyprolose [see: hydroxypropyl cellulose]

hypromellose INN, BAN *suspending and viscosity-increasing agent* [also: hydroxypropyl methylcellulose; hydroxypropylmethylcellulose]

Hyskon uterine infusion ℞ *hysteroscopy aid* [dextran 70; dextrose] 32%•10%

Hysone cream OTC *corticosteroidal anti-inflammatory; antifungal; antibacterial* [hydrocortisone; clioquinol] 10•30 mg/g

hyssop *(Hyssopus officinalis)* leaves *medicinal herb for chronic hay fever, congestion, cough, lung ailments, promoting expectoration, and sore throat*

hyssop, hedge *medicinal herb* [see: hedge hyssop]

hyssop, Indian; wild hyssop *medicinal herb* [see: blue vervain]

hyssop, prairie *medicinal herb* [see: wild hyssop]

HyTan oral suspension (discontinued 2009) ℞ *narcotic antitussive; antihistamine* [hydrocodone tannate; chlorpheniramine tannate] 5•4 mg/5 mL

Hytone cream, lotion, ointment ℞ *corticosteroidal anti-inflammatory* [hydrocortisone] 1%, 2.5%; 2.5%; 2.5%

Hytone 1% ointment, spray ℞ *corticosteroidal anti-inflammatory* [hydrocortisone] 1%

Hytrin soft capsules ℞ *alpha₁ blocker for hypertension and benign prostatic hyperplasia (BPH)* [terazosin (as HCl)] 1, 2, 5, 10 mg

Hyzaar 50-12.5; Hyzaar 100-12.5; Hyzaar 100-25 film-coated tablets ℞ *combination angiotensin receptor blocker (ARB) and diuretic for hypertension* [losartan potassium; hydrochlorothiazide] 50•12.5 mg; 100•12.5 mg; 100•25 mg

I Caps MV tablets OTC *vitamin/mineral supplement* [multiple vitamins and minerals; folic acid; biotin; lutein; zeaxanthin] ±•100 mcg•7.5 mcg•1.67 mg•0.83 mg

¹²³I [see: iodohippurate sodium I 123]

¹²³I [see: sodium iodide I 123]

¹²⁵I [see: albumin, iodinated I 125 serum]

¹²⁵I [see: diatrizoate sodium I 125]

¹²⁵I [see: diohippuric acid I 125]

¹²⁵I [see: diotyrosine I 125]

¹²⁵I [see: fibrinogen I 125]

¹²⁵I [see: insulin I 125]

¹²⁵I [see: iodohippurate sodium I 125]

¹²⁵I [see: iodopyracet I 125]

¹²⁵I [see: iomethin I 125]

¹²⁵I [see: iothalamate sodium I 125]

¹²⁵I [see: liothyronine I 125]

¹²⁵I [see: oleic acid I 125]

¹²⁵I [see: povidone I 125]

¹²⁵I [see: rose bengal sodium I 125]

¹²⁵I [see: sodium iodide I 125]

¹²⁵I [see: thyroxine I 125]

¹²⁵I [see: triolein I 125]

¹³¹I [see: albumin, aggregated iodinated I 131 serum]

¹³¹I [see: albumin, iodinated I 131 serum]

¹³¹I [see: diatrizoate sodium I 131]

^{131}I [see: diohippuric acid I 131]
^{131}I [see: diotyrosine I 131]
^{131}I [see: ethiodized oil I 131]
^{131}I [see: insulin I 131]
^{131}I [see: iodipamide sodium I 131]
^{131}I [see: iodoantipyrine I 131]
^{131}I [see: iodocholesterol I 131]
^{131}I [see: iodohippurate sodium I 131]
^{131}I [see: iodopyracet I 131]
^{131}I [see: iomethin I 131]
^{131}I [see: iothalamate sodium I 131]
^{131}I [see: iotyrosine I 131]
^{131}I [see: liothyronine I 131]
^{131}I [see: macrosalb (^{131}I)]
^{131}I [see: oleic acid I 131]
^{131}I [see: povidone I 131]
^{131}I [see: rose bengal sodium I 131]
^{131}I [see: sodium iodide I 131]
^{131}I [see: thyroxine I 131]
^{131}I [see: tolpovidone I 131]
^{131}I [see: triolein I 131]

ibacitabine INN

ibafloxacin USAN, INN, BAN *antibacterial*

ibandronate sodium USAN *bisphosphonate bone resorption inhibitor for the prevention and treatment of postmenopausal osteoporosis in women; also used for metastatic bone disease in breast cancer*

ibazocine INN

IBC (isobutyl cyanoacrylate) [see: bucrylate]

Iberet controlled-release Filmtabs (film-coated tablets) (discontinued 2008) OTC *vitamin/iron supplement* [iron (as ferrous sulfate); multiple B vitamins; vitamin C] 105•±•150 mg ⑫ eyebright

Iberet-500 controlled-release tablets (discontinued 2009) OTC *vitamin/iron supplement* [iron (as ferrous sulfate); multiple B vitamins; vitamin C] 95•±•500 mg ⑫ eyebright

Iberet-Folic-500 controlled-release Filmtabs (film-coated tablets) (discontinued 2008) Ɽ *hematinic* [iron (as ferrous sulfate); multiple B vitamins; vitamin C (as sodium ascorbate); folic acid] 105•±•500•0.8 mg

iboga *(Tabernanthe iboga) euphoric/hallucinogenic street drug, the root of which is chewed or chopped into a fine powder and mixed with other drugs; doses high enough to induce hallucinations are also likely to cause death*

ibopamine USAN, INN, BAN *peripheral dopaminergic agent; vasodilator*

ibritumomab tiuxetan USAN *radioimmunotherapy carrier; monoclonal antibody radiolabeled with indium In 111 and yttrium Y 90 to treat non-Hodgkin B-cell lymphoma (orphan)*

ibrotal [see: ibrotamide]

ibrotamide INN

IB-Stat oral spray Ɽ *pediatric anticholinergic "drying agent" for allergic rhinitis and hyperhidrosis* [hyoscyamine sulfate] 0.125 mg/mL

ibudilast INN

Ibudone film-coated tablets Ɽ *narcotic analgesic; antipyretic* [hydrocodone bitartrate; ibuprofen] 5•200, 10•200 mg ⑫ Iopidine

ibufenac USAN, INN, BAN *analgesic; anti-inflammatory*

ibuprofen USAN, USP, INN, BAN *analgesic; antipyretic; antiarthritic; nonsteroidal anti-inflammatory drug (NSAID) for mild to moderate pain, migraine headaches, and primary dysmenorrhea* 200, 400, 600, 800 mg oral; 100 mg/5 mL oral; 40 mg/mL oral

ibuprofen aluminum USAN *analgesic; antipyretic; antiarthritic; nonsteroidal anti-inflammatory drug (NSAID) for mild to moderate pain, migraine headaches, and primary dysmenorrhea*

Ibuprofen Children's Cold oral suspension OTC *decongestant; analgesic; antipyretic* [pseudoephedrine HCl; ibuprofen] 15•100 mg/5 mL

ibuprofen & diphenhydramine citrate *analgesic; antipyretic; antihistaminic sleep aid* 200•38 mg oral

ibuprofen & hydrocodone bitartrate *analgesic; narcotic antitussive* 200•5, 200•7.5, 200•10 mg oral

ibuprofen lysine *nonsteroidal anti-inflammatory drug (NSAID) used to* *close a significant patent ductus arteriosus (PDA) in premature infants (orphan)* (base=58.5%)

ibuprofen & oxycodone HCl *narcotic analgesic* 400•5 mg oral

ibuprofen piconol USAN *topical antiinflammatory*

ibuproxam INN

Ibutab tablets OTC *analgesic; antipyretic; antiarthritic; nonsteroidal anti-inflammatory drug (NSAID) for mild to moderate pain, migraine headaches, and primary dysmenorrhea* [ibuprofen] 200 mg

ibutamoren mesylate USAN *growth hormone for congenital growth hormone deficiency, musculoskeletal impairment, and hip fractures*

ibuterol INN

ibutilide INN *antiarrhythmic* [also: ibutilide fumarate]

ibutilide fumarate USAN *antiarrhythmic for atrial fibrillation/flutter* [also: ibutilide] 0.1 mg/mL injection

ibuverine INN

ibylcaine chloride [see: butethamine HCl]

ICA 17043 *investigational (Phase III) agent for sickle cell disease*

ICaps film-coated tablets OTC *vitamin/ mineral supplement* [vitamins A, B₂, C, and E; multiple minerals] 6000 IU•20 mg•200 mg•60 IU• ±

ICaps Plus tablets (discontinued 2008) OTC *vitamin/mineral supplement* [multiple vitamins & minerals]

Icar chewable tablets, oral suspension OTC *iron supplement* [carbonyl iron] 15 mg; 15 mg/1.25 mL ② agar; Wee Care

Icar Prenatal Therapy tablets + chewable tablets, softgels + chewable tablets (discontinued 2009) ℞ *prenatal vitamin/mineral/calcium/iron/omega-3 supplement* [tablets and softgels: multiple vitamins & minerals, iron (as carbonyl), folic acid, biotin, DHA, EPA; chewable tablets: calcium] ±• 29•1•0.03•120•180 mg; 600 mg

icatibant acetate USAN *competitive bradykinin receptor-2 antagonist for*

hereditary angioedema (HAE) (orphan)

ICE (idarubicin, cytarabine, etoposide) *chemotherapy protocol for acute myelocytic leukemia (AML)* [also known as: IDA-based BF12; idarubicin + cytarabine + etoposide]

ICE (ifosfamide, carboplatin, etoposide) [with mesna rescue] *chemotherapy protocol for osteosarcoma and lung cancer* [also known as: MICE]

Iceland moss (*Cetraria islandica*) plant *medicinal herb for anemia, bronchitis, hay fever, congestion, cough, digestive disorders, and lung disorders*

ICE-T (ifosfamide, carboplatin, etoposide, Taxol) [with mesna rescue] *chemotherapy protocol for sarcoma, breast cancer, and non–small cell lung cancer (NSCLC)* ② Aceta; Iosat

IC-Green powder for IV injection ℞ *diagnostic aid for ophthalmic angiography* [indocyanine green] 25 mg

ichthammol USP, BAN *topical anti-infective* 10%, 20%

iclazepam INN

icodextrin INN, BAN *peritoneal dialysis solution for end-stage renal disease (orphan)*

icopezil maleate USAN *acetylcholinesterase inhibitor; cognition adjuvant for Alzheimer disease*

icosapent INN *omega-3 marine triglyceride* [also: eicosapentaenoic acid (EPA)]

icospiramide INN ② oxiperomide

icotidine USAN *antagonist to histamine H₁ and H₂ receptors*

ictasol USAN *disinfectant*

Ictotest reagent tablets for professional use ℞ *in vitro diagnostic aid for bilirubin in the urine*

Icy Hot balm, cream OTC *analgesic; mild anesthetic; antipruritic; counterirritant* [methyl salicylate; menthol] 29%•7.6%; 30%•10%

Icy Hot Back Pain Relief; Icy Hot Pop & Peel; Icy Hot Pro-Therapy transdermal patch OTC *mild anesthetic; antipruritic; counterirritant* [menthol] 5%

Icy Hot Chill Stick OTC *analgesic; mild anesthetic; antipruritic; counterirritant* [methyl salicylate; menthol] 30%•10%

Icy Hot Pain Relieving Gel OTC *mild anesthetic; antipruritic; counterirritant* [menthol; alcohol 15%] 2.5%

Icy Hot PM Medicated lotion, patch OTC *mild anesthetic; antipruritic; counterirritant; analgesic for muscle and joint pain* [menthol; capsaicin] 7.5%• ⅐; 5%•0.025%

Icy Hot Roll transdermal patch OTC *mild anesthetic; antipruritic; counterirritant* [menthol] 7.5%

IDA-based BF12 (idarubicin, cytarabine, etoposide) *chemotherapy protocol for acute myelocytic leukemia (AML)* [also known as: ICE; idarubicin + cytarabine + etoposide]

Idamycin PFS powder for IV infusion ℞ *anthracycline antibiotic antineoplastic for acute myeloid leukemia (AML) (orphan); investigational (orphan) for myelodysplastic syndromes, acute and chronic myelogenous leukemia, and acute lymphoblastic leukemia in children* [idarubicin HCl] 5, 10, 20 mg/vial

idarubicin (IDR) INN, BAN *anthracycline antibiotic antineoplastic* [also: idarubicin HCl]

idarubicin HCl USAN, INN *anthracycline antibiotic antineoplastic for acute myeloid leukemia (AML) (orphan); investigational (orphan) for myelodysplastic syndromes, acute and chronic myelogenous leukemia, and acute lymphoblastic leukemia in children* [also: idarubicin] 5, 10, 20 mg/vial injection

idaverine INN

idazoxan INN, BAN

idebenone INN, JAN *investigational (orphan) for Friedreich ataxia, Duchenne muscular dystrophy, and Leber hereditary optic neuropathy*

idenast INN

Identi-Dose (trademarked packaging form) *unit dose package*

idoxifene USAN *antihormone antineoplastic; osteoporosis treatment; estrogen receptor antagonist for hormone replacement therapy*

idoxuridine (IDU) USAN, USP, INN, BAN, JAN *ophthalmic antiviral; investigational (orphan) for nonparenchymatous sarcomas*

IDR (idarubicin) [q.v.]

idralfidine INN

idremcinal USAN, INN *motilin agonist to stimulate gastrointestinal motility*

idrobutamine [see: butidrine]

idrocilamide INN

idropranolol INN

IDU (idoxuridine) [q.v.]

iduronidase [now: laronidase]

idursulfase *iduronate-2-sulfatase enzyme to improve walking capacity in patients with Hunter syndrome (mucopolysaccharidosis II; MPS II; orphan)*

IE (ifosfamide, etoposide) [with mesna rescue] *chemotherapy protocol for soft tissue sarcoma* [also: IfoVP (for osteosarcoma)]

ifenprodil INN

iFerex 150 capsules OTC *iron supplement* [iron] 150 mg

ifetroban USAN *antithrombotic; anti-ischemic; antivasospastic*

ifetroban sodium USAN *antithrombotic; anti-ischemic; antivasospastic*

Ifex powder for IV injection ℞ *antineoplastic for testicular cancer (orphan); investigational (orphan) for bone and soft tissue sarcomas* [ifosfamide] 1, 3 g

IFN (interferon) [q.v.]

IFN-alpha 2 (interferon alfa-2) [see: interferon alfa-2b, recombinant]

ifosfamide USAN, USP, INN, BAN *nitrogen mustard–type alkylating antineoplastic for testicular cancer (orphan); investigational (orphan) for bone and soft tissue sarcomas* 1, 3 g injection

IfoVP (ifosfamide, VePesid) [with mesna rescue] *chemotherapy protocol for osteosarcoma* [also: IE (for soft tissue sarcoma)]

ifoxetine INN

IG, Ig (immune globulin) [see: globulin, immune]

IgE pentapeptide [see: pentigetide]

Igel 56 ℞ *hydrophilic contact lens material* [hefilcon C] ⑨ OCL
IGF-1 (insulin-like growth factor-1) [now: mecasermin]
IGF-1/IGFBP-3 complex [see: mecasermin rinfabate]
IgG (immunoglobulin G) [see: globulin, immune]
IgG1 [see: immunoglobulin G1]
IGIM; IMIG (immune globulin intramuscular) [see: globulin, immune; Rh₀D immune globulin]
IGIV (immune globulin intravenous) [see: globulin, immune; Rh₀D immune globulin]
igmesine HCl USAN *sigma receptor ligand antidepressant*
IGSC, SCIG (immune globulin subcutaneous) [see: globulin, immune]
IL-1, IL-2, etc. [see: interleukin-1, interleukin-2, etc.]
IL-2 (interleukin-2) [see: aldesleukin; teceleukin; celmoleukin]
IL-4 pseudomonas toxin fusion protein *investigational (orphan) for astrocytic glioma*
IL-1 Trap [see: rilonacept]
IL-13-PE38QQR protein *investigational (orphan) for malignant glioma*
Ilaris powder for subcu injection ℞ *anti-inflammatory for cryopyrin-associated periodic syndrome (CAPS) and its variants, familial cold autoinflammatory syndrome (FCAS), and Muckle-Wells syndrome (orphan); investigational for systemic juvenile idiopathic arthritis (SJIA)* [canakinumab] 180 mg
ilepcimide USAN, INN *anticonvulsant; investigational (orphan) for drug-resistant generalized tonic-clonic epilepsy*
Iletin (U.S. products) [see: Lente Iletin II]
Ilex aquifolium; I. opaca; I. vomitoria medicinal herb [see: holly]
Ilex paraguariensis medicinal herb [see: yerba maté]
Ilex verticillata medicinal herb [see: winterberry]
Illicium anisatum; I. verum medicinal herb [see: star anise]

ilmofosine USAN, INN *antineoplastic*
ilodecakin USAN, INN *interleukin 10, human clone; immunomodulator for Crohn disease, ulcerative colitis, rheumatoid arthritis (RA), and psoriasis*
ilomastat USAN *matrix metalloproteinase (MMP) inhibitor for corneal ulcers, inflammation, and cancers*
ilonidap USAN, INN *anti-inflammatory*
Ilopan IM injection, IV infusion ℞ *GI stimulant for the prevention and treatment of postoperative paralytic ileus, intestinal atony, and decreased intestinal motility* [dexpanthenol] 250 mg/mL
iloperidone USAN, INN *selective serotonin and dopamine antagonist; atypical antipsychotic for schizophrenia*
iloprost INN, BAN *prostacyclin analogue; vasodilator for pulmonary arterial hypertension (PAH) (orphan); investigational (orphan) intravenous treatment for thrombocytopenia and Raynaud phenomenon associated with systemic sclerosis*
Ilotycin ophthalmic ointment (discontinued 2010) ℞ *antibiotic* [erythromycin] 0.5% ⑨ Altazine
Ilotycin Gluceptate IV injection ℞ *macrolide antibiotic* [erythromycin gluceptate] 1 g/vial
Iluvien *corticosteroidal anti-inflammatory; investigational (NDA filed) ocular implant for diabetic macular edema* [fluocinolone acetonide]
I-L-X elixir (discontinued 2008) OTC *vitamin/iron supplement* [multiple B vitamins; iron (as ferrous gluconate); liver concentrate 1:20] ≛•70•98 mg/15 mL ⑨ Aloxi; Olux
I-L-X B₁₂ caplets (discontinued 2008) OTC *vitamin/iron supplement* [multiple B vitamins; vitamin C; carbonyl iron; desiccated liver] ≛•120•37.5•130 mg
I-L-X B₁₂ elixir OTC *vitamin/iron supplement* [multiple B vitamins; ferric ammonium citrate; liver fraction 1] ≛•102•98 mg/15 mL
imafen INN *antidepressant* [also: imafen HCl] ⑨ Imovane
imafen HCl USAN *antidepressant* [also: imafen]

Imager ac rectal suspension ℞ *radiopaque contrast medium for gastrointestinal imaging* [barium sulfate] 100%

imanixil INN

imatinib mesylate USAN *antineoplastic for chronic myeloid leukemia (orphan), acute lymphoblastic leukemia, chronic eosinophilic leukemia, myelodysplastic disease, gastrointestinal stromal tumors (orphan), systemic mastocytosis, and dermatofibrosarcoma protuberans*

imazodan INN *cardiotonic* [also: imazodan HCl]

imazodan HCl USAN *cardiotonic* [also: imazodan]

imcarbofos USAN, INN *veterinary anthelmintic*

imciromab INN *monoclonal antibody Fab to myosin, murine* [also: imciromab pentetate]

imciromab pentetate USAN, BAN *monoclonal antibody Fab to myosin, murine* [also: imciromab; indium In 111 imciromab pentetate]

Imdur extended-release tablets ℞ *coronary vasodilator; antianginal* [isosorbide mononitrate] 30, 60, 120 mg ② imidurea

imexon INN *investigational (orphan) for multiple myeloma, metastatic malignant melanoma, pancreatic adenocarcinoma, and ovarian cancer*

imiclopazine INN

imidapril INN, BAN

imidazole carboxamide [see: dacarbazine]

imidazole salicylate INN

imidecyl iodine USAN *topical anti-infective*

imidocarb INN, BAN *antiprotozoal (Babesia)* [also: imidocarb HCl]

imidocarb HCl USAN *antiprotozoal (Babesia)* [also: imidocarb]

imidoline INN *antipsychotic* [also: imidoline HCl] ② amedalin; omidoline

imidoline HCl USAN *antipsychotic* [also: imidoline]

imidurea NF *antimicrobial* ② Imdur

IMIG; IGIM (intramuscular immune globulin) [see: globulin, immune; Rh₀D immune globulin]

imiglucerase USAN, INN *glucocerebrosidase enzyme replacement for type 1 Gaucher disease (orphan)*

imiloxan INN *antidepressant* [also: imiloxan HCl]

imiloxan HCl USAN *antidepressant* [also: imiloxan]

iminophenimide INN

iminostilbene anticonvulsants *a class of anticonvulsants with a chemical structure similar to tricyclic antidepressants*

imipemide [now: imipenem]

imipenem USAN, USP, INN, BAN, JAN *broad-spectrum carbapenem antibiotic*

imipramine INN, BAN *tricyclic antidepressant* [also: imipramine HCl] ② ampyrimine; embramine

imipramine HCl USP *tricyclic antidepressant; treatment for childhood enuresis* [also: imipramine] 10, 25, 50 mg oral

imipramine pamoate *tricyclic antidepressant* 75, 100, 125, 150 mg oral

imipraminoxide INN

imiquimod USAN, INN *topical immunomodulator for external genital and perianal warts (condylomata acuminata), actinic keratoses, and superficial basal cell carcinoma (sBCC)* 5% topical

imirestat INN

Imitrex film-coated tablets, nasal spray ℞ *vascular serotonin receptor agonist for the acute treatment of migraine headaches* [sumatriptan] 25, 50, 100 mg; 5, 20 mg/dose

Imitrex subcu injection in vials, prefilled syringes, or STATdose self-injector kits (two prefilled syringes) ℞ *vascular serotonin receptor agonist for the acute treatment of migraine and cluster headaches* [sumatriptan (as succinate)] 4, 6 mg/0.5 mL dose

ImmTher *investigational (orphan) immunostimulant for pulmonary and hepatic metastases of colorectal adenocarcinoma, Ewing sarcoma, and osteosarcoma* [disaccharide tripeptide glycerol dipalmitoyl]

ImmuDyn *investigational (orphan) agent to increase platelet count in immune thrombocytopenic purpura* [*Pseudomonas aeruginosa* purified extract]

Immun-Aid powder OTC *enteral nutritional therapy for immunocompromised patients* ② Emend

immune globulin (IG; Ig) [see: globulin, immune]

immune globulin intramuscular (IGIM; IgIM) [see: globulin, immune]

immune globulin intravenous (IGIV; IgIV) [see: globulin, immune]

immune globulin intravenous pentetate USAN *radiodiagnostic imaging agent for inflammation and infection* [also: indium In 111 IGIV pentetate]

immune globulin subcutaneous (IGSC; IgSC) [see: globulin, immune]

immune serum globulin (ISG) [see: globulin, immune]

Immunex CRP test kit for professional use ℞ *in vitro diagnostic aid for C-reactive protein (CRP) in blood to diagnose inflammatory conditions* [latex agglutination test]

Immuno-C *investigational (Phase II, orphan) treatment of cryptosporidiosis-induced diarrhea in immunocompromised patients* [*Cryptosporidium parvum* bovine colostrum IgG concentrate]

Immunocal powder for oral solution OTC *enteral nutritional therapy* [milk-based formula] 10 g/pouch

ImmunoCAP Specific IgE blood test kit for professional use ℞ *in vitro diagnostic aid for IgE detection* [316 different allergens]

immunoglobulin G1 (mouse monoclonal 7E11-C5.3 antihuman prostatic carcinoma cell) disulfide [see: capromab pendetide]

immunoglobulin G1 (mouse monoclonal ZCE025 antihuman antigen CEA) disulfide [see: indium In 111 altumomab pentetate; altumomab]

immunoglobulin G2 (human-mouse monoclonal HuM291 anti-CD3 antigen) disulfide [now: visilizumab]

immunosuppressants *a class of drugs used to suppress the immune response, used primarily after organ transplantation surgery*

Immupath *investigational (orphan) treatment for AIDS* [HIV-neutralizing antibodies]

ImmuRAID-AFP *investigational (orphan) for diagnostic aid for AFP-producing tumors, hepatoblastoma, and hepatocellular carcinoma* [monoclonal antibody to human alpha-fetoprotein (AFP), murine, radiolabeled with technetium Tc 99m]

ImmuRAID-hCG *investigational (orphan) diagnostic aid for hCG-producing tumors such as germ cell and trophoblastic cell tumors* [monoclonal antibody to human chorionic gonadotropin (hCG), murine, radiolabeled with technetium Tc 99m]

ImmuRAIT-LL2 *investigational (orphan) treatment for B-cell leukemia and lymphoma* [monoclonal antibody IgG_{2a} to B cell, murine, radiolabeled with iodine I 131]

Imodium capsules ℞ *antidiarrheal* [loperamide HCl] 2 mg

Imodium A-D caplets, oral liquid OTC *antidiarrheal* [loperamide HCl] 1 mg; 1 mg/5 mL, 1 mg/7.5 mL

Imodium Multi-Symptom Relief tablets, chewable tablets OTC *antidiarrheal; antiflatulent* [loperamide HCl; simethicone] 2•125 mg

Imogam Rabies-HT IM injection ℞ *passive immunizing agent for use after rabies exposure* [rabies immune globulin, heat treated] 150 IU/mL (300, 1500 IU/vial)

Imojev *investigational (NDA filed, orphan) active immunizing agent* [Japanese encephalitis (JE) virus vaccine]

imolamine INN, BAN

Imovax Rabies Vaccine IM injection ℞ *rabies vaccine for pre-exposure vaccination or post-exposure prophylaxis* [rabies vaccine, human diploid cell (HDCV)] ≥ 2.5 IU/mL

imoxiterol INN

impacarzine INN

Impact; Impact Advanced Recovery ready-to-use oral liquid OTC *enteral nutritional therapy* [lactose-free formula] 273 mL

Impact Rubella slide test for professional use ℞ *in vitro diagnostic aid for detection of rubella virus antibodies in serum* [latex agglutination test]

Impatiens balsamina; I. biflora; I. capensis medicinal herb [see: jewelweed]

IMPE [see: etipirium iodide]

Implanon subdermal polymer implant ℞ *progestin; long-term (3 years) contraceptive; also used as a male contraceptive* [etonogestrel] 68 mg

implitapide *investigational (orphan) for homozygous familial hypercholesterolemia and types I and V hyperlipoproteinemia*

impromidine INN, BAN *gastric secretion indicator* [also: impromidine HCl]

impromidine HCl USAN *gastric secretion indicator* [also: impromidine]

improsulfan INN

Improved Analgesic ointment (discontinued 2007) OTC *analgesic; mild anesthetic; antipruritic; counterirritant* [methyl salicylate; menthol] 18.3%•16%

Impruv Deep Moisturizing lotion OTC *moisturizer/emollient*

Impruv Natural Repair cream OTC *moisturizer/emollient*

imuracetam INN

Imuran tablets ℞ *immunosuppressant for organ transplantation (orphan) and rheumatoid arthritis; investigational (orphan) for graft-versus-host (GVH) disease of the oral mucosa* [azathioprine] 50 mg

Imuthiol *investigational (Phase II/III, orphan) immunomodulator for HIV and AIDS* [diethyldithiocarbamate]

Imuvert *investigational (orphan) for primary brain malignancies* [Serratia marcescens extract (polyribosomes)]

^{111}**In** [see: indium In 111 altumomab pentetate]

^{111}**In** [see: indium In 111 imciromab pentetate]

^{111}**In** [see: indium In 111 murine anti-CEA monoclonal antibody]

^{111}**In** [see: indium In 111 murine monoclonal antibody]

^{111}**In** [see: indium In 111 oxyquinoline]

^{111}**In** [see: indium In 111 pentetate]

^{111}**In** [see: indium In 111 pentetreotide]

^{111}**In** [see: indium In 111 satumomab pendetide]

^{111}**In** [see: pentetate indium disodium In 111]

^{113m}**In** [see: indium chlorides In 113m]

inactivated mumps vaccine [see: mumps virus vaccine, inactivated]

inactivated poliomyelitis vaccine (IPV) [see: poliovirus vaccine, inactivated]

inactivated poliovirus vaccine (IPV) [see: poliovirus vaccine, inactivated]

inamrinone USAN *cardiotonic* [also: amrinone]

inamrinone lactate *vasodilator for congestive heart failure*

inaperisone INN

Inapsine IV or IM injection (discontinued 2009) ℞ *general anesthetic; antiemetic* [droperidol] 2.5 mg/mL

Inatal Advance; Inatal Ultra tablets ℞ *prenatal vitamin/mineral/calcium/iron supplement* [multiple vitamins & minerals; calcium; iron (as carbonyl); folic acid] ≛•200•90•1 mg

Incivek film-coated caplets ℞ *hepatitis C virus (HCV) protease inhibitor for the treatment of HCV infections* [telaprevir] 375 mg

incobotulinumtoxin A *neurotoxin complex derived from Clostridium botulinum for blepharospasm and cervical dystonia; also used for achalasia, Frey syndrome, palmar hyperhidrosis, and Tourette syndrome*

Increlex subcu injection ℞ *recombinant human insulin-like growth factor-1 (rhIGF-1) for children with primary IGF deficiency without concomitant* growth hormone (GH) deficiency (orphan) [mecasermin] 10 mg/mL

incretin mimetic agents *a class of antidiabetic drugs that improve the body's normal glucose-sensing mechanisms by activating the glucagon-like peptide-1 (GLP-1) receptors*

indacaterol maleate *long-acting beta agonist; maintenance bronchodilator to improve pulmonary airflow in patients with COPD*

indacrinic acid [see: indacrinone]

indacrinone USAN, INN *antihypertensive; diuretic*

indalpine INN, BAN

Indamix DM oral suspension ℞ *antitussive; antihistamine; decongestant* [dextromethorphan tannate; dexchlorpheniramine tannate; pseudoephedrine tannate] 27.5•3•50 mg/5 mL

indanazoline INN

indanediones *a class of anticoagulants that interfere with vitamin K–dependent clotting factors*

indanidine INN

indanorex INN

indapamide USAN, INN, BAN *antihypertensive; diuretic for congestive heart failure* 1.25, 2.5 mg oral

indatraline INN

indecainide INN *antiarrhythmic* [also: indecainide HCl]

indecainide HCl USAN *antiarrhythmic* [also: indecainide]

indeloxazine INN *antidepressant* [also: indeloxazine HCl]

indeloxazine HCl USAN *antidepressant* [also: indeloxazine]

indenolol INN, BAN

Inderal IV injection (discontinued 2010) ℞ *beta-blocker; antiarrhythmic* [propranolol HCl] 1 mg/mL ⊠ Anadrol

Inderal tablets (discontinued 2008) ℞ *beta-blocker; antianginal; antiarrhythmic; antihypertensive* [propranolol HCl] 10, 20, 40, 60, 80 mg ⊠ Anadrol

Inderal LA long-acting capsules ℞ *beta-blocker; antianginal; antiarrhyth-*

mic; antihypertensive; also used for traumatic brain injury [propranolol HCl] 60, 80, 120, 160 mg ⊠ Anadrol

Inderide 40/25 tablets (discontinued 2008) ℞ *combination beta-blocker and diuretic for hypertension* [propranolol HCl; hydrochlorothiazide] 40•25 mg ⊠ Android; EndaRoid

Inderide 80/25 tablets (discontinued 2007) ℞ *combination beta-blocker and diuretic for hypertension* [propranolol HCl; hydrochlorothiazide] 80•25 mg ⊠ Android; EndaRoid

Indian apple *medicinal herb* [see: mandrake]

Indian arrow; Indian arrow wood *medicinal herb* [see: wahoo]

Indian bark *medicinal herb* [see: magnolia]

Indian bay *medicinal herb* [see: laurel]

Indian corn (Zea mays) styles (silk) *medicinal herb used as an analgesic, diuretic, demulcent, and litholytic*

Indian cress (Tropaeolum majus) flowers, leaves, and seeds *medicinal herb used as an antiseptic and expectorant*

Indian elm *medicinal herb* [see: slippery elm]

Indian frankincense *medicinal herb* [see: frankincense]

Indian hemp *medicinal herb* [see: marijuana]

Indian hyssop *medicinal herb* [see: blue vervain]

Indian paint, red *medicinal herb* [see: bloodroot]

Indian paint, yellow *medicinal herb* [see: goldenseal]

Indian pipe *medicinal herb* [see: fit root]

Indian plant *medicinal herb* [see: bloodroot; goldenseal]

Indian poke (Veratrum viride) *medicinal herb* [see: hellebore]

Indian root *medicinal herb* [see: spikenard; wahoo]

Indian shamrock *medicinal herb* [see: birthroot]

Indian tobacco *medicinal herb* [see: lobelia]

Indiana protocol (cisplatin, doxoru-bicin, cyclophosphamide) *chemotherapy protocol for ovarian cancer* [also known as: PAC-I]

indigo (*Indigofera* spp.) plant *medicinal herb for fever, hemorrhoids, inducing emesis, inflammation, liver cleansing, ovarian and stomach cancer, pain, scorpion stings, and worms; not generally regarded as safe and effective*

indigo, wild *medicinal herb* [see: wild indigo]

Indigo Carmine IV or IM injection ℞ *cystoscopy aid* [indigotindisulfonate sodium] 8 mg/mL

indigocarmine BAN, JAN *cystoscopy aid* [also: indigotindisulfonate sodium]

indigotindisulfonate sodium USP *cystoscopy aid* [also: indigocarmine]

indinavir USAN *antiretroviral protease inhibitor for HIV infection*

indinavir sulfate USAN *antiretroviral protease inhibitor for HIV infection* (base=80%)

indium *element (In)*

indium (^{111}In) diethylenetriamine pentaacetate JAN *radionuclide cisternography aid; radioactive agent* [also: indium In 111 pentetate]

indium chlorides In 113m USAN, USP *radioactive agent*

Indium DTPA In 111 intrathecal injection ℞ *radiodiagnostic imaging agent for radionuclide cisternograpy* [pentetate indium disodium In 111] 37 MBq (1 mCi)/mL

indium In 111 altumomab pentetate USAN *radiodiagnostic monoclonal antibody to carcinoembryonic antigen (CEA); investigational (orphan) for the detection of colorectal carcinoma* [also: altumomab]

indium In 111 antimelanoma antibody XMMME-0001-DTPA [see: antimelanoma antibody]

indium In 111 capromab *radiolabeled monoclonal antibody; imaging agent for new or recurrent prostate cancer and its metastases* [compare: capromab pendetide]

indium In 111 CYT-103 [now: indium In 111 satumomab pendetide]

indium In 111 ibritumomab tiuxetan *radioimmunotherapy for non-Hodgkin B-cell lymphoma (orphan)*

indium In 111 IGIV pentetate *radiodiagnostic imaging agent for inflammation and infection* [also: immune globulin intravenous pentetate]

indium In 111 imciromab pentetate *radiodiagnostic monoclonal antibody Fab to myosin, murine; investigational (orphan) imaging agent for cardiac necrosis and myocarditis*

indium In 111 oxyquinoline USAN, USP *radioactive agent; diagnostic aid*

indium In 111 pentetate USP *radionuclide cisternography aid; radioactive agent* [also: indium (^{111}In) diethylenetriamine pentaacetate]

indium In 111 pentetreotide USAN *radioactive imaging agent for SPECT scans of neuroendocrine tumors; investigational (orphan) radiotherapeutic agent for somatostatin receptor–positive neuroendocrine tumors*

indium In 111 satumomab pendetide USAN *radiodiagnostic imaging aid for ovarian (orphan) and colorectal carcinoma* [also: satumomab]

indobufen INN

indocate INN

Indocin oral suspension ℞ *nonsteroidal anti-inflammatory drug (NSAID) for moderate to severe osteoarthritis, rheumatoid arthritis, and ankylosing spondylitis, and acute bursitis/tendinitis* [indomethacin] 25 mg/5 mL

Indocin suppositories ℞ *nonsteroidal anti-inflammatory drug (NSAID) for moderate to severe osteoarthritis, rheumatoid arthritis, and ankylosing spondylitis, and acute bursitis/tendinitis* [indomethacin] 50 mg

Indocin I.V. powder for IV injection ℞ *prostaglandin synthesis inhibitor for neonatal closure of patent ductus arteriosus* [indomethacin sodium (trihydrate)] 1 mg

Indocin SR sustained-release capsules (discontinued 2010) ℞ *nonsteroidal anti-inflammatory drug (NSAID) for moderate to severe osteoarthritis, rheumatoid arthritis, and ankylosing spondylitis, and acute bursitis/tendinitis* [indomethacin] 75 mg

indocyanine green USP, JAN *in vivo diagnostic aid for cardiac output, hepatic function, and ophthalmic angiography* 25 mg injection

indolapril INN *antihypertensive* [also: indolapril HCl]

indolapril HCl USAN *antihypertensive* [also: indolapril]

indole 3-carbinol *natural phytochemical found in cruciferous vegetables; antioxidant and estrogen blocker shown effective against hormone-related cancers of the prostate, the uterus, and especially the breast; restores the p21 tumor suppressor gene*

indolidan USAN, INN, BAN *cardiotonic*

indolones *a class of dopamine receptor antagonists with conventional (typical) antipsychotic activity* [also called: dihydroindolones]

indometacin INN, JAN *antiarthritic; nonsteroidal anti-inflammatory drug (NSAID)* [also: indomethacin]

indometacin farnecil JAN *antiarthritic; nonsteroidal anti-inflammatory drug (NSAID)* [also: indomethacin]

indomethacin USAN, USP, BAN *nonsteroidal anti-inflammatory drug (NSAID) for moderate to severe osteoarthritis, rheumatoid arthritis, ankylosing spondylitis, and acute bursitis/tendinitis* [also: indometacin; indometacin farnecil] 25, 50, 75 mg oral; 50 mg rectal suppositories; 1 mg injection

indomethacin sodium USAN *anti-inflammatory; prostaglandin synthesis inhibitor for neonatal closure of patent ductus arteriosus* 1 mg injection

indopanolol INN

indopine INN

indoprofen USAN, INN, BAN *analgesic; anti-inflammatory*

indoramin USAN, INN, BAN *antihypertensive*

indoramin HCl USAN, BAN *antihypertensive*

indorenate INN *antihypertensive* [also: indorenate HCl]

indorenate HCl USAN *antihypertensive* [also: indorenate]

indoxole USAN, INN *antipyretic; anti-inflammatory*

indriline INN *CNS stimulant* [also: indriline HCl]

indriline HCl USAN *CNS stimulant* [also: indriline]

inductin [see: diphoxazide]

I-neb AAD (adaptive aerosol delivery) (trademarked delivery device) *oral inhalation solution dispenser*

InfaCare [see: Enfamil EnfaCare]

Infalyte oral solution OTC *electrolyte replacement* [sodium, potassium, and chloride electrolytes] ☒ Enfalyte

Infanrix IM injection ℞ *active immunizing agent for diphtheria, tetanus, and pertussis; Dtap (diphtheria predominant) vaccine used in the initial immunization series of infants and children 6 weeks to 6 years old* [diphtheria toxoid; tetanus toxoid; inactivated pertussis toxin] 25 Lf•10 Lf•25 mcg per 0.5 mL dose

Infantaire oral drops (discontinued 2011) OTC *analgesic; antipyretic* [acetaminophen] 100 mg/mL

Infasurf intratracheal suspension ℞ *agent for prophylaxis and treatment of respiratory distress syndrome (RDS) in premature infants (orphan)* [calfactant] 6 mL

Infatab (trademarked dosage form) *pediatric chewable tablet*

INFeD IV or IM injection ℞ *hematinic* [iron (as dextran)] 100 mg/dose ☒ Unifed

Infergen subcu injection ℞ *consensus interferon for the treatment of chronic hepatitis C virus (HCV) infections* [interferon alfacon-1] 9, 15 mcg/0.3 mL dose

infliximab *monoclonal antibody to TNFα (tumor necrosis factor alpha); anti-inflammatory for Crohn disease (orphan), ulcerative colitis, rheumatoid and psoriatic arthritis, ankylosing spondylitis, and plaque psoriasis*

influenza purified surface antigen [see: influenza split-virus vaccine]

influenza split-virus vaccine *subcategory of influenza virus vaccine*

influenza subvirion vaccine [see: influenza split-virus vaccine]

influenza virus vaccine, H1N1 (injectable) *(discontinued as a single-strain vaccine, but is included in the 2011–2012 seasonal flu vaccine) active immunizing agent for H1N1 influenza A (swine flu; Mexican pandemic flu) in adults and children ≥ 6 months* [virus strain: A/California/7/2009] 0.5 mL/dose in prefilled syringes (preservative-free), 0.5 mL/dose in multidose vials (contains mercury, 25 mcg/dose)

influenza virus vaccine, H1N1 (intranasal) *active immunizing agent for H1N1 influenza A (swine flu; Mexican pandemic flu) in adults and children 2–49 years* [virus strain: A/California/7/2009] 0.2 mL/dose (preservative-free)

influenza virus vaccine, H5N1 *active immunizing agent for H5N1 influenza A (avian flu; bird flu) in adults 18–64 years; this vaccine is not available commercially but has been stockpiled by the U.S. government for future outbreaks* [virus strain: A/Vietnam/1203/2004 (H5N1, clade 1)] 90 mcg/mL injection (with 98.2 mcg/dose thimerosal preservative=50mcg/dose mercury)

influenza virus vaccine, seasonal (inactivated injectable) USP *active immunizing agent for influenza* [virus strains for the 2011–2012 season: A/California/7/2009 (H1N1), A/Perth/16/2009 (H3N2), and B/Brisbane/60/2008]

influenza virus vaccine, seasonal (live intranasal) *active immunizing*

agent for influenza [virus strains for the 2011–2012 season: A/California/7/2009 (H1N1), A/Perth/16/2009 (H3N2), and B/Brisbane/60/2008]

influenza whole-virus vaccine *subcategory of influenza virus vaccine*

Infumorph 200; Infumorph 500 concentrate for continuous microinfusion ℞ *narcotic analgesic; intraspinal microinfusion for intractable chronic pain (orphan)* [morphine sulfate] 10 mg/mL (200 mg/vial); 25 mg/mL (500 mg/vial)

Infuvite Adult IV infusion ℞ *multivitamin adjunct for adults receiving parenteral nutrition* [multiple vitamins; folic acid; biotin] ± • 600 • 60 mcg

Infuvite Pediatric IV infusion ℞ *multivitamin adjunct for infants and children receiving parenteral nutrition* [multiple vitamins; folic acid; biotin] ± • 140 • 20 mcg

INH (isonicotinic acid hydrazide) [see: isoniazid]

INH-A00021 *investigational (orphan) agent to reduce or prevent staphylococci-induced nosocomial bacteremia in very low birthweight infants*

Inhal-Aid (trademarked delivery device) *portable inhalation device*

inhalants *a class of street drugs that include nitrous oxide, volatile nitrites, and petroleum distillates* [see: nitrous oxide; volatile nitrites; petroleum distillate inhalants]

InhibiZone surface treatment ℞ *prophylactic antibiotic treatment for penile prostheses before implantation* [minocycline; rifampin] 3–10 • 9–25 mg (depending on prosthesis size)

inicarone INN

iniparib *investigational (Phase III) antineoplastic for "triple-negative" breast cancers (those that have no estrogen receptors, no progesterone receptors, and very low levels of HER-2 protein)*

Inject-all (trademarked delivery form) *prefilled disposable syringe*

Inlay-Tabs (trademarked dosage form) *tablets with contrasting inlay*

Innohep deep subcu injection ℞ *anti-coagulant/antithrombotic for the prevention and treatment of deep vein thrombosis (DVT)* [tinzaparin sodium] 20 000 IU/mL

InnoLet prefilled disposable syringe OTC *device for self-administration of insulin* (available prefilled with **Novolin N** or **Novolin 70/30**) [insulin] 1–40 U/injection

InnoPran XL long-acting capsules ℞ *beta-blocker; antianginal; antiarrhythmic; antihypertensive; also used for traumatic brain injury* [propranolol HCl] 80, 120 mg

inocoterone INN *anti-acne* [also: inocoterone acetate]

inocoterone acetate USAN *anti-acne* [also: inocoterone]

inolimomab *investigational (orphan) for graft-versus-host disease*

INOmax inhalation gas ℞ *inhalation gas for neonatal hypoxic respiratory failure due to persistent pulmonary hypertension (orphan); investigational (orphan) for acute adult respiratory distress syndrome and to diagnose sarcoidosis* [nitric oxide] 100, 800 ppm

inosine INN, JAN ⧗ Anacin; Enzone; Unasyn

inosine pranobex BAN, JAN *investigational (orphan) immunomodulator for subacute sclerosing panencephalitis*

inosiplex [now: inosine pranobex]

Inositech capsules OTC *dietary lipotropic* [inositol] 324 mg

inositol NF *lipotropic supplement* 250, 500, 650 mg oral ⧗ anisatil

inositol niacinate USAN *peripheral vasodilator* [also: inositol nicotinate]

inositol nicotinate INN, BAN *peripheral vasodilator* [also: inositol niacinate]

inotropes *a class of drugs that affect the force or energy of muscle contractions*

Inova Acne Control Therapy Easy Pad cleansing pads ℞ *keratolytic for acne* [benzoyl peroxide; salicylic acid; tocopherol (vitamin E)] 4%•1%•5%, 8%•2%•5%

Inova Easy Pad cleansing pads ℞ *keratolytic for acne* [benzoyl peroxide; tocopherol (vitamin E)] 4%•5%, 8%•5%

inprochone [see: inproquone]

inproquone INN, BAN

INSH (isonicotinoyl-salicylidene-hydrazine) [see: salinazid]

InspirEase (trademarked delivery device) *portable inhalation device*

Inspra film-coated tablets ℞ *aldosterone receptor antagonist for hypertension and congestive heart failure (CHF); improves survival after a cardiovascular event* [eplerenone] 25, 50 mg

Insta-Glucose oral gel OTC *blood glucose elevating agent for hypoglycemia* [glucose] 40%

insulin USP, JAN *antidiabetic*

insulin, biphasic INN, BAN *antidiabetic*

insulin, biphasic isophane BAN *antidiabetic*

insulin, dalanated USAN, INN *antidiabetic*

insulin, globin zinc USP [also: globin zinc insulin]

insulin, human USAN, USP, INN, BAN, JAN *antidiabetic*

insulin, human, isophane USP *antidiabetic*

insulin, human zinc USP *antidiabetic*

insulin, human zinc, extended USP *antidiabetic*

insulin, isophane USP, BAN, INN, JAN *antidiabetic*

insulin, neutral USAN, JAN *antidiabetic* [also: neutral insulin]

insulin, NPH (neutral protamine Hagedorn) [see: insulin, isophane]

insulin, protamine zinc (PZI) USP *antidiabetic* [also: insulin zinc protamine; protamine zinc insulin]

insulin argine INN *antidiabetic*

insulin aspart USAN, INN *rapid-acting insulin analogue for diabetes*

insulin aspart protamine *intermediate-acting insulin analogue for diabetes*

insulin defalan INN *antidiabetic*

insulin detemir USAN *human-derived (rDNA) antidiabetic; long-acting insu-*

lin formulation intended to provide continuous basal insulin levels through once- or twice-daily subcu injections

insulin glargine INN *long-acting, once-daily basal insulin analogue for diabetes*

insulin glulisine *human-derived (rDNA) antidiabetic; rapid-onset, short-acting insulin analogue for diabetes*

insulin I 125 USAN *radioactive agent*

insulin I 131 USAN *radioactive agent*

insulin lispro USAN, INN, BAN *rapid-acting insulin analogue for diabetes*

insulin lispro protamine *intermediate-acting insulin analogue for diabetes*

Insulin Reaction oral gel OTC *blood glucose elevating agent for hypoglycemia* [glucose] 40%

insulin zinc USP, INN, BAN, JAN *antidiabetic*

insulin zinc, extended USP *antidiabetic* [also: insulin zinc suspension (crystalline)]

insulin zinc, prompt USP *antidiabetic* [also: insulin zinc suspension (amorphous)]

insulin zinc protamine JAN *antidiabetic* [also: insulin, protamine zinc; protamine zinc insulin]

insulin zinc suspension (amorphous) INN, BAN, JAN *antidiabetic* [also: insulin zinc, prompt]

insulin zinc suspension (crystalline) INN, BAN, JAN *antidiabetic* [also: insulin zinc, extended]

insulin-like growth factor-1, recombinant human (rhIGF-1) [now: mecasermin]

Intal aerosol spray ℞ *anti-inflammatory; mast cell stabilizer for prophylactic treatment of allergy, asthma, and bronchospasm* [cromolyn sodium] 800 mcg/dose

Intal solution for nebulization (discontinued 2008) ℞ *anti-inflammatory; mast cell stabilizer for prophylactic treatment of allergy, asthma, and bronchospasm* [cromolyn sodium] 20 mg/2 mL ampule

Integrilin IV injection ℞ *platelet aggregation inhibitor for acute coronary syn-*

drome, unstable angina, myocardial infarction, and cardiac surgery [eptifibatide] 0.75, 2 mg/mL

Intelence tablets ℞ *non-nucleoside reverse transcriptase inhibitor (NNRTI) for drug-resistant HIV-1 infections* [etravirine] 100, 200 mg

Intensol (trademarked dosage form) *concentrated oral solution*

α-2-interferon [see: interferon alfa-2b, recombinant]

interferon, fibroblast [now: interferon beta]

interferon, leukocyte [now: interferon alfa-n3]

interferon α2b [see: interferon alfa-2b]

interferon αA [see: interferon alfa-2a]

interferon alfa JAN *immunostimulant*

interferon alfa (BALL-1) JAN

interferon alfa-1b *investigational (orphan) antineoplastic for multiple myeloma*

interferon alfa-2a (IFN-αA; rIFN-A) USAN, INN, BAN, JAN *immunostimulant for hairy cell leukemia, hepatitis C, Kaposi sarcoma (orphan), and chronic myelogenous leukemia (orphan); investigational (orphan) for malignant melanoma and esophageal, renal, colorectal, and other cancers*

interferon alfa-2a & fluorouracil *investigational (orphan) for esophageal carcinoma and advanced colorectal cancer*

interferon alfa-2b (IFN-α2) USAN, INN, BAN *antineoplastic for hairy-cell leukemia, malignant melanoma, AIDS-related Kaposi sarcoma (orphan), and various other cancers; antiviral for condylomata acuminata and chronic hepatitis B and C infection*

interferon alfacon-1 USAN *bioengineered consensus interferon for the treatment of chronic hepatitis C virus (HCV) infections*

interferon alfa-n1 USAN, INN, BAN *antineoplastic; biological response modifier for chronic hepatitis C; investigational (orphan) for AIDS-related Kaposi* *sarcoma and human papillomavirus in severe respiratory papillomatosis*

interferon alfa-n3 USAN *immunomodulator and antiviral for condylomata acuminata*

interferon beta (IFN-B) BAN, JAN *antineoplastic; antiviral; immunomodulator*

interferon beta-1a USAN *immunomodulator for relapsing multiple sclerosis (orphan); investigational (orphan) for non-A, non-B hepatitis, juvenile rheumatoid arthritis, Kaposi sarcoma, brain tumors, and various other cancers*

interferon beta-1b USAN *immunomodulator for relapsing-remitting multiple sclerosis (orphan); investigational (orphan) for AIDS*

interferon gamma-1a JAN

interferon gamma-1b USAN, INN, BAN *immunoregulator for chronic granulomatous disease (orphan) and severe malignant osteopetrosis (orphan); investigational (orphan) for renal cell carcinoma and pulmonary fibrosis*

interferon gamma-2a [see: interferon gamma-1b]

α-interferons [see: interferon alfa-n1 and -n3]

Intergel irrigating solution ℞ *adhesion barrier for open gynecological and lower GI surgical procedures* [ferric hyaluronate] 0.5% ⑨ Antrocol

interleukin-1 alpha, recombinant human *investigational (orphan) hematopoietic potentiator for aplastic anemia and bone marrow transplants*

interleukin-1 receptor antagonist, recombinant human [now: anakinra]

interleukin-1 Trap [now: canakinumab]

interleukin-2 (aldesleukin) + interferon alfa-2 *chemotherapy protocol for renal cell carcinoma* [also known as: bio-chemotherapy]

interleukin-2, liposome-encapsulated recombinant *investigational (orphan) for brain, central nervous system, kidney, and pelvic cancers*

interleukin-2, recombinant (IL-2) [see: aldesleukin; teceleukin; celmoleukin]

interleukin-2 PEG [see: PEG-interleukin-2]

interleukin-3, recombinant human *investigational (orphan) adjunct to bone marrow transplants and Diamond-Blackfan anemia*

interleukin-10 (IL-10) [see: ilodecakin]

interleukin-11, recombinant human (rhIL-11) [see: oprelvekin]

interleukin-12 (IL-12) [see: edodekin alfa]

intermedine INN

Intermezzo sublingual tablet *investigational (NDA filed) doseform of the sedative/hypnotic used in* **Ambien** [zolpidem tartrate]

Intestinex capsules OTC *natural intestinal bacteria; probiotic; dietary supplement; fever blister treatment* [Lactobacillus acidophilus] 100 million CFU

intoplicine INN *antineoplastic; topoisomerase I and II inhibitor*

Intrachol *investigational (orphan) for choline deficiency of long-term parenteral nutrition* [choline chloride]

IntraDose injectable gel *investigational (NDA filed, orphan) alkylating antineoplastic for squamous cell carcinoma of the head and neck; investigational (orphan) for metastatic malignant melanoma* [cisplatin; epinephrine]

Intralipid 10% IV infusion (discontinued 2008) ℞ *nutritional therapy* [fat emulsion]

Intralipid 20%; Intralipid 30% IV infusion ℞ *nutritional therapy* [fat emulsion]

IntraSite gel OTC *wound dressing* [graft T starch copolymer] 2%

intravascular perfluorochemical emulsion *synthetic blood oxygen carrier for PTCA*

intravenous fat emulsion [see: fat emulsion, intravenous]

intrazole USAN, INN *anti-inflammatory*

intrinsic factor concentrate *antiane-mic to enhance the body's utilization of vitamin B₁₂*

intriptyline INN *antidepressant* [also: intriptyline HCl]

intriptyline HCl USAN *antidepressant* [also: intriptyline]

Introlan Half-Strength oral liquid OTC *enteral nutritional therapy* [lactose-free formula]

Introlite oral liquid OTC *enteral nutritional therapy* [lactose-free formula]

Intron A subc or IM injection (discontinued 2009) ℞ *antineoplastic for hairy cell leukemia, malignant melanoma, Kaposi sarcoma (orphan), and various other cancers; antiviral for condylomata acuminata and chronic hepatitis B and C infection* [interferon alfa-2b] 3, 5, 10, 18, 25, 50 million IU/vial ② Anturane

Intropaste oral paste ℞ *radiopaque contrast medium for esophageal imaging* [barium sulfate] 70%

Introvale tablets ℞ *monophasic oral contraceptive* [levonorgestrel; ethinyl estradiol] 0.15•0.03 mg

Intuniv extended-release tablets ℞ *nonstimulant treatment for attention-deficit/hyperactivity disorder (ADHD)* [guanfacine (as HCl)] 1, 2, 3, 4 mg

Inula helenium *medicinal herb* [see: elecampane]

inulin USP *diagnostic aid for renal function; dietary fiber supplement* 100 mg/mL injection ② Enlon

Invanz powder for IV or IM injection ℞ *broad-spectrum carbapenem antibiotic* [ertapenem (as sodium)] 1 g

Invega OROS (extended-release caplets) ℞ *once-daily novel (atypical) antipsychotic for schizophrenia; investigational (Phase III) for manic episodes of a bipolar disorder* [paliperidone] 1.5, 3, 6, 9 mg

Invega Sustenna extended-release IM injection in prefilled syringes ℞ *once-monthly antipsychotic for schizophrenia* [paliperidone (as palmitate)] 39, 78, 117, 156, 234 mg

invenol [see: carbutamide]

Inversine tablets (discontinued 2009) ℞ *antiadrenergic; ganglionic blocker for severe hypertension; investigational (orphan) for Tourette syndrome* [mecamylamine HCl] 2.5 mg

invert sugar [see: sugar, invert]

Invirase tablets, capsules ℞ *antiretroviral protease inhibitor for HIV* [saquinavir (as mesylate)] 500 mg; 200 mg

Invites RX film-coated tablets ℞ *vitamin/zinc supplement* [multiple vitamins; zinc; folic acid; biotin] ±• 12.5•1•0.3 mg

iobenguane (¹³¹I) INN *radioactive agent* [also: iobenguane I 131]

iobenguane I 123 USP *radioactive diagnostic aid*

iobenguane sulfate I 123 *radioactive diagnostic aid for the detection of metastatic pheochromocytoma or neuroblastoma (orphan)*

iobenguane sulfate I 131 USAN *diagnostic aid for pheochromocytoma (orphan)*

iobenzamic acid USAN, INN, BAN *radiopaque contrast medium for cholecystography*

Iobid DM sustained-release tablets ℞ *antitussive; expectorant* [dextromethorphan hydrobromide; guaifenesin] 30•600 mg

iobutoic acid INN

iocanlidic acid I 123 USAN *cardiac diagnostic aid*

Iocare Balanced Salt ophthalmic solution OTC *intraocular irrigating solution* [sodium chloride (balanced saline solution)]

iocarmate meglumine USAN *radiopaque contrast medium* [also: meglumine iocarmate]

iocarmic acid USAN, INN, BAN *radiopaque contrast medium*

iocetamic acid USAN, USP, INN, BAN *oral radiopaque contrast medium for cholecystography (62% iodine)*

iodamide USAN, INN, BAN *radiopaque contrast medium*

iodamide meglumine USAN *radiopaque contrast medium*

iodecimol INN

iodecol [see: iodecimol]

iodetryl INN

Iodex; Iodex-P ointment OTC *broad-spectrum antimicrobial* [povidone-iodine] 4.7%; 10% ⧈ ADEKs; Adoxa; Edex

Iodex with Methyl Salicylate ointment OTC *anti-infective; analgesic; counterirritant* [iodine; methyl salicylate] 4.7%•4.8%

iodinated (¹²⁵I) human serum albumin INN *radioactive agent; blood volume test* [also: albumin, iodinated I 125 serum]

iodinated (¹³¹I) human serum albumin INN, JAN *radioactive agent; intrathecal imaging agent; blood volume test* [also: albumin, iodinated I 131 serum]

iodinated glycerol [see: glycerol, iodinated]

iodinated I 125 albumin [see: albumin, iodinated I 125]

iodinated I 131 aggregated albumin [see: albumin, iodinated I 131 aggregated]

iodinated I 131 albumin [see: albumin, iodinated I 131]

iodine USP *broad-spectrum topical anti-infective; treatment for hyperthyroidism; thyroid saturation agent to block the uptake of radioactive iodine after a nuclear accident or attack; element (I)* 2% topical

iodine I 131 6B-iodomethyl-19-norcholesterol *investigational (orphan) for adrenal cortical imaging*

iodine I 131 metaiodobenzylguanidine sulfate [now: iobenguane sulfate I 131]

iodine I 131 tositumomab *monoclonal antibody to non-Hodgkin lymphoma (NHL), radiolabeled with iodine I 131, for the detection of NHL and targeted delivery of radiation (orphan)* [see also: tositumomab]

iodipamide USP, BAN *parenteral radiopaque contrast medium* [also: adipiodone]

iodipamide meglumine USP, BAN *parenteral radiopaque contrast medium (49.42% iodine)* [also: adipiodone meglumine]

iodipamide methylglucamine [see: iodipamide meglumine]

iodipamide sodium USP *parenteral radiopaque contrast medium*

iodipamide sodium I 131 USAN *radioactive agent*

iodisan [see: prolonium iodide]

iodixanol USAN, INN, BAN *parenteral radiopaque contrast medium (49.1% iodine)*

iodized oil NF

iodoalphionic acid NF [also: pheniodol sodium]

iodoantipyrine I 131 USAN *radioactive agent*

iodobehenate calcium NF

m-iodobenzylguanidine sulfate I 123 [see: iobenguane sulfate I 123]

iodocetylic acid (¹²³I) INN *diagnostic aid* [also: iodocetylic acid I 123]

iodocetylic acid I 123 USAN *diagnostic aid* [also: iodocetylic acid (¹²³I)]

iodochlorhydroxyquin [now: clioquinol]

iodocholesterol (¹³¹I) INN *radioactive agent* [also: iodocholesterol I 131]

iodocholesterol I 131 USAN *radioactive agent* [also: iodocholesterol (¹³¹I)]

iodoform NF

iodohippurate sodium I 123 USAN, USP *renal function test; radioactive agent*

iodohippurate sodium I 125 USAN *radioactive agent*

iodohippurate sodium I 131 USAN, USP *renal function test; radioactive agent* [also: sodium iodohippurate (¹³¹I)]

iodohydroxyquin [see: clioquinol]

iodol USP

iodomethamate sodium NF

iodopanoic acid [see: iopanoic acid]

Iodopen IV injection ℞ *iodine supplement; additive to IV solutions for total parenteral nutrition* [sodium iodide

(85% elemental iodine)] 118 mcg/mL (100 mcg/mL I)

iodophthalein, soluble [now: iodophthalein sodium]

iodophthalein sodium NF, INN

iodopyracet NF [also: diodone]

iodopyracet I 125 USAN *radioactive agent*

iodopyracet I 131 USAN *radioactive agent*

iodoquinol USAN, USP *antimicrobial; amebicide for intestinal amebiasis* [also: diiodohydroxyquinoline]

iodoquinol & hydrocortisone *amebicide; antimicrobial; corticosteroidal anti-inflammatory* 1%•1% topical

iodothiouracil INN, BAN

iodothymol [see: thymol iodide]

Iodotope capsules, oral solution (discontinued 2010) ℞ *radioactive antineoplastic for thyroid carcinoma; thyroid inhibitor for hyperthyroidism* [sodium iodide I 131] 8, 15, 30, 50, 100 mCi; 7.05 mCi/mL (7, 14, 28, 70, 106 mCi/vial)

iodoxamate meglumine USAN, BAN *radiopaque contrast medium*

iodoxamic acid USAN, INN, BAN *radiopaque contrast medium*

iodoxyl [see: iodomethamate sodium]

iofendylate INN *radiopaque contrast medium* [also: iophendylate]

iofetamine (^{123}I) INN *diagnostic aid; radioactive agent* [also: iofetamine HCl I 123] ② E-Vitamin

iofetamine HCl I 123 USAN *diagnostic aid; radioactive agent* [also: iofetamine (^{123}I)]

ioflupane I 123 *radiodiagnostic imaging agent for single photon emission computed tomography (SPECT) scans of the brain for the evaluation of parkinsonian syndromes*

Iofoam (trademarked dosage form) *topical foam*

ioglicic acid USAN, INN, BAN *radiopaque contrast medium*

ioglucol USAN, INN *radiopaque contrast medium*

ioglucomide USAN, INN *radiopaque contrast medium*

ioglunide INN

ioglycamic acid USAN, INN, BAN *radiopaque contrast medium for cholecystography*

iogulamide USAN *radiopaque contrast medium*

iohexol USAN, INN, BAN *parenteral radiopaque contrast medium (46.36% iodine)*

iolidonic acid INN

iolixanic acid INN

iomeglamic acid INN

iomeprol USAN, INN, BAN *radiopaque contrast medium*

iomethin I 125 USAN *neoplasm test; radioactive agent* [also: iometin (^{125}I)]

iomethin I 131 USAN *neoplasm test; radioactive agent* [also: iometin (^{131}I)]

iometin (^{125}I) INN *neoplasm test; radioactive agent* [also: iomethin I 125] ② emetine

iometin (^{131}I) INN *neoplasm test; radioactive agent* [also: iomethin I 131] ② emetine

iometopane I 123 USAN *diagnostic imaging aid for dopamine and serotonin transporter sites*

iomorinic acid INN

Ionamin capsules ℞ *anorexiant; CNS stimulant* [phentermine HCl resin complex] 15, 30 mg

Ionax foam OTC *medicated cleanser for acne* [benzalkonium chloride]

Ionax Astringent Skin Cleanser topical liquid OTC *keratolytic cleanser for acne* [salicylic acid; isopropyl alcohol]

Ionax Scrub OTC *abrasive medicated cleanser for acne* [benzalkonium chloride]

ionic contrast media *a class of older radiopaque agents that, in general, have a high osmolar concentration of iodine (the contrast agent), which corresponds to a higher incidence of adverse reactions* [also called: high osmolar contrast media (HOCM)]

Ionil shampoo OTC *antiseborrheic; keratolytic; antiseptic* [salicylic acid; benzalkonium chloride]

Ionil Plus shampoo (discontinued 2011) OTC *antiseborrheic; keratolytic* [salicylic acid] 2%

Ionil T shampoo OTC *antiseborrheic; antipsoriatic* [coal tar] 1%

Ionil-T Plus shampoo OTC *antiseborrheic; antipsoriatic; antipruritic; antibacterial* [coal tar] 2%

Ionosol B and 5% Dextrose IV infusion ℞ *intravenous nutritional/electrolyte therapy* [combined electrolyte solution; dextrose] 500, 1000 mg/dose

Ionosol T and 5% Dextrose IV infusion ℞ *intravenous nutritional/electrolyte therapy* [combined electrolyte solution; dextrose] 500, 1000 mL/dose

ionphylline [see: aminophylline]

Ionsys transdermal patch with a patient-controlled dose release button (discontinued 2010) ℞ *transdermal narcotic analgesic for short-term management of postoperative pain* [fentanyl (as HCl)] 40 mcg/actuation (maximum 3.2 mg/24 hr.)

iopamidol USAN, USP, INN, BAN *parenteral radiopaque contrast medium (49% iodine)*

iopanoic acid USP, INN, BAN *oral radiopaque contrast medium for cholecystography (66.68% iodine)*

iopentol USAN, INN, BAN *radiopaque contrast medium*

Iophen tablets, elixir, drops ℞ *expectorant* [iodinated glycerol] 30 mg; 60 mg/5 mL; 50 mg/mL ② Aviane

Iophen C-NR oral liquid ℞ *narcotic antitussive; expectorant* [codeine phosphate; guaifenesin] 10•100 mg/5 mL

Iophen DM-NR oral liquid ℞ *antitussive; expectorant* [dextromethorphan hydrobromide; guaifenesin] 10•100 mg/5 mL

Iophen NR oral liquid OTC *expectorant* [guaifenesin] 100 mg/5 mL

iophendylate USP, BAN *radiopaque contrast medium* [also: iofendylate]

iophenoic acid INN [also: iophenoxic acid]

iophenoxic acid USP [also: iophenoic acid]

Iophylline elixir (discontinued 2007) ℞ *antiasthmatic; bronchodilator; expectorant* [theophylline; iodinated glycerol] 120•30 mg/15 mL ② Avolean

Iopidine Drop-Tainers (eye drops) ℞ *sympathomimetic antiglaucoma agent* [apraclonidine HCl] 0.5%, 1%

ioprocemic acid USAN, INN *radiopaque contrast medium*

iopromide USAN, INN, BAN *parenteral radiopaque contrast medium (39% iodine)*

iopronic acid USAN, INN, BAN *radiopaque contrast medium for cholecystography*

iopydol USAN, INN, BAN *radiopaque contrast medium for bronchography*

iopydone USAN, INN, BAN *radiopaque contrast medium for bronchography* ② Ibudone

Iosal II sustained-release tablets ℞ *decongestant; expectorant* [pseudoephedrine HCl; guaifenesin] 60•600 mg ② Ocella; Wyseal

iosarcol INN

Iosat tablets OTC *thyroid saturation agent to block the uptake of radioactive iodine after a nuclear accident or attack* (orphan) [potassium iodide] 130 mg ② Aceta; ICE-T

iosefamic acid USAN, INN *radiopaque contrast medium*

ioseric acid USAN, INN *radiopaque contrast medium*

iosimide INN

iosulamide INN *radiopaque contrast medium* [also: iosulamide meglumine]

iosulamide meglumine USAN *radiopaque contrast medium* [also: iosulamide]

iosulfan blue *parenteral radiopaque contrast medium for lymphography*

iosumetic acid USAN, INN *radiopaque contrast medium*

iotalamic acid INN *radiopaque contrast medium* [also: iothalamic acid]

iotasul USAN, INN *radiopaque contrast medium*

iotetric acid USAN, INN *radiopaque contrast medium*

iothalamate meglumine USP *parenteral radiopaque contrast medium (47% iodine)* [also: meglumine iothalamate]

iothalamate sodium USP *parenteral radiopaque contrast medium (59.9% iodine)* [also: sodium iothalamate]

iothalamate sodium I 125 USAN *radioactive agent* [also: sodium iotalamate (^{125}I)]

iothalamate sodium I 131 USAN *radioactive agent* [also: sodium iotalamate (^{131}I)]

iothalamic acid USP, BAN *radiopaque contrast medium* [also: iotalamic acid]

iothiouracil sodium

iotranic acid INN

iotriside INN

iotrizoic acid INN

iotrol [now: iotrolan]

iotrolan USAN, INN, BAN *parenteral radiopaque contrast medium* 🔲 Atralin

iotroxic acid USAN, INN, BAN *radiopaque contrast medium*

iotyrosine I 131 USAN *radioactive agent*

ioversol USAN, INN, BAN *parenteral radiopaque contrast medium (47.3% iodine)*

ioxabrolic acid INN

ioxaglate meglumine USAN *parenteral radiopaque contrast medium* [also: meglumine ioxaglate]

ioxaglate sodium USAN *parenteral radiopaque contrast medium* [also: sodium ioxaglate]

ioxaglic acid USAN, INN, BAN *radiopaque contrast medium*

ioxilan USAN, INN *diagnostic aid* 🔲 Exelon

ioxitalamic acid INN

ioxotrizoic acid USAN, INN *radiopaque contrast medium*

iozomic acid INN

IPA (ifosfamide, Platinol, Adriamycin) *chemotherapy protocol for pediatric hepatoblastoma*

ipazilide fumarate USAN *antiarrhythmic*

ipecac USP *emetic*

ipecac, milk *medicinal herb* [see: birthroot; dogbane]

ipecac, powdered USP

ipexidine INN *dental caries preventative* [also: ipexidine mesylate]

ipexidine mesylate USAN, INN *dental caries preventative* [also: ipexidine]

ipilimumab *cytotoxic T-lymphocyte antigen 4 (CTLA-4)–blocking antibody for unresectable or metastatic melanoma; investigational (NDA filed) for non–small cell lung cancer (NSCLC)*

Iplex subcu injection (discontinued 2008) ℞ *recombinant human insulin-like growth factor-1 (rhIGF-1) for children with primary IGF deficiency without concomitant growth hormone (GH) deficiency (orphan)* [mecasermin rinfabate]

ipodate calcium USP *oral radiopaque contrast medium for cholecystography (61.7% iodine)*

ipodate sodium USAN, USP *oral radiopaque contrast medium for cholecystography (61.4% iodine)* [also: sodium ipodate; sodium iopodate]

IPOL subcu injection ℞ *vaccine for poliovirus types 1, 2, and 3* [poliovirus vaccine, inactivated] 0.5 mL 🔲 apple

Ipomoea pandurata *medicinal herb* [see: wild jalap]

Ipomoea violacea **(morning glory)** seeds contain *lysergic acid amide, chemically similar to LSD, which produces hallucinations when ingested as a street drug* [see also: LSD]

ipragratine INN

ipramidil INN

ipratropium bromide USAN, INN, BAN *anticholinergic bronchodilator for bronchospasm, emphysema, and chronic obstructive pulmonary disease (COPD); antisecretory for rhinorrhea 0.02% inhalation; 0.03%, 0.06% nasal spray*

ipratropium bromide & albuterol sulfate *bronchodilator combination for bronchospasm, emphysema, and chronic obstructive pulmonary disease (COPD) 0.017%•0.083% (0.5•3 mg/dose) inhaler*

iprazochrome INN
iprazone [see: isoprazone]
ipriflavone INN
iprindole USAN, INN, BAN *antidepressant*
Iprivasc powder for subcu injection ℞ *anticoagulant; thrombin inhibitor for the prevention of deep vein thrombosis (DVT) in elective hip replacement surgery* [desirudin] 15 mg/dose
iprocinodine HCl USAN, BAN *veterinary antibacterial*
iproclozide INN, BAN
iprocrolol INN
iprofenin USAN *hepatic function test*
iproheptine INN
iproniazid INN, BAN
ipronidazole USAN, INN, BAN *antiprotozoal (Histomonas)*
ipropethidine [see: properidine]
iproplatin USAN, INN, BAN *antineoplastic*
iprotiazem INN
iproxamine INN *vasodilator* [also: iproxamine HCl]
iproxamine HCl USAN *vasodilator* [also: iproxamine]
iprozilamine INN
ipsalazide INN, BAN
ipsapirone INN, BAN *anxiolytic* [also: ipsapirone HCl]
ipsapirone HCl USAN *anxiolytic* [also: ipsapirone]
Ipstyl (name changed to **Somatuline Depot** upon marketing release in 2007)
IPTD (isopropyl-thiadiazol) [see: glyprothiazol]
IPV (inactivated poliomyelitis vaccine) [see: poliovirus vaccine, inactivated]
IPV (inactivated poliovaccine) [see: poliovirus vaccine, inactivated]
iquindamine INN
Iquix eye drops ℞ *fluoroquinolone antibiotic for corneal ulcers* [levofloxacin] 1.5%
¹⁹²Ir [see: iridium Ir 192]
irbesartan USAN *angiotensin receptor blocker (ARB) for hypertension; treatment to delay the progression of diabetic nephropathy*

Ircon tablets OTC *iron supplement* [carbonyl iron] 66 mg ⊡ AeroCaine; argon
Ircon-FA tablets (discontinued 2008) OTC *vitamin/iron supplement* [iron (as carbonyl iron); folic acid] 82•0.8 mg
Iressa film-coated tablets ℞ *antineoplastic for advanced or metastatic non–small cell lung cancer (NSCLC)* [gefitinib] 250 mg ⊡ Aerius; Ear-Eze; Oracea; OROS; Urso
irgasan [see: triclosan]
iridium *element (Ir)*
iridium Ir 192 USAN *radioactive agent*
irindalone INN
irinotecan INN *topoisomerase I inhibitor; antineoplastic for metastatic colon and rectal cancers* [also: irinotecan HCl]
irinotecan HCl USAN, JAN *topoisomerase I inhibitor; antineoplastic for metastatic colorectal cancer* [also: irinotecan] 20 mg/mL injection
Iris florentina *medicinal herb* [see: orris root]
Iris versicolor *medicinal herb* [see: blue flag]
Irish broom *medicinal herb* [see: broom]
Irish moss (Chondrus crispus) plant *medicinal herb used as a demulcent*
irloxacin INN
irofulven USAN, INN *DNA synthesis inhibitor; apoptosis inducer; investigational (orphan) antineoplastic for renal cell carcinoma and ovarian cancer*
irolapride INN
Iromin-G film-coated tablets OTC *vitamin/calcium/iron supplement* [multiple vitamins; calcium (as gluconate, lactate, and carbonate); iron (as ferrous gluconate); folic acid] ≐•29.5•57•0.8 mg
iron *element (Fe)* ⊡ Errin
iron carbohydrate complex [see: polyferose]
Iron Chews chewable tablets OTC *iron supplement* [carbonyl iron] 15 mg
iron dextran USP *hematinic*
iron heptonate [see: gleptoferron]
iron hexacyanoferrate [see: ferric hexacyanoferrate]

iron hydroxide sucrose complex [see: iron sucrose; saccharated ferric oxide]

iron oxide, saccharated [see: iron sucrose; saccharated ferric oxide]

iron perchloride [see: ferric chloride]

iron polymalether [see: ferropolimaler]

Iron Protein Plus capsules OTC *iron supplement* [iron (as protein succinylate)] 15 mg

iron protein succinylate *hematinic (5% elemental iron)*

iron saccharate [see: iron sucrose; saccharated ferric oxide]

iron sorbitex USAN, USP *hematinic*

iron sucrose USAN *hematinic for iron deficiency in patients with non-dialysis-dependent chronic kidney disease (NDD-CKD), hemodialysis-dependent chronic kidney disease (HDD-CKD), and peritoneal dialysis-dependent chronic kidney disease (PDD-CKD)* [also: saccharated ferric oxide]

iron sugar [see: iron sucrose; saccharated ferric oxide]

Iron-Folic 500 tablets OTC *vitamin/calcium/iron supplement* [multiple B vitamins; calcium; iron (as ferrous fumarate); vitamin C (as sodium ascorbate); folic acid] ≜•105•28•500•0.8 mg

Irrigate eye wash OTC *extraocular irrigating solution* [sterile isotonic solution] ⎇ ergot

irritant laxatives *a subclass of laxatives that work by direct action on the intestinal mucosa and nerve plexus to increase peristaltic action* [more commonly called: stimulant laxatives]

irsogladine INN

irtemazole USAN, INN, BAN *uricosuric*

IS 5-MN (isosorbide 5-mononitrate) [see: isorbide mononitrate]

isaglidole INN

isamfazone INN

isamoltan INN

isamoxole USAN, INN, BAN *antiasthmatic*

isatoribine USAN *immunomodulator; cell growth regulator*

isaxonine INN

isbogrel INN

iseganan *antimicrobial* [also: iseganan HCl]

iseganan HCl USAN, INN *antimicrobial* [also: iseganan]

Isentress film-coated tablets ℞ *antiretroviral for drug-resistant HIV-1 infection* [raltegravir (as potassium)] 400 mg

isepamicin USAN, INN, BAN *aminoglycoside antibiotic*

isethionate USAN, BAN *combining name for radicals or groups* [also: isetionate]

isetionate INN *combining name for radicals or groups* [also: isethionate]

ISG (immune serum globulin) [see: globulin, immune]

Ismo film-coated tablets ℞ *coronary vasodilator; antianginal* [isosorbide mononitrate] 20 mg

Ismotic solution (discontinued 2010) ℞ *osmotic diuretic* [isosorbide] 45%

iso-alcoholic elixir NF

isoaminile INN, BAN

isoamyl p-methoxycinnamate [see: amiloxate]

isoamyl nitrate [see: amyl nitrite]

Iso-B capsules (discontinued 2008) OTC *vitamin supplement* [multiple B vitamins; folic acid; biotin] ≜•200•100 mcg

isobromindione INN

isobucaine HCl USP

isobutamben USAN, INN *topical anesthetic*

isobutane NF *aerosol propellant* ⎇ azapetine

isobutyl p-aminobenzoate [see: isobutamben]

isobutyl α-phenylcyclohexaneglycolate [see: ibuverine]

isobutyl 2-cyanoacrylate (IBC) [see: bucrylate]

isobutyl nitrite; butyl nitrite *amyl nitrite substitutes, sold as euphoric street drugs, which produce a quick but short-lived "rush"* [see also: amyl nitrite; volatile nitrites]

p-isobutylhydratropohydroxamic acid [see: ibuproxam]

isobutylhydrochlorothiazide [see: buthiazide]

isobutyramide *investigational (orphan) for sickle cell disease, beta-thalassemia syndrome, and beta-hemoglobinopathies*

isobuzole BAN [also: glysobuzole]

Isocal *oral liquid* OTC *enteral nutritional therapy* [lactose-free formula] ☒ Asacol; Os-Cal

Isocal HCN *ready-to-use oral liquid* OTC *enteral nutritional therapy* [lactose-free formula]

Isocal HN *oral liquid* OTC *enteral nutritional therapy* [lactose-free formula]

isocarboxazid USP, INN, BAN *monoamine oxidase (MAO) inhibitor for depression*

Isochron *extended-release tablets* ℞ *coronary vasodilator; antianginal* [isosorbide dinitrate] 40 mg

isoconazole USAN, INN, BAN *antibacterial; antifungal* ☒ azaconazole

isocromil INN

Isocult for Bacteriuria *culture paddles for professional use* ℞ *in vitro diagnostic aid for nitrate, uropathogens, or bacteria in the urine*

Isocult for Candida *culture paddles for professional use* ℞ *in vitro diagnostic aid for* Candida albicans *in the vagina*

Isocult for N. gonorrhoeae and Candida *culture test for professional use* ℞ *in vitro diagnostic aid for gonorrhea and Candida in various specimens*

Isocult for Neisseria gonorrhoeae *culture paddles for professional use* ℞ *in vitro diagnostic aid for gonorrhea*

Isocult for Staphylococcus aureus *culture paddles for professional use* ℞ *in vitro diagnostic aid for* Staphylococcus aureus *in exudate*

Isocult for Streptococcal pharyngitis *culture paddles for professional use* ℞ *in vitro diagnostic test for streptococcal pharyngitis in throat swabs*

Isocult for T. vaginalis and Candida *culture test for professional use* ℞ *in vitro diagnostic aid for* Trichomonas *and* Candida *in vaginal or urethral cultures*

isodapamide [see: zidapamide]

***d*-isoephedrine HCl** [see: pseudoephedrine HCl]

isoetarine INN *sympathomimetic bronchodilator* [also: isoetharine]

isoethadione [see: paramethadione]

isoetharine USAN, BAN *sympathomimetic bronchodilator* [also: isoetarine]

isoetharine HCl USP, BAN *sympathomimetic bronchodilator* 1% inhalation

isoetharine mesylate USP, BAN *sympathomimetic bronchodilator*

isofezolac INN

isoflupredone INN, BAN *anti-inflammatory* [also: isoflupredone acetate]

isoflupredone acetate USAN *anti-inflammatory* [also: isoflupredone]

isoflurane USAN, USP, INN, BAN *inhalation general anesthetic*

isoflurophate USP *antiglaucoma agent; irreversible cholinesterase inhibitor miotic* [also: dyflos]

Isoject (trademarked delivery form) *prefilled disposable syringe*

Isolan *oral liquid* OTC *enteral nutritional therapy* [lactose-free formula]

isoleucine (L-isoleucine) USAN, USP, INN, JAN *essential amino acid; symbols: Ile, I*

isoleucine & leucine & valine *investigational (orphan) for hyperphenylalaninemia*

Isolyte E; Isolyte S; Isolyte S pH 7.4 *IV infusion* ℞ *intravenous electrolyte therapy* [combined electrolyte solution] ☒ esilate; eysilate

Isolyte G (H; M; P; R; S) with 5% Dextrose *IV infusion* ℞ *intravenous nutritional/electrolyte therapy* [combined electrolyte solution; dextrose]

Isolyte S pH 7.4 *IV infusion* ℞ *intravenous electrolyte therapy* [combined electrolyte solution]

isomazole INN *cardiotonic* [also: isomazole HCl]

isomazole HCl USAN *cardiotonic* [also: isomazole]

isomeprobamate [see: carisoprodol]

isomer [def.] *One of a group of chemical compounds having the same molecular formula, but differing in either the arrangement of atoms or the bonds* *between atoms in the compound.* [see also: enantiomer]

isomerol USAN *antiseptic*

isometamidium BAN [also: isometamidium chloride]

isometamidium chloride INN [also: isometamidium]

isomethadone INN, BAN

isomethepdrine chloride [see: isomethepdrine]

isomethepdrine INN, BAN

isometheptene HCl [see: isomethepdrine]

isometheptene mucate USP *cerebral vasoconstrictor; "possibly effective" for migraine headaches*

isometheptene mucate & dichloralphenazone & acetaminophen *cerebral vasoconstrictor and analgesic for vascular and tension headaches; "possibly effective" for migraine headaches* 65•100•325 mg oral

Isomil oral liquid, powder for oral liquid OTC *hypoallergenic infant food* [soy protein formula] ☑ Esimil

Isomil DF ready-to-use oral liquid OTC *hypoallergenic infant food for management of diarrhea* [soy protein formula]

Isomil SF oral liquid OTC *hypoallergenic infant food* [soy protein formula, sucrose free]

isomolpan INN *antipsychotic; dopamine autoreceptor antagonist* [also: isomolpan HCl]

isomolpan HCl USAN *antipsychotic; dopamine autoreceptor antagonist* [also: isomolpan]

isomylamine HCl USAN *smooth muscle relaxant*

IsonaRif capsules ℞ *tuberculostatic* [rifampin; isoniazid] 300•150 mg

isoniazid USP, INN, BAN *bactericidal; primary tuberculostatic* 50, 100, 300 mg oral; 50 mg/5 mL oral; 100 mg/mL injection

isonicophen [see: aconiazide]

isonicotinic acid hydrazide (INH) [see: isoniazid]

isonicotinic acid vanillylidenehydrazide [see: ftivazide]

1-isonicotinoyl-2-salicylidenehydrazine (INSH) [see: salinazid]

isonicotinylhydrazine [see: isoniazid]

isonixin INN

isooctadecanol [see: isostearyl alcohol]

isooctadecyl alcohol [see: isostearyl alcohol]

Isopan oral liquid OTC *antacid* [magaldrate] 540 mg/5 mL ☑ azabon

Isopan Plus oral liquid OTC *antacid; antiflatulent* [magaldrate; simethicone] 540•40 mg/5 mL

isopentyl p-methoxycinnamate [see: amiloxate]

isopentyl nitrite [see: amyl nitrite]

isophenethanol [see: nifenalol]

isoprazone INN, BAN ☑ azaprocin

isoprednidene INN, BAN

isopregnenone [see: dydrogesterone]

isoprenaline INN, BAN *sympathomimetic bronchodilator; vasopressor for shock* [also: isoproterenol HCl]

L-isoprenaline [see: levisoprenaline]

isoprenaline HCl [see: isoproterenol HCl]

Isoprinosine *investigational (orphan) immunomodulator for subacute sclerosing panencephalitis* [inosine pranobex]

isoprofen INN

isopropamide iodide USP, INN, BAN *peptic ulcer adjunct*

isopropanol [see: isopropyl alcohol]

isopropicillin INN

isoproponum iodide [see: isopropamide iodide]

7-isopropoxyisoflavone [see: ipriflavone]

isopropyl alcohol USP *topical anti-infective/antiseptic; solvent*

isopropyl alcohol, rubbing USP *rubefacient*

N-isopropyl meprobamate [see: carisoprodol]

isopropyl myristate NF *emollient*

isopropyl palmitate NF *oleaginous vehicle*

isopropyl sebacate

isopropyl unoprostone [see: unoprostone isopropyl]

392   isopropylantipyrine

isopropylantipyrine [see: propyphenazone]

isopropylarterenol HCl [see: isoproterenol HCl]

isopropylarterenol sulfate [see: isoproterenol sulfate]

isoproterenol HCl USP *sympathomimetic bronchodilator; vasopressor for cardiac, hypovolemic, or septic shock; adjunct therapy for congestive heart failure (CHF)* [also: isoprenaline] 1:5000 (0.2 mg/mL) injection

isoproterenol sulfate USP *sympathomimetic bronchodilator*

Isoptin SR film-coated sustained-release tablets ℞ *antihypertensive; antianginal; antiarrhythmic; calcium channel blocker* [verapamil HCl] 120, 180, 240 mg

Isopto Atropine Drop-Tainers (eye drops) ℞ *cycloplegic; mydriatic* [atropine sulfate] 1%

Isopto Carbachol Drop-Tainers (eye drops) ℞ *antiglaucoma agent; direct-acting miotic* [carbachol] 1.5%, 3%

Isopto Carpine Drop-Tainers (eye drops) ℞ *antiglaucoma agent; direct-acting miotic* [pilocarpine HCl] 1%, 2%, 4%, 6%

Isopto Cetamide Drop-Tainers (eye drops) ℞ *antibiotic* [sulfacetamide sodium] 15%

Isopto Homatropine Drop-Tainers (eye drops) ℞ *cycloplegic; mydriatic* [homatropine hydrobromide] 2%, 5%

Isopto Hyoscine Drop-Tainers (eye drops) ℞ *cycloplegic; mydriatic* [scopolamine hydrobromide] 0.25%

Isopto Plain; Isopto Tears Drop-Tainers (eye drops) OTC *moisturizer/lubricant* [hydroxypropyl methylcellulose] 0.5%

Isordil Titradose (tablets) ℞ *coronary vasodilator; antianginal* [isosorbide dinitrate] 5, 10, 20, 30, 40 mg

isosorbide USAN, USP, INN, BAN *osmotic diuretic*

isosorbide dinitrate USAN, USP, INN, BAN *coronary vasodilator; antianginal* 2.5, 5, 10, 20, 30, 40 mg oral

isosorbide mononitrate USAN, INN, BAN *coronary vasodilator; antianginal* 10, 20, 30, 60, 120 mg oral

Isosource; Isosource HN; Isosource 1.5 Cal; Isosource VHN oral liquid OTC *enteral nutritional therapy* [lactose-free formula] 250, 1000, 1500 mL

isospaglumic acid INN

isospirilene [see: spirilene]

isostearyl alcohol USAN *emollient; solvent*

isosulfamerazine [see: sulfaperin]

isosulfan blue USAN *radiopaque contrast medium for lymphography* [also: sulphan blue] 1% injection

isosulpride INN

Isotein HN powder OTC *enteral nutritional therapy* [lactose-free formula]

3-isothiocyanato-1-propene [see: allyl isothiocyanate]

isothiocyanic acid, allyl ester [see: allyl isothiocyanate]

isothipendyl INN, BAN

isothipendyl HCl [see: isothipendyl]

isotiquimide USAN, INN, BAN *antiulcerative*

isotretinoin USAN, USP, INN, BAN *first generation retinoid; systemic keratolytic for severe recalcitrant cystic acne*

isotretinoin anisatil USAN *keratolytic for acne vulgaris*

Isovorin ℞ *chemotherapy "rescue" agent (orphan)* [L-leucovorin] ⊠ acifran

Isovue-200; Isovue-250; Isovue-300; Isovue-370 injection ℞ *radiopaque contrast medium* [iopamidol (49% iodine)] 408 mg/mL (200 mg/mL); 510 mg/mL (250 mg/mL); 612 mg/mL (300 mg/mL); 755 mg/mL (370 mg/mL)

Isovue-M 200; Isovue-M 300 intrathecal injection ℞ *radiopaque contrast medium for myelography* [iopamidol (49% iodine)] 408 mg/mL (200 mg/mL); 612 mg/mL (300 mg/mL)

isoxaprolol INN

isoxepac USAN, INN, BAN *anti-inflammatory*

isoxicam USAN, INN, BAN *nonsteroidal anti-inflammatory drug (NSAID); antiarthritic; analgesic; antipyretic*

isoxsuprine INN, BAN *peripheral vasodilator* [also: isoxsuprine HCl]

isoxsuprine HCl USP, JAN *peripheral vasodilator* [also: isoxsuprine] 10, 20 mg oral

I-Soyalac oral liquid OTC *hypoallergenic infant food* [soy protein formula]

isradipine USAN, INN, BAN *antihypertensive; dihydropyridine calcium channel blocker* 2.5, 5 mg oral

isrodipine [see: isradipine]

Istalol eye drops ℞ *antiglaucoma agent (beta-blocker)* [timolol maleate] 0.5%

Istodax IV infusion ℞ *antineoplastic for cutaneous T-cell lymphoma* [romidepsin] 10 mg

istradefylline *selective adenosine A_{2A} receptor antagonist; modified xanthine derivative; investigational (NDA filed) levodopa/carbidopa potentiator to reduce the severity of dyskinesia and improve motor function in Parkinson disease*

Isuprel IV injection or infusion (discontinued 2009) ℞ *vasopressor for cardiac, hypovolemic, or septic shock; adjunct therapy for congestive heart failure (CHF)* [isoproterenol HCl] 1:5000, 1:50 000 (0.2, 0.02 mg/mL) ② AspirLow

itanoxone INN

itasetron USAN *anxiolytic; antidepressant; antiemetic; serotonin 5-HT₃ receptor antagonist*

itazigrel USAN, INN *platelet antiaggregatory agent*

itazogrel [see: itazigrel]

Itch Relief Gel Spritz spray OTC *poison ivy treatment* [camphor] 0.5%

itchweed *(Veratrum viride)* *medicinal herb* [see: hellebore]

Itch-X topical foam ℞ *corticosteroidal anti-inflammatory* [hydrocortisone] 1%

Itch-X topical spray, gel OTC *anesthetic* [pramoxine HCl] 1%

Itchy Eye eye drops OTC *antihistamine and mast cell stabilizer for allergic conjunctivitis* [ketotifen (as fumarate)] 0.025%

itobarbital [see: butalbital]

itraconazole USAN, INN, BAN *systemic triazole antifungal* 100, 200 mg oral

itramin tosilate INN [also: itramin tosylate]

itramin tosylate BAN [also: itramin tosilate]

itrocainide INN

iturelix USAN, INN *gonadotropin releasing hormone antagonist; ovarian and testicular steroid suppressant*

I-Valex-1 powder OTC *formula for infants with leucine catabolism disorder* ② Avelox; Euflex

I-Valex-2 powder OTC *enteral nutritional therapy for leucine catabolism disorder* ② Avelox; Euflex

Ivarest cream OTC *poison ivy treatment* [calamine; diphenhydramine HCl] 14%•2%

ivarimod INN

Iveegam EN powder for IV infusion (discontinued 2010) ℞ *passive immunizing agent for HIV and Kawasaki syndrome; investigational (orphan) for acute myocarditis and juvenile rheumatoid arthritis; also used for Guillain-Barré syndrome, myasthenia gravis, and multiple sclerosis* [immune globulin (IGIV)] 5 g/dose

ivermectin USAN, INN, BAN *antiparasitic; anthelmintic for strongyloidiasis and onchocerciasis; also used to prevent the transmission of scabies to healthcare workers*

ivermectin component B_{1a}
ivermectin component B_{1b}

IVIG (intravenous immunoglobulin) [q.v.]

ivoqualine INN ② Evoclin

ivy *medicinal herb* [see: American ivy; English ivy; poison ivy]

Ivy Block lotion OTC *preventative for poison ivy, oak, or sumac; use before the risk of exposure* [bentoquatam] 5%

Ivy Cleanse medicated wipes OTC *to remove toxic oils from poison ivy, oak, or sumac* [isopropanol; cetyl alcohol]

Ivy Soothe cream OTC *poison ivy treatment; corticosteroidal anti-inflammatory* [hydrocortisone] 1%

Ivy Stat gel OTC *poison ivy treatment; corticosteroidal anti-inflammatory* [hydrocortisone] 1%

Ivy Super Dry topical liquid OTC *poison ivy treatment* [zinc acetate; isopropanol; benzyl alcohol] 2%•35%•10%

Ivy-Dry lotion OTC *poison ivy treatment* [zinc acetate; isopropanol] 2%•12.5%

ixabepilone *antibiotic antineoplastic; epothilone microtubule inhibitor for advanced or metastatic breast cancer*

Ixel (name changed to **Savella** upon marketing release in 2008)

Ixempra powder for IV infusion ℞ *antibiotic antineoplastic; epothilone microtubule inhibitor for advanced or metastatic breast cancer* [ixabepilone] 15, 45 mg/vial

Ixiaro suspension for injection ℞ *active immunizing agent* [Japanese encephalitis (JE) virus vaccine, inactivated] 6 mcg/0.5 mL dose ② OxyIR

izonsteride USAN *antineoplastic 5α-reductase inhibitor for prostate cancer*

JAK (janus-associated kinase) inhibitors *a class of agents that block the inflammatory and autoimmune action of the janus-associated kinase enzyme*

jalap (Ipomoea jalapa) *medicinal herb* [see: wild jalap]

Jalyn capsules ℞ *combination 5α-reductase blocker and alpha₁-adrenergic blocker for benign prostatic hyperplasia (BPH)* [dutasteride; tamsulosin HCl] 0.5•0.4 mg ② Alinia; aloin; ellaOne

Jamaica mignonette *medicinal herb* [see: henna (Lawsonia)]

Jamaica pepper *medicinal herb* [see: allspice]

Jamaica sarsaparilla *medicinal herb* [see: sarsaparilla]

Jamaica sorrel *medicinal herb* [see: hibiscus]

Jantoven tablets ℞ *coumarin-derivative anticoagulant for myocardial infarction, thromboembolic episodes, venous thrombosis, and pulmonary embolism* [warfarin sodium] 1, 2, 2.5, 3, 4, 5, 6, 7.5, 10 mg

Janumet film-coated caplets ℞ *combination product for type 2 diabetes that increases insulin production, decreases glucose production, and increases cellular response to insulin* [sitagliptin

phosphate; metformin HCl] 50•500, 50•1000 mg

janus-associated kinase (JAK) inhibitors *a class of agents that block the inflammatory and autoimmune action of the janus-associated kinase enzyme*

Januvia film-coated tablets ℞ *antidiabetic for type 2 diabetes that enhances the function of the body's incretin system to increase insulin production in the pancreas and reduce glucose production in the liver* [sitagliptin phosphate] 25, 50, 100 mg ② Gianvi

Japanese encephalitis (JE) virus vaccine, live attenuated *active immunizing agent (orphan)*

Japanese encephalitis (JE) virus vaccine, inactivated *active immunizing agent*

jasmine (Jasminum officinale) *flowers medicinal herb used as a calmative* ② Yasmin

jaundice berry *medicinal herb* [see: barberry]

jaundice root *medicinal herb* [see: goldenseal]

java pepper *medicinal herb* [see: cubeb]

Jay-Phyl syrup ℞ *antiasthmatic; bronchodilator; expectorant* [dyphylline; guaifenesin] 200•100 mg/10 mL ② Avail

J-Cof DHC oral liquid ℞ *narcotic antitussive; antihistamine; decongestant* [dihydrocodeine bitartrate; brompheniramine maleate; pseudoephedrine HCl] 7.5•3•15 mg/5 mL

Jeffersonia diphylla medicinal herb [see: twin leaf]

Jenloga tablets ℞ *antihypertensive; also used for ADHD, opioid and methadone withdrawal, and smoking cessation* [clonidine HCl] 0.1 mg

Jersey tea *medicinal herb* [see: New Jersey tea]

Jerusalem cowslip; Jerusalem sage *medicinal herb* [see: lungwort]

jessamine, yellow *medicinal herb* [see: gelsemium]

Jesuit's bark *medicinal herb* [see: quinine]

Jets chewable tablets OTC *dietary supplement* [lysine; multiple vitamins] 300• ± mg ⊠ A/T/S; oats

JE-VAX powder for subcu injection ℞ *active immunizing agent (orphan)* [Japanese encephalitis (JE) virus vaccine, live attenuated] 0.5 mL (1–3 years), 1 mL (≥ 4 years)

Jevity; Jevity 1.5 Cal ready-to-use oral liquid OTC *enteral nutritional therapy* [lactose-free formula] 237 mL/can ⊠ Avita

Jevtana IV infusion ℞ *antineoplastic for metastatic hormone-refractory prostate cancer (mHRPC)* [cabazitaxel] 40 mg/mL

jewelweed (*Impatiens balsamina; I. biflora; I. capensis*) *juice medicinal herb for prophylaxis and treatment of poison ivy rash*

Jew's harp plant *medicinal herb* [see: birthroot]

jiaogulan (*Gynostemma pentaphyllum*) leaves *medicinal herb used to regulate blood pressure and strengthen the immune system, and for its adaptogenic, antihyperlipidemic, antineoplastic, antioxidant, and cardio- and cerebrovascular protective effects* ⊠ equilin

jimsonweed (*Datura stramonium*) leaves and flowering tops *medicinal herb used as an analgesic, antiasthmatic, antispasmodic, hypnotic, and narcotic; also abused as a street drug*

Jinteli tablets (in packs of 28) ℞ *a mixture of synthetic and equine hormones; hormone replacement therapy for postmenopausal symptoms* [norethindrone acetate; ethinyl estradiol] 1 mg•5 mcg ⊠ Intal

J-Max extended-release tablets, syrup ℞ *decongestant; expectorant* [phenylephrine HCl; guaifenesin] 35•1200 mg; 5•200 mg/5 mL

J-Max DHC oral liquid ℞ *narcotic antitussive; expectorant* [dihydrocodeine bitartrate; guaifenesin] 7.5•100 mg/5 mL

jodphthalein sodium [see: iodophthalein sodium]

joe-pye weed *medicinal herb* [see: queen of the meadow]

jofendylate [see: iophendylate]

Johnson's Shea & Cocoa Butter Baby Lotion OTC *emollient/protectant* [shea butter; cocoa butter; glycerin; mineral oil]

Johnswort *medicinal herb* [see: St. John's wort]

Joint and Bone Vitality tablets OTC *dietary supplement* [vitamins C and D; multiple minerals; glucosamine HCl; chondroitin sulfate] 20 mg•66.67 IU• ± •500 mg•400 mg

Jolessa film-coated tablets (in packs of 91) ℞ *extended-cycle (3 month) monophasic oral contraceptive* [levonorgestrel; ethinyl estradiol] 0.15 mg•30 mcg × 84 days; counters × 7 days ⊠ Alesse

Jolivette tablets (in packs of 28) ℞ *oral contraceptive (progestin only)* [norethindrone] 0.35 mg

jopanoic acid [see: iopanoic acid]

josamycin USAN, INN *antibacterial*

jotrizoic acid [see: iotrizoic acid]

J-Tan oral suspension ℞ *antihistamine* [brompheniramine tannate] 4 mg/5 mL ⊠ Attain

J-Tan D oral suspension ℞ *decongestant; antihistamine* [phenylephrine tannate; brompheniramine tannate] 1.58•2.2 mg/5 mL

J-Tan D HC oral liquid (discontinued 2009) ℞ *narcotic antitussive; antihistamine; decongestant* [hydrocodone bitartrate; brompheniramine maleate; pseudoephedrine HCl] 2.5•3•15 mg/5 mL

J-Tan D PD oral drops ℞ *decongestant; antihistamine; for children 1–24 months* [pseudoephedrine HCl; brompheniramine maleate] 7.5•1 mg/mL

Juglans cinerea medicinal herb [see: butternut]

Juglans nigra medicinal herb [see: black walnut]

Juglans regia medicinal herb [see: English walnut]

Junel 21 Day 1/20; Junel 21 Day 1.5/30 tablets (in packs of 21) ℞ *monophasic oral contraceptive* [norethindrone acetate; ethinyl estradiol] 1 mg•20 mcg; 1.5 mg•30 mcg

Junel Fe 1/20 tablets (in packs of 28) ℞ *monophasic oral contraceptive; iron supplement* [norethindrone acetate; ethinyl estradiol; ferrous fumarate] 1 mg•20 mcg•75 mg × 21 days; 0•0•75 mg × 7 days

Junel Fe 1.5/30 tablets (in packs of 28) ℞ *monophasic oral contraceptive; iron supplement* [norethindrone acetate; ethinyl estradiol; ferrous fumarate] 1.5 mg•30 mcg•75 mg × 21 days; 0•0•75 mg × 7 days

"Junior Strength" products [see under product name]

juniper *(Juniperus communis)* berries *medicinal herb for arthritis, bleeding, bronchitis, colds, edema, infections, kidney infections, pancreatic disorders, uric acid build-up, urinary disorders, and water retention*

juniper, prickly *(Juniperus oxycedrus)* medicinal herb [see: juniper]

juniper tar USP *antieczematic*

Jurnista OROS (extended-release tablets) *investigational (Phase III) delivery form for a narcotic analgesic* [hydromorphone]

Just for Kids tooth gel OTC *dental caries preventative* [stannous fluoride] 0.4%

Just Tears eye drops OTC *moisturizer/lubricant* [polyvinyl alcohol] 1.4% ⚠ Estrace

Juvederm 18; Juvederm 24 subcu injection (discontinued 2007) ℞ *transparent dermal filler for wrinkles and facial folds; increasing numbers indicate increasing density, from fluid for superficial wrinkles to gel for deep folds* [hyaluronic acid] 24 mg/mL

Juvederm 24HV; Juvederm 30; Juvederm 30HV; Juvederm Ultra; Juvederm Ultra Plus subcu injection ℞ *transparent dermal filler for wrinkles and facial folds; increasing numbers indicate increasing density, from fluid for superficial wrinkles to gel for deep folds; "HV" indicates high viscosity* [hyaluronic acid] 24 mg/mL

Juvederm XC; Juvedern Ultra XC; Juvederm Ultra Plus XC subcu injectable gel ℞ *transparent dermal filler for severe wrinkles and facial folds; local anesthetic* [hyaluronic acid; lidocaine] 24 mg/mL•0.3%

K+ 8 film-coated extended-release tablets (discontinued 2007) ℞ *electrolyte replenisher* [potassium (as chloride)] 8 mEq (600 mg)

K+ 10 film-coated extended-release tablets ℞ *electrolyte replenisher* [potassium (as chloride)] 10 mEq (750 mg)

^{42}**K** [see: potassium chloride K 42]

k82 ImmunoCap test kit for professional use ℞ *in vitro diagnostic aid for specific latex allergies*

Kadian polymer-coated sustained-release pellets in capsules ℞ *narcotic analgesic* [morphine sulfate] 10, 20, 30, 50, 60, 80, 100, 200 mg ⊠ codeine; Quad Tann

kainic acid INN

Kala tablets OTC *natural intestinal bacteria; probiotic; dietary supplement; fever blister treatment; not generally regarded as safe and effective as an antidiarrheal* [*Lactobacillus acidophilus* (soy-based)] 200 million CFU

kalafungin USAN, INN *antifungal*

Kalbitor subcu injection ℞ *kallikrein inhibitor for acute attacks of hereditary angioedema (HAE) (orphan)* [ecallantide] 30 mg

Kaletra film-coated tablets, oral solution ℞ *antiretroviral protease inhibitor combination for HIV-1 infection* [lopinavir; ritonavir] 100•25, 200•50 mg; 80•20 mg/mL ⊠ Caltro; coal tar

Kalexate powder for rectal suspension ℞ *potassium-removing agent for hyperkalemia* [sodium polystyrene sulfonate] 454 g

kallidinogenase INN, BAN

Kalmia latifolia medicinal herb [see: mountain laurel]

kalmopyrin [see: calcium acetylsalicylate]

kalsetal [see: calcium acetylsalicylate]

Kaltostat; Kaltostat Fortex pads OTC *wound dressing* [calcium alginate fiber]

kalumb *medicinal herb* [see: colombo]

kanamycin INN, BAN *aminoglycoside antibiotic; tuberculosis retreatment* [also: kanamycin sulfate]

kanamycin B [see: bekanamycin]

kanamycin sulfate USP *aminoglycoside antibiotic; tuberculosis retreatment* [also: kanamycin] 75, 500, 1000 mg/ vial injection

Kank-a topical liquid/film OTC *mucous membrane anesthetic* [benzocaine] 20%

kanna *(Sceletium tortuosum)* plant *medicinal herb used as a antidepressant, anxiolytic, relaxant, and euphoriant*

Kantrex capsules (discontinued 2009) ℞ *aminoglycoside antibiotic* [kanamycin sulfate] 500 mg

Kantrex IV or IM injection, pediatric injection ℞ *aminoglycoside antibiotic* [kanamycin sulfate] 500, 1000 mg; 75 mg

Kao Lectrolyte powder for pediatric oral solution OTC *electrolyte replenisher*

Kaodene Non-Narcotic oral liquid OTC *antidiarrheal; GI adsorbent; antacid* [kaolin; pectin; bismuth subsalicylate] 130•6.48• ≜ mg/mL

kaolin USP clay *natural material used topically as an emollient and drying agent and ingested for binding gastrointestinal toxins and controlling diarrhea* ⊠ Calan; Clenia; Gilenya; khellin

Kaon elixir ℞ *electrolyte replenisher* [potassium (as gluconate)] 20 mEq/ 15 mL

Kaon-Cl; Kaon-Cl 10 extended-release tablets ℞ *electrolyte replenisher* [potassium (as chloride)] 6.7 mEq (500 mg); 10 mEq (750 mg)

Kaon-Cl 20% oral liquid ℞ *electrolyte replenisher* [potassium (as chloride); alcohol 5%] 40 mEq/15 mL

Kaopectate caplets, oral liquid OTC *antidiarrheal; antinauseant* [bismuth subsalicylate] 262 mg; 262, 575 mg/ 15 mL

Kaopectate Maximum Strength caplets OTC *antidiarrheal; GI adsorbent* [attapulgite] 750 mg

Kao-Spen oral suspension OTC *GI adsorbent; antidiarrheal* [kaolin; pectin] 5.2 g•260 mg per 30 mL ⊠ Gas-Ban

Kao-Tin oral liquid OTC *antidiarrheal; antinauseant* [bismuth subsalicylate] 262 mg/15 mL ⊠ K-Tan

Kapectolin oral liquid, oral suspension OTC *GI adsorbent; antidiarrheal* [bismuth subsalicylate] 262 mg/15 mL

Kapidex (name changed to **Dexilant** in 2010 to prevent confusion with **Casodex**)

Kapseal (trademarked dosage form) *capsules sealed with a band*

Kapvay extended-release tablets ℞ *adjunct to CNS stimulant medications for attention deficit-hyperactivity disorder (ADHD)* [clonidine HCl] 0.1, 0.2 mg

karaya gum *(Sterculia tragacantha; S. urens; S. villosa) medicinal herb used as a topical astringent and bulk laxative* ⍰ guar gum

Karidium tablets, chewable tablets, drops ℞ *dental caries preventative* [sodium fluoride] 2.2 mg; 2.2 mg; 0.275 mg/drop ⍰ Geridium

Karigel; Karigel-N gel ℞ *dental caries preventative* [fluoride (as sodium fluoride)] 0.5% (1.1%)

Kariva tablets (in packs of 28) ℞ *biphasic oral contraceptive* [desogestrel; ethinyl estradiol]
Phase 1 (21 days): 0.15 mg•20 mcg;
Phase 2 (5 days): 0•10 mcg;
Counters (2 days)

kasal USAN *food additive* ⍰ Kay Ciel; KCl

kaugoed; kougoed *medicinal herb* [see: kanna]

kava kava *(Piper methysticum) root medicinal herb for insomnia and nervousness*

Kay Ciel oral liquid, powder for oral solution (discontinued 2008) ℞ *electrolyte replenisher* [potassium (as chloride)] 20 mEq/15 mL; 20 mEq/pkt. ⍰ kasal; KCl

Kayexalate powder for oral or rectal suspension ℞ *potassium-removing agent for hyperkalemia* [sodium polystyrene sulfonate] 453.6 g

Kaylixir oral liquid ℞ *electrolyte replenisher* [potassium (as gluconate); alcohol 5%] 20 mEq/15 mL

K-C oral suspension OTC *antidiarrheal; GI adsorbent; antacid* [kaolin; pectin; bismuth subcarbonate] 5 g•260 mg• 260 mg per 30 mL

K+ Care powder for oral solution (discontinued 2007) ℞ *electrolyte replenisher* [potassium (as chloride)] 15, 20, 25 mEq/pkt.

K+ Care ET effervescent tablets (discontinued 2007) ℞ *electrolyte replenisher* [potassium (as bicarbonate)] 20, 25 mEq

KCl (potassium chloride) [q.v.]

K-Dur 10; K-Dur 20 controlled-release tablets ℞ *electrolyte replenisher* [potassium (as chloride)] 10 mEq (750 mg); 20 mEq (1500 mg)

kebuzone INN

Keflex Pulvules (capsules), oral suspension ℞ *first-generation cephalosporin antibiotic* [cephalexin] 250, 333, 500, 750 mg; 125, 250 mg/5 mL ⍰ GaviLAX

kellofylline [see: visnafylline]

Kelnor 1/35 tablets (in packs of 28) ℞ *monophasic oral contraceptive* [ethynodiol diacetate; ethinyl estradiol] 1 mg•35 mcg × 21 days; counters × 7 days

kelp *(Fucus versiculosus) plant medicinal herb for brittle fingernails, cleaning arteries, colitis, eczema, goiter, obesity, and toning adrenal, pituitary, and thyroid glands* ⍰ KLB

kelp *(Laminaria digitata; L. japonica) plant medicinal herb for cervical dilation and cervical ripening* ⍰ KLB

Kemadrin tablets (discontinued 2008) ℞ *anticholinergic; antiparkinsonian* [procyclidine HCl] 5 mg

Kemstro orally disintegrating tablets ℞ *skeletal muscle relaxant* [baclofen] 10, 20 mg

Kenaject-40 IM, intra-articular, intrabursal, intradermal injection (discontinued 2008) ℞ *corticosteroid; anti-inflammatory* [triamcinolone acetonide] 40 mg/mL

Kenalog lotion (discontinued 2008) ℞ *corticosteroidal anti-inflammatory* [triamcinolone acetonide] 0.025%, 0.1%

Kenalog ointment, cream, aerosol spray ℞ *corticosteroidal anti-inflammatory* [triamcinolone acetonide] 0.025%, 0.1%; 0.025%; ≟

Kenalog in Orabase oral paste ℞ *corticosteroidal anti-inflammatory* [triamcinolone acetonide] 0.1%

Kenalog-10; Kenalog-40 IM, intra-articular, intrabursal, intradermal injection ℞ *corticosteroid; anti-inflammatory* [triamcinolone acetonide] 10 mg/mL; 40 mg/mL

Kenalog-H cream (discontinued 2008) ℞ *corticosteroidal anti-inflammatory* [triamcinolone acetonide] 0.1%

Kendall compound A [see: dehydrocorticosterone]

Kendall compound B [see: corticosterone]

Kendall compound E [see: cortisone acetate]

Kendall compound F [see: hydrocortisone]

Kendall desoxy compound B [see: desoxycorticosterone acetate]

Kenonel cream ℞ *corticosteroidal anti-inflammatory* [triamcinolone acetonide] 1%

Kenwood Therapeutic oral liquid (discontinued 2008) OTC *vitamin/mineral supplement* [multiple vitamins & minerals]

keoxifene HCl [now: raloxifene HCl]

Kepivance powder for IV injection ℞ *keratinocyte growth factor (KGF) for radiation- and chemotherapy-induced oral mucositis* [palifermin] 6.25 mg/dose

Keppra film-coated tablets, oral solution, IV injection ℞ *anticonvulsant for myoclonic, partial-onset, and generalized tonic-clonic seizures; oral forms are also used to treat migraine headaches and bipolar disorder* [levetiracetam] 250, 500, 750, 1000 mg; 100 mg/mL; 100 mg/mL ⊠ copper

Keppra XR film-coated extended-release tablets ℞ *once-daily anticonvulsant for partial-onset seizures* [levetiracetam] 500, 750 mg

keracyanin INN

Kerafoam; Kerafoam 42 topical foam ℞ *moisturizer; emollient; keratolytic* [urea] 30%; 42% ⊠ CarraFoam

Keralac lotion, cream, ointment ℞ *moisturizer; emollient; keratolytic* [urea] 35%; 50%; 50% ⊠ garlic

Keralac Nail Gel ℞ *moisturizer; emollient; keratolytic* [urea] 50%

Keralac Nailstick topical solution ℞ *moisturizer; emollient; keratolytic* [urea] 50%

Keralyt gel ℞ *keratolytic* [salicylic acid] 3%

Kerasal ointment OTC *keratolytic and moisturizer/emollient for dry, rough, or cracked feet* [salicylic acid; urea] 5%•10% ⊠ Corzall; cresol; Cryselle

Kerasal AL cream OTC *moisturizer/emollient for dry, rough, or cracked feet* [ammonium lactate] ⊠ carazolol

Kerasal Ultra 20 cream OTC *keratolytic and moisturizer/emollient for dry, rough, or cracked feet* [urea; ammonium lactate] 20•5%

keratinocyte growth factor, recombinant human (rhKGF) *investigational (orphan) to reduce the incidence and severity of radiation-induced xerostomia*

Keratol HC cream ℞ *corticosteroidal anti-inflammatory; keratolytic; emollient* [hydrocortisone; urea] 1%•10%

keratolytics *a class of agents that cause sloughing of the horny layer of the epidermis and softening of the skin*

Keri Age Defy & Protect lotion OTC *moisturizer; emollient; sunscreen (SPF 15)* [octinoxate; oxybenzone] 7.5%•2%

Keri Long Lasting cream OTC *moisturizer; emollient*

Keri Original; Keri Advanced; Keri Nourishing Shea Butter; Keri Renewal Milk Body; Keri Renewal Skin Firming; Keri Sensitive Skin; Keri Shave lotion OTC *moisturizer; emollient*

KeriCort-10 cream OTC *corticosteroidal anti-inflammatory* [hydrocortisone] 1%

Kerlone film-coated tablets ℞ *beta-blocker for hypertension* [betaxolol HCl] 10, 20 mg

kernelwort *medicinal herb* [see: figwort]

Kerodex #51 cream OTC *skin protectant for dry or oily work* ⊠ cardiacs; Kredex

Kerodex #71 cream OTC *water repellant skin protectant for wet work* ⑨ cardiacs; Kredex

Kerol topical suspension, topical emulsion ℞ *moisturizer; emollient; keratolytic* [urea] 50% ⑨ caraway oil; coral

Kerol AD topical emulsion ℞ *moisturizer; emollient; keratolytic* [urea] 45%

Kerol ZX topical film ℞ *moisturizer; emollient; keratolytic* [urea] 50%

Ketalar IV or IM injection ℞ *rapid-acting general anesthetic; also abused as a street drug due to its "dissociative state" effects* [ketamine HCl] 10, 50, 100 mg/mL

ketamine INN, BAN *a rapid-acting general anesthetic; sometimes abused as a street drug due to its "dissociative state" effects* [also: ketamine HCl]

ketamine HCl USAN, USP, JAN *a rapid-acting general anesthetic; sometimes abused as a street drug due to its "dissociative state" effects* [also: ketamine] 10, 50, 100 mg/mL injection

ketanserin USAN, INN, BAN *serotonin antagonist*

ketazocine USAN, INN *analgesic*

ketazolam USAN, INN, BAN *minor tranquilizer*

Ketek film-coated tablets, Ketek Pak (10 film-coated tablets) ℞ *broad-spectrum ketolide antibiotic for community-acquired pneumonia (CAP); approval to treat other types of respiratory tract infections was withdrawn by the FDA in 2007* [telithromycin] 300, 400 mg; 400 mg

kethoxal USAN *antiviral* [also: ketoxal]

ketimipramine INN *antidepressant* [also: ketipramine fumarate]

ketimipramine fumarate [see: ketipramine fumarate]

ketipramine fumarate USAN *antidepressant* [also: ketimipramine]

7-KETO DHEA *investigational dehydroepiandrosterone (DHEA) derivative for Alzheimer disease*

ketobemidone INN, BAN

ketocaine INN ⑨ quatacaine

ketocainol INN

KetoCare reagent strips for home use OTC *in vitro diagnostic aid for acetone (ketones) in the urine*

ketocholanic acid [see: dehydrocholic acid]

ketoconazole USAN, USP, INN, BAN *broad-spectrum imidazole antifungal; topical treatment for tinea corporis, tinea cruris, tinea pedis, tinea versicolor, cutaneous candidiasis, and seborrheic dermatitis* 200 mg oral; 2% topical

ketoconazole & cyclosporine *investigational (orphan) to diminish nephrotoxicity from organ transplantation*

Keto-Diastix reagent strips (discontinued 2008) OTC *in vitro diagnostic aid for multiple urine products*

ketohexazine [see: cetohexazine]

ketolides *a class of oral antibiotics*

Ketonex-1 powder OTC *formula for infants with maple syrup urine disease (MSUD)*

Ketonex-2 powder ℞ *enteral nutritional therapy for maple syrup urine disease (MSUD)*

ketoprofen USAN, INN, BAN, JAN *analgesic; antipyretic; nonsteroidal anti-inflammatory drug (NSAID) for osteoarthritis, rheumatoid arthritis, and primary dysmenorrhea* 50, 75, 100, 150, 200 mg oral

ketorfanol USAN, INN *analgesic*

ketorolac INN, BAN *analgesic; nonsteroidal anti-inflammatory drug (NSAID) for moderately severe acute pain; investigational (NDA filed) intranasal formulation* [also: ketorolac tromethamine]

ketorolac tromethamine USAN *analgesic; nonsteroidal anti-inflammatory drug (NSAID) for moderately severe acute pain; ocular treatment for allergic conjunctivitis, cataract extraction, and corneal refractive surgery* [also: ketorolac] 0.4%, 0.5% eye drops; 10 mg oral; 15, 30 mg/mL injection

Ketostix reagent strips for home use (discontinued 2008) OTC *in vitro diagnostic aid for acetone (ketones) in the urine*

ketotifen INN, BAN *antihistamine; mast cell stabilizer* [also: ketotifen fumarate]

ketotifen fumarate USAN, JAN *antihistamine and mast cell stabilizer for allergic conjunctivitis* (base=71.4%) [also: ketotifen] 0.025% eye drops

Ketotransdel *investigational (Phase III) topical nonsteroidal anti-inflammatory drug (NSAID)*

ketotrexate INN

ketoxal INN *antiviral* [also: kethoxal]

Key-Pred 25; Key-Pred 50 IM injection (discontinued 2008) ℞ *corticosteroid; anti-inflammatory* [prednisolone acetate] 25 mg/mL; 50 mg/mL ⚕ capuride

Key-Pred-SP IV or IM injection (discontinued 2008) ℞ *corticosteroid; anti-inflammatory* [prednisolone sodium phosphate] 20 mg/mL

K-G Elixir ℞ *electrolyte replenisher* [potassium (as gluconate)] 20 mEq/ 15 mL

KGHB (potassium gamma hydroxy-butyrate) [see: gamma hydroxybutyrate (GHB)]

khellin INN ⚕ Calan; Clenia; Gilenya; kaolin

khelloside INN ⚕ Colazide

Kiacta oral *investigational (NDA filed, orphan) amyloid fibrinogen inhibitor for AA (secondary) amyloidosis* [eprodisate]

Kid Kare Children's Cough/Cold oral liquid OTC *antitussive; antihistamine; decongestant; for children 6–11 years* [dextromethorphan hydrobromide; chlorpheniramine maleate; pseudoephedrine HCl] 10•2•30 mg/10 mL

Kid Kare Nasal Decongestant oral drops OTC *nasal decongestant* [pseudoephedrine HCl] 7.5 mg/0.8 mL

kidney root *medicinal herb* [see: queen of the meadow]

KIE syrup (discontinued 2007) ℞ *bronchodilator; decongestant; expectorant* [ephedrine HCl; potassium iodide] 16•300 mg/10 mL

Kindercal oral liquid OTC *enteral nutritional therapy* [lactose-free formula]

Kinerase cream, lotion OTC *moisturizer; emollient* [N⁶-furfuryladenine] 0.1%

Kinerase Intensive Eye Cream OTC *moisturizer; emollient* [kinetin] 0.125%

Kineret subcu injection in prefilled syringes ℞ *interleukin-1 receptor antagonist (IL-1ra); nonsteroidal anti-inflammatory drug (NSAID) for rheumatoid arthritis (RA)* [anakinra] 100 mg

Kinevac powder for IV injection ℞ *diagnostic aid for gallbladder function* [sincalide] 1 mcg/mL

king's clover *medicinal herb* [see: melilot]

king's cure *medicinal herb* [see: pipsissewa]

king's fern *medicinal herb* [see: buckhorn brake]

kininase II inhibitors [see: angiotensin-converting enzyme inhibitors]

kinnikinnik *medicinal herb* [see: uva ursi]

Kinrix suspension for IM injection ℞ *active immunizing agent for diphtheria, tetanus, pertussis, hepatitis B and D, and three types of poliovirus* [diphtheria & tetanus toxoids & acellular pertussis (DTaP) vaccine; hepatitis B virus vaccine; inactivated poliovirus vaccine (IPV) Types 1, 2, and 3] 0.5 mL/dose

Kionex oral or rectal suspension, powder for oral or rectal suspension ℞ *potassium-removing agent for hyperkalemia* [sodium polystyrene sulfonate] 15 g/60 mL; 454 g ⚕ Cognex

kitasamycin USAN, INN, BAN, JAN *antibacterial* [also: acetylkitasamycin; kitasamycin tartrate]

kitasamycin tartrate JAN *antibacterial* [also: kitasamycin; acetylkitasamycin]

Klamath weed *medicinal herb* [see: St. John's wort]

Klaron lotion ℞ *antibiotic for acne* [sulfacetamide sodium] 10% ⚕ chlorine

KLB6; Ultra KLB6 softgels (discontinued 2008) OTC *dietary supplement* [vitamin B₆; multiple food supplements] 3.5•≜ mg; 16.7•≜ mg ⚕ kelp

Kleen-Handz solution (discontinued 2008) OTC *antiseptic* [ethyl alcohol] 62%

Klonopin tablets ℞ *anticonvulsant; anxiolytic for panic disorder; also used for parkinsonian dysarthria, neuralgias, multifocal tics, and manic episodes of a bipolar disorder; investigational (orphan) for hyperexplexia (startle disease)* [clonazepam] 0.5, 1, 2 mg

Klonopin Wafers (orally disintegrating tablets) (discontinued 2011) ℞ *anticonvulsant; anxiolytic for panic disorder; also used for parkinsonian dysarthria, neuralgias, multifocal tics, and manic episodes of a bipolar disorder* [clonazepam] 0.125, 0.25, 0.5, 1, 2 mg

K-Lor powder for oral solution ℞ *electrolyte replenisher* [potassium (as chloride)] 15, 20 mEq/pkt.

Klor-Con; Klor-Con/25 powder for oral solution ℞ *electrolyte replenisher* [potassium (as chloride)] 20 mEq/pkt.; 25 mEq/pkt. ⃞ chloroquine

Klor-Con M10; Klor-Con M15; Klor-Con M20 extended-release tablets ℞ *electrolyte replenisher* [potassium (as chloride)] 10 mEq (750 mg); 15 mEq (1125 mg); 20 mEq (1500 mg)

Klor-Con/EF effervescent tablets ℞ *electrolyte replenisher* [potassium (as bicarbonate and citrate)] 25 mEq

Klorvess oral liquid, effervescent granules, effervescent tablets ℞ *electrolyte replenisher* [potassium (as chloride)] 20 mEq/15 mL; 20 mEq/pkt.; 20 mEq ⃞ Claravis

Klotrix film-coated controlled-release tablets ℞ *electrolyte replenisher* [potassium (as chloride)] 10 mEq (750 mg) ⃞ Glutarex

Klout shampoo OTC *pesticide-free lice removal agent* [acetic acid; isopropanol; sodium laureth sulfate] ⃞ CoLyte; K-Lyte

K-Lyte; K-Lyte DS effervescent tablets ℞ *electrolyte replenisher* [potassium (as bicarbonate and citrate)] 25 mEq; 50 mEq ⃞ CoLyte; Klout

K-Lyte/Cl effervescent tablets (discontinued 2008) ℞ *electrolyte replenisher* [potassium (as chloride)] 25 mEq

K-Lyte/Cl powder for oral solution ℞ *electrolyte replenisher* [potassium (as chloride)] 25 mEq

K-Lyte/Cl 50 effervescent tablets ℞ *electrolyte replenisher* [potassium (as chloride)] 50 mEq

knitback; knitbone *medicinal herb* [see: comfrey]

knob grass; knob root *medicinal herb* [see: stone root]

knotted marjoram *medicinal herb* [see: marjoram]

knotweed (*Polygonum aviculare; P. hydropiper; P. persicaria; P. punctatum*) plant *medicinal herb used as an antiseptic, astringent, diaphoretic, diuretic, emmenagogue, rubefacient, and stimulant*

Koate-DVI (double viral inactivation) powder for IV injection ℞ *systemic hemostatic; antihemophilic for the prevention and control of bleeding in classical hemophilia (hemophilia A) and von Willebrand disease (orphan)* [antihemophilic factor concentrate, human] 250, 500, 1000 IU

Kof-Eze lozenges OTC *mild anesthetic; antipruritic; counterirritant* [menthol] 6 mg ⃞ Coughtuss

Kogenate FS powder for IV injection ℞ *systemic hemostatic; antihemophilic for the prevention and control of bleeding in classical hemophilia (hemophilia A) and von Willebrand disease (orphan)* [antihemophilic factor, recombinant] 250, 500, 1000, 2000, 3000 IU

KOH (potassium hydroxide) [q.v.]

kola nut (*Cola acuminata*) seed *medicinal herb used as a stimulant; natural source of caffeine* ⃞ Cal-Nate

Kolephrin caplets (discontinued 2007) OTC *decongestant; antihistamine; analgesic; antipyretic* [pseudoephedrine HCl; chlorpheniramine maleate; acetaminophen] 30•2•325 mg ⃞ Calphron; Claforan

Kolephrin GG/DM oral liquid OTC *antitussive; expectorant* [dextromethorphan hydrobromide; guaifenesin] 10•150 mg/5 mL

Kolephrin/DM caplets (discontinued 2007) OTC *antitussive; antihistamine; decongestant; analgesic; antipyretic* [dextromethorphan hydrobromide; chlorpheniramine maleate; pseudoephedrine HCl; acetaminophen] 10•2•30•325 mg

kolfocon A USAN *hydrophobic contact lens material*

kolfocon B USAN *hydrophobic contact lens material*

kolfocon C USAN *hydrophobic contact lens material*

kolfocon D USAN *hydrophobic contact lens material*

Kolyum oral liquid (discontinued 2008) ℞ *electrolyte replenisher* [potassium (as gluconate and chloride)] 20 mEq/15 mL ⃟ gallium

Kombiglyze XR film-coated extended-release caplets ℞ *combination treatment for type 2 diabetes that increases insulin production in the pancreas, reduces glucose production in the liver, and increases cellular response to insulin* [saxagliptin (as HCl); metformin HCl] 2.5•1000, 5•500, 5•1000 mg

kombucha (yeast/bacteria/fungus symbiont) fermented tea *natural treatment for aging, cancer, intestinal disorders, and rheumatism* ⃟ Compack

Kondremul Plain emulsion OTC *emollient laxative* [mineral oil]

Konsyl powder for oral solution OTC *bulk laxative* [psyllium] 6 g/tsp. or pkt. ⃟ Goniosol; Gynazole

Konsyl Easy Mix Formula powder for oral solution OTC *bulk laxative with electrolytes* [psyllium; electrolytes] 6•≛ g/tsp. or pkt.

Konsyl Fiber tablets OTC *bulk laxative; antidiarrheal* [calcium polycarbophil] 625 mg

Konsyl Orange powder for oral solution OTC *bulk laxative* [psyllium] 3.5 g/tbsp. or pkt.

Konsyl·D powder OTC *bulk laxative* [psyllium] 3.4 g/tsp.

Korean ginseng (Panax ginseng; P. shin-seng) *medicinal herb* [see: ginseng]

kougoed; kaugoed *medicinal herb* [see: kanna]

Kovia 6.5 ointment ℞ *proteolytic enzyme for débridement of necrotic tissue; vulnerary* [papain; urea] 650 000 IU/g•10%

Kovitonic oral liquid (discontinued 2008) OTC *vitamin/iron/amino acid supplement* [multiple B vitamins; iron (as ferric pyrophosphate); lysine; folic acid] ≛•42•10•0.1 mg/15 mL

K-Pax Immune Suport Protein Blend Powder powder for oral solution OTC *enteral nutritional therapy* [rice-based formula] 505 g.

K-Pax Immune Support capsules OTC *vitamin/mineral/calcium/iron supplement* [multiple vitamins & minerals; calcium; iron; folic acid; biotin] ≛•50•1.125•0.05•⃒ mg

K-Pax Protein Blend Powder powder for oral solution OTC *enteral nutritional therapy* [lactose-free formula] 908 g.

K-Pek oral suspension (discontinued 2007) OTC *antidiarrheal* [bismuth subsalicylate] 262 mg/15 mL ⃟ Gy-Pak

K-Pek II caplets OTC *antidiarrheal* [loperamide HCl] 2 mg ⃟ Gy-Pak

K-Phos M.F. tablets ℞ *urinary acidifier* [potassium acid phosphate; sodium acid phosphate] 155•350 mg (1.1 mEq K, 2.9 mEq Na)

K-Phos Neutral film-coated caplets ℞ *urinary acidifier; phosphorus supplement* [monobasic sodium phosphate; monobasic potassium phosphate; dibasic sodium phosphate] 250 mg (14.25 mEq) P

K-Phos No. 2 tablets ℞ *urinary acidifier* [potassium acid phosphate; sodium acid phosphate] 305•700 mg (2.3 mEq K, 5.8 mEq Na)

K-Phos Original tablets ℞ *urinary acidifier* [potassium acid phosphate] 500 mg (3.7 mEq K)

K.P.N. Prenatal with Extra Calcium tablets OTC *prenatal vitamin/mineral/calcium/iron supplement* [multiple vitamins & minerals; calcium; iron (as ferrous fumarate); folic acid; biotin] ±•333•9•0.27•0.01 mg

81mKr [see: krypton Kr 81m]

85Kr [see: krypton clathrate Kr 85]

Kristalose powder for oral solution ℞ *hyperosmotic laxative* [lactulose] 10, 20 g/pkt.

Kronocap (trademarked dosage form) *sustained-release capsule*

Kronofed-A sustained-release capsules (discontinued 2007) ℞ *decongestant; antihistamine* [pseudoephedrine HCl; chlorpheniramine maleate] 120•8 mg

Kronofed-A Jr. sustained-release capsules (discontinued 2007) ℞ *decongestant; antihistamine* [pseudoephedrine HCl; chlorpheniramine maleate] 60•4 mg

krypton *element (Kr)*

krypton clathrate Kr 85 USAN *radioactive agent*

krypton Kr 81m USAN, USP *radioactive agent*

Krystexxa IV infusion ℞ *uricase enzyme for hyperuricemia due to severe gout (orphan)* [pegloticase] 8 mg/mL

K-Tab film-coated extended-release tablets ℞ *electrolyte replenisher* [potassium (as chloride)] 10 mEq (750 mg) ⊘ Cotab; CTAB; Q-Tapp

K-Tan caplets (discontinued 2011) ℞ *decongestant antihistamine; sleep aid* [phenylephrine tannate; pyrilamine tannate] 25•60 mg ⊘ Kao-Tin

K-Tan 4 oral suspension (discontinued 2010) ℞ *decongestant; antihistamine; sleep aid* [phenylephrine tannate; pyrilamine tannate] 5•30 mg/5 mL ⊘ Kao-Tin

kudzu (Pueraria lobata; P. thunbergiana) root *medicinal herb for the management of alcoholism*

kunecatechins *a class of natural polyphenolic antioxidants; topical treatment for external genital and perianal warts (condyloma acuminatum) in immunocompromised adults* [also known as: sinecatechins; see also: catechins; epicatechins]

Kuric cream (discontinued 2011) ℞ *broad-spectrum antifungal for tinea corporis, tinea cruris, tinea pedis, tinea versicolor, cutaneous candidiasis, and seborrheic dermatitis* [ketoconazole] 2% ⊘ Carac; Coreg

Kutrase capsules ℞ *porcine-derived digestive enzymes* [pancrelipase (lipase; protease; amylase)] 2400•30 000•30 000 USP units

Kuvan tablets ℞ *phenylalanine hydroxylase (PAH) enzyme for mild to moderate phenylketonuria (PKU)* [sapropterin dihydrochloride] 100 mg ⊘ caffeine; C-Phen

Ku-Zyme capsules (discontinued 2009) ℞ *porcine-derived digestive enzymes* [pancrelipase (lipase; protease; amylase)] 1200•15 000•15 000 USP units

Ku-Zyme HP capsules (discontinued 2009) ℞ *porcine-derived digestive enzymes* [pancrelipase (lipase; protease; amylase)] 8000•30 000•30 000 USP units

K-vescent effervescent powder ℞ *electrolyte replenisher* [potassium (as chloride)] 20 mEq/pkt.

Kwelcof oral liquid (discontinued 2011) ℞ *narcotic antitussive; expectorant* [hydrocodone bitartrate; guaifenesin] 5•100 mg/5 mL

KwikPen (trademarked delivery device) *prefilled self-injection syringe for various* **Humalog** *products*

K-Y vaginal jelly OTC *moisturizer/lubricant* [glycerin; hydroxyethyl cellulose]

K-Y Plus vaginal gel OTC *spermicidal contraceptive (for use with a diaphragm)* [nonoxynol 9] 2.2%

kyamepromazin [see: cyamemazine]

Kybernin P IV *investigational (orphan) agent for thromboembolic episodes due*

to congenital AT-III deficiency [anti-
thrombin III concentrate]

Kynapid investigational (NDA filed)
selective ion channel blocker for the
acute conversion of atrial fibrillation
[vernakalant]

Kytril film-coated tablets (discontinued 2008) ℞ antiemetic to prevent

nausea and vomiting following chemotherapy, radiation, or surgery [granise-
tron (as HCl)] 1 mg

Kytril oral solution, IV infusion ℞
antiemetic to prevent nausea and vomiting following chemotherapy, radiation,
or surgery [granisetron (as HCl)] 1
mg/5 mL; 0.1, 1 mg/mL

L-5 hydroxytryptophan (L-5HTP)
natural precursor to serotonin; investigational (orphan) for tetrahydrobiopterin
deficiency; also used as a natural remedy
for depression

LAAM (l-acetyl-α-methadol [or] l-
alpha-acetyl-methadol) [see: levomethadyl acetate]

LABA (long-acting beta₂ agonist)
sympathomimetic bronchodilator for
asthma and bronchospasm, and for the
long-term treatment of COPD [see:
formoterol; salmeterol]

labetalol INN, BAN antiadrenergic
(alpha- and beta-blocker); antihypertensive [also: labetalol HCl]

labetalol HCl USAN, USP antiadrenergic
(alpha- and beta-blocker); antihypertensive [also: labetalol] 100, 200, 300
mg oral; 5 mg/mL injection

**Labrador tea (Ledum groenlandicum;
L. latifolium; L. palustre)** leaves
medicinal herb for bronchial infections,
cough, diarrhea, headache, kidney disorders, lung infections, malignancies,
rheumatism, and sore throat

Labstix reagent strips OTC in vitro diagnostic aid for multiple urine products

Lac-Dose caplets OTC digestive aid for
lactose intolerance [lactase enzyme]
3000 FCC units ⏢ Liqui-Doss

Lac-Hydrin cream, lotion ℞ moisturizer; emollient [ammonium lactate]
12%

Lac-Hydrin Five lotion OTC moisturizer; emollient [lactic acid]

LACI (lipoprotein-associated coagulation inhibitor) [see: tifacogin]

lacidipine USAN, INN, BAN antihypertensive; calcium channel blocker

LAC-Lotion ℞ moisturizer; emollient
[ammonium lactate] 12%

lacosamide adjunctive therapy for adults
with partial-onset seizures; investigational (Phase II) for diabetic neuropathy

Lacril eye drops OTC moisturizer/lubricant
[hydroxypropyl methylcellulose] 0.5%

Lacri-Lube NP; Lacri-Lube S.O.P.
ophthalmic ointment OTC moistur-
izer/lubricant [white petrolatum; mineral oil; lanolin]

Lacrisert ophthalmic insert OTC ophthalmic moisturizer/lubricant [hydroxy-
propyl cellulose] 5 mg

lactagogues a class of agents that promote or increase the flow of breast milk
[also called: galactagogues]

LactAid oral liquid, tablets OTC digestive aid for lactose intolerance [lactase
enzyme] 250 U/drop; 3000 U

lactalfate INN

lactase enzyme beta-D-galactosidase
digestive enzyme for lactose intolerance
9000 FCC units oral

lactated potassic saline [see: potassic
saline, lactated]

lactated Ringer (LR) injection [see:
Ringer injection, lactated]

lactated Ringer (LR) solution [see:
Ringer injection, lactated]

lactic acid USP pH adjusting agent;
investigational (orphan) for severe aph-

thous stomatitis in terminally immuno-compromised patients

Lactic Acid 10% E cream ℞ *emollient; moisturizer* [lactic acid; vitamin E] 10%•116.67 IU/g

lactic acid bacteria (*Lactobacillus, Bifidobacterium,* and *Streptococcus* sp.) *investigational (orphan) for chronic pouchitis*

LactiCare lotion OTC *emollient; moisturizer* [lactic acid]

LactiCare-HC lotion (discontinued 2010) ℞ *corticosteroidal anti-inflammatory* [hydrocortisone] 1%, 2.5%

Lactinex granules, chewable tablets OTC *natural intestinal bacteria; probiotic; dietary supplement; not generally regarded as safe and effective as an antidiarrheal* [*Lactobacillus acidophilus*; *L. bulgaricus*]

Lactinol lotion ℞ *emollient; moisturizer* [lactic acid] 10%

Lactinol-E cream (discontinued 2010) ℞ *emollient; moisturizer* [lactic acid; vitamin E] 10%•116.67 IU/g

lactitol INN, BAN

Lactobacillin Acidophilus capsules OTC *natural intestinal bacteria; probiotic; dietary supplement; fever blister treatment* [*Lactobacillus acidophilus*] 25 million CFU

Lactobacillus acidophilus *natural intestinal bacteria; probiotic; dietary supplement; fever blister treatment; not generally regarded as safe and effective as an antidiarrheal* [also: acidophilus]

Lactobacillus bifidus *natural intestinal bacteria; probiotic; dietary supplement; not generally regarded as safe and effective as an antidiarrheal*

Lactobacillus bulgaricus *natural intestinal bacteria; probiotic; dietary supplement; not generally regarded as safe and effective as an antidiarrheal*

Lactobacillus reuteri *natural intestinal bacteria; probiotic; dietary supplement*

Lactobacillus sp. *natural intestinal bacteria; probiotic; dietary supplement* [see also: lactic acid bacteria]

lactobin *investigational (orphan) for AIDS-related diarrhea*

lactobionic acid, calcium salt, dihydrate [see: calcium lactobionate]

Lactocal-F film-coated tablets ℞ *prenatal vitamin/mineral/calcium/iron supplement* [multiple vitamins & minerals; calcium; iron (as ferrous fumarate); folic acid] ≛•200•65•1 mg

lactoflavin [see: riboflavin]

LactoFree oral liquid, powder for oral liquid OTC *hypoallergenic infant formula* [milk-based formula, lactose free]

LactoFree LIPIL oral liquid, powder for oral liquid OTC *hypoallergenic infant formula fortified with omega-3 fatty acids* [milk-based formula, lactose free]

Lacto-Key-100; Lacto-Key-600 capsules OTC *natural intestinal bacteria; probiotic; dietary supplement; fever blister treatment* [*Lactobacillus acidophilus*] ≥ 1 billion CFU; ≥ 6 billion CFU

β-lactone [see: propiolactone]

γ-lactone D-glucofuranuronic acid [see: glucurolactone]

lactose NF *tablet and capsule diluent; dietary supplement*

Lactrase capsules OTC *digestive aid for lactose intolerance* [lactase enzyme] 250 mg

Lactrex 12% cream (discontinued 2010) ℞ *emollient; moisturizer* [lactic acid] 12%

Lactuca sativa *medicinal herb* [see: lettuce]

Lactuca virosa *medicinal herb* [see: wild lettuce]

lactulose USAN, USP, INN, BAN *hyperosmotic laxative; synthetic disaccharide used to prevent and treat portal-systemic encephalopathy* 10 g/15 mL oral or rectal

ladakamycin [now: azacitidine]

Lady Esther cream OTC *moisturizer; emollient* [mineral oil]

lady's mantle (*Alchemilla xanthochlora; A. vulgaris*) plant *medicinal herb for diarrhea and other digestive disorders; also used as an astringent,* anti-inflammatory agent, menstrual cycle regulator, and muscle relaxant

lady's slipper (*Cypripedium pubescens*) root medicinal herb for chorea, hysteria, insomnia, nervousness, and restlessness

Lagesic extended-release caplets ℞ analgesic; antipyretic; antihistamine; sleep aid [acetaminophen; phenyltoloxamine citrate] 600•66 mg ⊡ Luxiq

laidlomycin INN veterinary growth stimulant [also: laidlomycin propionate potassium]

laidlomycin propionate potassium USAN veterinary growth stimulant [also: laidlomycin]

Laki-Lorand factor [see: factor XIII]

L-All 12 oral suspension (discontinued 2008) ℞ antitussive; decongestant [carbetapentane tannate; phenylephrine tannate] 30•30 mg/5 mL

lamb mint medicinal herb [see: peppermint; spearmint]

lamb's quarter medicinal herb [see: birthroot]

Lamictal tablets, chewable/dispersible tablets ℞ anticonvulsant for partial seizures, Lennox-Gastaut syndrome (orphan), and primary generalized tonic-clonic (PGTC) seizures; maintenance treatment for bipolar disorder [lamotrigine] 25, 100, 150, 200 mg; 2, 5, 25 mg

Lamictal ODT (orally disintegrating tablets) ℞ anticonvulsant for partial seizures, Lennox-Gastaut syndrome (orphan), and primary generalized tonic-clonic (PGTC) seizures; maintenance treatment for bipolar disorder [lamotrigine] 25, 50, 100, 200 mg

Lamictal XR film-coated extended-release tablets ℞ once-daily adjunctive treatment for partial seizures and primary generalized tonic-clonic seizures [lamotrigine] 25, 50, 100, 200 mg

lamifiban USAN, INN glycoprotein (GP) IIb/IIIa receptor inhibitor; antiplatelet/ antithrombotic agent for unstable angina

lamifiban HCl USAN glycoprotein (GP) IIb/IIIa receptor inhibitor; antiplatelet/ antithrombotic agent for unstable angina

Laminaria digitata; L. japonica medicinal herb [see: kelp]

Lamisil tablets, granules for oral suspension ℞ systemic allylamine antifungal for onychomycosis and tinea capitis [terbinafine (as HCl)] 250 mg; 125, 187.5 mg/pkt

Lamisil AF Defense topical powder OTC antifungal [tolnaftate] 1%

Lamisil AT cream, gel, spray, drops OTC allylamine antifungal [terbinafine HCl] 1%

Lamium album medicinal herb [see: blind nettle]

lamivudine USAN, INN, BAN nucleoside reverse transcriptase inhibitor (NRTI); antiviral for HIV and chronic hepatitis B virus (HBV) infections

lamivudine & abacavir sulfate nucleoside reverse transcriptase inhibitor (NRTI) combination for HIV and AIDS 30•60 mg oral

lamivudine & abacavir sulfate & zidovudine nucleoside reverse transcriptase inhibitor (NRTI) combination for HIV and AIDS 150•300•300 mg oral

lamivudine & stavudine combination nucleoside reverse transcriptase inhibitor (NRTI) for HIV and AIDS 150•30, 150•40 mg oral

lamivudine & stavudine & nevirapine combination nucleoside reverse transcriptase inhibitor (NRTI) and non-nucleoside reverse transcriptase inhibitor (NNRTI) for HIV and AIDS 30•6•50, 60•12•100, 150•30•200, 150•40•200 mg oral

lamivudine & zidovudine nucleoside reverse transcriptase inhibitor (NRTI) combination for HIV and AIDS 30•60, 150•300, 200•200 mg oral

lamivudine & zidovudine & nevirapine combination nucleoside reverse transcriptase inhibitor (NRTI) and non-nucleoside reverse transcriptase *inhibitor (NNRTI) for HIV and AIDS* 30•60•50, 150•300•200 mg oral

lamotrigine USAN, INN, BAN *phenyltriazine anticonvulsant for partial seizures, Lennox-Gastaut syndrome (orphan), and primary generalized tonic-clonic (PGTC) seizures; maintenance treatment for bipolar disorder* 5, 25, 50, 100, 150, 200, 250 mg oral

Lampit (available only from the Centers for Disease Control) (discontinued 2011) ℞ *anti-infective for Chagas disease* [nifurtimox]

lamtidine INN, BAN

Lanabiotic ointment OTC *antibiotic; anesthetic* [polymyxin B sulfate; neomycin sulfate; bacitracin zinc; lidocaine] 10 000 U•3.5 mg•500 U•40 mg per g

Lanacane spray, cream OTC *anesthetic; antiseptic* [benzocaine; benzethonium chloride] 20%•0.1%; 6%•0.1% ⊡ lignocaine

Lanacaps (trademarked dosage form) *timed-release capsules*

Lanacort 5 cream, ointment OTC *corticosteroidal anti-inflammatory* [hydrocortisone acetate] 0.5% ⊡ lungwort

Lanacort 10 cream OTC *corticosteroidal anti-inflammatory* [hydrocortisone acetate] 1% ⊡ lungwort

Lanaphilic cream OTC *moisturizer; emollient; keratolytic* [urea] 20%

Lanaphilic ointment OTC *nontherapeutic base for compounding various dermatological preparations*

Lanaphilic with Urea ointment OTC *base for compounding various dermatological preparations; moisturizer; emollient* [urea] 10%

Lanatabs (trademarked dosage form) *sustained-release tablets*

lanatoside NF, INN, BAN

Laniazid C.T. tablets ℞ *tuberculostatic* [isoniazid] 300 mg

laninamivir *investigational (Phase III) inhaled vaccine for H5N1 (avian) influenza*

Laniseptic Therapeutic Cream OTC *moisturizer; emollient* [lanolin] 37%

lanolin USP *ointment base; water-in-oil emulsion; emollient/protectant*

lanolin, anhydrous USP *absorbent ointment base*

lanolin alcohols *ointment base ingredient*

Lanolor cream OTC *moisturizer; emollient*

Lanophyllin elixir (discontinued 2008) ℞ *antiasthmatic; bronchodilator* [theophylline] 80 mg/15 mL

Lan-O-Smooth cream OTC *moisturizer; emollient* [lanolin] 100%

lanoteplase USAN *thrombolytic; tissue plasminogen activator (tPA)*

Lanoxicaps capsules (discontinued 2008) ℞ *cardiac glycoside to increase cardiac output; antiarrhythmic* [digoxin] 0.05, 0.1, 0.2 mg

Lanoxin tablets, IV or IM injection ℞ *cardiac glycoside to increase cardiac output; antiarrhythmic* [digoxin] 0.125, 0.25 mg; 0.1, 0.25 mg/mL ⊡ Lincocin

lanreotide acetate USAN *somatostatin analogue; antineoplastic; reduces endogenous growth hormone (GH) and insulin growth factor-1 (IGF-1) levels to treat acromegaly (orphan)* (base=77%)

Lansinoh cream OTC *moisturizer; emollient* [lanolin] 100%

Lansinoh Diaper Rash ointment OTC *diaper rash treatment* [lanolin; zinc oxide; dimethicone] 15.5%•5/5%•5%

lansoprazole USAN, INN, BAN *proton pump inhibitor for gastric and duodenal ulcers, erosive esophagitis, gastroesophageal reflux disease (GERD), and other gastroesophageal disorders* 15, 30 mg oral

lanthanum *element (La)*

lanthanum carbonate *phosphate binder for hyperphosphatemia in end-stage renal disease (ESRD)*

Lantus vials, OptiClik cartridges, and SoloStar prefilled syringes for subcu injection ℞ *long-acting, once-daily basal insulin analogue for diabetes* [insulin glargine (rDNA)] 100 U/mL; 300 IU/3 mL; 300 U/3 mL

Lapacho colorado; L. morado medicinal herb [see: pau d'arco]

lapatinib ditosylate *tyrosine kinase inhibitor; antineoplastic for advanced or metastatic HER2-positive breast cancer; investigational for kidney, head, neck, and colon cancers* (base=63%)

lapirium chloride INN *surfactant* [also: lapyrium chloride]

laprafylline INN

lapyrium chloride USAN *surfactant* [also: lapirium chloride]

laquinimod *investigational (Phase III) once-daily oral therapy for relapsing-remitting multiple sclerosis*

laramycin [see: zorbamycin]

larch (*Larix americana; L. europaea*) bark, resin, young shoots, and needles *medicinal herb used as an anthelmintic, diuretic, laxative, and vulnerary; powdered bark is 98% arabinogalactans* [see also: arabinogalactans]

Lariam tablets (discontinued 2010) ℞ *antimalarial for acute chloroquine-resistant malaria (orphan)* [mefloquine HCl] 250 mg

Larix americana; L. europaea medicinal herb [see: larch]

Larodopa capsules (discontinued 2010) ℞ *dopamine precursor for Parkinson disease* [levodopa] 100, 250 mg

Larodopa tablets ℞ *dopamine precursor for Parkinson disease* [levodopa] 100, 250, 500 mg

laronidase *enzyme replacement therapy for mucopolysaccharidosis I (MPS I) (orphan)*

laropiprant *investigational (NDA filed) prostaglandin D_2 (PGD_2) inhibitor to reduce flushing during niacin therapy*

laroxyl [see: amitriptyline]

Larrea divaricata; L. glutinosa; L. tridentata medicinal herb [see: chaparral]

lasalocid USAN, INN, BAN *coccidiostat for poultry*

Lasix oral solution, IM or IV injection (discontinued 2011) ℞ *antihypertensive; loop diuretic for congestive heart failure, hepatic cirrhosis, and renal disease* [furosemide] 10 mg/mL; 10 mg/mL

Lasix tablets ℞ *antihypertensive; loop diuretic for congestive heart failure, hepatic cirrhosis, and renal disease* [furosemide] 20, 40, 80 mg

lasofoxifene tartrate USAN *second-generation selective estrogen receptor modulator (SERM); investigational (NDA filed) for osteoporosis; investigational for breast cancer*

Lassar paste [betanaphthol (q.v.) + zinc oxide (q.v.)]

Lastacaft eye drops ℞ *antihistamine for allergic conjunctivitis* [alcaftadine] 0.25%

latamoxef INN, BAN *anti-infective* [also: moxalactam disodium]

latamoxef disodium [see: moxalactam disodium]

latanoprost USAN, INN *topical prostaglandin agonist for glaucoma and ocular hypertension* [0.005% eye drops]

latex agglutination test *in vitro diagnostic aid*

Latisse topical ophthalmic solution ℞ *antihypertensive for glaucoma and ocular hypertension; used cosmetically to grow, thicken, and darken eyelashes* [bimatoprost] 0.03% ⓢ lettuce

latrepirdine *investigational (Phase III) mitochondria stabilizer to improve mental function in Alzheimer and Huntington diseases*

Latrix XM topical emulsion ℞ *keratolytic for the removal of dystrophic nails* [urea] 45%

Latrodectus **immune F(ab)2** *investigational (orphan) treatment for black widow spider bites*

Latuda tablets ℞ *once-daily atypical antipsychotic for schizophrenia* [lurasidone HCl] 40, 80 mg

laudexium methylsulfate [see: laudexium metilsulfate; laudexium methylsulphate]

laudexium methylsulphate BAN [also: laudexium metilsulfate]

laudexium metilsulfate INN [also: laudexium methylsulphate]

lauralkonium chloride INN

laurel (*Laurus nobilis*) leaves and fruit *medicinal herb used as an aromatic, astringent, carminative, and stomachic*

laurel, mountain; rose laurel; sheep laurel *medicinal herb* [see: mountain laurel]

laurel, red; swamp laurel *medicinal herb* [see: magnolia]

laurel, spurge; spurge olive *medicinal herb* [see: mezereon]

laureth 4 USAN *surfactant*

laureth 9 USAN *spermaticide; surfactant*

laureth 10S USAN *spermaticide*

lauril INN *combining name for radicals or groups*

laurilsulfate INN *combining name for radicals or groups* [also: sodium lauryl sulfate]

laurixamine INN

laurocapram USAN, INN *excipient*

laurocapram & methotrexate *investigational (orphan) for topical treatment of mycosis fungoides*

lauroguadine INN

laurolinium acetate INN, BAN

lauromacrogol 400 INN

Laurus nobilis *medicinal herb* [see: laurel]

Laurus persea *medicinal herb* [see: avocado]

lauryl isoquinolinium bromide USAN *anti-infective*

lavender (*Lavandula* spp.) flowers, leaves, and oil *medicinal herb for acne, bile flow stimulation, diabetes, edema, flatulence, hyperactivity, insomnia, intestinal spasms, migraine headache, and stimulating menstrual flow*

lavender oil NF

LaViv subcu injection ℞ *autologous cell dermal filler for moderate to severe nasolabial folds* [azficel-T]

lavoltidine INN *antiulcerative; histamine H_2-receptor blocker* [also: lavoltidine succinate; loxtidine]

lavoltidine succinate USAN *antiulcerative; histamine H_2-receptor blocker* [also: lavoltidine; loxtidine]

lawrencium *element* (Lr)

Lawsonia inermis *medicinal herb* [see: henna]

Laxative & Stool Softener softgels (discontinued 2007) OTC *stimulant laxative; stool softener* [casanthranol; docusate sodium] 30•100 mg

laxatives *a class of agents that promote evacuation of the bowels or have a mild purgative effect; subclasses: bulk-producing, emollient, hyperosmotic, saline, stimulant, and stool-softening* [see also: cathartics; purgatives; listed subclasses]

Lax-Lyte oral solution ℞ *pre-procedure bowel evacuant* [PEG 3350; sodium bicarbonate; sodium chloride; sodium sulfate; potassium chloride] 420•5.72•11.2•1.48 g/bottle

Lax-Pills tablets OTC *stimulant laxative* [sennosides] 15, 25 mg

lazabemide USAN, INN *antiparkinsonian*

lazabemide HCl USAN *antiparkinsonian*

Lazanda nasal spray ℞ *narcotic analgesic for breakthrough cancer pain* [fentanyl] 100, 400 mcg/spray

lazaroids *a class of potent antioxidants that can protect against oxygen radical–mediated lipid peroxidation and progressive neuronal degeneration following brain or spinal trauma, subarachnoid hemorrhage, or stroke* [also called: 21-aminosteroids]

Lazer Creme OTC *moisturizer; emollient* [vitamins A and E] 3333.3•116.67 U/g

Lazer Formalyde solution ℞ *anhidrotic for hyperhidrosis and bromhidrosis* [formaldehyde] 10%

LazerSporin-C ear drops ℞ *corticosteroidal anti-inflammatory; antibiotic* [hydrocortisone; neomycin sulfate; polymyxin B sulfate] 1%•5 mg•10 000 U per mL

LC-65 solution OTC *cleaning solution for hard, soft, or rigid gas permeable contact lenses*

L-Carnitine tablets, capsules OTC *dietary amino acid* [levocarnitine] 500 mg; 250 mg

LCD (liquor carbonis detergens) [see: coal tar]

LCR (leurocristine) [see: vincristine]

LCx Neisseria gonorrhoeae Assay reagent kit for professional use ℞ *in vitro diagnostic aid for* Neisseria gonorrhoeae *infection*

lead *element (Pb)*

lecimibide USAN *hypocholesterolemic; antihyperlipidemic*

lecithin NF *emulsifier; surfactant; natural phospholipid mixture of various phosphatidylcholines used as an antihypercholesterolemic and cognition enhancer for Alzheimer and other dementias* 420, 1200 mg oral

lecithol *natural remedy* [see: lecithin]

LED (liposome-encapsulated doxorubicin) [see: doxorubicin HCl, liposome-encapsulated]

Lederject (trademarked delivery form) *prefilled disposable syringe*

ledoxantrone trihydrochloride USAN *antineoplastic; topoisomerase II inhibitor*

Ledum groenlandicum; L. latifolium; L. palustre *medicinal herb* [see: Labrador tea]

leeches (Hirudo medicinalis) *natural adjunct to postsurgical wound management*

leek (Allium porrum) bulb, lower stem, and leaves *medicinal herb used as an appetite stimulant, decongestant, and diuretic*

Leena tablets (in packs of 28) ℞ *triphasic oral contraceptive* [norethindrone; ethinyl estradiol]
Phase 1 (7 days): 0.5 mg•35 mcg;
Phase 2 (9 days): 1 mg•35 mcg;
Phase 3 (5 days): 0.5 mg•35 mcg;
Counters (7 days)

lefetamine INN

leflunomide USAN, INN *immunomodulator for rheumatoid arthritis (RA); investigational (orphan) for malignant glioma, ovarian cancer, and prevention of organ transplant rejection* 10, 20 mg oral

Legalon *investigational (orphan) antitoxin for* Amanita phalloides *(mushroom) intoxication* [disodium silibinin dihemisuccinate]

Legatrin PM caplets OTC *prevention and treatment of nocturnal leg cramps* [diphenhydramine HCl; acetaminophen] 50•500 mg

legs, red *medicinal herb* [see: bistort]

leiopyrrole INN

lemidosul INN

lemon (Citrus limon) *fruit and peel medicinal herb used as an astringent, refrigerant, and source of vitamin C*

lemon, ground; wild lemon *medicinal herb* [see: mandrake]

lemon balm (Melissa officinalis) plant *medicinal herb used as an antispasmodic and sedative; also used for Graves disease and cold sores*

lemon oil NF

lemon verbena (Aloysiatriphylla spp.) leaves and flowers *medicinal herb for fever, flatulence, gastrointestinal spasms and other disorders, and sedation*

lemon walnut *medicinal herb* [see: butternut]

lemongrass (Andropogon citratus; Cymbopogon citratus) leaves *medicinal herb for colds, cough, fever, gastrointestinal spasm and other disorders, nervousness, pain, and rheumatism; also used as an antiemetic*

Lemotussin-DM oral liquid (discontinued 2007) ℞ *antitussive; antihistamine; decongestant; expectorant* [dextromethorphan hydrobromide; chlorpheniramine maleate; pseudoephedrine HCl; guaifenesin; potassium guaiacolsulfonate] 7.5•2•10•50•50 mg

Lemtrada *investigational (Phase III) immunosuppressant for multiple sclerosis* [alemtuzumab]

lenalidomide *immunomodulator for multiple myeloma and transfusion-dependent anemia in patients with myelodysplastic syndrome (orphan); thalidomide analogue*

lenampicillin INN

lenercept USAN *tumor necrosis factor (TNF) receptor antagonist for septic shock, multiple sclerosis, inflammatory bowel disease, and rheumatoid arthritis*

leniquinsin USAN, INN *antihypertensive*

lenitzol [see: amitriptyline]

lenograstim USAN, INN, BAN *immunomodulator; antineutropenic; hematopoietic stimulant*

lenperone USAN, INN *antipsychotic*

Lens Drops solution (discontinued 2010) OTC *rewetting solution for hard or soft contact lenses*

Lens Lubricant solution (discontinued 2010) OTC *rewetting solution for hard or soft contact lenses*

Lens Plus Daily Cleaner solution (discontinued 2010) OTC *surfactant cleaning solution for soft contact lenses*

Lens Plus Oxysept products [see: Oxysept]

Lens Plus Rewetting Drops (discontinued 2010) OTC *rewetting solution for soft contact lenses*

Lens Plus Sterile Saline aerosol solution OTC *rinsing/storage solution for soft contact lenses* [sodium chloride (saline solution)]

Lente Iletin II vials for subcu injection OTC *antidiabetic* [insulin zinc (pork)] 100 U/mL

lentin [see: carbachol]

lentinan JAN *immunomodulator*

Lentinula edodes medicinal herb [see: shiitake mushrooms]

Leontodon taraxacum medicinal herb [see: dandelion]

Leonurus cardiaca medicinal herb [see: motherwort]

leopard's bane *medicinal herb* [see: arnica]

Lepidium meyenii medicinal herb [see: maca]

lepirudin *anticoagulant for heparin-associated thrombocytopenia (orphan)*

leprostatics *a class of drugs effective against leprosy*

leptacline INN

leptandra; purple leptandra *medicinal herb* [see: Culver root]

lergotrile USAN, INN *prolactin enzyme inhibitor*

lergotrile mesylate USAN *prolactin enzyme inhibitor*

leridistim USAN *interleukin-3 and granulocyte colony-stimulating factor receptor agonist for chemotherapy-induced neutropenia and thrombocytopenia*

Lescol capsules ℞ *HMG-CoA reductase inhibitor for hypercholesterolemia, hypertriglyceridemia, mixed dyslipidemia, atherosclerosis, and coronary heart disease (CHD)* [fluvastatin (as sodium)] 20, 40 mg

Lescol XL film-coated extended-release tablets ℞ *HMG-CoA reductase inhibitor for hypercholesterolemia, hypertriglyceridemia, mixed dyslipidemia, atherosclerosis, and coronary heart disease (CHD)* [fluvastatin (as sodium)] 80 mg

lesopitron INN *anxiolytic*

lesser centaury *medicinal herb* [see: centaury]

Lessina film-coated tablets (in packs of 21 or 28) ℞ *monophasic oral contraceptive; emergency postcoital contraceptive* [levonorgestrel; ethinyl estradiol] 0.1 mg•20 mcg ⓓ leucine; lysine

Letairis film-coated tablets ℞ *vasodilator for pulmonary arterial hypertension (PAH)* [ambrisentan] 5, 10 mg ⓓ LTRAs

leteprinim potassium USAN *nerve growth factor*

letimide INN *analgesic* [also: letimide HCl]

letimide HCl USAN *analgesic* [also: letimide]

letosteine INN

letrazuril INN *investigational treatment for AIDS-related cryptosporidial diarrhea*

letrozole USAN, INN *aromatase inhibitor; estrogen antagonist; antineoplastic for early, advanced, or metastatic breast cancer in postmenopausal women* 2.5 mg oral

lettuce (*Lactuca sativa*) *juice and leaves medicinal herb used as an anodyne, antispasmodic, expectorant, and sedative (for herbal medical use, common garden lettuce is harvested after it has gone to seed, and a milky juice is extracted)* ⓓ Latisse

Leucanthemum parthenium medicinal herb [see: feverfew]

leucarsone [see: carbarsone]

leucine (L-leucine) USAN, USP, INN, JAN essential amino acid; symbols: Leu, L ⑦ Lessina; lysine

leucine & isoleucine & valine investigational (orphan) for hyperphenylalaninemia

L-leucine & L-tyrosine & L-serine investigational (orphan) for hepatocellular carcinoma

leucinocaine INN

leucocianidol INN

Leucomax ⑪ (available in 36 foreign countries) investigational (orphan) antineutropenic and hematopoietic stimulant for bone marrow transplants, chronic lymphocytic leukemia (CLL), myelodysplastic syndrome, aplastic anemia, and AIDS-related neutropenia [molgramostim]

leucomycin [see: kitasamycin; spiramycin]

L-leucovorin chemotherapy "rescue" agent (orphan)

leucovorin calcium USP antianemic; folate replenisher; antidote to folic acid antagonist; chemotherapy "rescue" agent (orphan) [also: calcium folinate] 5, 15, 25 mg oral; 10 mg/mL injection; 50, 100, 200, 350, 500 mg/vial injection

Leukeran film-coated tablets ℞ antineoplastic for multiple leukemias and lymphomas; also used for other malignancies [chlorambucil] 2 mg

Leukine IV infusion ℞ hematopoietic stimulant for graft delay (orphan) and bone marrow transplant in patients with acute lymphoblastic leukemia (ALL), Hodgkin disease, or non-Hodgkin lymphoma (NHL) [sargramostim] 250, 500 mcg/mL

leukocyte interferon [now: interferon alfa-n3]

leukocyte typing serum USP in vitro blood test

leukopoietin [see: sargramostim]

Leukotac investigational (orphan) for graft-versus-host disease [inolimomab]

leukotriene formation inhibitors a class of antiasthmatics that inhibit 5-lipoxygenase to suppress the formation of leukotrienes [also known as: 5-lipoxygenase inhibitors; compare to: leukotriene receptor antagonists (LTRAs)]

leukotriene receptor antagonists (LTRAs); leukotriene receptor inhibitors a class of antiasthmatics that inhibit the action of leukotrienes [compare to: leukotriene formation inhibitors]

leukotrienes (LT) a class of endogenous substances that cause inflammation, edema, mucus secretion, and smooth muscle contraction, which present as asthma and bronchoconstriction [also see: leukotriene formation inhibitors; leukotriene receptor antagonists (LTRAs)]

leupeptin investigational (orphan) aid to microsurgical peripheral nerve repair

leuprolide acetate USAN gonadotropin suppressant; antihormonal antineoplastic for various cancers; LHRH agonist for central precocious puberty (orphan), endometriosis, and uterine fibroids [also: leuprorelin] 5 mg/mL injection

leuprorelin INN, BAN testosterone suppressant; antihormonal antineoplastic for various cancers [also: leuprolide acetate]

leurocristine (LCR) [see: vincristine]

leurocristine sulfate [see: vincristine sulfate]

Leustatin IV infusion ℞ antineoplastic for hairy-cell leukemia (orphan); investigational (orphan) for chronic lymphocytic leukemia, myeloid leukemia, multiple sclerosis, and non-Hodgkin lymphoma [cladribine] 1 mg/mL

Levacet caplets OTC analgesic; antipyretic [aspirin; acetaminophen; salicylamide; caffeine] 500•250•150•40 mg

levacetylmethadol INN narcotic analgesic [also: levomethadyl acetate]

levalbuterol *sympathomimetic broncho-dilator; single isomer of albuterol*

levalbuterol HCl USAN *sympathomimetic bronchodilator; single isomer of albuterol* 1.25 mg/0.5 mL dose inhalation solution

levalbuterol sulfate USAN *sympathomimetic bronchodilator; single isomer of albuterol*

levalbuterol tartrate USAN *sympathomimetic bronchodilator; single isomer of albuterol*

Levall oral liquid ℞ *antitussive; decongestant; expectorant* [carbetapentane citrate; phenylephrine HCl; guaifenesin] 15•5•100 mg/5 mL ⌧ Livalo

Levall 5.0 oral liquid ℞ *narcotic antitussive; decongestant; expectorant* [hydrocodone bitartrate; phenylephrine HCl; guaifenesin] 2.5•5•100 mg/5 mL ⌧ Livalo

Levall 12 oral suspension ℞ *antitussive; decongestant* [carbetapentane tannate; phenylephrine tannate] 30•25 mg/5 mL ⌧ Livalo

levallorphan INN, BAN [also: levallorphan tartrate]

levallorphan tartrate USP [also: levallorphan]

levamfetamine INN *anorectic* [also: levamfetamine succinate; levamphetamine]

levamfetamine succinate USAN *anorectic* [also: levamfetamine; levamphetamine]

levamisole INN, BAN *biological response modifier; antineoplastic; veterinary anthelmintic* [also: levamisole HCl] ⌧ lofemizole

levamisole HCl USAN, USP *biological response modifier; antineoplastic; veterinary anthelmintic* [also: levamisole] ⌧ lofemizole HCl

levamphetamine BAN *anorectic* [also: levamfetamine succinate; levamfetamine]

levant berry (Anamirta cocculus; A. paniculata) leaves and berries *medicinal herb for epilepsy, lice, malaria, morphine poisoning, and worms; not*

generally regarded as safe and effective for ingestion or topical application on abraded skin

Levaquin film-coated tablets, oral solution, IV infusion ℞ *broad-spectrum fluoroquinolone antibiotic* [levofloxacin] 250, 500, 750 mg; 25 mg/mL; 250, 500, 750 mg

Levaquin Leva-pak (5 tablets) ℞ *broad-spectrum fluoroquinolone antibiotic for acute bacterial sinusitis* [levofloxacin] 750 mg

levarterenol [see: norepinephrine bitartrate]

levarterenol bitartrate [now: norepinephrine bitartrate]

Levatol caplets ℞ *beta-blocker for hypertension* [penbutolol sulfate] 20 mg

Levbid extended-release tablets ℞ *GI/GU antispasmodic; antiparkinsonian; anticholinergic "drying agent" for allergic rhinitis or hyperhidrosis* [hyoscyamine sulfate] 0.375 mg

levcromakalim USAN, INN, BAN *antiasthmatic; antihypertensive*

levcycloserine USAN, INN *enzyme inhibitor*

levdobutamine INN *cardiotonic* [also: levdobutamine lactobionate]

levdobutamine lactobionate USAN *cardiotonic* [also: levdobutamine]

levdropropizine INN

Levemir vials, prefilled syringes, and PenFill cartridges for subcu injection ℞ *antidiabetic; long-acting insulin formulation intended to provide continuous basal insulin levels through once- or twice-daily dosing* [insulin detemir, human (rDNA)] 100 U/mL; 300 U/3 mL; 300 U/3 mL

levemopamil INN *treatment for stroke*

levetiracetam USAN, INN *anticonvulsant for myoclonic, partial-onset, and generalized tonic-clonic seizures; oral forms are also used to treat migraine headaches and bipolar disorder* 250, 500, 750, 1000 mg oral; 100 mg/mL oral; 100 mg/mL infusion

levisoprenaline INN

Levisticum officinale medicinal herb [see: lovage]

Levitra film-coated tablets ℞ *selective vasodilator for erectile dysfunction (ED)* [vardenafil HCl] 2.5, 5, 10, 20 mg

Levlen tablets (in Slidecases of 28) (discontinued 2008) ℞ *monophasic oral contraceptive; emergency postcoital contraceptive* [levonorgestrel; ethinyl estradiol] 0.15 mg•30 mcg × 21 days; counters × 7 days ☑ Lufyllin

Levlite tablets (in Slidecases of 28) (discontinued 2008) ℞ *monophasic oral contraceptive* [levonorgestrel; ethinyl estradiol] 0.1 mg•20 mcg × 21 days; counters × 7 days ☑ Lypholyte

levlofexidine INN

levmetamfetamine USAN, USP *nasal decongestant*

levobetaxolol INN *topical antiglaucoma agent (beta-blocker)* [also: levobetaxolol HCl]

levobetaxolol HCl USAN *topical antiglaucoma agent (beta-blocker)* [also: levobetaxolol]

levobunolol INN, BAN *topical antiglaucoma agent (beta-blocker)* [also: levobunolol HCl]

levobunolol HCl USAN, USP *topical antiglaucoma agent (beta-blocker)* [also: levobunolol] 0.25%, 0.5% eye drops

levobupivacaine HCl USAN *long-acting local anesthetic*

levocabastine INN, BAN *antihistamine* [also: levocabastine HCl]

levocabastine HCl USAN *antihistamine; ophthalmic suspension for allergic conjunctivitis (orphan)* [also: levocabastine]

levocarbinoxamine tartrate [see: rotoxamine tartrate]

levocarnitine USAN, USP, INN *dietary amino acid for primary and secondary genetic carnitine deficiency (orphan) and end-stage renal disease (orphan); investigational (orphan) for pediatric cardiomyopathy* 330 mg oral; 100, 300 mg/mL oral; 200 mg/mL injection

levocetirizine dihydrochloride *second-generation piperazine antihistamine for allergic rhinitis and chronic idiopathic urticaria; isomer of cetirizine* 5 mg oral; 0.5 mg/mL oral

levodopa USAN, USP, INN, BAN, JAN *dopamine precursor for Parkinson disease*

levodopa & carbidopa *dopamine precursor plus potentiator for Parkinson disease (orphan)* 100•10, 100•25, 200•50, 250•25 mg oral

levodopa & carbidopa & entacapone *multi-modal treatment for Parkinson disease: dopamine precursor + decarboxylase inhibitor (levodopa potentiator) + COMT (catechol-O-methyltransferase) inhibitor* 100•25•200, 150•37.5•200 mg oral

Levo-Dromoran tablets; IV, IM, or subcu injection (discontinued 2011) ℞ *narcotic analgesic* [levorphanol tartrate] 2 mg; 2 mg/mL

levofacetoperane INN

levofenfluramine INN

levofloxacin USAN, INN, JAN *broad-spectrum fluoroquinolone antibiotic* 250, 500, 750 mg oral; 0.5% eye drops; 5, 25 mg/mL injection

levofuraltadone USAN, INN *antibacterial; antiprotozoal*

levoglutamide INN [now: glutamine]

Levolet tablets ℞ *synthetic thyroid hormone (T_4 fraction only)* [levothyroxine sodium] ☑ Lypholyte

levoleucovorin calcium USAN *antidote to folic acid antagonists; chemotherapy "rescue agent" for osteosarcoma and colorectal cancer* (base= 78%) 64 mg (50 mg base) injection

levomefolate; L-methylfolate *bioactive form of folic acid that crosses the blood-brain barrier* [see: folic acid]

levomenol INN

levomepate [see: atromepine]

levomepromazine INN *analgesic* [also: methotrimeprazine]

levomethadone INN

levomethadyl acetate USAN *narcotic analgesic* [also: levacetylmethadol]

levomethadyl acetate HCl USAN *narcotic analgesic for management of opiate addiction (orphan)*

levomethorphan INN, BAN

levometiomeprazine INN

levomoprolol INN

levomoramide INN, BAN

levonantradol INN, BAN *analgesic* [also: levonantradol HCl]

levonantradol HCl USAN *analgesic* [also: levonantradol]

levonordefrin USP *adrenergic; vasoconstrictor* [also: corbadrine]

levonorgestrel USAN, USP, INN, BAN *progestin; oral contraceptive; contraceptive intrauterine device (IUD); emergency postcoital ("morning after") contraceptive* 0.75 mg oral

levonorgestrel & ethinyl estradiol *monophasic oral contraceptive; extended-cycle (3 months) biphasic oral contraceptive* 50•30, 75•40, 90•20, 125•30 mcg; Phase 1: 150•30 mcg, Phase 2: 0•10 mcg

Levophed IV infusion ℞ *vasopressor for acute hypotensive shock* [norepinephrine bitartrate] 1 mg/mL

levophenacylmorphan INN, BAN

levopropicillin INN *antibacterial* [also: levopropylcillin potassium]

levopropicillin potassium [see: levopropylcillin potassium]

levopropoxyphene INN, BAN *antitussive* [also: levopropoxyphene napsylate]

levopropoxyphene napsylate USAN *antitussive* [also: levopropoxyphene]

levopropylcillin potassium USAN *antibacterial* [also: levopropicillin]

levopropylhexedrine INN

levoprotiline INN

Levora tablets (in packs of 28) ℞ *monophasic oral contraceptive* [levonorgestrel; ethinyl estradiol] 150•30 mcg × 21 days; counters × 7 days

levorin INN

levorotatory alkaloids of belladonna *a subclass of belladonna alkaloids (q.v.)* [also known as: belladonna L-alkaloids]

levorphanol INN, BAN *narcotic analgesic* [also: levorphanol tartrate]

levorphanol tartrate USP *narcotic analgesic* [also: levorphanol] 2 mg oral

levosimendan USAN *calcium sensitizer; vasodilator*

Levo-T tablets ℞ *synthetic thyroid hormone (T_4 fraction only)* [levothyroxine sodium] 25, 50, 75, 88, 100, 112, 125, 137, 150, 175, 200, 300 mcg

Levothroid caplets ℞ *synthetic thyroid hormone (T_4 fraction only)* [levothyroxine sodium] 25, 50, 75, 88, 100, 112, 125, 150, 175, 200, 300 mcg

levothyroxine sodium USP, INN *synthetic thyroid hormone (T_4 fraction only)* [also: thyroxine] 25, 50, 75, 88, 100, 112, 125, 137, 150, 175, 200, 300 mcg oral; 100, 200, 500 mcg injection

levoxadrol INN *local anesthetic; smooth muscle relaxant* [also: levoxadrol HCl]

levoxadrol HCl USAN *local anesthetic; smooth muscle relaxant* [also: levoxadrol]

Levoxyl tablets ℞ *synthetic thyroid hormone (T_4 fraction only)* [levothyroxine sodium] 25, 50, 75, 88, 100, 112, 125, 137, 150, 175, 200, 300 mcg

LEV/PSE/GG extended-release capsules ℞ *decongestant; expectorant* [pseudoephedrine HCl; guaifenesin] 90•400 mg

Levsin drops, elixir (discontinued 2008) ℞ *GI/GU antispasmodic; antiparkinsonian; anticholinergic "drying agent" for allergic rhinitis and hyperhidrosis* [hyoscyamine sulfate] 0.125 mg/mL; 0.125 mg/5 mL

Levsin IV, IM, or subcu injection ℞ *GI/GU antispasmodic to reduce motility during radiologic imaging; preoperative antimuscarinic to reduce salivary and gastric secretions* [hyoscyamine sulfate] 0.5 mg/mL

Levsin tablets ℞ *GI/GU antispasmodic; antiparkinsonian; anticholinergic "drying agent" for allergic rhinitis and hyperhidrosis* [hyoscyamine sulfate] 0.125 mg

Levsin PB drops (discontinued 2008) ℞ *GI/GU anticholinergic/antispasmodic; sedative* [hyoscyamine sulfate;

phenobarbital; alcohol 5%] 0.125•
15 mg/mL

Levsin with Phenobarbital tablets ℞
GI/GU antispasmodic; anticholinergic;
sedative [hyoscyamine sulfate; phe-
nobarbital] 0.125•15 mg

Levsinex Timecaps (timed-release capsules) ℞ GI/GU antispasmodic; antiparkinsonian; anticholinergic "drying
agent" for allergic rhinitis or hyperhidrosis [hyoscyamine sulfate] 0.375 mg

Levsin/SL sublingual tablets (also may
be chewed or swallowed) ℞ GI/GU
antispasmodic; anticholinergic [hyoscy-
amine sulfate] 0.125 mg

Levulan Kerastick topical solution ℞
photosensitizer for photodynamic therapy
of precancerous actinic keratoses of the
face and scalp (used with the **BLU-U
Blue Light Photodynamic Therapy
Illuminator**) [aminolevulinic acid
HCl] 20%

levulose BAN nutrient; caloric replacement [also: fructose]

Lexapro film-coated tablets, oral solution ℞ selective serotonin reuptake
inhibitor (SSRI) for major depressive
disorder (MDD) and generalized anxiety disorder (GAD); also used for post-
traumatic stress disorder (PTSD) [esci-
talopram (as oxalate)] 5, 10, 20 mg;
5 mg/5 mL

lexipafant USAN platelet activating factor (PAF) antagonist

Lexiscan IV injection in vials and
prefilled syringes ℞ coronary vasodilator to induce pharmacological stress
for myocardial perfusion imaging [rega-
denoson] 0.4 mg/5 mL

lexithromycin USAN, INN antibacterial

Lexiva film-coated caplets, oral suspension ℞ antiretroviral; HIV-1 protease inhibitor [fosamprenavir calcium
(converts to amprenavir)] 700 mg
(600 mg); 50 mg/mL (43 mg/mL)

lexofenac INN

Lexuss 210 oral liquid ℞ antihistamine; narcotic antitussive [chlorphen-
iramine maleate; codeine phosphate]
2•10 mg/5 mL

Lexxel film-coated dual-release tablets
(discontinued 2008) ℞ antihypertensive; angiotensin-converting enzyme
(ACE) inhibitor; calcium channel
blocker [enalapril maleate (immediate release); felodipine (extended
release)] 5•2.5, 5•5 mg

LH (luteinizing hormone) [see:
lutropin alfa]

**LH-RF (luteinizing hormone–releas-
ing factor) acetate hydrate** [see:
gonadorelin acetate]

LH-RF diacetate tetrahydrate [now:
gonadorelin acetate]

LH-RF dihydrochloride [now:
gonadorelin HCl]

LH-RF HCl [see: gonadorelin HCl]

**LH-RH (luteinizing hormone–
releasing hormone)** an endogenous
hormone, produced in the hypothalamus, which stimulates the release of
luteinizing hormone (LH) and follicle-
stimulating hormone (FSH) from the
pituitary [also known as: gonadotropin-releasing hormone (Gn-RH)]

Lialda film-coated delayed-release tablets ℞ once-daily anti-inflammatory
for mild to moderate ulcerative colitis
[mesalamine (5-aminosalicylic acid)]
1.2 g

liarozole INN, BAN antipsoriatic; aromatase inhibitor [also: liarozole fumarate]
② Lioresal

liarozole fumarate USAN antipsoriatic;
aromatase inhibitor; investigational
(orphan) for congenital ichthyosis [also:
liarozole]

liarozole HCl USAN antineoplastic for
prostate cancer; aromatase inhibitor

liatermin USAN dopaminergic neuronal
growth stimulator for Parkinson disease

**Liatris scariosa; L. spicata; L. squar-
rosa** medicinal herb [see: blazing star]

libecillide INN

libenzapril USAN, INN antihypertensive;
angiotensin-converting enzyme (ACE)
inhibitor

LibiGel gel androgen; investigational
(Phase III) for female sexual dysfunc-

tion (FSD) and hypoactive sexual desire disorder (HSDD) [testosterone]

Librax capsules ℞ GI/GU *anticholinergic/antispasmodic; anxiolytic* [clidinium bromide; chlordiazepoxide HCl] 2.5•5 mg Ⓓ Loprox

Librium capsules ℞ *benzodiazepine anxiolytic; sedative; alcohol withdrawal aid; also abused as a street drug* [chlordiazepoxide HCl] 10 mg Ⓓ Lipram

Librium powder for IM or IV injection (discontinued 2009) ℞ *benzodiazepine anxiolytic; sedative; alcohol withdrawal aid; also abused as a street drug* [chlordiazepoxide HCl] 100 mg Ⓓ Lipram

Lice Asphyxiator liquid emulsion *investigational (Phase III) nontoxic, insecticide-free treatment for head lice*

Lice Treatment shampoo OTC *pediculicide for lice* [pyrethrins; piperonyl butoxide] 0.33%•4%

Licide Complete Lice Treatment shampoo + gel OTC *pediculicide for lice* [pyrethrins; piperonyl butoxide] 0.33%•4%

licorice *(Glycyrrhiza glabra; G. pallidiflora; G. uralensis)* root *medicinal herb for Addison disease, blood cleansing, colds, cough, drug withdrawal, female disorders, hoarseness, hypoglycemia, lung disorders, sore throat, and stomach ulcers; also used as an expectorant and to increase energy*

licostinel USAN *NMDA receptor antagonist*

licryfilcon A USAN *hydrophilic contact lens material*

licryfilcon B USAN *hydrophilic contact lens material*

LidaMantle cream ℞ *anesthetic* [lidocaine HCl] 3%

LidaMantle HC cream, lotion ℞ *corticosteroidal anti-inflammatory; anesthetic* [hydrocortisone acetate; lidocaine] 0.5%•3%

LidaMantle HC Relief Pad ℞ *corticosteroidal anti-inflammatory; anesthetic* [hydrocortisone acetate; lidocaine] 2%•2%

lidamidine INN *antiperistaltic* [also: lidamidine HCl]

lidamidine HCl USAN *antiperistaltic* [also: lidamidine]

Lidex cream, ointment, topical solution ℞ *corticosteroidal anti-inflammatory* [fluocinonide] 0.05%

Lidex-E cream ℞ *corticosteroidal anti-inflammatory; emollient* [fluocinonide] 0.05%

lidimycin INN *antifungal* [also: lydimycin]

lidocaine USP, INN *topical/local anesthetic; transdermal delivery for postherpetic neuralgia (orphan)* [also: lignocaine]

lidocaine benzyl benzoate [see: denatonium benzoate]

lidocaine HCl USP *topical/local anesthetic; mucous membrane anesthetic; antiarrhythmic for acute ventricular arrhythmias* [also: lignocaine HCl] 2%, 3%, 4%, 5% topical; 0.5%, 1%, 2% IV injection; 4%, 10%, 20% IV admixture

Lidocaine HCl in Dextrose injection, IV infusion ℞ *local anesthetic for obstetric use; IV infusion for acute ventricular arrhythmias* [lidicaine HCl; dextrose] 1.5%•7.5%, 5%•7.5%; 0.2%, 0.4%, 0.8%

lidocaine HCl & epinephrine *injectable local anesthetic; vasoconstrictor* 0.5%•1:200 000, 1%•1:100 000, 1%•1:200 000, 1.5%•1:200 000, 2%•1:50 000, 2%•1:100 000, 2%•1:200 000 injection

lidocaine HCl & hydrocortisone acetate *local anesthetic; corticosteroidal anti-inflammatory* 0.5%•3%, 0.55%•2.8%, 3%•2.5% topical

lidocaine & prilocaine *local anesthetic* 2.5%•2.5% topical

Lidocaine/Hydrocortisone Rectal cream in prefilled applicators (discontinued 2007) ℞ *corticosteroidal anti-inflammatory; anesthetic* [hydrocortisone acetate; lidocaine HCl] 0.5%•3%

LidoCort anorectal gel in prefilled applicators ℞ *corticosteroidal anti-inflammatory; anesthetic* [hydrocortisone acetate; lidocaine HCl] 2.5%•3%

Lidoderm transdermal patch ℞ *anesthetic for post-herpetic neuralgia (orphan)* [lidocaine] 5%

lidofenin USAN, INN *hepatic function test*

lidofilcon A USAN *hydrophilic contact lens material*

lidofilcon B USAN *hydrophilic contact lens material*

lidoflazine USAN, INN, BAN *coronary vasodilator*

LidoPen auto-injector (automatic IM injection device) ℞ *emergency injection for cardiac arrhythmias* [lidocaine HCl] 300 mg/3 mL dose

Lidosite Topical System transdermal patch (discontinued 2009) ℞ *local anesthetic* [lidocaine HCl; epinephrine] 10%•0.1%

lifarizine USAN, INN, BAN *platelet aggregation inhibitor*

life everlasting *medicinal herb* [see: everlasting]

Life Extension Booster; Life Extension Super Booster softgels OTC *vitamin/mineral supplement* [multiple vitamins & minerals]

Life Extension Herbal Mix powder for oral solution OTC *dietary supplement*

Life Extension Mix; Life Extension Mix with Niacin; Life Extension Mix without Copper caplets, capsules, powder for oral solution OTC *vitamin/mineral supplement* [multiple vitamins & minerals]

Life Extension Two-Per-Day tablets OTC *vitamin/mineral supplement* [multiple vitamins & minerals]

life root (*Senecio aureus; S. jacoboea; S. vulgaris*) *medicinal herb for childbirth pain, diaphoresis, edema, fever, and stimulation of labor and menses; not generally regarded as safe and effective for ingestion because of hepatotoxicity*

LifeCare bags (delivery form) *premixed IV infusion bags*

life-of-man *medicinal herb* [see: spikenard]

lifibrate USAN, INN *antihyperlipoproteinemic*

lifibrol USAN, INN *antihyperlipidemic*

LIG (lymphocyte immune globulin) [see: antithymocyte globulin (ATG)]

light mineral oil [see: mineral oil, light]

lignocaine BAN *topical/local anesthetic* [also: lidocaine] ⓢ Lanacane

lignocaine HCl BAN *local anesthetic; antiarrhythmic* [also: lidocaine HCl]

lignosulfonic acid, sodium salt [see: polignate sodium]

lilopristone INN

lily, conval; May lily *medicinal herb* [see: lily of the valley]

lily, ground *medicinal herb* [see: birthroot]

lily, white pond; sweet water lily; sweet-scented pond lily; sweet-scented water lily; white water lily; toad lily *medicinal herb* [see: white pond lily]

lily of the valley (*Convallaria majalis*) flower, leaves, and rhizome *medicinal herb for arrhythmias, edema, epilepsy, and heart disorders*

limaprost INN

limarsol [see: acetarsone]

Limbitrol; Limbitrol DS tablets ℞ *antidepressant; anxiolytic* [chlordiazepoxide; amitriptyline HCl] 5•12.5 mg; 10•25 mg

Limbrel capsules ℞ *natural COX-2 inhibitor; analgesic and anti-inflammatory for the dietary management of osteoarthritis* [flavocoxid] 250, 500 mg

lime USP *pharmaceutic necessity*

lime, sulfurated (calcium polysulfide, calcium thiosulfate) USP *wet dressing/soak for cystic acne and seborrhea*

lime tree *medicinal herb* [see: linden tree]

linagliptin *dipeptidyl peptidase-4 (DPP-4) inhibitor; oral antidiabetic that enhances the function of the body's incretin system to increase insulin pro-*

*duction in the pancreas and reduce glu-
cose production in the liver*

linarotene USAN, INN *antikeratinizing
agent*

Lincocin capsules (discontinued 2008)
℞ *lincosamide antibiotic* [lincomycin
(as HCl)] 500 mg ⊠ Lanoxin

Lincocin IV or IM injection ℞ *lincosamide antibiotic* [lincomycin (as
HCl)] 300 mg/mL ⊠ Lanoxin

lincomycin USAN, INN, BAN *lincosamide antibiotic*

lincomycin HCl USP *lincosamide antibiotic*

Lincorex IV or IM injection (discontinued 2008) ℞ *lincosamide antibiotic*
[lincomycin (as HCl)] 300 mg/mL

lincosamides *a class of antimicrobial
antibiotics with potentially serious side
effects, to which bacterial resistance has
been shown*

lindane USAN, USP, INN, BAN *pediculicide for lice; scabicide* 1% topical

linden tree *(Tilia americana; T. cordata; T. europaea; T. platyphyllos)*
flowers *medicinal herb for diaphoresis,
diarrhea, headache, hypertension, indigestion, nasal congestion, nervousness,
skin moisturizer, stomach disorders,
and throat irritation*

linezolid USAN *oxazolidinone antibiotic
for gram-positive bacterial infections,
including community-acquired or nosocomial pneumonia, skin and skin structure infections, and vancomycin-resis-
tant enterococcal infections*

Linguets (trademarked dosage form)
buccal tablets

Linjeta subcu injection *investigational
(Phase III) fast-acting insulin for dia-
betes* (previously investigational as
VIAject)

**Linker protocol (daunorubicin,
vincristine, prednisone, asparaginase, teniposide, cytarabine,
methotrexate, leucovorin [res-
cue])** *chemotherapy protocol for acute
lymphocytic leukemia (ALL)*

linogliride USAN, INN *antidiabetic*

linogliride fumarate USAN *antidiabetic*

linolexamide [see: clinolamide]

Linomide *investigational (orphan) bone
marrow transplant adjunct for leukemia*
[roquinimex]

linopiridine USAN, INN *cognition
enhancer for Alzheimer disease*

linseed *medicinal herb* [see: flaxseed]

linsidomine INN

lint bells *medicinal herb* [see: flaxseed]

lintopride INN

lintuzumab *investigational (orphan) for
acute myelogenous leukemia*

Linum usitatissimum *medicinal herb*
[see: flaxseed]

lion's ear; lion's tail *medicinal herb*
[see: motherwort]

lion's tooth *medicinal herb* [see: dande-
lion]

Lioresal caplets ℞ *skeletal muscle relaxant* [baclofen] 10, 20 mg ⊠ liarozole

Lioresal intrathecal injection ℞ *skeletal muscle relaxant for intractable spasticity due to multiple sclerosis, cerebral
palsy, or spinal cord injury (orphan);
investigational (orphan) for trigeminal
neuralgia* [baclofen] 0.05 mg/0.5 mL
(50 mcg/mL), 10 mg/20 mL (500
mcg/mL), 10 mg/5 mL (2000 mcg/mL)

liothyronine INN, BAN *radioactive
agent* [also: liothyronine I 125]

liothyronine I 125 USAN *radioactive
agent* [also: liothyronine]

liothyronine I 131 USAN *radioactive
agent*

liothyronine sodium USP, BAN *synthetic thyroid hormone (T_3 fraction
only); treatment of myxedema coma or
precoma (orphan)* 5, 25, 50 mcg oral;
10 mcg injection

liotrix USAN, USP *synthetic thyroid hormone (a 4:1 mixture of T_4 and T_3)*

Lip Medex oral ointment OTC *mild
mucous membrane anesthetic; antipruritic; counterirritant* [camphor; phe-
nol] 1%•0.54%

lipancreatin [see: pancrelipase]

lipase *digestive enzyme (digests fats)* [24
IU/mg in pancrelipase; 2 IU/mg in
pancreatin]

lipase of pancreas [see: pancrelipase]

lipase triacylglycerol [see: pancrelipase]

lipid/DNA human cystic fibrosis gene *investigational (orphan) for cystic fibrosis*

Lipil [see: Enfamil LIPIL; LactoFree LIPIL; ProSobee LIPIL]

Lipisorb powder OTC *enteral nutritional therapy* [lactose-free formula]

Lipitor film-coated tablets ℞ *HMG-CoA reductase inhibitor for hypercholesterolemia, dysbetalipoproteinemia, hypertriglyceridemia, mixed dyslipidemia, and the prevention of cardiovascular disease and stroke in high-risk patients* [atorvastatin calcium] 10, 20, 40, 80 mg

Lipofen capsules ℞ *antihyperlipidemic for primary hypercholesterolemia, hypertriglyceridemia, and mixed dyslipidemia; also used for hyperuricemia* [fenofibrate] 50, 150 mg

Lipo-Flavonoid caplets OTC *dietary lipotropic; vitamin supplement* [choline; inositol; multiple B vitamins; vitamin C; lemon bioflavonoids] 111.3•111.3• ± •100•100 mg

Lipogen capsules, caplets (discontinued 2008) OTC *dietary lipotropic; vitamin supplement* [choline; inositol; multiple vitamins] 111•111• ± mg

α-lipoic acid; lipoicin *natural antioxidant* [see: alpha lipoic acid]

Lipomul oral liquid (discontinued 2010) OTC *dietary fat supplement* [corn oil] 10 g/15 mL

Lipo-Nicin/100 tablets ℞ *peripheral vasodilator; antihyperlipidemic* [niacin; niacinamide; multiple vitamins] 100•75• ± mg

Lipo-Nicin/300 timed-release capsules ℞ *peripheral vasodilator; antihyperlipidemic* [niacin; multiple vitamins] 300• ± mg

Liponol capsules (discontinued 2008) OTC *dietary lipotropic; vitamin supplement* [choline; inositol; methionine; multiple B vitamins] 115•83•110• ± mg

lipopeptides [see: cyclic lipopeptides]

lipoprotein-associated coagulation inhibitor (LACI) [see: tifacogin]

liposomal amphotericin B [see: amphotericin B lipid complex (ABLC)]

liposomal cyclosporin A [see: cyclosporine, liposomal]

liposomal gentamicin [see: gentamicin liposome]

liposome-encapsulated doxorubicin HCl (LED) [see: doxorubicin HCl, liposome-encapsulated]

liposome-encapsulated T4 endonuclease V (T4N5) [see: T4 endonuclease V, liposome encapsulated]

Liposyn II 10%; Liposyn II 20%; Liposyn III 10%; Liposyn III 20%; Liposyn III 30% IV infusion ℞ *nutritional therapy* [fat emulsion]

Lipotriad extended-release caplets OTC *vitamin/mineral supplement* [multiple vitamins and minerals; lutein] ± • 250 mcg

lipotropics *a class of oral nutritional supplements*

5-lipoxygenase inhibitors [see: leukotriene formation inhibitors]

Lipram 4500 delayed-release capsules containing enteric-coated microspheres (discontinued 2009) ℞ *porcine-derived digestive enzymes* [pancrelipase (lipase; protease; amylase)] 4500•25 000•20 000 USP units ☑ Librium

Lipram-CR5; Lipram-CR10; Lipram-CR20 delayed-release capsules containing enteric-coated microspheres ℞ *porcine-derived digestive enzymes* [pancrelipase (lipase; protease; amylase)] 5000•18 750•16 600 USP units; 10 000•37 500•33 200 USP units; 20 000•75 000•66 400 USP units ☑ Librium

Lipram-PN10; Lipram-PN16; Lipram-PN20 delayed-release capsules containing enteric-coated microspheres (discontinued 2009) ℞ *porcine-derived digestive enzymes* [pancrelipase (lipase; protease; amylase)] 10 000•30 000•30 000 USP units;

16 000•48 000•48 000 USP units;
20 000•44 000•56 000 USP units ☑
Librium

**Lipram-UL12; Lipram-UL18;
Lipram-UL20** delayed-release capsules containing enteric-coated microspheres (discontinued 2010) ℞ *porcine-derived digestive enzymes* [pancrelipase (lipase; protease; amylase)] 12 000•39 000•39 000 USP units; 18 000•58 500•58 500 USP units; 20 000•65 000•65 000 USP units ☑ Librium

liprotamase *investigational (NDA filed) non-porcine derived enzyme replacement therapy for patients with pancreatic insufficiency*

Li-Q-Nol *natural enzyme cofactor; investigational (orphan) for Huntington disease, pediatric CHF, and mitochondrial cytopathies* [coenzyme Q10 (as ubiquinol)]

Liquadd oral solution (discontinued 2009) ℞ *CNS stimulant for attention-deficit/hyperactivity disorder (ADHD)* [dextroamphetamine sulfate] 5 mg/5 mL ☑ Locoid

liquefied phenol [see: phenol, liquefied]

Liquibid sustained-release tablet ℞ *expectorant* [guaifenesin] 400 mg

Liquibid-D dual-release caplets ℞ *decongestant; expectorant* [phenylephrine HCl (extended release); guaifenesin (38% immediate release; 62% extended release)] 40•650 mg

Liquibid-D 1200 dual-release caplets (discontinued 2008) ℞ *decongestant; expectorant* [phenylephrine HCl (25% immediate release; 75% extended release); guaifenesin (33% immediate release; 67% extended release)] 40•1200 mg

Liquibid-PD dual-release tablets ℞ *decongestant; expectorant* [phenylephrine HCl; guaifenesin] 20•315 mg (5•120 mg immediate release; 15• 195 mg extended release)

Liquibid PD-R tablets ℞ *decongestant; expectorant* [phenylephrine HCl; guaifenesin] 5•200 mg

LiquiCaps; Liqui-caps (dosage form) *soft liquid-filled gelcaps*

Liquicet oral liquid ℞ *narcotic analgesic; antipyretic* [hydrocodone bitartrate; acetaminophen] 10•500 mg/15 mL

Liqui-Char oral liquid OTC *adsorbent antidote for poisoning* [activated charcoal] 12.5 g/60 mL, 15 g/75 mL, 25 g/120 mL, 30 g/120 mL, 50 g/240 mL

Liqui-Coat HD concentrated oral suspension ℞ *radiopaque contrast medium for gastrointestinal imaging* [barium sulfate] 210%

Liquicough DM oral liquid OTC *antitussive; decongestant; expectorant* [dextromethorphan hydrobromide; pseudoephedrine HCl; guaifenesin] 15•32•175 mg/5 mL

Liquid Caps (dosage form) *soft liquid-filled gelcaps*

liquid glucose [see: glucose, liquid]

liquid petrolatum [see: mineral oil]

Liquid Pred syrup (discontinued 2008) ℞ *corticosteroid; anti-inflammatory* [prednisone; alcohol 5%] 5 mg/5 mL

Liquid Tabs (dosage form) *liquid-filled tablets*

Liquidambar orientalis; L. styraciflua *medicinal herb* [see: storax]

Liqui-Doss emulsion OTC *emollient laxative* [mineral oil] ☑ Lac-Dose

Liquifilm Tears; Liquifilm Forte eye drops (discontinued 2010) OTC *moisturizer/lubricant* [polyvinyl alcohol] 1.4%; 3%

Liquifilm Wetting solution (discontinued 2010) OTC *wetting solution for hard contact lenses*

Liqui-Gels; Liqui-gels (trademarked dosage form) *soft liquid-filled gelcaps*

Liquimat lotion OTC *antiseptic and keratolytic for acne* [sulfur] 4%

Liquiprin Drops for Children (discontinued 2008) OTC *analgesic; antipyretic* [acetaminophen] 80 mg/1.66 mL

Liquitab (trademarked dosage form) *chewable tablet*

LiquiVent *investigational (Phase III, orphan) treatment for acute respiratory distress syndrome (ARDS) in adults* [perflubron]

liquor carbonis detergens (LCD)
[see: coal tar]

liraglutide *glucagon-like peptide-1 (GLP-1); antidiabetic for type 2 diabetes; investigational (Phase II) for weight loss*

liroldine INN

lisadimate USAN, INN *sunscreen*

lisdexamfetamine dimesylate *CNS stimulant; oral treatment for attention-deficit/hyperactivity disorder (ADHD)*

lisinopril USAN, INN, BAN *antihypertensive; angiotensin-converting enzyme (ACE) inhibitor; adjunctive treatment for congestive heart failure (CHF)* 2.5, 5, 10, 20, 30, 40 mg oral

lisinopril & hydrochlorothiazide *combination angiotensin-converting enzyme (ACE) inhibitor and diuretic for hypertension* 10•12.5, 20•12.5, 20•25 mg oral

lisofylline (LSF) USAN *acetyltransferase inhibitor; investigational (Phase III, orphan) immunomodulator and cytokine inhibitor for acute myeloid leukemia*

lissamine green *diagnostic aid for ophthalmic abnormalities* 1.5 mg strips

Listerine; Cool-Mint Listerine; FreshBurst Listerine; Natural Citrus Listerine; Tartar Control Listerine *mouthwash/gargle* OTC *analgesic; mild anesthetic; antipruritic; counterirritant; antiseptic* [methyl salicylate; eucalyptol; thymol; menthol; alcohol 22%–26%] 0.06%•0.09%•0.06%•0.04% ℞ Loestrin

Listerine Tooth Defense *oral rinse* OTC *dental caries preventative* [sodium fluoride; alcohol 21.6%] 0.0221% (0.01% fluoride) ℞ Loestrin

Listermint Arctic Mint *mouthwash/gargle* OTC *oral antiseptic*

lisuride INN [also: lysuride]

lithium *element (Li); antipsychotic for manic episodes* 8 mEq/5 mL oral

lithium benzoate NF

lithium carbonate USAN, USP *antimanic; immunity booster in chemotherapy and AIDS* (150 mg=4 mEq lithium) 150, 300, 450, 600 mg oral

lithium citrate USP *antimanic; immunity booster in chemotherapy and AIDS* 300 mg/5 mL oral

lithium hydroxide USP *antimanic*

lithium hydroxide monohydrate
[see: lithium hydroxide]

Lithium QD *investigational (Phase III) once-daily antipsychotic for manic episodes of a bipolar disorder* [lithium carbonate]

lithium salicylate NF

Lithobid *slow-release tablets* ℞ *antipsychotic for manic episodes* [lithium (as carbonate)] 8 mEq (300 mg)

litholytics *a class of agents that dissolve stones or calculi* [see also: antilithics]

Lithonate *capsules* ℞ *antipsychotic for manic episodes* [lithium carbonate] 300 mg

Lithostat *tablets* ℞ *adjunctive therapy in chronic urea-splitting urinary tract infections* [acetohydroxamic acid] 250 mg

Lithotabs *film-coated tablets* ℞ *antipsychotic for manic episodes* [lithium carbonate] 300 mg

litracen INN ℞ Lotrisone

Little Colds Cough Formula *oral drops* OTC *antitussive for children 2–3 years* [dextromethorphan hydrobromide] 7.5 mg/mL

Little Colds Decongestant Plus Cough *oral drops* OTC *antitussive; decongestant; for children 4–12 years* [dextromethorphan hydrobromide; phenylephrine HCl] 5•2.5 mg/mL

Little Colds for Infants and Children *oral drops* OTC *nasal decongestant* [phenylephrine HCl] 0.25%

Little Fevers *oral drops (discontinued 2011)* OTC *analgesic; antipyretic* [acetaminophen] 80 mg/mL

Little Noses Gentle Formula, Infants and Children *nose drops* OTC *nasal decongestant* [phenylephrine HCl] 0.125%

Little Tummys Laxative oral drops OTC *stimulant laxative* [sennosides] 8.8 mg/mL

Livalo film-coated tablets ℞ *HMG-CoA reductase inhibitor for hyperlipidemia and mixed dyslipidemia* [pitavastatin (as calcium)] 1, 2, 4 mg ⊡ Levall

liver, desiccated; liver extracts *source of vitamin* B_{12}

liver lily *medicinal herb* [see: blue flag]

liverleaf; liverwort *medicinal herb* [see: hepatica]

LiveTan DM oral suspension (discontinued 2009) ℞ *antitussive; antihistamine; sleep aid; decongestant* [dextromethorphan tannate; diphenhydramine tannate; phenylephrine tannate] 75•25•7.5 mg/5 mL

lividomycin INN

Livitrinsic-f capsules (discontinued 2009) ℞ *hematinic* [iron (as ferrous fumarate); vitamin B_{12}; vitamin C; intrinsic factor concentrate; folic acid] 110•0.015•75•240•0.5 mg

lixazinone sulfate USAN *cardiotonic; phosphodiesterase inhibitor*

lixisenatide *glucagon-like peptide-1 (GLP-1); investigational (Phase III) antidiabetic for type 2 diabetes*

lixivaptan USAN *selective vasopressin V_2–receptor antagonist for nonhypovolemic hyponatremia*

LKV Infant Drops powder + liquid (discontinued 2008) OTC *vitamin supplement* [multiple vitamins; biotin] ≟•75 mcg/0.6 mL

LLD factor [see: cyanocobalamin]

10% LMD IV injection ℞ *plasma volume expander for shock due to hemorrhage, burns, or surgery* [dextran 40] 10%

LMD (low molecular weight dextran) [see: dextran 40]

LMWD (low molecular weight dextran) [see: dextran 40]

L-M-X4 cream OTC *anesthetic* [lidocaine, liposome-encapsulated] 4%

L-M-X5 anorectal cream OTC *anesthetic* [lidocaine, liposome-encapsulated] 5%

Lo Loestrin Fe tablets (in packs of 28) ℞ *biphasic oral contraceptive; iron supplement* [norethindrone acetate; ethinyl estradiol; ferrous fumarate]
Phase 1 (24 days): 1 mg•10 mcg•75 mg
Phase 2 (2 days): 0•10 mcg•75 mg;
Counters (2 days) 0•0•75 mg

Lobac capsules (discontinued 2009) ℞ *skeletal muscle relaxant; antihistamine; sleep aid; analgesic; antipyretic* [salicylamide; phenyltoloxamine; acetaminophen] 200•20•300 mg

Lobana Body lotion OTC *moisturizer; emollient*

Lobana Body Shampoo; Lobana Liquid Lather topical liquid OTC *soap-free therapeutic skin cleanser* [chloroxylenol]

Lobana Derm-Ade cream OTC *moisturizer; emollient* [vitamins A, D, and E]

Lobana Peri-Garde ointment OTC *moisturizer; emollient; antiseptic* [vitamins A, D, and E; chloroxylenol]

lobelia *(Lobelia inflata)* plant (tincture) *medicinal herb for arthritis, asthma, bronchitis, hay fever, colds, cough, ear infections, epilepsy, fever, food poisoning, lockjaw, nervousness, pain, pneumonia, preventing miscarriage, whooping cough, and worms*

lobeline INN *nicotine withdrawal aid* [also: lobeline HCl]

lobeline HCl JAN *nicotine withdrawal aid* [also: lobeline]

lobendazole USAN, INN *veterinary anthelmintic*

lobenzarit INN *antirheumatic* [also: lobenzarit sodium]

lobenzarit sodium USAN *antirheumatic* [also: lobenzarit]

lobradimil USAN *receptor-mediated permeabilizer; blood-brain barrier permeability-enhancing agent*

lobucavir USAN, INN *antiviral*

lobuprofen INN

locicortolone dicibate INN

locicortone [see: locicortolone dicibate]

Locoid cream, ointment, solution, lotion ℞ *corticosteroidal anti-inflam-*

matory [hydrocortisone butyrate] 0.1% ☒ Liquadd

Locoid Lipocream ℞ *corticosteroidal anti-inflammatory* [hydrocortisone butyrate (in an oil-in-water emulsion)] 0.1% (70% oil•30% water)

locust plant *medicinal herb* [see: senna]

lodaxaprine INN

lodazecar INN

lodelaben USAN, INN *antiarthritic; emphysema therapy adjunct*

lodenosine USAN *reverse transcriptase antiviral*

lodinixil INN

lodiperone INN

Lodosyn tablets ℞ *potentiator of levo-dopa for Parkinson disease (no effect when given alone)* [carbidopa] 25 mg

lodoxamide INN, BAN *antiallergic; antiasthmatic* [also: lodoxamide ethyl]

lodoxamide ethyl USAN *antiallergic; antiasthmatic* [also: lodoxamide]

lodoxamide trometamol BAN *antiallergic; antiasthmatic* [also: lodoxamide tromethamine]

lodoxamide tromethamine USAN *antiasthmatic; ophthalmic mast cell stabilizer for vernal keratoconjunctivitis (orphan)* [also: lodoxamide trometamol]

Lodrane oral liquid ℞ *decongestant; antihistamine* [pseudoephedrine HCl; brompheniramine maleate] 60•4 mg/5 mL

Lodrane 12 D; Lodrane 24 D sustained-release tablets ℞ *decongestant; antihistamine* [pseudoephedrine HCl; brompheniramine maleate] 45•6 mg; 90•12 mg

Lodrane 12 Hour extended-release tablets ℞ *antihistamine* [brompheniramine maleate] 6 mg

Lodrane 24 extended-release capsules ℞ *antihistamine* [brompheniramine maleate] 12 mg

Lodrane D oral suspension ℞ *decongestant; antihistamine* [pseudoephedrine tannate; brompheniramine tannate] 90•8 mg/5 mL

Lodrane LD sustained-release capsules (discontinued 2007) ℞ *decongestant;*

antihistamine [pseudoephedrine HCl; brompheniramine maleate] 60•6 mg

Lodrane XR oral suspension ℞ *antihistamine* [brompheniramine tannate] 8 mg/5 mL

Loestrin 21 1/20; Loestrin 21 1.5/30 tablets (in packs of 21) ℞ *monophasic oral contraceptive* [norethindrone acetate; ethinyl estradiol] 1 mg•20 mcg; 1.5 mg•30 mcg ☒ Listerine

Loestrin 24 Fe tablets (in packs of 28) ℞ *monophasic oral contraceptive; iron supplement* [norethindrone acetate; ethinyl estradiol; ferrous fumarate] 1•0.02•75 mg × 24 days; 0•0•75 mg × 4 days

Loestrin Fe 1/20 tablets (in packs of 28) ℞ *monophasic oral contraceptive; iron supplement* [norethindrone acetate; ethinyl estradiol; ferrous fumarate] 1 mg•20 mcg•75 mg × 21 days; 0•0•75 mg × 7 days

Loestrin Fe 1.5/30 tablets (in packs of 28) ℞ *monophasic oral contraceptive; iron supplement* [norethindrone acetate; ethinyl estradiol; ferrous fumarate] 1.5 mg•30 mcg•75 mg × 21 days; 0•0•75 mg × 7 days

lofemizole INN *anti-inflammatory; analgesic; antipyretic* [also: lofemizole HCl] ☒ levamisole

lofemizole HCl USAN *anti-inflammatory; analgesic; antipyretic* [also: lofemizole] ☒ levamisole HCl

lofendazam INN, BAN

lofentanil INN, BAN *narcotic analgesic* [also: lofentanil oxalate]

lofentanil oxalate USAN *narcotic analgesic* [also: lofentanil]

lofepramine INN, BAN *antidepressant* [also: lofepramine HCl]

lofepramine HCl USAN *antidepressant* [also: lofepramine]

lofexidine INN, BAN *antihypertensive* [also: lofexidine HCl]

lofexidine HCl USAN *centrally acting alpha-2-adrenergic agonist for hypertension; investigational (Phase III) treatment for opiate withdrawal syndrome* [also: lofexidine]

Lofibra capsules, tablets ℞ *antihyper-lipidemic for primary hypercholesterol-emia, hypertriglyceridemia, and mixed dyslipidemia; also used for hyperurice-mia* [fenofibrate] 67, 134, 200 mg; 54, 160 mg

loflucarban INN

Logen tablets ℞ *antidiarrheal* [diphen-oxylate HCl; atropine sulfate] 2.5•0.025 mg

LoHist oral drops OTC *decongestant; antihistamine; for children 2–12 years* [phenylephrine HCl; chlorphenir-amine maleate] 2.5•1 mg/mL

LoHist 12 Hour extended-release tablets ℞ *antihistamine* [bromphenir-amine tannate] 6 mg

LoHist 12D extended-release tablets ℞ *decongestant; antihistamine* [pseu-doephedrine HCl; brompheniramine maleate] 45•6 mg

LoHist-D oral liquid ℞ *decongestant; antihistamine* [pseudoephedrine HCl; chlorpheniramine maleate] 30•2 mg/5 mL

LoHist-DM syrup ℞ *antitussive; anti-histamine; decongestant* [dextrometh-orphan hydrobromide; bromphenir-amine maleate; phenylephrine HCl] 10•2•5 mg/5 mL

LoHist-LQ oral liquid ℞ *decongestant; antihistamine* [pseudoephedrine HCl; brompheniramine maleate] 60•4 mg/5 mL

LoHist-PD Pediatric oral drops (dis-continued 2010) ℞ *decongestant; antihistamine; for children 1–24 months* [pseudoephedrine HCl; brompheniramine maleate] 12.5•1 mg/mL

LoHist-PEB oral liquid OTC *decongestant; antihistamine* [phenylephrine HCl; brompheniramine maleate] 10•4 mg/5 mL

LoHist-PSB oral liquid OTC *decongestant; antihistamine* [pseudoephedrine HCl; brompheniramine maleate] 20•4 mg/5 mL

LoKara lotion ℞ *corticosteroidal anti-inflammatory* [desonide] 0.05%

Lomanate oral liquid ℞ *antidiarrheal* [diphenoxylate HCl; atropine sulfate] 2.5•0.025 mg/5 mL

lombazole INN, BAN

lomefloxacin USAN, INN, BAN *broad-spectrum fluoroquinolone antibiotic*

lomefloxacin HCl USAN *broad-spec-trum fluoroquinolone antibiotic*

lomefloxacin mesylate USAN *antibac-terial*

lometraline INN *antipsychotic; antipar-kinsonian* [also: lometraline HCl]

lometraline HCl USAN *antipsychotic; antiparkinsonian* [also: lometraline]

lometrexol INN *antineoplastic* [also: lometrexol sodium]

lometrexol sodium USAN *antineoplas-tic* [also: lometrexol]

lomevactone INN

lomifylline INN

lomitapide *investigational (Phase III, orphan) treatment for hypertriglyceride-mia due to familial chylomicronemia*

lomofungin USAN *antifungal*

Lomotil tablets, oral liquid ℞ *antidiar-rheal* [diphenoxylate HCl; atropine sulfate] 2.5•0.025 mg; 2.5•0.025 mg/5 mL

lomustine USAN, INN, BAN *nitrosourea-type alkylating antineoplastic for brain tumors and Hodgkin disease*

Lonalac powder OTC *enteral nutritional therapy* [milk-based formula]

lonapalene USAN *antipsoriatic*

lonaprofen INN

lonazolac INN

Long-Acting Cough Suppressant oral liquid OTC *antitussive* [dextromethor-phan hydrobromide] 15 mg/5 mL

lonidamine INN, BAN *indazole-3-car-boxylic acid*

Lonox tablets ℞ *antidiarrheal* [diphen-oxylate HCl; atropine sulfate] 2.5•0.025 mg

loop diuretics *a class of diuretic agents that inhibit the reabsorption of sodium and chloride*

Lo/Ovral tablets (in Pilpaks of 21 or 28) ℞ *monophasic oral contraceptive; emergency postcoital contraceptive* [norgestrel; ethinyl estradiol] 0.3 mg•30 mcg

loperamide INN, BAN *antiperistaltic; antidiarrheal* [also: loperamide HCl]

loperamide HCl USAN, USP, JAN *antiperistaltic; antidiarrheal* [also: loperamide] 2 mg oral; 1 mg/5 mL oral

loperamide oxide INN, BAN *antiperistaltic; antidiarrheal*

Lophophora williamsii a flowering Mexican cactus whose heads (mescal buttons) are used to produce mescaline, a hallucinogenic street drug

Lopid film-coated tablets ℞ *triglyceride-lowering antihyperlipidemic for hypertriglyceridemia (types IV and V hyperlipidemia) and coronary heart disease* [gemfibrozil] 600 mg (300 mg capsules available in Canada)

lopinavir USAN *antiviral protease inhibitor for HIV infection*

lopirazepam INN

loprazolam INN, BAN

lopremone [now: protirelin]

Lopressor tablets, IV injection ℞ *antianginal; antihypertensive; beta-blocker* [metoprolol tartrate] 50, 100 mg; 1 mg/mL

Lopressor HCT 50/25; Lopressor HCT 100/25; Lopressor HCT 100/50 tablets ℞ *combination beta-blocker and diuretic for hypertension* [metoprolol tartrate; hydrochlorothiazide] 50•25 mg; 100•25 mg; 100•50 mg

loprodiol INN

Loprox cream, gel, topical suspension, shampoo ℞ *antifungal for tinea pedis, tinea cruris, tinea corporis, tinea versicolor, candidiasis, and seborrheic dermatitis* [ciclopirox] 0.77% ⊡ Librax

Lorabid Pulvules (capsules), powder for oral suspension (discontinued 2007) ℞ *second-generation cephalosporin antibiotic* [loracarbef] 200, 400 mg; 100, 200 mg/5 mL

loracarbef USAN, INN *second-generation cephalosporin antibiotic*

lorajmine INN *antiarrhythmic* [also: lorajmine HCl]

lorajmine HCl USAN *antiarrhythmic* [also: lorajmine]

Loramyc ⓔ buccal tablet (available in France) *investigational (Phase III) antifungal for oropharyngeal candidiasis* [miconazole]

lorapride INN

loratadine USAN, INN, BAN *second-generation peripherally selective piperidine antihistamine for allergic rhinitis; also used for chronic idiopathic urticaria* 10 mg oral; 5 mg/5 mL oral

Loratadine D extended-release tablets OTC *nonsedating antihistamine; decongestant* [loratadine; pseudoephedrine HCl] 10•240 mg

Loratadine Hive Relief syrup OTC *nonsedating antihistamine for hives* [loratadine] 5 mg/5 mL

lorazepam USAN, USP, INN, BAN *benzodiazepine anxiolytic; preanesthetic sedative; anticonvulsant* 0.5, 1, 2 mg oral; 2 mg/mL oral; 2, 4 mg/mL injection

Lorazepam Intensol oral drops ℞ *benzodiazepine anxiolytic; sedative; anticonvulsant* [lorazepam] 2 mg/mL

lorbamate USAN, INN *muscle relaxant*

lorcainide INN, BAN *antiarrhythmic* [also: lorcainide HCl]

lorcainide HCl USAN *antiarrhythmic* [also: lorcainide]

lorcaserin HCl *investigational (NDA filed) selective serotonin 5-HT$_{2c}$ receptor agonist for the treatment of obesity*

Lorcet Plus; Lorcet 10/650 tablets ℞ *narcotic analgesic; antipyretic* [hydrocodone bitartrate; acetaminophen] 7.5•650 mg; 10•650 mg

Lorcet-HD capsules (discontinued 2009) ℞ *narcotic analgesic; antipyretic* [hydrocodone bitartrate; acetaminophen] 5•500 mg

lorcinadol USAN, INN, BAN *analgesic*

loreclezole USAN, INN, BAN *antiepileptic*

Lorenzo oil (erucic acid and oleic acid) *natural treatment for childhood adrenoleukodystrophy and adrenomyeloneuropathy in adults*

lorglumide INN

lormetazepam USAN, INN, BAN *sedative; hypnotic*

lornoxicam USAN, INN, BAN *analgesic; anti-inflammatory*

Lorothidol (available only from the Centers for Disease Control) (discontinued 2011) ℞ *anti-infective for paragonimiasis and fascioliasis* [bithionol]

lorpiprazole INN

Lortab elixir ℞ *narcotic analgesic; antipyretic* [hydrocodone bitartrate; acetaminophen] 2.5•167 mg/5 mL

Lortab 2.5/500 tablets (discontinued 2009) ℞ *narcotic analgesic; antipyretic* [hydrocodone bitartrate; acetaminophen] 2.5•500 mg

Lortab 5/500; Lortab 7.5/500; Lortab 10/500 tablets ℞ *narcotic analgesic; antipyretic* [hydrocodone bitartrate; acetaminophen] 5•500 mg; 7.5•500 mg; 10•500 mg

Lortab ASA tablets (discontinued 2009) ℞ *narcotic analgesic; antipyretic* [hydrocodone bitartrate; aspirin] 5•500 mg

lortalamine USAN, INN *antidepressant*

Lortuss DM oral liquid OTC *antitussive; antihistamine; sleep aid; decongestant* [dextromethorphan hydrobromide; doxylamine succinate; pseudoephedrine HCl] 15•6.25•30 mg/5 mL

Lortuss EX oral suspension ℞ *narcotic antitussive; decongestant; expectorant* [codeine phosphate; pseudoephedrine HCl; guaifenesin] 10•22.5•100 mg/5 mL

Lortuss HC oral liquid (discontinued 2009) ℞ *narcotic antitussive; decongestant* [hydrocodone bitartrate; phenylephrine HCl] 3.75•7.5 mg/5 mL

Lortuss LQ oral liquid OTC *decongestant; antihistamine; sleep aid* [pseudoephedrine HCl; doxylamine succinate] 30•6.25 mg/5 mL

lorvotuzumab mertansine *investigational (orphan) antineoplastic for Merkel cell carcinoma and small cell lung cancer*

Loryna film-coated tablets (in packs of 28) ℞ *monophasic oral contraceptive in a novel 24-day regimen* [drospirenone; ethinyl estradiol] 3 mg•20 mcg × 24 days; counters × 4 days

lorzafone USAN, INN *minor tranquilizer*

losartan INN *angiotensin receptor blocker (ARB) for hypertension; treatment to delay the progression of diabetic nephropathy* [also: losartan potassium]

losartan potassium USAN *angiotensin receptor blocker (ARB) for hypertension; treatment to delay the progression of diabetic nephropathy* [also: losartan] 25, 50, 100 mg oral

losartan potassium & hydrochlorothiazide *combination angiotensin receptor blocker (ARB) and diuretic for hypertension* 50•12.5, 100•12.5, 100•25 mg

LoSeasonique film-coated tablets (in packs of 91) ℞ *extended-cycle (3 months) biphasic oral contraceptive* [levonorgestrel; ethinyl estradiol] Phase 1 (84 days): 0.1 mg•20 mcg; Phase 2 (7 days): 0•10 mcg

losigamone INN

losindole INN

losmiprofen INN

losoxantrone INN *antineoplastic* [also: losoxantrone HCl]

losoxantrone HCl USAN *antineoplastic* [also: losoxantrone]

losulazine INN *antihypertensive* [also: losulazine HCl]

losulazine HCl USAN *antihypertensive* [also: losulazine]

Lotemax eye drop suspension, ophthalmic ointment ℞ *corticosteroidal anti-inflammatory* [loteprednol etabonate] 0.5%

Lotensin tablets ℞ *angiotensin-converting enzyme (ACE) inhibitor for hypertension; also used for heart failure, nondiabetic nephropathy, and the prevention of recurrent stroke* [benazepril HCl] 10, 20, 40 mg

Lotensin HCT tablets ℞ *combination angiotensin-converting enzyme (ACE) inhibitor and diuretic for hypertension* [benazepril HCl; hydrochlorothiazide] 10•12.5, 20•12.5, 20•25 mg

loteprednol INN *corticosteroidal anti-inflammatory* [also: loteprednol etabonate]

loteprednol etabonate USAN *topical ophthalmic corticosteroidal anti-inflammatory* [also: loteprednol]

lotifazole INN

lotrafiban HCl USAN *platelet aggregation inhibitor; GP IIb/IIIa receptor antagonist*

Lotrel capsules ℞ *combination angiotensin-converting enzyme (ACE) inhibitor and calcium channel blocker for hypertension* [amlodipine besylate; benazepril HCl] 2.5•10, 5•10, 5•20, 5•40, 10•20, 10•40 mg

lotrifen INN

Lotrimin AF cream, topical solution, lotion OTC *antifungal* [clotrimazole] 1%

Lotrimin AF powder, spray powder, spray liquid OTC *antifungal for tinea pedis, tinea cruris, and tinea corporis* [miconazole nitrate] 2%

Lotrimin Ultra cream OTC *benzylamine antifungal* [butenafine HCl] 1%

Lotrisone lotion ℞ *corticosteroidal anti-inflammatory; antifungal* [betamethasone dipropionate; clotrimazole] 0.05%•1% ② litracen

Lotronex film-coated tablets ℞ *twice-daily treatment for diarrhea-predominant irritable bowel syndrome (IBS) in women* [alosetron (as HCl)] 0.5, 1 mg

lotucaine INN

lousewort *medicinal herb* [see: betony; feverweed]

lovage (Angelica levisticum; Levisticum officinale) leaves and roots *medicinal herb for bad breath, boils, edema, flatulence, and sore throat; also used topically as a skin emollient*

lovastatin USAN, INN, BAN HMG-CoA *reductase inhibitor for hypercholesterolemia, hyperlipidemia, atherosclerosis, and the prevention and treatment of coronary heart disease (CHD)* 10, 20, 40 mg oral

Lovaza gelcaps ℞ *adjunct to diet restriction for hypertriglyceridemia; investiga-*

tional (orphan) for immunoglobulin A nephropathy [omega-3 acid ethyl esters (eicosapentaenoic acid and docosahexanoic acid)] 1000 mg (465 mg EPA; 375 mg DHA)

Lovenox deep subcu injection, pre-filled syringes ℞ *anticoagulant/antithrombotic for prevention of deep vein thrombosis (DVT) following knee, hip, or abdominal surgery, unstable angina, and myocardial infarction* [enoxaparin sodium] 100 mg/mL; 30, 40, 60, 80, 100, 120, 150 mg

loviride USAN, INN *non-nucleoside reverse transcriptase inhibitor (NNRTI) antiviral*

low molecular weight dextran (LMD; LMWD) [see: dextran 40]

low molecular weight heparins *a class of anticoagulants used for the prophylaxis or treatment of thromboembolic complications of surgery and ischemic complications of unstable angina or myocardial infarction*

low osmolar contrast media (LOCM) *a class of newer radiopaque agents that have a low osmolar concentration of iodine (the contrast agent), which corresponds to a lower incidence of adverse reactions* [also called: nonionic contrast media]

Lowila Cake bar OTC *soap-free therapeutic skin cleanser*

Low-Ogestrel tablets (in packs of 28) ℞ *monophasic oral contraceptive; emergency postcoital contraceptive* [norgestrel; ethinyl estradiol] 0.3 mg•30 mcg × 21 days; counters × 7 days

Lowsium Plus oral suspension OTC *antacid; antiflatulent* [magaldrate; simethicone] 540•40 mg/5 mL

loxanast INN

loxapine USAN, INN, BAN *minor tranquilizer; conventional (typical) dibenzoxazepine antipsychotic for schizophrenia*

loxapine HCl *minor tranquilizer; conventional (typical) dibenzoxazepine antipsychotic for schizophrenia*

loxapine succinate USAN *minor tranquilizer; conventional (typical) dibenz-*

oxazepine antipsychotic for schizophrenia (base=73.4%) 6.8, 13.6, 34, 68.1 mg oral (5, 10, 25, 50 mg base)

loxiglumide INN

Loxitane capsules ℞ conventional (typical) dibenzoxazepine antipsychotic for schizophrenia [loxapine (as succinate)] 5, 10, 25, 50 mg

loxoprofen INN

loxoribine USAN, INN immunostimulant; vaccine adjuvant; investigational (orphan) for common variable immunodeficiency

loxotidine [now: lavoltidine succinate]

loxtidine BAN antiulcerative; histamine H_2-receptor blocker [also: lavoltidine succinate; lavoltidine]

lozilurea INN

Lozi-Tabs (trademarked dosage form) lozenges

Lozol film-coated tablets (discontinued 2008) ℞ antihypertensive; diuretic for congestive heart failure [indapamide] 1.25, 2.5 mg

L-PAM (L-phenylalanine mustard) [see: melphalan]

LR (lactated Ringer) solution [see: Ringer injection, lactated]

LSD (lysergic acid diethylamide) hallucinogenic street drug associated with disorders of sensory and temporal perception, depersonalization, and ataxia [medically known as lysergide]

LSF (lisofylline) [q.v.]

LTA 360 Kit topical solution ℞ anesthetic [lidocaine HCl] 4%

LTRAs (leukotriene receptor antagonists) a class of antiasthmatics ⑨ Letairis

Lu texaphyrin [see: motexafin lutetium]

lubeluzole USAN, INN neuroprotector

lubiprostone selective chloride channel activator to increase fluid secretion in the small intestine for the treatment of chronic idiopathic constipation in adults and irritable bowel syndrome (IBS) in women

Lubricating Jelly OTC vaginal moisturizer/lubricant [glycerin; propylene glycol]

Lubricoat (trademarked ingredient) surgical aid [ferric hyaluronate]

Lubriderm Daily Moisture with SPF 15 lotion OTC moisturizer; emollient; sunscreen [octinoxate; octisalate; oxybenzone] 7.5%•4%•3%

Lubriderm Intense Skin Repair cream OTC moisturizer; emollient

Lubriderm Skin Nourishing with Sea Kelp Extract lotion OTC moisturizer; emollient

LubriFresh P.M. ophthalmic ointment OTC ocular moisturizer/lubricant [white petrolatum; mineral oil] 83%•15%

Lubrin vaginal inserts OTC lubricant for sexual intercourse [glycerin; caprylic triglyceride] ⑨ Lupron

Lubriskin lotion OTC moisturizer; emollient

LubriTears eye drops OTC moisturizer/lubricant [hydroxypropyl methylcellulose] 0.3%

LubriTears ophthalmic ointment OTC ocular moisturizer/lubricant [white petrolatum; mineral oil; lanolin]

lucanthone INN, BAN antischistosomal [also: lucanthone HCl]

lucanthone HCl USAN, USP antischistosomal [also: lucanthone]

lucartamide INN

Lucassin investigational (NDA filed, orphan) hormone to improve renal function in patients with hepatorenal syndrome (HRS) [terlipressin]

lucensomycin [see: lucimycin]

Lucentis ophthalmic intravitreal injection ℞ vascular endothelial growth factor (VEGF-A) inhibitor for neovascular (wet) age-related macular degeneration (AMD); investigational for diabetic retinopathy [ranibizumab] 10 mg/mL (0.5 mg/dose)

Lucilia caesar natural treatment [see: maggots]

lucimycin INN

lucinactant *investigational (NDA filed, orphan) for respiratory distress syndrome in adults and premature infants and meconium aspiration in newborn infants* [also: KL4 surfactant]

Ludent chewable tablets ℞ *dental caries preventative* [fluoride] 0.25, 0.5, 1 mg

Luer-lock (trademarked delivery form) *prefilled self-injection syringe*

lufironil USAN, INN *collagen inhibitor*

lufuradom INN

Lufyllin tablets ℞ *antiasthmatic; bronchodilator* [dyphylline] 200 mg ⓢ Levlen

Lufyllin 400 tablets ℞ *antiasthmatic; bronchodilator* [dyphylline] 400 mg ⓢ Levlen

Lufyllin-EPG tablets, elixir (discontinued 2007) ℞ *antiasthmatic; bronchodilator; decongestant; expectorant; sedative* [dyphylline; ephedrine HCl; guaifenesin; phenobarbital] 100•16•200•16 mg; 150•24•300•24 mg/15 mL

Lufyllin-GG elixir ℞ *antiasthmatic; bronchodilator; expectorant* [dyphylline; guaifenesin] 100•100 mg/15 mL

Lufyllin-GG tablets (discontinued 2007) ℞ *antiasthmatic; bronchodilator; expectorant* [dyphylline; guaifenesin] 200•200 mg

Lugol oral solution ℞ *treatment for hyperthyroidism* [iodine; potassium iodide] 5%•10%

lumefantrine *treatment for malaria*

Lumigan eye drops ℞ *antihypertensive for glaucoma and ocular hypertension; used cosmetically to grow, thicken, and darken eyelashes* [bimatoprost] 0.01%, 0.03%

lumiliximab *investigational (Phase III) antineoplastic for leukemia*

Luminal Sodium IV or IM injection ℞ *long-acting barbiturate sedative, hypnotic, and anticonvulsant; also abused as a street drug* [phenobarbital (as sodium); alcohol 10%] 60, 130 mg/mL

Lumitene capsules OTC *vitamin A precursor* [beta carotene] 30 mg (50 000 IU)

Lumizyme IV infusion ℞ *enzyme replacement therapy for patients with Pompe disease (glycogenosis type 2; glycogen storage disease type II; GSDII)* [alglucosidase alfa] 2.5 mg/mL

Lunelle IM injection (discontinued 2010) ℞ *once-monthly injectable contraceptive* [estradiol cypionate; medroxyprogesterone acetate] 5•25 mg/0.5 mL

Lunesta film-coated tablets ℞ *nonbarbiturate sedative and hypnotic for chronic insomnia* [eszopiclone] 1, 2, 3 mg

lung surfactant, synthetic [see: colfosceril palmitate]

lungwort (*Pulmonaria officinalis*) flowering plant *medicinal herb used as an astringent, demulcent, emollient, expectorant, and pectoral* ⓢ Lanacort

2,6-lupetidine [see: nanofin]

lupitidine INN *veterinary antagonist to histamine H_2 receptors* [also: lupitidine HCl]

lupitidine HCl USAN *veterinary antagonist to histamine H_2 receptors* [also: lupitidine]

Lupron; Lupron Pediatric subcu injection (daily) (discontinued 2011) ℞ *hormonal antineoplastic for prostatic cancer and central precocious puberty (orphan)* [leuprolide acetate] 5 mg/mL ⓢ Lubrin

Lupron Depot microspheres for IM injection (monthly) ℞ *hormonal antineoplastic for prostatic cancer, endometriosis, and uterine fibroids* [leuprolide acetate] 3.75, 7.5 mg

Lupron Depot–3 month; Lupron Depot–4 month; Lupron Depot–6 month microspheres for IM injection ℞ *hormonal antineoplastic for prostatic cancer, endometriosis, and uterine fibroids* [leuprolide acetate] 11.5, 22.5 mg; 30 mg; 45 mg

Lupron Depot-Ped microspheres for IM injection (monthly) ℞ *hormonal antineoplastic for central precocious puberty (orphan)* [leuprolide acetate] 7.5, 11.25, 15 mg

luprostiol INN, BAN

lurasidone HCl *atypical antipsychotic for schizophrenia*

Luride Lozi-Tabs (chewable tablets), drops, gel ℞ *dental caries preventative* [sodium fluoride] 0.25, 1.1, 2.2 mg; 1.1 mg/mL; 1.2%

Luride SF Lozi-Tabs (lozenges) ℞ *dental caries preventative* [sodium fluoride] 2.2 mg

lurosetron mesylate USAN *antiemetic*

lurtotecan dihydrochloride USAN *antineoplastic; topoisomerase I inhibitor*

Lusedra IV injection ℞ *general anesthetic* [fospropofol disodium] 35 mg/mL

Lusonal oral liquid ℞ *nasal decongestant; expectorant* [pseudoephedrine HCl; guaifenesin] 7.5•100 mg/5 mL

Lustra; Lustra-AF cream ℞ *hyperpigmentation bleaching agent* [hydroquinone] 4%

lutein *natural carotenoid used to prevent and treat age-related macular degeneration (AMD), retinitis pigmentosa (RP), and other retinal dysfunction*

luteinizing hormone, recombinant human (rhLH) [see: lutropin alfa]

luteinizing hormone–releasing factor acetate hydrate [see: gonadorelin acetate]

luteinizing hormone–releasing factor diacetate tetrahydrate [now: gonadorelin acetate]

luteinizing hormone–releasing factor dihydrochloride [now: gonadorelin HCl]

luteinizing hormone–releasing factor HCl [see: gonadorelin HCl]

luteinizing hormone–releasing hormone (LH-RH) *an endogenous hormone, produced in the hypothalamus, which stimulates the release of luteinizing hormone (LH) and follicle-stimulating hormone (FSH) from the pituitary* [also known as: gonadotropin-releasing hormone (Gn-RH)]

Lutera tablets (in packs of 28) ℞ *monophasic oral contraceptive* [levonorgestrel; ethinyl estradiol] 0.1 mg• 20 mcg × 21 days; counters × 7 days

lutetium *element (Lu)*

lutetium texaphyrin [now: motexafin lutetium]

lutrelin INN *luteinizing hormone-releasing hormone (LHRH) agonist* [also: lutrelin acetate]

lutrelin acetate USAN *luteinizing hormone-releasing hormone (LHRH) agonist* [also: lutrelin]

Lutrepulse powder for continuous ambulatory infusion (discontinued 2007) ℞ *gonadotropin-releasing hormone for the induction of ovulation in women with hypothalamic amenorrhea (orphan)* [gonadorelin acetate] 0.8, 3.2 mg

lutropin alfa USAN *gonadotropin; recombinant human luteinizing hormone (rhLH) for the induction of ovulation in hypogonadal women (orphan)*

Luveris powder for subcu injection ℞ *gonadotropin; recombinant human luteinizing hormone (rhLH) for the induction of ovulation in hypogonadal women (orphan)* [lutropin alfa] 75 IU/dose

Luvox film-coated tablets ℞ *selective serotonin reuptake inhibitor (SSRI) for obsessive-compulsive disorder (OCD); also used for depression, bulimia nervosa, and panic disorder* [fluvoxamine maleate] 25, 50, 100 mg

Luvox CR extended-release capsules ℞ *selective serotonin reuptake inhibitor (SSRI) for obsessive-compulsive disorder (OCD) and social anxiety disorder; also used for depression, bulimia nervosa, and panic disorder* [fluvoxamine maleate] 100, 150 mg

luxabendazole INN, BAN

Luxiq foam ℞ *corticosteroidal anti-inflammatory for scalp dermatoses* [betamethasone valerate] 0.12%

lyapolate sodium USAN *anticoagulant* [also: sodium apolate]

Lybrel film-coated tablets ℞ *non-cyclic (continuous-use) oral contraceptive that completely eliminates menstrual cycles; investigational (Phase III) for premenstrual dysphoric disorder*

(PMDD) [levonorgestrel; ethinyl estradiol] 0.9 mg•20 mcg

lycetamine USAN *topical antimicrobial*

lycine HCl [see: betaine HCl]

lycopene *natural substance found in high concentration in ripe tomatoes; a member of the carotene family; used as an antineoplastic and antioxidant*

Lycopodium clavatum medicinal herb [see: club moss]

Lycopus virginicus medicinal herb [see: bugleweed]

lydimycin USAN *antifungal* [also: lidimycin]

lymecycline INN, BAN

Lymphazurin 1% subcu injection ℞ *radiopaque contrast medium for lymphography* [isosulfan blue] 10 mg/mL (1%)

LymphoCide *investigational (Phase III, orphan) monoclonal antibody for AIDS-related non-Hodgkin lymphoma* [epratuzumab, radiolabeled with yttrium Y 90]

lymphocyte immune globulin (LIG) [see: antithymocyte globulin (ATG)]

lymphogranuloma venereum antigen USP

LymphoScan *monoclonal antibody IgG$_{2a}$ to B cell, murine; investigational (Phase III, orphan) diagnostic aid for non-Hodgkin B-cell lymphoma, AIDS-related lymphomas, and other acute and chronic B-cell leukemias* [technetium Tc 99m bectumomab]

lynestrenol USAN, INN *progestin* [also: lynoestrenol]

lynoestrenol BAN *progestin* [also: lynestrenol]

Lyo-Ject (trademarked delivery form) *prefilled dual-chambered syringe with lyophilized powder and diluent*

Lypholized Vitamin B Complex & Vitamin C with B$_{12}$ injection ℞ *parenteral vitamin therapy* [multiple B vitamins; vitamin C] ±•50 mg/mL

Lypholyte; Lypholyte II IV admixture ℞ *intravenous electrolyte therapy* [combined electrolyte solution] ② Levlite

lypressin USAN, USP, INN, BAN *posterior pituitary hormone; antidiuretic; vasoconstrictor*

Lyrica capsules, oral solution ℞ *anticonvulsant for partial-onset seizures; agent for the management of neuropathic pain from diabetic peripheral neuropathy (DPN), postherpetic neuralgia (PHN), and fibromyalgia; investigational (NDA filed) for generalized anxiety disorder (GAD)* [pregabalin] 25, 50, 75, 100, 150, 200, 225, 300 mg; 20 mg/mL

lysergic acid diethylamide (LSD) *street drug* [see: LSD; lysergide]

lysergide INN, BAN

lysine (L-lysine) USAN, INN *essential amino acid; symbols: Lys, K; natural remedy for the prophylaxis and treatment of recurrent oral and genital herpes simplex outbreaks; inhibits HSV replication* 312, 500, 1000 mg oral ② Lessina; leucine

lysine acetate USP *amino acid*

DL-lysine acetylsalicylate [see: aspirin DL-lysine]

lysine HCl USAN, USP *amino acid*

L-lysine monoacetate [see: lysine acetate]

L-lysine monohydrochloride [see: lysine HCl]

8-L-lysine vasopressin [see: lypressin]

Lysiplex Plus oral liquid OTC *vitamin/mineral/iron supplement* [multiple vitamins & minerals; iron (as ferric ammonium citrate); folic acid] ±• 10•0.8 mg/15 mL

Lysodase *investigational (orphan) chronic enzyme replacement therapy for Gaucher disease* [PEG-glucocerebrosidase]

Lysodren tablets ℞ *antibiotic antineoplastic for inoperable adrenal cortical carcinoma and Cushing syndrome* [mitotane] 500 mg

lysostaphin USAN *antibacterial enzyme*

Lysteda tablets ℞ *systemic hemostatic for menorrhagia* [tranexamic acid] 650 mg

lysuride BAN [also: lisuride]

M-2 protocol (vincristine, carmustine, cyclophosphamide, prednisone, melphalan) *chemotherapy protocol for multiple myeloma*

MAA (macroaggregated albumin) [see: albumin, aggregated]

Maalox; Maalox Advanced; Maalox Advanced Maximum Strength; Maalox Multi-Symptom oral liquid OTC *antacid; antiflatulent* [aluminum hydroxide; magnesium hydroxide; simethicone] 200•200•20 mg/5 mL; 200•200•20 mg/5 mL; 400•400•40 mg/5 mL; 400•400•40 mg/5 mL

Maalox Advanced Strength; Maalox Plus Antacid Junior chewable tablets OTC *antacid; antiflatulent; calcium supplement* [calcium (as carbonate); simethicone] 400 (1000)•60 mg; 160 (400)•24 mg

Maalox Antacid Barrier chewable tablets OTC *antacid; calcium supplement* [calcium (as carbonate)] 200 mg (500 mg)

Maalox Children's chewable tablets OTC *antacid; calcium supplement* [calcium (as carbonate)] 160 mg (400 mg)

Maalox Max chewable tablets OTC *antacid; antiflatulent; calcium supplement* [calcium (as carbonate); simethicone] 400 (1000)•60 mg

Maalox Total Stomach Relief oral suspension OTC *antidiarrheal; antinauseant* [bismuth subsalicylate] 525 mg/15 mL

MAb; MAB (monoclonal antibodies) [q.v.]

mabuterol INN

MAC; MAC III (methotrexate, actinomycin D, cyclophosphamide) *chemotherapy protocol for gestational trophoblastic neoplasm*

maca (*Lepidium meyenii*) root *medicinal herb used as an adaptogen, aphrodisiac in males, fertility aid in females, and to relieve stress*

MACC (methotrexate, Adriamycin, cyclophosphamide, CCNU) *chemotherapy protocol for non–small cell lung cancer (NSCLC)*

mace (*Myristica fragrans*) dried nutmeg aril (the fleshy network surrounding the seed) *medicinal herb* [see: nutmeg]

MACOP-B (methotrexate, Adriamycin, cyclophosphamide, Oncovin, prednisone, bleomycin) [with ketoconazole or Bactrim antibiotic] *chemotherapy protocol for non-Hodgkin lymphoma* ☑ Mega-B

macroaggregated albumin (MAA) [see: albumin, aggregated]

macroaggregated iodinated (^{131}I) human albumin [see: macrosalb (^{131}I)]

Macrobid capsules R̶ *urinary antibiotic* [nitrofurantoin (macrocrystals); nitrofurantoin monohydrate] 25•75 mg

Macrodantin capsules R̶ *urinary antibiotic* [nitrofurantoin (macrocrystals)] 25, 50, 100 mg

Macrodex IV infusion R̶ *plasma volume expander for shock due to hemorrhage, burns, or surgery* [dextran 70] 6%

macrogol 4000 INN, BAN [also: polyethylene glycol 4000]

macrogol ester 2000 INN *surfactant* [also: polyoxyl 40 stearate]

macrogol ester 400 INN *surfactant* [also: polyoxyl 8 stearate]

macrolides *a class of antibiotics that are bacteriostatic or bactericidal, depending on drug concentration*

macrophage colony-stimulating factor (M-CSF) [now: cilmostim]

macrophage-targeted β-glucocerebrosidase [now: alglucerase]

macrosalb (^{131}I) INN, BAN

macrosalb (^{99m}Tc) INN, BAN [also: technetium (^{99m}Tc) labeled macroaggregated human ...]

Macrotys actaeoides *medicinal herb* [see: black cohosh]

Macugen intravitreous injection in prefilled syringes ℞ *pegylated VEGF (vascular endothelial growth factor) antagonist for neovascular (wet) age-related macular degeneration (AMD); also used for diabetic macular edema* [pegaptanib sodium] 0.3 mg/dose ② Mycogen

MacuTrition softgels + tablets OTC *vitamin/mineral supplement* [vitamins C, D, and E; multiple minerals and herbs; fish oil; lutein; zeaxanthin] 500 mg•1332 U•76 U• ± •800 mg• 8 mg•2 mg

mad-dog weed; mad weed *medicinal herb* [see: skullcap]

madnep; madness *medicinal herb* [see: masterwort]

maduramicin USAN, INN *anticoccidal*

mafenide USAN, INN, BAN *bacteriostatic; adjunct to burn therapy*

mafenide acetate USP *broad-spectrum bacteriostatic to prevent meshed autograft loss on second- and third-degree burns (orphan)*

mafenide HCl

mafilcon A USAN *hydrophilic contact lens material* ② mefloquine

mafoprazine INN

mafosfamide INN *investigational (orphan) for neoplastic meningitis*

Mag-200 tablets OTC *magnesium supplement* [magnesium oxide] 200 mg Mg

magaldrate USAN, USP, INN *antacid* 540 mg/5 mL oral

Magaldrate Plus oral suspension OTC *antacid; antiflatulent* [magaldrate; simethicone] 540•40 mg/5 mL

Magalox Plus chewable tablets OTC *antacid; antiflatulent* [aluminum hydroxide; magnesium hydroxide; simethicone] 200•200•25 mg

Magan tablets ℞ *analgesic; antirheumatic* [magnesium salicylate] 545 mg ② Makena

Mag-Cal tablets (discontinued 2008) OTC *calcium/mineral supplement* [calcium (as carbonate); multiple minerals; vitamin D] 416.7 mg• ± •66.7 IU

Mag-Cal Mega tablets OTC *mineral supplement* [magnesium; calcium] 166.7•133.3 mg

Mag-Caps capsules (discontinued 2008) OTC *magnesium supplement* [magnesium (as oxide)] 85 mg

Mag-G tablets OTC *magnesium supplement* [magnesium (as gluconate dihydrate)] 27 mg

maggots *(Lucilia caesar; Phaenicia sericata; Pharmia regina) natural treatment for debriding necrotic tissue in abscesses, burns, cellulitis, gangrene, osteomyelitis, and ulcers*

magic mouthwash *a slang term for the combination of a local anesthetic plus one or more of the following: an antihistamine, a corticosteroid, an antifungal, an antibiotic—with or without an antacid used as a carrier*

Maginex enteric-coated tablets OTC *magnesium supplement* [magnesium (as L-aspartate HCl)] 61 mg

Maginex DS tablets OTC *magnesium/calcium/phosphorus supplement* [magnesium (as gluconate dihydrate); calcium (as dibasic calcium phosphate); phosphorus (as dibasic calcium phosphate)] 27•87.5•66 mg

Magnacal ready-to-use oral liquid OTC *enteral nutritional therapy* [lactose-free formula] ② Monocal

Magnacet caplets ℞ *narcotic analgesic; antipyretic* [oxycodone HCl; acetaminophen] 5•400, 7.5•400, 10•400 mg ② Menest

Magnaprin; Magnaprin Arthritis Strength Captabs film-coated tablets (discontinued 2007) OTC *analgesic; antipyretic; anti-inflammatory; antirheumatic* [aspirin (buffered with aluminum hydroxide, magnesium hydroxide, and calcium carbonate)] 325 mg ② minaprine

MagneBind 200; MagneBind 300 tablets OTC *calcium/magnesium supplement that binds dietary phosphate* [calcium carbonate; magnesium carbonate] 400•200 mg; 250•300 mg

MagneBind 400 Rx tablets ℞ *calcium/magnesium supplement that binds dietary phosphate* [calcium carbonate; magnesium carbonate; folic acid] 200•400•1 mg

magnesia, milk of USP *antacid; saline laxative* [also: magnesium hydroxide] 400 mg/5 mL oral

magnesia magma [now: magnesia, milk of]

magnesium *element (Mg)*

magnesium aluminosilicate hydrate [see: almasilate]

magnesium aluminum silicate NF *suspending agent*

magnesium amino acid chelate *dietary magnesium supplement*

magnesium aspartate [see: potassium aspartate & magnesium aspartate]

magnesium carbonate USP *antacid; dietary magnesium supplement*

magnesium carbonate hydrate [see: magnesium carbonate]

magnesium chloride USP *electrolyte replenisher* 1.97 mEq/mL (20%) injection

magnesium chloride hexahydrate [see: magnesium chloride]

magnesium citrate USP *dietary magnesium supplement; saline laxative* 100 mg Mg oral; 1.75 g/30 mL oral

magnesium clofibrate INN

magnesium D-gluconate dihydrate [see: magnesium gluconate]

magnesium D-gluconate hydrate [see: magnesium gluconate]

magnesium EDTA (ethylene diamine tetraacetic acid) [see: edetate magnesium disodium]

magnesium gluconate USP *dietary magnesium supplement* 12.7 mg Mg oral

magnesium glycinate USAN

magnesium hydroxide USP *antacid; saline laxative* [also: magnesia, milk of]

magnesium hydroxycarbonate *antiurolithic*

magnesium oxide USP *antacid; sorbent; magnesium supplement* (base=

60.3%) 250, 400 mg (150.75, 241.3 mg Mg) oral

magnesium phosphate USP *antacid*

magnesium phosphate pentahydrate [see: magnesium phosphate]

magnesium salicylate (MS) USP *analgesic; antipyretic; anti-inflammatory; antirheumatic*

magnesium salicylate tetrahydrate [see: magnesium salicylate]

magnesium silicate NF *tablet excipient*

magnesium silicate hydrate [see: magnesium trisilicate]

magnesium stearate NF *tablet and capsule lubricant*

magnesium sulfate USP, JAN *anticonvulsant used for eclampsia or preeclampsia; controls hypertension and convulsions due to acute nephritis in children; saline laxative; electrolyte replenisher; magnesium supplement; also used as a tocolytic for preterm labor* 4%, 8%, 12.5%, 50% (0.325, 0.65, 1, 4 mEq/mL) injection

magnesium sulfate heptahydrate [see: magnesium sulfate]

magnesium trisilicate USP *antacid*

magnesium-L-aspartate HCl *dietary magnesium supplement*

Magnevist IV injection ℞ *paramagnetic contrast medium for imaging of the head and neck, and to enhance MRIs of the brain, spine, and other CNS tissue* [gadopentetate dimeglumine] 469 mg/mL

magnolia (Magnolia glauca) bark *medicinal herb used as an antiperiodic, aromatic, astringent, diaphoretic, febrifuge, stimulant, and tonic*

Magnox oral suspension OTC *antacid* [aluminum hydroxide; magnesium hydroxide] 225•200 mg/5 mL ⊡ Minox

Magonate oral liquid OTC *magnesium supplement* [magnesium (as gluconate dihydrate)] 27, 54 mg/5 mL

Magonate tablets OTC *magnesium/calcium/phosphorus supplement* [magnesium (as gluconate dihydrate); calcium (as dibasic calcium phosphate);

phosphorus (as dibasic calcium phosphate)] 27•87.5•66 mg

Magonate Natal pediatric oral drops OTC *magnesium supplement* [magnesium gluconate] 3.52 mg Mg/mL

Mag-Ox 400 tablets OTC *antacid; magnesium supplement* [magnesium oxide] 400 mg (241 mg Mg)

Mag-SR tablets OTC *calcium/magnesium supplement* [calcium; magnesium] 106•64 mg ② Maxair

Mag-Tab SR sustained-release caplets OTC *magnesium supplement* [magnesium (as lactate dihydrate)] 84 mg

Magtrate tablets OTC *magnesium supplement* [magnesium gluconate] 500 mg (29 mg Mg)

mahogany birch; mountain mahogany *medicinal herb* [see: birch]

Mahonia aquifolium medicinal herb [see: Oregon grape]

ma-huang *medicinal herb* [see: ephedra]

MAID (mesna [rescue], Adriamycin, ifosfamide, dacarbazine) *chemotherapy protocol for soft tissue and bone sarcomas*

maitake mushrooms *(Grifola frondosa)* cap and stem *medicinal herb for cancer, diabetes, hypercholesterolemia, hypertension, obesity, and stimulation of the immune system*

maitansine INN *antineoplastic* [also: maytansine]

Maitec injection *investigational (orphan) agent for disseminated* Mycobacterium avium-intracellulare *infection* [gentamicin sulfate, liposomal]

Majorana hortensis medicinal herb [see: marjoram]

Major-Con chewable tablets OTC *antiflatulent* [simethicone] 80 mg

Major-gesic tablets (discontinued 2007) OTC *antihistamine; sleep aid; analgesic; antipyretic* [phenyltoloxamine citrate; acetaminophen] 30•325 mg

Makena IM injection ℞ *synthetic progesterone; once-weekly therapy to prevent preterm birth in women with a history of spontaneous preterm delivery*

[hydroxyprogesterone caproate] 250 mg/mL ② Magan

malaleuca *medicinal herb* [see: tea tree oil]

Malarone; Malarone Pediatric film-coated tablets ℞ *malaria prophylaxis and treatment* [atovaquone; proguanil HCl (chloroguanide HCl)] 250•100 mg; 62.5•25 mg ② Myleran

malathion USP, BAN *pediculicide for lice* 0.5% topical ② Miltown

maletamer INN *antiperistaltic* [also: malethamer]

malethamer USAN *antiperistaltic* [also: maletamer]

maleylsulfathiazole INN

malic acid NF *acidifying agent*

malidone [see: aloxidone]

Mallamint chewable tablets OTC *antacid* [calcium carbonate] 420 mg

mallow *(Malva rotundifolia; M. sylvestris)* plant *medicinal herb used as an astringent, demulcent, emollient, and expectorant*

mallow, marsh *(Althaea officinalis) medicinal herb* [see: marsh mallow]

malonal [see: barbital]

malotilate USAN, INN *liver disorder treatment* ② Multilyte

Malpighia glabra; M. punicifolia medicinal herb [see: acerola]

Maltsupex powder OTC *bulk laxative* [barley malt soup extract] 8 g/scoop

Malva rotundifolia; M. sylvestris medicinal herb [see: mallow]

Mammol ointment OTC *emollient for nipples of nursing mothers* [bismuth subnitrate] 40%

m-**AMSA (acridinylamine methanesulphon anisidide)** [see: amsacrine]

Mandameth enteric-coated tablets (discontinued 2009) ℞ *urinary antibiotic* [methenamine mandelate] 0.5, 1 g

Mandelamine film-coated tablets (discontinued 2009) ℞ *urinary antibiotic* [methenamine mandelate] 0.5, 1 g

mandelic acid NF

mandrake *(Mandragora officinarium; Podophyllum peltatum)* root and resin *medicinal herb for cancer, condy-*

lomata, constipation, fever, indigestion, liver disorders, lower bowel disorders, warts, and worms; not generally regarded as safe and effective for children or pregnant women

mangafodipir trisodium USAN *parenteral radiopaque contrast agent to enhance MRIs of the liver*

manganese *element (Mn)*

manganese chloride USP *dietary manganese supplement; additive to IV solutions for total parenteral nutrition (28% elemental manganese)* 0.36 mg/mL (0.1 mg/mL Mn) injection

manganese chloride tetrahydrate [see: manganese chloride]

manganese citrate *dietary manganese supplement (30% elemental manganese)*

manganese gluconate (manganese D-gluconate) USP *dietary manganese supplement*

manganese glycerophosphate NF

manganese hypophosphite NF

manganese phosphinate [see: manganese hypophosphite]

manganese sulfate USP *dietary manganese supplement; additive to IV solutions for total parenteral nutrition (32% elemental manganese)* 0.308 mg/mL (0.1 mg/mL Mn) injection

manganese sulfate monohydrate [see: manganese sulfate]

Mangimin caplets OTC *mineral supplement* [manganese] 10 mg

mangofodipir trisodium *MRI contrast medium for liver imaging*

manidipine 6300 INN

manna sugar [see: mannitol]

mannite [see: mannitol]

mannitol (D-mannitol) USP *renal function test aid; antihypertensive; osmotic diuretic; urologic irrigant; mucolytic for bronchiectasis and cystic fibrosis (orphan)* 10%, 15%, 20%, 25% injection ☒ Mynatal

mannitol hexanitrate INN

mannityl nitrate [see: mannitol hexanitrate]

D-mannoheptulose *the active principle in avocado that suppresses excess insulin*

production by the pancreas; investigational treatment for obesity and type 2 diabetes [also: avocado sugar extract]

mannomustine INN, BAN

mannopentaose phosphate sulfate *investigational (orphan) for high-risk, advanced melanoma*

mannosulfan INN

manozodil INN

Mantoux test [see: tuberculin]

MAO inhibitors (monoamine oxidase inhibitors) [q.v.]

Maolate tablets (discontinued 2007) ℞ *skeletal muscle relaxant* [chlorphenesin carbamate] 400 mg

Maox 420 tablets OTC *antacid* [magnesium oxide] 420 mg ☒ Megace; M-oxy

Māpap tablets, caplets, capsules, rapid-release gelcaps, oral liquid OTC *analgesic; antipyretic* [acetaminophen] 325 mg; 500 mg; 500 mg; 500 mg; 166.67 mg/5 mL ☒ MOBP

Māpap, Children's chewable tablets, elixir OTC *analgesic; antipyretic* [acetaminophen] 80 mg; 160 mg/5 mL

Māpap, Junior chewable tablets OTC *analgesic; antipyretic* [acetaminophen] 160 mg

Māpap Arthritis Pain extended-release tablets OTC *analgesic; antipyretic* [acetaminophen] 650 mg

Māpap Cold Formula Multi-Symptom tablets OTC *antitussive; decongestant; analgesic; antipyretic* [dextromethorphan hydrobromide; phenylephrine HCl; acetaminophen] 10•5•325 mg

Māpap Infant Drops (discontinued 2011) OTC *analgesic; antipyretic* [acetaminophen] 100 mg/mL

Māpap Sinus geltabs OTC *decongestant; analgesic; antipyretic* [pseudoephedrine HCl; acetaminophen] 30•500 mg

Māpap Sinus Congestion and Pain caplets OTC *decongestant; analgesic; antipyretic* [phenylephrine HCl; acetaminophen] 5•325 mg

maple lungwort *medicinal herb* [see: lungwort]

Marlin Salt System 439

maprotiline USAN, INN *tetracyclic anti-depressant*

maprotiline HCl USP *tetracyclic antide-pressant* 25, 50, 75 mg oral

Maranox tablets (discontinued 2008) OTC *analgesic; antipyretic* [acetaminophen] 325 mg

maraviroc *cellular chemokine receptor 5 (CCR5) inhibitor; twice-daily oral antiretroviral for early-stage HIV-1 infections*

Marax tablets (discontinued 2007) ℞ *antiasthmatic; bronchodilator; decongestant* [theophylline; ephedrine sulfate] 130•25 mg

Marax-DF pediatric syrup (discontinued 2007) ℞ *antiasthmatic; bronchodilator; decongestant; antihistamine* [theophylline; ephedrine sulfate; hydroxyzine HCl] 97.5•18.75•7.5 mg/15 mL

Marblen tablets, oral liquid OTC *antacid* [calcium carbonate; magnesium carbonate] 520•400 mg; 540•400 mg/5 mL

Marcaine injection ℞ *local anesthetic* [bupivacaine HCl] 0.25%, 0.5%, 0.75%

Marcaine with Epinephrine injection ℞ *local anesthetic* [bupivacaine HCl; epinephrine] 0.25%•1:200 000, 0.5%•1:200 000, 0.75%•1:200 000

Mar-Cof BP oral liquid ℞ *narcotic antitussive; antihistamine; decongestant* [codeine phosphate; brompheniramine maleate; pseudoephedrine HCl] 7.5•2•30 mg/5 mL

Mar-Cof CG oral liquid ℞ *narcotic antitussive; expectorant* [codeine phosphate; guaifenesin] 7.5•225 mg/5 mL

Mar-Cof Expectorant syrup (discontinued 2011) ℞ *narcotic antitussive; expectorant* [hydrocodone bitartrate; potassium guaiacolsulfonate] 5•350 mg/5 mL

mare's tail *medicinal herb* [see: fleabane; horseweed]

Marezine tablets OTC *antiemetic; anticholinergic; antihistamine; motion sickness preventative* [cyclizine HCl] 50 mg ⃞ morazone

Margesic capsules ℞ *barbiturate sedative; analgesic; antipyretic* [butalbital; acetaminophen; caffeine] 50•325•40 mg

Margesic H capsules ℞ *narcotic analgesic; antipyretic* [hydrocodone bitartrate; acetaminophen] 5•500 mg

maribavir USAN *investigational (Phase III) benzimidazole riboside antiviral for cytomegalovirus disease in stem cell transplants*

maridomycin INN

marigold (Calendula officinalis) florets *medicinal herb for bruises, cuts, dysmenorrhea, eye infections, fever, and skin diseases; not generally regarded as safe and effective*

marijuana; marihuana (Cannabis sativa) *euphoric/hallucinogenic street drug made from the dried leaves and flowering tops of the cannabis plant; medicinal herb for asthma, analgesia, leprosy, and loss of appetite; investigational (orphan) for HIV-wasting syndrome*

marijuana extracts ⃝ *analgesic for pain associated with cancer and multiple sclerosis* [see: delta-9-tetrahydrocannabinol (THC); cannabidiol (CBD)]

marimastat USAN *antineoplastic; matrix metalloproteinase (MMP) inhibitor*

Marine Lipid Concentrate softgels (discontinued 2008) OTC *dietary supplement* [omega-3 fatty acids (eicosapentaenoic acid and docosahexaenoic acid)] 1200 mg (360 mg EPA; 240 mg DHA)

Marinol oil-filled gelcaps ℞ *antiemetic for chemotherapy; appetite stimulant for AIDS patients (orphan)* [dronabinol] 2.5, 5, 10 mg ⃞ Moranyl

mariptiline INN

marjoram (Majorana hortensis; Origanum vulgare) plant *medicinal herb for abdominal cramps, colic, headache, indigestion, respiratory problems, and violent cough*

Marlin Salt System tablets (discontinued 2010) OTC *rinsing/storage solution* *for soft contact lenses* [sodium chloride (normal saline solution)] 250 mg

Marlin Salt System II tablets OTC *rinsing/storage solution for soft contact lenses* [sodium chloride (normal saline solution)] 250 mg

Marmine IV or IM injection ℞ *antinauseant; antiemetic; antivertigo; motion sickness preventative* [dimenhydrinate] 50 mg/mL

Marmine tablets OTC *antinauseant; antiemetic; antivertigo; motion sickness preventative* [dimenhydrinate] 50 mg

Marnatal-F Plus Duo Pack film-coated tablets + softgels ℞ *prenatal vitamin/mineral/calcium/iron/omega-3 supplement* [multiple vitamins & minerals; calcium; iron (as polysaccharide iron complex); folic acid + EPA; DHA] ±•250•60•1 mg (tablets) + 150•100 mg (softgels)

Marogen *investigational (orphan) hematinic for anemia of end-stage renal disease* [epoetin beta]

maroxepin INN

Marplan tablets ℞ *monoamine oxidase (MAO) inhibitor for depression* [isocarboxazid] 10 mg

Marpres tablets (discontinued 2007) ℞ *antihypertensive; vasodilator; diuretic* [hydrochlorothiazide; reserpine; hydralazine HCl] 15•0.1•25 mg

Marrubium vulgare medicinal herb [see: horehound]

marsh clover; marsh trefoil *medicinal herb* [see: buckbean]

marsh mallow (Althaea officinalis) root *medicinal herb for asthma, boils, bronchial infections, cough, emphysema, infected wounds, kidney disorders, lung congestion, sore throat, and urinary bleeding*

Mar-Spas orally disintegrating caplets ℞ *GI antispasmodic; anticholinergic "drying agent" for allergic rhinitis* [L-hyoscyamine sulfate] 0.25 mg

MARstem *investigational (orphan) agent for myelodysplastic syndrome and neutropenia due to bone marrow transplantation* [angiotensin 1-7]

Marten-Tab caplets ℞ *barbiturate sedative; analgesic; antipyretic* [butalbital; acetaminophen] 50•325 mg

Marthritic tablets ℞ *analgesic; antipyretic; anti-inflammatory; antirheumatic* [salsalate] 750 mg

Masophen tablets, capsules OTC *analgesic; antipyretic* [acetaminophen] 325, 500 mg; 500 mg

masoprocol USAN, INN *antineoplastic for actinic keratoses (AK)*

Massé Breast cream OTC *moisturizer and emollient for nipples of nursing women*

Massengill Baking Soda Freshness vaginal solution OTC *cleanser and deodorizer; acidity modifier* [sodium bicarbonate]

Massengill Disposable Douche vaginal solution OTC *antiseptic/germicidal cleanser and deodorizer; acidity modifier* [cetylpyridinium chloride; lactic acid; sodium lactate]

Massengill Disposable Douche; Massengill Vinegar & Water Extra Mild vaginal solution OTC *acidity modifier; cleanser and deodorizer* [vinegar (acetic acid)]

Massengill Douche solution concentrate OTC *vaginal cleanser and deodorizer; acidity modifier* [lactic acid; sodium lactate; sodium bicarbonate]

Massengill Douche vaginal powder OTC *cleanser and deodorizer; analgesic; mild anesthetic; antipruritic; counterirritant* [methyl salicymate; ammonium alum; phenol; menthol; thymol]

Massengill Feminine Cleansing Wash topical liquid OTC *for external perivaginal cleansing*

Massengill Medicated towelettes OTC *corticosteroidal anti-inflammatory* [hydrocortisone] 0.5%

Massengill Medicated Douche with Cepticin; Massengill Medicated Disposable Douche with Cepticin vaginal solution OTC *antiseptic/germicidal cleanser and deodorizer* [povidone-iodine] 12%; 10%

Massengill Vinegar & Water Extra Cleansing with Puraclean vaginal solution OTC *antiseptic/germicidal cleanser and deodorizer; acidity modifier* [cetylpyridinium chloride; vinegar (acetic acid)]

mast cell stabilizers *a class of topical agents that inhibit the antigen-induced release of inflammatory mediators (e.g., various histamines and leukotrienes) from human mast cells; used on nasal, ophthalmological, and gastrointestinal mucosa* [also known as: mediator release inhibitors]

masterwort (Heracleum lanatum) root and seed *medicinal herb used as an antispasmodic, carminative, and stimulant*

Mastisol topical liquid OTC *adhesive for securing dressings, IV lines, etc. on the skin*

maté *medicinal herb* [see: yerba maté]

Matricaria chamomilla medicinal herb [see: chamomile]

matrix metalloproteinase (MMP) inhibitors *a class of investigational (orphan) agents to treat corneal ulcers*

Matulane capsules ℞ *antineoplastic for Hodgkin disease; investigational (orphan) for malignant glioma; also used for other lymphomas, melanoma, brain tumors, and lung cancer* [procarbazine HCl] 50 mg

Matzim LA extended-release caplets ℞ *antihypertensive; antianginal; calcium channel blocker* [diltiazem HCl] 120, 180, 240, 300, 360, 420 mg

Mavik tablets ℞ *antihypertensive; angiotensin-converting enzyme (ACE) inhibitor; treatment for congestive heart failure* [trandolapril] 1, 2, 4 mg ⑦ MVAC

maxacalcitol USAN *vitamin D_3 analogue*

Maxair Autohaler (breath-activated metered-dose inhaler) ℞ *sympathomimetic bronchodilator for asthma and bronchospasm* [pirbuterol (as acetate)] 0.2 mg/dose ⑦ Mag-SR

Maxalt caplets ℞ *vascular serotonin 5-$HT_{1B/1D}$ receptor agonist for the acute treatment of migraine* [rizatriptan benzoate] 5, 10 mg

Maxalt-MLT orally disintegrating tablets ℞ *vascular serotonin 5-$HT_{1B/1D}$ receptor agonist for the acute treatment of migraine* [rizatriptan benzoate] 5, 10 mg

Maxamine *investigational (NDA filed, orphan) adjuvant to interleukin-2 for stage IV malignant melanoma and acute myeloid leukemia (AML)* [histamine dihydrochloride]

Maxaquin film-coated tablets (discontinued 2009) ℞ *broad-spectrum fluoroquinolone antibiotic* [lomefloxacin HCl] 400 mg

Maxaron Forte capsules ℞ *hematinic* [iron (as elemental iron, elemental ferrous bisglycinate, and polysaccharide iron); vitamin B_{12}; vitamin C; folic acid] 150•0.025•60•1 mg

MaxEPA soft capsules (discontinued 2008) OTC *dietary supplement* [multiple vitamins & minerals; omega-3 fatty acids (eicosapentaenoic acid and docosahexaenoic acid)] ≛•1000 mg (180 mg EPA; 120 mg DHA)

Maxibolin *an anabolic steroid abused as a street drug* [see: ethylestrenol]

Maxichlor PEH DM caplets ℞ *decongestant; antihistamine; antitussive* [phenylephrine HCl; chlorpheniramine maleate; dextromethorphan hydrobromide] 10•4•20 mg

Maxidex Drop-Tainers (eye drop/ear drop suspension) ℞ *corticosteroidal anti-inflammatory for corneal injury, ophthalmic inflammation, and otic inflammation* [dexamethasone] 0.1%

Maxidone caplets ℞ *narcotic analgesic; antipyretic* [hydrocodone bitartrate; acetaminophen] 10•750 mg ⑦ mixidine

Maxifed caplets ℞ *decongestant; expectorant* [pseudoephedrine HCl; guaifenesin] 60•400 mg

Maxifed DM sustained-release caplets, oral liquid OTC *antitussive; decongestant; expectorant* [dextromethorphan hydrobromide; pseudoephedrine HCl; guaifenesin] 20•40•400 mg; 10•20•200 mg/5 mL

Maxifed DMX sustained-release caplets OTC *antitussive; decongestant; expectorant* [dextromethorphan hydrobromide; pseudoephedrine HCl; guaifenesin] 20•60•400 mg

Maxifed-G sustained-release caplets OTC *decongestant; expectorant* [pseudoephedrine HCl; guaifenesin] 60• 580 mg

Maxiflor cream, ointment ℞ *corticosteroidal anti-inflammatory* [diflorasone diacetate] 0.05%

Maxiflu DM caplets ℞ *antitussive; decongestant; expectorant; analgesic; antipyretic* [dextromethorphan hydrobromide; pseudoephedrine HCl; guaifenesin; acetaminophen] 20•60•400•500 mg

Maxiflu G tablets (discontinued 2008) ℞ *antitussive; decongestant; expectorant; analgesic; antipyretic* [dextromethorphan hydrobromide; pseudoephedrine HCl; guaifenesin; acetaminophen] 30•60•600•500 mg

Maxilube vaginal jelly OTC *moisturizer/lubricant*

Maximum Blue Label; Maximum Green Label tablets (discontinued 2008) OTC *vitamin/mineral supplement* [multiple vitamins & minerals; folic acid; biotin] ±•130•50 mcg

Maximum D3 capsules OTC *vitamin supplement* [cholecalciferol (vitamin D_3)] 10 000 IU

Maximum Red Label tablets OTC *vitamin/mineral/iron supplement* [multiple vitamins & minerals; iron (as ferrous succinate and iron chelate); folic acid; biotin] ±•3.3•0.13•0.05 mg

"Maximum Strength" products [see under product name]

Maxiphen DM; Maxiphen-G DM extended-release caplets ℞ *antitussive; decongestant; expectorant* [dextromethorphan hydrobromide; phenylephrine HCl; guaifenesin] 20•10•400 mg; 30•20•1000 mg

Maxiphen-G extended-release caplets (discontinued 2008) ℞ *decongestant; expectorant* [phenylephrine HCl; guaifenesin] 20•1000 mg

Maxipime powder for IV or IM injection (discontinued 2011) ℞ *fourth-generation cephalosporin antibiotic* [cefepime HCl] 0.5, 1, 2 g

Maxitrol eye drop suspension, ophthalmic ointment ℞ *corticosteroidal anti-inflammatory; antibiotic* [dexamethasone; neomycin sulfate; polymyxin B sulfate] 0.1%•0.35%•10 000 U/mL; 0.1%•0.35%•10 000 U/g

Maxi-Tuss DM oral liquid (discontinued 2007) ℞ *antitussive; expectorant* [dextromethorphan hydrobromide; guaifenesin] 20•200 mg/5 mL

Maxi-Tuss HC oral liquid (discontinued 2007) ℞ *narcotic antitussive; antihistamine; decongestant* [hydrocodone bitartrate; chlorpheniramine maleate; phenylephrine HCl] 2.5•4•10 mg/5 mL

Maxi-Tuss HCG oral liquid (discontinued 2011) ℞ *narcotic antitussive; expectorant* [hydrocodone bitartrate; guaifenesin] 6•200 mg/5 mL

Maxi-Tuss HCX oral liquid (discontinued 2009) ℞ *narcotic antitussive; antihistamine; decongestant* [hydrocodone bitartrate; chlorpheniramine maleate; phenylephrine HCl] 6•2•12 mg/5 mL

Maxivate ointment, cream ℞ *corticosteroidal anti-inflammatory* [betamethasone dipropionate] 0.05%

Maxi-Vite tablets (discontinued 2008) OTC *vitamin/mineral/calcium/iron supplement* [multiple vitamins & minerals; calcium; iron; folic acid; biotin] ±•53.5•1.5•0.4•0.001 mg

Maxolon tablets (discontinued 2010) ℞ *antiemetic for chemotherapy and postoperative nausea and vomiting; GI stimulant for diabetic gastroparesis and gastroesophageal reflux* [metoclopramide (as HCl)] 10 mg

Maxovite sustained-release tablets (discontinued 2008) OTC *vitamin/mineral supplement* [multiple vitamins & minerals; folic acid; biotin] ± • 330 • 11.7 mcg

Maxzide tablets ℞ *antihypertensive; diuretic* [triamterene; hydrochlorothiazide] 37.5 • 25, 75 • 50 mg

May apple *medicinal herb* [see: mandrake]

May bells; May lily *medicinal herb* [see: lily of the valley]

May bush; May tree *medicinal herb* [see: hawthorn]

May lily *medicinal herb* [see: lily of the valley]

maytansine USAN *antineoplastic; clinical trials discontinued 1990 due to toxicity* [also: maitansine]

mazapertine succinate USAN *antipsychotic; dopamine receptor antagonist*

mazaticol INN

mazindol USAN, USP, INN, BAN *anorexiant; CNS stimulant; investigational (orphan) treatment for Duchenne muscular dystrophy*

mazipredone INN

MB (methylene blue) [q.v.]

m-BACOD; M-BACOD (methotrexate, bleomycin, Adriamycin, cyclophosphamide, Oncovin, dexamethasone) *chemotherapy protocol for non-Hodgkin lymphoma* ("m" is 200 mg/m²; "M" is 3 g/m²)

m-BACOD (methotrexate, bleomycin, Adriamycin, cyclophosphamide, Oncovin, dexamethasone), reduced dose *chemotherapy protocol for HIV-associated non-Hodgkin lymphoma* ("reduced dose" refers to a lower dosage of cyclophosphamide and dexamethasone than m-BACOD)

MBC (methotrexate, bleomycin, cisplatin) *chemotherapy protocol for head and neck cancer*

MBR (methylene blue, reduced) [see: methylene blue]

MC (mitoxantrone, cytarabine) *chemotherapy protocol for acute myelocytic leukemia (AML)*

M-Caps capsules ℞ *urinary acidifier to control ammonia production* [racemethionine] 200 mg

MCH (microfibrillar collagen hemostat) [q.v.]

M-Clear capsules ℞ *narcotic antitussive; expectorant* [codeine phosphate; guaifenesin] 9 • 200 mg

M-Clear Jr syrup (discontinued 2007) ℞ *narcotic antitussive; expectorant* [hydrocodone bitartrate; potassium guaiacolsulfonate] 2.5 • 175 mg/5 mL

M-Clear WC oral liquid ℞ *narcotic antitussive; expectorant* [codeine phosphate; guaifenesin] 6.3 • 100 mg/5 mL

M-CSF (macrophage colony-stimulating factor) [now: cilmostim]

MCT oil OTC *dietary fat supplement* [medium-chain triglycerides from coconut oil]

MCT (medium chain triglycerides) [q.v.]

MD-76 R injection ℞ *radiopaque contrast medium* [diatrizoate meglumine; diatrizoate sodium (48.7% total iodine)] 660 • 100 mg/mL (370 mg/mL)

MDA (methylenedioxyamphetamine) [see: MDMA, MDEA]

MDEA (3,4-methylenedioxyethamphetamine) *a hallucinogenic amphetamine derivative closely related to MDMA, abused as a street drug, which causes dependence* [see also: amphetamines; MDMA]

MDI (delivery device) *metered-dose inhaler*

MDMA (3,4-methylenedioxymethamphetamine) *widely abused hallucinogenic and euphoric street drug that is chemically related to amphetamines and mescaline and causes dependence; investigational treatment for post-traumatic stress disorder (PTSD)* [see also: amphetamines; mescaline; MDEA]

MDP (methylene diphosphonate) [now: medronate disodium]

MEA (mercaptoethylamine) [see: mercaptamine]

meadow cabbage *medicinal herb* [see: skunk cabbage]

meadow sorrel *medicinal herb* [see: sorrel]

meadowsweet *(Filipendula ulmaria)* plant *medicinal herb used for ulcers and upper respiratory problems; also used as an astringent, diaphoretic, and diuretic*

mealberry *medicinal herb* [see: uva ursi]

mealy starwort *medicinal herb* [see: star grass]

measles immune globulin USP

measles virus vaccine, live USP *active immunizing agent for measles (rubeola)*

measles & rubella virus vaccine, live USP *active immunizing agent for measles (rubeola) and rubella*

measles, mumps, & rubella virus vaccine, live USP *active immunizing agent for measles (rubeola), mumps, and rubella*

measles, mumps, rubella, & varicella virus vaccine, live attenuated *active immunizing agent for measles (rubeola), mumps, rubella, and varicella*

Mebadin (available only from the Centers for Disease Control) (discontinued 2011) ℞ *investigational anti-infective for amebiasis and amebic dysentery* [dehydroemetine]

meballymal [see: secobarbital]

mebamoxine [see: benmoxin]

mebanazine INN, BAN

Mebaral tablets ℞ *long-acting barbiturate sedative, hypnotic, and anticonvulsant* [mephobarbital] 32, 50, 100 mg

mebendazole USAN, USP, INN *anthelmintic for trichuriasis, enterobiasis, ascariasis, and uncinariasis* 100 mg oral

mebenoside INN

mebeverine INN *smooth muscle relaxant* [also: mebeverine HCl]

mebeverine HCl USAN *smooth muscle relaxant* [also: mebeverine]

mebezonium iodide INN, BAN

mebhydrolin INN, BAN

mebiquine INN

mebolazine INN

mebrofenin USAN, INN *hepatobiliary function test*

mebrophenhydramine HCl [see: embramine HCl]

mebubarbital [see: pentobarbital]

mebumal [see: pentobarbital]

mebutamate USAN, INN *antihypertensive*

mebutizide INN

mecamylamine INN *antiadrenergic; ganglionic blocker for severe hypertension* [also: mecamylamine HCl]

mecamylamine HCl USP *antiadrenergic; ganglionic blocker for severe hypertension; investigational (orphan) for Tourette syndrome* [also: mecamylamine]

mecamylamine HCl & nicotine *investigational (Phase III) transdermal patch for smoking cessation*

mecarbinate INN

mecarbine [see: mecarbinate]

mecasermin USAN, INN, BAN *recombinant human insulin-like growth factor-1 (rhIGF-1) for children with primary IGF deficiency without concomitant growth hormone (GH) deficiency (growth hormone insensitivity syndrome); investigational (NDA filed, orphan) for amyotrophic lateral sclerosis*

mecasermin & insulin-like growth factor binding protein-3 (IGF-1/IGFBP-3) *recombinant human insulin-like growth factor-1 (rhIGF-1) plus a binding protein; investigational (orphan) for severe burns* [now: mecasermin rinfabate]

mecasermin rinfabate *recombinant human insulin-like growth factor-1 (rhIGF-1) for children with primary IGF deficiency without concomitant growth hormone (GH) deficiency; investigational (orphan) for GH-insensitivity syndrome and extreme insulin-resistance syndromes*

MeCCNU (methyl chloroethyl-cyclohexyl-nitrosourea) [see: semustine]

mecetronium ethylsulfate USAN *antiseptic* [also: mecetronium etilsulfate]

mecetronium etilsulfate INN *antiseptic* [also: mecetronium ethylsulfate]

mechlorethamine HCl USP *nitrogen mustard–type alkylating antineoplastic for various leukemias, lymphomas, and carcinomas, polycythemia vera, and mycosis fungoides (orphan)* [also:

chlormethine; mustine; nitrogen mustard N-oxide HCl]

meciadanol INN

mecillinam INN, BAN *antibacterial* [also: amdinocillin]

mecinarone INN

meclizine HCl USP *antiemetic; antihistamine; anticholinergic; motion sickness relief* [also: meclozine] 12.5, 25, 50 mg oral

meclocycline USAN, INN, BAN *topical antibiotic* ◻ meglucycline

meclocycline sulfosalicylate USAN, USP *topical antibiotic*

meclofenamate sodium USAN, USP *analgesic; antiarthritic; nonsteroidal anti-inflammatory drug (NSAID) for osteoarthritis, rheumatoid arthritis, primary dysmenorrhea, and other mild to moderate pain* 50, 100 mg oral

meclofenamic acid USAN, INN *nonsteroidal anti-inflammatory drug (NSAID)*

meclofenoxate INN, BAN

meclonazepam INN

mecloqualone USAN, INN *sedative; hypnotic*

mecloralurea INN

meclorisone INN, BAN *topical anti-inflammatory* [also: meclorisone dibutyrate]

meclorisone dibutyrate USAN *topical anti-inflammatory* [also: meclorisone]

mecloxamine INN

meclozine INN, BAN *antiemetic; antihistamine; anticholinergic; motion sickness relief* [also: meclizine HCl] ◻ Miacalcin

mecobalamin USAN, INN *vitamin; hematopoietic*

mecrilate INN *tissue adhesive* [also: mecrylate]

mecrylate USAN *tissue adhesive* [also: mecrilate]

mecysteine INN

Medacote lotion (discontinued 2008) OTC *antihistamine; astringent* [pyrilamine maleate; zinc oxide] 1%•⅖ ◻ Modecate

Medalone 40; Medalone 80 [see: depMedalone 40; depMedalone 80]

medazepam INN *minor tranquilizer* [also: medazepam HCl]

medazepam HCl USAN *minor tranquilizer* [also: medazepam]

medazomide INN

medazonamide [see: medazomide]

Medebar Plus rectal suspension R̸ *radiopaque contrast medium for gastrointestinal imaging* [barium sulfate] 100%

Medent-DM sustained-release tablets (discontinued 2011) R̸ *antitussive; decongestant; expectorant* [dextromethorphan hydrobromide; pseudoephedrine HCl; guaifenesin] 30•60•800 mg

Medent-DMI tablets OTC *antitussive; decongestant; expectorant* [dextromethorphan hydrobromide; pseudoephedrine HCl; guaifenesin] 20•60•400 mg

Medent-PE extended-release tablets R̸ *decongestant; expectorant* [phenylephrine HCl; guaifenesin] 12.5•600 mg

Mederma gel OTC *moisturizer and emollient for scars* [PEG-4; onion extract; xanthan gum; allantoin]

Medescan oral suspension R̸ *radiopaque contrast medium for gastrointestinal imaging* [barium sulfate] 2.3%

medetomidine INN, BAN *veterinary analgesic; veterinary sedative* [also: medetomidine HCl]

medetomidine HCl USAN *veterinary analgesic; veterinary sedative* [also: medetomidine]

mediator release inhibitors *a class of topical agents that inhibit the antigen-induced release of inflammatory mediators (e.g., various histamines and leukotrienes) from human mast cells; used on nasal, ophthalmological, and gastrointestinal mucosa* [also known as: mast cell stabilizers]

medibazine INN

Medicago sativa medicinal herb [see: alfalfa]

medical air [see: air, medical]

Medicated Acne Cleanser OTC *antiseptic, antifungal, and keratolytic for acne* [colloidal sulfur; resorcinol] 4%•2%

Medicated Body Powder OTC *mild anesthetic; antipruritic; counterirritant; astringent; emollient; drying agent* [menthol; zinc oxide; talc] 0.15%•1%• ⚲

Medicidin-D tablets OTC *decongestant; antihistamine; analgesic; antipyretic* [phenylephrine HCl; chlorpheniramine maleate; acetaminophen] 5• 2•325 mg

medicinal zinc peroxide [see: zinc peroxide, medicinal]

Medicone anorectal ointment (discontinued 2010) OTC *anesthetic* [benzocaine] 20% ⃞ Modicon

Medi-Derm cream OTC *analgesic; mild anesthetic; antipruritic; counterirritant* [methyl salicylate; menthol; capsaicin] 20%•5%•0.035%

Medi-First Extra Strength Pain Relief tablets OTC *analgesic; antipyretic; anti-inflammatory* [aspirin; acetaminophen; salicylamide; caffeine] 162•110•152•32.4 mg

Medi-First Sinus Decongestant tablets (discontinued 2009) OTC *nasal decongestant* [pseudoephedrine HCl] 30 mg

medifoxamine INN

Medigesic capsules (discontinued 2010) ℞ *barbiturate sedative; analgesic; antipyretic* [butalbital; acetaminophen; caffeine] 50•325•40 mg

medinal [see: barbital sodium]

Mediotic-HC ear drops ℞ *corticosteroidal anti-inflammatory; local anesthetic; antiseptic* [hydrocortisone; pramoxine HCl; chloroxylenol; benzalkonium chloride] 1%•1%•0.1%•0.01%

Mediplast plaster OTC *keratolytic* [salicylic acid] 40%

Mediplex Tabules (tablets) (discontinued 2008) OTC *vitamin/mineral supplement* [multiple vitamins & minerals]

Mediplex Plus tablets (discontinued 2008) OTC *vitamin/mineral supplement* [multiple vitamins & minerals; folic acid] ⚲•0.4 mg

Medi-Quik topical spray, topical aerosol spray OTC *anesthetic; antiseptic*

[lidocaine; benzalkonium chloride] 2%•0.13%

medium-chain triglycerides (MCT) *dietary lipid supplement*

medorinone USAN, INN *cardiotonic*

medorubicin INN

Medotar ointment OTC *antipsoriatic; antiseborrheic; astringent; antiseptic* [coal tar; zinc oxide] 1%• ⚲

medrogestone USAN, INN, BAN *progestin*

Medrol tablets, Dosepak (unit of use package) ℞ *corticosteroid; anti-inflammatory; immunosuppressant* [methylprednisolone] 2, 4, 8, 16, 24, 32 mg ⃞ Mydral

medronate disodium USAN *pharmaceutic aid*

medronic acid USAN, INN, BAN *pharmaceutic aid*

Medrox ointment, topical patch OTC *analgesic; mild anesthetic; antipruritic; counterirritant* [methyl salicylate; menthol; capsaicin] 20%•5%•0.0375%

medroxalol USAN, INN, BAN *antihypertensive*

medroxalol HCl USAN *antihypertensive*

medroxiprogesterone acetate [see: medroxyprogesterone acetate]

medroxyprogesterone INN, BAN *synthetic progestin for secondary amenorrhea or abnormal uterine bleeding; hormonal antineoplastic* [also: medroxyprogesterone acetate]

medroxyprogesterone acetate USP *synthetic progestin for secondary amenorrhea, abnormal uterine bleeding, and endometrial hyperplasia; hormonal antineoplastic; investigational (orphan) for immune thrombocytopenic purpura* [also: medroxyprogesterone] 2.5, 5, 10 mg oral; 150 mg/mL injection

medrylamine INN

medrysone USAN, USP, INN *ophthalmic corticosteroidal anti-inflammatory*

mefeclorazine INN

mefenamic acid USAN, USP, INN, BAN *analgesic; nonsteroidal anti-inflammatory drug (NSAID) for mild to moderate pain and primary dysmenorrhea* 250 mg oral

mefenidil USAN, INN *cerebral vasodilator*
mefenidil fumarate USAN *cerebral vasodilator*
mefenidramium metilsulfate INN
mefenorex INN *anorectic* [also: mefenorex HCl]
mefenorex HCl USAN *anorectic* [also: mefenorex]
mefeserpine INN
mefexamide USAN, INN *CNS stimulant*
mefloquine USAN, INN, BAN *antimalarial* ⊠ mafilcon
mefloquine HCl USAN *antimalarial for acute chloroquine-resistant malaria (orphan)* 250 mg oral
Mefoxin powder or frozen premix for IV or IM injection (discontinued 2010) ℞ *cephamycin antibiotic* [cefoxitin sodium] 1, 2, 10 g
mefruside USAN, INN *diuretic*
Mega VM-80 tablets OTC *vitamin/mineral/calcium/iron/herbal supplement* [multiple vitamins & minerals; calcium (as carbonate and dicalcium phosphate); iron (as ferrous gluconate); folic acid; biotin; multiple herbs] ≛•19•2•0.4•0.08• ≛ mcg
Mega-B tablets (discontinued 2008) OTC *vitamin supplement* [multiple B vitamins; folic acid; biotin] ≛•100• 100 mcg ⊠ MACOP-B
Megace tablets ℞ *synthetic progestin; hormonal antineoplastic for advanced carcinoma of the breast or endometrium* [megestrol acetate] 40 mg ⊠ Maox
Megace; Megace ES oral suspension ℞ *synthetic progestin for the treatment of AIDS-related anorexia and cachexia (orphan)* [megestrol acetate] 40 mg/mL; 125 mg/mL ⊠ Maox
Megagen *investigational (orphan) adjunct to hematopoietic stem cell transplantation* [megakaryocyte growth and development factor, pegylated, recombinant human]
megakaryocyte growth and development factor, pegylated, recombinant human *investigational (orphan) adjunct to hematopoietic stem cell transplantation*

megallate INN *combining name for radicals or groups*
megalomicin INN *antibacterial* [also: megalomicin potassium phosphate]
megalomicin potassium phosphate USAN *antibacterial* [also: megalomicin]
megestrol INN, BAN *synthetic progestin; hormonal antineoplastic for breast or endometrial cancer* [also: megestrol acetate] ⊠ Maxitrol
megestrol acetate USAN, USP *synthetic progestin; hormonal antineoplastic for breast or endometrial cancer; treatment of AIDS-related anorexia and cachexia (orphan)* [also: megestrol] 20, 40 mg oral; 40 mg/mL oral
meglitinide INN
meglitinides *a class of antidiabetic agents that stimulate insulin production in the pancreas*
meglucycline INN ⊠ meclocycline
meglumine USP, INN *radiopaque contrast medium*
meglumine diatrizoate BAN *oral/parenteral radiopaque contrast medium (46.67% iodine)* [also: diatrizoate meglumine]
meglumine iocarmate BAN *radiopaque contrast medium* [also: iocarmate meglumine]
meglumine iothalamate BAN *parenteral radiopaque contrast medium (47% iodine)* [also: iothalamate meglumine]
meglumine ioxaglate BAN *radiopaque contrast medium* [also: ioxaglate meglumine]
meglutol USAN, INN *antihyperlipoproteinemic* ⊠ miglitol
mel B [see: melarsoprol]
mel W [see: melarsonyl potassium]
Melacine *investigational (NDA filed, orphan) theraccine (therapeutic vaccine) for invasive stage IIB–IV melanoma* [melanoma vaccine]
meladrazine INN, BAN
melafocon A USAN *hydrophobic contact lens material*
melagatran *parenteral anticoagulant and direct thrombin inhibitor*

Melaleuca alternifolia *medicinal herb*
[see: tea tree oil]

Melanocid *investigational (orphan)
treatment for invasive malignant melanoma* [pegylated arginine deiminase]

melanoma vaccine *investigational
(NDA filed, orphan) theraccine (thera-
peutic vaccine) for invasive stage IIB–
IV melanoma*

melarsonyl potassium INN, BAN

melarsoprol INN, BAN *investigational
anti-infective for trypanosomiasis*

Melatonex *time-release tablets* OTC
natural supplement to aid the sleep cycle
[melatonin; vitamin B₆; calcium;
iron] 3•10•31•1 mg

melatonin *natural sleep aid; investigational (orphan) for circadian rhythm
sleep disorders in blind people with no
light perception*

melengestrol INN *antineoplastic; progestin* [also: melengestrol acetate]

melengestrol acetate USAN *antineoplastic; progestin* [also: melengestrol]

meletimide INN

melfalan [see: melphalan]

Melfiat-105 Unicelles (sustained-
release capsules) ℞ *CNS stimulant;
anorexiant* [phendimetrazine tartrate]
105 mg

Melia azedarach *medicinal herb* [see:
pride of China]

melilot (*Melilotus alba; M. officinalis*)
*flowering plant medicinal herb used as
an antispasmodic, diuretic, emollient,
expectorant, and vulnerary*

Melimmune *investigational (orphan) for
invasive cutaneous melanoma* [mono-
clonal antibody to anti-idiotype melanoma-associated antigen, murine]

melinamide INN

Melissa officinalis *medicinal herb* [see:
lemon balm]

melitracen INN *antidepressant* [also:
melitracen HCl]

melitracen HCl USAN *antidepressant*
[also: melitracen]

melizame USAN, INN *sweetener*

meloxicam USAN, INN, BAN *COX-2
inhibitor; analgesic; antipyretic; nonste-*

*roidal anti-inflammatory drug (NSAID)
for osteoarthritis, rheumatoid arthritis,
and juvenile rheumatoid arthritis; also
used for ankylosing spondylitis and acute
bursitis/tendinitis* 7.5, 15 mg oral; 7.5
mg/5 mL oral

Melpaque HP *cream* ℞ *hyperpigmentation bleaching agent* [hydroquinone
(in a sunscreen base)] 4%

melperone INN, BAN

melphalan (MPL) USAN, USP, INN,
BAN, JAN *nitrogen mustard-type alkylating antineoplastic for multiple myeloma
(orphan) and ovarian cancer; investigational (orphan) for metastatic melanoma;
also used for breast and testicular cancers and bone marrow transplantation*
50 mg/vial injection

Melquin HP *cream* ℞ *hyperpigmentation bleaching agent* [hydroquinone] 4%

memantine INN *NMDA (N-methyl-D-
aspartate) antagonist; neuroprotective
agent; investigational (Phase III) once-
daily dosing* [also: memantine HCl]

memantine HCl *NMDA (N-methyl-
D-aspartate) antagonist to suppress the
symptoms of Alzheimer disease* [also:
memantine]

MembraneBlue *ophthalmic injection
in prefilled syringes* ℞ *surgical aid for
staining ophthalmic tissue during vitrectomy* [trypan blue] 0.15%

Memoir (trademarked delivery device)
*a battery-powered self-injector for insulin
with a memory chip that tracks the last
16 doses*

Memorette (trademarked packaging
form) *patient compliance package*

memotine INN *antiviral* [also: memotine HCl]

memotine HCl USAN *antiviral* [also:
memotine]

menabitan INN *analgesic* [also: menabitan HCl]

menabitan HCl USAN *analgesic* [also:
menabitan]

Menactra IM injection ℞ *meningitis
vaccine for children, adolescents, and
adults 2–55 years* [meningococcal
polysaccharide vaccine, groups A, C,

Y, and W-135, conjugated to diphtheria toxoid] 4•4•4•4•48 mcg per 0.5 mL dose

menadiol BAN *vitamin K₄; prothrombogenic* [also: menadiol sodium diphosphate]

menadiol sodium diphosphate USP *vitamin K₄; prothrombogenic* [also: menadiol]

menadiol sodium sulfate INN

menadione USP *vitamin K₃; prothrombogenic* ② Minidyne

menadione sodium bisulfite USP, INN

Menadol captabs (discontinued 2009) OTC *analgesic; antipyretic; antiarthritic; nonsteroidal anti-inflammatory drug (NSAID) for mild to moderate pain, migraine headaches, and primary dysmenorrhea* [ibuprofen] 200 mg

menaphthene [see: menadione]

menaphthone [see: menadione]

menaphthone sodium bisulfite [see: menadione sodium bisulfite]

menaquinone *vitamin K₂; prothrombogenic*

menatetrenone INN

menbutone INN, BAN

M-End oral liquid (discontinued 2009) ℞ *narcotic antitussive; antihistamine; decongestant* [hydrocodone bitartrate; brompheniramine maleate; pseudoephedrine HCl] 2.5•2•15 mg/5 mL

M-End Max oral liquid (discontinued 2009) ℞ *narcotic antitussive; antihistamine; decongestant* [hydrocodone bitartrate; brompheniramine maleate; phenylephrine HCl] 5•2•7.5 mg/5 mL

M-End PE oral liquid ℞ *narcotic antitussive; decongestant; antihistamine* [codeine phosphate; phenylephrine HCl; brompheniramine maleate] 19•10•4 mg/15 mL

M-End WC oral liquid ℞ *narcotic antitussive; decongestant; antihistamine* [codeine phosphate; pseudoephedrine HCl; brompheniramine maleate] 19•30•4 mg/15 mL

mendelevium *element (Md)*

Menest film-coated tablets ℞ *a mixture of equine estrogens for the treatment of postmenopausal symptoms; palliative therapy for prostate and breast cancers* [esterified estrogens] 0.3, 0.625, 1.25, 2.5 mg ② Magnacet

menfegol INN

menglytate INN

menichlopholan [see: niclofolan]

Meni-D capsules (discontinued 2010) ℞ *anticholinergic; antivertigo agent; motion sickness preventative* [meclizine HCl] 25 mg

meningococcal polysaccharide vaccine, group A USP *active bacterin for meningitis (Neisseria meningitidis)*

meningococcal polysaccharide vaccine, group C USP *active bacterin for meningitis (Neisseria meningitidis)*

meningococcal polysaccharide vaccine, group W-135 *active bacterin for meningitis (Neisseria meningitidis)*

meningococcal polysaccharide vaccine, group Y *active bacterin for meningitis (Neisseria meningitidis)*

Menispermum cocculus; M. lacunosum medicinal herb [see: levant berry]

menitrazepam INN

menoctone USAN, INN *antimalarial*

menogaril USAN, INN *antibiotic antineoplastic*

Menomune-A/C/Y/W-135 powder for subcu injection ℞ *meningitis vaccine* [meningococcal polysaccharide vaccine, groups A, C, Y, and W-135] 50 mcg of each group per 0.5 mL dose

Menopur powder or pellet for IM injection ℞ *gonadotropin; follicle-stimulating hormone (FSH) and luteinizing hormone (LH) for the induction of ovulation in women and spermatogenesis in men; adjunct to assisted reproductive technologies (ART)* [menotropins] 75 FSH units + 75 LH units

Menostar transdermal patch ℞ *estrogen replacement therapy for postmenopausal symptoms* [estradiol-17β] 14 mcg/day

menotropins USAN, USP *gonadotropin; follicle-stimulating hormone (FSH) and* *luteinizing hormone (LH) for the induction of ovulation in women and spermatogenesis in men; adjunct to assisted reproductive technologies (ART)* [also: follitropin beta]

Men-Phor lotion OTC *mild anesthetic; antipruritic; counterirritant* [menthol; camphor] 0.5%•0.5%

Mentax cream ℞ *benzylamine antifungal* [butenafine HCl] 1% ⑫ Metanx; Mintox

Mentha piperita medicinal herb [see: peppermint]

Mentha pulegium medicinal herb [see: pennyroyal]

Mentha spicata medicinal herb [see: spearmint]

Menthoderm gel OTC *analgesic; mild anesthetic; antipruritic; counterirritant* [methyl salicylate; menthol] 15%• 10%

menthol USP *mild topical anesthetic; antipruritic; counterirritant* ⑫ mannitol; Mynatal

Menthol Cough Drops lozenges OTC *mild anesthetic; antipruritic; counterirritant* [menthol] 6.5 mg

Mentholatum vaporizing ointment OTC *mild anesthetic; antipruritic; counterirritant* [menthol; camphor] 9%•1.3%

Mentholatum Cherry Chest Rub for Kids vaporizing ointment OTC *mild anesthetic; antipruritic; counterirritant; antiseptic* [menthol; camphor; eucalyptus oil] 4.7%•2.6%•1.2%

menthyl anthranilate [see: meradimate]

Menveo powder for IM injection ℞ *meningitis vaccine for children, adolescents, and adults 11–55 years; investigational (NDA filed) for children 2–10 years* [meningococcal polysaccharide vaccine, groups A, C, Y, and W-135, conjugated to diphtheria toxoid CRM$_{197}$] 10•5•5•5 mcg per 0.5 mL/0.5 mL dose

Menyanthes trifoliata medicinal herb [see: buckbean]

meobentine INN *antiarrhythmic* [also: meobentine sulfate]

meobentine sulfate USAN *antiarrhythmic* [also: meobentine]

mepacrine INN *anthelmintic; antimalarial* [also: quinacrine HCl]

mepacrine HCl [see: quinacrine HCl]

meparfynol [see: methylpentynol]

mepartricin USAN, INN *antifungal; antiprotozoal*

mepazine acetate [see: pecazine]

mepenzolate bromide USP, INN *GI anticholinergic/antispasmodic; adjunctive treatment for peptic ulcers*

mepenzolate methylbromide [see: mepenzolate bromide]

mepenzolone bromide [see: mepenzolate bromide]

meperidine HCl USP *narcotic analgesic; also abused as a street drug* [also: pethidine] 50, 75, 100, 150 mg oral; 50 mg/5 mL oral; 10, 25, 50, 75, 100 mg/mL injection

meperidine HCl & promethazine HCl *narcotic analgesic; sedative* 50• 25 mg oral

Mephaquin ℞ *antimalarial for acute chloroquine-resistant malaria (orphan)* [mefloquine HCl]

mephenesin NF, INN

mephenhydramine [see: moxastine]

mephenoxalone INN

mephentermine INN *adrenergic; vasoconstrictor; vasopressor for hypotensive shock* [also: mephentermine sulfate]

mephentermine sulfate USP *adrenergic; vasoconstrictor; vasopressor for hypotensive shock* [also: mephentermine]

mephenytoin USAN, USP, INN *hydantoin anticonvulsant* [also: methoin]

mephobarbital USP, JAN *anticonvulsant; sedative* [also: methylphenobarbital; methylphenobarbitone]

Mephyton tablets ℞ *coagulant to correct anticoagulant-induced prothrombin deficiency; vitamin K supplement* [phytonadione] 5 mg

mepicycline [see: pipacycline]

MEPIG (mucoid exopolysaccharide *Pseudomonas* **[hyper]immune globulin)** [q.v.]

mepindolol INN, BAN

mepiperphenidol bromide

mepiprazole INN, BAN

mepirizole [see: epirizole]

mepiroxol INN

mepitiostane INN

mepivacaine INN *local anesthetic* [also: mepivacaine HCl]

mepivacaine HCl USP *local anesthetic* [also: mepivacaine] 3% injection

mepivacaine HCl & levonordefrin *injectable local anesthetic; vasoconstrictor* 2%•1:20 000 injection

mepixanox INN

mepolizumab USAN, INN *immunomodulator; investigational (orphan) for asthma due to hypereosinophilic syndrome*

mepramidil INN

meprednisone USAN, USP, INN

meprobamate USP, INN, BAN, JAN *anxiolytic; sedative; hypnotic; minor tranquilizer; also abused as a street drug* 200, 400 mg oral

Mepron *oral suspension* ℞ *antiprotozoal for AIDS-related* Pneumocystis pneumonia (PCP) *(orphan); investigational (orphan) for AIDS-related* Toxoplasma gondii *encephalitis* [atovaquone] 750 mg/5 mL

meproscillarin INN, BAN

meprothixol BAN [also: meprotixol]

meprotixol INN [also: meprothixol]

Meprozine *capsules* ℞ *narcotic analgesic; sedative* [meperidine HCl; promethazine HCl] 50•25 mg ⑨ mupirocin

meprylcaine INN *local anesthetic* [also: meprylcaine HCl]

meprylcaine HCl USP *local anesthetic* [also: meprylcaine]

meptazinol INN, BAN *analgesic* [also: meptazinol HCl]

meptazinol HCl USAN *analgesic* [also: meptazinol]

mepyramine INN, BAN *antihistamine* [also: pyrilamine maleate]

mepyramine maleate [see: pyrilamine maleate]

mepyrium [see: amprolium]

mepyrrotazine [see: dimelazine]

mequidox USAN, INN *antibacterial*

mequinol USAN, INN *hyperpigmentation bleaching agent* ⑨ Micanol; Myconel

mequitamium iodide INN

mequitazine INN, BAN

mequitazium iodide [see: mequitamium iodide]

meradimate USAN *ultraviolet A sunscreen*

meragidone sodium

meralein sodium USAN, INN *topical anti-infective*

meralluride NF, INN

merbaphen USP

merbromin NF, INN *general antiseptic*

mercaptamine INN *antiurolithic* [also: cysteamine]

mercaptoarsenical [see: arsthinol]

mercaptoarsenol [see: arsthinol]

mercaptoethylamine (MEA) [see: mercaptamine]

mercaptomerin (MT6) INN [also: mercaptomerin sodium]

mercaptomerin sodium USP [also: mercaptomerin]

mercaptopurine (6-MP) USP, INN, BAN, JAN *antimetabolite antineoplastic for acute lymphocytic, lymphoblastic, myelogenous, and myelomonocytic leukemias* 50 mg oral

mercuderamide INN

mercufenol chloride USAN *topical anti-infective*

mercumatilin sodium INN

mercuric oxide, yellow NF *ophthalmic antiseptic (FDA ruled it "not safe and effective" in 1992)*

mercuric salicylate NF

mercuric succinimide NF

mercurobutol INN

mercurophylline NF, INN

mercurous chloride [see: calomel]

mercury *element (Hg)*

mercury, ammoniated USP *topical antiseptic; antipsoriatic*

mercury amide chloride [see: mercury, ammoniated]

mercury oleate NF

merethoxylline procaine

mergocriptine INN

Meridia capsules (discontinued 2010) ℞ *anorexiant for the treatment of obesity* [sibutramine HCl] 5, 10, 15 mg

merisoprol acetate Hg 197 USAN *radioactive agent*

merisoprol acetate Hg 203 USAN *radioactive agent*

merisoprol Hg 197 USAN *renal function test; radioactive agent*

Meritene powder OTC *enteral nutritional therapy* [milk-based formula]

meropenem USAN, INN, BAN *broad-spectrum carbapenem antibiotic for bacterial meningitis in children, intra-abdominal infections, and complicated skin and skin structure infections (SSSIs); investigational (orphan) for acute pulmonary episodes in cystic fibrosis* 500, 1000 mg injection

Merrem I.V. powder for IV infusion ℞ *broad-spectrum carbapenem antibiotic for bacterial meningitis in children, intra-abdominal infections, and complicated skin and skin structure infections (SSSIs); investigational (orphan) for acute pulmonary episodes in cystic fibrosis* [meropenem] 500, 1000 mg

mersalyl INN

mersalyl sodium [see: mersalyl]

Mersol solution OTC *antiseptic; antibacterial; antifungal* [thimerosal] 1:1000 ⊘ Murocel

Mersol tincture (discontinued 2008) OTC *antiseptic; antibacterial; antifungal* [thimerosal] 1:1000 ⊘ Murocel

mertiatide INN

Meruvax II powder for subcu injection (discontinued 2011) ℞ *rubella vaccine* [rubella virus vaccine, live] 0.5 mL

mesabolone INN

Mesafem *investigational (Phase III) selective serotonin reuptake inhibitor (SSRI) for postmenopausal hot flashes and other vasomotor symptoms* [paroxetine mesylate]

mesalamine USAN *anti-inflammatory for ulcerative colitis and proctitis* [also: mesalazine] 4 g/60 mL enema ⊘ mezilamine; muzolimine

mesalazine INN, BAN *anti-inflammatory; treatment of ulcerative colitis and proctitis* [also: mesalamine]

mescaline *hallucinogenic street drug derived from the flowering heads (mescal buttons) of a Mexican cactus*

meseclazone USAN, INN *anti-inflammatory*

Mesehist DM oral liquid ℞ *antitussive; antihistamine; decongestant* [dextromethorphan hydrobromide; chlorpheniramine maleate; pseudoephedrine HCl] 15•2•15 mg/5 mL

Mesehist WC oral liquid ℞ *narcotic antitussive; decongestant; antihistamine* [codeine phosphate; pseudoephedrine HCl; brompheniramine maleate] 6.3•10•1.3 mg/5 mL

mesembryanthemum *medicinal herb* [see: kanna]

mesifilcon A USAN *hydrophilic contact lens material*

mesilate INN *combining name for radicals or groups* [also: mesylate]

mesna USAN, INN, BAN *prophylaxis for ifosfamide-induced hemorrhagic cystitis (orphan); investigational (orphan) treatment for cyclophosphamide-induced hemorrhagic cystitis* 1, 100 mg/mL injection, 400 mg oral

Mesnex film-coated caplets, IV injection ℞ *prophylaxis for ifosfamide-induced hemorrhagic cystitis (orphan); investigational (orphan) treatment for cyclophosphamide-induced hemorrhagic cystitis* [mesna] 400 mg; 100 mg/mL

mesocarb INN

meso-inositol [see: inositol]

meso-NDGA (nordihydroguaiaretic acid) [see: masoprocol]

meso-nordihydroguaiaretic acid (NDGA) [see: masoprocol]

mesoridazine USAN, INN *phenothiazine antipsychotic*

mesoridazine besylate USP *conventional (typical) phenothiazine antipsychotic for schizophrenia*

mespiperone C 11 USAN *radiopharmaceutical imaging aid for PET scans of the* brain (produced at bedside for immediate administration)

mespirenone INN

mestanolone INN, BAN

mestenediol [see: methandriol]

mesterolone USAN, INN, BAN androgen; also abused as a street drug

Mestinon IM or IV injection (discontinued 2010) ℞ muscle stimulant for myasthenia gravis; antidote to muscle relaxants [pyridostigmine bromide] 5 mg/mL

Mestinon tablets, Timespan (extended-release tablets), syrup ℞ muscle stimulant for myasthenia gravis; antidote to muscle relaxants [pyridostigmine bromide] 60 mg; 180 mg; 60 mg/5 mL

mestranol USAN, USP, INN estrogen

mesudipine INN

mesulergine INN

mesulfamide INN

mesulfen INN [also: mesulphen]

mesulphen BAN [also: mesulfen]

mesuprine INN vasodilator; smooth muscle relaxant [also: mesuprine HCl]

mesuprine HCl USAN vasodilator; smooth muscle relaxant [also: mesuprine]

mesuximide INN succinimide anticonvulsant for petit mal (absence) seizures [also: methsuximide]

mesylate USAN, USP, BAN combining name for radicals or groups [also: mesilate]

metabromsalan USAN, INN disinfectant

metabutethamine HCl NF

metabutoxycaine HCl NF

metacetamol INN, BAN

metaclazepam INN

metacycline INN antibacterial [also: methacycline]

Metadate CD dual-release capsules (30% immediate release, 70% extended release) ℞ CNS stimulant; once-daily treatment for attention-deficit/hyperactivity disorder (ADHD) [methylphenidate HCl] 10, 20, 30, 40, 50, 60 mg

Metadate ER extended-release tablets ℞ CNS stimulant for attention-deficit/

hyperactivity disorder (ADHD) and narcolepsy [methylphenidate HCl] 10, 20 mg

Metafolin (trademarked ingredient) OTC bioactive form of folic acid that crosses the blood-brain barrier [folic acid (as L-methylfolate)]

Metaglip film-coated tablets ℞ antidiabetic combination for type 2 diabetes that stimulates insulin secretion in the pancreas, decreases hepatic glucose production, and increases cellular response to insulin [glipizide; metformin HCl] 2.5•250

metaglycodol INN

metahexamide INN

metahexanamide [see: metahexamide]

metalkonium chloride INN

metallibure INN anterior pituitary activator for swine [also: methallibure]

metalol HCl USAN antiadrenergic (beta-blocker)

metamelfalan INN

metamfazone INN [also: methamphazone]

metamfepramone INN [also: dimepropion]

metamfetamine INN CNS stimulant; often abused as a street drug [also: methamphetamine HCl]

metamizole sodium INN analgesic; antipyretic [also: dipyrone]

metampicillin INN

Metamucil capsules OTC bulk laxative [psyllium husk] 520 mg

Metamucil effervescent powder OTC bulk laxative; antacid [psyllium hydrophilic mucilloid; sodium bicarbonate; potassium bicarbonate] 3.4• 2•2 g/pkt.

Metamucil wafers OTC bulk laxative [psyllium husk] 3.4 g

Metamucil Original Texture; Metamucil Smooth Texture; Berry Burst! Metamucil powder OTC bulk laxative [psyllium husk] 3.4 g/dose

metandienone INN [also: methandrostenolone; methandienone]

metanixin INN

Metanx tablets OTC *vitamin B supplement* [vitamins B_6 and B_{12}; folic acid (as L-methylfolate)] 35•2•3 mg ⑨ Mentax

metaoxedrine chloride [see: phenylephrine HCl]

metaphosphoric acid, potassium salt [see: potassium metaphosphate]

metaphosphoric acid, trisodium salt [see: sodium trimetaphosphate]

metaphyllin [see: aminophylline]

metapramine INN

metaproterenol polistirex USAN *sympathomimetic bronchodilator* [also: orciprenaline]

metaproterenol sulfate USAN, USP *sympathomimetic bronchodilator* 10, 20 mg oral; 10 mg/5 mL oral

metaradrine bitartrate [see: metaraminol bitartrate]

metaraminol INN *adrenergic; vasopressor for acute hypotensive shock, anaphylaxis, or traumatic shock* [also: metaraminol bitartrate]

metaraminol bitartrate USP *adrenergic; vasopressor for acute hypotensive shock, anaphylaxis, or traumatic shock* [also: metaraminol]

Metaret injection *investigational (NDA filed, orphan) growth factor antagonist for prostate cancer* [suramin hexasodium] 600 mg

Metastron IV injection ℞ *analgesic for metastatic bone pain* [strontium chloride Sr 89] 10.9–22.6 mg/mL (4 mCi)

Metatensin #2; Metatensin #4 tablets (discontinued 2007) ℞ *antihypertensive* [trichlormethiazide; reserpine] 2•0.1 mg; 4•0.1 mg

metaterol INN

metaxalone USAN, INN, BAN *skeletal muscle relaxant* 800 mg oral

metazamide INN

metazepium iodide [see: buzepide metiodide]

metazide INN

metazocine INN, BAN

metbufen INN

metcaraphen HCl

metembonate INN *combining name for radicals or groups*

meteneprost USAN, INN *oxytocic; prostaglandin*

metenolone INN *anabolic steroid; also abused as a street drug* [also: methenolone acetate; methenolone; metenolone acetate]

metenolone acetate JAN *anabolic steroid; also abused as a street drug* [also: methenolone acetate; metenolone; methenolone]

metenolone enanthate JAN *anabolic steroid; also abused as a street drug* [also: methenolone enanthate]

metergoline INN, BAN

metergotamine INN

metescufylline INN

metesculetol INN

metesind glucuronate USAN *specific thymidylate synthase (TS) inhibitor antineoplastic*

metethoheptazine INN

metetoin INN *anticonvulsant* [also: methetoin] ⑨ mitotane

metformin USAN, INN, BAN *biguanide antidiabetic for type 2 diabetes that decreases hepatic glucose production and increases cellular response to insulin* [also: metformin HCl]

Metformin ER extended-release caplets (discontinued 2007) ℞ *biguanide antidiabetic that decreases hepatic glucose production and increases cellular response to insulin* [metformin HCl] 500 mg

metformin HCl USAN, JAN *biguanide antidiabetic for type 2 diabetes that decreases hepatic glucose production and increases cellular response to insulin* [also: metformin] 500, 750, 850, 1000 mg oral

metformin HCl & glipizide *antidiabetic combination for type 2 diabetes that stimulates insulin secretion in the pancreas, decreases hepatic glucose production, and increases cellular response to insulin* 250•2.5, 500•2.5, 500•5 mg

metformin HCl & glyburide *antidiabetic combination for type 2 diabetes* that decreases hepatic glucose production, increases cellular response to insulin, and stimulates insulin secretion in the pancreas 250•1.25, 500•2.5, 500•5 mg oral

metformin HCl & pioglitazone HCl combination biguanide and thiazolidinedione (TZD)/peroxisome proliferator–activated receptor–gamma (PPARγ) agonist antidiabetic that decreases hepatic production of glucose and increases cellular response to insulin 500•15, 850•15 mg oral

methacholine bromide NF

methacholine chloride USP, INN cholinergic; bronchoconstrictor for in vivo pulmonary challenge tests

methacrylic acid copolymer NF tablet-coating agent

methacycline USAN antibacterial [also: metacycline]

methacycline HCl USP gram-negative and gram-positive bacteriostatic; antirickettsial

methadol [see: dimepheptanol]

methadone INN narcotic analgesic; narcotic addiction detoxicant; often abused as a street drug [also: methadone HCl]

methadone HCl USP narcotic analgesic; narcotic addiction detoxicant; often abused as a street drug [also: methadone] 5, 10, 40 mg oral; 5, 10 mg/5 mL oral; 10 mg/mL oral; 10 mg/mL injection

methadonium chloride [see: methadone HCl]

Methadose tablets, dispersible tablets, oral concentrate ℞ narcotic analgesic; narcotic addiction detoxicant; often abused as a street drug [methadone HCl] 5, 10 mg; 40 mg; 10 mg/mL

methadyl acetate USAN narcotic analgesic [also: acetylmethadol]

methafilcon B USAN hydrophilic contact lens material

Methagual OTC analgesic; counterirritant [methyl salicylate; guaiacol] 8%•2%

Methalgen cream (discontinued 2007) OTC analgesic; mild anesthetic; antipruritic; counterirritant [methyl salicylate; menthol; camphor; mustard oil]

methallenestril INN

methallenestrol [see: methallenestril]

methallibure USAN anterior pituitary activator for swine [also: metallibure]

methalthiazide USAN diuretic; antihypertensive

methamoctol

methamphazone BAN [also: metamfazone]

methamphetamine HCl USP CNS stimulant; often abused as a street drug [also: metamfetamine] 5 mg oral

methampyrone [now: dipyrone]

methanabol [see: methandriol]

methandienone BAN [also: methandrostenolone; metandienone]

methandriol

methandrostenolone USP steroid; discontinued for human use, but the veterinary product is still available and sometimes abused as a street drug [also: metandienone; methandienone]

methaniazide INN

methanol [see: methyl alcohol]

methantheline bromide USP peptic ulcer adjunct [also: methanthelinium bromide]

methanthelinium bromide INN, BAN anticholinergic [also: methantheline bromide]

methaphenilene INN, BAN [also: methaphenilene HCl]

methaphenilene HCl NF [also: methaphenilene]

methapyrilene INN [also: methapyrilene fumarate]

methapyrilene fumarate USP [also: methapyrilene]

methapyrilene HCl USP

methaqualone USAN, USP, INN, BAN hypnotic; sedative; often abused as a street drug, which leads to dependence

methaqualone HCl USP

metharbital USP, INN, JAN anticonvulsant [also: metharbitone]

metharbitone BAN anticonvulsant [also: metharbital]

methastyridone INN

Methatropic capsules (discontinued 2008) OTC *dietary lipotropic; vitamin supplement* [choline; inositol; methionine; multiple B vitamins] 115• 83•110• ± mg

methazolamide USP, INN *carbonic anhydrase inhibitor for glaucoma* 25, 50 mg oral ☒ mitozolomide

Methblue 65 tablets ℞ *urinary anti-infective and antiseptic; antidote to cyanide poisoning* [methylene blue] 65 mg

methcathinone *a highly addictive manufactured street drug similar to cathinone, with amphetamine-like effects* [see also: cathinone; *Catha edulis*]

methdilazine USP, INN *phenothiazine antihistamine; antipruritic*

methdilazine HCl USP *phenothiazine antihistamine; antipruritic*

methenamine USP, INN *urinary antibiotic*

methenamine hippurate USAN, USP *urinary antibiotic* [also: hexamine hippurate] 1 g oral

methenamine mandelate USP *urinary antibiotic*

methenamine sulfosalicylate *topical antipsoriatic*

methenolone BAN *anabolic steroid; also abused as a street drug* [also: methenolone acetate; metenolone; metenolone acetate]

methenolone acetate USAN *anabolic steroid; also abused as a street drug* [also: metenolone; methenolone; metenolone acetate]

methenolone enanthate USAN *anabolic steroid; also abused as a street drug* [also: metenolone enanthate]

metheptazine INN

Methergine coated tablets, IV or IM injection ℞ *oxytocic for induction of labor, control of postpartum uterine atony, and postpartum hemorrhage* [methylergonovine maleate] 0.2 mg; 0.2 mg/mL

methestrol INN

methetharimide [see: bemegride]

methetoin USAN *anticonvulsant* [also: metetoin] ☒ mitotane

methicillin sodium USAN, USP *penicillinase-resistant penicillin antibiotic* [also: meticillin]

methimazole USP *thyroid inhibitor for hyperthyroidism* [also: thiamazole] 5, 10 mg oral

methindizate BAN [also: metindizate]

methiodal sodium USP, INN

methiomeprazine INN

methiomeprazine HCl [see: methiomeprazine]

methionine (DL-methionine) NF, JAN *urinary acidifier* [also: racemethionine] 500 mg oral

methionine (L-methionine) USAN, USP, INN, JAN *essential amino acid; symbols: Met, M; investigational (orphan) for AIDS myelopathy*

methionyl neurotropic factor, brain-derived, recombinant *investigational (orphan) for amyotrophic lateral sclerosis (ALS)*

N-methionylleptin (human) [see: metreleptin]

methiothepin [see: metitepine]

methisazone USAN *antiviral* [also: metisazone]

methisoprinol [now: inosine pranobex]

Methitest tablets ℞ *synthetic androgen for hypogonadism or testosterone deficiency in men, delayed puberty in boys, and metastatic breast cancer in women; hormone replacement therapy (HRT) for postandropausal symptoms; also abused as a street drug* [methyltestosterone] 10 mg

methitural INN

methixene HCl USAN *smooth muscle relaxant* [also: metixene]

methocamphone methylsulfate [see: trimethidinium methosulfate]

methocarbamol USP, INN, BAN, JAN *skeletal muscle relaxant* 500, 750 mg oral

methocidin INN

methohexital USP, INN *barbiturate general anesthetic* [also: methohexitone]

methohexital sodium USP *barbiturate general anesthetic*

methohexitone BAN *barbiturate general anesthetic* [also: methohexital]

methoin BAN *anticonvulsant* [also: mephenytoin]

methonaphthone [see: menbutone]

methophedrine [see: methoxyphedrine]

methophenazine [see: metofenazate]

methopholine USAN *analgesic* [also: metofoline]

methoprene INN

methopromazine INN

methopromazine maleate [see: methopromazine]

methopyrimazole [see: epirizole]

d-**methorphan** [see: dextromethorphan]

d-**methorphan hydrobromide** [see: dextromethorphan hydrobromide]

methoserpidine INN, BAN

methotrexate (MTX) USAN, USP, INN, BAN, JAN *antimetabolite antineoplastic for leukemia, lymphoma, and various solid tumors; systemic antipsoriatic; antirheumatic for adult and juvenile rheumatoid arthritis (orphan)* 2.5 mg oral

methotrexate & laurocapram *investigational (orphan) for topical treatment of mycosis fungoides*

Methotrexate LPF Sodium *preservative-free injection* ℞ *antimetabolite antineoplastic for leukemia, lymphoma, various solid tumors, and osteogenic sarcoma (orphan); systemic antipsoriatic; antirheumatic* [methotrexate sodium] 2.5 mg/mL

methotrexate sodium USP *antirheumatic; systemic antipsoriatic; antimetabolite antineoplastic for leukemia, lymphoma, various solid tumors, and osteogenic sarcoma (orphan)* 20, 50, 250, 1000 mg/vial injection; 2.5, 25 mg/mL injection

methotrimeprazine USAN, USP *central analgesic; CNS depressant* [also: levomepromazine]

methotrimeprazine maleate *CNS depressant; neuroleptic*

methoxamine INN *adrenergic; vasoconstrictor; vasopressor for hypotensive shock during surgery* [also: methoxamine HCl]

methoxamine HCl USP *adrenergic; vasoconstrictor; vasopressor for hypotensive shock during surgery* [also: methoxamine]

methoxiflurane [see: methoxyflurane]

methoxsalen (8-methoxsalen) USP *repigmentation agent for vitiligo; antipsoriatic; palliative treatment for cutaneous T-cell lymphoma (CTCL); investigational (orphan) for diffuse systemic sclerosis and cardiac allografts*

methoxy polyethylene glycol [see: polyethylene glycol monomethyl ether]

2-methoxyestradiol *investigational (orphan) for multiple myeloma, ovarian cancer, and pulmonary arterial hypertension*

methoxyfenoserpin [see: mefeserpine]

methoxyflurane USAN, USP, INN, BAN *inhalation general anesthetic*

methoxyphedrine INN

p-**methoxyphenacyl** [see: anisatil]

methoxyphenamine INN [also: methoxyphenamine HCl]

methoxyphenamine HCl USP [also: methoxyphenamine]

4-methoxyphenol [see: mequinol]

o-**methoxyphenyl salicylate acetate** [see: guacetisal]

methoxypromazine maleate [see: methopromazine]

8-methoxypsoralen (8-MOP) [see: methoxsalen]

5-methoxyresorcinol [see: flamenol]

methphenoxydiol [see: guaifenesin]

methscopolamine bromide USP *anticholinergic; GI antispasmodic; adjunctive treatment for peptic ulcers* [also: hyoscine methobromide] 2.5, 5 mg oral

methscopolamine nitrate *anticholinergic; respiratory antisecretory*

methsuximide USP, BAN *succinimide anticonvulsant for petit mal (absence) seizures* [also: mesuximide]

methyclothiazide USAN, USP, INN *antihypertensive; diuretic* 2.5, 5 mg oral

methydromorphine [see: methyldihydromorphine]

methyl alcohol NF *solvent*

methyl aminolevulinate HCl *photosensitizer for photodynamic therapy of precancerous actinic keratoses of the face and scalp; for use with* **CureLight BroadBand Model 01** *(red light illumination)*

methyl benzoquate BAN *coccidiostat for poultry* [also: nequinate]

methyl cresol [see: cresol]

methyl cysteine [see: mecysteine]

methyl *p*-hydroxybenzoate [see: methylparaben]

methyl isobutyl ketone NF *alcohol denaturant*

methyl nicotinate USAN

methyl palmoxirate USAN *antidiabetic*

methyl phthalate [see: dimethyl phthalate]

methyl salicylate NF *topical analgesic; mild topical anesthetic; counterirritant; flavoring agent*

methyl sulfoxide [see: dimethyl sulfoxide]

methyl violet [see: gentian violet]

***l*-methylaminoethanolcatechol** [see: epinephrine]

methylaminopterin [see: methotrexate]

methylandrostenediol [see: methandriol]

methylatropine nitrate USAN *anticholinergic* [also: atropine methonitrate]

methylbenactyzium bromide INN

methylbenzethonium chloride USP, INN *topical anti-infective/antiseptic*

α-methylbenzylhydrazine [see: mebanazine]

methylcarbamate of salicylanilide [see: anilamate]

methyl-CCNU (chloroethyl-cyclohexyl-nitrosourea) [see: semustine]

methylcellulose USP, INN *ophthalmic moisturizer; suspending and viscosity-increasing agent; bulk laxative*

methylcellulose, propylene glycol ether of [see: hydroxypropyl methylcellulose]

methylchromone INN, BAN

N-methyl-D-aspartate (NMDA) *an endogenous neurotransmitter similar to glutamate; an NMDA inhibitor blocks the action of glutamate, which can overstimulate the receptors and become neurotoxic in excessive amounts, causing various dementias and CNS disorders*

methyldesorphine INN, BAN

methyldigoxin [see: metildigoxin]

methyldihydromorphine INN

methyldihydromorphinone HCl [see: metopon]

methyldinitrobenzamide [see: dinitolmide]

methyldioxatrine [see: meletimide]

N-methyldiphenethylamine [see: demelverine]

α-methyl-DL-thyroxine ethyl ester [see: etiroxate]

methyldopa USAN, USP, INN, BAN, JAN *centrally acting antiadrenergic antihypertensive* 250, 500 mg oral

α-methyldopa [now: methyldopa]

methyldopa & hydrochlorothiazide *combination central antiadrenergic and diuretic for hypertension* 250•15, 250•25, 500•30, 500•50 mg oral

methyldopate BAN *centrally acting antiadrenergic antihypertensive* [also: methyldopate HCl]

methyldopate HCl USAN, USP *centrally acting antiadrenergic antihypertensive* [also: methyldopate] 50 mg/mL injection

methylene blue (MB) USP *antimethemoglobinemic; GU antiseptic; antidote to cyanide poisoning; diagnostic aid for gastric secretions* [also: methylthioninium chloride] 65 mg oral; 10 mg/mL injection

methylene chloride NF *solvent*

methylene diphosphonate (MDP) [now: medronate disodium]

methylenedioxyamphetamine (MDA) [see: MDMA, MDEA]

3,4-methylenedioxyethamphetamine (MDEA) [q.v.]

3,4-methylenedioxymethamphetamine (MDMA) [q.v.]

6-methyleneoxytetracycline (MOTC) [see: methacycline]

methylenprednisolone [see: prednylidene]

methylergometrine INN *oxytocic* [also: methylergonovine maleate]

methylergometrine maleate [see: methylergonovine maleate]

methylergonovine maleate USP *oxytocic for induction of labor, control of postpartum uterine atony, and postpartum hemorrhage* [also: methylergometrine] 0.2 mg oral; 0.2 mg/mL injection

methylergonovinium bimaleate [see: methylergonovine maleate]

methylergotamine [see: metergotamine]

methylestrenolone [see: normethandrone]

L-methylfolate; levomefolate *bioactive form of folic acid that crosses the blood-brain barrier* [see: folic acid]

methyl-GAG (methylglyoxal-*bis*-guanylhydrazone) [see: mitoguazone]

methylglyoxal-*bis*-guanylhydrazone (methyl-GAG; MGBG) [see: mitoguazone]

1-methylhexylamine [see: tuaminoheptane]

1-methylhexylamine sulfate [see: tuaminoheptane sulfate]

N-methylhydrazine [see: procarbazine]

Methylin tablets, chewable tablets, oral liquid ℞ *CNS stimulant for attention-deficit/hyperactivity disorder (ADHD) and narcolepsy* [methylphenidate HCl] 5, 10, 20 mg; 2.5, 5, 10 mg; 5, 10 mg/5 mL

Methylin ER extended-release tablets ℞ *CNS stimulant for attention-deficit/ hyperactivity disorder (ADHD) and narcolepsy* [methylphenidate HCl] 10, 20 mg

methylmorphine [see: codeine]

methylnaltrexone bromide *opioid receptor antagonist for opioid-induced constipation (orphan); investigational (NDA filed) for postoperative ileus*

methyl-nitro-imidazole [see: carnidazole]

methylnortestosterone [see: normethandrone]

methylparaben USAN, NF *antifungal agent; preservative*

methylparaben sodium USAN, NF *antimicrobial preservative*

methylparafynol [see: meparfynol]

methylpentynol INN, BAN

methylperidol [see: moperone]

(+)-methylphenethylamine [see: dextroamphetamine]

(–)-methylphenethylamine [see: levamphetamine]

methylphenethylamine HCl [see: amphetamine HCl]

methylphenethylamine phosphate [see: amphetamine phosphate]

(–)-methylphenethylamine succinate [see: levamfetamine succinate]

methylphenethylamine sulfate [see: amphetamine sulfate]

(+)-methylphenethylamine sulfate [see: dextroamphetamine sulfate]

methylphenidate INN, BAN *CNS stimulant for attention-deficit/hyperactivity disorder (ADHD) and narcolepsy; also abused as a street drug* [also: methylphenidate HCl]

methylphenidate HCl (MPH) USP, JAN *CNS stimulant for attention-deficit/hyperactivity disorder (ADHD) and narcolepsy; also abused as a street drug* [also: methylphenidate] 5, 10, 18, 20, 27, 36, 54 mg oral; 5, 10 mg/5 mL oral

methylphenobarbital INN *anticonvulsant; sedative* [also: mephobarbital; methylphenobarbitone]

methylphenobarbitone BAN *anticonvulsant; sedative* [also: mephobarbital; methylphenobarbital]

d-methylphenylamine sulfate [see: dextroamphetamine sulfate]

methylphytyl napthoquinone [see: phytonadione]

methylprednisolone USP, INN, BAN, JAN *corticosteroid; anti-inflammatory;*

immunosuppressant 4, 8, 16, 32 mg oral

methylprednisolone aceponate INN

methylprednisolone acetate USP, JAN *corticosteroid; anti-inflammatory; immunosuppressant* 20, 40, 80 mg/mL injection

methylprednisolone hemisuccinate USP *corticosteroid; anti-inflammatory*

methylprednisolone sodium phosphate USAN *corticosteroid; anti-inflammatory* 40, 125, 500, 1000 mg/ vial injection

methylprednisolone sodium succinate USP, JAN *corticosteroid; anti-inflammatory; immunosuppressant* 40, 125, 500, 1000, 2000 mg injection

methylprednisolone suleptanate USAN, INN *corticosteroid; anti-inflammatory*

methylpromazine

4-methylpyrazole (4-MP) [see: fomepizole]

methylrosaniline chloride [now: gentian violet]

methylrosanilinium chloride INN *topical anti-infective* [also: gentian violet]

methylscopolamine bromide [see: methscopolamine bromide]

methylsulfate USP *combining name for radicals or groups* [also: metilsulfate]

methylsulfonylmethane (MSM) *natural source of sulfur; promotes an increase in collagen and the endogenous antioxidant glutathione*

methyltestosterone USP, INN, BAN *synthetic androgen for hypogonadism or testosterone deficiency in men, delayed puberty in boys, and metastatic breast cancer in women; hormone replacement therapy (HRT) for postandropausal symptoms; also abused as a street drug* 10, 25 mg oral

methyltestosterone & esterified estrogens *combination synthetic androgen and equine estrogen; hormone replacement therapy for postmenopausal symptoms* 1.25•0.625, 2.5•1.25 mg oral

L-**5-methyltetrahydrofolate (L-5-MTHF)** [see: levomefolate; L-methylfolate]

methyltheobromine [see: caffeine]

methylthionine chloride [see: methylene blue]

methylthionine HCl [see: methylene blue]

methylthioninium chloride INN *antimethemoglobinemic; antidote to cyanide poisoning* [also: methylene blue]

methylthiouracil USP, INN

methyltrienolone [see: metribolone]

methynodiol diacetate USAN *progestin* [also: metynodiol]

methyprylon USP, INN *sedative; hypnotic* [also: methprylone]

methyprylone BAN *sedative* [also: methyprylon]

methyridene BAN [also: metyridine]

methysergide USAN, INN, BAN *migraine-specific vasoconstrictor and peripheral serotonin antagonist for the prophylaxis of vascular headaches*

methysergide maleate USP *migraine-specific vasoconstrictor and peripheral serotonin antagonist for the prophylaxis of vascular headaches*

metiamide USAN, INN *antagonist to histamine H_2 receptors*

metiapine USAN, INN *antipsychotic*

metiazinic acid INN

metibride INN

meticillin INN *penicillinase-resistant penicillin antibiotic* [also: methicillin sodium]

meticillin sodium *penicillinase-resistant penicillin antibiotic* [see: methicillin sodium]

Meticorten tablets (discontinued 2008) ℞ *corticosteroid; anti-inflammatory; immunosuppressant* [prednisone] 1 mg

meticrane INN

metildigoxin INN

metilsulfate INN *combining name for radicals or groups* [also: methylsulfate]

Metimyd eye drop suspension (discontinued 2009) ℞ *corticosteroidal anti-inflammatory; antibiotic* [prednisolone acetate; sulfacetamide sodium] 0.5%•10%

Metimyd ophthalmic ointment ℞ *corticosteroidal anti-inflammatory; antibiotic* [prednisolone acetate; sulfacetamide sodium] 0.5%•10%

metindizate INN [also: methindizate]

metioprim USAN, INN, BAN *antibacterial*

metioxate INN

metipirox INN

metipranolol USAN, INN, BAN *topical antiglaucoma agent (beta-blocker)*

metipranolol HCl *topical antiglaucoma agent (beta-blocker)* 0.3% eye drops

metiprenaline INN

metirosine INN *antihypertensive* [also: metyrosine]

metisazone INN *antiviral* [also: methisazone]

metitepine INN

metixene INN *smooth muscle relaxant* [also: methixene HCl]

metixene HCl [see: methixene HCl]

metizoline INN *adrenergic; vasoconstrictor* [also: metizoline HC]

metizoline HCl USAN *adrenergic; vasoconstrictor* [also: metizoline]

metkefamide INN *analgesic* [also: metkephamid acetate]

metkefamide acetate [see: metkephamid acetate]

metkephamid acetate USAN *analgesic* [also: metkefamide]

metochalcone INN

metocinium iodide INN

metoclopramide INN, BAN, JAN *antiemetic for chemotherapy; GI stimulant; antidopaminergic; radiosensitizer* [also: metoclopramide HCl]

metoclopramide HCl USAN, USP, JAN *antidopaminergic; antiemetic for chemotherapy and postoperative nausea and vomiting; GI stimulant for diabetic gastroparesis, gastroesophageal reflux, small bowel intubation, and radiological examination of the intestine* [also: metoclopramide] 5, 10 mg oral; 5 mg/5 mL oral; 5 mg/mL injection

metoclopramide monohydrochloride monohydrate [see: metoclopramide HCl]

metocurine iodide USAN, USP *neuromuscular blocker; muscle relaxant*

metofenazate INN

metofoline INN *analgesic* [also: methopholine]

metogest USAN, INN *hormone*

metolazone USAN, INN *antihypertensive; diuretic for congestive heart failure and renal disease; also used for osteoporosis and diabetes insipidus* 2.5, 5, 10 mg oral

metomidate INN, BAN

metopimazine USAN, INN *antiemetic*

Metopirone softgels ℞ *diagnostic aid for testing hypothalamic-pituitary adrenocorticotropic hormone (ACTH) function* [metyrapone] 250 mg

metopon INN

metopon HCl [see: metopon]

metoprine USAN *antineoplastic*

metoprolol USAN, INN, BAN *antianginal; antihypertensive; antiadrenergic (beta-blocker)*

metoprolol fumarate USAN *antianginal; antihypertensive; antiadrenergic (beta-blocker)*

metoprolol succinate USAN *antianginal; antihypertensive; antiadrenergic (beta-blocker)* 25, 50, 100, 200 mg oral

metoprolol tartrate USAN, USP *antianginal; antihypertensive; antiadrenergic (beta-blocker)* 25, 50, 100 mg oral; 1 mg/mL injection

metoprolol tartrate & hydrochlorothiazide *combination beta-blocker and diuretic for hypertension* 50•25, 100•25, 100•50 mg oral

metoquizine USAN, INN *anticholinergic*

metoserpate INN *veterinary sedative* [also: metoserpate HCl]

metoserpate HCl USAN *veterinary sedative* [also: metoserpate]

metostilenol INN

metoxepin INN

metoxiestrol [see: moxestrol]

Metozolv ODT (orally disintegrating tablets) ℞ *antiemetic for chemother-*

apy and postoperative nausea and vomiting; GI stimulant for diabetic gastroparesis, gastroesophageal reflux, small bowel intubation, and radiological examination of the intestine; also used for hiccups [metoclopramide (as HCl)] 5, 10 mg

metrafazoline INN

metralindole INN

metrazifone INN

metreleptin USAN, INN *metabolic regulator for obesity; investigational (NDA filed, orphan) for metabolic disorders due to generalized or familial lipodystrophy*

metrenperone USAN, INN, BAN *veterinary myopathic*

metribolone INN

metrifonate USAN, INN *veterinary anthelmintic* [also: trichlorfon; metriphonate]

metrifudil INN

metriphonate BAN *veterinary anthelmintic* [also: trichlorfon; metrifonate]

metrizamide USAN, INN *parenteral radiopaque contrast medium (48.25% iodine)*

metrizoate sodium USAN *radiopaque contrast medium* [also: sodium metrizoate]

Metro I.V. ready-to-use injection ℞ *antibiotic; antiprotozoal; amebicide* [metronidazole] 500 mg/100 mL

MetroCream; MetroGel; MetroLotion ℞ *antibiotic for rosacea (orphan); investigational (orphan) for decubitus ulcers and perioral dermatitis* [metronidazole] 0.75%

MetroGel gel ℞ *antibacterial for rosacea; investigational (orphan) for perioral dermatitis* [metronidazole] 1%

MetroGel 1% Kit gel + skin cleanser ℞ *antibacterial for rosacea* [metronidazole; Cetaphil cleansing solution (q.v.)] 1%•4 oz.

MetroGel Vaginal gel ℞ *antibacterial for bacterial vaginosis* [metronidazole] 0.75%

MetroLotion lotion ℞ *antibacterial for rosacea* [metronidazole] 0.75%

metronidazole USAN, USP, INN, BAN *antibiotic; antiprotozoal/amebicide; acne rosacea treatment (orphan); investigational (orphan) for perioral dermatitis, advanced decubitus ulcers, and perianal Crohn disease* 250, 375, 500, 750 mg oral; 500 mg/100 mL injection; 0.75%, 1% topical/vaginal

metronidazole benzoate *antiprotozoal (Trichomonas)*

metronidazole HCl USAN *antibiotic; antiprotozoal; amebicide*

metronidazole phosphate USAN *antibacterial; antiprotozoal*

metuclazepam [see: metaclazepam]

meturedepa USAN, INN *antineoplastic*

Metvixia cream ℞ *photosensitizer for photodynamic therapy of precancerous actinic keratoses of the face and scalp; for use with* **CureLight BroadBand Model 01** *(red light illumination)* [methyl aminolevulinate HCl] 16.8%

metynodiol INN *progestin* [also: methynodiol diacetate]

metynodiol diacetate [see: methynodiol diacetate]

metyrapone USAN, USP, INN *diagnostic aid for testing hypothalamic-pituitary adrenocorticotropic hormone (ACTH) function*

metyrapone tartrate USAN *pituitary function test*

metyridine INN [also: methyridene]

metyrosine USAN, USP *antihypertensive; pheochromocytomic agent*

Mevacor tablets ℞ *HMG-CoA reductase inhibitor for hypercholesterolemia, atherosclerosis, and the prevention and treatment of coronary heart disease (CHD)* [lovastatin] 20, 40 mg

mevastatin INN

mevinolin [now: lovastatin]

mexafylline INN

mexazolam INN

mexenone INN, BAN

mexiletine INN, BAN *antiarrhythmic* [also: mexiletine HCl]

mexiletine HCl USAN, USP *antiarrhythmic* [also: mexiletine] 150, 200, 150 mg

mexiprostil INN

Mexitil capsules ℞ *antiarrhythmic* [mexiletine HCl] 150, 200, 250 mg

mexoprofen INN

mexrenoate potassium USAN, INN *aldosterone antagonist*

Mexsana Medicated powder OTC *diaper rash treatment* [kaolin; zinc oxide; eucalyptus oil; camphor; cornstarch]

mezacopride INN

mezepine INN

mezereon *(Daphne mezereum)* bark *medicinal herb used as a cathartic, diuretic, emetic, and rubefacient; eating the berries can be fatal, and people have been poisoned by eating birds that ate the berries*

mezilamine INN ☒ mesalamine; muzolimine

mezlocillin USAN, INN *extended-spectrum penicillin antibiotic*

mezlocillin sodium USP *extended-spectrum penicillin antibiotic*

MF (methotrexate, fluorouracil) [with leucovorin rescue] *chemotherapy protocol for breast cancer*

MFF (mometasone furoate & formoterol) [q.v.]

MG Cold Sore Formula topical solution OTC *mucous membrane anesthetic; antipruritic; counterirritant* [lidocaine; menthol] 2•1%

MG217 Medicated ointment OTC *antipsoriatic; antiseborrheic; antifungal; keratolytic; antiseptic* [coal tar solution; colloidal sulfur; salicylic acid] 2%•1.1%•1.5%

MG217 Medicated Tar lotion, ointment OTC *antipsoriatic; antiseborrheic* [coal tar solution] 1%; 2%

MG217 Medicated Tar shampoo OTC *antiseborrheic; antipsoriatic; antipruritic; antibacterial* [coal tar] 3%

MG217 Medicated Tar-Free shampoo OTC *antiseborrheic; keratolytic; antiseptic* [sulfur; salicylic acid] 5%•3%

MG217 Sal-Acid ointment OTC *antipsoriatic; keratolytic* [salicylic acid] 3%

MG400 shampoo OTC *antiseborrheic; keratolytic; antiseptic* [salicylic acid; sulfur] 3%•5%

MGA (melengestrol acetate) [q.v.]

MGBG (methylglyoxal-*bis*-guanylhydrazone) [see: mitoguazone]

MGW (magnesium sulfate + glycerin + water) enema [q.v.]

MHP-A tablets ℞ *urinary antibiotic; antiseptic; analgesic; antispasmodic* [methenamine; phenyl salicylate; methylene blue; benzoic acid; atropine sulfate; hyoscyamine sulfate] 40.8•18.1•5.4•4.5•0.03•0.03 mg

Miacalcin metered-dose nasal spray ℞ *calcium regulator for postmenopausal osteoporosis; investigational (orphan) for Paget disease* [calcitonin (salmon)] 200 IU/0.09 mL dose

Miacalcin subcu or IM injection ℞ *calcium regulator for Paget disease (orphan), hypercalcemia, and postmenopausal osteoporosis* [calcitonin (salmon)] 200 IU/mL ☒ meclozine

Mi-Acid gelcaps OTC *antacid* [calcium carbonate; magnesium carbonate] 311•232 mg

Mi-Acid; Mi-Acid II oral liquid OTC *antacid; antiflatulent* [aluminum hydroxide; magnesium hydroxide; simethicone] 200•200•20 mg/5 mL; 400•400•40 mg/5 mL

mianserin INN, BAN *serotonin inhibitor; antihistamine* [also: mianserin HCl]

mianserin HCl USAN, JAN *serotonin inhibitor; antihistamine* [also: mianserin]

mibefradil INN *vasodilator and calcium channel blocker for hypertension and chronic stable angina* [also: mibefradil dihydrochloride]

mibefradil dihydrochloride USAN *vasodilator and calcium channel blocker for hypertension and chronic stable angina* [also: mibefradil]

M¹³¹IBG [now: iobenguane sulfate I 131]

MIBG-I-123 [see: iobenguane sulfate I 123]

mibolerone USAN, INN *anabolic; androgen*

micafungin sodium *systemic echino-candin antifungal for prophylaxis and treatment of esophageal candidiasis and prophylaxis of candidiasis in patients undergoing hemopoietic stem cell transplantation (HSCT)*

Micardis tablets ℞ *angiotensin receptor blocker (ARB) for hypertension* [telmisartan] 20, 40, 80 mg

Micardis HCT tablets ℞ *combination angiotensin receptor blocker (ARB) and diuretic for hypertension* [telmisartan; hydrochlorothiazide] 40•12.5, 80•12.5, 80•25 mg

Micatin cream, powder, spray powder, spray liquid OTC *antifungal for tinea pedis, tinea cruris, and tinea corporis* [miconazole nitrate] 2%

MICE (mesna [rescue], ifosfamide, carboplatin, etoposide) *chemotherapy protocol for osteosarcoma and lung cancer* [also known as: ICE]

micinicate INN

miconazole USP, INN, BAN, JAN *imidazole antifungal for oropharyngeal candidiasis*

Miconazole 7 vaginal suppositories (discontinued 2007) OTC *antifungal* [miconazole nitrate] 100 mg

miconazole nitrate USAN, USP, JAN *imidazole antifungal; topical treatment for tinea pedis, tinea cruris, and tinea corporis; vaginal treatment for candidiasis* 2% topical/vaginal

Micrainin tablets (discontinued 2009) ℞ *analgesic; antipyretic; anti-inflammatory; anxiolytic; sedative* [aspirin; meprobamate] 325•200 mg

MICRhoGAM Ultra-Filtered Plus IM injection, prefilled syringes ℞ *obstetric Rh factor immunity suppressant* [Rh$_O$(D) immune globulin] 50 mcg (250 IU)

microbubble contrast agent *investigational (orphan) neurosonographic diagnostic aid for intracranial tumors*

Microcaps (trademarked dosage form) *fast-melting tablets*

microcrystalline cellulose [see: cellulose, microcrystalline]

microcrystalline wax [see: wax, microcrystalline]

microfibrillar collagen hemostat (MCH) *topical hemostat for surgery*

Microgestin Fe 1/20 tablets (in packs of 28) ℞ *monophasic oral contraceptive; iron supplement* [norethindrone acetate; ethinyl estradiol; ferrous fumarate] 1 mg•20 mcg•75 mg × 21 days; 0•0•75 mg × 7 days

Microgestin Fe 1.5/30 tablets (in packs of 28) ℞ *monophasic oral contraceptive; iron supplement* [norethindrone acetate; ethinyl estradiol; ferrous fumarate] 1.5 mg•30 mcg•75 mg × 21 days; 0•0•75 mg × 7 days

Micro-K; Micro-K 10 Extencaps (controlled-release capsules) ℞ *electrolyte replenisher* [potassium (as chloride)] 8 mEq (600 mg); 10 mEq (750 mg)

Micro-K LS extended-release powder for oral solution (discontinued 2008) ℞ *electrolyte replenisher* [potassium (as chloride)] 20 mEq/pkt.

MicroKlenz topical liquid OTC *antiseptic wound cleanser* [acemannan]

Microlipid emulsion OTC *dietary fat supplement* [safflower oil] 50%

Micronase tablets (discontinued 2009) ℞ *sulfonylurea antidiabetic that stimulates insulin secretion in the pancreas* [glyburide] 1.25, 2.5, 5 mg

microNefrin solution for inhalation (discontinued 2009) OTC *sympathomimetic bronchodilator for bronchial asthma and COPD; vasopressor for shock* [epinephrine HCl] 1.125%

micronized aluminum *astringent*

micronomicin INN

Micronor [see: Ortho Micronor]

microplasmin, recombinant human *investigational (orphan) adjunct to vitrectomy in pediatric patients*

Microstix-3 reagent strips for professional use ℞ *in vitro diagnostic aid for nitrate, uropathogens, or bacteria in the urine*

MicroTrak *Chlamydia trachomatis* slide test for professional use ℞ *in* *vitro diagnostic aid for* Chlamydia trachomatis

MicroTrak HSV 1/HSV 2 Culture Identification/Typing Test culture test for professional use ℞ *in vitro diagnostic aid for herpes simplex virus in tissue cultures*

MicroTrak HSV 1/HSV 2 Direct Specimen Identification/Typing Test slide test for professional use ℞ *in vitro diagnostic aid for herpes simplex virus in external lesions*

MicroTrak *Neisseria gonorrhoeae* **Culture Confirmation Test** reagent kit for professional use ℞ *in vitro diagnostic aid for* Neisseria gonorrhoeae

Microzide capsules ℞ *antihypertensive; diuretic* [hydrochlorothiazide] 12.5 mg

mictine [see: aminometradine]

midaflur USAN, INN *sedative*

midaglizole INN

midalcipran [see: milnacipran]

midamaline INN

Midamor tablets ℞ *antihypertensive; potassium-sparing diuretic for congestive heart failure; investigational (orphan) inhalant for cystic fibrosis; also used for lithium-induced polyuria* [amiloride HCl] 5 mg

midazogrel INN

midazolam INN, BAN, JAN *short-acting benzodiazepine general anesthetic* [also: midazolam HCl]

midazolam HCl USAN *short-acting benzodiazepine general anesthetic* [also: midazolam] 2 mg/mL oral; 1, 5 mg/mL injection

midazolam maleate USAN *intravenous anesthetic*

midecamycin INN

midodrine INN, BAN *antihypotensive; vasoconstrictor; vasopressor for orthostatic hypotension (OH)* [also: midodrine HCl]

midodrine HCl USAN, JAN *antihypotensive; vasoconstrictor; vasopressor for orthostatic hypotension (orphan); also used for urinary incontinence* [also: midodrine] 2.5, 5, 10 mg oral

Midol Cramp Formula tablets OTC *analgesic; antipyretic; nonsteroidal anti-inflammatory drug (NSAID) for mild to moderate pain of primary dysmenorrhea* [ibuprofen] 200 mg

Midol Extended Relief caplets OTC *analgesic; nonsteroidal anti-inflammatory drug (NSAID) for osteoarthritis, rheumatoid arthritis, juvenile arthritis, ankylosing spondylitis, primary dysmenorrhea, bursitis/tendinitis, and other mild to moderate pain* [naproxen (as sodium)] 200 mg

Midol Maximum Strength Menstrual caplets, gelcaps OTC *analgesic; antipyretic; antihistamine; sleep aid* [acetaminophen; caffeine; pyrilamine maleate] 500•60•15 mg

Midol PM caplets OTC *analgesic; antipyretic; antihistamine; sleep aid* [acetaminophen; diphenhydramine] 500•25 mg

Midol PMS caplets, gelcaps OTC *analgesic; antipyretic; diuretic; antihistamine; sleep aid* [acetaminophen; pamabrom; pyrilamine maleate] 500•25•15 mg

Midol Teen caplets OTC *analgesic; antipyretic; diuretic* [acetaminophen; pamabrom] 500•25 mg

Midrin capsules ℞ *cerebral vasoconstrictor and analgesic for vascular and tension headaches; "possibly effective" for migraine headaches* [isometheptene mucate; dichloralphenazone; acetaminophen] 65•100•325 mg ⚕ Mudrane

Midstream Pregnancy Test kit for home use OTC *in vitro diagnostic aid; urine pregnancy test*

mifamurtide *liposomal muramyl tripeptide phosphatidylethanolamine (MTP-PE); investigational (NDA filed, orphan) for high-grade osteosarcoma following surgical resection*

mifarmonab [see: imciromab pentetate]

mifentidine INN

Mifeprex tablets ℞ (not available in pharmacies; administered only by a physician in an office, clinic, or hospital setting) *abortifacient for intrauterine pregnancy; postcoital contra-*

ceptive; progesterone antagonist; also used for uterine leiomyomata [mifepristone] 200 mg

mifepristone USAN, INN, BAN progesterone antagonist; GR-II antagonist; abortifacient for the termination of intrauterine pregnancy; postcoital contraceptive; investigational (orphan) for Cushing syndrome

mifobate USAN, INN antiatherosclerotic

Migergot suppositories ℞ migraine treatment; vasoconstrictor [ergotamine tartrate; caffeine] 2•100 mg

miglitol USAN, INN, BAN antidiabetic agent for type 2 diabetes; alpha-glucosidase inhibitor that delays the digestion of dietary carbohydrates ② meglutol

miglustat glucosylceramide synthase inhibitor; substrate reduction therapy (SRT) to reduce the glycosphingolipid (GSL) production in type I Gaucher disease (orphan); investigational (NDA filed) for Niemann-Pick type C (NP-C) dementia

mignonette, Jamaica medicinal herb [see: henna (Lawsonia)]

Migragesic IDA capsules ℞ cerebral vasoconstrictor and analgesic for vascular and tension headaches; "possibly effective" for migraine headaches [isometheptene mucate; dichloralphenazone; acetaminophen] 65•100•325 mg

Migranal nasal spray ℞ ergot alkaloid for the rapid control of migraine and other vascular headaches [dihydroergotamine mesylate] 0.5 mg/spray

MigraTen capsules ℞ cerebral vasoconstrictor and analgesic for migraine and tension headaches [isometheptene mucate; acetaminophen; caffeine] 65•325•100 mg

Migratine capsules (discontinued 2008) ℞ cerebral vasoconstrictor and analgesic for vascular and tension headaches; "possibly effective" for migraine headaches [isometheptene mucate; dichloralphenazone; acetaminophen] 65•100•325 mg

Migrazone capsules ℞ cerebral vasoconstrictor and analgesic for vascular

and tension headaches; "possibly effective" for migraine headaches [isometheptene mucate; dichloralphenazone; acetaminophen] 65•100•325 mg ② Myochrysine

mikamycin INN, BAN

milacemide INN anticonvulsant; antidepressant [also: milacemide HCl]

milacemide HCl USAN anticonvulsant; antidepressant [also: milacemide]

Mil-Adregen tablets OTC vitamin/mineral supplement [vitamins B₅, B₅, and C; multiple minerals and glandular concentrates; citrus bioflavonoids] 60•50•250• ± •25 mg

milameline HCl USAN partial muscarinic agonist for Alzheimer disease

mild silver protein [see: silver protein, mild]

milenperone USAN, INN, BAN antipsychotic

Miles Nervine caplets OTC antihistamine; sleep aid [diphenhydramine HCl] 25 mg

milfoil medicinal herb [see: yarrow]

milipertine USAN, INN antipsychotic

milk ipecac medicinal herb [see: birthroot; dogbane]

milk of bismuth [see: bismuth, milk of]

milk of magnesia (MOM) [see: magnesia, milk of]

Milk of Magnesia, Concentrated oral suspension OTC antacid; saline laxative [milk of magnesia (magnesium hydroxide)] 2400 mg/10 mL

Milk of Magnesia-Cascara, Concentrated oral suspension OTC antacid; saline/stimulant laxative [milk of magnesia; aromatic cascara fluidextract; alcohol 7%] 30•5 mL/15 mL

milk thistle (Silybum marianum) seeds medicinal herb for Amanita mushroom poisoning, bronchitis, gallbladder disorders, hemorrhage, liver damage, peritonitis, spleen disorders, stomach disorders, and varicose veins

milkweed (Asclepias syriaca) roots medicinal herb used as a diuretic, emetic, purgative, and tonic

Millipred tablets, oral solution ℞ *corticosteroid; anti-inflammatory* [prednisolone] 5 mg; 15 mg/5 mL

milnacipran INN *selective serotonin and norepinephrine reuptake inhibitor*

milnacipran HCl *selective serotonin and norepinephrine reuptake inhibitor antidepressant for fibromyalgia syndrome*

milodistim USAN *antineutropenic; hematopoietic stimulant; granulocyte macrophage colony-stimulating factor (GM-CSF) + interleukin 3*

Milophene tablets ℞ *ovulation stimulant* [clomiphene citrate] 50 mg

miloxacin INN

milrinone USAN, INN, BAN *cardiotonic*

milrinone lactate *vasodilator for congestive heart failure* 20, 40 mg injection

miltefosine INN *anthelmintic for leishmaniasis; investigational for HIV infections*

Miltown tablets ℞ *anxiolytic; also abused as a street drug* [meprobamate] 200, 400 mg

milverine INN

mimbane INN *analgesic* [also: mimbane HCl]

mimbane HCl USAN *analgesic* [also: mimbane]

Mimvey film-coated tablets (in packs of 28) ℞ *a mixture of natural and synthetic hormones; hormone replacement therapy for postmenopausal symptoms* [estradiol; norethindrone acetate] 1•0.5 mg

Mimyx cream ℞ *moisturizer; emollient* [betaine; olive oil; glycerin]

minalrestat USAN *aldose reductase inhibitor for diabetic neuropathy and other long-term diabetic complications*

minaprine USAN, INN, BAN *psychotropic* ⧉ Magnaprin

minaprine HCl USAN *antidepressant*

minaxolone USAN, INN *anesthetic*

mindodilol INN

mindolic acid [see: clometacin]

mindoperone INN

MINE (mesna [rescue], ifosfamide, Novantrone, etoposide) *chemotherapy protocol for non-Hodgkin lymphoma*

MINE-ESHAP (alternating cycles of MINE and ESHAP) *chemotherapy protocol for non-Hodgkin lymphoma*

minepentate INN, BAN

Mineral Freez gel OTC *mild anesthetic; antipruritic; counterirritant* [menthol] 2%

Mineral Ice [see: Therapeutic Mineral Ice]

mineral oil USP *emollient/protectant; moisturizer/lubricant; laxative; solvent*

mineral oil, light NF *tablet and capsule lubricant; vehicle*

Mineral Zinc tablets OTC *calcium/zinc supplement* [calcium; zinc] 122•10 mg

mineralocorticoids *a class of adrenal cortical steroids that are used for partial replacement therapy in adrenocortical insufficiency*

Minerin lotion OTC *emollient/protectant* [lanolin; glyceryl; mineral oil; PEG; propylene glycol]

Mini Two-Way Action tablets (discontinued 2007) OTC *bronchodilator; decongestant; expectorant* [ephedrine HCl; guaifenesin] 12.5•200, 25•200 mg

MiniAdFVIII *investigational (orphan) agent for hemophilia A* [adenovirus-based vector Factor VIII complementary DNA to somatic cells]

mini-BEAM (BCNU, etoposide, ara-C, melphalan) *chemotherapy protocol for Hodgkin lymphoma*

Minidyne solution OTC *broad-spectrum antimicrobial* [povidone-iodine] 10% ⧉ menadione

Min-I-Mix (delivery form) *dual-chambered prefilled syringe*

Minipress capsules ℞ *antihypertensive; alpha$_1$ blocker* [prazosin (as HCl)] 1, 2, 5 mg

Miniprin Low Dose chewable tablets OTC *analgesic; antipyretic; anti-inflammatory* [aspirin] 81 mg

Minirin nasal spray (discontinued 2008) ℞ *posterior pituitary hormone for hemophilia A (orphan), von Willebrand disease (orphan), central diabetes insipidus, and nocturnal enuresis* [desmopressin acetate; chlorobutanol] 10•500 mcg/dose

Minitran transdermal patch ℞ *coronary vasodilator; antianginal; also used for acute myocardial infarction, erectile dysfunction, and Raynaud disease* [nitroglycerin] 0.1, 0.2, 0.4, 0.6 mg/hr. (9, 18, 36, 54 mg total)

Minit-Rub OTC *analgesic; mild anesthetic; antipruritic; counterirritant* [methyl salicylate; menthol; camphor] 15%•3.5%•2.3%

Minizide 1; Minizide 2; Minizide 5 capsules (discontinued 2007) ℞ *antihypertensive; alpha-blocker; diuretic* [prazosin HCl; polythiazide] 1•0.5 mg; 2•0.5 mg; 5•0.5 mg

Minocin pellet-filled capsules, oral suspension, powder for IV injection ℞ *tetracycline antibiotic for gram-negative and gram-positive bacteria; antirickettsial; investigational (orphan) for chronic malignant pleural effusion and sarcoidosis* [minocycline (as HCl)] 50, 100 mg; 50 mg/5 mL

Minocin PAC (Professional Acne Care) 60 capsules plus 3 skin care products ℞ *tetracycline antibiotic for acne* [minocycline HCl] 50, 100 mg

minocromil USAN, INN, BAN *prophylactic antiallergic*

minocycline USAN, INN, BAN *tetracycline antibiotic for gram-negative and gram-positive bacteria; antirickettsial; adjunct to scaling and root planing for periodontitis*

minocycline HCl USP *tetracycline antibiotic for gram-negative and gram-positive bacteria; antirickettsial; investigational (orphan) for chronic malignant pleural effusion and sarcoidosis* 45, 50, 75, 90, 100, 135 mg oral

Min-O-Ear ear drops OTC *emollient* [mineral oil]

minoxidil USAN, USP, INN, BAN *antihypertensive; peripheral vasodilator; topical hair growth stimulant* 2.5, 10 mg oral

Minoxidil for Men topical solution OTC *hair growth stimulant* [minoxidil; alcohol] 2%•60%, 5%•30%

mint; lamb mint; mackerel mint; Our Lady's mint *medicinal herb* [see: spearmint]

mint, brandy; lamb mint *medicinal herb* [see: peppermint]

mint, mountain *medicinal herb* [see: marjoram; Oswego tea]

mint, squaw *medicinal herb* [see: pennyroyal]

Mintezol chewable tablets (discontinued 2010) ℞ *anthelmintic for strongyloidiasis (threadworm), larva migrans, and trichinosis* [thiabendazole] 500 mg

Mintezol oral suspension (discontinued 2009) ℞ *anthelmintic for strongyloidiasis (threadworm), larva migrans, and trichinosis* [thiabendazole] 500 mg/5 mL

Mintox chewable tablets OTC *antacid* [aluminum hydroxide; magnesium hydroxide] 200•200, 300•150 mg ☑ Mentax

Mintox oral suspension OTC *antacid; antiflatulent* [aluminum hydroxide; magnesium hydroxide; simethicone] 200•200•20 mg/5 mL ☑ Mentax

Mintox Plus oral liquid OTC *antacid; antiflatulent* [aluminum hydroxide; magnesium hydroxide; simethicone] 500•450•40 mg/5 mL

Mintuss MR syrup (discontinued 2007) ℞ *narcotic antitussive; antihistamine; sleep aid; decongestant* [hydrocodone bitartrate; pyrilamine maleate; phenylephrine HCl] 10•10•10 mg/10 mL

Minute-Gel ℞ *dental caries preventative* [acidulated phosphate fluoride] 1.23%

Miochol-E solution ℞ *direct-acting miotic for ophthalmic surgery* [acetylcholine chloride] 1:100

mioflazine INN, BAN *coronary vasodilator* [also: mioflazine HCl]

mioflazine HCl USAN *coronary vasodilator* [also: mioflazine]

Mi-Omega capsules ℞ *dietary supplement* [omega-3 fatty acids (eicosapentaenoic acid and docosahexaenoic acid); vitamin B_6; vitamin B_{12};

folic acid] 500•12.5•0.5•1 mg (35 mg EPA; 350 mg DHA)

Miostat solution ℞ *direct-acting miotic for ophthalmic surgery* [carbachol] 0.01%

miotics *a class of drugs that cause the pupil of the eye to contract*

mipafilcon A USAN *hydrophilic contact lens material*

mipimazole INN

mipomersen *investigational (NDA filed) treatment for heterozygous familial hypercholesterolemia*

MiraFlow solution OTC *cleaning solution for hard or soft contact lenses*

MiraForte [see: Super MiraForte with Chrysin]

MiraLAX powder for oral solution OTC (previously ℞) *hyperosmotic laxative; pre-procedure bowel evacuant* [polyethylene glycol 3350] 17 g/dose

Mirapex tablets ℞ *dopamine agonist for idiopathic Parkinson disease; treatment for primary restless legs syndrome (RLS)* [pramipexole dihydrochloride] 0.125, 0.25, 0.5, 0.75, 1, 1.5 mg

Mirapex ER extended-release tablets ℞ *dopamine agonist for idiopathic Parkinson disease* [pramipexole dihydrochloride] 0.375, 0.75, 1.5, 2.25, 3, 3.75, 4.5 mg

Miraphen PSE extended-release tablets (discontinued 2007) ℞ *decongestant; expectorant* [pseudoephedrine HCl; guaifenesin] 120•600 mg

MiraSept Step 2 solution (discontinued 2010) OTC *rinsing/storage solution for soft contact lenses* [sodium chloride (preserved saline solution)]

MiraSept System solutions (discontinued 2010) OTC *two-step chemical disinfecting system for soft contact lenses* [hydrogen peroxide–based]

Miraxion *investigational (Phase III) for Huntington disease* [semi-synthetic derivative of eicosapentaenoic acid (EPA)]

Mircera IV injection in single-use vials and prefilled syringes ℞ *erythropoiesis-stimulating agent (ESA) for the treat-*

ment of anemia due to chronic renal failure (orphan) [epoetin beta (in methoxy PEG)] 50, 75, 100, 150, 200, 250, 300, 400, 600, 800, 1000 mcg

Mircette tablets (in packs of 28) ℞ *biphasic oral contraceptive* [desogestrel; ethinyl estradiol]
Phase 1 (21 days): 0.15 mg•20 mcg;
Phase 2 (5 days): 0•10 mcg;
Counters (2 days)

Mirena intrauterine device (IUD) ℞ *long-term (5 year) T-shaped contraceptive insert* [levonorgestrel] 20 mcg/day ⍰ Murine

mirfentanil INN *analgesic* [also: mirfentanil HCl]

mirfentanil HCl USAN *analgesic* [also: mirfentanil]

mirincamycin INN *antibacterial; antimalarial* [also: mirincamycin HCl]

mirincamycin HCl USAN *antibacterial; antimalarial* [also: mirincamycin]

mirisetron maleate USAN *anxiolytic*

miristalkonium chloride INN

miroprofen INN

mirosamicin INN

mirostipen USAN *myeloprotectant*

mirtazapine USAN, INN *serotonin 5-HT_{1A} agonist; tetracyclic antidepressant* 7.5, 15, 30, 45 mg oral

misonidazole USAN, INN *antiprotozoal (Trichomonas)*

misoprostol USAN, INN, BAN *prevents NSAID-induced gastric ulcers; has been used for cervical ripening and induction of labor; use by pregnant women can cause abortion, premature birth, or birth defects; investigational (orphan) for complete expulsion of the products of conception* 100, 200 mcg oral

Mission Prenatal; Mission Prenatal F.A.; Mission Prenatal H.P. film-coated tablets OTC *prenatal vitamin/calcium/iron supplement* [multiple vitamins; calcium; iron (as ferrous gluconate); folic acid] ≛•50•30•0.4 mg; ≛•50•30•0.8 mg; ≛•50•30•0.8 mg

Mission Prenatal Rx tablets (discontinued 2008) ℞ *vitamin/calcium/iron supplement* [multiple vitamins; cal-

cium; iron; folic acid] ≜•175•29.5•
1 mg

Mission Surgical Supplement tablets
(discontinued 2008) OTC *vitamin/iron
supplement* [multiple vitamins; iron
(as ferrous gluconate)] ≜•27 mg

mistletoe (*Phoradendron flavescens;
P. serotinum; P. tomentosum; Viscum album***)** plant *medicinal herb for
cancer, chorea, epilepsy, hypertension,
internal hemorrhages, menstrual disorders, nervousness, poor circulation, and
spleen disorders; not generally regarded
as safe and effective for ingestion as it
is highly toxic*

Mistometer (trademarked delivery
form) *metered-dose inhalation aerosol*

Mitchella repens medicinal herb [see:
squaw vine]

mithramycin [now: plicamycin]

mitindomide USAN, INN *antineoplastic*

mitobronitol INN, BAN

mitocarcin USAN, INN *antineoplastic*

mitoclomine INN, BAN

mitocromin USAN *antineoplastic*

mitoflaxone INN

mitogillin USAN, INN *antineoplastic*

mitoguazone INN *investigational
(orphan) antineoplastic for non-Hodgkin lymphoma*

mitolactol INN *investigational (orphan)
antineoplastic for brain tumors and
recurrent or metastatic cervical squamous cell carcinoma*

mitomalcin USAN, INN *antineoplastic*

mitomycin USAN, USP, INN, BAN *antibiotic antineoplastic for disseminated
adenocarcinoma of the stomach or pancreas; investigational (orphan) for refractory glaucoma and glaucoma surgery* 5,
20, 40 mg injection

mitomycin C (MTC) [see: mitomycin]

mitonafide INN

mitopodozide INN, BAN

mitoquidone INN, BAN

mitosper USAN, INN *antineoplastic*

mitotane USAN, USP, INN *antibiotic antineoplastic for inoperable adrenal cortical carcinoma and Cushing syndrome*
⨂ metetoin

mitotenamine INN, BAN

mitotic inhibitors *a class of antineoplastics that inhibit cell division (mitosis)*

mitoxantrone INN *antibiotic antineoplastic* [also: mitoxantrone HCl;
mitozantrone]

mitoxantrone HCl USAN, USP, JAN
*antibiotic antineoplastic for prostate
cancer (orphan) and acute nonlymphocytic leukemia (ANLL) (orphan);
immunomodulator for progressive and
relapsing-remitting multiple sclerosis
(orphan)* [also: mitoxantrone; mito-
zantrone] 2 mg/mL injection

mitozantrone BAN *antineoplastic* [also:
mitoxantrone HCl; mitoxantrone]

mitozolomide INN, BAN

mitronal [see: cinnarizine]

mitumomab USAN *antineoplastic monoclonal antibody for* G_{D3} *ganglioside–
expressing tumors*

mivacurium chloride USAN, INN,
BAN *neuromuscular blocking agent* 2
mg/mL injection

mivobulin isethionate USAN *antineoplastic; mitotic inhibitor; tubulin binder*

Mixed E 400; Mixed E 1000 softgels
OTC *vitamin supplement* [vitamin E]
400 IU; 1000 IU

mixed tocopherols [see: vitamin E]

mixidine USAN, INN *coronary vasodilator* ⨂ Maxidone

Mix-O-Vial (trademarked delivery
form) *two-compartment vial*

mizoribine INN

**MMP (matrix metalloproteinase)
inhibitors** [q.v.]

**MMR (measles, mumps & rubella
vaccines)** [q.v.]

M-M-R II powder for subcu injection
R̶ *measles, mumps, and rubella vaccine* [measles, mumps, and rubella
virus vaccine, live; neomycin] 1000
U•20 000 U•1000 U•25 mcg/0.5
mL dose

Moban tablets (discontinued 2010) R̶
*conventional (typical) dihydroindolone
antipsychotic for schizophrenia* [molin-
done HCl] 5, 10, 25, 50 mg

mobecarb INN

mobenzoxamine INN

Mobic tablets, oral suspension ℞ *once-daily analgesic; antipyretic; nonsteroidal anti-inflammatory drug (NSAID) for osteoarthritis, rheumatoid arthritis, and juvenile rheumatoid arthritis; also used for ankylosing spondylitis and acute bursitis/tendinitis* [meloxicam] 7.5, 15 mg; 7.5 mg/5 mL ② MBC

Mobidin tablets ℞ *analgesic; antipyretic; anti-inflammatory; antirheumatic* [magnesium salicylate] 600 mg

Mobigesic tablets (discontinued 2008) OTC *analgesic; antipyretic; anti-inflammatory; antihistamine; sleep aid* [magnesium salicylate; phenyltoloxamine citrate] 325•30 mg

Mobisyl Creme OTC *analgesic* [trolamine salicylate] 10%

MOBP (mitomycin, Oncovin, bleomycin, Platinol) *chemotherapy protocol for cervical cancer* ② Māpap

moccasin snake antivenin [see: antivenin (Crotalidae) polyvalent]

mocimycin INN

mociprazine INN

mock pennyroyal *medicinal herb* [see: pennyroyal]

moclobemide USAN, INN, BAN *antidepressant; MAO inhibitor*

moctamide INN

modafinil USAN, INN *analeptic for excessive daytime sleepiness due to narcolepsy (orphan), obstructive sleep apnea, or shift work sleep disorder (SWSD); also used for fatigue associated with multiple sclerosis*

modaline INN *antidepressant* [also: modaline sulfate]

modaline sulfate USAN *antidepressant* [also: modaline]

Modane enteric-coated tablets OTC *stimulant laxative* [bisacodyl] 5 mg

modecainide USAN, INN *antiarrhythmic*

Modicon tablets (in Dialpaks and Veridates of 28) ℞ *monophasic oral contraceptive* [norethindrone; ethinyl estradiol] 0.5 mg•35 mcg × 21 days; counters × 7 days ② Medicone

modified Bagshawe protocol *chemotherapy protocol for gestational trophoblastic neoplasm* [see: CHAMOCA]

modified bovine lung surfactant extract [see: beractant]

modified Burow solution [see: aluminum acetate solution]

modified cellulose gum [now: croscarmellose sodium]

modified Shohl solution (sodium citrate & citric acid) *urinary alkalinizer; compounding agent*

Moducal powder OTC *carbohydrate caloric supplement* [glucose polymers]

Moduretic tablets ℞ *antihypertensive; diuretic* [amiloride HCl; hydrochlorothiazide] 5•50 mg

moexipril INN *antihypertensive; angiotensin-converting enzyme (ACE) inhibitor*

moexipril HCl USAN *antihypertensive; angiotensin-converting enzyme (ACE) inhibitor* 7.5, 15 mg oral

moexipril HCl & hydrochlorothiazide *combination angiotensin-converting enzyme (ACE) inhibitor and diuretic for hypertension* 7.5•12.5, 15•12.5, 15•25 mg oral

moexiprilat INN

mofebutazone INN

mofedione [see: oxazidione]

mofegiline INN *antiparkinsonian* [also: mofegiline HCl]

mofegiline HCl USAN *antiparkinsonian* [also: mofegiline]

mofetil USAN, INN *combining name for radicals or groups*

mofloverine INN

mofoxime INN

moguisteine INN

Moist Again vaginal gel OTC *moisturizer/lubricant* [glycerin; aloe vera]

Moi-Stir throat spray, Swabsticks OTC *saliva substitute*

Moisture Drops eye drops OTC *moisturizer/lubricant* [hydroxypropyl methylcellulose] 0.5%

Moisture Eyes eye drops OTC *moisturizer/lubricant* [propylene glycol] 0.95%

mold allergenic extracts *diagnosis and treatment of allergies*

molfarnate INN

molgramostim USAN, INN, BAN *antineutropenic and hematopoietic stimulant; investigational (orphan) for bone marrow transplants, chronic lymphocytic leukemia (CLL), myelodysplastic syndrome, aplastic anemia, and AIDS-related neutropenia*

molinazone USAN, INN *analgesic*

molindone INN *conventional (typical) dihydroindolone antipsychotic for schizophrenia* [also: molindone HCl]

molindone HCl USAN *conventional (typical) dihydroindolone antipsychotic for schizophrenia* [also: molindone]

Mollifene Ear Wax Removing Formula ear drops OTC *cerumenolytic to emulsify and disperse ear wax* [carbamide peroxide] 6.5%

molracetam INN

molsidomine USAN, INN *antianginal; coronary vasodilator*

molybdenum *element (Mo)*

Molypen IV injection (discontinued 2011) Ⅎ *intravenous nutritional therapy* [ammonium molybdate tetrahydrate] 25 mcg/mL

MOM (milk of magnesia) [see: magnesia, milk of]

Momentum caplets OTC *analgesic; antipyretic; anti-inflammatory; antihistamine; sleep aid* [aspirin; phenyltoloxamine citrate] 500•15 mg

Momentum Muscular Backache Formula caplets OTC *analgesic; antipyretic; anti-inflammatory* [magnesium salicylate] 580 mg

mometasone INN, BAN *topical corticosteroidal anti-inflammatory* [also: mometasone furoate]

mometasone furoate USAN *topical corticosteroidal anti-inflammatory; oral inhalation aerosol for chronic asthma; nasal aerosol for seasonal or perennial allergic rhinitis and nasal polyps* [also: mometasone] 0.1% topical

mometasone furoate & formoterol (MFF) *investigational (Phase III)* *inhaled combination therapy for asthma and chronic obstructive pulmonary disease (COPD)*

Momexin cream Ⅎ *corticosteroidal anti-inflammatory* [mometasone furoate] 0.1%

Momordica charantia *medicinal herb* [see: bitter melon]

monalazone disodium INN

monalium hydrate [see: magaldrate]

Monarc-M powder for IV injection (discontinued 2008) Ⅎ *systemic hemostatic; antihemophilic for the prevention and control of bleeding in classical hemophilia (hemophilia A) and von Willebrand disease (orphan)* [antihemophilic factor concentrate] 2–15 IU/mg

Monarda didyma *medicinal herb* [see: Oswego tea]

Monarda fistulosa *medicinal herb* [see: wild bergamot]

Monarda punctata *medicinal herb* [see: horsemint]

monarsen *investigational (orphan) for myasthenia gravis*

monascus yeast (*Monascus purpureus*) *natural remedy for gastric disorders, indigestion, lowering cholesterol, and poor circulation*

monatepil INN *antianginal; antihypertensive* [also: monatepil maleate]

monatepil maleate USAN *antianginal; antihypertensive* [also: monatepil]

monensin USAN, INN *antiprotozoal; antibacterial; antifungal*

Monistat cream OTC *antifungal* [miconazole nitrate] 2%

Monistat 1 vaginal ointment in prefilled applicator OTC *antifungal* [tioconazole] 6.5%

Monistat 1 Combination Pack vaginal inserts + cream OTC *antifungal* [miconazole nitrate] 200 mg + 2%

Monistat 1-Day vaginal ointment in prefilled applicator OTC *antifungal* [tioconazole] 6.5%

Monistat 3 vaginal cream, combination pack (vaginal inserts + cream), cream combination pak (vaginal cream in prefilled applicators +

external cream) OTC *antifungal* [miconazole nitrate] 2%; 200 mg + 2%; 4% + 2%

Monistat 7 vaginal inserts, vaginal cream, combination pack (inserts + cream) OTC *antifungal* [miconazole nitrate] 100 mg; 2%; 100 mg + 2%

Monistat-Derm cream (discontinued 2008) ℞ *antifungal for tinea pedis, tinea cruris, and tinea corporis* [miconazole nitrate] 2%

mono- & di-acetylated monoglycerides NF *plasticizer*

mono- & di-glycerides NF *emulsifying agent*

monoamine oxidase (MAO) inhibitors (MAOIs) *a class of antidepressants that increase CNS monoamine neurotransmitters (epinephrine, norepinephrine, and serotonin)*

monobactams *a class of bactericidal antibiotics effective against gram-negative aerobic pathogens*

monobasic potassium phosphate [see: potassium phosphate, monobasic]

monobasic sodium phosphate [see: sodium phosphate, monobasic]

monobenzone USP, INN *depigmenting agent for vitiligo*

monobenzyl ether of hydroquinone [see: monobenzone]

monobromated camphor [see: camphor, monobromated]

Monocal tablets OTC *calcium/fluoride supplement* [calcium; fluoride] 250• 3 mg ② Magnacal

monocalcium phosphate [see: calcium phosphate, dibasic]

Monocaps tablets OTC *vitamin/mineral/calcium/iron supplement* [multiple vitamins & minerals; calcium (as carbonate and ascorbate); iron (as ferrous fumarate); folic acid; biotin] ±•50•14•0.4•0.015 mg

Monocete EZ Swabs medicated swabs ℞ *cauterant; keratolytic* [monochloroacetic acid] 80%

Mono-Chlor topical liquid (discontinued 2009) ℞ *cauterant; keratolytic* [monochloroacetic acid] 80%

monochloroacetic acid *strong keratolytic/cauterant*

monochlorothymol [see: chlorothymol]

monochlorphenamide [see: clofenamide]

Monoclate P powder for IV injection ℞ *systemic hemostatic; antihemophilic for the prevention and control of bleeding in classical hemophilia (hemophilia A) and von Willebrand disease (orphan)* [antihemophilic factor concentrate, human] 250, 500, 1000, 1500 IU

monoclonal antibodies (MAb; MAB) *a class of biological agents that have been cloned (exact copies produced asexually in vitro or in vivo) from a single cell harvested from a human, mouse, or rat; cloning multiplies the number of antibodies attacking the target* [compare: chimeric, human, humanized, and murine variants]

monoclonal antibody 1D10, humanized *investigational (orphan) agent for non-Hodgkin B-cell lymphoma*

monoclonal antibody 5A8 to CD4 *investigational (orphan) for post-exposure prophylaxis to occupational HIV exposure*

monoclonal antibody 5c8, recombinant humanized [now: ruplizumab]

monoclonal antibody 5G1.1, humanized *investigational (orphan) C5 complement inhibitor for dermatomyositis*

monoclonal antibody 7E3 [see: abciximab]

monoclonal antibody to alpha-fetoprotein (AFP), murine, radiolabeled with iodine I 123 *investigational (orphan) diagnostic aid for AFP-producing tumors, hepatocellular carcinoma, and hepatoblastoma*

monoclonal antibody to alpha-fetoprotein (AFP), murine, radiolabeled with iodine I 131 *investigational (orphan) for AFP-producing* *tumors, hepatocellular carcinoma, and hepatoblastoma*

monoclonal antibody to alpha-feto-protein (AFP), murine, radiola-beled with technetium Tc 99m *investigational (orphan) diagnostic aid for AFP-producing tumors, hepatoblastoma, and hepatocellular carcinoma*

monoclonal antibody to anti-idio-type melanoma-associated anti-gen, murine *investigational (orphan) for invasive cutaneous melanoma*

monoclonal antibody to B4, ricin (blocked) conjugated murine *investigational (orphan) for B-cell lymphoma, leukemia, and treatment of bone marrow in non-T-cell acute lymphocytic leukemia*

monoclonal antibody B43.13 *investigational (orphan) for epithelial ovarian cancer*

monoclonal antibody to B-cell lymphoma, murine or human *investigational (orphan) for B-cell lymphoma*

monoclonal antibody to cA2, chimeric [see: infliximab]

monoclonal antibody to carcinoembryonic antigen (CEA), chimeric (sheep-human), radiolabeled with yttrium Y 90 [now: yttrium Y 90 labetuzumab]

monoclonal antibody to carcinoembryonic antigen (CEA), humanized [now: altumomab; altumomab pentetate]

monoclonal antibody to carcinoembryonic antigen (CEA), humanized, radiolabeled with indium In 111 [now: indium In 111 altumomab pentetate]

monoclonal antibody to CD2, humanized *investigational (orphan) for graft-versus-host disease and prevention of renal transplant rejection*

monoclonal antibody to CD3 [see: muromonab-CD3; teplizumab; visilizumab]

monoclonal antibody to CD4, human *investigational (orphan) for mycosis fungoides*

monoclonal antibody to CD6, ricin (blocked) conjugated murine *investigational (orphan) for T-cell leukemias, lymphomas, and other mature T-cell malignancies*

monoclonal antibody to CD16, humanized *investigational (Phase III, orphan) for adult immune thrombocytopenic purpura (ITP)*

monoclonal antibody to CD22 antigen on B-cells [now: epratuzumab]

monoclonal antibody to CD23 immunoglobulin G1 (IgG1) kappa *investigational (orphan) for chronic lymphocytic leukemia*

monoclonal antibody to CD30, human *investigational (orphan) for Hodgkin disease and T-cell lymphomas*

monoclonal antibody to CD40 *investigational (orphan) for multiple myeloma*

monoclonal antibody to CD45 *investigational (orphan) to prevent acute graft rejection of human organ transplants*

monoclonal antibody to CD55 *investigational (orphan) for gastric tumors*

monoclonal antibody to cytomegalovirus (CMV), human *investigational (orphan) to prevent or treat CMV retinitis and other CMV infections due to bone marrow transplants, organ transplants, or AIDS*

monoclonal antibody to endotoxin E5 [now: edobacomab]

monoclonal antibody to epidermal growth factor receptor (EGFR) protein [see: cetuximab; gefitinib; panitumumab]

monoclonal antibody Fab to myosin, murine [now: imciromab pentetate]

monoclonal antibody Fab to myosin, murine, radiolabeled with indium In 111 [now: indium In 111 imciromab pentetate]

monoclonal antibody to fibrin [now: biciromab]

monoclonal antibody G250 to IgG, chimeric (human-murine) *investigational (orphan) agent for renal cell carcinoma*

monoclonal antibody to gpIIb/IIIa [now: abciximab]

monoclonal antibody to hepatitis B virus, human [now: tuvirumab]

monoclonal antibody to hsp90, recombinant human [now: efungumab]

monoclonal antibody HuM291, chimeric (human-mouse) [now: visilizumab]

monoclonal antibody to human chorionic gonadotropin (hCG), murine, radiolabeled with iodine I 123 *investigational (orphan) diagnostic aid for hCG-producing tumors*

monoclonal antibody to human chorionic gonadotropin (hCG), murine, radiolabeled with iodine I 131 *investigational (orphan) for hCG-producing tumors*

monoclonal antibody to human chorionic gonadotropin (hCG), murine, radiolabeled with technetium Tc 99m *investigational (orphan) diagnostic aid for hCG-producing tumors such as germ cell and trophoblastic cell tumors*

monoclonal antibody to human epidermal growth factor receptor 2 (HER2) protein [see: trastuzumab]

monoclonal antibody IDEC-131 to CD40L, humanized *investigational (Phase II, orphan) for systemic lupus erythematosus (SLE)*

monoclonal antibody IgG$_{1k}$ to CTLA-4, human *investigational (orphan) for high-risk stages II, III, and IV melanoma*

monoclonal antibody IgG$_{2a}$ to B cell, murine [now: bectumomab]

monoclonal antibody IgG$_{2a}$ to B cell, murine, radiolabeled with iodine I 131 *investigational (orphan) for B-cell leukemia and lymphoma*

monoclonal antibody IgG$_{2a}$ to B cell, murine, radiolabeled with technetium Tc 99m [now: technetium Tc 99m bectumomab]

monoclonal antibody IgM (C-58) to cytomegalovirus (CMV) *investigational (orphan) treatment and prophylaxis of CMV infections in allogenic bone marrow transplants*

monoclonal antibody to integrin receptor avb3/avb5, human *investigational (orphan) for high-risk stages II, III, and IV malignant melanoma*

monoclonal antibody to interleukin-6 receptors, humanized [see: tocilizumab]

monoclonal antibody to leukocyte function–associated antigen-1 (LFA-1), recombinant humanized [now: efalizumab]

monoclonal antibody LL2, humanized [now: epratuzumab]

monoclonal antibody to lupus nephritis *investigational (orphan) for immunization against lupus nephritis*

monoclonal antibody to Lym-1, radiolabeled with iodine I 131 *investigational (Phase III, orphan) treatment for non-Hodgkin B-cell lymphoma*

monoclonal antibody to melanoma, murine, radiolabeled with technetium Tc 99m *investigational (orphan) for diagnostic imaging agent for metastases of malignant melanoma*

monoclonal antibody M-T412 IgG to CD4, chimeric (human-murine) [now: priliximab]

monoclonal antibody to MY9, ricin (blocked) conjugated murine *investigational (orphan) for myeloid leukemia (including acute myelogenous leukemia [AML]), ex vivo treatment of autologous bone marrow in AML, and blast crisis in chronic myeloid leukemia (CML)*

monoclonal antibody to N901, ricin (blocked) conjugated murine *investigational (orphan) for small cell lung cancer*

monoclonal antibody to non-Hodgkin lymphoma (NHL) [now: tositumomab]

monoclonal antibody to non-Hodgkin lymphoma (NHL), radiolabeled with iodine I 131 [now: iodine I 131 tositumomab]

monoclonal antibody to pan T lymphocyte [now: zolimomab aritox]

monoclonal antibody to platelet-derived growth factor D, human *investigational (orphan) to slow the progression of IgA nephropathy and delay kidney failure*

monoclonal antibody to polymorphic epithelial mucin, murine *investigational (Phase III, orphan) adjunctive treatment for ovarian cancer*

monoclonal antibody SC-1 [see: monoclonal antibody to CD55]

monoclonal antibody to Shiga-like toxin II, humanized *investigational (orphan) for the treatment of hemolytic uremic syndrome due to Shiga-like toxin–producing E. coli*

monoclonal antibody to Staphylococcus, chimeric, humanized *investigational (orphan) prophylaxis of S. epidermidis sepsis in low birthweight infants*

monoclonal antibody to TNF (tumor necrosis factor) [now: nerelimomab]

monoclonal antibody to TNF, chimeric A2 (human-murine) IgG [now: infliximab]

monoclonal antibody to TNFα (tumor necrosis factor alpha) [now: infliximab]

monoclonal antibody to transforming growth factor beta 1, human *investigational (orphan) for systemic sclerosis* [compare: anti–transforming growth factor B1,2,3]

monoclonal antibody tumor necrosis treatment (TNT-1B), chimeric, radiolabeled with iodine I 131 *investigational (orphan) treatment for malignant glioblastoma multiforme and anaplastic astrocytoma*

monoclonal antibody to vascular endothelial growth factor, recombinant human (rhuMAb-VEGF) [now: bevacizumab]

monoclonal antibody vehicles [see: targeted monoclonal antibody vehicles (T-MAVs)]

monoclonal antibody XMMEn-0e5 to endotoxin [now: edobacomab]

monoclonal factor IX [see: factor IX complex]

monoctanoin USAN, BAN *anticholelithogenic for dissolution of cholesterol gallstones (orphan)*

monoctanoin component A

monoctanoin component B

monoctanoin component C

monoctanoin component D

Mono-Diff reagent kit for professional use ℞ *in vitro diagnostic aid for mononucleosis*

Monodox capsules ℞ *tetracycline antibiotic* [doxycycline monohydrate] 50, 100 mg

Mono-Drop (trademarked delivery form) *prefilled eye drop dispenser*

monoethanolamine NF *surfactant*

monoethanolamine oleate INN *sclerosing agent* [also: ethanolamine oleate]

Monoket tablets ℞ *coronary vasodilator; antianginal* [isosorbide mononitrate] 10, 20 mg

Mono-Latex reagent kit for professional use ℞ *in vitro diagnostic aid for mononucleosis*

monolaurin *investigational (Phase III, orphan) for nonbullous congenital ichthyosiform erythroderma (a.k.a. congenital primary ichthyosis)*

monometacrine INN

Mononessa tablets (in packs of 28) ℞ *monophasic oral contraceptive* [norgestimate; ethinyl estradiol] 0.25 mg• 35 mcg × 21 days; counters × 7 days

Mononine powder for IV infusion ℞ *systemic hemostatic; antihemophilic for factor IX deficiency (hemophilia B; Christmas disease) (orphan)* [factor IX, human] 500, 1000 U/vial

monooctanoin [see: monoctanoin]

monophenylbutazone [see: mofebutazone]

monophosphothiamine INN

Mono-Plus reagent kit for professional use ℞ *in vitro diagnostic aid for mononucleosis*

monopotassium 4-aminosalicylate [see: aminosalicylate potassium]

monopotassium carbonate [see: potassium bicarbonate]

monopotassium D-gluconate [see: potassium gluconate]

monopotassium monosodium tartrate tetrahydrate [see: potassium sodium tartrate]

monopotassium phosphate [see: potassium phosphate, monobasic]

Monopril tablets ℞ *antihypertensive; angiotensin-converting enzyme (ACE) inhibitor; adjunctive treatment for congestive heart failure (CHF)* [fosinopril sodium] 10, 20, 40 mg

Monopril-HCT tablets ℞ *combination angiotensin-converting enzyme (ACE) inhibitor and diuretic for hypertension* [fosinopril sodium; hydrochlorothiazide] 10•12.5, 20•12.5 mg

monosodium p-aminohippurate [see: aminohippurate sodium]

monosodium 4-aminosalicylate dihydrate [see: aminosalicylate sodium]

monosodium carbonate [see: sodium bicarbonate]

monosodium D-gluconate [see: sodium gluconate]

monosodium D-thyroxine hydrate [see: dextrothyroxine sodium]

monosodium glutamate NF *flavoring agent; perfume*

monosodium L-ascorbate [see: sodium ascorbate]

monosodium L-thyroxine hydrate [see: levothyroxine sodium]

monosodium phosphate dihydrate [see: sodium phosphate, monobasic]

monosodium phosphate monohydrate [see: sodium phosphate, monobasic]

monosodium salicylate [see: sodium salicylate]

monosodium sulfite [see: sodium bisulfite]

Monospot slide test for professional use ℞ *in vitro diagnostic aid for mononucleosis*

monostearin [see: glyceryl monostearate]

Monosticon Dri-Dot slide test for professional use ℞ *in vitro diagnostic aid for mononucleosis*

monosulfiram BAN [also: sulfiram]

Mono-Sure slide test for professional use ℞ *in vitro diagnostic aid for mononucleosis*

Mono-Test slide test for professional use ℞ *in vitro diagnostic aid for mononucleosis*

monothioglycerol NF *preservative*

Monotropa uniflora medicinal herb [see: fit root]

Monovial (trademarked packaging form) *single-use vial with transfer needle set*

monoxerutin INN

monoxychlorosene *germicidal mouthwash*

Monsel solution [see: ferric subsulfate]

montelukast sodium USAN *leukotriene receptor antagonist (LTRA) for allergic rhinitis, exercise-induced bronchoconstriction (EIB), and the prophylaxis and long-term treatment of asthma* (base=96%)

monteplase INN ☑ Mynate Plus

montirelin INN

montmorillonite (redmond clay) *natural remedy for bug bites and stings and other skin problems*

Montreal BCG vaccine [see: BCG vaccine]

Monurol granules for oral solution ℞ *broad-spectrum bactericidal antibiotic for urinary tract infections* [fosfomycin tromethamine] 3 g/pkt.

moose elm *medicinal herb* [see: slippery elm]

8-MOP capsules ℞ *systemic psoralens for psoriasis, repigmentation of idiopathic vitiligo, and cutaneous T-cell lymphoma (CTCL); used to increase tolerance to sunlight and enhance pigmentation* [methoxsalen] 10 mg

MOP (mechlorethamine, Oncovin, procarbazine) *chemotherapy protocol for pediatric brain tumors*

8-MOP (8-methoxypsoralen) [see: methoxsalen]

moperone INN

mopidamol INN

mopidralazine INN

MOPP (mechlorethamine, Oncovin, procarbazine, prednisone) *chemotherapy protocol for Hodgkin lymphoma and brain cancer (medulloblastoma)*

MOPP/ABV (mechlorethamine, Oncovin, procarbazine, prednisone; Adriamycin, bleomycin, vinblastine) *chemotherapy protocol for Hodgkin lymphoma*

MOPP/ABVD (alternating cycles of MOPP and ABVD) *chemotherapy protocol for Hodgkin lymphoma* [also known as: ABVD/MOPP]

moprolol INN

moquizone INN

MORAb-009 *investigational (orphan) monoclonal antibody to mesothelin for the treatment of pancreatic cancer*

moracizine INN, BAN *antiarrhythmic* [also: moricizine]

morantel INN *anthelmintic* [also: morantel tartrate]

morantel tartrate USAN *anthelmintic* [also: morantel]

Moranyl (available only from the Centers for Disease Control) (discontinued 2011) ℞ *antiparasitic for African trypanosomiasis and onchocerciasis* [suramin sodium] ② Marinol

morazone INN, BAN ② Marezine

morclofone INN

More-Dophilus powder OTC *natural intestinal bacteria; probiotic; dietary supplement; fever blister treatment; not generally regarded as safe and effective as an antidiarrheal* [Lactobacillus acidophilus] *4 billion CFU/g*

morforex INN

moricizine USAN *antiarrhythmic* [also: moracizine]

moricizine HCl *antiarrhythmic for severe ventricular arrhythmias*

morinamide INN

Morinda citrifolia *medicinal herb* [see: noni]

Mormon tea *medicinal herb* [see: ephedra]

morniflumate USAN, INN *anti-inflammatory*

morning glory (Ipomoea violacea) *seeds contain lysergic acid amide, chemically similar to LSD, which produce hallucinations when ingested as a street drug* [see also: LSD]

morocromen INN

moroxydine INN, BAN

morphazinamide [see: morinamide]

morpheridine INN, BAN

morphine BAN *narcotic analgesic; widely abused as a street drug, which leads to dependence* [also: morphine sulfate] ② myrophine

morphine dinicotinate ester [see: nicomorphine]

Morphine ER extended-release tablets ℞ *narcotic analgesic* [morphine sulfate] *100, 200 mg*

morphine HCl USP *narcotic analgesic preferred in Germany and England; often abused as a street drug, which leads to dependence*

morphine sulfate (MS) USP *narcotic analgesic preferred in the U.S.; intraspinal microinfusion for intractable chronic pain (orphan); often abused as a street drug, which leads to dependence* [also: morphine] *15, 30, 60, 100, 200 mg oral; 2, 4, 20 mg/mL oral; 0.5, 1, 2, 4, 5, 8, 10, 15, 25, 50 mg/mL injection; 5, 10, 20, 30 mg rectal*

Morphine Sulfate in 5% Dextrose IV, IM, or subcu injection ℞ *narcotic analgesic* [morphine sulfate] *1 mg/mL*

4-morpholinecarboximidoylguanidine [see: moroxydine]

2-morpholinoethylrutin [see: ethoxazorutoside]

3-morpholinosydnoneimine [see: linsidomine]

morpholinyl succinimide [see: morsuximide]

morpholinylethyl morphine [see: pholcodine]

morrhuate sodium USP *sclerosing agent for varicose veins* [also: sodium morrhuate] 50 mg/mL injection

morsuximide INN

morsydomine [see: molsidomine]

mortification root *medicinal herb* [see: marsh mallow]

Morton Salt Substitute; Morton Seasoned Salt Substitute OTC *salt substitute; electrolyte replenisher* [potassium chloride] 64 mEq K/5 g; 56 mEq K/5 g

Morus nigra; M. rubra medicinal herb [see: mulberry]

Moschus moschiferus natural remedy [see: deer musk]

Mosco topical liquid OTC *keratolytic* [salicylic acid in flexible collodion] 17.6%

mosquito plant *medicinal herb* [see: pennyroyal]

motapizone INN

motavizumab *investigational (NDA filed) monoclonal antibody to respiratory syncytial virus (RSV)*

MOTC (methyleneoxytetracycline) [see: methacycline]

motesanib *investigational (Phase III) antineoplastic for non–squamous cell lung cancer*

motexafin gadolinium USAN *investigational (NDA filed, orphan) radiosensitizer for non-small cell lung cancer patients with brain metastases*

motexafin lutetium USAN *radiosensitizer*

mother of thyme *medicinal herb* [see: thyme]

motherwort (*Leonurus cardiaca*) flowering tops and leaves *medicinal herb used as an antispasmodic, astringent, calmative, cardiac, emmenagogue, hepatic, laxative, nervine, and stomachic*

Motofen tablets ℞ *antidiarrheal* [difenoxin HCl; atropine sulfate] 1•0.025 mg

motrazepam INN

motretinide USAN, INN *keratolytic*

Motrin, Children's chewable tablets, oral suspension OTC *analgesic; antipyretic; nonsteroidal anti-inflammatory drug (NSAID) for minor aches and pains* [ibuprofen] 50 mg; 100 mg/5 mL

Motrin, Infants' oral drops OTC *analgesic; antipyretic; nonsteroidal anti-inflammatory drug (NSAID) for minor aches and pains* [ibuprofen] 40 mg/mL

Motrin, Junior Strength tablets, chewable tablets OTC *analgesic; antipyretic; nonsteroidal anti-inflammatory drug (NSAID) for minor aches and pains* [ibuprofen] 100 mg

Motrin Children's Cold oral suspension OTC *decongestant; analgesic; antipyretic* [pseudoephedrine HCl; ibuprofen] 15•100 mg/5 mL

Motrin IB tablets, gelcaps OTC *analgesic; antipyretic; antiarthritic; nonsteroidal anti-inflammatory drug (NSAID) for mild to moderate pain, migraine headaches, and primary dysmenorrhea* [ibuprofen] 200 mg

Motrin Migraine Pain caplets OTC *analgesic; antipyretic; nonsteroidal anti-inflammatory drug (NSAID) for mild to moderate pain of migraine headaches* [ibuprofen] 200 mg

mountain ash (*Sorbus americana; S. aucuparia*) fruit *medicinal herb used as an aperient, astringent, and diuretic*

mountain balm *medicinal herb* [see: yerba santa]

mountain box; mountain cranberry *medicinal herb* [see: uva ursi]

mountain laurel (*Kalmia latifolia*) leaves *medicinal herb used as an astringent and sedative*

mountain mahogany *medicinal herb* [see: birch]

mountain mint *medicinal herb* [see: marjoram; Oswego tea]

mountain snuff; mountain tobacco *medicinal herb* [see: arnica]

mountain sorrel *medicinal herb* [see: wood sorrel]

mountain strawberry *medicinal herb* [see: strawberry]

mountain sumach *medicinal herb* [see: sumach]

mountain sweet *medicinal herb* [see: New Jersey tea]

mountain tea *medicinal herb* [see: wintergreen]

mouse ear *(Hieracium pilosella)* plant *medicinal herb used as an astringent, cholagogue, and diuretic* 🔾 MSIR

MouthKote throat spray OTC *saliva substitute*

MouthKote O/R mouthwash OTC *mild anesthetic; antipruritic; counterirritant; antiseptic* [menthol; benzyl alcohol]

MouthKote O/R oral solution OTC *topical antihistamine* [diphenhydramine] 1.25%

mouthroot *medicinal herb* [see: gold thread]

Movectro oral (available in Russia) *investigational (orphan) disease-modifying agent for chronic progressive multiple sclerosis* [cladribine]

moveltipril INN

MoviPrep oral liquid ℞ *pre-procedure bowel evacuant for colonoscopy* [PEG 3350; sodium sulfate; sodium chloride; potassium chloride; ascorbic acid; sodium ascorbate] 100•7.5• 2.691•1.015•4.7•5.9 g/2 L dose

moxadolen INN

moxalactam disodium USAN, USP *cephalosporin antibiotic* [also: latamoxef]

moxantrazole [now: teloxantrone HCl]

moxaprindine INN

moxastine INN

Moxatag extended-release film-coated tablets ℞ *aminopenicillin antibiotic* [amoxicillin (as trihydrate)] 775 mg

moxaverine INN, BAN

moxazocine USAN, INN *analgesic; antitussive*

moxestrol INN

Moxeza Drop-Tainer (eye drops) ℞ *broad-spectrum fluoroquinolone antibiotic* [moxifloxacin (as HCl)] 0.5%

moxicoumone INN

moxidectin USAN, INN *veterinary antiparasitic*

moxifloxacin HCl USAN *broad-spectrum fluoroquinolone antibiotic*

moxilubant maleate USAN *leukotriene B_4 receptor antagonist for rheumatoid arthritis and psoriasis*

moxipraquine INN, BAN

moxiraprine INN

moxisylyte INN [also: thymoxamine]

moxnidazole USAN, INN *antiprotozoal (Trichomonas)*

moxonidine USAN, INN *centrally acting sympatholytic for hypertension, congestive heart failure, and type 2 diabetes*

M-oxy tablets ℞ *narcotic analgesic* [oxycodone HCl] 5 mg 🔾 Maox

Mozobil subcu injection ℞ *stem cell mobilizer for autologous stem cell transplants in patients with non-Hodgkin lymphoma and multiple myeloma* [plerixafor] 20 mg/mL

MP (melphalan, prednisone) *chemotherapy protocol for multiple myeloma*

MP (mitoxantrone, prednisone) *chemotherapy protocol for prostate cancer*

4-MP (4-methylpyrazole) [see: fomepizole]

6-MP (6-mercaptopurine) [see: mercaptopurine]

MPA (medroxyprogesterone acetate) [q.v.]

MPA (mycophenolic acid) [q.v.]

MPF [see: Mucoprotective Factor]

MPH (methylphenidate HCl) [q.v.]

MPIF-1 (myeloid progenitor inhibitory factor 1) [see: mirostipen]

MPL (melphalan) [q.v.]

MRV (mixed respiratory vaccine) [q.v.]

MS (magnesium salicylate) [q.v.]

MS (morphine sulfate) [q.v.]

MS Contin controlled-release tablets ℞ *narcotic analgesic; preoperative sedative and anxiolytic* [morphine sulfate] 15, 30, 60, 100, 200 mg

MSIR oral solution, oral concentrate ℞ *narcotic analgesic; preoperative sedative and anxiolytic* [morphine sulfate] 10, 20 mg/5 mL; 20 mg/mL 🔾 mouse ear

MSM (methylsulfonylmethane) *natural source of sulfur; promotes an increase in collagen and the endogenous antioxidant glutathione*

MSTA (Mumps Skin Test Antigen) intradermal injection (discontinued 2008) ℞ *diagnostic aid to assess immune system competency (not effective in testing immunity to mumps virus)* [mumps skin test antigen] 0.1 mL (4 U/0.1 mL)

MT6 (mercaptomerin) [q.v.]

M·Tabs (trademarked dosage form) *orally disintegrating tablets*

MTC (mitomycin C) [see: mitomycin]

MTC-DOX (magnetically targeted carrier with doxorubicin) *investigational (orphan) delivery system for hepatocellular carcinoma*

M.T.E.-4; M.T.E.-4 Concentrated; M.T.E.-5; M.T.E.-5 Concentrated; M.T.E.-6; M.T.E.-6 Concentrated; M.T.E.-7 IV injection (discontinued 2008) ℞ *intravenous nutritional therapy* [multiple trace elements (metals)]

L-5-MTHF (L-5-methyltetrahydrofolate) [see: levomefolate; L-methylfolate]

mTHPC [see: temoporfin]

mTOR (mammalian target of rapamycin) *a class of antineoplastics that target the same receptors as* **rapamycin** *(now* **sirolimus**)*, a natural bacteriaderived antifungal drug, but with greater cytotoxic effect*

MTP-PE (muramyl tripeptide phosphatidylethanolamine) [see: mifamurtide]

MTX (methotrexate) [q.v.]

MTX/6-MP (methotrexate, mercaptopurine) [with or without leucovorin rescue] *chemotherapy protocol for acute lymphocytic leukemia (ALL); ongoing continuation protocol* [also see: 1DMTX; 1DMTX/6-MP (first-day initiation protocols)]

MTX/6-MP/VP (methotrexate, mercaptopurine, vincristine, prednisone) *chemotherapy protocol for acute lymphocytic leukemia (ALL)*

MTX-CDDPAdr (methotrexate, CDDP, Adriamycin) [with leucovorin rescue] *chemotherapy protocol for pediatric osteosarcoma*

Mucinex extended-release tablets, dual-release tablets OTC *expectorant* [guaifenesin] 600, 1200 mg; 600 mg (100 mg immediate release, 500 mg extended release)

Mucinex Children's oral liquid OTC *expectorant* [guaifenesin] 100 mg/5 mL

Mucinex Cold for Kids oral liquid OTC *expectorant; decongestant* [guaifenesin; phenylephrine HCl] 100•2.5 mg/5 mL

Mucinex Cough for Kids oral liquid OTC *expectorant; antitussive* [guaifenesin; dextromethorphan hydrobromide] 100•5 mg/5 mL

Mucinex Cough Mini-Melts for Kids oral granules OTC *expectorant; antitussive* [guaifenesin; dextromethorphan hydrobromide] 100•5 mg/packet

Mucinex D extended-release tablets OTC *expectorant; decongestant* [guaifenesin; pseudoephedrine HCl] 600•60, 1200•120 mg

Mucinex DM extended-release tablets OTC *expectorant; antitussive* [guaifenesin; dextromethorphan hydrobromide] 600•30, 1200•60 mg

Mucinex Mini-Melts Children's; Mucinex Mini-Melts Junior oral granules (name changed to **Mucinex Mini-Melts for Kids** in 2009)

Mucinex Mini-Melts for Kids oral granules OTC *expectorant* [guaifenesin] 50, 100 mg/packet

Mucinex with Codeine extended-release tablets *investigational (NDA filed) expectorant; narcotic antitussive* [guaifenesin; codeine phosphate] 600•30, 1200•60 mg

Muco-Fen DM sustained-release tablets (discontinued 2007) ℞ *antitussive; expectorant* [dextromethorphan hydrobromide; guaifenesin] 60•1000 mg

mucoid exopolysaccharide *Pseudomonas* **hyperimmune globulin (MEPIG)** *investigational (orphan) for the prevention and treatment of pulmonary infections of cystic fibrosis*

mucolytics *a class of respiratory inhalant drugs that destroy or inhibit mucin*

Mucomyst solution for nebulization or intratracheal instillation (discontinued 2011) ℞ *mucolytic* [acetylcysteine sodium] 10%, 20%

Mucoprotective Factor (MPF) (trademarked ingredient) *aromatic flavored syrup* [eriodictyon]

MucusRelief tablets OTC *expectorant* [guaifenesin] 400 mg

MucusRelief DM caplets OTC *antitussive; expectorant* [dextromethorphan hydrobromide; guaifenesin] 20•400 mg

MucusRelief Sinus tablets OTC *decongestant; expectorant* [phenylephrine HCl; guaifenesin] 10•400 mg

Mudrane tablets (discontinued 2007) ℞ *antiasthmatic; bronchodilator; decongestant; expectorant; sedative* [aminophylline; ephedrine HCl; potassium iodide; phenobarbital] 111•16•195•8 mg ⑫ Midrin

Mudrane GG tablets (discontinued 2007) ℞ *antiasthmatic; decongestant; expectorant; sedative* [theophylline; ephedrine HCl; guaifenesin; phenobarbital] 111•16•100•8 mg

Mudrane GG-2 tablets (discontinued 2007) ℞ *antiasthmatic; bronchodilator; expectorant* [theophylline; guaifenesin] 111•100 mg

MuGard oral rinse ℞ *mucus membrane protectant*

mugwort (Artemisia vulgaris) root and plant *medicinal herb used as a diaphoretic, emmenagogue, and laxative*

muira puama (Ptychopetalum olacoides) stem *medicinal herb used as an aphrodisiac and treatment for impotence in South America; clinical trials in France confirm these effects*

mulberry (Morus nigra; M. rubra) bark *medicinal herb used as an anthelmintic and cathartic*

mullein (Verbascum nigrum; V. phlomoides; V. thapsiforme; V. thapsus) plant *medicinal herb for asthma, bleeding in bowel and lungs, bronchitis, pain, bruises, cough, croup, diarrhea, hemorrhoids, earache, gout, insomnia, lymphatic system, nervousness, pleurisy, sinus congestion, and tuberculosis* ⑫ Myolin

Multaq film-coated tablets ℞ *antiarrhythmic for atrial fibrillation and atrial flutter* [dronedarone (as HCl)] 400 mg

MulTE-Pak-4; MulTE-Pak-5 IV injection (discontinued 2010) ℞ *intravenous nutritional therapy* [multiple trace elements (metals)]

Multi 75 timed-release tablets (discontinued 2008) OTC *vitamin/mineral supplement* [multiple vitamins & minerals; folic acid; biotin] ±•0.4•⦥ mg ⑫ Maolate

Multi Vit with Iron drops OTC *vitamin/iron supplement* [multiple vitamins; iron] ±•10 mg/mL

Multi VitaBets with Fluoride chewable tablets OTC *vitamin supplement; dental caries preventative* [multiple vitamins; fluoride; folic acid] ±•250•300 mcg

Multi Vitamin Concentrate injection ℞ *parenteral vitamin supplement* [multiple vitamins]

Multi-Day Multivitamin Plus Iron tablets OTC *vitamin/iron supplement* [multiple vitamins; iron (as ferrous fumarate); folic acid] ±•18•0.4 mg

Multi-Day plus Minerals tablets OTC *vitamin/mineral/calcium/iron supplement* [multiple vitamins & minerals; calcium (as carbonate and dicalcium phosphate); iron (as ferrous fumarate); folic acid; biotin] ±•162•18•0.4•0.03 mg

Multi-Day with Beta-Carotene tablets OTC *vitamin supplement* [multiple vitamins; folic acid] ±•400 mcg

Multi-Day with Calcium and Extra Iron tablets (discontinued 2008) OTC *vitamin/calcium/iron supplement* [multiple vitamins; calcium; iron; folic acid] ±•⦥•27•0.4 mg

Multifol; Multifol Plus caplets ℞ *vitamin/calcium/iron supplement* [multiple vitamins; calcium (as carbonate); iron (as ferrous fumarate); folic acid] ±•125•65•1 mg; ±•100•65•1 mg

Multigen film-coated tablets ℞ *hematinic* [iron; vitamin B$_{12}$; vitamin C; desiccated stomach substance; succinic acid] 70•0.01•152•50•75 mg

MultiHance IV injection ℞ *paramagnetic contrast agent to enhance MRIs of the brain, spine, and other CNS tissue* [gadobenate dimeglumine] 529 mg/mL

Multilex film-coated tablets OTC *vitamin/mineral supplement* [multiple vitamins & minerals]

Multilex T & M tablets OTC *vitamin/mineral/iron supplement* [multiple vitamins & minerals; iron (as ferrous fumarate)] ±•15 mg

Multilyte-20; Multilyte-40 IV admixture ℞ *intravenous electrolyte therapy* [combined electrolyte solution] ☑ malotilate

Multi-Mineral tablets (discontinued 2008) OTC *mineral supplement* [multiple minerals]

Multinatal Plus film-coated tablets ℞ *vitamin/mineral/calcium/iron supplement* [multiple vitamins & minerals; calcium; iron; folic acid] ±•200•30•1 mg

Multiple Trace Element Neonatal IV injection (discontinued 2011) ℞ *intravenous nutritional therapy* [multiple trace elements (metals)]

Multiple Trace Element with Selenium; Multiple Trace Element with Selenium Concentrated IV injection (discontinued 2010) ℞ *intravenous nutritional therapy* [multiple trace elements (metals)]

Multistix; Multistix 2; Multistix 7; Multistix 8 SG; Multistix 9; Multistix 9 SG; Multistix 10 SG reagent strips OTC *in vitro diagnostic aid for multiple urine products*

Multistix PRO reagent strips for professional use ℞ *in vitro diagnostic aid for urine protein/creatinine ratio*

Multistix SG reagent strips (discontinued 2008) OTC *in vitro diagnostic aid for multiple urine products*

Multitrace-4; Multitrace-4 Concentrate; Multitrace-4 Neonatal; Multitrace-4 Pediatric; Multitrace-5; Multitrace-5 Concentrate IV injection ℞ *intravenous nutritional therapy* [multiple trace elements (metals)]

Multi-Vit with Fluoride oral drops ℞ *vitamin supplement; dental caries preventative* [multiple vitamins; fluoride] ±•0.25 mg/mL

multivitamin infusion, neonatal formula *investigational (orphan) total parenteral nutrition for very low birthweight infants*

multivitamin infusion without vitamin K *parenteral vitamin supplement for patients receiving anticoagulant therapy (orphan)*

Multivitamin Iron and Fluoride oral drops ℞ *vitamin/iron supplement; dental caries preventative* [multiple vitamins; iron (as ferrous sulfate); fluoride] ±•10•? mg/mL

Multi-Vitamin Mineral with Beta-Carotene tablets (discontinued 2008) OTC *vitamin/mineral/iron supplement* [multiple vitamins & minerals; iron (as ferrous fumarate); folic acid; biotin] ±•27•0.4•0.45 mg

Multi-Vitamin with Fluoride chewable tablets OTC *vitamin supplement; dental caries preventative* [multiple vitamins; fluoride; folic acid] ±•250•300, ±•500•300, ±•1000•300 mcg

Multivitamin with Fluoride pediatric oral drops (discontinued 2008) ℞ *vitamin supplement; dental caries preventative* [multiple vitamins; fluoride] ±•250, ±•500 mcg/mL

Multivitamins with A, B, D, E and K Plus Zinc chewable tablets, softgels, oral drops OTC *vitamin supplement* [multiple vitamins; folic acid; biotin] ±•200•100 mcg; ±•200•100 mcg; ±•0•15 mcg

Multivite with FL chewable tablets OTC *vitamin supplement; dental caries preventative* [multiple vitamins; fluoride; folic acid] ±•500•300 mcg

Mulvidren-F Softabs (pediatric chewable tablets) (discontinued 2008) R *vitamin supplement; dental caries preventative* [multiple vitamins; fluoride] ≟•1 mg

mumps skin test antigen (MSTA) USP *diagnostic aid to assess immune system competency*

mumps vaccine [see: mumps virus vaccine, inactivated]

mumps virus vaccine, inactivated NF

mumps virus vaccine, live USP *active immunizing agent for mumps*

Mumpsvax powder for subcu injection (discontinued 2011) R *mumps vaccine* [mumps virus vaccine, live] 0.5 mL

mupirocin USAN, INN, BAN *topical antibiotic* 2% topical ⑨ Meprozine

mupirocin calcium USAN *topical antibiotic* (base=93%)

muplestim USAN *progenitor cell stimulator for neutropenia and thrombocytopenia*

murabutide INN

muraglitazar *peroxisome proliferator–activated receptor (PPAR)–alpha and –gamma agonist; antidiabetic to control blood glucose levels, lower triglycerides, and raise HDL*

muramyl tripeptide phosphatidylethanolamine (MTP-PE) [see: mifamurtide]

Murine eye drops OTC *moisturizer/lubricant* [polyvinyl alcohol] 0.5% ⑨ Mirena

Murine Ear ear drops OTC *cerumenolytic to emulsify and disperse ear wax; antiseptic* [carbamide peroxide; alcohol] 6.5%•6.3%

Murine Earigate spray OTC *ear wash* [purified water]

murine monoclonal antibodies *antibodies cloned from a single mouse or rat cell* [see: monoclonal antibodies]

Murine Plus eye drops OTC *decongestant; vasoconstrictor; moisturizer/lubricant* [tetrahydrozoline HCl; polyvinyl alcohol; povidone] 0.05%•0.5%•0.6%

Muro 128 eye drops, ophthalmic ointment OTC *corneal edema-reducing agent* [sodium chloride (hypertonic saline solution)] 2%, 5%; 5%

murocainide INN

Murocel eye drops OTC *moisturizer/lubricant* [methylcellulose] 1% ⑨ Mersol

Murocoll-2 eye drops (discontinued 2010) R *cycloplegic; mydriatic* [scopolamine hydrobromide; phenylephrine HCl] 0.3%•10%

murodermin INN

muromonab-CD3 USAN, INN *monoclonal antibody to CD3; immunosuppressant for renal, hepatic, and cardiac transplants; also used for graft-versus-host disease following bone marrow transplants*

Muroptic-5 eye drops OTC *corneal edema-reducing agent* [sodium chloride (hypertonic saline solution)] 5%

muscarinic agonists *a class of investigational analgesics*

Muse single-use intraurethral suppository R *vasodilator for erectile dysfunction* [alprostadil] 125, 150, 500, 1000 mcg

musk *natural remedy* [see: deer musk]

mustaral oil [see: allyl isothiocyanate]

mustard (Brassica alba; Sinapis alba) seeds and oil *medicinal herb for indigestion and liver and lung disorders; also used as an appetizer, diuretic, emetic, and soak for aching feet, arthritis, and rheumatism*

mustard oil [see: allyl isothiocyanate]

Mustargen powder for IV or intracavitary injection R *nitrogen mustard–type alkylating antineoplastic for various leukemias, lymphomas, and carcinomas, polycythemia vera, and mycosis fungoides (orphan)* [mechlorethamine HCl] 10 mg

Musterole Deep Strength Rub OTC *analgesic; mild anesthetic; antipruritic; counterirritant* [methyl salicylate; methyl nicotinate; menthol] 30%•0.5%•3%

Musterole Extra Strength OTC *mild topical anesthetic; antipruritic; counterirritant* [camphor; menthol] 5%•3%

mustine BAN *nitrogen mustard-type alkylating antineoplastic* [also: mechlorethamine HCl; chlormethine; nitrogen mustard N-oxide HCl]

mustine HCl [see: mechlorethamine HCl]

Mutamycin powder for IV injection (discontinued 2008) R *antibiotic antineoplastic for disseminated adenocarcinoma of the stomach or pancreas* [mitomycin] 5, 20, 40 mg

muzolimine USAN, INN *diuretic; antihypertensive* ⑦ mesalamine; mezilamine

MV (mitomycin, vinblastine) *chemotherapy protocol for breast cancer*

MV (mitoxantrone, VePesid) *chemotherapy protocol for acute myelocytic leukemia (ALL)*

MVAC; M-VAC (methotrexate, vinblastine, Adriamycin, cisplatin) *chemotherapy protocol for bladder cancer* ⑦ Mavik

M-Vax *investigational (Phase III, orphan) theraccine for postsurgical stage III malignant melanoma* [autologous DNP-conjugated tumor vaccine]

M.V.I. Neonatal IV infusion *investigational (orphan) total parenteral nutrition for very low birthweight infants* [multivitamin infusion, neonatal formula]

M.V.I. Pediatric injection R *parenteral vitamin supplement* [multiple vitamins; folic acid; biotin] ±•140•20 mcg/5 mL

M.V.I.-12 injection R *parenteral vitamin supplement without vitamin K for patients receiving anticoagulant therapy (orphan)* [multiple vitamins; folic acid; biotin] ±•400•60 mcg/5 mL

M.V.M. capsules (discontinued 2008) OTC *vitamin/mineral/iron supplement* [multiple vitamins & minerals; iron; folic acid; biotin] ±•3.6 mg•0.08 mg•160 mcg

MVP (mitomycin, vinblastine, Platinol) *chemotherapy protocol for non–small cell lung cancer (NSCLC)*

MVPP (mechlorethamine, vinblastine, procarbazine, prednisone/prednisolone) *chemotherapy protocol for Hodgkin lymphoma* (note: prednisone is preferred in the U.S.; prednisolone is preferred in the U.K.)

Mx-dnG1 retroviral vector *investigational (NDA filed, orphan) tumor-targeted gene therapy for pancreatic cancer*

Myadec tablets OTC *vitamin/mineral/calcium/iron supplement* [multiple vitamins & minerals; calcium (as dicalcium phosphate); iron (as ferrous fumarate); folic acid; biotin] ±•162•18•0.4•0.03 mg

Myambutol film-coated tablets R *tuberculostatic* [ethambutol HCl] 100, 400 mg

Mycamine powder for IV infusion R *systemic echinocandin antifungal for prophylaxis and treatment of esophageal candidiasis and prophylaxis of candidiasis in patients undergoing hemopoietic stem cell transplantation (HSCT)* [micafungin sodium] 50, 100 mg/dose

Mycelex troches R *antifungal; oral candidiasis prophylaxis or treatment* [clotrimazole] 10 mg

Mycelex-3 vaginal cream in prefilled applicator OTC *antifungal* [butoconazole nitrate] 2%

Mycelex-7 vaginal cream, combination pack (vaginal inserts + cream) OTC *antifungal* [clotrimazole] 1%; 100 mg + 1%

Mycifradin Sulfate oral solution R *aminoglycoside antibiotic* [neomycin sulfate] 125 mg/5 mL

Myci-GC oral liquid R *narcotic antitussive; expectorant* [codeine phosphate; guaifenesin] 10•100 mg/5 mL

Mycinaire Saline Mist nasal spray OTC *nasal moisturizer* [sodium chloride (saline solution)] 0.65%

Mycinette throat spray OTC *mild mucous membrane anesthetic; antiseptic; astringent* [phenol; alum] 1.4%•0.3%

Mycinettes lozenges OTC *mucous membrane anesthetic* [benzocaine] 15 mg

"mycins" *brief term for a class of antibiotics derived from various strains of the fungus-like bacteria* Streptomyces, *or their synthetic analogues, whose generic names end in "mycin," such as lincomycin* [properly called: aminoglycosides]

Myci-Spray nasal spray OTC *decongestant; antihistamine* [phenylephrine HCl; pyrilamine maleate] 0.25%•0.15%

Mycobacterium avium **sensitin RS-10** *investigational (orphan) diagnostic aid for* Mycobacterium avium *infection in immunocompromised patients*

Myco-Biotic II cream ℞ *corticosteroidal anti-inflammatory; antibiotic; antifungal* [triamcinolone acetonide; neomycin sulfate; nystatin] 0.1%•0.5%•100 000 U per g

Mycobutin capsules ℞ *antiviral/antibacterial for prevention of* Mycobacterium avium *complex (MAC) in advanced HIV patients (orphan)* [rifabutin] 150 mg

Mycocide NS topical solution OTC *antiseptic* [benzalkonium chloride]

Mycogen II cream, ointment ℞ *corticosteroidal anti-inflammatory; antifungal* [triamcinolone acetonide; nystatin] 0.1%•100 000 U per g ⧉ Macugen

Mycograb *investigational (Phase III, orphan) for invasive candidiasis and other severe fungal infections* [efungumab]

Mycolog-II cream, ointment ℞ *corticosteroidal anti-inflammatory; antifungal* [triamcinolone acetonide; nystatin] 0.1%•100 000 U per g

Myconel cream ℞ *corticosteroidal anti-inflammatory; antifungal* [triamcinolone acetonide; nystatin] 0.1%•100 000 U per g ⧉ mequinol; Micanol

mycophenolate mofetil USAN *purine biosynthesis inhibitor; immunosuppressant for allogenic renal, hepatic, or cardiac transplants (orphan); investigational (orphan) for pemphigus vulgaris* 250, 500 mg oral

mycophenolate mofetil HCl USAN *purine biosynthesis inhibitor; immuno-*

suppressant for allogenic renal, hepatic, or cardiac transplants

mycophenolate sodium [see: mycophenolic acid]

mycophenolic acid (MPA) USAN, INN *immunosuppressant for allogenic renal transplants*

Mycostatin cream, ointment, powder ℞ *antifungal* [nystatin] 100 000 U/g

Mycostatin film-coated tablets ℞ *systemic antifungal* [nystatin] 500 000 U

Mycostatin Pastilles (troches) ℞ *antifungal; oral candidiasis treatment* [nystatin] 200 000 U

Myco-Triacet II cream, ointment ℞ *corticosteroidal anti-inflammatory; antifungal* [triamcinolone acetonide; nystatin] 0.1%•100 000 U per g

mydeton [see: tolperisone]

MyDex extended-release caplets ℞ *decongestant; expectorant* [phenylephrine HCl; guaifenesin] 30•900 mg

Mydfrin 2.5% eye drops ℞ *decongestant; vasoconstrictor; mydriatic* [phenylephrine HCl] 2.5%

Mydral eye drops ℞ *cycloplegic; mydriatic* [tropicamide] 0.5%, 1% ⧉ Medrol

Mydriacyl Drop-Tainers (eye drops) ℞ *cycloplegic; mydriatic* [tropicamide] 1%

mydriatics *a class of drugs that cause the pupil of the eye to dilate*

myelin *investigational (orphan) for multiple sclerosis*

myeloid progenitor inhibitory factor 1 (MPIF-1) [see: mirostipen]

myelosan [see: busulfan]

myfadol INN

Myferon 150 capsules OTC *iron supplement* [iron (as polysaccharide-iron complex)] 150 mg

Myfortic film-coated delayed-release tablets ℞ *immunosuppressant for allogenic renal transplant* [mycophenolic acid] 180, 360 mg

Mygel; Mygel II oral suspension OTC *antacid; antiflatulent* [aluminum hydroxide; magnesium hydroxide; simethicone] 200•200•20 mg/5 mL; 400•400•40 mg/5 mL

MyHist-DM oral liquid ℞ *antitussive; antihistamine; sleep aid; decongestant* [dextromethorphan hydrobromide; pyrilamine maleate; phenylephrine HCl] 15•12.5•7.5 mg/5 mL

MyHist-PD oral liquid ℞ *decongestant; antihistamine; sleep aid* [phenylephrine 7.5•2•12.5 mg/5 mL

Mykrox tablets (discontinued 2008) ℞ *antihypertensive; diuretic* [metolazone] 0.5 mg

Mylagen gelcaps OTC *antacid* [calcium carbonate; magnesium carbonate] 311•232 mg

Mylagen; Mylagen II oral liquid OTC *antacid; antiflatulent* [aluminum hydroxide; magnesium hydroxide; simethicone] 200•200•20 mg/5 mL; 400•400•40 mg/5 mL

Mylanta lozenges OTC *antacid* [calcium carbonate] 600 mg

Mylanta oral liquid OTC *antacid; antiflatulent* [aluminum hydroxide; magnesium hydroxide; simethicone] 200•200•20, 400•400•40 mg/5 mL

Mylanta, Children's oral liquid, chewable tablets OTC *antacid; calcium supplement* [calcium (as carbonate)] 160 mg/5 mL (400 mg/5 mL); 160 mg (400 mg)

Mylanta Antacid gelcaps OTC *antacid* [calcium carbonate; magnesium hydroxide] 550•125 mg

Mylanta Gas chewable tablets, softgels OTC *antiflatulent* [simethicone] 80, 125 mg; 125 mg

Mylanta Ultra chewable tablets OTC *antacid* [calcium carbonate; magnesium hydroxide] 700•300 mg

Myleran film-coated tablets ℞ *alkylating antineoplastic for chronic myelogenous leukemia (CML)* [busulfan] 2 mg ▣ Malarone

Mylicon drops OTC *antiflatulent* [simethicone] 40 mg/0.6 mL

Mylocel film-coated caplets ℞ *antineoplastic for melanoma, squamous cell carcinoma, myelocytic leukemia, and ovarian cancer; also adjunctive therapy for HIV infections* [hydroxyurea] 1000 mg

Mylotarg powder for IV infusion (discontinued 2010) ℞ *monoclonal antibody–targeted chemotherapy agent for acute myeloid leukemia (orphan)* [gemtuzumab ozogamicin] 5 mg

Mynatal capsules (discontinued 2008) ℞ *vitamin/mineral/calcium/iron supplement* [multiple vitamins & minerals; calcium; iron; folic acid; biotin] ≛•300•65•1•0.03 mg ▣ mannitol

Mynatal FC caplets (discontinued 2008) ℞ *vitamin/mineral/calcium/iron supplement* [multiple vitamins & minerals; calcium; iron; folic acid; biotin] ≛•250•60•1•0.03 mg

Mynatal P.N. captabs (discontinued 2008) ℞ *vitamin/calcium/iron supplement* [multiple vitamins; calcium; iron; folic acid] ≛•125•60•1 mg

Mynatal P.N. Forte caplets (discontinued 2008) ℞ *vitamin/mineral/calcium/iron supplement* [multiple vitamins & minerals; calcium; iron; folic acid] ≛•250•60•1 mg

Mynatal Rx caplets (discontinued 2008) ℞ *vitamin/mineral/calcium/iron supplement* [multiple vitamins & minerals; calcium; iron; folic acid; biotin] ≛•200•60•1•0.03 mg

Mynate 90 Plus delayed-release caplets (discontinued 2008) ℞ *vitamin/calcium/iron supplement* [multiple vitamins; calcium; iron; folic acid] ≛•250•90•1 mg ▣ monteplase

Myobloc injection ℞ *neurotoxin complex for the symptomatic treatment of cervical dystonia (orphan)* [rimabotulinumtoxin B] 5000 U/mL

Myochrysine IM injection ℞ *antirheumatic* [gold sodium thiomalate] 50 mg/mL ▣ Migrazone

Myocide NS topical solution OTC *antiseptic* [benzalkonium chloride]

Myoflex Creme OTC *analgesic* [trolamine salicylate] 10%

Myolin IV or IM injection ℞ *skeletal muscle relaxant* [orphenadrine citrate] 30 mg/mL ▣ mullein

Myoscint ⓔ (approved in Europe) *investigational (orphan) imaging agent*

for cardiac necrosis and myocarditis [indium In 111 imciromab pentetate]

Myotrophin injection *investigational (NDA filed, orphan) for amyotrophic lateral sclerosis* [mecasermin]

Myoview ℞ *cardiovascular imaging aid* [technetium Tc 99m tetrofosmin]

Myozyme IV infusion ℞ *enzyme replacement therapy for patients with Pompe disease (glycogenosis type 2; glycogen storage disease type II; GSDII) (orphan)* [alglucosidase alfa] 50 mg ⧉ MSM; MZM

Myphetane DX Cough syrup (discontinued 2009) ℞ *antitussive; antihistamine; decongestant* [dextromethorphan hydrobromide; brompheniramine maleate; pseudoephedrine HCl; alcohol 1%] 10•2•30 mg/5 mL

Myrac film-coated tablets ℞ *tetracycline antibiotic for gram-negative and gram-positive bacteria; antirickettsial* [minocycline (as HCl)] 50, 75, 100 mg

myralact INN, BAN

Myrica cerifera medicinal herb [see: bayberry]

myricodine [see: myrophine]

Myristica fragrans medicinal herb [see: nutmeg; mace]

myristica oil [see: nutmeg oil]

myristyl alcohol NF *stiffening agent*

myristyltrimethylammonium bromide *antiseborrheic*

myrophine INN, BAN ⧉ morphine

Myroxylon balsamum; M. pereirae medicinal herb [see: Peruvian balsam]

myrrh *(Commiphora abssynica; C. molmol; C. myrrha)* seeds *medicinal herb for bad breath, bronchitis, cancer, constipation, hay fever, hemorrhoids, leprosy, lung diseases, mouth and skin sores, sore throat, syphilis, and stimulating menses; also used as an antiseptic and astringent*

myrtecaine INN

Myrtilli fructus medicinal herb [see: bilberry]

myrtle *medicinal herb* [see: periwinkle]

myrtle, bog *medicinal herb* [see: buckbean]

myrtle, wax *medicinal herb* [see: bayberry]

myrtle flag; grass myrtle; sweet myrtle *medicinal herb* [see: calamus]

Mysoline tablets ℞ *anticonvulsant for grand mal, psychomotor, and focal epileptic seizures; also used for essential tremor and benign familial tremor* [primidone] 50, 250 mg

myspamol [see: proquamezine]

Mytelase caplets ℞ *muscle stimulant for myasthenia gravis* [ambenonium chloride] 10 mg

Mytussin AC Cough syrup ℞ *narcotic antitussive; expectorant* [codeine phosphate; guaifenesin; alcohol 3.5%] 10•100 mg/5 mL

Mytussin DAC oral liquid ℞ *narcotic antitussive; decongestant; expectorant* [codeine phosphate; pseudoephedrine HCl; guaifenesin; alcohol 1.7%] 10•30•100 mg/5 mL

Mytussin DM syrup (discontinued 2007) OTC *antitussive; expectorant* [dextromethorphan hydrobromide; guaifenesin] 10•100 mg/5 mL

myuizone [see: thioacetazone; thiacetazone]

My-Vitalife capsules (discontinued 2008) OTC *vitamin/mineral/calcium/ iron supplement* [multiple vitamins & minerals; calcium; iron; folic acid; biotin] ≟•130•27•0.4•0.03 mg

MZM tablets ℞ *carbonic anhydrase inhibitor for glaucoma* [methazolamide] 25, 50 mg

MZM (methazolamide) [q.v.]

M-Zole 3 Combination Pack vaginal suppositories + cream (discontinued 2009) OTC *antifungal* [miconazole nitrate] 200 mg; 2%

M-Zole 7 Dual Pack vaginal suppositories + cream (discontinued 2009) OTC *antifungal* [miconazole nitrate] 100 mg; 2%

N₂ (nitrogen) [q.v.]

N-3 polyunsaturated fatty acids
[see: doconexent; icosapent; omega-3 marine triglycerides]

Na PCA; sodium PCA (sodium pyrrolidone carboxylic acid) [q.v.]

²²Na [see: sodium chloride Na 22]

nabazenil USAN, INN *anticonvulsant*

Nabi-HB IM injection ℞ *immunizing agent following exposure to hepatitis B surface antigen; investigational (orphan) prophylaxis against hepatitis B reinfection in liver transplant patients* [hepatitis B immune globulin] 1, 5 mL

nabilone USAN, INN, BAN *synthetic cannabinoid; antiemetic for nausea and vomiting associated with cancer chemotherapy; restricted use due to the high possibility of disturbing psychomimetic reactions and psychological dependence*

nabitan INN *analgesic* [also: nabitan HCl]

nabitan HCl USAN *analgesic* [also: nabitan]

naboctate INN *antiglaucoma agent; antinauseant* [also: naboctate HCl]

naboctate HCl USAN *antiglaucoma agent; antinauseant* [also: naboctate]

nabumetone USAN, INN, BAN *analgesic; nonsteroidal anti-inflammatory drug (NSAID) for osteoarthritis and rheumatoid arthritis* 500, 750 mg oral

nabutan HCl [now: nabitan HCl]

NAC (N-acetyl cysteine) *natural source of cysteine; promotes an increase in the endogenous antioxidant glutathione* [see also: acetylcysteine]

nacartocin INN

N¹-acetylsulfanilamide [see: sulfacetamide]

NaCl (sodium chloride) [q.v.]

Nacystelyn dry powder for inhalation *investigational (orphan) for cystic fibrosis* [N-acetylcysteinate lysine]

NAD (nicotinamide-adenine dinucleotide) [see: nadide]

nadide USAN, INN *antagonist to alcohol and narcotics*

nadisan [see: carbutamide]

nadolol USAN, USP, INN, BAN *antiadrenergic (beta-blocker); antianginal; antihypertensive; also used for migraine prophylaxis* 20, 40, 80, 120, 160 mg oral

nadolol & bendroflumethiazide *combination beta-blocker and diuretic for hypertension* 40•5, 80•5 mg oral

nadoxolol INN

nadroparin calcium INN, BAN *low molecular weight heparin; anticoagulant/antithrombotic for prevention of deep vein thrombosis (DVT) after surgery, clotting during hemodialysis, unstable angina, and myocardial infarction*

naepaine HCl NF

nafamostat INN *anticoagulant; antifibrinolytic* [also: nafamostat mesylate; nafamostat mesilate]

nafamostat mesilate JAN *anticoagulant; antifibrinolytic* [also: nafamostat mesylate; nafamostat]

nafamostat mesylate USAN *anticoagulant; antifibrinolytic* [also: nafamostat; nafamostat mesilate]

nafarelin INN, BAN *luteinizing hormone-releasing hormone (LHRH) agonist* [also: nafarelin acetate]

nafarelin acetate USAN *luteinizing hormone-releasing hormone (LHRH) agonist for central precocious puberty (orphan) and endometriosis* [also: nafarelin]

nafazatrom INN, BAN

nafcaproic acid INN

nafcillin INN *penicillinase-resistant penicillin antibiotic* [also: nafcillin sodium] Ⓩ naphazoline

nafcillin sodium USAN, USP *penicillinase-resistant penicillin antibiotic* [also: nafcillin] 1, 2, 10 g IV infusion

nafenodone INN

nafenopin USAN, INN *antihyperlipoproteinemic*

nafetolol INN

nafimidone INN *anticonvulsant* [also: nafimidone HCl]

490 nafimidone HCl

nafimidone HCl USAN *anticonvulsant* [also: nafimidone]

nafiverine INN

naflocort USAN, INN *topical adrenocortical steroid*

nafomine INN *muscle relaxant* [also: nafomine malate] ② Novamine

nafomine malate USAN *muscle relaxant* [also: nafomine]

nafoxadol INN

nafoxidine HCl USAN, INN *antiestrogen*

nafronyl oxalate USAN *vasodilator* [also: naftidrofuryl]

naftalofos USAN, INN *veterinary anthelmintic*

naftazone INN, BAN

naftidrofuryl INN *vasodilator* [also: nafronyl oxalate]

naftifine INN, BAN *broad-spectrum antifungal* [also: naftifine HCl]

naftifine HCl USAN *broad-spectrum antifungal; topical treatment for tinea pedis, tinea cruris, and tinea corporis* [also: naftifine]

Naftin cream, gel ℞ *broad-spectrum antifungal for tinea pedis, tinea cruris, and tinea corporis* [naftifine HCl] 1%

naftopidil INN

naftoxate INN

naftypramide INN *antibacterial*

naganol [see: suramin sodium]

NaGHB (sodium gamma hydroxybutyrate) [see: gamma hydroxybutyrate (GHB); sodium oxybate]

Naglazyme IV infusion ℞ *recombinant human enzyme for the treatment of mucopolysaccharidosis VI (MPS VI; Maroteaux-Lamy syndrome) (orphan)* [galsulfase] 1 mg/mL

nagrestipen USAN *stem cell inhibitory protein*

nalazosulfamide [see: salazosulfamide]

nalbuphine INN, BAN *narcotic agonist-antagonist analgesic for moderate to severe pain; adjunct to obstetric and surgical analgesia* [also: nalbuphine HCl]

nalbuphine HCl USAN *narcotic agonist-antagonist analgesic for moderate to severe pain; adjunct to obstetric and*

surgical analgesia [also: nalbuphine] 10, 20 mg/mL injection

Naldecon Senior EX oral liquid OTC *expectorant* [guaifenesin] 200 mg/5 mL

NalDex caplets (discontinued 2009) ℞ *decongestant; antihistamine* [phenylephrine HCl; dexchlorpheniramine maleate] 18.5•3.5 mg

Nalex AC syrup ℞ *narcotic antitussive; antihistamine* [codeine phosphate; brompheniramine maleate] 10•2 mg/5 mL

Nalex Expectorant oral liquid ℞ *narcotic antitussive; decongestant; expectorant* [hydrocodone bitartrate; pseudoephedrine HCl; guaifenesin; alcohol 12.5%] 5•60•200 mg/5 mL

Nalex-A caplets, oral liquid ℞ *decongestant; antihistamine; sleep aid* [phenylephrine HCl; chlorpheniramine maleate; phenyltoloxamine citrate] 20•4•40 mg; 5•2.5•7.5 mg/5 mL

Nalex-A 12 oral suspension ℞ *decongestant; antihistamine; sleep aid* [phenylephrine tannate; chlorpheniramine tannate; pyrilamine tannate] 5•2•12.5 mg/5 mL

Nalex-DH oral liquid ℞ *narcotic antitussive; decongestant* [hydrocodone bitartrate; phenylephrine HCl] 5•10 mg/10 mL

Nalfon Pulvules (capsules) ℞ *analgesic; nonsteroidal anti-inflammatory drug (NSAID) for osteoarthritis, rheumatoid arthritis, and other mild to moderate pain; also used for juvenile rheumatoid arthritis, migraine headaches, and sunburn pain* [fenoprofen calcium] 200, 400 mg

Nalfrx oral suspension ℞ *decongestant; antihistamine; sleep aid* [pseudoephedrine tannate; dexchlorpheniramine tannate; pyrilamine tannate] 75•2.5•12.5 mg/5 mL

nalidixane [see: nalidixic acid]

nalidixate sodium USAN *antibacterial*

nalidixic acid USAN, USP, INN *quinolone antibiotic for urinary tract infections (UTIs)*

nalmefene USAN, INN, BAN *narcotic antagonist; antidote to opioid overdose; postanesthesia "stir-up"; investigational (Phase III) treatment for alcoholism*

nalmefene HCl *narcotic antagonist; antidote to opioid overdose; postanesthesia "stir-up"*

nalmetrene [now: nalmefene]

nalmexone INN *analgesic; narcotic antagonist* [also: nalmexone HCl]

nalmexone HCl USAN *analgesic; narcotic antagonist* [also: nalmexone]

nalorphine INN [also: nalorphine HCl]

nalorphine HCl USP [also: nalorphine]

naloxiphane tartrate [see: levallorphan tartrate]

naloxone INN, BAN *narcotic antagonist* [also: naloxone HCl] ☒ Nyloxin

naloxone HCl USAN, USP, JAN *narcotic antagonist* [also: naloxone] 0.4, 1 mg/mL injection

naloxone HCl & pentazocine *narcotic agonist-antagonist analgesic; also abused as a street drug* 0.5•50 mg oral

naltrexone USAN, INN, BAN *narcotic antagonist*

naltrexone HCl *narcotic antagonist for opiate dependence or overdose (orphan) and alcoholism; also used for pruritus and irritable bowel syndrome* 50 mg oral

Namenda film-coated caplets, oral solution R̲ *NMDA (N-methyl-D-aspartate) antagonist to suppress the symptoms of Alzheimer disease* [memantine HCl] 5, 10 mg; 2 mg/mL

Namenda XR extended-release capsules R̲ *NMDA (N-methyl-D-aspartate) antagonist to suppress the symptoms of Alzheimer disease* [memantine HCl] 7, 14, 21, 28 mg

naminterol INN

[¹³N] ammonia [see: ammonia N 13]

namoxyrate USAN, INN *analgesic*

namuron [see: cyclobarbitone]

nanafrocin INN

nandrolone BAN *anabolic* [also: nandrolone cyclotate]

nandrolone cyclotate USAN *anabolic* [also: nandrolone]

nandrolone decanoate USAN, USP *androgen/anabolic steroid for anemia of renal insufficiency; also used for AIDS-wasting syndrome; sometimes abused as a street drug* 200 mg/mL injection

nandrolone phenpropionate USP *androgen/anabolic steroid for metastatic breast cancer in women; sometimes abused as a street drug*

naniopine [see: nanofin]

NanobacTEST-S for professional use R̲ *blood serum test for the presence of nanobacterial antigens and antibodies*

NanobacTEST-U/A for professional use R̲ *rapid screening urine test for the presence of live, uncalcified nanobacteria by visual color comparison* [ELISA test]

nanofin INN

nanterinone INN, BAN

nantradol INN *analgesic* [also: nantradol HCl]

nantradol HCl USAN *analgesic* [also: nantradol]

NAPA (N-acetyl-*p*-aminophenol) [see: acetaminophen]

NAPA (N-acetyl-procainamide) [see: acecainide HCl]

napactadine INN *antidepressant* [also: napactadine HCl]

napactadine HCl USAN *antidepressant* [also: napactadine]

napadisilate INN *combining name for radicals or groups* [also: napadisylate]

napadisylate BAN *combining name for radicals or groups* [also: napadisilate]

napamezole INN *antidepressant* [also: napamezole HCl]

napamezole HCl USAN *antidepressant* [also: napamezole]

Na-PCA topical spray OTC *natural skin moisturizing factor; humectant* [sodium pyrrolidone carboxylic acid; aloe vera]

naphazoline INN, BAN *topical ophthalmic decongestant and vasoconstrictor; nasal decongestant* [also: naphazoline HCl; naphazoline nitrate] ☒ nafcillin

naphazoline HCl USP *topical ophthalmic decongestant/vasoconstrictor; nasal decongestant* [also: naphazoline; naphazoline nitrate] 0.1% eye drops

naphazoline HCl & antazoline phosphate *topical ophthalmic decongestant and antihistamine* 0.05%•0.5%

naphazoline HCl & pheniramine maleate *topical ophthalmic decongestant and antihistamine* 0.025%•0.3% eye drops

naphazoline nitrate JAN *topical ophthalmic vasoconstrictor; nasal decongestant* [also: naphazoline HCl; naphazoline]

Naphazoline Plus eye drops (discontinued 2010) OTC *decongestant; antihistamine* [naphazoline HCl; pheniramine maleate] 0.025%•0.3%

Naphcon eye drops OTC *decongestant; vasoconstrictor* [naphazoline HCl] 0.012% ☒ nefocon; Novocain

Naphcon-A Drop-Tainers (eye drops) OTC *decongestant; antihistamine* [naphazoline HCl; pheniramine maleate] 0.025%•0.3% ☒ nefocon; Novocain

Naphoptic-A eye drops (discontinued 2011) ℞ *decongestant; antihistamine* [naphazoline HCl; pheniramine maleate] 0.025%•0.3%

2-naphthol [see: betanaphthol]

naphthonone INN

naphthypramide [see: naftypramide]

Naphuride (available only from the Centers for Disease Control) (discontinued 2011) ℞ *antiparasitic for African trypanosomiasis and onchocerciasis* [suramin sodium]

napirimus INN

napitane mesylate USAN *antidepressant; alpha-adrenergic blocker; norepinephrine uptake antagonist*

Naprelan controlled-release caplets ℞ *once-daily analgesic; nonsteroidal antiinflammatory drug (NSAID) for osteoarthritis, rheumatoid arthritis, juvenile arthritis, and ankylosing spondylitis* [naproxen (as sodium)] 375, 500, 750 mg

naprodoxime INN

Naprosyn tablets, oral suspension ℞ *analgesic; nonsteroidal anti-inflammatory drug (NSAID) for osteoarthritis, rheumatoid arthritis, juvenile arthritis,* ankylosing spondylitis, primary dysmenorrhea, bursitis/tendinitis, and other mild to moderate pain [naproxen] 250, 375, 500 mg; 125 mg/5 mL ☒

niaprazine

Naprosyn EC [see: EC-Naprosyn]

naproxcinod *investigational (Phase III) cyclooxygenase-inhibiting nitric oxide–donor (CINOD) for osteoarthritis*

naproxen USAN, USP, INN, BAN, JAN *analgesic; nonsteroidal anti-inflammatory drug (NSAID) for osteoarthritis, rheumatoid arthritis, juvenile arthritis, ankylosing spondylitis, primary dysmenorrhea, bursitis/tendinitis, and other mild to moderate pain* 250, 375, 500 mg oral; 125 mg/5 mL oral ☒ nibroxane

naproxen sodium USAN, USP *analgesic; nonsteroidal anti-inflammatory drug (NSAID) for osteoarthritis, rheumatoid arthritis, juvenile arthritis, ankylosing spondylitis, primary dysmenorrhea, bursitis/tendinitis, and other mild to moderate pain* (base=91%) 220, 275, 550 mg oral

naproxol USAN, INN *anti-inflammatory; analgesic; antipyretic*

napsagatran USAN, INN *antithrombotic*

napsilate INN *combining name for radicals or groups* [also: napsylate]

napsylate USAN, BAN *combining name for radicals or groups* [also: napsilate]

naranol INN *antipsychotic* [also: naranol HCl] ☒ Norinyl

naranol HCl USAN *antipsychotic* [also: naranol]

narasin USAN, INN, BAN *coccidiostat; veterinary growth stimulant*

naratriptan INN, BAN *vascular serotonin 5-HT$_{1D}$ receptor agonist for the acute treatment of migraine* [also: naratriptan HCl]

naratriptan HCl USAN *vascular serotonin 5-HT$_{1D}$ receptor agonist for the acute treatment of migraine* [also: naratriptan] 1, 2.5 mg oral

Narcan IV, IM, or subcu injection ℞ *narcotic antagonist for opiate depend-*

*ence or overdose; hypotension treat-
ment* [naloxone HCl] 0.4 mg/mL

narcotic agonist-antagonists *a class
of opioid or morphine-like analgesics
with lower abuse potential than pure
narcotic agonist analgesics*

narcotic agonists; narcotics *a class of
opioid or morphine-like analgesics that
relieve pain and induce sleep*

narcotine [see: noscapine]

narcotine HCl [see: noscapine HCl]

nard *medicinal herb* [see: spikenard]

Nardil film-coated tablets ℞ *MAO
inhibitor for atypical, nonendogenous,
or neurotic depression; also used for
bulimia, post-traumatic stress disorder
(PTSD), chronic migraine, and social
anxiety disorder (SAD)* [phenelzine
sulfate] 15 mg

Nariz oral liquid ℞ *decongestant; expectorant* [phenylephrine HCl; guaifen-
esin] 15•400 mg/10 mL

Naropin injection ℞ *long-acting local
or regional anesthetic for surgery; epidural block for cesarean section* [ropiva-
caine HCl] 0.2%, 0.5%, 0.75%, 1%

narrow dock *medicinal herb* [see: yellow dock]

Nasabid SR long-acting tablets (discontinued 2009) ℞ *decongestant;
expectorant* [pseudoephedrine HCl;
guaifenesin] 90•600 mg

Nasacort AQ nasal spray in a metered-
dose pump ℞ *corticosteroidal anti-
inflammatory for seasonal or perennial
allergic rhinitis* [triamcinolone aceto-
nide] 55 mcg/dose

Nasacort HFA pressurized metered-
dose inhaler (pMDI) with a CFC-free
propellant (discontinued 2008) ℞
*corticosteroidal anti-inflammatory for
seasonal or perennial allergic rhinitis* [tri-
amcinolone acetonide] 55 mcg/dose

NāSal nasal spray, nose drops OTC *nasal
moisturizer* [sodium chloride (saline
solution)] 0.65% ☒ Neosol

Nasal Decongestant pediatric oral
drops OTC *nasal decongestant* [pseudo-
ephedrine HCl] 7.5 mg/0.8 mL

Nasal Decongestant spray OTC *nasal
decongestant* [oxymetazoline HCl]
0.05%

**Nasal Decongestant, Children's
Non-Drowsy** oral liquid OTC *nasal
decongestant* [pseudoephedrine HCl]
15 mg/5 mL

**Nasal Decongestant Sinus Non-
Drowsy** tablets (discontinued 2007)
OTC *decongestant; analgesic; antipyretic* [pseudoephedrine HCl; aceta-
minophen] 30•500 mg

Nasal Moist nasal spray OTC *nasal
moisturizer* [sodium chloride (saline
solution)] 0.65%

Nasal Relief nasal spray OTC *nasal
decongestant* [oxymetazoline HCl]
0.05%

Nasal Spray OTC *nasal moisturizer*
[sodium chloride (saline solution)]

NasalCrom nasal spray OTC *anti-
inflammatory/mast cell stabilizer for the
prophylaxis of allergic rhinitis* [cromo-
lyn sodium] 4% (5.2 mg/dose)

NasalCrom A nasal spray + tablets
OTC *anti-inflammatory/mast cell stabilizer for the prophylaxis of allergic rhinitis; antihistamine* [cromolyn sodium;
chlorpheniramine maleate] 4% (5.2
mg/dose); 4 mg

NasalCrom CA nasal spray + tablets
OTC *anti-inflammatory/mast cell stabilizer for the prophylaxis of allergic rhinitis; decongestant; analgesic; antipyretic*
[cromolyn sodium; pseudoephedrine
HCl; acetaminophen] 4% (5.2 mg/
dose); 30 mg•500 mg

Nasal-Ease with Zinc nasal gel OTC
nasal moisturizer and anti-infective
[zinc acetate]

Nasal-Ease with Zinc Gluconate
nasal spray OTC *nasal moisturizer and
anti-infective* [zinc gluconate]

Nasarel metered dose nasal spray (discontinued 2009) ℞ *corticosteroidal
anti-inflammatory for seasonal or
perennial rhinitis* [flunisolide] 0.025%
(29 mcg/dose) ☒ Nizoral

Nasatab LA long-acting caplets ℞
decongestant; expectorant [pseudo-

ephedrine HCl; guaifenesin] 120•
500 mg

Nascobal nasal gel in metered-dose
applicator (discontinued 2007) ℞
*maintenance administration following
intramuscular vitamin B*$_{12}$ *therapy* [cya-
nocobalamin] 500 mcg/0.1 mL dose

Nascobal nasal spray ℞ *once-weekly
maintenance administration following
intramuscular vitamin B*$_{12}$ *therapy* [cya-
nocobalamin] 500 mcg/0.1 mL dose

Nasex; Nasex-G extended-release
caplets (discontinued 2008) ℞ *decongestant; expectorant* [phenylephrine
HCl; guaifenesin] 25•650 mg; 25•
835 mg

**NASHA (non-animal stabilized
hyaluronic acid)** [see: hyaluronic
acid]

**Nashville Rabbit Antithymocyte
Serum** *investigational* (*orphan*) *passive
immunizing agent to prevent allograft
rejection of solid organ and bone marrow
transplants* [antithymocyte globulin,
rabbit]

Nasofed oral suspension (discontinued
2010) ℞ *decongestant* [pseudoephed-
rine tannate] 50 mg/5 mL

Nasohist oral drops ℞ *decongestant;
antihistamine* [phenylephrine HCl;
chlorpheniramine maleate] 2•1
mg/mL

Nasohist DM oral drops ℞ *antitussive;
antihistamine; decongestant* [dextro-
methorphan hydrobromide; chlorpheniramine maleate; phenylephrine HCl] 3•1•2 mg/mL

Nasonex nasal spray in a metered-
dose pump ℞ *corticosteroidal anti-
inflammatory for seasonal or perennial
allergic rhinitis and nasal polyps*
[mometasone furoate] 50 mcg/dose

Nasop orally disintegrating tablets
(discontinued 2009) ℞ *nasal decongestant* [phenylephrine HCl] 10 mg

Nasotuss oral liquid ℞ *narcotic antitussive; decongestant; antihistamine*
[codeine phosphate; phenylephrine
HCl; chlorcyclizine HCl] 10•10•25
mg/5 mL ⊡ NiaStase

Nasturtium officinale medicinal herb
[see: watercress]

NAT (novel acting thrombolytic)
[q.v.]

NataCaps capsules (discontinued
2009) ℞ *prenatal vitamin/mineral/iron
supplement* [multiple vitamins &
minerals; iron (as ferrous fumarate);
folic acid] ≐•324•1 mg

NataChew chewable tablets ℞ *prenatal vitamin/mineral/iron supplement*
[multiple vitamins & minerals; iron
(as ferrous fumarate); folic acid] ≐•
29•1 mg

Natacyn eye drop suspension ℞ *antifungal* [natamycin] 5%

NataFort film-coated tablets ℞ *prenatal vitamin/iron supplement* [multiple
vitamins; iron (as ferrous sulfate and
carbonyl); folic acid] ≐•60•1 mg

**NatalCare Advanced; NatalCare
Advanced-RF** tablets (discontinued
2009) ℞ *prenatal vitamin/mineral/cal-
cium/iron supplement; stool softener*
[multiple vitamins & minerals; calcium; iron (as carbonyl); folic acid;
docusate sodium] ≐•200•90•1•50
mg

NatalCare GlossTabs tablets (discontinued 2009) ℞ *prenatal vitamin/min-
eral/calcium/iron supplement; stool softener* [multiple vitamins & minerals;
calcium; iron (as carbonyl); folic
acid; biotin; docusate sodium] ≐•
200•90•1•0.03•50 mg

NatalCare PIC film-coated tablets ℞
*prenatal vitamin/mineral/calcium/iron
supplement* [multiple vitamins &
minerals; calcium; iron (as polysaccharide iron complex); folic acid;
hydrogenated oil] ≐•125•60•1 mg;
≐•250•60•1 mg

NatalCare PIC Forte film-coated tablets (discontinued 2009) ℞ *prenatal
vitamin/mineral/calcium/iron supplement* [multiple vitamins & minerals;
calcium; iron (as polysaccharide iron
complex); folic acid; hydrogenated
oil] ≐•250•60•1 mg

NatalCare Plus film-coated tablets (discontinued 2009) ℞ *prenatal vitamin/mineral/calcium/iron supplement* [multiple vitamins & minerals; calcium; iron (as ferrous fumarate); folic acid; hydrogenated oil] ≛•200•27•1 mg

NatalCare Rx film-coated tablets ℞ *prenatal vitamin/mineral/calcium/iron supplement* [multiple vitamins & minerals; calcium; iron (as ferrous gluconate); folic acid; biotin; hydrogenated oil] ≛•100•27•0.8•0.015 mg

NatalCare Three film-coated tablets ℞ *prenatal vitamin/mineral/calcium/iron supplement* [multiple vitamins & minerals; calcium; iron (as ferrous fumarate); folic acid; hydrogenated oil] ≛•200•28•1 mg

NatalCare Ultra [see: Ultra NatalCare]

natalizumab *humanized monoclonal antibody (huMAb) anti-inflammatory for the treatment of multiple sclerosis and Crohn disease; availability restricted due to an increased risk of progressive multifocal leukoencephalopathy (PML)*

natamycin USAN, USP, INN, BAN *ophthalmic fungicidal antibiotic* [also: pimaricin]

Natarex Prenatal tablets (discontinued 2008) ℞ *prenatal vitamin/calcium/iron supplement* [multiple vitamins; calcium; iron; folic acid; biotin] ≛•200•60•1•0.03 mg

NataTab CFe film-coated tablets ℞ *prenatal vitamin/mineral/calcium/iron supplement* [multiple vitamins & minerals; calcium; iron (as carbonyl); folic acid; hydrogenated oil] ≛•200•50•1 mg

NataTab FA film-coated tablets ℞ *prenatal vitamin/mineral/calcium/iron supplement* [multiple vitamins & minerals; calcium; iron (as ferrous fumarate); folic acid; hydrogenated oil] ≛•200•29•1 mg

NataTab Rx film-coated tablets ℞ *prenatal vitamin/mineral/calcium/iron supplement* [multiple vitamins & minerals; calcium; iron (as caronyl); folic acid; biotin; hydrogenated oil] ≛•200•29•1•0.03 mg

Natazia tablets (28-day package) ℞ *quadriphasic oral contraceptive* [estradiol valerate; dienogest] ② NeoTuss
Phase 1 (2 days): 3•0 mg;
Phase 2 (5 days): 2•2 mg;
Phase 3 (17 days): 2•3 mg;
Phase 4 (2 days): 1•0 mg

nateglinide USAN *meglitinide antidiabetic for type 2 diabetes that stimulates the release of insulin from the pancreas; amino acid–derivative* 60, 120 mg oral

Natelle-EZ caplets ℞ *prenatal vitamin/mineral/calcium/iron supplement* [multiple vitamins & minerals; calcium; iron (as ferrous bisglycinate chelate); folic acid; biotin; choline bitartrate] ≛•100•25•0.8•0.03•55 mg

Natrecor powder for IV injection ℞ *human B-type natriuretic peptide (hBNP); vasodilator for acute congestive heart failure* [nesiritide citrate] 1.58 mg/vial

Natroba topical suspension OTC *pediculicide for lice* [spinosad] 0.9%

Natural E 200; Natural E 400 softgels OTC *vitamin supplement* [vitamin E] 200 U; 400 U

Natural Fiber Laxative powder OTC *bulk laxative* [psyllium hydrophilic mucilloid] 3.4 g/dose

natural killer cell stimulatory factor [see: edodekin alfa]

Natural Psyllium Fiber powder OTC *bulk laxative* [psyllium hydrophilic mucilloid] 3.4 g/tsp.

Natural Vitamin E oral liquid OTC *vitamin supplement; also used as a skin conditioner* [vitamin E] 1150 IU/1.25 mL

Naturalyte oral solution OTC *electrolyte replacement* [sodium, potassium, and chloride electrolytes] 240 mL, 1 L ② Nutrilyte

Nature Throid tablets ℞ *natural thyroid replacement for hypothyroidism or thyroid cancer* [thyroid, desiccated (porcine)] 16.25, 32.4, 48.75, 64.8, 81.25, 97.5, 113.75, 129.6, 146.25, 162.5, 194.4, 260, 325 mg (64.8 mg=1 gr.)

Nature's Remedy tablets (discontinued 2009) OTC *stimulant laxative* [cascara sagrada; aloe] 150•100 mg

Nature's Tears eye drops OTC *moisturizer/lubricant* [hydroxypropyl methylcellulose] 0.4%

Naturetin tablets (discontinued 2008) ℞ *antihypertensive; diuretic* [bendroflumethiazide] 5 mg

Naturvus ℞ *hydrophilic contact lens material* [hefilcon B] ⑨ Neutra-Phos

Nausatrol oral solution OTC *antiemetic for nausea associated with influenza, morning sickness, motion sickness, inhalation anesthesia, or food and drink indiscretions* [phosphorated carbohydrate solution (dextrose, fructose, and phosphoric acid)] 1.87 g•1.87 g•21.5 mg per 15 mL dose

Nausea Relief oral solution OTC *antiemetic for nausea associated with influenza, morning sickness, motion sickness, inhalation anesthesia, or food and drink indiscretions* [phosphorated carbohydrate solution (dextrose, fructose, and phosphoric acid)] 1.87 g• 1.87 g•21.5 mg per dose

Nausetrol oral solution OTC *antiemetic for nausea associated with influenza, morning sickness, motion sickness, inhalation anesthesia, or food and drink indiscretions* [phosphorated carbohydrate solution (fructose, dextrose, and orthophosphoric acid)] 118 mL (44•44•5 g)

Navane capsules ℞ *conventional (typical) thioxanthene antipsychotic for schizophrenia* [thiothixene] 1, 2, 5, 10, 20 mg

Navane oral concentrate ℞ *conventional (typical) thioxanthene antipsychotic for schizophrenia* [thiothixene HCl] 5 mg/mL

Navelbine IV injection ℞ *antineoplastic for Hodgkin disease and lung, breast and ovarian cancer* [vinorelbine tartrate] 10 mg/mL

naxagolide INN *antiparkinsonian; dopamine agonist* [also: naxagolide HCl]

naxagolide HCl USAN *antiparkinsonian; dopamine agonist* [also: naxagolide]

naxaprostene INN

naxifylline USAN *treatment of edema due to congestive heart failure*

Nazarin oral liquid (discontinued 2008) ℞ *decongestant; expectorant* [phenylephrine HCl; guaifenesin] 15•400 mg/10 mL

Nazarin HC oral liquid ℞ *narcotic antitussive; decongestant; expectorant* [hydrocodone bitartrate; phenylephrine HCl; guaifenesin] 2.5•7.5•150 mg/5 mL

9-NC (9-nitrocamptothecin) [see: rubitecan]

ND Clear sustained-release capsules (discontinued 2007) ℞ *decongestant; antihistamine* [pseudoephedrine HCl; chlorpheniramine maleate] 120•8 mg

nealbarbital INN [also: nealbarbitone]

nealbarbitone BAN [also: nealbarbital]

nebacumab USAN, INN, BAN *antiendotoxin monoclonal antibody; investigational (orphan) for gram-negative bacteremia in endotoxin shock*

Nebido injection *investigational (NDA filed) long-acting hormone replacement for male hypogonadism* [testosterone]

nebidrazine INN

nebivolol HCl USAN, INN *beta-blocker for hypertension*

nebracetam INN

nebramycin USAN, INN *antibacterial*

nebramycin factor 6 [see: tobramycin]

NebuPent inhalation aerosol ℞ *antiprotozoal; treatment and prophylaxis of Pneumocystis pneumonia (PCP) (orphan)* [pentamidine isethionate] 300 mg

Necon 0.5/35; Necon 1/35 tablets (in packs of 21 or 28) ℞ *monophasic oral contraceptive* [norethindrone; ethinyl estradiol] 0.5 mg•35 mcg; 1 mg•35 mcg

Necon 1/50 tablets (in packs of 21 or 28) ℞ *monophasic oral contraceptive* [norethindrone; mestranol] 1 mg• 50 mcg

Necon 10/11 tablets (in packs of 21 or 28) ℞ *biphasic oral contraceptive* [norethindrone; ethinyl estradiol] Phase 1 (10 days): 0.5 mg•35 mcg; Phase 2 (11 days): 1 mg•35 mcg

Necon 7/7/7 tablets (in packs of 28) ℞ *triphasic oral contraceptive* [norethindrone; ethinyl estradiol] Phase 1 (7 days): 0.5 mg•35 mcg; Phase 2 (7 days): 0.75 mg•35 mcg; Phase 3 (7 days): 1 mg•35 mcg; Counters (7 days)

nedocromil USAN, INN, BAN *anti-inflammatory; mast cell stabilizer; anti-asthmatic*

nedocromil calcium USAN *anti-inflammatory; mast cell stabilizer; anti-asthmatic*

nedocromil sodium USAN *ophthalmic mast cell stabilizer for allergic conjunctivitis*

neem tree (*Azadirachta indica*) fruit, leaves, root, and oil *medicinal herb for contraception, diabetes, heart disease, malaria, skin diseases, ulcers, and worms; also used as a pesticide and insect repellent; not generally regarded as safe and effective for infants as it may cause death*

Néevo coated caplets ℞ *prenatal vitamin/mineral/calcium/iron supplement* [multiple vitamins and minerals; calcium (as carbonate); iron (as polysaccharide iron complex); folic acid (as L-methylfolate); biotin] ±•200•29•1•0.03 mg

Néevo DHA capsule ℞ *prenatal vitamin/calcium/iron/omega-3 supplement* [multiple vitamins; calcium (as tricalcium phosphate); iron (as ferrous fumarate); folic acid (as L-methylfolate); docosahexaenoic acid (DHA)] ±•75•27•1•250 mg

nefazodone INN *antidepressant; selective serotonin and norepinephrine reuptake inhibitor (SSNRI)* [also: nefazodone HCl]

nefazodone HCl USAN *antidepressant; selective serotonin and norepinephrine reuptake inhibitor (SSNRI); FDA*

approval for use in children and adolescents was withdrawn in 2004 due to safety concerns [also: nefazodone] 50, 100, 150, 200, 250 mg oral

neflumozide INN *antipsychotic* [also: neflumozide HCl]

neflumozide HCl USAN *antipsychotic* [also: neflumozide]

nefocon A USAN *hydrophobic contact lens material* ② Naphcon; Novocain

nefopam INN *analgesic* [also: nefopam HCl]

nefopam HCl USAN *analgesic* [also: nefopam]

nefrolan [see: clorexolone]

Negaban *investigational (orphan) antibiotic for pulmonary Burkholderia cepacia infections* [temocillin sodium]

NegGram caplets ℞ *quinolone antibiotic for urinary tract infections (UTIs)* [nalidixic acid] 500 mg

nelarabine USAN *DNA synthesis inhibitor; antineoplastic for T-cell acute lymphoblastic leukemia (T-ALL; orphan) and T-cell lymphoblastic lymphoma (T-LBL; orphan); nucleoside analogue; prodrug of ara-G*

neldazosin INN

nelezaprine INN *muscle relaxant* [also: nelezaprine maleate]

nelezaprine maleate USAN *muscle relaxant* [also: nelezaprine]

nelfilcon A USAN *hydrophilic contact lens material*

nelfinavir mesylate USAN *antiretroviral; protease inhibitor for HIV-1 infection*

nemadectin USAN, INN *veterinary antiparasitic*

nemazoline INN *nasal decongestant* [also: nemazoline HCl]

nemazoline HCl USAN *nasal decongestant* [also: nemazoline]

Nembutal Sodium capsules, IV or IM injection, suppositories ℞ *sedative; hypnotic; also abused as a street drug* [pentobarbital sodium] 50, 100 mg; 50 mg/mL; 30, 60, 120, 200 mg

Neo DM oral drops ℞ *antitussive; antihistamine; decongestant; for children 3–24 months* [dextromethorphan hydrobromide; chlorpheniramine maleate; phenylephrine HCl] 2.75•0.75•1.75 mg/mL

Neo DM oral suspension ℞ *antitussive; antihistamine; decongestant* [dextromethorphan tannate; brompheniramine tannate; phenylephrine tannate] 30•10•25 mg/5 mL

Neo DM syrup, oral liquid ℞ *antitussive; antihistamine; decongestant* [dextromethorphan hydrobromide; brompheniramine maleate; pseudoephedrine HCl] 30•3•50 mg/5 mL

Neo HC syrup ℞ *narcotic antitussive; decongestant; antihistamine* [hydrocodone bitartrate; phenylephrine HCl; chlorpheniramine maleate] 5•7.5•3 mg/5 mL

neoarsphenamine NF, INN

Neoasma caplets (discontinued 2007) ℞ *antiasthmatic; bronchodilator; expectorant* [theophylline; guaifenesin] 125•100 mg

NeoBenz Micro; NeoBenz Micro SD cream ℞ *keratolytic for acne* [benzoyl peroxide] 3.5%, 5.5%, 8.5%

NeoBenz Micro Wash ℞ *keratolytic for acne* [benzoyl peroxide] 7%

neocarzinostatin [now: zinostatin]

Neocate One + ready-to-use pediatric oral liquid OTC *enteral nutritional therapy* [lactose-free formula] 237 mL 🔲 nicotine

Neocera (trademarked ingredient) suppository *nontherapeutic base for compounding various dermatological preparations* [polyethylent glycol 400, 1450, and 8000; polysorbate 60]

neocid [see: chlorophenothane]

neocinchophen NF, INN

NeoDecadron Ocumeter (eye drops), ophthalmic ointment (discontinued 2008) ℞ *corticosteroidal anti-inflammatory; antibiotic* [dexamethasone sodium phosphate; neomycin sulfate] 0.1%•0.35%; 0.05%•0.35%

Neo-Dexair eye drops ℞ *corticosteroidal anti-inflammatory; antibiotic* [dexamethasone sodium phosphate; neomycin sulfate] 0.1%•0.35%

Neo-Dexameth eye drops (discontinued 2008) ℞ *corticosteroidal anti-inflammatory; antibiotic* [dexamethasone sodium phosphate; neomycin sulfate] 0.1%•0.35%

Neo-Diaral capsules OTC *antidiarrheal* [loperamide] 2 mg

neodymium *element (Nd)*

Neo-fradin oral solution ℞ *aminoglycoside antibiotic* [neomycin sulfate] 125 mg/5 mL 🔲 nifuradene

Neofrin eye drops ℞ *decongestant; vasoconstrictor; mydriatic* [phenylephrine HCl] 2.5%, 10% 🔲 Nephron

Neohaler (delivery device) *oral inhalation device for encapsulated powder*

Neoloid oral emulsion (discontinued 2009) OTC *stimulant laxative* [castor oil] 36.4%

Neomark *investigational (NDA filed, orphan) radiosensitizer for primary brain tumors* [broxuridine]

neo-mercazole [see: carbimazole]

neomycin INN, BAN *antibacterial* [also: neomycin palmitate] 🔲 nimazone; Numoisyn

neomycin B [see: framycetin]

neomycin palmitate USAN *antibacterial* [also: neomycin]

neomycin & polymyxin B sulfate *antibiotic* 40 mg•200 000 U per mL intravesical solution

neomycin sulfate USP *aminoglycoside antibiotic* 500 mg oral

neomycin sulfate & polymyxin B sulfate & bacitracin zinc *topical antibiotic* 5 mg•10 000 U•400 U per g ophthalmic

neomycin sulfate & polymyxin B sulfate & dexamethasone *topical ophthalmic antibiotic and corticosteroidal anti-inflammatory* 0.35%•10 000 U/mL•0.1% eye drops

neomycin sulfate & polymyxin B sulfate & gramicidin *topical antibiotic* 1.75 mg•10 000 U•0.025 mg per mL eye drops

neomycin sulfate & polymyxin B sulfate & hydrocortisone *topical ophthalmic/otic antibiotic and cortico-*

steroidal anti-inflammatory 0.35% •
10 000 U/mL • 1% eye drops; 5
mg/mL • 10 000 U/mL • 1% ear drops

neomycin undecenoate [see: neomycin undecylenate]

neomycin undecylenate USAN *antibacterial; antifungal*

neon *element (Ne)*

Neopap suppositories (discontinued 2008) OTC *analgesic; antipyretic* [acetaminophen] 125 mg

neopenyl [see: clemizole penicillin]

NeoProfen IV injection ℞ *nonsteroidal anti-inflammatory drug (NSAID) for neonatal closure of patent ductus arteriosus (orphan)* [ibuprofen (as lysine)] 10 mg/mL

neoquate [see: nequinate]

Neoral gelcaps, oral solution ℞ *immunosuppressant for allogenic kidney, liver, and heart transplants (orphan), rheumatoid arthritis, and psoriasis* [cyclosporine; alcohol 11.9%] 25, 100 mg; 100 mg/mL ② Norel

Neosalus cream OTC *emollient/protectant* [dimethicone; glycerin] ② Neusalus

Neosar powder for IV injection (discontinued 2008) ℞ *antineoplastic for a wide variety of malignancies* [cyclophosphamide] 100 mg

Neosol orally disintegrating tablets ℞ *GI/GU antispasmodic; antiparkinsonian; anticholinergic "drying agent" for allergic rhinitis and hyperhidrosis* [hyoscyamine sulfate] 0.125 mg ② NāSal

Neosporin Drop Dose (eye drops) ℞ *antibiotic* [polymyxin B sulfate; neomycin sulfate; gramicidin] 10 000 U • 1.75 mg • 0.025 mg per mL

Neosporin ophthalmic ointment (discontinued 2010) ℞ *antibiotic* [polymyxin B sulfate; neomycin sulfate; bacitracin zinc] 10 000 U • 5 mg • 400 U per g

Neosporin AF cream, spray liquid OTC *antifungal for tinea pedis, tinea cruris, and tinea corporis* [miconazole nitrate] 2%

Neosporin G.U. Irrigant solution ℞ *antibiotic* [neomycin sulfate; polymyxin B sulfate] 40 mg • 200 000 U per mL

Neosporin Original ointment OTC *antibiotic* [polymyxin B sulfate; neomycin sulfate; bacitracin zinc] 5000 U • 3.5 mg • 400 U per g

Neosporin Plus Pain Relief cream OTC *antibiotic; local anesthetic* [polymyxin B sulfate; neomycin sulfate; pramoxine HCl] 10 000 U • 3.5 mg • 10 mg per g

Neosporin Plus Pain Relief ointment OTC *antibiotic; local anesthetic* [polymyxin B sulfate; neomycon sulfate; bacitracin zinc; pramoxine HCl] 10 000 U • 3.5 mg • 500 U • 10 mg per g

neostigmine BAN *cholinergic/anticholinesterase muscle stimulant* [also: neostigmine bromide]

neostigmine bromide USP, INN, BAN *oral anticholinesterase muscle stimulant for myasthenia gravis* [also: neostigmine]

neostigmine methylsulfate USP *injectable anticholinesterase muscle stimulant for myasthenia gravis; urinary stimulant for postsurgical urinary retention; antidote to neuromuscular blockers* 1:1000 (1 mg/mL), 1:2000 (0.5 mg/mL), 1:4000 (0.25 mg/mL) injection

Neostrata Skin Lightening gel (discontinued 2011) OTC *hyperpigmentation bleaching agent* [hydroquinone] 2%

Neo-Synephrine IV, IM, or subcu injection ℞ *vasopressor for hypotensive or cardiac shock* [phenylephrine HCl] 1% (10 mg/mL)

Neo-Synephrine 4-Hour Mild Formula nasal spray (name changed to **Neo-Synephrine Mild Strength** in 2008)

Neo-Synephrine 12-Hour nasal spray (discontinued 2008) OTC *nasal decongestant* [oxymetazoline HCl] 0.05%

Neo-Synephrine 12-Hour Extra Moisturizing nasal spray OTC *nasal*

decongestant [oxymetazoline HCl] 0.05%

Neo-Synephrine Mild Strength; Neo-Synephrine Regular Strength; Neo-Synephrine Extra Strength nasal spray, nose drops OTC *nasal decongestant* [phenylephrine HCl] 0.25%; 0.5%; 1%

Neo-Tabs tablets ℞ *aminoglycoside antibiotic* [neomycin sulfate] 500 mg

Neotic ear drops OTC *anesthetic; analgesic; emollient; for acute otitis media and the removal of cerumen* [benzocaine; antipyrine; glycerin; zinc acetate dihydrate] 1%•5.4%•2%•1%

Neotrace-4 IV injection (discontinued 2011) ℞ *intravenous nutritional therapy* [multiple trace elements (metals)] ⍰ Nu-Tears

Neotricin HC ophthalmic ointment ℞ *corticosteroidal anti-inflammatory; antibiotic* [hydrocortisone acetate; neomycin sulfate; bacitracin zinc; polymyxin B sulfate] 1%•3.5%•400 U/g•10 000 U/g

NeoTuss oral liquid OTC *antitussive; expectorant* [dextromethorphan hydrobromide; guaifenesin] 30•200 mg/5 mL ⍰ Natazia

NeoTuss-D oral liquid OTC *antitussive; decongestant; expectorant* [dextromethorphan hydrobromide; phenylephrine HCl; guaifenesin] 30•7.5•200 mg/5 mL

nepafenac USAN *nonsteroidal anti-inflammatory drug (NSAID) for pain and inflammation following cataract extraction surgery*

Nepeta cataria *medicinal herb* [see: catnip]

Nephplex tablets ℞ *vitamin/zinc supplement* [multiple B vitamins; vitamin C; folic acid; biotin; zinc] ±•60•1•0.3•12.5 mg

NephrAmine 5.4% IV infusion ℞ *nutritional therapy for renal failure* [multiple essential amino acids; electrolytes]

nephritics *a class of agents that affect the kidney (a term used in folk medicine)*

Nephro-Calci tablets OTC *calcium supplement* [calcium (as carbonate)] 600 mg (1500 mg)

Nephrocaps capsules (discontinued 2008) ℞ *vitamin supplement* [multiple B vitamins; vitamin C; folic acid; biotin] ±•100 mg•1 mg•150 mcg

Nephro-Fer tablets (discontinued 2009) OTC *iron supplement* [iron (as ferrous fumarate)] 115 mg

Nephron solution for inhalation (discontinued 2009) OTC *sympathomimetic bronchodilator; vasopressor for shock* [epinephrine HCl] 1.125% ⍰ Neofrin

Nephron FA tablets ℞ *hematinic* [iron (as ferrous fumarate); multiple B vitamins; ascorbic acid; folic acid; biotin; docusate sodium] 200•±•40•1•0.3•75 mg

Nephronex oral liquid OTC *vitamin supplement* [multiple B vitamins; vitamin C; folic acid; biotin] ±•60•0.9•0.3 mg/5 mL

Nephro-Vite tablets OTC *vitamin supplement* [multiple B vitamins; vitamin C; folic acid; biotin] ±•60•0.8•0.3 mg

Nephro-Vite Rx film-coated tablets ℞ *vitamin supplement* [multiple B vitamins; vitamin C; folic acid; biotin] ±•60•1•0.3 mg

Nephro-Vite Vitamin B Complex and C Supplement tablets (discontinued 2008) OTC *vitamin supplement* [multiple B vitamins; vitamin C; folic acid; biotin] ±•60•0.8•0.3 mg

Nephrox oral suspension OTC *antacid; laxative* [aluminum hydroxide; mineral oil 10%] 320 mg/5 mL ⍰ Niferex

nepicastat HCl USAN *dopamine beta-hydroxylase inhibitor for congestive heart failure*

Nepro oral liquid OTC *enteral nutritional therapy for acute or chronic renal failure* [lactose-free formula] 240 mL

neptamustine INN *antineoplastic* [also: pentamustine]

neptunium *element (Np)*

nequinate USAN, INN *coccidiostat for poultry* [also: methyl benzoquate] ⊡ Nu-knit

neraminol INN

nerbacadol INN

nerelimomab USAN *monoclonal antibody to tumor necrosis factor (TNF); cytokine modulator*

neridronic acid INN

Nerium indicum; N. oleander *medicinal herb* [see: oleander]

nerve growth factor, recombinant human (rhNGF) *investigational (orphan) for HIV-associated sensory neuropathy*

nervines *a class of agents that have a calming or soothing effect on the nerves (a term used in folk medicine)*

Nesacaine; Nesacaine MPF injection ℞ *local anesthetic; central or peripheral nerve block, including lumbar and epidural block* [chloroprocaine HCl] 1%, 2%; 2%, 3% ⊡ New-Skin

nesapidil INN

Nesina tablets (available in Japan) *investigational (NDA filed) dipeptidyl peptidase-4 (DPP-4) inhibitor antidiabetic* [alogliptin] 25 mg

nesiritide USAN *human B-type natriuretic peptide (hBNP); vasodilator for acute congestive heart failure*

nesiritide citrate *human B-type natriuretic peptide (hBNP); vasodilator for acute congestive heart failure*

nesosteine INN

Nestabs CBF; Nestabs FA tablets (discontinued 2008) ℞ *vitamin/calcium/iron supplement for pregnancy and lactation* [multiple vitamins; calcium; iron (as ferrous fumarate); folic acid] ≐•200•50•1 mg; ≐•200•29•1 mg

Nestlé Good Start [see: Good Start]

Nestlé VHC 2.25 oral liquid OTC *enteral nutritional therapy* [soy-based formula] 250 mL/can

nethalide [see: pronetalol]

netilmicin INN, BAN *aminoglycoside antibiotic* [also: netilmicin sulfate]

netilmicin sulfate USAN, USP *aminoglycoside antibiotic* [also: netilmicin]

netobimin USAN, INN, BAN *veterinary anthelmintic*

netrafilcon A USAN *hydrophilic contact lens material*

nettle (*Urtica dioica; U. urens*) leaves and root *medicinal herb for blood cleansing, bronchitis, diarrhea, edema, hypertension, bleeding, and rheumatism; competitively binds to sex hormone–binding globulin (SHBG) to increase the level of free testosterone* ⊡ Nytol

nettle, hemp; bee nettle; dog nettle; hemp dead nettle *medicinal herb* [see: hemp nettle]

nettle flowers; dead nettle; stingless nettle; white nettle *medicinal herb* [see: blind nettle]

netupitant *selective NK1 receptor antagonist; investigational (NDA filed) antiemetic to prevent chemotherapy-induced nausea and vomiting (CINV)*

Neulasta subcu injection in prefilled syringe ℞ *hematopoietic stimulant for severe chronic neutropenia (SCN) following cancer chemotherapy* [pegfilgrastim] 10 mg/mL ⊡ Nulecit

Neumega powder for subcu injection ℞ *platelet growth factor for prevention of thrombocytopenia following chemotherapy or radiation (orphan)* [oprelvekin] 5 mg

Neupogen IV or subcu injection, prefilled syringes ℞ *hematopoietic stimulant for severe chronic neutropenia (orphan), acute myeloid leukemia (AML), and bone marrow transplants; investigational (Phase III, orphan) cytokine for AIDS-related cytomegalovirus retinitis; investigational (orphan) for myelodysplastic syndrome* [filgrastim] 300 mcg/mL; 300, 480 mcg

Neuprex injection *investigational (Phase III, orphan) agent for meningococcemia* [bactericidal and permeability-increasing protein, recombinant (rBPI-21)]

neural dopaminergic cells (or precursors), porcine fetal *investiga-*

tional (orphan) intracerebral implant for stage 4 and 5 Parkinson disease

neural gabaergic cells (or precursors), porcine fetal *investigational (orphan) intracerebral implant for Huntington disease*

NeuRecover-DA; NeuRecover-SA capsules OTC *dietary supplement* [multiple vitamins & minerals; multiple amino acids; folic acid] ± •0.067 mg; ± •0.067 mg

Neurelan *investigational (orphan) agent for multiple sclerosis and spinal cord injury* [fampridine]

NeuroCell-HD *investigational (orphan) intracerebral implant for Huntington disease* [neural gabaergic cells, porcine fetal]

NeuroCell-PD *investigational (Phase II/III, orphan) intracerebral implant for advanced Parkinson disease* [neural dopaminergic cells, porcine fetal]

Neurodep injection ℞ *parenteral vitamin therapy* [multiple B vitamins; vitamin C] ± •50 mg/mL

Neurodep Caps capsules OTC *vitamin supplement* [vitamins B_1, B_6, and B_{12}] 125•125•1 mg

Neurolite injection ℞ *imaging aid for SPECT brain scans* [technetium Tc 99m bicisate]

Neurontin capsules, film-coated caplets, oral solution ℞ *anticonvulsant for partial-onset seizures; treatment for postherpetic neuralgia; investigational (orphan) for amyotrophic lateral sclerosis* [gabapentinhydrocod] 100, 300, 400 mg; 600, 800 mg; 250 mg/5 mL

neurosin [see: calcium glycerophosphate]

NeuroSlim capsules OTC *dietary supplement* [multiple vitamins & minerals; multiple amino acids; folic acid; biotin] ± •0.066•0.05 mg

neurotrophic growth factor [see: methionyl neurotrophic factor]

neurotrophin-1 *investigational (orphan) for motor neuron disease and amyotrophic lateral sclerosis*

Neusalus aerosol foam OTC *emollient/ protectant* [dimethicone; glycerin] ⊠ Neosalus

neustab [see: thioacetazone; thiacetazone]

Neut IV or subcu injection ℞ *pH buffer for metabolic acidosis; urinary alkalinizer* [sodium bicarbonate] 4% (0.48 mEq Na/mL)

Neutra-Caine liquid ℞ *mixed with injectable local anesthetics to reduce stinging pain at the injection site* [sodium bicarbonate] 7.5% ⊠ Nutricon

NeutraGard Advanced tooth gel ℞ *dental caries preventative* [fluoride (as sodium fluoride)] 0.5% (1.1%)

Neutrahist oral drops ℞ *decongestant; antihistamine; for children 6–36 months* [pseudoephedrine HCl; chlorpheniramine maleate] 9•0.8 mg/mL

Neutrahist PDX oral drops OTC *antitussive; antihistamine; decongestant; analgesic; for children 6–11 years* [dextromethorphan hydrobromide; chlorpheniramine maleate; pseudoephedrine HCl] 3•0.8•9 mg/mL

neutral acriflavine [see: acriflavine]

neutral insulin INN, BAN, JAN *antidiabetic* [also: insulin, neutral]

neutramycin USAN, INN *antibacterial*

Neutra-Phos powder for oral solution (discontinued 2009) OTC *phosphorus supplement* [monobasic sodium phosphate; monobasic potassium phosphate; dibasic sodium phosphate; dibasic potassium phosphate] 250 mg (14.25 mEq) P/pkt. ⊠ Naturvus

Neutra-Phos-K powder for oral solution (discontinued 2009) OTC *phosphorus supplement* [monobasic potassium phosphate; dibasic potassium phosphate] 250 mg (14.25 mEq) P/ pkt.

NeutraSal powder for oral solution OTC *saline laxative; electrolytes* [monobasic sodium phosphate; dibasic sodium phosphate; calcium chloride; sodium chloride; sodium bicarbonate; silicon dioxide] 10•10•50•450• 16•2 mg ⊠ Nutr-E-Sol

NeuTrexin powder for IV injection (discontinued 2008) ℞ *antiprotozoal for AIDS-related* Pneumocystis *pneumonia (PCP) (orphan); investigational (orphan) antineoplastic for multiple cancers* [trimetrexate glucuronate] 25 mg

neutroflavine [see: acriflavine]

Neutrogena Antiseptic Cleanser for Acne-Prone Skin topical liquid OTC *cleanser for acne* [benzethonium chloride]

Neutrogena Baby Cleansing Formula Soap bar (discontinued 2010) OTC *therapeutic skin cleanser*

Neutrogena Body lotion, oil OTC *moisturizer; emollient*

Neutrogena Clear Pore topical liquid OTC *keratolytic cleansing mask for acne* [benzoyl peroxide] 3.5%

Neutrogena Drying gel (discontinued 2009) OTC *astringent and antiseptic for acne* [hamamelis water (witch hazel); isopropyl alcohol]

Neutrogena Moisture lotion OTC *moisturizer; emollient* 🔁 nitrogen mustard

Neutrogena Non-Drying Cleansing lotion OTC *soap-free therapeutic skin cleanser*

Neutrogena Norwegian Formula Hand cream OTC *moisturizer; emollient*

Neutrogena Oil-Free Acne Wash topical liquid OTC *keratolytic cleanser for acne* [salicylic acid] 2%

Neutrogena Soap; Neutrogena Cleansing for Acne-Prone Skin; Neutrogena Dry Skin Soap; Neutrogena Oily Skin Soap bar OTC *therapeutic skin cleanser*

Neutrogena T/Gel Original shampoo OTC *antiseborrheic; antipsoriatic; antipruritic; antibacterial* [coal tar extract] 2%

Neutrogena T/Sal shampoo OTC *antiseborrheic; antipsoriatic; antipruritic; antibacterial* [salicylic acid; coal tar] 2%•2%

neutrophil inhibitor, recombinant human (rhNI) *investigational (orphan) for cystic fibrosis*

Nevanac eye drop suspension ℞ *nonsteroidal anti-inflammatory drug (NSAID) for pain and inflammation following cataract extraction surgery* [nepafenac] 0.1%

nevirapine USAN, INN *oral antiviral non-nucleoside reverse transcriptase inhibitor (NNRTI) for HIV-1 infections*

nevirapine & lamivudine & stavudine *combination nucleoside reverse transcriptase inhibitor (NRTI) and non-nucleoside reverse transcriptase inhibitor (NNRTI) for HIV and AIDS* 50•30•6, 100•60•12, 200•150•30, 200•150•40 mg oral

nevirapine & lamivudine & zidovudine *combination nucleoside reverse transcriptase inhibitor (NRTI) and non-nucleoside reverse transcriptase inhibitor (NNRTI) for HIV and AIDS* 50•30•60, 200•150•300 mg oral

New Jersey tea (*Ceanothus americanus***)** root bark *medicinal herb used as an astringent, expectorant, and sedative*

New Zealand green-lipped mussel (*Perna canaliculus***)** freeze-dried body or gonads *natural treatment for osteoarthritis and rheumatoid arthritis*

new-estranol 1 [see: diethylstilbestrol]

new-oestranol 1 [see: diethylstilbestrol]

new-oestranol 11 [see: diethylstilbestrol dipropionate]

NewPaks (trademarked delivery form) *ready-to-use closed system containers*

NewPhase Complete caplets OTC *natural/herbal supplement for the relief or postmenopausal symptoms* [multiple vitamins and minerals; isoflavones; phytoestrogens]

New-Skin topical liquid, spray OTC *skin protectant; antiseptic* [hydroxyquinoline] 🔁 Nesacaine

NexACT (trademarked delivery device) *topical delivery system*

Nexavar film-coated tablets ℞ *antineoplastic for advanced renal cell carcinoma (orphan) and hepatocellular carcinoma* [sorafenib (as tosylate)] 200 mg

Nexcede orally disintegrating film ℞ *analgesic; nonsteroidal anti-inflamma-*

tory drug (NSAID) for mild aches and pains [ketoprofen] 12.5 mg

nexeridine INN *analgesic* [also: nexeridine HCl]

nexeridine HCl USAN *analgesic* [also: nexeridine]

Nexiclon XR extended-release oral suspension ℞ *adjunct to stimulant treatment of ADHD* [clonidine HCl] 0.09 mg/mL

Nexium delayed-release enteric-coated pellets in capsules ℞ *proton pump inhibitor for gastric and duodenal ulcers, erosive esophagitis, GERD, and other gastroesophageal disorders* [esomeprazole magnesium] 20, 40 mg

Nexium delayed-release oral suspension ℞ *proton pump inhibitor for gastric and duodenal ulcers, erosive esophagitis, GERD, and other gastroesophageal disorders* [esomeprazole magnesium] 10, 20, 40 mg

Nexium I.V. powder for infusion ℞ *proton pump inhibitor for the short-term treatment of GERD in patients who cannot take the drug orally* [esomeprazole sodium] 20, 40 mg

Nexrutine capsules OTC *dietary supplement; selective COX-2 inhibitor; anti-inflammatory; antipyretic* [Phellodendron amurense extract] 250 mg

Next Choice tablets OTC ≥ 17 years; ℞ ≤ 16 years *emergency progestin-only postcoital contraceptive* [levonorgestrel] 0.75 mg

Nexterone IV infusion ℞ *antiarrhythmic for acute ventricular tachycardia and fibrillation* [amiodarone HCl] 150, 180, 300, 360 mg/bag

NFL (Novantrone, fluorouracil, leucovorin [rescue]) *chemotherapy protocol for breast cancer*

NG-29 *investigational (orphan) diagnostic aid for pituitary release of growth hormone*

N-Graft *investigational (orphan) intracerebral implant for advanced Parkinson disease (for co-implantation with fetal neural cells)* [Sertoli cells, porcine]

N.G.T. cream ℞ *corticosteroidal anti-inflammatory; antifungal* [triamcinolone acetonide; nystatin] 0.1%• 100 000 U per g

NI (neutrophil inhibitor) [q.v.]

niacin (vitamin B₃) USP *water-soluble vitamin; peripheral vasodilator; antihyperlipidemic for hypertriglyceridemia (types IV and V hyperlipidemia) and hypercholesterolemia* [also: nicotinic acid] 50, 100, 125, 250, 400, 500 mg oral

Niacin Flush-Free capsules OTC *vitamin B₃ supplement; antihyperlipidemic* [niacin] 750 mg

Niacin Flush-Free tablets OTC *vitamin B₃ supplement; antihyperlipidemic* [niacin] 400 mg

Niacin No Flush tablets OTC *vitamin B₃ supplement; antihyperlipidemic* [niacin] 100, 250 mg

niacinamide (vitamin B₃) USP *water-soluble vitamin; enzyme cofactor; treatment for vitamin B₃ deficiency; also used for several dermatologic conditions, including psoriasis* [also: nicotinamide] 100, 500 mg oral

niacinamide hydroiodide *expectorant*

Niacor immediate-release tablets ℞ *vitamin B₃ therapy; peripheral vasodilator; antihyperlipidemic for hypertriglyceridemia (types IV and V hyperlipidemia) and hypercholesterolemia* [niacin] 500 mg

nialamide NF, INN

niaprazine INN ⊘ Naprosyn

Niaspan enteric-coated, extended-release caplets ℞ *vitamin B₃ therapy; peripheral vasodilator; antihyperlipidemic for hypertriglyceridemia (types IV and V hyperlipidemia) and hypercholesterolemia* [niacin] 500, 750, 1000 mg ⊘ NuSpin

nibroxane USAN, INN *topical antimicrobial* ⊘ naproxen

nicafenine INN

nicainoprol INN

nicametate INN, BAN

nicaraven INN

nicarbazin BAN

nicardipine INN, BAN *vasodilator for chronic stable angina; calcium channel blocker for hypertension* [also: nicardipine HCl]

nicardipine HCl USAN *vasodilator for chronic stable angina; calcium channel blocker for hypertension* [also: nicardipine] 20, 30 mg oral; 2.5 mg/mL injection

NicCheck I reagent strips OTC *in vitro diagnostic aid for urine nicotine, used to determine the smoking status of the subject*

N'Ice throat spray OTC *mild anesthetic; antipruritic; counterirritant* [menthol] 0.12%

N'Ice; N'Ice 'n Clear lozenges OTC *mild anesthetic; antipruritic; counterirritant* [menthol] 5 mg

N'Ice Vitamin C Drops (lozenges) OTC *vitamin C supplement* [ascorbic acid] 60 mg

nicergoline USAN, INN *vasodilator*

niceritrol INN, BAN

nicethamide BAN [also: nikethamide]

niceverine INN

nickel *element (Ni)*

niclofolan INN, BAN

niclosamide USAN, INN *anthelmintic for cestodiasis (tapeworm)*

nicoboxil INN

nicoclonate INN

nicocodine INN, BAN

nicocortonide INN

NicoDerm CQ Step 1; NicoDerm CQ Step 2; NicoDerm CQ Step 3 transdermal patch OTC *smoking cessation aid for the relief of nicotine withdrawal symptoms* [nicotine] 21 mg/day; 14 mg/day; 7 mg/day

nicodicodine INN, BAN

nicoduozide (isoniazid + nicothiazone)

nicofibrate INN

nicofuranose INN

nicofurate INN

nicogrelate INN

Nicomide tablets (discontinued 2010) ℞ *vitamin/mineral supplement* [nicoti-namide; zinc oxide; cupric oxide; folic acid] 750•25•1.5•0.5 mg

nicomol INN

nicomorphine INN, BAN

nicopholine INN

nicorandil USAN, INN *coronary vasodilator*

Nicorette chewing gum, lozenges OTC *smoking cessation aid for the relief of nicotine withdrawal symptoms* [nicotine (as polacrilex)] 2, 4 mg ② NuCort

nicothiazone INN

nicotinaldehyde thiosemicarbazone [see: nicothiazone]

nicotinamide (vitamin B₃) INN, BAN, JAN *water-soluble vitamin; enzyme cofactor; treatment for vitamin B₃ deficiency; also used for several dermatologic conditions, including psoriasis* [also: niacinamide] 100, 500 mg oral

Nicotinamide with Zinc-Copper and Folic Acid tablets ℞ *vitamin/mineral supplement* [nicotinamide; zinc oxide; cupric oxide; folic acid] 750•25•1.5•0.5 mg

nicotinamide-adenine dinucleotide (NAD) [now: nadide]

nicotine *a poisonous alkaloid used as an insecticide and external parasiticide; the active principle in tobacco; smoking cessation aid for the relief of nicotine withdrawal symptoms* [see also: tobacco] 7, 14, 21 mg/day transdermal ② Neocate One

nicotine bitartrate USAN *smoking cessation aid for the relief of nicotine withdrawal symptoms*

nicotine conjugate vaccine *investigational (Phase III) vaccine for nicotine addiction*

nicotine & mecamylamine HCl *investigational (Phase III) transdermal patch for smoking cessation*

nicotine polacrilex USAN *smoking cessation aid for the relief of nicotine withdrawal symptoms* 2, 4 mg oral

nicotine resin complex [see: nicotine polacrilex]

nicotinic acid (vitamin B₃) INN, BAN, JAN *water-soluble vitamin; peripheral* *vasodilator; antihyperlipidemic for hyper-triglyceridemia (types IV and V hyper-lipidemia) and hypercholesterolemia* [also: niacin] 50, 100, 125, 250, 400, 500, 1000 mg oral

nicotinic acid amide [see: niacinamide; nicotinamide]

nicotinic acid 1-oxide [see: oxiniacic acid]

nicotinohydroxamic acid [see: nicoxamat]

6-nicotinoyl dihydrocodeine [see: nicodicodine]

6-nicotinoylcodeine [see: nicocodine]

4-nicotinoylmorpholine [see: nicopholine]

nicotinyl alcohol USAN, BAN *peripheral vasodilator*

nicotinyl tartrate

Nicotrol oral inhaler ℞ *smoking cessation aid for the relief of nicotine withdrawal symptoms* [nicotine] 10 mg (4 mg delivered) per cartridge

Nicotrol NS nasal spray ℞ *smoking cessation aid for the relief of nicotine withdrawal symptoms* [nicotine] 0.5 mg/spray

Nicotrol Step 1; Nicotrol Step 2; Nicotrol Step 3 transdermal patch OTC *smoking cessation aid for the relief of nicotine withdrawal symptoms* [nicotine] 15 mg/day; 10 mg/day; 5 mg/day

nicotylamide [see: niacinamide]

nicoumalone BAN [also: acenocoumarol]

nicoxamat INN

nictiazem INN

nictindole INN

NicVAX *investigational (Phase III) vaccine for nicotine addiction* [nicotine conjugate vaccine]

Nidran ℞ *alkylating antineoplastic* [nimustin HCl]

nidroxyzone INN

Nifediac CC film-coated extended-release tablets ℞ *calcium channel blocker for hypertension; also used for anal fissures and Raynaud phenomenon* [nifedipine] 30, 60, 90 mg

Nifedical XL film-coated sustained-release tablets ℞ *coronary vasodilator for angina with or without vasospasm; calcium channel blocker for hypertension; also used for anal fissures and Raynaud phenomenon* [nifedipine] 30, 60 mg

nifedipine USAN, USP, INN, BAN *coronary vasodilator for angina with or without vasospasm; calcium channel blocker for hypertension; also used for anal fissures and Raynaud phenomenon; investigational (orphan) for interstitial cystitis* 10, 20, 30, 60, 90 mg oral

nifenalol INN

nifenazone INN, BAN

Niferex tablets, elixir OTC *iron supplement* [iron (as polysaccharide-iron complex)] 50, 100 mg/5 mL ☑ Nephrox

Niferex Gold film-coated tablets ℞ *hematinic* [iron (as ferrous bis-glycinate chelate and polysaccharide-iron complex); vitamin B_{12}; vitamin C; folic acid] 200•0.025•110•1 mg

Niferex-150 capsules OTC *vitamin/iron supplement* [vitamin C (as calcium ascorbate and calcium threonate); iron (as ferrous aspartoglycinate and polysaccharide-iron complex); succinic acid] 50•150•50 mg ☑ Nephrox

Niferex-150 Forte capsules ℞ *hematinic* [iron (as elemental iron, elemental polysaccharide iron, and ferric aspartoglycinate); vitamin B_{12}; vitamin C; folic acid] 150•0.025•60•1 mg

Niferex-PN film-coated tablets ℞ *prenatal vitamin/iron supplement* [iron (as polysaccharide-iron complex); multiple vitamins & minerals; folic acid] 60•±•1 mg

Niferex-PN Forte film-coated tablets (discontinued 2008) ℞ *prenatal vitamin/mineral/calcium/iron supplement* [multiple vitamins & minerals; calcium; polysaccharide-iron complex; folic acid] ±•250•60•1 mg

niflumic acid INN

nifluridide USAN *ectoparasiticide*
nifungin USAN, INN
nifuradene USAN, INN *antibacterial* 🄰
Neo-fradin
nifuralazine [see: furalazine]
nifuraldezone USAN, INN *antibacterial*
nifuralide INN
nifuramizone [see: nifurethazone]
nifuratel USAN, INN *antibacterial; antifungal; antiprotozoal (Trichomonas)*
nifuratrone USAN, INN *antibacterial*
nifurazolidone [see: furazolidone]
nifurdazil USAN, INN *antibacterial*
nifurethazone INN
nifurfoline INN
nifurhydrazone [see: nihydrazone]
nifurimide USAN, INN *antibacterial*
nifurizone INN
nifurmazole INN
nifurmerone USAN, INN *antifungal*
nifuroquine INN
nifuroxazide INN
nifuroxime NF, INN
nifurpipone (NP) INN
nifurpirinol USAN, INN *antibacterial*
nifurprazine INN
nifurquinazol USAN, INN *antibacterial*
nifursemizone USAN, INN *antiprotozoal for poultry (Histomonas)*
nifursol USAN, INN *antiprotozoal for poultry (Histomonas)*
nifurthiazole USAN, INN *antibacterial*
nifurthiline [see: thiofuradene]
nifurtimox INN, BAN *anti-infective for Chagas disease* (available only from the Centers for Disease Control and Prevention)
nifurtoinol INN
nifurvidine INN
nifurzide INN
Night Time Multi-Symptom Cold/Flu Relief liquid-filled gelcaps OTC *antitussive; antihistamine; sleep aid; decongestant; analgesic; antipyretic* [dextromethorphan hydrobromide; doxylamine succinate; pseudoephedrine HCl; acetaminophen] 15•6.25•30•325 mg
nightshade; nightshade vine *medicinal herb* [see: bittersweet nightshade]

nightshade, American *medicinal herb* [see: pokeweed]
nightshade, deadly *medicinal herb* [see: belladonna]
nightshade, fetid; stinking nightshade *medicinal herb* [see: henbane]
nightshade, three-leaved *medicinal herb* [see: birthroot]
Nighttime Cold softgels (discontinued 2007) OTC *antitussive; antihistamine; sleep aid; decongestant; analgesic; antipyretic* [dextromethorphan hydrobromide; doxylamine succinate; pseudoephedrine HCl; acetaminophen] 10•6.25•30•250 mg
niguldipine INN
nihydrazone INN
nikethamide NF, INN [also: nicethamide]
Nilandron tablets ℞ *antiandrogen antineoplastic for metastatic prostate cancer* [nilutamide] 150 mg
nileprost INN
nilestriol INN *estrogen* [also: nylestriol]
nilotinib HCl *protein-tyrosine kinase inhibitor antineoplastic for Philadelphia chromosome–positive chronic myeloid leukemia (CML)*
nilprazole INN
Nilstat cream (discontinued 2010) ℞ *antifungal* [nystatin] 100 000 U/g
Nilstat ointment ℞ *antifungal* [nystatin] 100 000 U/g
Nilstat oral suspension, bulk powder for oral suspension ℞ *antifungal; oral candidiasis treatment* [nystatin] 100 000 U/mL; 150 million, 1 billion, 2 billion U
niludipine INN
nilutamide USAN, INN, BAN *antiandrogen antineoplastic adjunct to surgical or chemical castration for metastatic prostate cancer*
nilvadipine USAN, INN, JAN *calcium channel antagonist*
nimazone USAN, INN *anti-inflammatory* 🄰 neomycin; Numoisyn
Nimbex IV infusion ℞ *nondepolarizing neuromuscular blocking agent for anes-*

thesia [cisatracurium besylate] 2, 10 mg/mL

Nimbus; Nimbus Quick Strip test kit for home use OTC *in vitro diagnostic aid; urine pregnancy test* [monoclonal antibody-based enzyme immunoassay]

Nimbus Plus test kit for professional use ℞ *in vitro diagnostic aid; urine pregnancy test*

nimesulide INN, BAN

nimetazepam INN

nimidane USAN, INN *veterinary acaricide*

nimodipine USAN, INN, BAN *vasodilator; calcium channel blocker for subarachnoid hemorrhage (SAH)* 30 mg oral

nimorazole INN, BAN

Nimotop soft liquid-filled capsules (discontinued 2008) ℞ *calcium channel blocker for subarachnoid hemorrhage (SAH)* [nimodipine] 30 mg

nimotuzumab *investigational (orphan) monoclonal antibody for malignant glioma*

nimustine INN *alkylating neoplastic*

nimustine HCl *alkylating neoplastic*

niobium *element (Nb)*

niometacin INN ⑨ Pneumotussin

Nion B Plus C caplets (discontinued 2008) OTC *vitamin supplement* [multiple B vitamins; vitamin C] ≟•300 mg

Nipent powder for IV injection ℞ *antibiotic antineoplastic for hairy cell leukemia (orphan); investigational (orphan) for chronic lymphocytic leukemia and cutaneous and peripheral T-cell lymphomas* [pentostatin] 10 mg

niperotidine INN

nipradilol INN

Nipride (brand discontinued 1992) [see: sodium nitroprusside]

niprisan *investigational (orphan) for sickle cell disease*

niprofazone INN

Niravam orally disintegrating tablets ℞ *benzodiazepine anxiolytic; sedative; treatment for panic disorders and agoraphobia* [alprazolam] 0.25, 0.5, 1, 2 mg

niridazole USAN, INN *antischistosomal*

nisbuterol INN *bronchodilator* [also: nisbuterol mesylate]

nisbuterol mesylate USAN *bronchodilator* [also: nisbuterol]

nisobamate USAN, INN *minor tranquilizer*

nisoldipine USAN, INN, BAN, JAN *coronary vasodilator; calcium channel blocker for hypertension* 8.5, 17, 25.5, 34 mg oral

nisoxetine USAN, INN *antidepressant*

nisterime INN *androgen* [also: nisterime acetate]

nisterime acetate USAN *androgen* [also: nisterime]

nitarsone USAN, INN *antiprotozoal (Histomonas)*

nitazoxanide (NTZ) INN *antiprotozoal for pediatric diarrhea due to* Cryptosporidium parvum *and* Giardia lamblia *infections (orphan); investigational (orphan) for intestinal amebiasis*

Nite Time Children's Liquid (discontinued 2007) OTC *antitussive; antihistamine; decongestant* [dextromethorphan hydrobromide; chlorpheniramine maleate; pseudoephedrine HCl] 15•2•30 mg/15 mL

Nite Time Cold Formula for Adults oral liquid (discontinued 2007) OTC *antitussive; antihistamine; sleep aid; decongestant; analgesic; antipyretic* [dextromethorphan hydrobromide; doxylamine succinate; pseudoephedrine HCl; acetaminophen; alcohol 10%] 30•12.5•60•1000 mg/30 mL

nithiamide USAN *veterinary antibacterial* [also: aminitrozole; acinitrazole]

Nithiodote IV injection ℞ *antidote to acute cyanide poisoning* [sodium nitrite; sodium thiosulfate] 30•250 mg/mL

nitisinone *adjunctive treatment for hereditary tyrosinemia type 1 (HT-1), a pediatric liver disease (orphan); investigational (orphan) for alkaptonuria*

nitracrine INN

nitrafudam INN *antidepressant* [also: nitrafudam HCl]

nitrafudam HCl USAN *antidepressant* [also: nitrafudam]

nitralamine HCl USAN *antifungal*

nitramisole INN *anthelmintic* [also: nitramisole HCl]

nitramisole HCl USAN *anthelmintic* [also: nitramisole]

nitraquazone INN

nitrates *a class of antianginal agents that cause the relaxation of vascular smooth muscles*

nitratophenylmercury [see: phenylmercuric nitrate]

nitrazepam USAN, INN, BAN, JAN *benzodiazepine sedative; anxiolytic; anticonvulsant; hypnotic*

nitre, sweet spirit of [see: ethyl nitrite]

nitrefazole INN, BAN

Nitrek transdermal patch ℞ *coronary vasodilator; antianginal; also used for acute myocardial infarction, erectile dysfunction, and Raynaud disease* [nitroglycerin] 0.2, 0.4, 0.6 mg/hr. (22.4, 44.8, 67.2 mg total)

nitrendipine USAN, INN, BAN, JAN *antihypertensive; calcium channel blocker*

nitric acid NF *acidifying agent*

nitric oxide *inhalation gas for neonatal hypoxic respiratory failure due to persistent pulmonary hypertension (orphan); investigational (orphan) for acute adult respiratory distress syndrome and to diagnose sarcoidosis*

nitricholine perchlorate INN

"nitro paste"; "nitropaste" *a brief term for "nitroglycerin paste"* [properly called: nitroglycerin ointment]

***p*-nitrobenzenearsonic acid** [see: nitarsone]

Nitro-Bid ointment ℞ *coronary vasodilator; antianginal; also used for acute myocardial infarction, chronic anal fissure pain, erectile dysfunction, and Raynaud disease* [nitroglycerin] 2% (15 mg/inch)

9-nitrocamptothecin (9-NC); 9-nitro-20-(S)-camptothecin [now: rubitecan]

nitroclofene INN

nitrocycline USAN, INN *antibacterial*

nitrodan USAN, INN *anthelmintic*

Nitro-Dur transdermal patch ℞ *coronary vasodilator; antianginal; also used for acute myocardial infarction, erectile dysfunction, and Raynaud disease* [nitroglycerin] 0.1, 0.2, 0.3, 0.4, 0.6, 0.8 mg/hr. (20, 40, 60, 80, 120, 160 mg total)

nitroethanolamine [see: aminoethyl nitrate]

nitrofuradoxadone [see: furmethoxadone]

nitrofural INN *broad-spectrum bactericidal; adjunct to burn treatment* [also: nitrofurazone]

nitrofurantoin USP, INN *urinary antibiotic* 50, 100 mg oral; 25 mg/5 mL oral

nitrofurantoin sodium *urinary antibiotic*

nitrofurazone USP, BAN *broad-spectrum bactericidal; adjunct to burn treatment and skin grafting* [also: nitrofural] 0.2% topical

nitrofurmethone [see: furaltadone]

nitrofuroxizone [see: nidroxyzone]

nitrogen (N₂) NF *air displacement agent; element (N)* ⑫ Neutra-Caine; Nutricon

nitrogen monoxide [see: nitrous oxide]

nitrogen mustard N-oxide HCl JAN *alkylating antineoplastic* [also: mechlorethamine HCl; chlormethine; mustine] ⑫ Neutrogena Moisture

nitrogen mustards *a class of alkylating antineoplastics* ⑫ Neutrogena Moisture

nitrogen oxide (N₂O) [see: nitrous oxide]

nitroglycerin USP *coronary vasodilator; antianginal; antihypertensive* [also: glyceryl trinitrate] 0.3, 0.4, 0.6 mg sublingual; 2.5, 6.5, 9 mg oral; 5 mg/mL injection; 0.1, 0.2, 0.4, 0.6 mg/hr. transdermal; 2% topical

Nitroglycerin in Dextrose injection ℞ *coronary vasodilator; antianginal; antihypertensive* [nitroglycerin] 100 mcg/mL•5%, 200 mcg/mL•5%, 400 mcg/mL•5%

nitrohydroxyquinoline [see: nitroxoline]

Nitrolan oral liquid OTC *enteral nutritional therapy* [lactose-free formula] ☑ Nutrilan

Nitrolingual Pumpspray CFC-free translingual aerosol ℞ *coronary vasodilator; emergency antianginal* [nitroglycerin; alcohol 20%] 0.4 mg/metered dose

nitromannitol [see: mannitol hexanitrate]

nitromersol USP *topical anti-infective*

nitromide USAN *coccidiostat for poultry; antibacterial*

nitromifene INN

nitromifene citrate USAN *antiestrogen*

NitroMist translingual aerosol ℞ *coronary vasodilator; emergency antianginal* [nitroglycerin] 0.4 mg/spray

"nitropaste"; "nitro paste" *a brief term for "nitroglycerin paste"* [properly called: nitroglycerin ointment]

Nitropress powder for IV injection, flip-top vials ℞ *vasodilator for hypertensive emergency* [sodium nitroprusside] 50 mg/dose

nitroprusside sodium [see: sodium nitroprusside]

NitroQuick sublingual tablets (discontinued 2009) ℞ *coronary vasodilator; emergency antianginal* [nitroglycerin] 0.3, 0.4, 0.6 mg (1/200, 1/150, 1/100 gr.)

nitroscanate USAN, INN *veterinary anthelmintic*

nitrosoureas *a class of alkylating antineoplastics*

Nitrostat sublingual tablets ℞ *coronary vasodilator; emergency antianginal* [nitroglycerin] 0.3, 0.4, 0.6 mg (1/200, 1/150, 1/100 gr.)

nitrosulfathiazole INN [also: paranitrosulfathiazole]

NitroTab sublingual tablets (discontinued 2007) ℞ *coronary vasodilator; emergency antianginal* [nitroglycerin] 0.3, 0.4, 0.6 mg (1/200, 1/150, 1/100 gr.)

Nitro-Time extended-release capsules ℞ *coronary vasodilator; antianginal;*

antihypertensive [nitroglycerin] 2.5, 6.5, 9 mg

nitrous acid, sodium salt [see: sodium nitrite]

nitrous oxide (N₂O) USP *a weak inhalation general anesthetic; sometimes abused as a street drug to create a dreamy or floating sensation*

nitroxinil INN

nitroxoline INN, BAN

nivacortol INN *corticosteroid; anti-inflammatory* [also: nivazol]

nivadipine [see: nilvadipine]

nivaquine [see: chloroquine phosphate]

nivazol USAN *corticosteroid; anti-inflammatory* [also: nivacortol] ☑ Novasal

Nivea After Tan; Nivea Moisturizing; Nivea Moisturizing Extra Enriched lotion OTC *moisturizer; emollient*

Nivea Moisturizing; Nivea Skin oil OTC *moisturizer; emollient*

Nivea Moisturizing Creme Soap bar OTC *therapeutic skin cleanser*

Nivea Ultra Moisturizing Creme OTC *moisturizer; emollient*

nivimedone sodium USAN *antiallergic*

Nix cream OTC *parasiticide for scabies and lice; also used for papulopustular rosacea* [permethrin] 1%

Nix Complete Lice Treatment System topical liquid OTC *parasiticide for scabies and lice; also used for papulopustular rosacea* [permethrin; alcohol 20%] 1%

nixylic acid INN

nizatidine USAN, USP, INN, BAN, JAN *histamine H₂ antagonist for gastric and duodenal ulcers and gastroesophageal reflux disease (GERD); also used to prevent NSAID-induced gastric ulcers* 150, 300 mg oral; 15 mg/mL oral

nizofenone INN

Nizoral cream ℞ *antifungal for tinea corporis, tinea cruris, tinea pedis, tinea versicolor, cutaneous candidiasis, and seborrheic dermatitis* [ketoconazole] 2% ☑ Nasarel

Nizoral shampoo ℞ (available OTC in Canada) *antifungal for dandruff* [ketoconazole] 2% ⊠ Nasarel

Nizoral tablets (discontinued 2008) ℞ *systemic imidazole antifungal* [ketoconazole] 200 mg ⊠ Nasarel

Nizoral A-D shampoo OTC *antifungal for dandruff* [ketoconazole] 1%

NMDA (N-methyl-D-aspartate) [q.v.]

N-Multistix; N-Multistix SG reagent strips (discontinued 2008) OTC *in vitro diagnostic aid for multiple urine products*

NNRTIs (non-nucleoside reverse transcriptase inhibitors) [see: reverse transcriptase inhibitors]

No Pain-HP roll-on liquid OTC *counterirritant; analgesic for muscle and joint pain* [capsaicin] 0.075%

nobelium *element (No)*

noberastine USAN, INN, BAN *antihistamine*

Noble Formula cream, topical spray OTC *antibacterial; antifungal* [pyrithione zinc] 0.25%

noble yarrow *medicinal herb* [see: yarrow]

nocebo effect [L. I will harm] *a perceived adverse effect from an inert substance* [compare to: placebo effect]

nocloprost INN

nocodazole USAN, INN *antineoplastic*

nodding wakerobin *medicinal herb* [see: birthroot]

Nodolor capsules ℞ *cerebral vasoconstrictor and analgesic for vascular and tension headaches; "possibly effective" for migraine headaches* [isomethep-tene mucate; dichloralphenazone; acetaminophen] 65•100•325 mg

NōDōz coated caplets OTC *CNS stimulant; analeptic* [caffeine] 200 mg

nofecainide INN

nofetumomab merpentan *monoclonal antibody imaging agent for small cell lung cancer*

nogalamycin USAN, INN *antineoplastic*

NoHist extended-release caplets ℞ *decongestant; antihistamine* [phenyl-

ephrine HCl; chlorpheniramine maleate] 20•8 mg ⊠ Nuhist

NoHist A oral liquid ℞ *decongestant; antihistamine; sleep aid* [phenylephrine HCl; chlorpheniramine maleate; phenyltoloxamine citrate] 5•2.5•7.5 mg/5 mL ⊠ Nuhist

NoHist DMX extended-release caplets ℞ *decongestant; antihistamine; antitussive* [phenylephrine HCl; chlorpheniramine maleate; dextromethorphan hydrobromide] 20•8•30 mg

NoHist EXT extended-release tablets ℞ *antihistamine; anticholinergic to dry mucosal secretions* [chlorpheniramine maleate; methscopolamine nitrate] 8•2.5 mg

NoHist LQ oral liquid OTC *decongestant; antihistamine* [phenylephrine HCl; chlorpheniramine maleate] 10•4 mg/5 mL

NoHist PDX oral drops ℞ *decongestant; antihistamine; antitussive; for children 2–11 years* [phenylephrine HCl; chlorpheniramine maleate; dextromethorphan hydrobromide] 1.75•0.75•2.75 mg/mL

NoHist Plus chewable caplets ℞ *decongestant; antihistamine; anticholinergic to dry mucosal secretions* [phenylephrine HCl; chlorpheniramine maleate; methscopolamine nitrate] 10•2•1.25 mg

Nolahist tablets (discontinued 2009) OTC *nonselective piperidine antihistamine for allergic rhinitis* [phenindamine tartrate] 25 mg

nolinium bromide USAN, INN *antisecretory; antiulcerative*

nomegestrol acetate (NOMAC) INN *progestin*

nomelidine INN

nomifensine INN *antidepressant* [also: nomifensine maleate]

nomifensine maleate USAN *antidepressant* [also: nomifensine]

Nomuc-PE extended-release capsules ℞ *decongestant; expectorant* [pseudoephedrine HCl; guaifenesin] 60•200 mg

nonabine INN, BAN

nonabsorbable surgical suture [see: suture, nonabsorbable surgical]

nonachlazine [now: azaclorzine HCl]

nonacog alfa USAN, INN *synthetic human blood coagulation factor IX; antihemophilic for hemophilia B and Christmas disease (orphan)* [also: factor IX complex]

nonanedioic acid [see: azelaic acid]

nonaperone INN

nonapyrimine INN

Non-Aspirin caplets OTC *analgesic; antipyretic* [acetaminophen] 500 mg

nonathymulin INN

nondestearinated cod liver oil [see: cod liver oil, nondestearinated]

Non-Drowsy Allergy Relief orally disintegrating tablets OTC *nonsedating antihistamine for allergic rhinitis* [loratadine] 10 mg

Non-Drowsy Allergy Relief for Kids syrup OTC *nonsedating antihistamine for allergic rhinitis* [loratadine] 5 mg/5 mL

Non-Habit Forming Stool Softener capsules OTC *laxative; stool softener* [docusate sodium] 100 mg

noni (Morinda citrifolia) berries *medicinal herb for arthritis, bacterial infections, diabetes, drug addiction, headache, hypertension, liver and skin disorders, pain, and slowing aging; also used as an antioxidant*

nonionic contrast media *a class of newer radiopaque agents that, in general, have a low osmolar concentration of iodine (the contrast agent), which corresponds to a lower incidence of adverse reactions* [also called: low osmolar contrast media (LOCM)]

nonivamide INN

non-nucleoside reverse transcriptase inhibitors (NNRTIs) [see: reverse transcriptase inhibitors]

nonoxinol 4 INN *surfactant* [also: nonoxynol 4]

nonoxinol 9 INN *wetting and solubilizing agent; spermicide* [also: nonoxynol 9]

nonoxinol 15 INN *surfactant* [also: nonoxynol 15]

nonoxinol 30 INN *surfactant* [also: nonoxynol 30]

nonoxynol 4 USAN *surfactant* [also: nonoxinol 4]

nonoxynol 9 USAN, USP *wetting and solubilizing agent; spermicide* [also: nonoxinol 9]

nonoxynol 10 NF *surfactant*

nonoxynol 15 USAN *surfactant* [also: nonoxinol 15]

nonoxynol 30 USAN *surfactant* [also: nonoxinol 30]

nonsteroidal anti-inflammatory drugs (NSAIDs) *a class of anti-inflammatory drugs that have analgesic and antipyretic effects*

nonylphenoxypolyethoxyethanol [see: nonoxynol 4, 9, 15, & 30]

Nootropil ℞ *cognition adjuvant; investigational (orphan) for myoclonus* [piracetam]

nopal plant *medicinal herb for cleansing the lymphatic system, diabetes, digestion, obesity, neutralizing toxins, and preventing arteriosclerosis*

Nora-BE tablets (in packs of 28) ℞ *oral contraceptive (progestin only)* [norethindrone] 0.35 mg

noracymethadol INN *analgesic* [also: noracymethadol HCl]

noracymethadol HCl USAN *analgesic* [also: noracymethadol]

noradrenaline bitartrate [see: norepinephrine bitartrate]

noramidopyrine methanesulfonate sodium [see: dipyrone]

norandrostenolone phenylpropionate [see: nandrolone phenpropionate]

norbolethone USAN *anabolic* [also: norboletone]

norboletone INN *anabolic* [also: norbolethone]

norbudrine INN [also: norbutrine]

norbutrine BAN [also: norbudrine]

norclostebol INN

Norco tablets ℞ *narcotic analgesic; antipyretic* [hydrocodone bitartrate; acetaminophen] 5•325, 7.5•325, 10•325 mg

norcodeine INN, BAN

Norcuron powder for IV injection ℞ *nondepolarizing neuromuscular blocker; adjunct to anesthesia* [vecuronium bromide] 10, 20 mg/vial

norcycline [see: sancycline]

nordazepam INN

nordefrin HCl NF

Nordette-28 tablets (in Pilpaks of 28) ℞ *monophasic oral contraceptive; emergency postcoital contraceptive* [levonorgestrel; ethinyl estradiol] 0.15 mg• 30 mcg

nordinone INN

NordiPen (trademarked delivery device) *subcu self-injector for* **Norditropin**

Norditropin powder for subcu injection (discontinued 2008) ℞ *growth hormone for children and adults with congenital or endogenous growth hormone deficiency (GHD), short bowel syndrome, or AIDS-wasting syndrome; for children with Turner syndrome, Prader-Willi syndrome, or renal-induced growth failure* [somatropin] 4, 8 mg (12, 24 IU) per vial

Norditropin prefilled cartridges for **NordiPen** (self-injection device) ℞ *growth hormone for children and adults with congenital or endogenous growth hormone deficiency (GHD), short bowel syndrome, or AIDS-wasting syndrome; for children with Turner syndrome, Prader-Willi syndrome, or renal-induced growth failure* [somatropin] 5, 15 mg (15, 45 IU) per 1.5 mL cartridge

Norditropin NordiFlex pen (self-injection device) ℞ *growth hormone for children and adults with congenital or endogenous growth hormone deficiency (GHD), short bowel syndrome, or AIDS-wasting syndrome; for children with Turner syndrome, Prader-Willi syndrome, or renal-induced growth failure* [somatropin] 5, 10, 15, 30 mg (15, 30, 45, 90 IU)

Norel DM oral liquid (discontinued 2010) ℞ *antitussive; antihistamine; decongestant* [dextromethorphan

hydrobromide; chlorpheniramine maleate; phenylephrine HCl] 15•4• 10 mg/5 mL

Norel EX dual-release caplets ℞ *decongestant; expectorant* [phenylephrine HCl (extended release); guaifenesin (50% immediate release; 50% extended release)] 40•800 mg

Norel LA extended-release tablets (discontinued 2007) ℞ *decongestant; antihistamine* [phenylephrine HCl; carbinoxamine maleate] 40•8 mg ⚗

Neoral

Norel SR extended-release tablets ℞ *decongestant; antihistamine; sleep aid; analgesic* [phenylephrine HCl; chlorpheniramine maleate; phenyltoloxamine citrate; acetaminophen] 40• 8•50•325 mg

norelgestromin USAN *progestin-type contraceptive*

norephedrine HCl [see: phenylpropanolamine HCl]

norepinephrine INN *adrenergic; vasoconstrictor; vasopressor for shock* [also: norepinephrine bitartrate]

norepinephrine bitartrate USAN, USP *adrenergic; vasoconstrictor; vasopressor for acute hypotensive shock* [also: norepinephrine] 1 mg/mL injection

norethandrolone NF, INN

norethindrone USP *synthetic progestin for amenorrhea, abnormal uterine bleeding, and endometriosis* [also: norethisterone] 0.35 mg oral

norethindrone acetate USP *synthetic progestin for amenorrhea, abnormal uterine bleeding, and endometriosis* 5 mg oral

norethindrone acetate & estradiol *a mixture of synthetic and natural hormones; hormone replacement therapy for postmenopausal symptoms* 0.5•1 mg oral

norethindrone acetate & ethinyl estradiol *monophasic oral contraceptive* 0.4•0.035, 0.5•0.035, 0.75• 0.035, 0.8•0.25, 1•0.005, 1•0.02, 1•0.03, 1•0.035 mg

norethisterone INN, BAN, JAN *progestin* [also: norethindrone]

norethynodrel USAN, USP *progestin* [also: noretynodrel]

noretynodrel INN *progestin* [also: norethynodrel]

noreximide INN

norfenefrine INN

Norflex IV or IM injection ℞ *skeletal muscle relaxant; analgesic; anticholinergic* [orphenadrine citrate] 30 mg/mL

norfloxacin USAN, USP, INN, BAN, JAN *broad-spectrum fluoroquinolone antibiotic*

norfloxacin succinil INN

norflurane USAN, INN *inhalation anesthetic*

Norforms vaginal suppositories OTC *moisturizer/lubricant* [polyethylene glycol]

Norgesic; Norgesic Forte tablets (discontinued 2009) ℞ *skeletal muscle relaxant; analgesic; antipyretic* [orphenadrine citrate; aspirin; caffeine] 25•385•30 mg; 50•770•60 mg

norgesterone INN

norgestimate USAN, INN, BAN *progestin*

norgestimate & ethinyl estradiol *monophasic oral contraceptive* 180•25, 215•25, 215•35, 250•25, 250•35 mcg

norgestomet USAN, INN *progestin*

norgestrel USAN, USP, INN *progestin*

d-norgestrel *(incorrect enantiomer designation)* [now: levonorgestrel]

D-norgestrel [see: levonorgestrel]

norgestrienone INN

Norinyl 1 + 35 tablets (in Wallettes of 28) ℞ *monophasic oral contraceptive* [norethindrone; ethinyl estradiol] 1 mg•35 mcg × 21 days; counters × 7 days ☒ naranol

Norinyl 1 + 50 tablets (in Wallettes of 28) ℞ *monophasic oral contraceptive* [norethindrone; mestranol] 1 mg•50 mcg × 21 days; counters × 7 days ☒ naranol

Noritate cream ℞ *antibiotic for rosacea* [metronidazole] 1%

norletimol INN

norleusactide INN [also: pentacosactride]

norlevorphanol INN, BAN

norlupinanes *a class of antibiotics* [also called: quinolizidines]

½ normal saline (½ NS; 0.45% sodium chloride) *electrolyte replacement*

normal saline (NS; 0.9% sodium chloride) *electrolyte replacement* [also: saline solution]

normal serum albumin [see: albumin, human]

normethadone INN, BAN

normethandrolone [see: normethandrone]

normethandrone

normethisterone [see: normethandrone]

Normix *investigational (orphan) antibacterial for hepatic encephalopathy* [rifaximin]

Normodyne IV infusion (discontinued 2009) ℞ *alpha- and beta-blocker; antihypertensive* [labetalol HCl] 5 mg/mL

normorphine INN, BAN

Normosang *investigational (orphan) for acute symptomatic porphyria and myelodysplastic syndrome* [heme arginate]

Normosol-M IV infusion ℞ *intravenous electrolyte therapy* [combined electrolyte solution] 1000 mL

Normosol-M and 5% Dextrose; Normosol-R and 5% Dextrose IV infusion ℞ *intravenous nutritional/electrolyte therapy* [combined electrolyte solution; dextrose]

Normosol-R; Normosol-R pH 7.4 IV infusion ℞ *intravenous electrolyte therapy* [combined electrolyte solution]

Noroxin film-coated tablets ℞ *broad-spectrum fluoroquinolone antibiotic* [norfloxacin] 400 mg

Norpace capsules ℞ *antiarrhythmic* [disopyramide phosphate] 100, 150 mg

Norpace CR controlled-release capsules ℞ *antiarrhythmic* [disopyramide phosphate] 100, 150 mg

norpipanone INN, BAN

Norpramin film-coated tablets ℞ *tricyclic antidepressant* [desipramine HCl] 10, 25, 50, 75, 100, 150 mg

norpseudoephedrine [see: cathine]

Nor-QD tablets (in packs of 28) ℞ *oral contraceptive (progestin only)* [norethindrone] 0.35 mg

Nortemp, Children's oral suspension OTC *analgesic; antipyretic* [acetaminophen] 160 mg/5 mL

nortestosterone phenylpropionate [see: nandrolone phenpropionate]

Nor-Tet capsules ℞ *broad-spectrum antibiotic* [tetracycline HCl] 250, 500 mg

nortetrazepam INN

Northera *investigational (NDA filed, orphan) synthetic precursor of norepinephrine for neurogenic orthostatic hypotension* [droxidopa]

Northyx tablets ℞ *thyroid inhibitor for hyperthyroidism* [methimazole] 5, 10, 15, 20 mg

Nortrel 0.5/35; Nortrel 1/35 tablets (in packs of 21 or 28) ℞ *monophasic oral contraceptive* [norethindrone; ethinyl estradiol] 0.5 mg•35 mcg; 1 mg•35 mcg

nortriptyline HCl USAN, USP, INN *tricyclic antidepressant* [10, 25, 50, 75 mg oral; 10 mg/5 mL oral]

Norvasc tablets ℞ *antianginal; antihypertensive; calcium channel blocker* [amlodipine besylate] 2.5, 5, 10 mg

norvinisterone INN

norvinodrel [see: norgesterone]

Norvir film-coated tablets, softgels, oral solution ℞ *antiretroviral protease inhibitor for HIV infection* [ritonavir] 100 mg; 100 mg; 80 mg/mL

Norway pine; Norway spruce *medicinal herb* [see: spruce]

Norwich coated tablets OTC *analgesic; antipyretic; anti-inflammatory; antirheumatic* [aspirin] 325, 500 mg

nosantine INN, BAN

noscapine USP, INN *antitussive*

noscapine HCl NF *antitussive*

Nose Better gel OTC *emollient; moisturizer; protectant; mild anesthetic; antipruritic; counterirritant* [allantoin; camphor; menthol] 0.5%•0.75%•0.5%

nosebleed *medicinal herb* [see: yarrow]

nosiheptide USAN, INN *veterinary growth stimulant*

Nōstrilla Complete Congestion Relief; Nōstrilla 12-Hour nasal spray OTC *nasal decongestant* [oxymetazoline HCl] 0.05%

Nōstrilla Conditioning Double Moisture nasal spray OTC *nasal moisturizer; bacteriostatic antiseptic* [sodium chloride (saline solution); benzalkonium chloride]

notensil maleate [see: acepromazine]

Notuss-AC oral liquid (discontinued 2009) ℞ *narcotic antitussive; antihistamine* [codeine phosphate; chlorpheniramine maleate] 10•2 mg/5 mL

Notuss-DC oral liquid (discontinued 2009) ℞ *narcotic antitussive; decongestant* [codeine phosphate; pseudoephedrine HCl] 10•30 mg/5 mL

Notuss-Forte syrup ℞ *narcotic antitussive; decongestant; antihistamine* [hydrocodone bitartrate; pseudoephedrine HCl; chlorpheniramine maleate] 5•40•4 mg/5 mL

Notuss-NX oral liquid ℞ *narcotic antitussive; antihistamine* [codeine phosphate; chlorcyclizine HCl] 10•9.375 mg/5 mL

Notuss-NXD oral liquid ℞ *narcotic antitussive; decongestant; antihistamine* [codeine phosphate; pseudoephedrine HCl; chlorcyclizine HCl] 10•30•9.375 mg/5 mL

Notuss-PD oral liquid (discontinued 2007) ℞ *narcotic antitussive; decongestant; antihistamine* [hydrocodone bitartrate; phenylephrine HCl; dexchlorpheniramine maleate] 4•5•2 mg/5 mL

Notuss-PE oral liquid ℞ *narcotic antitussive; decongestant* [codeine phosphate; phenylephrine HCl] 10•10 mg/5 mL

Nouriva Repair cream OTC *emollient/ protectant* [petrolatum; paraffin; mineral oil]

NovaCare film-coated tablets ℞ *prenatal vitamin/mineral/calcium/iron supplement* [multiple vitamins & minerals; calcium; iron; folic acid] ±•250•40•1 mg

Novacet lotion (discontinued 2008) ℞ *antibiotic and keratolytic for acne* [sulfacetamide sodium; sulfur] 10%•5%

Novacort gel ℞ *corticosteroidal anti-inflammatory; local anesthetic* [hydrocortisone acetate; pramoxine] 2%•1%

Nova-Dec tablets (discontinued 2008) OTC *vitamin/mineral/iron supplement* [multiple vitamins & minerals; iron; folic acid; biotin] ±•30 mg•0.4 mg•30 mcg

Novagest Expectorant with Codeine oral liquid (discontinued 2007) ℞ *narcotic antitussive; decongestant; expectorant* [codeine phosphate; pseudoephedrine HCl; guaifenesin; alcohol 1.4%] 10•30•100 mg/5 mL

Novahistine DH oral liquid ℞ *narcotic antitussive; antihistamine; decongestant* [dihydrocodeine bitartrate; chlorpheniramine maleate; phenylephrine HCl] 7.25•5•2 mg/5 mL

Novahistine DMX oral liquid (discontinued 2007) OTC *antitussive; decongestant; expectorant* [dextromethorphan hydrobromide; pseudoephedrine HCl; guaifenesin; alcohol 5%] 10•30•100 mg/5 mL

novamidon [see: aminopyrine]

Novamine; Novamine 15% IV infusion ℞ *total parenteral nutrition; peripheral parenteral nutrition* [multiple essential and nonessential amino acids] ⊡ nafomine

Novantrone IV infusion ℞ *antibiotic antineoplastic for prostate cancer (orphan) and acute nonlymphocytic leukemia (ANLL) (orphan); immunomodulator for progressive and relapsing-remitting multiple sclerosis (orphan)* [mitoxantrone (as HCl)] 2 mg/mL

Novarel powder for IM injection ℞ *a human-derived hormone used for prepubertal cryptorchidism or hypogonadism and to induce ovulation in anovulatory women* [chorionic gonadotropin] 1000 U/mL

Novasal film-coated tablets (discontinued 2008) ℞ *analgesic; antipyretic; anti-inflammatory* [magnesium salicylate tetrahydrate] 600 mg ⊡ nivazol

NovaSource Renal oral liquid in **Tetra Brik** packs OTC *enteral nutritional therapy for renal failure* [milk-based formula] 237 mL/pack

Novasus oral suspension ℞ *narcotic antitussive; antihistamine* [hydrocodone tannate; chlorpheniramine tannate] 5•4 mg/5 mL

novel (atypical) antipsychotics *a class of agents with a high affinity to the serotonin receptors and varying degrees of affinity to other neurotransmitter receptors; "atypical" due to the low incidence of extrapyramidal side effects (EPS)* [compare to: conventional (typical) antipsychotics]

novel acting thrombolytic (NAT) *investigational (orphan) for peripheral arterial occlusion*

novobiocin INN, BAN *bacteriostatic antibiotic* [also: novobiocin calcium]

novobiocin calcium USP *bacteriostatic antibiotic* [also: novobiocin]

novobiocin sodium USP *bacteriostatic antibiotic*

Novocain injection ℞ *local anesthetic for central or peripheral nerve block* [procaine HCl] 1%, 10% ⊡ Naphcon; nefocon

Novolin 70/30 vials for subcu injection OTC *antidiabetic* [isophane human insulin (rDNA); human insulin (rDNA)] 100 U/mL

Novolin 70/30 PenFill NovoPen cartridge (discontinued 2009) OTC *antidiabetic* [isophane human insulin (rDNA); human insulin (rDNA)] 150 U/1.5 mL, 300 U/3 mL

Novolin 70/30 Prefilled syringes (discontinued 2009) OTC *antidiabetic* [isophane human insulin (rDNA); human insulin (rDNA)] 150 U/1.5 mL

Novolin N vials for subcu injection OTC *antidiabetic* [isophane human insulin (rDNA)] 100 U/mL

Novolin N PenFill NovoPen cartridge (discontinued 2009) OTC *antidiabetic* [isophane human insulin (rDNA)] 150 U/1.5 mL, 300 U/3 mL

Novolin N Prefilled syringes (discontinued 2009) OTC *antidiabetic* [isophane human insulin (rDNA)] 150 U/1.5 mL

Novolin R vials for subcu injection OTC *antidiabetic* [human insulin (rDNA)] 100 U/mL

Novolin R PenFill NovoPen cartridge (discontinued 2009) OTC *antidiabetic* [human insulin (rDNA)] 150 U/1.5 mL, 300 U/3 mL

Novolin R Prefilled syringes (discontinued 2009) OTC *antidiabetic* [human insulin (rDNA)] 150 U/1.5 mL

NovoLog vials for subcu injection ℞ *rapid-acting insulin analogue for diabetes* [insulin aspart, human (rDNA)] 100 U/mL

NovoLog FlexPen self-injector for subcu injection ℞ *rapid-acting insulin analogue for diabetes* [insulin aspart, human (rDNA)] 300 U/3 mL

NovoLog Mix 50/50 subcu injection ℞ *dual-acting insulin analogue for diabetes* [insulin aspart protamine; insulin aspart, human (rDNA)] 50%•50% (100 U/mL total)

NovoLog Mix 70/30 vials for subcu injection ℞ *dual-acting insulin analogue for diabetes* [insulin aspart protamine; insulin aspart, human (rDNA)] 70%•30% (100 U/mL total)

NovoLog Mix 70/30 FlexPen self-injector for subcu injection ℞ *dual-acting insulin analogue for diabetes* [insulin aspart protamine; insulin aspart, human (rDNA)] 70%•30% (100 U/mL total)

NovoLog PenFill NovoPen cartridges for subcu injection ℞ *rapid-acting insulin analogue for diabetes* [insulin aspart, human (rDNA)] 300 U/3 mL

NovoPen 1.5; NovoPen Junior (trademarked delivery device) *pre-filled reusable syringe for* **Novolin PenFill** *cartridges with* **NovoFine** *30-gauge disposable needles* [insulin (several types available)] 1–40 U/injection

NovoSeven powder for IV injection (discontinued 2008) ℞ *coagulant for hemophilia A and B (orphan); investigational (orphan) for Glanzmann thrombasthenia* [factor VIIa, recombinant] 1.2, 2.4, 4.8 mg/vial

NovoSeven RT powder for IV injection ℞ *coagulant for hemophilia A and B (orphan); investigational (orphan) for Glanzmann thrombasthenia* [factor VIIa, recombinant] 1, 2, 5 mg/vial

NovoTwist (trademarked delivery device) *single-twist needle for use with a* **FlexPen** *insulin self-injector*

NOVP (Novantrone, Oncovin, vinblastine, prednisone) *chemotherapy protocol for Hodgkin lymphoma*

Noxafil oral suspension ℞ *broad-spectrum antifungal for the treatment of oropharyngeal candidiasis and prophylaxis of serious invasive fungal infections in immunocompromised patients* [posaconazole] 200 mg/5 mL

noxiptiline INN [also: noxiptyline]

noxiptyline BAN [also: noxiptiline]

noxythiolin BAN [also: noxytiolin]

noxytiolin INN [also: noxythiolin]

NP (nifurpipone) [q.v.]

NP Thyroid tablets ℞ *natural thyroid replacement for hypothyroidism or thyroid cancer* [thyroid, desiccated (porcine)] 30, 60, 90 mg (0.5, 1, 1.5 gr.)

NPH (neutral protamine Hagedorn) insulin [see: insulin, isophane]

NPI 32101 *investigational (Phase III) nanocrystalline silver for use as a topical antimicrobial barrier*

Nplate subcu injection ℞ *hematopoietic; oral thrombopoietin (TPO) receptor agonist to increase platelet production in immune thrombocytopenic purpura (ITP)* [romiplostim] 250, 500 mcg

NRTIs (nucleoside reverse transcriptase inhibitors) [see: reverse transcriptase inhibitors]

NS (normal saline) [q.v.]

NSAIDs (nonsteroidal anti-inflammatory drugs) [q.v.]

NTZ (nitazoxanide) [q.v.]

Nubain IV, IM, or subcu injection ℞ *narcotic agonist-antagonist analgesic for moderate to severe pain; adjunct to obstetric and surgical analgesia* [nalbuphine HCl] 10, 20 mg/mL

nucleoside reverse transcriptase inhibitors (NRTI) *a class of antiretroviral drugs that inhibits the activity of reverse transcriptase (polymerase) in viral cells, causing a termination of DNA chain elongation, which prevents replication of the cells* [see: reverse transcriptase inhibitors]

nuclomedone INN

nuclotixene INN

Nucofed capsules ℞ *narcotic antitussive; decongestant* [codeine phosphate; pseudoephedrine HCl] 20•60 mg

NuCort lotion ℞ *corticosteroidal anti-inflammatory* [hydrocortisone] 2% 🔊 Nicorette

Nucynta film-coated tablets ℞ *central analgesic for moderate to severe pain* [tapentadol (as HCl)] 50, 75, 100 mg

Nucynta ER extended-release tablets ℞ *central analgesic for moderate to severe pain* [tapentadol (as HCl)] 50, 100, 150, 200, 250 mg

Nuedexta capsules ℞ *NMDA inhibitor and sigma-1 agonist plus potentiator for involuntary emotional expression disorder (pseudobulbar affect); investigational (Phase III) treatment for diabetic neuropathic pain* [dextromethorphan (as hydrobromide); quinidine (as sulfate)] 20•10 mg

nufenoxole USAN, INN *antiperistaltic*

Nuhist oral suspension (discontinued 2007) ℞ *decongestant; antihistamine* [phenylephrine tannate; chlorpheniramine tannate] 5•4.5 mg/5 mL 🔊 NoHist

Nu-Iron 150 capsules OTC *iron supplement* [iron (as polysaccharide-iron complex)] 150 mg

Nu-Iron Plus elixir (discontinued 2008) ℞ *hematinic* [iron (as polysaccharide-iron complex); vitamin B$_{12}$; folic acid] 300•0.075•3 mg/15 mL

Nu-Iron V film-coated tablets (discontinued 2008) ℞ *hematinic; vitamin/iron supplement* [iron (as polysaccharide-iron complex); multiple vitamins; folic acid] 60• ± •1 mg

Nu-knit (trademarked dosage form) *oxidized cellulose hemostatic pad* 🔊 nequinate

Nulecit IV infusion ℞ *hematinic for iron deficiency due to chronic hemodialysis with erythropoietin therapy* [iron (as sodium ferric gluconate)] 12.5 mg/mL 🔊 Neulasta

NuLev orally disintegrating tablets ℞ *GI/GU antispasmodic; antiparkinsonian; anticholinergic "drying agent" for allergic rhinitis* [hyoscyamine sulfate] 0.125 mg

Nulojix powder for IV infusion ℞ *immunosuppressant to prevent kidney transplant rejection* [belatacept] 250 mg/vial

NuLytely powder for oral solution ℞ *pre-procedure bowel evacuant* [polyethylene glycol–electrolyte solution (PEG 3350, potassium chloride, sodium bicarbonate, sodium chloride)]

Numby Stuff topical liquid ℞ *anesthetic* [lidocaine HCl; epinephrine] 2%•1:100 000

Numoisyn lozenges, oral suspension ℞ *saliva substitute* 🔊 neomycin; nimazone

Numorphan IV, IM, or subcu injection (name changed to **Opana** in 2007)

Numzident oral gel (discontinued 2008) OTC *mucous membrane anesthetic* [benzocaine] 10%

Numzit Teething lotion (discontinued 2008) OTC *mucous membrane anesthetic; antiseptic* [benzocaine; alcohol 12.1%] 0.2%

Numzit Teething oral gel OTC *mucous membrane anesthetic* [benzocaine] 7.5%

Nu-Natal Advanced film-coated tablets ℞ *vitamin/mineral/calcium/iron supplement; stool softener* [multiple vitamins & minerals; calcium; iron (as carbonyl); folic acid; docusate sodium] ±•200•90•1•50 mg

NuOx gel ℞ *antiseptic and keratolytic for acne* [benzoyl peroxide; sulfur] 6%•3• ⓡ Nix

Nupercainal ointment OTC *anesthetic* [dibucaine] 1%

Nupercainal rectal suppositories OTC *emollient; astringent* [cocoa butter; zinc oxide] 2.1•0.25 g

Nuprin tablets, caplets OTC *analgesic; antiarthritic; antipyretic; nonsteroidal anti-inflammatory drug (NSAID) for mild to moderate pain, migraine headaches, and primary dysmenorrhea* [ibuprofen] 200 mg

Nuquin HP cream ℞ *hyperpigmentation bleaching agent* [hydroquinone (in a sunscreen base)] 4%

Nursette (trademarked delivery form) *prefilled disposable bottle*

Nu-Salt OTC *salt substitute; electrolyte replenisher* [potassium chloride] 68 mEq K/5 g

NuSpin (trademarked delivery device) *prefilled multidose self-injector for* **Nutropin AQ** ⓡ Niaspan

nut, oil *medicinal herb* [see: butternut]

Nu-Tears eye drops OTC *moisturizer/lubricant* [polyvinyl alcohol] 1.4% ⓡ Neotrace

Nu-Tears II eye drops OTC *moisturizer/lubricant* [polyvinyl alcohol; polyethylene glycol 400] 1%•1% ⓡ Neotrace

nutmeg (*Myristica fragrans*) seed and aril *medicinal herb for diarrhea, flatulence, inducing expectoration, insomnia, mouth sores, rheumatism, salivary stimulation, and stimulating menstruation*

nutmeg oil NF

Nutracort cream ℞ *corticosteroidal anti-inflammatory* [hydrocortisone] 1%

Nutraderm cream, lotion OTC *moisturizer; emollient*

Nutraderm lotion OTC *nontherapeutic base for compounding various dermatological preparations*

Nutraderm Bath Oil OTC *bath emollient*

Nutraloric powder OTC *enteral nutritional therapy* [milk-based formula]

Nutrament oral liquid OTC *enteral nutritional therapy* [milk-based formula] 12 oz./can

Nutramigen oral liquid, powder for oral liquid OTC *hypoallergenic infant food* [enzymatically hydrolyzed protein formula]

Nutraplus cream, lotion OTC *moisturizer; emollient; keratolytic* [urea] 10%

Nutra-Soothe bath oil OTC *bath emollient* [colloidal oatmeal; light mineral oil]

Nutravance film-coated tablets ℞ *vitamin/mineral supplement* [multiple vitamins & minerals; folic acid; biotin] ±•1•0.1 mg

Nutren 1.0 oral liquid OTC *enteral nutritional therapy* [lactose-free formula]

Nutren 1.5 oral liquid OTC *enteral nutritional therapy* [lactose-free formula]

Nutren 2.0 ready-to-use oral liquid OTC *enteral nutritional therapy* [lactose-free formula] 1 L

Nutr-E-Sol oral liquid OTC *vitamin supplement* [vitamin E] 798 IU/30 mL ⓡ NeutraSal

NutreStore *investigational (orphan) agent used with human growth hormone (hGH) to treat short bowel syndrome* [glutamine]

Nutricon tablets (discontinued 2008) OTC *vitamin/mineral/calcium/iron supplement* [multiple vitamins & minerals; calcium; iron; folic acid; biotin] ±•200•20•0.4•0.15 mg ⓡ Neutra-Caine

NutriDox capsules ℞ *tetracycline antibiotic* [doxycycline] 75 mg

Nutrifac ZX caplets ℞ *vitamin/mineral supplement* [multiple vitamins & minerals; folic acid; biotin] ±•1•0.2 mg

NutriFocus ready-to-use oral liquid OTC *enteral nutritional therapy* [milk- and soy-based formula] 237 mL/can

NutriHeal ready-to-use oral liquid OTC *enteral nutritional therapy* [milk-based formula] 250 mL/can

Nutrilan ready-to-use oral liquid OTC *enteral nutritional therapy* [lactose-free formula] ⑨ Nitrolan

Nutrilyte; Nutrilyte II IV admixture ℞ *intravenous electrolyte therapy* [combined electrolyte solution] ⑨ Naturalyte

NutriNate chewable tablets (discontinued 2009) ℞ *prenatal vitamin/mineral/iron supplement* [multiple vitamins & minerals; iron (as ferrous fumarate); folic acid] ±•29•1 mg

Nutrineal *investigational (orphan) nutritional supplement for continuous ambulatory peritoneal dialysis patients* [peritoneal dialysis solution with 1.1% amino acids]

NutriSpire film-coated caplets (discontinued 2009) OTC *vitamin/mineral/calcium/iron supplement* [multiple vitamins & minerals; calcium (as carbonate); iron (as carbonyl iron); folic acid] ±•200•29•1 mg

Nutropin powder for subcu injection ℞ *growth hormone for children and adults with congenital or endogenous growth hormone deficiency (GHD), short bowel syndrome, or AIDS-wasting syndrome; for children with Turner syndrome, Prader-Willi syndrome, or renal-induced growth failure* [somatropin] 5, 10 mg (15, 30 IU) per vial

Nutropin AQ subcu injection, prefilled cartridge for self-injector ℞ *growth hormone for children and adults with congenital or endogenous growth hormone deficiency (GHD), short bowel syndrome, or AIDS-wasting syndrome; for children with Turner syndrome, Prader-Willi syndrome, or renal-induced growth failure* [somatropin] 10, 20 mg (30, 60 IU) per vial; 10, 20 mg (30, 60 IU) per 2 mL cartridge

Nutropin AQ NuSpin 5; Nutropin AQ NuSpin 10; Nutropin AQ NuSpin 20 prefilled multidose self-injector ℞ *growth hormone for children and adults with congenital or endogenous growth hormone deficiency (GHD), short bowel syndrome, or AIDS-wasting syndrome; for children with Turner syndrome, Prader-Willi syndrome, or renal-induced growth failure* [somatropin] 5 mg (15 IU); 10 mg (30 IU); 20 mg (60 IU)

Nutrox capsules (discontinued 2008) OTC *vitamin/mineral/amino acid supplement* [multiple vitamins & minerals; multiple amino acids]

NuvaRing vaginal ring ℞ *self-administered one-month contraceptive insert* [ethinyl estradiol; etonogestrel] 15• 120 mcg/day

nuvenzepine INN

Nuvigil tablets ℞ *analeptic for excessive daytime sleepiness due to narcolepsy (orphan), obstructive sleep apnea, or shift work sleep disorder (SWSD); investigational (NDA filed) for jet lag* [armodafinil] 50, 150, 250 mg

nyctal [see: carbromal]

nydrane [see: benzchlorpropamid]

Nydrazid IM injection ℞ *tuberculostatic* [isoniazid] 100 mg/mL

nylestriol USAN *estrogen* [also: nilestriol]

nylidrin HCl USP *peripheral vasodilator* [also: buphenine]

Nyloxin oral spray, topical gel OTC *a natural pain reliever made to homeopathic standards for chronic pain* [cobra venom (a neurotoxin)] ⑨ naloxone

Nyloxin Rx oral spray, topical gel ℞ *a natural pain reliever made to homeopathic standards for stage 3 pain due to adrenomyeloneuropathy (AMN) and multiple sclerosis (MS)* [cobra venom (a neurotoxin)]

Nymphaea odorata medicinal herb [see: white pond lilly]

Nyotran *investigational (NDA filed, orphan) systemic antifungal for Aspergillus fumigatus and other invasive fungal infections* [nystatin, liposomal]

NyQuil Cough syrup OTC *antitussive; antihistamine; sleep aid* [dextromethorphan hydrobromide; doxylamine succinate] 30•12.5 mg/30 mL

NyQuil Multi-Symptom Cold & Flu Relief LiquiCaps (liquid-filled gelcaps) OTC *antitussive; antihistamine; sleep aid; analgesic; antipyretic* [dextromethorphan hydrobromide; doxylamine succinate; acetaminophen] 15•6.25•325 mg

NyQuil Multi-Symptom Cold/Flu Relief oral liquid OTC *antitussive; antihistamine; sleep aid; analgesic; antipyretic* [dextromethorphan hydrobromide; doxylamine succinate; acetaminophen] 30•12.5•1000 mg/30 mL

NyQuil Sinex LiquiCaps (liquid-filled gelcaps) OTC *antitussive; antihistamine; sleep aid; decongestant; analgesic; antipyretic* [doxylamine succinate; phenylephrine HCl; acetaminophen] 6.25•5•325 mg

nystatin USP, INN, BAN, JAN *polyene antifungal* 500 000 U oral; 100 000 U/mL oral; 100 000 mg vaginal; 100 000 U/g topical; 50, 150, 500 million, 1, 2, 5 billion U bulk

nystatin, liposomal *investigational (NDA filed, orphan) systemic antifungal for* Aspergillus fumigatus *and other invasive fungal infections*

Nystop powder ℞ *antifungal* [nystatin] 100 000 U/g

Ny-Tannic caplets ℞ *decongestant; antihistamine* [phenylephrine tannate; chlorpheniramine tannate] 25•9 mg

Nytol tablets OTC *antihistamine; sleep aid* [diphenhydramine HCl] 25, 50 mg ⑨ nettle

NZ-1002 *investigational (orphan) enzyme replacement therapy for mucopolysaccharidosis I*

NZGLM (New Zealand green-lipped mussel) [q.v.]

O₂ (oxygen) [q.v.]

oak *medicinal herb* [see: white oak]

Oasis mouthwash, throat spray OTC *saliva substitute*

oatmeal, colloidal *demulcent*

oats (Avena sativa) grain and straw *medicinal herb for dry itchy skin, hyperlipidemia, indigestion, insomnia, nervousness, opium addiction, reducing the desire to smoke, and strengthening the heart* ⑨ A/T/S

OB Complete caplets ℞ *prenatal vitamin/mineral/iron supplement* [multiple vitamins & minerals; iron (as micronized ferronyl); folic acid] ±•50•1.25 mg

OB Complete chewable tablets ℞ *prenatal vitamin/mineral/calcium/iron/omega-3 supplement* [multiple vitamins & minerals; calcium; iron; folic acid; docosahexaenoic acid (DHA)] ±•20•20•1•100 mg

OB Complete with DHA softgels ℞ *prenatal vitamin/mineral/iron/omega-3 supplement* [multiple vitamins & minerals; iron (as ferrous fumarate); folic acid; docosahexaenoic acid (DHA)] ±•28•1.25•200 mg

obecalp *placebo (spelled backward)* [q.v.]

obidoxime chloride USAN, INN *cholinesterase reactivator*

oblimersen sodium *antisense antineoplastic; investigational (NDA filed, orphan) for malignant melanoma; investigational (Phase III, orphan) for multiple myeloma and chronic lymphocytic leukemia (CLL)*

Obstetrix-100 tablets ℞ *prenatal vitamin/mineral/calcium/iron supplement; stool softener* [multiple vitamins; calcium; iron; folic acid; zinc; docusate sodium] ±•250•100•1•25•50 mg

Obtrex enteric-coated tablets ℞ *prenatal vitamin/mineral/iron supplement; stool softener* [multiple vitamins and minerals; iron (as carbonyl); docusate sodium] ⚕•29•50 mg

O-Cal F.A. film-coated tablets ℞ *vitamin/mineral/calcium/iron supplement* [multiple vitamins & minerals; calcium (as carbonate); iron (as ferrous fumarate); folic acid] ⚕•200•27•1 mg

O-Cal Prenatal tablets ℞ *vitamin/mineral/calcium/iron supplement* [multiple vitamins & minerals; calcium; iron; folic acid] ⚕•200•15•1 mg

ocaperidone USAN, INN, BAN *antipsychotic*

Occlusal-HP topical liquid OTC *keratolytic* [salicylic acid in polyacrylic vehicle] 17%

Ocean; Ocean for Kids nasal spray OTC *nasal moisturizer* [sodium chloride (saline solution)] 0.65% ⚕ Aceon; Aczone

Ocella film-coated tablets (in packs of 28) ℞ *monophasic oral contraceptive* [drospirenone; ethinyl estradiol] 3 mg•30 mcg × 21 days; counters × 7 days ⚕ Iosal

ocfentanil INN *narcotic analgesic* [also: ocfentanil HCl]

ocfentanil HCl USAN *narcotic analgesic* [also: ocfentanil]

ociltide INN

Ocimum basilicum medicinal herb [see: basil]

ocinaplon USAN *anxiolytic*

OCL oral solution ℞ *pre-procedure bowel evacuant* [polyethylene glycol–electrolyte solution (PEG 3350)] 60 g/L

ocrase INN ⚕ Eucrease

ocrilate INN *tissue adhesive* [also: ocrylate]

ocrylate USAN *tissue adhesive* [also: ocrilate]

OCT (22-oxacalcitriol) [see: maxacalcitol]

octabenzone USAN, INN *ultraviolet screen*

octacaine INN

octacosactrin BAN [also: tosactide]

octacosanol *natural extract of wheat germ used to treat hypercholesterolemia;* *effective for lowering LDL-cholesterol, raising HDL-cholesterol, stopping the formation of arterial lesions and plaque deposits, and inhibiting clot formation*

octadecafluorodecehydronaphthalene [see: perflunafene]

octadecanoic acid, calcium salt [see: calcium stearate]

octadecanoic acid, sodium salt [see: sodium stearate]

octadecanoic acid, zinc salt [see: zinc stearate]

1-octadecanol [see: stearyl alcohol]

9-octadecenylamine hydrofluoride [see: dectaflur]

octafonium chloride INN

Octagam IV infusion (discontinued 2010) ℞ *passive immunizing agent for primary (inherited) immunodeficiency disorders; also used for Guillain-Barré syndrome, myasthenia gravis, and multiple sclerosis* [immune globulin (IGIV)] 5% (1, 2.5, 5, 10 g/dose)

Octamide PFS IV or IM injection (discontinued 2010) ℞ *antiemetic for chemotherapy and postoperative nausea and vomiting; GI stimulant for diabetic gastroparesis, gastroesophageal reflux, small bowel intubation, and radiological examination of the intestine; also used for hiccups* [metoclopramide (as HCl)] 5 mg/mL

octamoxin INN

octamylamine INN

octanoic acid USAN, INN *antifungal*

octapinol INN

Octastatin *antineoplastic; synthetic octapeptide analogue of somatostatin; investigational (orphan) for GI and pancreatic fistulas* [vapreotide acetate]

octastine INN

octatropine methylbromide INN, BAN *anticholinergic; peptic ulcer adjunct* [also: anisotropine methylbromide]

octatropone bromide [see: anisotropine methylbromide]

octaverine INN, BAN

octazamide USAN, INN *analgesic* ⚕ actisomide

octenidine INN, BAN *topical anti-infective* [also: octenidine HCl]

octenidine HCl USAN *topical anti-infective* [also: octenidine]

octenidine saccharin USAN *dental plaque inhibitor*

Octicare ear drops, ear drop suspension (discontinued 2007) ℞ *corticosteroidal anti-inflammatory; antibiotic* [hydrocortisone; neomycin sulfate; polymyxin B sulfate] 1%•5 mg• 10 000 U per mL

octicizer USAN *plasticizer*

octil INN *combining name for radicals or groups*

octimibate INN

octinoxate USAN *ultraviolet B sunscreen*

octisalate USAN *ultraviolet sunscreen*

octisamyl [see: octamylamine]

Octocaine HCl injection ℞ *local anesthetic* [lidocaine HCl; epinephrine] 2%•1:50 000, 2%•1:100 000

octoclothepine [see: clorotepine]

octocrilene INN *ultraviolet screen* [also: octocrylene]

octocrylene USAN *ultraviolet screen* [also: octocrilene]

octodecactide [see: codactide]

octodrine USAN, INN *adrenergic; vasoconstrictor; local anesthetic*

octopamine INN

octotiamine INN

octoxinol INN *surfactant/wetting agent* [also: octoxynol 9]

octoxynol 9 USAN, NF *surfactant/wetting agent; spermicide* [also: octoxinol]

OctreoScan injection ℞ *radioactive imaging agent for SPECT scans of neuroendocrine tumors* [indium In 111 pentetreotide] 10 mcg/vial

octreotide USAN, INN, BAN *somatostatin analogue; gastric antisecretory for acromegaly and severe diarrhea due to VIPomas and other tumors* (orphan)

octreotide acetate USAN *somatostatin analogue; gastric antisecretory for acromegaly and severe diarrhea due to VIPomas and other tumors* (orphan) (base= 89.3%) 0.05, 0.1, 0.2, 0.5, 1 mg/mL injection

octreotide pamoate USAN *antineoplastic*

octriptyline INN *antidepressant* [also: octriptyline phosphate]

octriptyline phosphate USAN *antidepressant* [also: octriptyline]

octrizole USAN, INN *ultraviolet screen*

octyl methoxycinnamate [see: octinoxate]

octyl salicylate [see: octisalate]

S-octyl thiobenzoate [see: tioctilate]

octyl-2-cyanoacrylate [see: ocrylate]

octyldodecanol NF *oleaginous vehicle*

OcuCaps caplets (discontinued 2008) OTC *vitamin/mineral supplement* [vitamins A, C, and E; multiple minerals] 5000 IU•400 mg•182 mg• ±

OcuCoat prefilled syringe OTC *ophthalmic surgical aid* [hydroxypropyl methylcellulose] 2%

OcuCoat; OcuCoat PF eye drops (discontinued 2009) OTC *moisturizer/ lubricant* [hydroxypropyl methylcellulose] 0.8%

Ocudose (trademarked delivery form) *single-use eye drop dispenser*

Ocudox capsules ℞ *antibiotic for periodontal disease* [doxycycline hyclate] 50 mg ⊘ AquADEKs

Ocufen eye drops ℞ *nonsteroidal anti-inflammatory drug (NSAID); intraoperative miosis inhibitor* [flurbiprofen sodium] 0.03% ⊘ Aquavan

ocufilcon A USAN *hydrophilic contact lens material*

ocufilcon B USAN *hydrophilic contact lens material*

ocufilcon C USAN *hydrophilic contact lens material*

ocufilcon D USAN *hydrophilic contact lens material*

ocufilcon F USAN *hydrophilic contact lens material*

Ocuflox eye drops ℞ *fluoroquinolone antibiotic for bacterial conjunctivitis and corneal ulcers* (orphan) [ofloxacin] 0.3%

Ocumeter (trademarked delivery form) *prefilled eye drop dispenser*

OCuSOFT solution OTC *eyelid cleanser for blepharitis or contact lenses*

OcuSoft VMS film-coated tablets OTC *vitamin/mineral supplement* [vitamins A, C, and E; multiple minerals] 5000 IU•60 mg•30 mg• ±

Ocusulf-10 eye drops (discontinued 2010) ℞ *antibiotic* [sulfacetamide sodium] 10% ② AK-Sulf

Ocuvite film-coated tablets OTC *vitamin/mineral supplement* [vitamins A, C, and E; multiple minerals; lutein] 1000 IU•200 mg•60 IU• ± •2 mg ② Aquavit

Ocuvite Adult; Ocuvite Adult 50+ softgels OTC *vitamin/mineral/EFA supplement* [vitamins C and E; multiple minerals; omega-3 fatty acids; lutein] 100 mg•15 IU• ± •100 mg•2 mg; 150 mg•30 IU• ± •150 mg•6 mg

Ocuvite DF tablets OTC *vitamin supplement* [multiple vitamins; alpha-lipoic acid] ± •140 mg

Ocuvite Extra tablets OTC *vitamin/mineral supplement* [vitamins A, C, and E; multiple B vitamins; multiple minerals; lutein] 1000 IU•300 mg• 100 IU• ± • ± •2 mg

Ocuvite Lutein capsules OTC *vitamin/mineral supplement* [vitamins C and E; multiple minerals; lutein] 60 mg• 30 IU• ± •6 mg

Ocuvite PreserVision film-coated tablets, softgels OTC *vitamin/mineral supplement* [vitamins A, C, and E; multiple minerals] 7160 IU•113 mg•100 IU• ± ; 14 300 IU•226 mg•200 IU• ±

odanacatib *investigational (NDA filed) agent for osteoporosis*

Odor Free ArthriCare [see: ArthriCare, Odor Free]

Oenothera biennis medicinal herb [see: evening primrose]

OEP (oil of evening primrose) [see: evening primrose]

oestradiol BAN *estrogen replacement therapy for the treatment of postmenopausal disorders and prevention of postmenopausal osteoporosis; palliative therapy for prostatic and breast cancers* [also: estradiol]

oestradiol benzoate BAN [also: estradiol benzoate]

oestradiol valerate BAN *estrogen* [also: estradiol valerate]

oestriol succinate BAN *estrogen* [also: estriol; estriol succinate]

oestrogenine [see: diethylstilbestrol]

oestromenin [see: diethylstilbestrol]

oestrone BAN *estrogen replacement therapy for postmenopausal disorders; palliative therapy for prostatic and breast cancers* [also: estrone]

ofatumumab *monoclonal antibody to B-cell malignancies; treatment for chronic lymphocytic leukemia (CLL)*

Off-Ezy Corn & Callus Remover kit (topical liquid + cushion pads) OTC *keratolytic* [salicylic acid in a collodion-like vehicle] 17%

Off-Ezy Wart Remover topical liquid OTC *keratolytic* [salicylic acid in a collodion-like vehicle] 17%

Ofirmev IV infusion ℞ *analgesic; antipyretic* [acetaminophen] 10 mg/mL (1000 mg/vial)

ofloxacin USAN, INN, BAN, JAN *broad-spectrum fluoroquinolone antibiotic; topical corneal ulcer treatment (orphan)* 200, 300, 400 mg oral; 0.3% eye drops; 0.3% ear drops

ofornine USAN, INN *antihypertensive*

Oforta film-coated caplets ℞ *antineoplastic for chronic lymphocytic leukemia (CLL)* [fludarabine phosphate] 10 mg

oftasceine INN

Ogen tablets (discontinued 2010) ℞ *bioidentical human estrogen replacement therapy for the treatment of postmenopausal symptoms and prevention of postmenopausal osteoporosis* [estrone (from estropipate)] 0.625, 1.25 (0.75, 1.5) mg ② Acanya; A.C.N.; Yocon

Ogestrel 0.5/50 tablets (in packs of 28) ℞ *monophasic oral contraceptive; emergency postcoital contraceptive* [norgestrel; ethinyl estradiol] 0.5 mg• 50 mcg × 21 days; counters × 7 days ② Oxytrol

oglufanide disodium USAN *immunomodulator; investigational (orphan)* angiogenesis inhibitor antineoplastic for ovarian cancer

oil nut medicinal herb [see: butternut]

oil of evening primrose (OEP) [see: evening primrose]

oil of mustard [see: allyl isothiocyanate]

Oil of Olay Foaming Face Wash topical liquid OTC cleanser for acne

oil ricini [see: castor oil]

Oilatum Soap bar OTC therapeutic skin cleanser

ointment, hydrophilic USP ointment base; oil-in-water emulsion

ointment, white USP oleaginous ointment base

ointment, yellow USP ointment base

olaflur USAN, INN, BAN dental caries preventative

olamine USAN, INN combining name for radicals or groups

olanexidine HCl USAN topical antibiotic for nosocomial or wound infections

olanzapine USAN, INN rapid-acting novel (atypical) thienobenzodiazepine antipsychotic for schizophrenia, treatment-resistant depression, and manic or depressive episodes of a bipolar disorder; also used for obsessive-compulsive disorder (OCD) (available as a generic drug in Canada) ⊠ elanzepine

olanzapine pamoate long-acting novel (atypical) thienobenzodiazepine antipsychotic for schizophrenia (base=43.5%)

olaquindox INN, BAN

old man's beard medicinal herb [see: fringe tree; woodbine]

old tuberculin (OT) [see: tuberculin]

Olea europaea medicinal herb [see: olive]

oleander (Nerium indicum; N. oleander) plant medicinal herb for asthma, cancer, corns, epilepsy, and heart disease; not generally regarded as safe and effective in any form as it is very toxic

oleandomycin INN [also: oleandomycin phosphate]

oleandomycin, triacetate ester [see: troleandomycin]

oleandomycin phosphate NF [also: oleandomycin]

oleic acid NF emulsion adjunct

oleic acid I 125 USAN radioactive agent

oleic acid I 131 USAN radioactive agent

oleovitamin A [now: vitamin A]

oleovitamin A & D USP source of vitamins A and D

oleovitamin D, synthetic [now: ergocalciferol]

Oleptro extended-release film-coated caplets ℞ antidepressant; also used for insomnia, prevention of migraine headaches, aggressive behavior, alcoholism, and cocaine withdrawal [trazodone HCl] 150, 300 mg

olethytan 20 [see: polysorbate 80]

oletimol INN

oleum caryophylii [see: clove oil]

oleum gossypii seminis [see: cottonseed oil]

oleum maydis [see: corn oil]

oleum ricini [see: castor oil]

oleyl alcohol NF emulsifying agent; emollient

oligomycin D [see: rutamycin]

olive (Olea europaea) leaves, bark, and fruit medicinal herb used as an antiseptic, astringent, cholagogue, demulcent, emollient, febrifuge, hypoglycemic, laxative, and tranquilizer ⊠ Aleve; Aluvia; ELF

olive, spurge; spurge laurel medicinal herb [see: mezereon]

olive oil NF pharmaceutic aid

olivomycin INN

olmesartan USAN angiotensin receptor blocker (ARB) for hypertension

olmesartan medoxomil USAN, INN angiotensin receptor blocker (ARB) for hypertension

olmidine INN

olopatadine INN antiallergic; antiasthmatic

olopatadine HCl USAN antihistamine and mast cell stabilizer for allergic conjunctivitis and seasonal allergic rhinitis (base=90.2%) 0.2% eye drops

olpimedone INN

olsalazine INN, BAN GI anti-inflammatory [also: olsalazine sodium]

olsalazine sodium USAN *anti-inflammatory for ulcerative colitis* [also: olsalazine]

oltipraz INN

Olux; Olux-E topical foam ℞ *corticosteroidal anti-inflammatory for scalp dermatoses and plaque psoriasis* [clobetasol propionate; alcohol 60%] 0.05% ▣ Aloxi; I-L-X

olvanil USAN, INN *analgesic*

OM 401 *investigational (orphan) for sickle cell disease*

omacetaxine mepesuccinate *investigational (NDA filed) antineoplastic for chronic myeloid leukemia (CML)*

omaciclovir USAN *antiviral DNA polymerase inhibitor for herpes zoster*

Omacor gelcaps (U.S. name changed to **Lovaza** in 2008) ▣ Amicar

omalizumab *recombinant humanized monoclonal antibody (rhuMAb) to immunoglobulin E (anti-IgE) for the treatment of moderate to severe asthma*

Omapro *investigational (NDA filed) antineoplastic for chronic myeloid leukemia (CML)* [omacetaxine mepesuccinate]

omega-3 (N-3) fatty acids [see: docosahexaenoic acid (DHA); doconexent; eicosapentaenoic acid (EPA); icosapent]

omega-3 acid ethyl esters *ethyl esters of docosahexaenoic acid (q.v.) and eicosapentaenoic acid (q.v.); adjunct to diet restriction for hypertriglyceridemia; investigational (orphan) for immunoglobulin A nephropathy*

Omega-3 Complex softgels OTC *dietary supplement* [eicosapentaenoic acid (EPA); docosahexaenoic acid (DHA); vitamin E] 251 mg•192 mg•11 IU

omega-3 fatty acids with all double bonds in the *cis* **configuration** *investigational (orphan) preventative for organ graft rejection*

Omega-3 Fish Oil softgels OTC *dietary supplement* [omega-3 fatty acids (eicosapentaenoic acid and docosahexaenoic acid)] 340 mg (216 mg EPA; 120 mg DHA)

omega-3 marine triglycerides BAN [12% docosahexaenoic acid (q.v.) + 18% eicosapentaenoic acid (q.v.)]

Omega-3 Norwegian Cod Liver Oil softgels OTC *vitamin/EFA supplement* [vitamins A and D; eicosapentaenoic acid; docosahexaenoic acid] 1250 IU•135 IU•34 mg•32, 2664 IU•200 IU•110•100 mg

omeprazole USAN, INN, BAN, JAN *proton pump inhibitor for gastric and duodenal ulcers, erosive esophagitis, gastroesophageal reflux disease (GERD), upper GI bleeding, and other gastroesophageal disorders; also used for laryngitis* 10, 20, 40 mg oral

omeprazole magnesium USAN *proton pump inhibitor for acid indigestion and heartburn; also used for laryngitis* (base=97%)

omeprazole sodium USAN *gastric antisecretory*

omeprazole & sodium bicarbonate *combination proton pump inhibitor and antacid for gastric and duodenal ulcers, erosive esophagitis, GERD, and other gastroesophageal disorders* 20•1100, 20•1680, 40•1100, 40•1680 mg oral

omeprazole & sodium bicarbonate & magnesium hydroxide *combination proton pump inhibitor and antacid for gastric and duodenal ulcers, erosive esophagitis, GERD, and other gastroesophageal disorders* 20•750•343, 40•750•343 mg oral

omidoline INN ▣ amedalin; imidoline

Omnaris nasal spray ℞ *once-daily corticosteroidal anti-inflammatory for seasonal or perennial allergic rhinitis* [ciclesonide] 50 mcg/spray

Omnicef capsules, oral suspension ℞ *third-generation cephalosporin antibiotic* [cefdinir] 300 mg; 125, 250 mg/5 mL

Omnigest EZ caplets OTC *herbal supplement to aid digestion* [multiple plant-derived digestive enzymes]

OMNIhist L.A. II long-acting tablets ℞ *decongestant; antihistamine; anticholinergic to dry mucosal secretions* [phenylephrine HCl; chlorpheniramine maleate; methscopolamine nitrate] 25•8•2.5 mg

Omnipaque 140; Omnipaque 240; Omnipaque 300; Omnipaque 350 injection ℞ *radiopaque contrast medium* [iohexol (46.36% iodine)] 302 mg/mL (140 mg/mL); 518 mg/mL (240 mg/mL); 647 mg/mL (300 mg/mL); 755 mg/mL (350 mg/mL)

Omnipaque 180 injection (discontinued 2008) ℞ *radiopaque contrast medium* [iohexol (46.36% iodine)] 388 mg/mL (180 mg/mL)

Omnipred eye drop suspension ℞ *corticosteroidal anti-inflammatory* [prednisolone acetate] 1% ② emonapride

Omniscan IV injection ℞ *radiopaque contrast medium for thoracic, abdominal, pelvic, and retroperitoneal imaging and to enhance MRIs of the brain, spine, and other CNS tissue* [gadodiamide] 287 mg/mL

Omnitrope powder for subcu injection, prefilled cartridges for self-injector ℞ *growth hormone for children and adults with congenital or endogenous growth hormone deficiency (GHD), short bowel syndrome, or AIDS-wasting syndrome; for children with Turner syndrome, Prader-Willi syndrome, or renal-induced growth failure* [somatropin] 1.5, 5.8 mg (4.5, 17.4 IU) per vial; 5, 10 mg (15, 30 IU) per cartridge

omoconazole INN *antifungal*

omoconazole nitrate USAN *antifungal*

omonasteine INN

Omr-IgG-am 5% [WNV] *investigational (orphan) passive immunizing agent for the West Nile virus* [immune globulin with high titers of West Nile virus antibodies]

onabotulinumtoxin A *neurotoxin complex derived from* Clostridium botulinum; *treatment for blepharospasm and strabismus of dystonia (orphan), cervical dystonia (orphan), migraine headaches, spasticity, hyperhidrosis, and facial wrinkles* [also: abobotulinumtoxin A]

onapristone INN *antineoplastic for hormone-dependent cancers*

Oncaspar IV or IM injection ℞ *antineoplastic for acute lymphocytic leukemia (orphan) and acute lymphoblastic leukemia* [pegaspargase] 750 IU/mL

Once Daily; Once Daily Regular Formula tablets OTC *vitamin supplement* [multiple vitamins]

Once Daily Multivitamin with Iron tablets OTC *vitamin/iron supplement* [multiple vitamins; iron (as ferrous sulfate)] ±•18 mg

OncoGel *antineoplastic; investigational (orphan) for esophageal cancer* [paclitaxel]

Oncolym *investigational (Phase III, orphan) treatment for non-Hodgkin B-cell lymphoma* [monoclonal antibody to Lym-1, radiolabeled with iodine I 131]

Onconase *investigational (Phase III) antineoplastic for unresectable malignant mesothelioma (UMM)* [ranpirnase]

OncoTrac imaging kit *investigational (orphan) for diagnostic imaging agent for metastasis of malignant melanoma* [monoclonal antibodies to melanoma, murine, radiolabeled with technetium Tc 99m]

Oncovin IV injection, Hyporets (prefilled syringes) ℞ *antineoplastic for lung and breast cancers, various leukemias, lymphomas, and sarcomas* [vincristine sulfate] 1 mg/mL

Oncovite film-coated tablets OTC *vitamin supplement* [multiple vitamins; folic acid] ±•400 mcg

ondansetron INN, BAN *serotonin 5-HT₃ receptor antagonist; antiemetic to prevent nausea and vomiting following chemotherapy, radiation, or surgery* [also: ondansetron HCl] 4, 8, 24 mg oral; 4 mg/5 mL oral

ondansetron HCl USAN *serotonin 5-HT₃ receptor antagonist; antiemetic to prevent nausea and vomiting following chemotherapy, radiation, or surgery* [also: ondansetron] 4, 8, 16, 24 mg oral; 4 mg/5 mL oral; 0.64, 2 mg/mL injection

Ondrox sustained-release tablets (discontinued 2008) OTC *vitamin/mineral/calcium supplement* [multiple vitamins & minerals; multiple amino acids; calcium; folic acid; biotin] ± • ± • 50•0.2•0.015 mg ⑨ Androxy

1+1-F Creme ℞ *corticosteroidal anti-inflammatory; antifungal; antibacterial; anesthetic* [hydrocortisone; clioquinol; pramoxine] 1%•3%•1%

1% HC ointment ℞ *corticosteroidal anti-inflammatory* [hydrocortisone] 1%

One Touch reagent strips for home use OTC *in vitro diagnostic aid for blood glucose* ⑨ Ontak

166Ho-DOTMP *investigational (orphan) for multiple myeloma*

One-A-Day 55 Plus tablets (discontinued 2008) OTC *vitamin/mineral supplement* [multiple vitamins & minerals; folic acid; biotin] ± •400•30 mcg

One-A-Day Active; One-A-Day All-Day Energy tablets OTC *vitamin/mineral/calcium/iron supplement* [multiple vitamins & minerals; calcium (as carbonate); iron (as ferrous fumarate); folic acid] ± •110•9•0.4 mg; ± •250•9•0.4 mg

One-A-Day Essential tablets OTC *vitamin supplement* [multiple vitamins; folic acid] ± •400 mcg

One-A-Day Extras Antioxidant softgel capsules (discontinued 2008) OTC *vitamin/mineral supplement* [vitamins A, C, and E; multiple minerals] 5000 IU•250 mg•200 IU• ±

One-A-Day Kids Complete Bugs Bunny & Friends; One-A-Day Kids Complete Scooby Doo chewable tablets OTC *vitamin/mineral/calcium/iron supplement* [multiple vitamins & minerals; calcium; iron (as ferrous fumarate); folic acid; biotin; hydrogenated oil] ± •100•18• 0.4•0.03 mg

One-A-Day Kids Scooby Doo Gummies OTC *vitamin/mineral supplement*

[multiple vitamins and minerals; folic acid; biotin] ± •100•37.5 mcg

One-A-Day Kids Scooby Doo Plus Calcium chewable tablets OTC *vitamin/mineral supplement* [multiple vitamins and minerals; folic acid] ± •300 mcg

One-A-Day Maximum Formula tablets OTC *vitamin/mineral/calcium/iron supplement* [multiple vitamins & minerals; calcium (as carbonate and dicalcium phosphate); iron (as ferrous fumarate); folic acid; biotin] ± •18•0.4•0.03 mg

One-A-Day Men's Health Formula; One-A-Day Men's 50+ Advantage; One-A-Day Women's 50+ Advantage tablets OTC *vitamin/mineral supplement* [multiple vitamins and minerals; folic acid; biotin] ± • 400•30 mcg

One-A-Day Women's Formula tablets OTC *vitamin/calcium/iron supplement* [multiple vitamins; calcium (as carbonate); iron (as ferrous fumarate); folic acid] ± •450•18•0.4 mg

one.click (trademarked delivery device) *subcutaneous auto-injector*

One-Daily tablets OTC *vitamin/iron supplement* [multiple vitamins; iron] ± •18 mg

One-Daily Multi-Vitamin with Minerals tablets OTC *vitamin/mineral/calcium/iron supplement* [multiple vitamins & minerals; calcium; iron] ± •19•4.5 mg

1DMTX/6-MP (methotrexate, mercaptopurine) [with leucovorin rescue] *chemotherapy protocol for acute lymphocytic leukemia (ALL); the first-day initiation protocol* [followed by: MTX/6-MP (the ongoing continuation protocol)]

One-Tablet-Daily OTC *vitamin supplement* [multiple vitamins; folic acid] ± •400 mcg

One-Tablet-Daily with Iron OTC *vitamin/iron supplement* [multiple vitamins; iron (as ferrous fumarate); folic acid] ± •18•0.4 mg

One-Tablet-Daily with Minerals OTC *vitamin/mineral/calcium/iron supplement* [multiple vitamins & minerals; calcium (as carbonate and dicalcium phosphate) iron (as ferrous fumarate); folic acid; biotin] ±•162•18•0.4•0.03 mg

Onfi (available in Canada as **Alti-Clobazam**) *investigational (NDA filed) benzodiazepine tranquilizer used as an anticonvulsant for seizures associated with Lennox-Gastaut syndrome (LGS)* [clobazam]

Onglyza film-coated tablets ℞ *antidiabetic for type 2 diabetes that enhances the function of the body's incretin system to increase insulin production in the pancreas and reduce glucose production in the liver* [saxagliptin (as HCl)] 2.5, 5 mg

onion *(Allium cepa)* bulb *medicinal herb used as an anthelmintic, antiseptic, antispasmodic, carminative, diuretic, expectorant, and stomachic*

Onkolox *investigational (orphan) for renal cell carcinoma* [coumarin]

Onset Forte micro-coated tablets OTC *decongestant; antihistamine; analgesic; antipyretic* [phenylphrine HCl; chlorpheniramine maleate; acetaminophen] 5•2•162.5 mg

Onsolis orally disintegrating film ℞ *transmucosal narcotic analgesic for chronic pain in opioid-tolerant cancer patients* [fentanyl (as citrate)] 200, 400, 600, 800, 1200 mcg

Ontak frozen solution for IV injection ℞ *antineoplastic for recurrent or persistent cutaneous T-cell lymphoma (orphan); also used for chronic lymphocytic leukemia and non-Hodgkin lymphoma* [denileukin diftitox] 150 mcg/mL ⑨ One Touch

ontazolast USAN *antiasthmatic; leukotriene biosynthesis inhibitor*

ontianil INN

Onxol IV infusion ℞ *antineoplastic for AIDS-related Kaposi sarcoma (orphan), breast and ovarian cancers, and non–small cell lung cancer (NSCLC)* [paclitaxel] 6 mg/mL

OPA (Oncovin, prednisone, Adriamycin) *chemotherapy protocol for pediatric Hodgkin lymphoma*

Opana tablets, IV, IM, or subcu injection ℞ *narcotic analgesic for moderate to severe pain and for preoperative support of anesthesia; investigational (orphan) for intractable pain in narcotic-tolerant patients* [oxymorphone HCl] 5, 10 mg; 1 mg/mL

Opana ER extended-release film-coated tablets ℞ *narcotic analgesic for long-term treatment of moderate to severe pain* [oxymorphone HCl] 5, 7.5, 10, 15, 20, 30, 40 mg

Opaxio *investigational (Phase III) taxane antineoplastic for non–small cell lung cancer (NSCLC)* [polyglutamate paclitaxel]

Opcon-A eye drops OTC *decongestant; antihistamine; moisturizer/lubricant* [naphazoline HCl; pheniramine maleate; hydroxypropyl methylcellulose] 0.027%•0.315%•0.5% ⑨ Apokyn

Operand solution, prep pads, swab sticks, surgical scrub, perineal wash concentrate, aerosol, Iofoam skin cleanser, ointment OTC *broad-spectrum antimicrobial* [povidone-iodine] 1%; 1%; 1%; 7.5%; 1%; 0.5%; 1%; 1%

Operand Douche vaginal concentrate OTC *antiseptic/germicidal cleanser and deodorizer* [povidone-iodine]

Ophena *investigational (Phase III) selective estrogen receptor modulator (SERM) for the relief of postmenopausal symptoms* [ospemifene]

Ophthetic eye drops ℞ *topical anesthetic* [proparacaine HCl] 0.5%

Ophthifluor antecubital venous injection (discontinued 2008) ℞ *ophthalmic diagnostic agent* [fluorescein sodium] 10%

opiniazide INN

opipramol INN *antidepressant; antipsychotic* [also: opipramol HCl]

opipramol HCl USAN *antidepressant; antipsychotic* [also: opipramol]

opium USP *narcotic analgesic; antiperistaltic; used in neonatal opioid withdrawal programs; often abused as a street drug, which is highly addictive* 10 mg/mL oral

opium, powdered USP *narcotic analgesic*

Opium Tincture, Deodorized oral liquid ℞ *narcotic analgesic; antiperistaltic; used in neonatal opioid withdrawal programs; often abused as a street drug, which is highly addictive* [opium; alcohol 19%] 10 mg/mL

Oplopanax horridus medicinal herb [see: devil's club]

OPPA (Oncovin, prednisone, procarbazine, Adriamycin) *chemotherapy protocol for pediatric Hodgkin lymphoma*

oprelvekin USAN *platelet growth factor for prevention of thrombocytopenia following chemotherapy or radiation (orphan)* [also: interleukin 11, recombinant human]

Optaflu ⓔᵁᴿ IM injection (available in Europe) *investigational seasonal influenza virus vaccine grown in dog kidney cells instead of chicken eggs*

Optase gel ℞ *proteolytic enzyme for débridement of necrotic tissue; vulnerary* [trypsin; Peruvian balsam; castor oil] 0.12•87•788 mg/g

Opteform moldable bone paste ℞ *human allograft material for orthopedic surgery* [demineralized bone powder; cortical bone chips]

Opticare PMS tablets (discontinued 2008) OTC *vitamin/mineral supplement; digestive enzymes* [multiple vitamins & minerals; iron; folic acid; biotin; pancrelipase (amylase; protease; lipase)] ≛•2.5 mg•0.033 mg•10.4 mcg•2500 U•2500 U•200 U

Opti-Clean II solution (discontinued 2010) OTC *cleaning solution for hard or soft contact lenses*

Opti-Clean II Especially for Sensitive Eyes solution OTC *cleaning solution for rigid gas permeable contact lenses*

Opti-Clear eye drops OTC *decongestant; vasoconstrictor* [tetrahydrozoline HCl] 0.05%

OptiClik (trademarked insulin delivery device) *cartridge-type subcu injector for* **Lantus**

Opticrom 4% eye drops ℞ *mast cell stabilizer for vernal keratoconjunctivitis (orphan)* [cromolyn sodium]

Opticyl eye drops (discontinued 2011) ℞ *cycloplegic; mydriatic* [tropicamide] 0.5%, 1%

Opti-Free solution OTC *chemical disinfecting solution for soft contact lenses* (note: multiple products with the same name)

Opti-Free solution OTC *rewetting solution for soft contact lenses* (note: multiple products with the same name)

Opti-Free solution OTC *surfactant cleaning solution for soft contact lenses* (note: multiple products with the same name)

Opti-Free tablets (discontinued 2010) OTC *enzymatic cleaner for soft contact lenses* [pork pancreatin] (note: multiple products with the same name)

Opti-Free Express Multi-Purpose solution OTC *chemical disinfecting solution for soft contact lenses* [myristamidopropyl dimethylamine; polyquaternium-1] 0.0005%•0.001%

Opti-gen tablets OTC *vitamin/mineral supplement* [vitamins A, C, and E; multiple minerals] 5000 IU•60 mg•30 mg• ≛ ⓩ Apetigen; aptocaine

Optigene ophthalmic solution OTC *extraocular irrigating solution* [sterile isotonic solution] ⓩ Apetigen; aptocaine

Optigene 3 eye drops OTC *decongestant; vasoconstrictor* [tetrahydrozoline HCl] 0.05% ⓩ Apetigen; aptocaine

Optilets-500 Filmtabs (film-coated tablets) (discontinued 2008) OTC *vitamin supplement* [multiple vitamins]

Optilets-M-500 Filmtabs (film-coated tablets) (discontinued 2008) OTC *vitamin/mineral/iron supplement* [multiple vitamins & minerals; iron] ≛•20 mg

OptiMARK IV injection ℞ *paramagnetic contrast agent to enhance MRIs of the brain, head, and spine and liver structure and vascularity* [gadoversetamide] 330.9 mg

Optimental oral liquid OTC *enteral nutritional therapy* 237 mL

Optimmune *investigational (orphan) tear stimulant for severe keratoconjunctivitis sicca in Sjögren syndrome* [cyclosporine]

Optimox Prenatal tablets (discontinued 2008) OTC *vitamin/mineral/calcium/iron supplement* [multiple vitamins & minerals; calcium; iron; folic acid] ± • 100 • 5 • 0.133 mg

Optinate film-coated tablets + capsules (discontinued 2009) ℞ *prenatal calcium/iron/omega-3 supplement* [multiple vitamins & minerals; calcium (as citrate); iron (as carbonyl); folic acid; biotin; docusate sodium + docosahexaenoic acid (DHA)] ± • 200 • 90 • 1 • 0.03 • 50 mg (tablets) + 250 mg (capsules)

Opti-One solution OTC *rewetting solution for soft contact lenses*

Opti-One Multi-Purpose solution OTC *chemical disinfecting solution for soft contact lenses* [EDTA; polyquaternium-1] 0.05% • 0.001%

OptiPen One (trademarked insulin delivery device) *cartridge-type subcu injector*

OptiPranolol eye drops ℞ *antiglaucoma agent (beta-blocker)* [metipranolol HCl] 0.3%

Optiray 160; Optiray 240; Optiray 300; Optiray 320; Optiray 350 injection ℞ *radiopaque contrast medium* [ioversol (47.3% iodine)] 339 mg/mL (160 mg/mL); 509 mg/mL (240 mg/mL); 636 mg/mL (300 mg/mL); 678 mg/mL (320 mg/mL); 741 mg/mL (350 mg/mL)

Opti-Soft Especially for Sensitive Eyes solution (discontinued 2010) OTC *rinsing/storage solution for soft contact lenses* [sodium chloride (preserved saline solution)]

Optison suspension for IV injection ℞ *radiopaque contrast medium to enhance echocardiography* [perflutren protein] 0.33–1 mg/3 mL vial

Opti-Tears solution (discontinued 2010) OTC *rewetting solution for hard or soft contact lenses*

Optivar eye drops ℞ *antihistamine and mast cell stabilizer for allergic conjunctivitis* [azelastine HCl] 0.05%

Optive eye drops OTC *moisturizer; emollient* [carboxymethylcellulose sodium; glycerin] 0.5% • 0.9%

Optivite P.M.T. tablets OTC *vitamin/mineral/calcium/iron supplement* [multiple vitamins & minerals; calcium; iron (as amino acid chelate); folic acid] ± • 20.8 • 2.5 • 0.03 mg

OptiZen eye drops OTC *moisturizer/lubricant* [polysorbate 80] 0.5%

Opti-Zyme Enzymatic Cleaner Especially for Sensitive Eyes tablets (discontinued 2010) OTC *enzymatic cleaner for soft or rigid gas permeable contact lenses* [pork pancreatin]

OPV (oral poliovirus vaccine) [see: poliovirus vaccine, live oral]

ORA5 topical liquid OTC *oral anti-infective* [copper sulfate; iodine; potassium iodide]

Orabase oral gel (discontinued 2007) OTC *mucous membrane anesthetic* [benzocaine] 15%

Orabase; Orabase-B oral paste OTC *mucous membrane anesthetic* [benzocaine] 20%

Orabase Baby oral gel OTC *mucous membrane anesthetic* [benzocaine] 7.5%

Orabase HCA oral paste ℞ *corticosteroidal anti-inflammatory* [hydrocortisone acetate] 0.5%

Orabase Lip Healer cream OTC *mucous membrane anesthetic; antipruritic; counterirritant; vulnerary* [benzocaine; menthol; allantoin] 5% • 0.5% • 1.5%

Orabase Soothe-N-Seal topical liquid OTC *mucous membrane sealant and protectant for canker and mouth sores* [cyanoacrylate]

Orabase-Plain oral paste OTC *relief from minor oral irritations* [plasticized hydrocarbon gel]

Oracea dual-release capsules (75% immediate release, 25% delayed release) ℞ *tetracycline antibiotic for the once-daily treatment for rosacea* [doxycycline] 40 mg ⚕ Aerius; Ear-Eze; Iressa; OROS; Urso

Oracit solution ℞ *urinary alkalinizing agent* [sodium citrate; citric acid] 490•640 mg/5 mL

Orajel topical liquid OTC *mucous membrane anesthetic* [benzocaine; alcohol 44.2%] 20% ⚕ Erygel

Orajel; Orajel Brace-aid; Orajel/d; Denture Orajel; Baby Orajel Nighttime Formula oral gel OTC *mucous membrane anesthetic* [benzocaine] 10%, 20%; 20%; 10%; 10%; 10% ⚕ Erygel

Orajel, Baby topical liquid, oral gel OTC *mucous membrane anesthetic* [benzocaine] 7.5%

Orajel Mouth-Aid topical liquid, oral gel OTC *mucous membrane anesthetic* [benzocaine] 20%

Orajel Perioseptic oral liquid OTC *antiseptic for braces* [carbamide peroxide] 15%

Orajel P.M. Nighttime Formula Toothache Pain Relief cream OTC *mucous membrane anesthetic* [benzocaine] 20%

Orajel Tooth & Gum Cleanser, Baby gel OTC *removes plaque-like film* [poloxamer 407; simethicone] 2%• 0.12%

Oral Pain Relief oral gel OTC *mucous membrane anesthetic* [benzocaine] 20%

Oral Wound Rinse mouthwash OTC *hydrogel wound treatment* [acemannan]

Oralet (trademarked dosage form) *oral lozenge/lollipop* ⚕ Aurolate

Oral-lyn (approved in India and Ecuador) *investigational (Phase III) oral insulin spray*

Oralone Dental paste (discontinued 2009) ℞ *corticosteroidal anti-inflammatory* [triamcinolone acetonide] 0.1%

OraMagic Plus oral rinse OTC *mucous membrane anesthetic* [benzocaine] 10%

Oramorph SR sustained-release tablets ℞ *narcotic analgesic* [morphine sulfate] 15, 30, 60, 100 mg

orange flower oil NF *flavoring agent; perfume*

orange flower water NF

orange oil NF

orange peel tincture, sweet NF

orange root *medicinal herb* [see: goldenseal]

orange spirit, compound NF

orange swallow wort *medicinal herb* [see: pleurisy root]

orange syrup NF

Orap tablets ℞ *antispasmodic/antidyskinetic for Tourette syndrome* [pimozide] 1, 2 mg (4 mg available in Canada)

Oraphen-PD elixir (discontinued 2008) OTC *analgesic; antipyretic* [acetaminophen] 120 mg/5 mL

Orapred oral solution ℞ *corticosteroidal anti-inflammatory for asthma* [prednisolone (as sodium phosphate); alcohol 2%] 15 mg/5 mL

Orapred ODT (orally disintegrating tablets) ℞ *corticosteroidal anti-inflammatory for asthma* [prednisolone (as sodium phosphate)] 10, 15, 30 mg

Oraqix oral gel OTC *mucous membrane anesthetic* [lidocaine; prilocaine] 2.5%•2.5%

OraQuick Advance HIV-1/2 Antibody Test reagent kit for professional use ℞ *in vitro diagnostic aid for HIV-1 and HIV-2 antibodies in oral fluid, whole blood, or plasma*

OraQuick Rapid HIV-1 Antibody Test reagent kit for home use OTC *in vitro diagnostic aid for HIV-1 and HIV-2 antibodies in a fingerstick blood sample and HIV-1 antibodies in oral fluid*

orarsan [see: acetarsone]

Orasept throat spray OTC *mucous membrane anesthetic; antiseptic* [benzocaine; methylbenzethonium chloride] 0.996%•1.037% ⚕ Aricept

Orasept topical liquid OTC *oral astringent; antiseptic* [tannic acid; methylbenzethonium chloride; alcohol 53.31%] 12.16%•1.53% ⊡ Aricept

Orasol topical liquid OTC *mucous membrane anesthetic; antipruritic; counterirritant; antiseptic* [benzocaine; phenol; alcohol 70%] 6.3%•0.5% ⊡ Eryzole; uracil

Orasone tablets (discontinued 2008) ℞ *corticosteroid; anti-inflammatory; immunosuppressant* [prednisone] 1, 5, 10, 20, 50 mg ⊡ AeroZoin; Ureacin

OraSure reagent kit for home use OTC *in vitro diagnostic aid for HIV antibodies* ⊡ Arzerra

OraSure HIV-1 reagent kit for professional use ℞ *in vitro diagnostic aid for HIV antibodies using oral mucosal transudate* [single-sample, three-test kit: two ELISA assays + Western Blot assay]

OraVerse oral injection in prefilled cartridges ℞ *alpha-blocker to reverse soft-tissue anesthesia following oral surgery* [phentolamine mesylate] 0.4 mg/1.7 mL ⊡ Aerofreeze

Oravig buccal tablet ℞ *antifungal for oropharyngeal candidiasis* [miconazole] 50 mg

Oravig buccal tablets ℞ *antifungal for oropharyngeal candidiasis (OPC), also known as thrush* [miconazole] 50 mg

Oraxyl capsules ℞ *antimicrobial adjunct to scaling and root planing to reduce pocket depth in periodontitis* [doxycycline (as hyclate)] 20 mg

orazamide INN

Orazinc capsules, tablets OTC *zinc supplement* [zinc sulfate] 220 mg; 110 mg ⊡ arsenic

orBec investigational (Phase III, orphan) *oral treatment for intestinal graft vs. host disease* [beclomethasone dipropionate]

Orbivan capsules ℞ *barbiturate sedative; analgesic; antipyretic* [butalbital; acetaminophen; caffeine] 50•300•40 mg

orbofiban acetate USAN *platelet aggregation inhibitor; fibrinogen receptor antagonist*

orbutopril INN

orchanet *medicinal herb* [see: henna (Alkanna)]

orciprenaline INN, BAN *bronchodilator* [also: metaproterenol polistirex]

orciprenaline polistirex [see: metaproterenol polistirex]

orciprenaline sulfate [see: metaproterenol sulfate]

orconazole INN *antifungal* [also: orconazole nitrate]

orconazole nitrate USAN *antifungal* [also: orconazole]

oregano *medicinal herb* [see: marjoram]

Oregon grape *(Mahonia aquifolium)* rhizome and root *medicinal herb for acne, blood disorders, eczema, jaundice, liver disorders, promoting digestion, psoriasis, and staphylococcal infections*

Orencia powder for IV infusion, prefilled syringes for subcu injection ℞ *immunomodulator for rheumatoid arthritis (RA) and juvenile idiopathic arthritis* [abatacept] 250 mg; 125 mg/mL ⊡ Orinase

orestrate INN

orestrol [see: diethylstilbestrol dipropionate]

Orexin chewable tablets (discontinued 2008) OTC *vitamin supplement* [vitamins B_1, B_6, and B_{12}] 8.1 mg•4.1 mg•25 mcg

Orfadin capsules ℞ *adjunctive treatment for hereditary tyrosinemia type 1 (HT-1), a pediatric liver disease (orphan); investigational (orphan) for alkaptonuria* [nitisinone] 2, 5, 10 mg

Organ-I NR tablets OTC *expectorant* [guaifenesin] 200 mg

Organidin NR oral liquid (discontinued 2010) ℞ *expectorant* [guaifenesin] 100 mg/5 mL

Organidin NR tablets ℞ *expectorant* [guaifenesin] 200 mg

organoclay [see: bentoquatam]

orgotein USAN, INN, BAN *anti-inflammatory; antirheumatic; investigational (orphan) for amyotrophic lateral sclerosis and to prevent donor organ reperfusion injury* [previously known as superoxide dismutase (SOD)]

orienticine A; orienticine D [see: orientiparcin]

orientiparcin INN [a mixture of orienticine A and orienticine D]

Origanum vulgare medicinal herb [see: marjoram]

Orinase tablets Ŗ *sulfonylurea antidiabetic that stimulates insulin secretion in the pancreas* [tolbutamide] 500 mg ⧅ errhines; Orencia

Orinase Diagnostic powder for IV injection (discontinued 2010) Ŗ *in vivo diagnostic aid for pancreatic islet cell adenoma* [tolbutamide sodium] 1 g

oritavancin diphosphate USAN *investigational (NDA filed) peptidoglycan synthesis inhibitor antibiotic for complicated skin and skin structure infections (cSSSI)*

orlipastat [see: orlistat]

orlistat USAN, INN *lipase inhibitor to suppress the absorption of dietary fats, leading to weight loss; preventative for type 2 diabetes*

ormaplatin USAN *antineoplastic*

ormetoprim USAN, INN *antibacterial*

Ornex No Drowsiness caplets OTC *decongestant; analgesic; antipyretic* [pseudoephedrine HCl; acetaminophen] 30•325, 30•500 mg

ornidazole USAN, INN *anti-infective*

Ornidyl IV injection concentrate Ŗ *antiprotozoal for* Trypanosoma brucei gambiense *(sleeping sickness) infection (orphan); investigational (orphan) for AIDS-related* Pneumocystis pneumonia *(PCP)* [eflornithine HCl] 200 mg/mL

ornipressin INN

ornithine (L-ornithine) INN ⧅ aranotin

ornithine vasopressin [see: ornipressin]

ornoprostil INN

OROS (trademarked dosage form) *extended- or patterned-release tablets* ⧅ Aerius; Ear-Eze; Iressa; Oracea; Urso

orotic acid INN

orotirelin INN

orpanoxin USAN, INN *anti-inflammatory*

orphenadine citrate [see: orphenadrine citrate]

orphenadrine INN, BAN *skeletal muscle relaxant; analgesic; anticholinergic* [also: orphenadrine citrate]

orphenadrine citrate USP *skeletal muscle relaxant; analgesic; anticholinergic; also used at bedtime for quinine-resistant leg cramps* [also: orphenadrine] 100 mg oral; 30 mg/mL injection

Orphenadrine Compound; Orphenadrine Compound-DS tablets Ŗ *skeletal muscle relaxant; analgesic; antipyretic* [orphenadrine citrate; aspirin; caffeine] 25•385•30 mg; 50•770•60 mg

orphenadrine HCl *anticholinergic; antiparkinsonian*

Orphengesic; Orphengesic Forte tablets (discontinued 2009) Ŗ *skeletal muscle relaxant; analgesic; antipyretic* [orphenadrine citrate; aspirin; caffeine] 25•385•30 mg; 50•770•60 mg

orpressin [see: ornipressin]

orris root *(Iris florentina) medicinal herb used as a diuretic and stomachic*

Orsythia tablets (in packs of 28) Ŗ *monophasic oral contraceptive* [levonorgestrel; ethinyl estradiol] 0.1 mg•20 mcg ⧅ Oracit

ortetamine INN

orthesin [see: benzocaine]

Ortho Evra transdermal patch Ŗ *once-weekly contraceptive* [norelgestromin; ethinyl estradiol] 150•20 mcg/day

Ortho Micronor tablets (in Dialpaks of 28) Ŗ *oral contraceptive (progestin only)* [norethindrone] 0.35 mg

Ortho Tri-Cyclen tablets (in Dialpaks and Veridates of 28) Ŗ *triphasic oral contraceptive; treatment for acne vulgaris in females* [norgestimate; ethinyl estradiol]
Phase 1 (7 days): 0.18 mg•35 mcg;
Phase 2 (7 days): 0.215 mg•35 mcg;
Phase 3 (7 days): 0.25•35 mcg;
Counters (7 days)

Ortho Tri-Cyclen Lo tablets (in Dialpaks and Veridates of 28) Ŗ *triphasic oral contraceptive* [norgestimate; ethi-

nyl estradiol]
Phase 1 (7 days): 0.18 mg•25 mcg;
Phase 2 (7 days): 0.215 mg•25 mcg;
Phase 3 (7 days): 0.25 mg•25 mcg;
Counters (7 days)

Ortho-Cept tablets (in Dialpaks and Veridates of 28) ℞ *monophasic oral contraceptive* [desogestrel; ethinyl estradiol] 0.15 mg•30 mcg × 21 days; counters × 7 days

Orthoclone OKT3 IV injection ℞ *immunosuppressant for renal, hepatic, and cardiac transplants; also used for graft-versus-host disease following bone marrow transplants* [muromonab-CD3] 5 mg/5 mL

orthocresol NF

Ortho-Cyclen tablets (in Dialpaks and Veridates of 28) ℞ *monophasic oral contraceptive* [norgestimate; ethinyl estradiol] 0.25 mg•35 mcg × 21 days; counters × 7 days

Ortho-Est tablets (discontinued 2008) ℞ *bioidentical human estrogen replacement therapy for the treatment of postmenopausal symptoms and prevention of postmenopausal osteoporosis* [estrone (from estropipate)] 0.625, 1.25 (0.75, 1.5) mg

Ortho-Gynol vaginal gel OTC *spermicidal contraceptive (for use with a diaphragm)* [octoxynol 9] 1%

Ortho-Novum 1/35 tablets (in Dialpaks and Veridates of 28) ℞ *monophasic oral contraceptive* [norethindrone; ethinyl estradiol] 1 mg•35 mcg × 21 days; counters × 7 days

Ortho-Novum 1/50 tablets (in Dialpaks of 28) ℞ *monophasic oral contraceptive* [norethindrone; mestranol] 1 mg•50 mcg × 21 days; counters × 7 days

Ortho-Novum 7/7/7 tablets (in Dialpaks and Veridates of 28) ℞ *triphasic oral contraceptive* [norethindrone; ethinyl estradiol]
Phase 1 (7 days): 0.5 mg•35 mcg;
Phase 2 (7 days): 0.75 mg•35 mcg;
Phase 3 (7 days): 1 mg•35 mcg;
Counters (7 days)

Ortho-Novum 10/11 tablets (in Dialpaks of 28) ℞ *biphasic oral contraceptive* [norethindrone; ethinyl estradiol]
Phase 1 (10 days): 500•35 mcg;
Phase 2 (11 days): 1000•35 mcg;
Counters (7 days)

Ortho-Prefest [see: Prefest]

orthotolidine

Orthovisc intra-articular injection in prefilled syringes ℞ *viscoelastic lubricant and "shock absorber" for osteoarthritis of the knee* [hyaluronan] 30 mg/2 mL

OrthoWash oral rinse ℞ *dental caries preventative* [sodium fluoride (as acidulated phosphate solution)] 0.044%

Or-Tyl IM injection (discontinued 2011) ℞ *gastrointestinal anticholinergic/antispasmodic for irritable bowel syndrome (IBS)* [dicyclomine HCl] 10 mg/mL

oryzanol A, B, and C *medicinal herb* [see: rice bran oil]

osalmid INN

osarsal [see: acetarsone]

Os-Cal film-coated caplets, film-coated tablets, chewable tablets OTC *calcium supplement* [calcium (as carbonate); vitamin D] ≜•200 IU; ≜•400 IU; ≜•400 IU ② Asacol; Isocal

Os-Cal 250+D film-coated tablets (discontinued 2008) OTC *calcium supplement* [calcium (as carbonate); vitamin D] 250 mg•125 IU

Os-Cal 500 tablets, chewable tablets OTC *calcium supplement* [calcium (as carbonate)] 500 mg (1250 mg) ② Asacol; Isocal

Os-Cal 500+D film-coated tablets OTC *calcium supplement* [calcium (as carbonate); vitamin D] 500 mg•200 IU

Os-Cal Extra D caplets OTC *calcium/vitamin D supplement* [calcium (as carbonate); vitamin D] 500 mg•500 IU

Os-Cal Fortified tablets (discontinued 2008) OTC *vitamin/mineral/calcium/iron supplement* [multiple vitamins & minerals; calcium (as carbonate); iron (as ferrous fumarate)] ≜•250•5 mg

Os-Cal Ultra tablets OTC *vitamin/min-eral/calcium supplement* [vitamins C, D, and E; multiple minerals; calcium (as carbonate)] 60 mg•200 IU•15 IU• ± •600 mg

oseltamivir phosphate USAN *antiviral neuraminidase inhibitor for the prophy-laxis and treatment of influenza A and B infections; also used for the prophy-laxis and treatment of H1N1 influenza A (swine flu; Mexican pandemic flu) infections*

osmadizone INN

Osmitrol IV infusion ℞ *antihyperten-sive; osmotic diuretic* [mannitol] 5%, 10%, 15%, 20%

osmium *element (Os)*

Osmoglyn solution (discontinued 2010) ℞ *osmotic diuretic* [glycerin] 50%

Osmolite; Osmolite HN oral liquid OTC *enteral nutritional therapy* [lac-tose-free formula]

OsmoPrep tablets ℞ *saline laxative; pre-procedure bowel evacuant* [sodium phosphate (monobasic and dibasic)] 1.5 g

Osmorhiza longistylis medicinal herb [see: sweet cicely]

osmotic diuretics *a class of diuretics that increase excretion of sodium and chloride and decrease tubular absorption of water*

Osmunda cinnamomea; O. regalis medicinal herb [see: buckhorn brake]

ospemifene *investigational (Phase III) selective estrogen receptor modulator (SERM) for the relief of postmenopau-sal symptoms*

Ostavir *investigational (orphan) prophy-laxis of hepatitis B reinfection following liver transplants* [tuvirumab]

Osteo-D *investigational (orphan) calcium regulator for familial hypophosphatemic rickets* [secalciferol]

Osteofil injectable bone paste ℞ *human allograft material for orthopedic surgery* [demineralized bone powder]

OsteoMax effervescent powder for oral solution OTC *dietary supplement*

[calcium citrate; vitamin D; magne-sium] 500 mg•200 IU•200 mg

Osteo-Mins powder (discontinued 2008) OTC *vitamin/mineral/calcium supplement* [vitamins C and D; cal-cium; magnesium; potassium] 500 mg•100 IU•250 mg•250 mg•45 mg per 4.5 g

Ostiderm lotion OTC *for hyperhidrosis and bromhidrosis* [aluminum sulfate; zinc oxide] 14.5• ± mg/g

Ostiderm roll-on OTC *for hyperhidrosis and bromhidrosis* [aluminum chloro-hydrate; camphor; alcohol]

OstiGen Melts orally disintegrating tablets OTC *calcium supplement; vita-min and mineral supplement* [calcium; vitamin D; multiple vitamins & minerals] 350 mg•150 IU• ±

ostreogrycin INN, BAN

osvarsan [see: acetarsone]

Oswego tea (Monarda didyma) leaves and flowers *medicinal herb used as a calmative, rubefacient, and stimulant*

OT (old tuberculin) [see: tuberculin]

otamixaban *investigational (Phase III) factor Xa coagulation inhibitor for acute coronary events*

otelixizumab *investigational (Phase III) monoclonal antibody treatment for type 1 diabetes*

Otic Domeboro ear drops ℞ *antibac-terial; antifungal; antiseptic; astringent* [acetic acid; aluminum acetate] 2%• ±

Otic Edge ear drops (discontinued 2011) ℞ *anesthetic and analgesic for acute otitis media and the removal of cerumen* [benzocaine; antipyrine; acetic acid; polycosanol] 1.4%• 5.4%•0.01%•0.01%

Oticair ear drop suspension ℞ *cortico-steroidal anti-inflammatory; antibiotic* [hydrocortisone; neomycin sulfate; polymyxin B sulfate] 1%•5 mg• 10 000 U per mL

Oticin ear drops ℞ *anesthetic; antibac-terial; antiseptic* [proxazocain HCl; parachlorometaxylenol] 0.1%• 0.01% ⓓ Otozin

Oticin HC ear drops ℞ *anesthetic; antibacterial; antiseptic; steroidal anti-inflammatory* [proxazocain HCl; parachlorometaxylenol; hydrocortisone] 0.1%•0.01%•0.1%

otilonium bromide INN, BAN

otimerate sodium INN

Otocain ear drops ℞ *anesthetic* [benzocaine] 20%

Oto-End ear drops ℞ *corticosteroidal anti-inflammatory; local anesthetic; antiseptic* [hydrocortisone; pramoxine HCl; chloroxylenol] 10•10•1 mg/mL

Otomar-HC ear drops ℞ *corticosteroidal anti-inflammatory; local anesthetic; antiseptic* [hydrocortisone; pramoxine HCl; chloroxylenol] 10•10•1 mg/mL

Otosporin ear drops ℞ *corticosteroidal anti-inflammatory; antibiotic* [hydrocortisone; neomycin sulfate; polymyxin B sulfate] 1%•5 mg•10 000 U per mL

Otozin ear drops ℞ *antiseptic; anesthetic; analgesic; emollient* [zinc acetate; benzocaine; antipyrine; glycerin] 1%•1%•5.4%•2% ⓢ Oticin

Otrivin nasal spray, nose drops, pediatric nose drops OTC *nasal decongestant* [xylometazoline HCl] 0.1%; 0.1%; 0.05% ⓢ etorphine; Etrafon

ouabain USP

Our Lady's mint *medicinal herb* [see: spearmint]

Outgro solution OTC *pain relief for ingrown toenails* [tannic acid; chlorobutanol; isopropyl alcohol 83%] 25%•5%

Ovace foam ℞ *antibiotic for acute and chronic seborrheic dermatitis and secondary bacterial infections of the scalp and skin* [sulfacetamide sodium] 10%

Ovace Plus cream, shampoo ℞ *antibiotic for acute and chronic seborrheic dermatitis and secondary bacterial infections of the scalp and skin* [sulfacetamide sodium] 10%

Ovace Plus Wash soap ℞ *antibiotic for acute and chronic seborrheic dermatitis and secondary bacterial infections* [sulfacetamide sodium] 10%

ovandrotone albumin INN, BAN

OvaRex *investigational (Phase II, orphan) therapeutic vaccine for epithelial ovarian cancer* [monoclonal antibody B43.13]

Ovastat *investigational (orphan) for ovarian cancer* [treosulfan]

O-Vax *investigational (Phase III, orphan) theraccine for adjuvant treatment of ovarian cancer* [autologous DNP-modified tumor vaccine]

Ovcon 35 caplets, chewable tablets (in packs of 21 or 28) ℞ *monophasic oral contraceptive* [norethindrone; ethinyl estradiol] 0.4 mg•35 mcg

Ovcon 35 Fe chewable tablets (name changed to **Femcon Fe** in 2007)

Ovcon 50 caplets (in packs of 28) ℞ *monophasic oral contraceptive* [norethindrone; ethinyl estradiol] 1 mg•50 mcg × 21 days; counters × 7 days

Ovide lotion ℞ *pediculicide for lice* [malathion; isopropyl alcohol 78%] 0.5% ⓢ Ovoid

Ovidrel prefilled syringes for subcu injection ℞ *fertility stimulant for anovulatory women; adjuvant therapy for cryptorchidism* [choriogonadotropin alfa] 250 mcg/0.5 mL

ovine corticotropin-releasing hormone [see: corticorelin ovine triflutate]

Ovoid (trademarked dosage form) *sugar-coated tablet* ⓢ Ovide

Ovral tablets (in Pilpaks of 21 and 28) ℞ *monophasic oral contraceptive; emergency postcoital contraceptive* [norgestrel; ethinyl estradiol] 0.5 mg•50 mcg

Ovrette tablets (in Pilpaks of 28) (discontinued 2008) ℞ *oral contraceptive (progestin only)* [norgestrel] 0.075 mg

Ovulation Scope kit for home use OTC *in vitro diagnostic aid to predict ovulation time from a saliva sample*

OvuLite kit for home use OTC *in vitro diagnostic aid to predict ovulation time from a saliva sample*

[^{15}O] water [see: water O 15]

ox bile extract [see: bile salts]

oxabolone cipionate INN

oxabrexine INN
22-oxacalcitriol (OCT) [see: maxacalcitol]
oxaceprol INN
oxacillin INN *penicillinase-resistant penicillin antibiotic* [also: oxacillin sodium]
oxacillin sodium USAN, USP *penicillinase-resistant penicillin antibiotic* [also: oxacillin] 0.5, 1, 2, 10 g injection
oxadimedine INN
oxadimedine HCl [see: oxadimedine]
oxadoddy *medicinal herb* [see: Culver root]
oxaflozane INN
oxaflumazine INN
oxafuradene [see: nifuradene]
oxagrelate USAN, INN *platelet antiaggregatory agent*
oxalinast INN
oxaliplatin USAN, INN *alkylating antineoplastic for advanced or metastatic colorectal cancers; also used for non-Hodgkin lymphoma and advanced ovarian cancer (orphan); investigational (orphan) for primary hyperoxaluria* 50, 100 mg/vial injection
Oxalis acetosella *medicinal herb* [see: wood sorrel]
oxamarin INN *hemostatic* [also: oxamarin HCl]
oxamarin HCl USAN *hemostatic* [also: oxamarin]
oxametacin INN
oxamisole INN *immunoregulator* [also: oxamisole HCl]
oxamisole HCl USAN *immunoregulator* [also: oxamisole]
oxamniquine USAN, USP, INN *antischistosomal; anthelmintic for schistosomiasis (flukes)*
oxamphetamine hydrobromide [see: hydroxyamphetamine hydrobromide]
oxamycin [see: cycloserine]
oxanamide INN
Oxandrin caplets ℞ *anabolic steroid for bone pain due to osteoporosis; investigational (Phase III, orphan) for AIDS-wasting syndrome; investigational (orphan) for muscular dystrophy and*

growth delay; also abused as a street drug [oxandrolone] 2.5, 10 mg
oxandrolone USAN, USP, INN, BAN, JAN *anabolic steroid for bone pain due to osteoporosis; investigational (Phase III, orphan) for AIDS-wasting syndrome; investigational (orphan) for muscular dystrophy, alcoholic hepatitis, and growth delay; also abused as a street drug to increase muscle mass* 2.5, 10 mg oral
oxantel INN *anthelmintic* [also: oxantel pamoate]
oxantel pamoate USAN *anthelmintic* [also: oxantel]
oxantrazole HCl [see: piroxantrone HCl]
oxapadol INN
oxapium iodide INN
oxaprazine
oxapropanium iodide INN
oxaprotiline INN *antidepressant* [also: oxaprotiline HCl]
oxaprotiline HCl USAN *antidepressant* [also: oxaprotiline]
oxaprozin USAN, INN, BAN *analgesic; nonsteroidal anti-inflammatory drug (NSAID) for osteoarthritis and rheumatoid arthritis* 600 mg oral
oxaprozin potassium *analgesic; nonsteroidal anti-inflammatory drug (NSAID) for osteoarthritis and rheumatoid arthritis* (base=88.5%)
oxarbazole USAN, INN *antiasthmatic*
oxarutine [see: ethoxazorutoside]
oxatomide USAN, INN *antiallergic; antiasthmatic*
oxazafone INN
oxazepam USAN, USP, INN *benzodiazepine anxiolytic; sedative; alcohol withdrawal aid* 10, 15, 30 mg oral
oxazidione INN
oxazolam INN
oxazolidin [see: oxyphenbutazone]
oxazolidinediones *a class of anticonvulsants (no longer used)*
oxazorone INN ② oxisuran
oxcarbazepine INN *anticonvulsant for partial seizures in adults or children; also used for bipolar disorder and diabetic*

neuropathy 150, 300, 600 mg oral; 60 mg/mL oral

oxdralazine INN

Oxecta tablets ℞ *immediate-release opioid analgesic for moderate-to-severe pain; incorporates abuse-deterrent technology to prevent its conversion to a street drug* [oxycodone HCl; niacin] 5, 7.5 mg ⓘ Exact

oxeladin INN, BAN

oxendolone USAN, INN *antiandrogen for benign prostatic hypertrophy*

Oxepa oral liquid OTC *nutritional therapy for modulating inflammation due to systemic inflammatory response syndrome (SIRS), sepsis, trauma, burns, acute lung injury, and acute respiratory distress syndrome (ARDS)* [multiple vitamins and minerals; eicosapentaenoic acid (EPA); gamma-linolenic acid (GLA)] ±•4.6•4 g/L

oxepinac INN

oxerutins BAN

oxetacaine INN *topical anesthetic* [also: oxethazaine]

oxetacillin INN

2-oxetanone [see: propiolactone]

oxethazaine USAN, BAN *topical anesthetic* [also: oxetacaine] ⓘ oxytocin

oxetorone INN *migraine-specific analgesic* [also: oxetorone fumarate]

oxetorone fumarate USAN *migraine-specific analgesic* [also: oxetorone]

oxfenamide [see: oxiramide]

oxfendazole USAN, INN *anthelmintic*

oxfenicine USAN, INN, BAN *vasodilator*

oxibendazole USAN, INN *anthelmintic*

oxibetaine INN

oxibuprocaine chloride [see: benoxinate HCl]

oxichlorochine sulfate [see: hydroxychloroquine sulfate]

oxicinchophen [see: oxycinchophen]

oxiconazole INN, BAN *broad-spectrum topical antifungal* [also: oxiconazole nitrate]

oxiconazole nitrate USAN *broad-spectrum topical antifungal* [also: oxiconazole]

oxicone [see: oxycodone]

oxidized cellulose [see: cellulose, oxidized]

oxidized cholic acid [see: dehydrocholic acid]

oxidized regenerated cellulose [see: cellulose, oxidized regenerated]

oxidopamine USAN, INN *ophthalmic adrenergic*

oxidronic acid USAN, INN, BAN *calcium regulator*

oxifenamate [see: hydroxyphenamate]

oxifentorex INN

Oxi-Freeda tablets OTC *vitamin/mineral/amino acid supplement* [multiple vitamins & minerals; multiple amino acids; folic acid] ±•±•100 mcg

oxifungin INN *antifungal* [also: oxifungin HCl]

oxifungin HCl USAN *antifungal* [also: oxifungin]

oxilorphan USAN, INN *narcotic antagonist*

oximetazoline HCl [see: oxymetazoline HCl]

oximetholone [see: oxymetholone]

oximonam USAN, INN *antibacterial*

oximonam sodium USAN *antibacterial*

oxindanac INN

oxiniacic acid INN

oxiperomide USAN, INN *antipsychotic* ⓘ icospiramide

oxipertine [see: oxypertine]

oxipethidine [see: hydroxypethidine]

oxiphenbutazone [see: oxyphenbutazone]

oxiphencyclimine chloride [see: oxyphencyclimine HCl]

Oxiplen capsules OTC *vitamin/mineral supplement* [vitamins A, C, and E; multiple minerals; multiple amino acids] 5000 IU•2500 mg•100 mg• ±•±

Oxipor VHC lotion OTC *antipsoriatic; antiseborrheic; keratolytic* [coal tar; alcohol 79%] 5%

oxiprocaine [see: hydroxyprocaine]

oxiprogesterone caproate [see: hydroxyprogesterone caproate]

oxipurinol INN *xanthine oxidase inhibitor* [also: oxypurinol]

oxiracetam INN, BAN *treatment for Alzheimer disease*

oxiramide USAN, INN *antiarrhythmic*

oxisopred INN

Oxistat cream, lotion ℞ *broad-spectrum antifungal* [oxiconazole nitrate] 1%

oxistilbamidine isethionate [see: hydroxystilbamidine isethionate]

oxisuran USAN, INN *antineoplastic* ⑨ oxazorone

oxitefonium bromide INN

oxitetracaine [see: hydroxytetracaine]

oxitetracycline [see: oxytetracycline]

oxitriptan INN

oxitriptyline INN

oxitropium bromide INN, BAN

oxmetidine INN, BAN *antagonist to histamine H_2 receptors* [also: oxmetidine HCl]

oxmetidine HCl USAN *antagonist to histamine H_2 receptors* [also: oxmetidine]

oxmetidine mesylate USAN *antagonist to histamine H_2 receptors*

oxodipine INN

oxogestone INN *progestin* [also: oxogestone phenpropionate]

oxogestone phenpropionate USAN *progestin* [also: oxogestone]

oxoglurate INN *combining name for radicals or groups*

oxolamine INN

oxolinic acid USAN, INN *antibacterial*

oxomemazine INN

oxonazine INN

4-oxopentanoic acid, calcium salt [see: calcium levulinate]

oxophenarsine INN [also: oxophenarsine HCl]

oxophenarsine HCl USP [also: oxophenarsine]

5-oxoproline [see: pidolic acid]

oxoprostol INN, BAN

oxothiazolidine carboxylate (L-2-oxothiazolidine-4-carboxylic acid) *investigational (orphan) immunomodulator for adult respiratory distress syndrome and amyotrophic lateral sclerosis*

oxozepam [see: oxazepam]

oxpentifylline BAN *peripheral vasodilator; hemorheologic agent* [also: pentoxifylline]

oxpheneridine INN

oxprenoate potassium INN

oxprenolol INN *coronary vasodilator* [also: oxprenolol HCl]

oxprenolol HCl USAN, USP *coronary vasodilator* [also: oxprenolol]

OxSODrol *anti-inflammatory; antirheumatic; investigational (orphan) to prevent donor organ reperfusion injury* [orgotein (previously known as superoxide dismutase, or SOD)]

Oxsoralen lotion ℞ *psoralens for repigmentation of idiopathic vitiligo* [methoxsalen] 1%

Oxsoralen-Ultra softgels ℞ *systemic psoralens for the treatment of severe recalcitrant psoriasis* [methoxsalen] 10 mg

oxtriphylline USP *bronchodilator* (theophylline=64%) [also: choline theophyllinate] 100, 200 mg oral; 50, 100 mg/5 mL oral

Oxy Medicated Cleanser & Pads OTC *keratolytic cleanser for acne* [salicylic acid; alcohol] 0.5%•22%, 0.5%•40%, 2%•50%

Oxy Medicated Soap bar OTC *disinfectant/antiseptic; medicated cleanser for acne* [triclosan] 1%

Oxy Night Watch; Oxy Night Watch for Sensitive Skin lotion OTC *keratolytic for acne* [salicylic acid] 2%; 1%

Oxy Oil-Free Acne Wash topical liquid OTC *keratolytic for acne* [benzoyl peroxide] 10%

oxybenzone USAN, USP, INN *ultraviolet screen*

oxybuprocaine INN, BAN *topical anesthetic* [also: benoxinate HCl; oxybuprocaine HCl]

oxybuprocaine HCl JAN *topical anesthetic* [also: benoxinate HCl; oxybuprocaine]

oxybutynin USAN, INN, BAN *anticholinergic; smooth muscle relaxant; uri-*

nary antispasmodic [also: oxybutynin chloride]

oxybutynin chloride USAN, USP *anticholinergic; smooth muscle relaxant; urinary antispasmodic for urge urinary incontinence and frequency* [also: oxybutynin] 5, 10, 15 mg oral; 5 mg/5 mL oral

oxybutynin HCl *investigational (Phase III) topical gel delivery form for overactive bladder*

Oxycel pads, pledgets, strips ℞ *local hemostat for surgery* [cellulose, oxidized] ⧉ Oxizole

oxychlorosene USAN *topical antiseptic*

oxychlorosene sodium USAN *topical antiseptic*

oxycinchophen INN, BAN

oxyclipine INN *anticholinergic* [also: propenzolate HCl]

oxyclipine HCl [see: propenzolate HCl]

oxyclozanide INN, BAN

oxycodone USAN, INN, BAN *narcotic analgesic; also abused as a street drug*

oxycodone HCl USAN, USP *narcotic analgesic; also abused as a street drug* 5, 10, 15, 20, 30, 40, 80 mg oral; 5, 100 mg/5 mL oral; 20 mg/mL oral drops

oxycodone HCl & acetaminophen *narcotic analgesic* 2.5•325, 5•325, 7.5•325, 7.5•500, 10•325, 7.5•500, 10•650 mg oral

oxycodone HCl & aspirin *narcotic analgesic* 4.8355•325 mg oral

oxycodone HCl & ibuprofen *narcotic analgesic* 5•400 mg oral

oxycodone terephthalate USP *narcotic analgesic; also abused as a street drug*

OxyContin controlled-release tablets ℞ *narcotic analgesic* [oxycodone HCl] 10, 15, 20, 30, 40, 60, 80, 160 mg

Oxydess II tablets ℞ *CNS stimulant; amphetamine* [dextroamphetamine sulfate] 10 mg

oxydimethylquinazine [see: antipyrine]

oxydipentonium chloride INN

oxyethyltheophylline [see: etofylline]

OxyFast oral drops ℞ *narcotic analgesic* [oxycodone HCl] 20 mg/mL

oxyfedrine INN, BAN

oxyfenamate INN *minor tranquilizer* [also: hydroxyphenamate]

oxyfilcon A USAN *hydrophilic contact lens material*

oxygen (O₂) USP *medicinal gas; element (O)*

oxygen, polymeric *investigational (orphan) for sickle cell anemia*

oxygen 93 percent USP *medicinal gas*

OxyIR immediate-release capsules ℞ *narcotic analgesic* [oxycodone HCl] 5 mg ⧉ Ixiaro

oxymesterone INN, BAN

oxymetazoline INN, BAN *topical ocular vasoconstrictor; nasal decongestant* [also: oxymetazoline HCl]

oxymetazoline HCl USAN, USP *topical ocular decongestant/vasoconstrictor; nasal decongestant* [also: oxymetazoline] 0.05% nasal

oxymetholone USAN, USP, INN, BAN *androgen; anabolic steroid for anemia; also abused as a street drug*

oxymethylene urea [see: polynoxylin]

oxymorphone INN, BAN *narcotic analgesic* [also: oxymorphone HCl]

oxymorphone HCl USP *narcotic analgesic for moderate to severe pain and for preoperative support of anesthesia; investigational (orphan) for intractable pain in narcotic-tolerant patients* [also: oxymorphone] 5, 7.5, 10, 15, 20, 30, 40 mg oral

oxypendyl INN

oxypertine USAN, INN *antidepressant*

oxyphenbutazone USP, INN *antiinflammatory; antirheumatic; antipyretic; analgesic*

oxyphencyclimine INN *anticholinergic* [also: oxyphencyclimine HCl]

oxyphencyclimine HCl USP *peptic ulcer adjunct* [also: oxyphencyclimine]

oxyphenhydrazine [see: carsalam]

oxyphenisatin BAN *laxative* [also: oxyphenisatin acetate; oxyphenisatine]

oxyphenisatin acetate USAN *laxative* [also: oxyphenisatine; oxyphenisatin]

oxyphenisatine INN *laxative* [also: oxyphenisatin acetate; oxyphenisatin]

oxyphenonium bromide

oxyphylline [see: etofylline]

oxypurinol USAN *xanthine oxidase inhibitor for hyperuricemia; metabolite of allopurinol* [also: oxipurinol]

oxypurinol sodium *investigational (NDA filed, orphan) xanthine oxidase inhibitor for hyperuricemia; metabolite of allopurinol*

oxypyrronium bromide INN

oxyquinoline USAN *disinfectant/antiseptic*

oxyquinoline benzoate [see: benzoxiquine]

oxyquinoline sulfate USAN, NF *complexing agent; antiseptic*

oxyridazine INN

Oxysept solution + tablets (discontinued 2010) OTC *two-step chemical disinfecting system for soft contact lenses* [hydrogen peroxide–based]

Oxysept 2 solution (discontinued 2010) OTC *rinsing/storage solution for soft contact lenses* [sodium chloride (saline solution)]

oxysonium iodide INN

oxytetracycline USP, INN *broad-spectrum tetracycline antibiotic; antirickettsial*

oxytetracycline calcium USP *tetracycline antibiotic; antirickettsial*

oxytetracycline HCl USP *tetracycline antibiotic; antirickettsial*

oxytocics *a class of posterior pituitary hormones that stimulate contraction of the myometrium (uterine muscle)*

oxytocin USP, INN *posterior pituitary hormone; oxytocic for induction of labor* 10 U/mL injection

Oxytrol transdermal patch ℞ *urinary antispasmodic for urge urinary incontinence and frequency* [oxybutynin chloride] 36 mg (3.9 mg/day)

Oxyzal Wet Dressing topical liquid OTC *antiseptic dressing for minor infections* [oxyquinoline sulfate; benzalkonium chloride]

Oysco 500 chewable tablets OTC *calcium supplement* [calcium (as carbonate)] 500 mg (1250 mg)

Oysco D; Oysco 500 + D tablets OTC *calcium supplement* [calcium (as carbonate); vitamin D] ≟•125 IU; 500 mg•200 IU

Oyst-Cal 500 film-coated tablets OTC *calcium supplement* [calcium (as carbonate)] 500 mg (1250 mg)

Oyst-Cal-D film-coated tablets OTC *calcium supplement* [calcium (as carbonate); vitamin D] 250 mg•125 IU

Oyster Calcium tablets (discontinued 2008) OTC *calcium supplement* [calcium (as carbonate); vitamins A and D] 375 mg•800 IU•200 IU

Oyster Calcium 500 + D tablets (discontinued 2008) OTC *calcium supplement* [calcium (as carbonate); vitamin D] 500 mg•125 IU

Oyster Calcium with Vitamin D tablets (discontinued 2008) OTC *calcium supplement* [calcium (as carbonate); vitamin D] 250 mg•125 IU

Oyster Shell Calcium tablets OTC *calcium supplement* [calcium (as carbonate)] 500 mg (1250 mg)

Oyster Shell Calcium 500 + D tablets OTC *calcium supplement* [calcium (as carbonate); vitamin D] 500 mg• 200 IU

Oyster Shell Calcium with Vitamin D tablets OTC *calcium supplement* [calcium (as carbonate); vitamin D] 250 mg•125 IU

Oystercal-D 250 tablets (discontinued 2008) OTC *calcium supplement* [calcium (as carbonate); vitamin D] 250 mg•125 IU

oz; gamma-oz *medicinal herb* [see: rice bran oil]

ozagrel INN *antiasthmatic* [also: ozagrel sodium] ⊚ Ascor L

ozagrel sodium JAN *antiasthmatic* [also: ozagrel]

ozolinone USAN, INN *diuretic*

Ozurdex injectable ocular implant ℞ *corticosteroidal anti-inflammatory for macular edema* [dexamethasone] 0.7 mg

P **Chlor DM** oral drops ℞ *antitussive; decongestant; antihistamine* [dextromethorphan hydrobromide; phenylephrine HCl; chlorpheniramine maleate] 3•3.5•1 mg/mL

P **Chlor GG** oral drops ℞ *decongestant; antihistamine; expectorant; for children 2–24 months* [phenylephrine HCl; chlorpheniramine maleate; guaifenesin] 2•1•20 mg/mL

P & S shampoo OTC *antiseborrheic; keratolytic* [salicylic acid] 2%

P & S shampoo OTC *keratolytic* [salicylic acid] 2%

P & S topical liquid OTC *antimicrobial hair dressing* [phenol]

^{32}**P** [see: chromic phosphate P 32]

^{32}**P** [see: polymetaphosphate P 32]

^{32}**P** [see: sodium phosphate P 32]

PA MAb *investigational (orphan) treatment for anthrax exposure* [now: raxibacumab]

PAB (para-aminobenzoate) [see: aminobenzoic acid]

PABA (para-aminobenzoic acid) [now: aminobenzoic acid]

PABA sodium [see: aminobenzoate sodium]

pabestrol D [see: diethylstilbestrol dipropionate]

PAC; PAC-I (Platinol, Adriamycin, cyclophosphamide) *chemotherapy protocol for ovarian cancer, endometrial cancer, and thymoma; "I" stands for "Indiana protocol," used for ovarian cancer only*

P-A-C Analgesic tablets OTC *analgesic; antipyretic; anti-inflammatory* [aspirin; caffeine] 400•32 mg

Pacerone tablets ℞ *antiarrhythmic for acute ventricular tachycardia and fibrillation (orphan)* [amiodarone HCl] 100, 200 mg

PA-CI (pegylated Adriamycin, cisplatin) *chemotherapy protocol for pediatric hepatoblastoma*

Packer's Pine Tar soap OTC *antiseborrheic; antipsoriatic; antipruritic; antibacterial* [pine tar]

paclitaxel USAN, INN, BAN *antineoplastic for AIDS-related Kaposi sarcoma (orphan), breast and ovarian cancers, and non–small cell lung cancer; derived from the Pacific yew tree; investigational (orphan) for esophageal cancer* 6 mg/mL injection

paclitaxel + carboplatin + etoposide *chemotherapy protocol for primary adenocarcinoma and small cell lung cancer (SCLC)*

paclitaxel & docosahexaenoic acid (DHA) *investigational (orphan) taxane for hormone-refractory prostate cancer*

paclitaxel tocosol *investigational (Phase III) formulation of paclitaxel in a vitamin E–based emulsion for the treatment of metastatic breast cancer*

paclitaxel + vinorelbine *chemotherapy protocol for breast and non–small cell lung cancer*

Pacnex LP; Pacnex HP medicated pads ℞ *keratolytic for acne* [benzoyl peroxide] 4.25%; 7%

pacrinolol INN

padimate INN *ultraviolet screen* [also: padimate A]

padimate A USAN *ultraviolet screen* [also: padimate]

padimate O USAN *ultraviolet screen*

Paeonia officinalis medicinal herb [see: peony]

pafenolol INN ☒ befunolol

paflufocon A USAN *hydrophobic contact lens material*

paflufocon B USAN *hydrophobic contact lens material*

paflufocon C USAN *hydrophobic contact lens material*

paflufocon D USAN *hydrophobic contact lens material*

paflufocon E USAN *hydrophobic contact lens material*

pagoclone USAN *nonsedating anxiolytic*

PAH (para-aminohippurate) [see: aminohippuric acid]

PAHA (para-aminohippuric acid) [see: aminohippuric acid]

Pain and Fever tablets, caplets OTC *analgesic; antipyretic* [acetaminophen] 325, 500 mg; 500 mg

Pain and Fever, Children's chewable tablets, oral liquid OTC *analgesic; antipyretic* [acetaminophen] 80 mg; 160 mg/5 mL

Pain and Fever, Children's oral drops (discontinued 2011) OTC *analgesic; antipyretic* [acetaminophen] 100 mg/mL

Pain Bust-R II cream OTC *analgesic; mild anesthetic; antipruritic; counterirritant* [methyl salicylate; menthol] 17%•12%

Pain Doctor cream OTC *mild anesthetic; antipruritic; counterirritant; analgesic for muscle and joint pain* [methyl salicylate; menthol; capsaicin] 25%•10%•0.025%

Pain Gel Plus OTC *mild anesthetic; antipruritic; counterirritant* [menthol] 4%

Pain Relief caplets OTC *analgesic; antipyretic* [acetaminophen] 500 mg

Pain Reliever tablets OTC *analgesic; antipyretic* [acetaminophen] 325, 500 mg

Pain Relieving Rub cream OTC *analgesic; mild anesthetic; antipruritic; counterirritant* [methyl salicylate; menthol] 15%•10%

Painaid tablets OTC *analgesic; antipyretic; anti-inflammatory* [acetaminophen; aspirin; salicylamide; caffeine] 110•162•152•32.4 mg

Painaid BRF (Back Relief Formula) tablets OTC *analgesic; antipyretic; anti-inflammatory* [magnesium salicylate tetrahydrate; acetaminophen] 250•250 mg

Painaid ESF (Extra Strength Formula) tablets OTC *analgesic; antipyretic; anti-inflammatory* [acetaminophen; aspirin; caffeine] 250•250•65 mg

Painaid PMF (Premenstrual Formula) tablets OTC *analgesic; antipyretic;*

diuretic [acetaminophen; pamabrom] 500•25 mg

Pain-gesic tablets OTC *analgesic; antipyretic; antihistamine; sleep aid* [acetaminophen; phenyltoloxamine citrate] 325•30 mg

paint, Indian *medicinal herb* [see: bloodroot]

paint, yellow Indian *medicinal herb* [see: goldenseal]

paint root, red *medicinal herb* [see: bloodroot]

Pain-X gel (discontinued 2011) OTC *counterirritant; analgesic for muscle and joint pain; mild anesthetic; antipruritic* [capsaicin; menthol; camphor] 0.05%•5%•4% ② Panokase; Pin-X

PALA disodium [see: sparfosate sodium]

Paladin ointment OTC *diaper rash treatment* [zinc oxide; petrolatum; lanolin; vitamins A & D] ② belladonna; Polydine

palatrigine INN, BAN

Palcaps 10; Palcaps 20 delayed-release capsules ℞ *porcine-derived digestive enzymes* [pancrelipase (lipase; protease; amylase)] 10 000•37 500•33 200 USP units; 20 000•75 000•66 400 USP units

paldimycin USAN, INN *antibacterial*

paldimycin A [see: paldimycin]

paldimycin B [see: paldimycin]

pale gentian *medicinal herb* [see: gentian]

palestrol [see: diethylstilbestrol]

Palgic tablets, oral liquid ℞ *antihistamine for allergic rhinitis* [carbinoxamine maleate] 4 mg; 4 mg/5 mL

Palgic-D extended-release caplets (discontinued 2007) ℞ *decongestant; antihistamine* [pseudoephedrine HCl; carbinoxamine maleate] 80•8 mg

Palgic-DS syrup (discontinued 2007) ℞ *decongestant; antihistamine* [pseudoephedrine HCl; carbinoxamine maleate] 25•2 mg/5 mL

palifermin *keratinocyte growth factor (KGF) for radiation- and chemotherapy-induced oral mucositis*

palifosfamide *investigational (orphan) antineoplastic for soft-tissue sarcomas*

palinavir USAN *antiviral; HIV-1 protease inhibitor*

palinum [see: cyclobarbitone]

paliperidone *dopamine D_2 and serotonin 5-HT$_{2A}$ receptor antagonist; novel (atypical) benzisoxazole antipsychotic for schizophrenia; investigational (Phase III) for manic episodes of a bipolar disorder; active metabolite of* risperidone

paliperidone palmitate *dopamine D_2 and serotonin 5-HT$_{2A}$ receptor antagonist; long-acting injectable antipsychotic for schizophrenia; active metabolite of* risperidone

palivizumab *monoclonal antibody for prophylaxis of respiratory syncytial virus (RSV) in infants*

palladium *element (Pd)*

palladium Pd 103 *radioactive "seeds" for ultrasound-guided brachytherapy for adenocarcinoma of the prostate*

palm, dwarf; dwarf palmetto; pan palm *medicinal herb* [see: saw palmetto]

palmidrol INN

Palmitate-A 5000 tablets (discontinued 2009) OTC *vitamin supplement* [vitamin A palmitate] 5000 IU

palmitic acid USAN *ultrasound contrast medium for echocardiography*

palmoxirate sodium USAN *antidiabetic* [also: palmoxiric acid]

palmoxiric acid INN *antidiabetic* [also: palmoxirate sodium]

Palomar "E" ointment OTC *emollient* [vitamin E]

palonosetron HCl USAN *selective serotonin 5-HT$_3$ antagonist; antiemetic to prevent chemotherapy-induced and postoperative nausea and vomiting* (base=89%)

PALS coated tablets OTC *systemic deodorant for ostomy, breath, and body odors* [chlorophyllin copper complex] 100 mg

PAM; L-PAM (phenylalanine mustard) [see: melphalan]

2-PAM (2-pyridine aldoxime methylchloride) [see: pralidoxime chloride]

pamabrom USAN *nonprescription diuretic*

pamaqueside USAN *hypocholesterolemic; cholesterol absorption inhibitor; antiatherosclerotic*

pamaquine naphthoate NF

pamatolol INN *antiadrenergic (beta-blocker)* [also: pamatolol sulfate]

pamatolol sulfate USAN *antiadrenergic (beta-blocker)* [also: pamatolol]

Pamelor capsules ℞ *tricyclic antidepressant* [nortriptyline HCl] 10, 25, 50, 75 mg

Pamelor oral solution (discontinued 2010) ℞ *tricyclic antidepressant* [nortriptyline HCl] 10 mg/5 mL

pamidronate disodium USAN *bisphosphonate bone resorption inhibitor for the prevention and treatment of postmenopausal osteoporosis; also used for bone metastases of breast cancer* 30, 60, 90 mg/vial injection

pamidronic acid INN, BAN

Pamine; Pamine Forte tablets ℞ *anticholinergic; GI antispasmodic; adjunctive treatment for peptic ulcers* [methscopolamine bromide] 2.5 mg; 5 mg

Pamine FQ Kit tablets + capsules ℞ *anticholinergic; GI antispasmodic; natural intestinal bacteria; probiotic; adjunctive treatment for peptic ulcers* [methscopolamine bromide (tablets); **Flora-Q** (capsules)] 5 mg; 8 million CFU

Pamisyl *investigational (orphan) for ulcerative colitis* [aminosalicylic acid]

pamoate USAN, USP *combining name for radicals or groups* [also: embonate]

Pamprin, Nighttime powder OTC *antihistamine; sleep aid; analgesic; antipyretic* [diphenhydramine HCl; acetaminophen] 50•650 mg

Pamprin Maximum Pain Relief caplets OTC *analgesic; antipyretic; diuretic* [acetaminophen; magnesium salicylate; pamabrom] 250•250•25 mg

Pamprin Multi-Symptom caplets, tablets OTC *analgesic; antipyretic; diuretic; antihistamine; sleep aid* [acetaminophen; pamabrom; pyrilamine maleate] 500•25•15 mg

Pan C Ascorbate tablets (discontinued 2007) OTC *vitamin C supplement with multiple bioflavonoids* [vitamin C; citrus bioflavonoids; hesperidin] 200•100•100 mg

Pan C-500 tablets OTC *vitamin C supplement with multiple bioflavonoids* [vitamin C; citrus bioflavonoids; hesperidin] 500•100•100 mg

PAN-2400 capsules OTC *digestive enzymes* [pancrelipase (lipase; protease; amylase)] 9816•60 214•75 900 U

Panacet 5/500 tablets (discontinued 2009) ℞ *narcotic analgesic; antipyretic* [hydrocodone bitartrate; acetaminophen] 5•500 mg ⊞ boneset; poinsettia

panadiplon USAN, INN *anxiolytic*

Panadol tablets, caplets (discontinued 2008) OTC *analgesic; antipyretic* [acetaminophen] 500 mg

Panadol, Children's chewable tablets, oral liquid (discontinued 2008) OTC *analgesic; antipyretic* [acetaminophen] 80 mg; 160 mg/5 mL

Panadol, Infants' drops (discontinued 2008) OTC *analgesic; antipyretic* [acetaminophen] 100 mg/mL

Panadol, Junior caplets (discontinued 2008) OTC *analgesic; antipyretic* [acetaminophen] 160 mg

Panafil ointment, spray ℞ *proteolytic enzyme for débridement of necrotic tissue; vulnerary; wound deodorant* [papain; urea; chlorophyllin copper complex] 521 700 U/g•10%•0.5% ⊞ PenFill

Panafil SE spray ℞ *proteolytic enzyme for débridement of necrotic tissue; vulnerary; wound deodorant* [papain; urea; chlorophyllin copper complex] 405 900 U/g•10%•0.5%

Panafil White ointment ℞ *enzyme for wound débridement; vulnerary* [papain; urea] 10%•10%

Panalgesic cream (discontinued 2008) OTC *analgesic; mild anesthetic; antipruritic; counterirritant* [methyl salicylate; menthol] 35%•4%

Panalgesic Gold liniment OTC *analgesic; mild anesthetic; antipruritic; counterirritant; antiseptic* [methyl salicylate; camphor; menthol; alcohol 22%] 55%•3.1%•1.25%

Panasal 5/500 tablets (discontinued 2008) ℞ *narcotic analgesic; antipyretic* [hydrocodone bitartrate; aspirin] 5•500 mg ⊞ Banzel

Panasol-S tablets (discontinued 2008) ℞ *corticosteroid; anti-inflammatory; immunosuppressant* [prednisone] 1 mg

Panatuss DXP syrup ℞ *decongestant; antihistamine; antitussive* [phenylephrine HCl; dexbrompheniramine maleate; dextromethorphan hydrobromide] 10•2•15•20 mg/5 mL

Panax ginseng; P. shin-seng (**Korean ginseng**) *medicinal herb* [see: ginseng]

Panax horridum medicinal herb [see: devil's club]

Panax pseudoginseng (**Chikusetsu ginseng; Himalayan ginseng; Sanchi ginseng; Zhuzishen**) *medicinal herb* [see: ginseng]

Panax quinquefolia (**American ginseng**) *medicinal herb* [see: ginseng]

Panax spp. medicinal herb [see: ginseng]

Panax trifolius (**dwarf ginseng**) *medicinal herb* [see: ginseng]

Pancof-PD syrup (discontinued 2009) ℞ *narcotic antitussive; antihistamine; decongestant* [dihydrocodeine bitartrate; chlorpheniramine maleate; phenylephrine HCl] 3•2•7.5 mg/5 mL

pancopride USAN, INN *antiemetic; anxiolytic; peristaltic stimulant*

Pancrease MT 4; Pancrease MT 16; Pancrease MT 20 capsules containing enteric-coated microtablets ℞ *porcine-derived digestive enzymes* [pancrelipase (lipase; protease; amylase)]

4•12•12; 16•48•48; 20•44•56 thousand USP units

Pancrease MT 10 capsules containing enteric-coated microtablets (discontinued 2010) ℞ *porcine-derived digestive enzymes* [pancrelipase (lipase; protease; amylase)] 10•30•30 thousand USP units

pancreatin USP *porcine-derived digestive enzymes; a combination of lipase, protease, and amylase* [also see: amylase; lipase; protease]

Pancreaze delayed-release capsules ℞ *porcine-derived digestive enzymes* [pancrelipase (amylase; lipase; protease)] 17.5•4.2•10, 43.75•10.5•25, 61•21•37, 70•16.8•40 thousand USP units

Pancrecarb MS-4; Pancrecarb MS-8; Pancrecarb MS-16 delayed-release capsules containing enteric-coated microspheres ℞ *porcine-derived digestive enzymes* [pancrelipase (lipase; protease; amylase)] 4000•25 000•25 000 USP units; 8000•45 000•40 000 USP units; 16 000•52 000•52 000 USP units

pancrelipase USAN, USP *porcine-derived digestive enzymes; a combination of lipase, protease, and amylase* [also see: amylase; lipase; protease] 4.5•25•20, 5•17•27, 8•30•30, 16•48•48, 16•60•60 thousand USP units oral

pancuronium bromide USAN, INN *nondepolarizing neuromuscular blocking agent; muscle relaxant; adjunct to tracheal intubation for general anesthesia or mechanical ventilation* 1, 2 mg/mL injection

Pandel cream ℞ *corticosteroidal anti-inflammatory* [hydrocortisone probutate] 0.1%

Panenza injection *investigational (NDA filed) active immunizing agent for H1N1 influenza A (swine flu; Mexican pandemic flu)* [influenza virus vaccine, H1N1 (non-adjuvanted)] 15 mcg

Panfil G capsules, syrup (discontinued 2007) ℞ *antiasthmatic; bronchodilator; expectorant* [dyphylline; guaifenesin] 200•100 mg; 100•50 mg/5 mL

pangamic acid [now: dimethylglycine HCl]

Pangestyme CN-10 delayed-release capsules (discontinued 2009) ℞ *porcine-derived digestive enzymes* [pancrelipase (lipase; protease; amylase)] 10 000•37 500•33 200 USP units

Pangestyme CN-20 delayed-release capsules (discontinued 2009) ℞ *porcine-derived digestive enzymes* [pancrelipase (lipase; protease; amylase)] 20 000•75 000•66 400 USP units

Pangestyme EC delayed-release capsules (discontinued 2009) ℞ *porcine-derived digestive enzymes* [pancrelipase (lipase; protease; amylase)] 4500•25 000•20 000 USP units

Pangestyme MT16 delayed-release capsules (discontinued 2009) ℞ *porcine-derived digestive enzymes* [pancrelipase (lipase; protease; amylase)] 16 000•48 000•48 000 USP units

Pangestyme UL12 delayed-release capsules (discontinued 2009) ℞ *porcine-derived digestive enzymes* [pancrelipase (lipase; protease; amylase)] 12 000•39 000•39 000 USP units

Pangestyme UL18 delayed-release capsules (discontinued 2009) ℞ *porcine-derived digestive enzymes* [pancrelipase (lipase; protease; amylase)] 18 000•58 500•58 500 USP units

Pangestyme UL20 delayed-release capsules (discontinued 2009) ℞ *porcine-derived digestive enzymes* [pancrelipase (lipase; protease; amylase)] 20 000•65 000•65 000 USP units

Panglobulin NF powder for IV infusion (discontinued 2007) ℞ *passive immunizing agent for HIV and idiopathic thrombocytopenic purpura (ITP)* [immune globulin] 1, 3, 6, 12 g

Panhematin powder for IV injection ℞ *enzyme inhibitor for acute intermittent porphyria (AIP), porphyria variegata, and hereditary coproporphyria (orphan)* [hemin] 301 mg/vial

panidazole INN, BAN

Panitone-500 tablets (discontinued 2008) OTC *analgesic; antipyretic* [acetaminophen] 500 mg

panitumumab *monoclonal antibody IgG2 to human epidermal growth factor receptor (EGFR) for metastatic colorectal cancer*

Panixine DisperDose tablets for oral suspension ℞ *first-generation cephalosporin antibiotic* [cephalexin] 125, 250 mg

Panlor DC capsules (discontinued 2010) ℞ *narcotic antitussive; analgesic; antipyretic* [dihydrocodeine bitartrate; acetaminophen; caffeine] 16•356.4•30 mg

Panlor SS tablets (discontinued 2011) ℞ *narcotic analgesic; antipyretic* [dihydrocodeine bitartrate; acetaminophen; caffeine] 32•712.8•60 mg

PanMist-DM extended-release caplets, syrup (discontinued 2007) ℞ *antitussive; decongestant; expectorant* [dextromethorphan hydrobromide; pseudoephedrine HCl; guaifenesin] 32•48•595 mg; 15•40•100 mg/5 mL

PanMist-JR extended-release caplets (discontinued 2007) ℞ *decongestant; expectorant* [pseudoephedrine HCl; guaifenesin] 48•595 mg

PanMist-LA extended-release caplets (discontinued 2007) ℞ *decongestant; expectorant* [pseudoephedrine HCl; guaifenesin] 85•795 mg

PanMist-S syrup (discontinued 2007) ℞ *decongestant; expectorant* [pseudoephedrine HCl; guaifenesin] 40•200 mg/5 mL

Pannaz sustained-release tablets (discontinued 2007) ℞ *decongestant; antihistamine; anticholinergic to dry mucosal secretions* [pseudoephedrine HCl; carbinoxamine maleate; methscopolamine bromide] 90•8•2.5 mg

Pannaz S syrup (discontinued 2007) ℞ *decongestant; antihistamine; anticholinergic to dry mucosal secretions* [pseudoephedrine HCl; carbinoxamine maleate; methscopolamine nitrate] 15•2•1.25 mg/5 mL

Panocaps; Panocaps MT 16; Panocaps MT 20 delayed-release capsules ℞ *porcine-derived digestive enzymes* [pancrelipase (lipase; protease; amylase)] 4500•25 000•20 000 USP units; 16 000•48 000•48 000 USP units; 20 000•44 000•56 000 USP units

Panokase tablets ℞ *porcine-derived digestive enzymes* [pancrelipase (lipase; protease; amylase)] 8000•30 000•30 000 USP units ⨂ Pain-X; Pin-X

panomifene INN

Panorex *investigational (orphan) antineoplastic adjunct for pancreatic cancer* [edrecolomab]

Panoxyl cleansing bar OTC *keratolytic for acne* [benzoyl peroxide] 5%, 10%

Panoxyl 5; Panoxyl 10 gel (discontinued 2010) ℞ *keratolytic and antiseptic for acne* [benzoyl peroxide; alcohol] 5%•12%; 10%•20%

Panoxyl AQ 2½; Panoxyl AQ 5; Panoxyl AQ 10 gel ℞ *keratolytic for acne* [benzoyl peroxide] 2.5%; 5%; 10%

Panretin capsules *investigational (Phase III, orphan) treatment for acute promyelocytic leukemia (APL); investigational (orphan) to prevent retinal detachment due to proliferative vitreoretinopathy* [alitretinoin]

Panretin gel ℞ *retinoid for cutaneous lesions of AIDS-related Kaposi sarcoma (orphan)* [alitretinoin] 0.1%

Panscol lotion, ointment OTC *keratolytic* [salicylic acid] 3%

pansy (Viola tricolor) plant *medicinal herb used as an anodyne, demulcent, diaphoretic, diuretic, expectorant, laxative, and vulnerary*

pantenicate INN

panthenol USAN, USP, INN *B complex vitamin*

D-panthenol [see: dexpanthenol]

Panthoderm cream OTC *antipruritic; vulnerary; emollient* [dexpanthenol] 2%

pantoprazole USAN, INN, BAN *proton pump inhibitor for erosive esophagitis* associated with gastroesophageal reflux disease (GERD)

pantoprazole sodium USAN *proton pump inhibitor for erosive esophagitis associated with gastroesophageal reflux disease (GERD) and Zollinger-Ellison syndrome* (base=89%) 20, 40 mg oral

pantothenic acid (vitamin B₅) BAN *water-soluble vitamin; coenzyme A precursor* [also: calcium pantothenate] 92, 200, 500 mg oral

DL-pantothenic acid [see: calcium pantothenate, racemic]

pantothenol [see: dexpanthenol]

pantothenyl alcohol [see: panthenol]

D-pantothenyl alcohol [see: dexpanthenol]

panuramine INN, BAN

Panzem *investigational (orphan) for multiple myeloma* [2-methoxyestradiol]

Panzem NCD *investigational (orphan) for ovarian cancer* [2-methoxyestradiol]

papain USP *topical proteolytic enzyme for debridement of necrotic tissue*

papain & trypsin & chymotrypsin *investigational (orphan) enzyme combination adjunct to chemotherapy for multiple myeloma*

papain & urea & chlorophyllin *proteolytic enzyme for debridement of necrotic tissue; vulnerary; wound deodorant* 521 700 U/g•10%•0.5% topical

papaverine BAN *peripheral vasodilator; smooth muscle relaxant* [also: papaverine HCl]

papaverine HCl USP *peripheral vasodilator; smooth muscle relaxant for cerebral, myocardial, and peripheral ischemias; investigational (orphan) topical treatment for sexual dysfunction due to spinal cord injury* [also: papaverine] 150 mg oral; 30 mg/mL

papaveroline INN, BAN

papaya (Carica papaya) leaves, fruit, juice, and seeds *medicinal herb for aiding digestion, gas, insect bites, and intestinal worms*

Paplex Ultra topical solution ℞ *keratolytic* [salicylic acid in flexible collodion] 26%

papoose root *medicinal herb* [see: blue cohosh]

Papryll topical foam ℞ *proteolytic enzyme for débridement of necrotic tissue; vulnerary; wound deodorant* [papain; urea; chlorophyllin copper complex] 520 000 U•100 mg•5 mg per g

Pap-Urea ointment (discontinued 2008) ℞ *proteolytic enzyme for débridement of necrotic tissue; vulnerary* [papain; urea] 830 000 IU/g•10%

Par Glycerol elixir ℞ *expectorant* [iodinated glycerol] 60 mg/5 mL

para-aminobenzoate (PAB) [see: aminobenzoic acid]

Para-Aminobenzoic Acid tablets, powder OTC *water-soluble vitamin; "possibly effective" for scleroderma and other skin diseases and Peyronie disease* [aminobenzoic acid] 100, 500 mg; 120 g

para-aminobenzoic acid (PABA) [now: aminobenzoic acid]

para-aminohippurate (PAH) [see: aminohippuric acid]

para-aminohippurate sodium [see: aminohippurate sodium]

para-aminohippuric acid (PAHA) [see: aminohippuric acid]

para-aminosalicylate (PAS) [see: aminosalicylic acid]

para-aminosalicylic acid (PASA) [see: aminosalicylic acid]

Parabolan *brand name for trenbolone hexahydrobenzylcarbonate, a European veterinary anabolic steroid abused as a street drug*

parabromdylamine maleate [see: brompheniramine maleate]

Paracaine eye drops ℞ *topical anesthetic* [proparacaine HCl] 0.5% ② procaine; pyrrocaine

paracetaldehyde [see: paraldehyde]

paracetamol INN, BAN *analgesic; antipyretic* [also: acetaminophen]

parachlorometaxylenol (PCMX) *topical antiseptic; broad-spectrum antibacterial*

parachlorophenol (PCP) USP *topical antibacterial*

parachlorophenol, camphorated USP *topical dental anti-infective*

paracodin [see: dihydrocodeine]

paraffin NF *stiffening agent* ⊘ Preven; Privine

paraffin, liquid [see: mineral oil]

paraffin, synthetic NF *stiffening agent*

Paraflex caplets ℞ *skeletal muscle relaxant* [chlorzoxazone] 250 mg

paraflutizide INN

Parafon Forte DSC caplets ℞ *skeletal muscle relaxant* [chlorzoxazone] 500 mg ⊘ Profen Forte

paraformaldehyde USP

Paraguay tea *medicinal herb* [see: yerba maté]

parahydrecin [now: isomerol]

Paral oral liquid, rectal liquid (discontinued 2008) ℞ *sedative; hypnotic* [paraldehyde] ⊘ perilla; Prelu; Prolia

paraldehyde USP *hypnotic; sedative; anticonvulsant* 1 g/mL oral or rectal

paramethadione USP, INN, BAN *anticonvulsant*

paramethasone INN *corticosteroid; anti-inflammatory* [also: paramethasone acetate] ⊘ perimetazine; promethazine

paramethasone acetate USAN, USP *corticosteroid; anti-inflammatory* [also: paramethasone]

para-nitrosulfathiazole NF [also: nitrosulfathiazole]

paranyline HCl USAN *anti-inflammatory* [also: renytoline]

parapenzolate bromide USAN, INN *anticholinergic*

Paraplatin injection (discontinued 2007) ℞ *alkylating antineoplastic for ovarian and other cancers* [carboplatin] 10 mg/mL

Paraplatin powder for IV injection ℞ *alkylating antineoplastic for ovarian and other cancers* [carboplatin] 50, 150, 450 mg

parapropamol INN

pararosaniline embonate INN *antischistosomal* [also: pararosaniline pamoate]

pararosaniline pamoate USAN *antischistosomal* [also: pararosaniline embonate]

parasympathomimetics *a class of agents that produce effects similar to those of the parasympathetic nervous system* [also called: cholinergic agonists]

parathesin [see: benzocaine]

parathiazine INN

parathyroid USP *hormone*

parathyroid hormone (1-34), biosynthetic human [see: teriparatide]

paraxazone INN

parbendazole USAN, INN *anthelmintic* ⊘ propenidazole

parconazole INN *antifungal* [also: parconazole HCl] ⊘ pirquinozol

parconazole HCl USAN *antifungal* [also: parconazole]

Parcopa RapiTabs (orally disintegrating tablets) ℞ *dopamine precursor for Parkinson disease; decarboxylase inhibitor (levodopa potentiator)* [levodopa; carbidopa] 100•10, 100•25, 250•25 mg

parecoxib USAN, INN *COX-2 inhibitor; anti-inflammatory; analgesic*

parecoxib sodium USAN *COX-2 inhibitor; anti-inflammatory; analgesic*

paregoric (PG) (a preparation of opium, anise oil, benzoic acid, camphor, alcohol, and glycerin) USP *antiperistaltic; narcotic analgesic; used in neonatal opioid withdrawal programs; sometimes abused as a street drug* 2 mg opium/5 mL oral

Paremyd eye drops ℞ *mydriatic; weak cycloplegic* [hydroxyamphetamine hydrobromide; tropicamide] 1%•0.25% ⊘ PerioMed; ProMod

parenabol [see: boldenone undecylenate]

Parepectolin concentrated oral liquid (discontinued 2008) OTC *GI adsorbent; antidiarrheal* [attapulgite] 600 mg/15 mL

Parvlex 551

pareptide INN *antiparkinsonian* [also: pareptide sulfate]

pareptide sulfate USAN *antiparkinsonian* [also: pareptide]

parethoxycaine INN

parethoxycaine HCl [see: parethoxycaine]

Par-F tablets (discontinued 2008) ℞ *vitamin/mineral/calcium/iron supplement* [multiple vitamins & minerals; calcium; iron; folic acid] ≛•250•60•1 mg

pargeverine INN

Pargluva tablets ℞ *antidiabetic to control blood glucose levels, lower triglycerides, and raise HDL* [muraglitazar] 5 mg

pargolol INN ⊘ pyrogallol

pargyline INN *antihypertensive* [also: pargyline HCl]

pargyline HCl USAN, USP *antihypertensive* [also: pargyline]

paricalcitol USAN *fat-soluble vitamin; synthetic vitamin D analogue for hyperparathyroidism secondary to chronic kidney disease (CKD)* 2, 5 mcg/mL injection

paridocaine INN ⊘ piridocaine

Parlodel SnapTabs (scored tablets), capsules ℞ *dopamine agonist for Parkinson disease; lactation preventative; treatment for acromegaly, infertility, and hypogonadism* [bromocriptine (as mesylate)] 2.5 mg; 5 mg

Par-Natal Plus 1 Improved tablets (discontinued 2008) ℞ *vitamin/calcium/iron supplement* [multiple vitamins; calcium; iron; folic acid] ≛•200•65•1 mg ⊘ Prenatal Plus

Parnate film-coated tablets ℞ *MAO inhibitor for major depression; also used for migraine prevention, social anxiety disorder (SAD), panic disorder, bipolar depression, and Alzheimer and Parkinson disease* [tranylcypromine sulfate] 10 mg ⊘ burnet

parodilol INN

parodyne [see: antipyrine]

paroleine [see: mineral oil]

paromomycin INN, BAN *aminoglycoside antibiotic; amebicide* [also: paromomycin sulfate]

Paromomycin investigational (orphan) *agent for visceral leishmaniasis* [aminosidine]

paromomycin sulfate USP *aminoglycoside antibiotic; amebicide for acute and chronic intestinal amebiasis; investigational (orphan) for cutaneous leishmaniasis* [also: paromomycin] 250 mg oral

paroxetine USAN, INN, BAN *selective serotonin reuptake inhibitor (SSRI) for depression, obsessive-compulsive disorder, and panic disorder*

paroxetine HCl *selective serotonin reuptake inhibitor (SSRI) for depression, obsessive-compulsive disorder, panic disorder, social anxiety disorder, generalized anxiety disorder, post-traumatic stress disorder, and premenstrual dysphoric disorder* 10, 12.5, 20, 25, 30, 37.5, 40 mg oral; 10 mg/5 mL oral

paroxetine mesylate *selective serotonin reuptake inhibitor (SSRI) for depression, obsessive-compulsive disorder, and panic disorder*

paroxyl [see: acetarsone]

paroxypropione INN

parpanit HCl [see: caramiphen HCl]

parsalmide INN

parsley (Petroselinum sativum) leaves and root *medicinal herb for amenorrhea, bladder infections, blood building and cleansing, body lice, colic, dysmenorrhea, flatulence, gallstones, inducing abortion, jaundice, nephritis, prostate disorder, and urinary retention*

parsley fern *medicinal herb* [see: tansy]

parsnip, cow; wooly parsnip *medicinal herb* [see: masterwort]

Parthenocissus quinquefolia *medicinal herb* [see: American ivy]

partricin USAN, INN *antifungal; antiprotozoal*

partridge berry *medicinal herb* [see: squaw vine; wintergreen]

parvaquone INN, BAN ⊘ porofocon

Parvlex tablets OTC *vitamin/mineral/iron supplement* [multiple B vitamins &

minerals; iron (as ferrous fumarate); vitamin C; folic acid] ≛•29•60•0.4 mg

parvovirus B19 vaccine, recombinant *investigational (orphan) prevention of transient aplastic anemia due to sickle cell disease*

PAS (para-aminosalicylate) [see: aminosalicylic acid]

PASA (para-aminosalicylic acid) [see: aminosalicylic acid]

Paser delayed-release granules for oral solution ℞ *treatment for multidrug-resistant tuberculosis (MDR-TB) (orphan)* [aminosalicylic acid] 4 g/pkt.

pasiniazid INN

pasque flower *(Anemone patens)* plant *medicinal herb used as a diaphoretic, diuretic, and rubefacient; not generally regarded as safe and effective due to toxicity*

passion flower *(Passiflora incarnata)* plant *medicinal herb for asthma, bronchitis, eye infections, fever, inflamed hemorrhoids, insomnia, menopause, nervousness, pain related to neurasthenia, and attention-deficit disorder, nervousness, and excitability in children*

Pastilles (dosage form) *troches*

Pataday Drop-Tainers (eye drops) ℞ *once-daily antihistamine and mast cell stabilizer for allergic conjunctivitis* [olopatadine HCl] 0.2%

Patanase nasal spray in a metered-dose pump ℞ *antihistamine and mast cell stabilizer for seasonal allergic rhinitis* [olopatadine (as HCl)] 0.6% (600 mcg/spray)

Patanol Drop-Tainers (eye drops) ℞ *antihistamine and mast cell stabilizer for allergic conjunctivitis* [olopatadine HCl] 0.1% ☒ Botanol

patience, garden *medicinal herb* [see: yellow dock]

patience dock *medicinal herb* [see: bistort]

pau d'arco *(Lapacho colorado; L. morado)* inner bark *medicinal herb for boils, blood cleansing, cancer, Candida albicans infections, chlorosis, diabetes,* *leukemia, skin wounds, syphilis, and pain*

Paullinia cupana; P. sorbilis *medicinal herb* [see: guarana]

paulomycin USAN, INN *antibacterial* ☒ peliomycin

Pausinystalia johimbe *medicinal herb* [see: yohimbe]

pauson *medicinal herb* [see: bloodroot]

Pavagen TD timed-release capsules ℞ *peripheral vasodilator; smooth muscle relaxant for cerebral, myocardial, and peripheral ischemias* [papaverine HCl] 150 mg

pawpaw *(Asimina triloba)* fruit *medicinal herb used as an antimicrobial and antineoplastic*

paxamate INN

Paxene *investigational (Phase III, orphan) antineoplastic for AIDS-related Kaposi sarcoma* [paclitaxel]

Paxil film-coated tablets, oral suspension ℞ *selective serotonin reuptake inhibitor (SSRI) for depression, obsessive-compulsive disorder, panic disorder, social anxiety disorder, generalized anxiety disorder, and post-traumatic stress disorder* [paroxetine HCl] 10, 20, 30, 40 mg; 10 mg/5 mL ☒ piquizil

Paxil CR enteric-coated controlled-release tablets ℞ *selective serotonin reuptake inhibitor (SSRI) for depression, panic disorder, premenstrual dysphoric disorder (PMDD), and social anxiety disorder (SAD)* [paroxetine HCl] 12.5, 25, 37.5 mg

pazelliptine INN

pazinaclone USAN *anxiolytic*

Pazo Hemorrhoid ointment OTC *temporary relief of hemorrhoidal symptoms; vasoconstrictor; antipruritic; counterirritant; astringent* [ephedrine sulfate; camphor; zinc oxide] 0.2%•2%•5%

Pazo Hemorrhoid suppositories OTC *temporary relief of hemorrhoidal symptoms; vasoconstrictor; astringent; emollient* [ephedrine sulfate; zinc oxide] 3.8•96.5 mg

pazopanib HCl *vascular endothelial growth factor (VEGF) inhibitor; anti-*

neoplastic for advanced renal cell carcinoma; investigational for thyroid cancer (base=92.3%)

pazoxide USAN, INN antihypertensive

PB·Hyos elixir ℞ GI/GU anticholinergic/antispasmodic; sedative [atropine sulfate; scopolamine hydrobromide; hyoscyamine hydrobromide; phenobarbital; alcohol 23%] 0.0194•0.0065•0.1037•16.2 mg/5 mL

PBM Allergy syrup ℞ antitussive; antihistamine; decongestant [dextromethorphan hydrobromide; brompheniramine maleate; pseudoephedrine HCl] 15•3•30 mg/5 mL

PC (paclitaxel, carboplatin) [with or without filgrastim hematopoietic] chemotherapy protocol for bladder, esophageal, cervical, and non–small cell lung cancer (NSCLC) [also: Carbo-Tax; CaT]

PC (paclitaxel, cisplatin) chemotherapy protocol for head, neck, and endometrial cancer [also: CT]

PC (phosphatidylcholine) [see: lecithin]

PC Tar shampoo OTC antiseborrheic; antipsoriatic; antipruritic; antibacterial [coal tar] 1%

PCE Dispertabs (delayed-release tablets) ℞ macrolide antibiotic [erythromycin] 333, 500 mg

PCE (polymer-coated erythromycin) [see: erythromycin]

PCM chewable tablets ℞ decongestant; antihistamine; anticholinergic to dry mucosal secretions [phenylephrine HCl; chlorpheniramine maleate; methscopolamine nitrate] 10•2•1.25 mg

PCM Allergy extended-release tablets (discontinued 2009) ℞ decongestant; antihistamine; anticholinergic to dry mucosal secretions [phenylephrine HCl; chlorpheniramine maleate; methscopolamine nitrate] 20•12•2.5 mg

PCMX (parachlorometaxylenol) [q.v.]

PCOs (procyanidolic oligomers) [q.v.]

PCP (parachlorophenol) [q.v.]

PCP (phenylcyclohexyl piperidine) a powerful veterinary analgesic/anesthetic; often abused as a hallucinogenic street drug [medically known as phencyclidine HCl]

PCV (pneumococcal vaccine) [q.v.]

PCV (procarbazine, CCNU, vincristine) chemotherapy protocol for brain tumors

PD·COF oral drops (discontinued 2010) ℞ antitussive; antihistamine; decongestant; for children 6–24 months [dextromethorphan hydrobromide; chlorpheniramine maleate; phenylephrine HCl] 3•1•3.5 mg/mL

PD·COF syrup ℞ antitussive; antihistamine; decongestant [dextromethorphan hydrobromide; chlorpheniramine maleate; phenylephrine HCl] 15•4•12.5 mg/5 mL

PDE III (phosphodiesterase III) inhibitors a class of platelet aggregation inhibitors

PDGA (pteroyldiglutamic acid)

PD·Hist D syrup, oral drops (discontinued 2011) ℞ decongestant; antihistamine; drops for children 6–24 months [phenylephrine HCl; chlorpheniramine maleate] 12.5•4 mg/5 mL; 3.5•1 mg/mL ⑫ Bidhist

PDLA (phosphinicodilactic acid) [see: foscolic acid]

PE (paclitaxel, estramustine) chemotherapy protocol for prostate cancer

PE (phenylephrine) [q.v.]

PE (polyethylene) [q.v.]

PE·CPM·MSN 8·2·0.75 syrup ℞ decongestant; antihistamine; anticholinergic to dry mucosal secretions [phenylephrine HCl; chlorpheniramine maleate; methscopolamine nitrate] 8•2•0.75 mg/5 mL

PE·HCL·CPM·MSN 10·2·0.75 syrup ℞ decongestant; antihistamine; anticholinergic to dry mucosal secretions [phenylephrine HCl; chlorpheniramine maleate; methscopolamine nitrate] 10•2•0.75 mg/5 mL

PE Tann 20 mg/CP Tann 4 mg oral suspension ℞ *decongestant; antihistamine* [phenylephrine tannate; chlorpheniramine tannate] 20•4 mg/5 mL

pea, ground squirrel *medicinal herb* [see: twin leaf]

pea, turkey; wild turkey pea *medicinal herb* [see: turkey corn]

peach (Prunus persica) bark and leaves *medicinal herb for bladder disorders, chest congestion, chronic bronchitis, nausea, and water retention*

peanut oil NF *solvent*

PEB (Platinol, etoposide, bleomycin) *chemotherapy protocol for testicular cancer, germ call tumors, and adenocarcinoma* [also known as: BEP]

pecazine INN, BAN 🔲 Bicozene

pecazine acetate [see: pecazine]

pecilocin INN, BAN 🔲 bizelesin

pecocycline INN

pectin USP *suspending agent; protectant; GI adsorbent*

pectorals *a class of agents that relieve disorders of the respiratory tract, such as expectorants*

Pedia Relief Cough-Cold oral liquid ℞ *antitussive; antihistamine; decongestant; for children 6–11 years* [dextromethorphan hydrobromide; chlorpheniramine maleate; pseudoephedrine HCl] 5•1•15 mg/5 mL

Pedia Relief Decongestant Plus Cough oral drops (discontinued 2007) OTC *antitussive; decongestant; for children 2–3 years* [dextromethorphan hydrobromide; pseudoephedrine HCl] 5•15 mg/1.6 mL

PediaCare Children's Decongestant oral solution OTC *nasal decongestant* [phenylephrine HCl] 2.5 mg/5 mL

PediaCare Children's Long-Acting Cough freezer pops, oral solution OTC *antitussive for children 2–11 years* [dextromethorphan hydrobromide] 7.5 mg/pop; 7.5 mg/5 mL

PediaCare Children's NightRest Multi-Symptom Cold oral liquid OTC *decongestant; antihistamine; sleep aid; for children 6–11 years* [phenylephrine HCl; diphenhydramine HCl] 5•12.5 mg/5 mL

PediaCare Children's Nighttime Cough oral solution OTC *antihistamine; antitussive; sleep aid* [diphenhydramine HCl] 12.5 mg/5 mL

PediaCare Fever oral suspension, oral drops OTC *analgesic; antipyretic; nonsteroidal anti-inflammatory drug (NSAID) for minor aches and pains* [ibuprofen] 100 mg/5 mL; 40 mg/mL

PediaCare Infant Decongestant & Cough (PE) oral drops OTC *antitussive; decongestant; for children 2–5 years* [dextromethorphan hydrobromide; phenylephrine HCl] 5•2.5 mg/1.6 mL

PediaCare Infant Decongestant & Cough (PSE) oral drops OTC *antitussive; decongestant; for children 2–5 years* [dextromethorphan hydrobromide; pseudoephedrine HCl] 5•15 mg/1.6 mL

PediaCare Infant's Decongestant oral drops (discontinued 2009) OTC *nasal decongestant* [pseudoephedrine HCl] 7.5 mg/0.8 mL

PediaCare Infants' Long-Acting Cough oral drops OTC *antitussive for children 2–3 years* [dextromethorphan hydrobromide] 3.75 mg/0.8 mL

Pediaderm AF cream ℞ *antifungal* [nystatin] 100 000 U/g

Pediaderm TA cream ℞ *corticosteroidal anti-inflammatory* [triamcinolone acetonide] 0.1%

Pediaflor drops (discontinued 2010) ℞ *dental caries preventative* [sodium fluoride] 1.1 mg/mL

Pediahist DM oral drops ℞ *antitussive; antihistamine; decongestant; for children 1–18 months* [dextromethorphan hydrobromide; brompheniramine maleate; pseudoephedrine HCl] 4•1•15 mg/mL

Pediahist DM syrup ℞ *antitussive; decongestant; antihistamine; expectorant* [dextromethorphan hydrobromide; pseudoephedrine HCl; brompheniramine maleate; guaifenesin] 5•30•2•50/5 mL

Pedia-Lax chewable tablets OTC *saline laxative; antacid* [magnesium hydroxide] 400 mg

Pedialyte oral solution, freezer pops OTC *electrolyte replacement* [sodium, potassium, and chloride electrolytes]

Pediamist low-pressure nasal spray OTC *nasal moisturizer for children* [sodium chloride (saline solution)]

PediaPhyl D oral suspension ℞ *decongestant; antihistamine* [phenylephrine tannate; chlorpheniramine tannate] 10•8 mg/5 mL

Pediapred oral solution ℞ *corticosteroid; anti-inflammatory* [prednisolone (as sodium phosphate)] 5 mg/5 mL

Pediarix IM injection in vials and prefilled syringes ℞ *active immunizing agent for diphtheria, tetanus, pertussis, hepatitis B and D, and three types of poliovirus* [diphtheria & tetanus toxoids & acellular pertussis (DTaP) vaccine; hepatitis B virus vaccine; inactivated poliovirus vaccine Types 1, 2, and 3] 0.5 mL/dose

PediaSure; PediaSure with Fiber ready-to-use oral liquid OTC *total or supplementary infant feeding* 240 mL

PediaTan oral suspension (discontinued 2009) ℞ *antihistamine* [chlorpheniramine tannate] 8 mg/5 mL

PediaTan D oral suspension (discontinued 2009) ℞ *decongestant; antihistamine* [phenylephrine tannate; chlorpheniramine tannate] 10•8 mg/5 mL

Pediatex oral liquid ℞ *antihistamine for allergic rhinitis* [carbinoxamine maleate] 1.67 mg/5 mL

Pediatex 12 oral suspension ℞ *antihistamine for allergic rhinitis* [carbinoxamine tannate] 3.2 mg/5 mL

Pediatex-CT chewable tablets ℞ *decongestant; antihistamine; sleep aid* [phenylephrine HCl; diphenhydramine HCl] 5•12.5 mg/5 mL

Pediatric Cough & Cold Medicine oral liquid OTC *antitussive; antihistamine; decongestant; for children 6–11 years* [dextromethorphan hydrobromide; chlorpheniramine maleate; pseudoephedrine HCl] 10•2•30 mg/10 mL

Pediatric Decongestant and Cough oral drops (discontinued 2008) OTC *antitussive; decongestant; for children 2–5 years* [dextromethorphan hydrobromide; phenylephrine HCl] 2.5•7.5 mg/0.8 mL

Pediatric Electrolyte oral solution OTC *electrolyte replacement* [dextrose; multiple electrolytes] 1 L

pediatric VAC *chemotherapy protocol for pediatric sarcomas* [see: VAC pediatric]

Pediazole oral suspension (discontinued 2009) ℞ *antibiotic* [erythromycin ethylsuccinate; sulfisoxazole acetyl] 200•600 mg/5 mL

Pedi-Boro Soak Paks powder packets (discontinued 2010) OTC *astringent wet dressing (modified Burow solution)* [aluminum sulfate; calcium acetate]

pediculicides *a class of agents effective against head and pubic lice*

Pedi-Dri powder ℞ *antifungal* [nystatin] 100 000 U/g

Pediotic ear drop suspension (discontinued 2009) ℞ *corticosteroidal anti-inflammatory; antibiotic* [hydrocortisone; neomycin sulfate; polymyxin B sulfate] 1%•5 mg•10 000 U per mL

Pediox pediatric chewable tablets (discontinued 2007) ℞ *decongestant; antihistamine* [pseudoephedrine HCl; chlorpheniramine maleate] 15•2 mg

Pediox-S oral suspension ℞ *antihistamine* [chlorpheniramine maleate] 4 mg/5 mL

Pedi-Pro foot powder OTC *antifungal; anhidrotic* [benzalkonium chloride] 1%

Pedi-Vit-A Creme OTC *moisturizer; emollient* [vitamin A] 100 000 U/30 g

Pedotic otic suspension ℞ *corticosteroidal anti-inflammatory; antibiotic* [hydrocortisone; neomycin sulfate;

polymyxin B sulfate] 1%•5 mg•
10 000 U per mL

PedTE-Pak-4 IV injection (discontinued 2011) ℞ *intravenous nutritional therapy* [multiple trace elements (metals)]

Pedtrace-4 IV injection (discontinued 2011) ℞ *intravenous nutritional therapy* [multiple trace elements (metals)]

PedvaxHIB IM injection ℞ *vaccine for H. influenzae type b (HIB) infections in children 2–71 months* [*Haemophilus influenzae* b conjugate vaccine; *Neisseria meningitidis* OMPC] 7.5•125 mcg/dose

pefloxacin USAN, INN, BAN *antibacterial*

pefloxacin mesylate USAN *antibacterial*

PEG (polyethylene glycol) [q.v.]

pegacaristim USAN *megakaryocyte stimulating factor for thrombocytopenia*

PEG-ADA (polyethylene glycol–adenosine deaminase) [see: pegademase bovine]

pegademase INN *adenosine deaminase (ADA) replacement* [also: pegademase bovine]

pegademase bovine USAN *adenosine deaminase (ADA) replacement for severe combined immunodeficiency disease (orphan)* [also: pegademase]

PEG-adenosine deaminase (PEG-ADA) [see: pegademase bovine]

Peganone tablets ℞ *hydantoin anticonvulsant* [ethotoin] 250 mg

pegaptanib sodium *pegylated VEGF (vascular endothelial growth factor) antagonist for neovascular (wet) age-related macular degeneration (AMD); also used for diabetic macular edema*

pegaspargase (PEG-L-asparaginase) USAN, INN *antineoplastic for acute lymphocytic leukemia (orphan) and acute lymphoblastic leukemia*

Pegasys subcu injection, prefilled syringes ℞ *immunomodulator for chronic hepatitis B virus (HBV) and chronic hepatitis C virus (HCV) infection; investigational (orphan) for renal cell carcinoma and chronic myelogen-* *ous leukemia* [peginterferon alfa-2a] 180 mcg/mL

PEG-ES (polyethylene glycol–electrolyte solution) [q.v.]

pegfilgrastim *recombinant human granulocyte colony-stimulating factor (G-CSF) in polyethylene glycol (PEG); hematopoietic stimulant for severe chronic neutropenia (SCN) following cancer chemotherapy*

PE/GG 7.5/100 oral liquid ℞ *decongestant; expectorant* [phenylephrine HCl; guaifenesin] 7.5•100 mg/5 mL

PEG-glucocerebrosidase *investigational (orphan) chronic enzyme replacement therapy for Gaucher disease*

peginesatide *investigational (NDA filed) synthetic peptide–based erythropoiesis-stimulating agent (ESA) to increase RBC production for anemia due to chronic renal failure*

peginterferon alfa-2a *immunomodulator for chronic hepatitis B virus (HBV) and chronic hepatitis C virus (HCV) infection; investigational (orphan) for renal cell carcinoma and chronic myelogenous leukemia*

peginterferon alfa-2b *immunomodulator for chronic hepatitis C and malignant melanoma; also used for chronic myelogenous leukemia and renal cell carcinoma*

PEG-interleukin-2 *investigational (orphan) for primary immunodeficiencies associated with T-cell defects*

PegIntron powder for subcu injection ℞ *immunomodulator for chronic hepatitis C; also used for chronic myelogenous leukemia and renal cell carcinoma* [peginterferon alfa-2b] 100, 160, 240, 300 mcg/mL

peglicol 5 oleate USAN *emulsifying agent*

pegloticase *recombinant uricase enzyme for hyperuricemia due to severe gout (orphan); investigational (Phase III, orphan) agent for cancer-related tumor lysis syndrome*

pegnartograstim USAN *immunostimulant adjunct to cancer chemotherapy*

pegorgotein USAN, INN *free-radical scavenger*

pegoterate USAN, INN *suspending agent*

pegoxol 7 stearate USAN *emulsifying agent*

PEG-SOD (polyethylene glycol–superoxide dismutase) [see: pegorgotein]

PEG-uricase (polyethylene glycol–urate oxidase) [see: pegloticase]

pegvisomant USAN *growth hormone receptor antagonist for acromegaly (orphan)*

pegylated [def.] *bound to polyethylene glycol (PEG), an inactive solvent used as a carrier for an active ingredient*

pegylated doxorubicin [see: doxorubicin HCl, liposome-encapsulated]

pegylated interferon alfa-2b *investigational (Phase III) treatment for malignant melanoma*

PE-Hist DM syrup ℞ *decongestant; antihistamine; antitussive* [phenylephrine HCl; chlorpheniramine maleate; dextromethorphan hydrobromide] 5•2•15 mg/5 mL

pelanserin INN *antihypertensive; vasodilator; serotonin adrenergic blocker* [also: pelanserin HCl]

pelanserin HCl USAN *antihypertensive; vasodilator; serotonin adrenergic blocker* [also: pelanserin]

peldesine USAN *purine nucleoside phosphorylase inhibitor for psoriasis; investigational (orphan) for cutaneous T-cell lymphoma*

PeleVerus Clear ointment OTC *antiseptic* [zinc acetate] 0.9%

peliomycin USAN, INN *antineoplastic* ② bleomycin

pellants *a class of agents that purify or cleanse the system, particularly the blood* [also called: depurants; depuratives]

pelretin USAN, INN *antikeratinizing agent*

pelrinone INN *cardiotonic* [also: pelrinone HCl]

pelrinone HCl USAN *cardiotonic* [also: pelrinone]

pemedolac USAN, INN *analgesic*

pemerid INN *antitussive* [also: pemerid nitrate]

pemerid nitrate USAN *antitussive* [also: pemerid]

pemetrexed disodium USAN *folic acid antagonist; inhibitor of thymidylate synthase, dihydrofolate reductase, and glycinamide ribonucleotide formyl transferase; antineoplastic for malignant pleural mesothelioma (orphan) and non–small cell lung cancer (NSCLC)*

pemirolast INN *ophthalmic antiallergic; mast cell stabilizer* [also: pemirolast potassium]

pemirolast potassium USAN *ophthalmic mast cell stabilizer for allergic conjunctivitis* [also: pemirolast]

pemoline USAN, INN, BAN, JAN *CNS stimulant for attention-deficit/hyperactivity disorder (ADHD) and narcolepsy*

pempidine INN, BAN

penamecillin USAN, INN, BAN *antibacterial*

penbutolol INN, BAN *beta-blocker for hypertension* [also: penbutolol sulfate]

penbutolol sulfate USAN *beta-blocker for hypertension* [also: penbutolol]

penciclovir USAN, INN, BAN *topical antiviral for recurrent herpes labialis*

penciclovir sodium USAN *antiviral for herpes infections*

PENcream OTC *moisturizer/emollient*

pendecamaine INN, BAN

pendiomide [see: azamethonium bromide]

Penecare cream, lotion OTC *moisturizer; emollient* [lactic acid] ② Benicar

Penecort cream, solution ℞ *corticosteroidal anti-inflammatory* [hydrocortisone] 1% ② Bencort

"penems" *brief term for a class of broad-spectrum antibiotics that include doripenem, fropenem, ertapenem, imipenem, and meropenem* [properly called: carbapenems]

PenFill (trademarked delivery form) *insulin injector refill cartridge* ② Panafil

penfluridol USAN, INN *antipsychotic*

penflutizide INN

pengitoxin INN

penicillamine USAN, USP, INN *metal chelating agent; antirheumatic*

penicillin aluminum

penicillin benzathine phenoxymethyl [now: penicillin V benzathine]

penicillin calcium USP

penicillin G benzathine USP *natural penicillin antibiotic* [also: benzathine benzylpenicillin; benzathine penicillin; benzylpenicillin benzathine]

penicillin G hydrabamine *natural penicillin antibiotic*

penicillin G potassium USP *natural penicillin antibiotic* [also: benzylpenicillin potassium] 1, 2, 3, 5, 10, 20 million U/vial injection

penicillin G procaine USP *natural penicillin antibiotic* [also: procaine penicillin]

penicillin G redox [see: redox-penicillin G]

penicillin G sodium USP *natural penicillin antibiotic* [also: benzylpenicillin sodium] 5 000 000 U injection

penicillin hydrabamine phenoxymethyl [now: penicillin V hydrabamine]

penicillin N [see: adicillin]

penicillin O [see: almecillin]

penicillin O chloroprocaine

penicillin O potassium

penicillin O sodium

penicillin phenoxymethyl [now: penicillin V]

penicillin potassium G [see: penicillin G potassium]

penicillin potassium phenoxymethyl [now: penicillin V potassium]

penicillin V USAN, USP *natural penicillin antibiotic* [also: phenoxymethylpenicillin]

penicillin V benzathine USAN, USP *natural penicillin antibiotic*

penicillin V hydrabamine USAN, USP *natural penicillin antibiotic*

penicillin V potassium USAN, USP *natural penicillin antibiotic* 250, 500 mg oral

Penicillin VK tablets, powder for oral solution ℞ *natural penicillin antibiotic* [penicillin V potassium] 250, 500 mg; 125, 250 mg/5 mL

penicillin-152 potassium [see: phenethicillin potassium]

penicillinase INN, BAN

penicillinase-resistant penicillins *a subclass of penicillins (q.v.)*

penicillinphenyrazine [see: phenyracillin]

penicillins *a class of bactericidal antibiotics, divided into natural, penicillinase-resistant, aminopenicillin, and extended-spectrum penicillins, and effective against both gram-positive and gram-negative bacteria* [also called: "cillins"]

penidural [see: benzathine penicillin]

penimepicycline INN

penimocycline INN

PenInject (trademarked delivery form) *prefilled self-injection syringe*

penirolol INN

Pen-Kera cream OTC *moisturizer; emollient*

Penlac Nail Lacquer topical solution ℞ *antifungal for onychomycosis* [ciclopirox] 8%

penmesterol INN

Pennsaid topical liquid ℞ *anti-inflammatory for osteoarthritis of the hands and knees* [diclofenac sodium] 1.5% (16.05 mg/mL)

pennyroyal *(Hedeoma pulegeoides; Mentha pulegium)* plant *medicinal herb for childbirth pain, colds, colic, fever, gas, inducing abortion and menstruation, mouth sores, respiratory illnesses, and venomous bites; also used as an insect repellent; not generally regarded as safe and effective for ingestion due to toxicity* ⚲ Benuryl

penoctonium bromide INN

penprostene INN

penta tea *medicinal herb* [see: jiaogulan]

pentabamate USAN, INN *minor tranquilizer*

Pentacarinat IV or IM injection ℞ *antiprotozoal; treatment and prophylaxis of Pneumocystis pneumonia (PCP)* *(orphan)* [pentamidine isethionate] 300 mg

Pentacel powder for IM injection ℞ *vaccine for diphtheria, pertussis, tetanus (DPT), polio, and* H. influenzae *type* b (HIB) *infections* [diphtheria and tetanus toxoids and acellular pertussis, adsorbed; poliovirus, inactivated; *Haemophilus* b conjugate vaccine (DTaP-IPV/Hib)] 0.5 mL/dose

pentacosactride BAN [also: norleusactide]

pentacynium chloride INN

pentacyone chloride [see: pentacynium chloride]

pentaerithritol tetranicotinate [see: niceritrol]

pentaerithrityl tetranitrate INN *vasodilator* [also: pentaerythritol tetranitrate]

pentaerythritol tetranitrate (PETN) USP *coronary vasodilator; antianginal* [also: pentaerithrityl tetranitrate]

pentaerythritol trinitrate [see: pentrinitrol]

pentafilcon A USAN *hydrophilic contact lens material*

pentafluranol INN, BAN

pentagastrin USAN, INN, JAN *gastric secretion indicator*

pentagestrone INN

pentalamide INN, BAN

pentalyte USAN, USP, NF *electrolyte combination*

Pentam 300 IV or IM injection ℞ *antiprotozoal; treatment and prophylaxis of* Pneumocystis *pneumonia (PCP) (orphan)* [pentamidine isethionate] 300 mg

pentamethazene [see: azamethonium bromide]

pentamethonium bromide INN, BAN

pentamethylenetetrazol [see: pentylenetetrazol]

pentamidine INN, BAN

pentamidine isethionate *antiprotozoal; treatment and prophylaxis of* Pneumocystis *pneumonia (PCP) (orphan)* 300 mg injection

pentamin [see: azamethonium bromide]

pentamorphone USAN, INN *narcotic analgesic*

pentamoxane INN

pentamoxane HCl [see: pentamoxane]

pentamustine USAN *antineoplastic* [also: neptamustine]

pentanedial [see: glutaral]

pentanitrol [see: pentaerythritol tetranitrate]

pentaphonate

pentapiperide INN

pentapiperium methylsulfate USAN *anticholinergic* [also: pentapiperium metilsulfate]

pentapiperium metilsulfate INN *anticholinergic* [also: pentapiperium methylsulfate]

pentaquine INN [also: pentaquine phosphate] ② Pontocaine

pentaquine phosphate USP [also: pentaquine]

Pentasa controlled-release capsules ℞ *anti-inflammatory for active ulcerative colitis, proctosigmoiditis, and proctitis* [mesalamine (5-aminosalicylic acid)] 250, 500 mg

pentasodium colistinmethanesulfonate [see: colistimethate sodium]

Pentaspan *investigational (orphan) leukapheresis adjunct to improve leukocyte yield* [pentastarch]

PentaStaph *investigational multi-component active bacterin against methicillin-resistant* S. aureus *(MRSA)* [*Staphylococcus aureus* vaccine, pentavalent]

pentastarch USAN, BAN *red cell sedimenting agent; investigational (orphan) leukapheresis adjunct to improve leukocyte yield*

pentavalent gas gangrene antitoxin

pentazocine USAN, USP, INN, BAN *narcotic agonist-antagonist analgesic; also abused as a street drug*

pentazocine HCl USAN, USP *narcotic agonist-antagonist analgesic; also abused as a street drug*

pentazocine HCl & acetaminophen *narcotic agonist-antagonist analgesic; antipyretic* 25•650 mg oral

pentazocine lactate USAN, USP *narcotic agonist-antagonist analgesic for moderate to severe pain; adjunct to surgical anesthesia; also abused as a street drug*

pentazocine & naloxone HCl *narcotic agonist-antagonist analgesic; also abused as a street drug* 50•0.5 mg oral

pentetate calcium trisodium (Ca-DTPA) USAN *chelating agent for plutonium, americium, and curium; approved to treat contamination from radioactive materials (e.g., radiation sickness from "dirty bombs") (orphan)* [also: calcium trisodium pentetate] 200 mg/mL (1 g/dose) injection

pentetate calcium trisodium Yb 169 USAN *radioactive agent*

pentetate indium disodium In 111 USAN *radiodiagnostic imaging agent for radionuclide cisternography*

pentetate trisodium [see: pentetate calcium trisodium; pentetate zinc trisodium]

pentetate zinc trisodium (Zn-DTPA) *chelating agent for plutonium, americium, and curium; approved to treat contamination from radioactive materials (e.g., radiation sickness from "dirty bombs") (orphan)* 200 mg/mL (1 g/dose) injection

pentethylcyclanone [see: cyclexanone]

pentetic acid USAN, BAN *diagnostic aid; chelating agent for radioactive plutonium, americium, or curium ingestion (orphan)*

pentetrazol INN [also: pentylenetetrazol]

pentetreotide [see: indium In 111 pentetreotide]

penthanil diethylenetriamine penta-acetic acid (DTPA) [see: pentetic acid]

penthienate bromide NF

penthrichloral INN, BAN

pentiapine INN *antipsychotic* [also: pentiapine maleate]

pentiapine maleate USAN *antipsychotic* [also: pentiapine]

penticide [see: chlorophenothane]

pentifylline INN, BAN

pentigetide USAN, INN *antiallergic*

pentisomicin USAN, INN *anti-infective*

pentisomide INN

pentizidone INN *antibacterial* [also: pentizidone sodium]

pentizidone sodium USAN *antibacterial* [also: pentizidone]

pentobarbital USP, INN *sedative; hypnotic; also abused as a street drug* [also: pentobarbitone; pentobarbital calcium]

pentobarbital calcium JAN *sedative; hypnotic; also abused as a street drug* [also: pentobarbital; pentobarbitone]

pentobarbital sodium USP, JAN *sedative; hypnotic; also abused as a street drug* [also: pentobarbitone sodium] 50 mg/mL injection

pentobarbitone BAN *sedative; hypnotic; also abused as a street drug* [also: pentobarbital]

pentobarbitone sodium BAN *sedative; hypnotic; also abused as a street drug* [also: pentobarbital sodium]

Pentolair eye drops (discontinued 2011) ℞ *mydriatic; cycloplegic* [cyclopentolate HCl] 1%

pentolinium tartrate NF [also: pentolonium tartrate]

pentolonium tartrate INN [also: pentolinium tartrate]

pentolonum bitartrate [see: pentolinium tartrate]

pentomone USAN, INN *prostate growth inhibitor*

pentopril USAN, INN *antihypertensive; angiotensin-converting enzyme (ACE) inhibitor*

pentorex INN

pentosalen BAN

pentosan polysulfate sodium USAN, INN *urinary tract anti-inflammatory and analgesic for interstitial cystitis (orphan)* [also: pentosan polysulphate sodium]

pentosan polysulphate sodium BAN *urinary tract anti-inflammatory and analgesic* [also: pentosan polysulfate sodium]

Pentostam (available only from the Centers for Disease Control) (discontinued 2011) ℞ *investigational anti-infective for leishmaniasis* [sodium stibogluconate]

pentostatin USAN, INN *antibiotic antineoplastic for hairy cell leukemia (orphan); investigational (orphan) for chronic lymphocytic leukemia and cutaneous and peripheral T-cell lymphomas* 10 mg injection

Pentothal powder for IV injection ℞ *barbiturate general anesthetic* [thiopental sodium] 2%, 2.5% (20, 25 mg/mL)

pentoxifylline USAN, INN *peripheral vasodilator; hemorheologic agent* [also: oxpentifylline] 400 mg oral

pentoxiverine citrate [see: carbetapentane citrate]

pentoxyverine INN [also: carbetapentane citrate]

pentoxyverine citrate [see: carbetapentane citrate]

Pentrax shampoo OTC *antiseborrheic; antipsoriatic; antipruritic; antibacterial* [coal tar] 5%

pentrinitrol USAN, INN *coronary vasodilator*

***tert*-pentyl alcohol** [see: amylene hydrate]

6-pentyl-*m*-cresol [see: amylmetacresol]

pentylenetetrazol NF [also: pentetrazol]

pentymal [see: amobarbital]

Pen-Vee K tablets, powder for oral solution (discontinued 2002) ℞ *natural penicillin antibiotic* [penicillin V potassium] 250, 500 mg; 125, 250 mg/5 mL

peony (*Paeonia officinalis*) root (other parts are poisonous) *medicinal herb used as an antispasmodic, diuretic, and sedative*

Pepcid film-coated tablets, powder for oral suspension ℞ *histamine H_2 antagonist for gastric and duodenal ulcers, gastroesophageal reflux disease (GERD), and gastric hypersecretory conditions* [famotidine] 20, 40 mg; 40 mg/5 mL

Pepcid IV injection, IV infusion (discontinued 2008) ℞ *histamine H_2 antagonist for gastric and duodenal ulcers, gastroesophageal reflux disease (GERD), and gastric hypersecretory conditions* [famotidine] 10 mg/mL; 20 mg/50 mL

Pepcid AC ("acid controller") tablets, chewable tablets, gelcaps OTC *histamine H_2 antagonist for acid indigestion and heartburn* [famotidine] 10, 20 mg; 10 mg; 10 mg

Pepcid AC EZ Chews chewable tablets OTC *histamine H_2 antagonist for acid indigestion and heartburn* [famotidine] 20 mg

Pepcid Complete chewable tablets OTC *combination antacid and histamine H_2 antagonist for acid indigestion and heartburn* [calcium carbonate; magnesium hydroxide; famotidine] 800•165•10 mg

Pepcid RPD orally disintegrating tablets ℞ *histamine H_2 antagonist for gastric and duodenal ulcers, gastroesophageal reflux disease (GERD), and gastric hypersecretory conditions* [famotidine] 20, 40 mg

pepleomycin [see: peplomycin sulfate]

peplomycin INN *antineoplastic* [also: peplomycin sulfate]

peplomycin sulfate USAN *antineoplastic* [also: peplomycin]

pepper, African red; American red pepper; bird pepper; cayenne pepper; chili pepper; cockspur pepper; garden pepper; red pepper; Spanish pepper *medicinal herb* [see: cayenne]

pepper, Jamaica *medicinal herb* [see: allspice]

pepper, java; tailed pepper *medicinal herb* [see: cubeb]

pepper, water *medicinal herb* [see: knotweed]

pepper, wild *medicinal herb* [see: mezereon]

pepperidge bush *medicinal herb* [see: barberry]

peppermint NF *flavoring agent; perfume*

peppermint *(Mentha piperita)* leaves *medicinal herb for appetite stimulation, colds, colic, indigestion, fever, gas and heartburn, headache, shock, sore throat, and toothache*

peppermint oil NF *flavoring agent*

peppermint spirit USP *flavoring agent; perfume*

peppermint water NF *flavored vehicle*

pepsin *digestive aid*

pepstatin USAN, INN *pepsin enzyme inhibitor*

Peptamen ready-to-use oral liquid OTC *enteral nutritional therapy for GI impairment*

Peptic Relief chewable tablets, oral liquid OTC *antidiarrheal; antinauseant* [bismuth subsalicylate] 262 mg; 262 mg/15 mL

peptide YY (PYY) *endogenous peptides manufactured in the GI tract postprandially in proportion to the caloric content of a meal; subdivided into PYY 1-36 (PYY-I) and PYY 3-36 (PYY-II); exogenous administration of PYY-II is investigational for weight loss*

Peptinex; Peptinex DT oral liquid in **Tetra Brik** packs OTC *enteral nutritional treatment for patients with GI impairment* [whey protein formula] 8 oz./pack

Pepto Children's chewable tablets OTC *antacid; calcium supplement* [calcium (as carbonate)] 160 mg (400 mg)

Pepto Diarrhea Control oral solution OTC *antidiarrheal* [loperamide HCl] 1 mg/5 mL

Pepto-Bismol chewable tablets, caplets, oral liquid OTC *antidiarrheal; antinauseant* [bismuth subsalicylate] 262 mg; 262 mg; 262, 524 mg/15 mL

peraclopone INN

peradoxime INN

perafensine INN

peralopride INN

peramivir USAN *influenza neuraminidase inhibitor for the prophylaxis and treatment of influenza A and B virus infections*

Peranex HC anorectal cream ℞ *local anesthetic and corticosteroidal anti-inflammatory for hemorrhoids* [lidocaine HCl; hydrocortisone acetate] 2%•2%

peraquinsin INN

perastine INN ⊡ prazitone; Proseon

peratizole INN, BAN

perbufylline INN

Percocet tablets ℞ *narcotic analgesic; antipyretic* [oxycodone HCl; acetaminophen] 2.5•325, 5•325, 7.5•325, 7.5•500, 10•325, 10•650 mg ⊡ Pyrroxate

Percodan tablets ℞ *narcotic analgesic; antipyretic; also abused as a street drug* [oxycodone HCl; oxycodone terephthalate; aspirin] 4.5•0.38•325 mg

Percodan-Demi tablets (discontinued 2007) ℞ *narcotic analgesic; antipyretic; also abused as a street drug* [oxycodone HCl; oxycodone terephthalate; aspirin] 2.25•0.19•325 mg

Percogesic tablets OTC *antihistamine; sleep aid; analgesic; antipyretic* [diphenhydramine HCl; acetaminophen] 12.5•325 mg

Percogesic Extra Strength caplets OTC *antihistamine; sleep aid; analgesic; antipyretic* [diphenhydramine HCl; acetaminophen] 12.5•500 mg

Perdiem granules OTC *bulk laxative* [psyllium] 4.03 g/tsp. ⊡ Prodium

Perdiem Overnight Relief granules (discontinued 2009) OTC *bulk laxative; stimulant laxative* [psyllium; senna] 3.25•0.74 g/tsp.

perfilcon A USAN *hydrophilic contact lens material*

perflenapent USAN *ultrasound contrast medium*

perflexane USAN *ultrasound contrast medium*

perflisopent USAN *ultrasound contrast medium*

perfluamine INN, BAN

perflubron USAN, INN *oral MRI contrast medium; investigational (Phase III, orphan) treatment for acute respiratory distress syndrome (ARDS) in adults*

perflunafene INN, BAN

perflutren USAN *parenteral radiopaque contrast medium to enhance echocardiography*

perfomedil INN

Perforomist *solution for inhalation* ℞ *twice-daily bronchodilator for asthma, COPD, and emphysema* [formoterol fumarate] 20 mcg/2 mL dose

perfosfamide USAN *investigational (orphan) antineoplastic for the ex vivo treatment of autologous bone marrow in acute myelogenous/nonlymphocytic leukemia*

Pergamid *investigational (orphan) antineoplastic for the ex vivo treatment of autologous bone marrow in acute myelogenous/nonlymphocytic leukemia* [perfosfamide]

pergolide INN, BAN *dopamine agonist; antiparkinsonian; also used for restless legs syndrome (RLS)* [also: pergolide mesylate]

pergolide mesylate USAN *dopamine agonist; antiparkinsonian; also used for restless legs syndrome (RLS); investigational (orphan) for Tourette syndrome; removed from the market in 2007 due to safety concerns* [also: pergolide]

perhexiline INN *coronary vasodilator* [also: perhexiline maleate] ② pyroxylin

perhexiline maleate USAN *coronary vasodilator* [also: perhexiline]

periciazine INN *phenothiazine antipsychotic* [also: pericyazine]

PeriColace *tablets (discontinued 2010)* OTC *stimulant laxative; stool softener* [sennosides; docusate sodium] 8.6•50 mg

pericyazine BAN *phenothiazine antipsychotic* [also: periciazine]

Peridex *mouth rinse* ℞ *antimicrobial; gingivitis treatment; investigational (orphan) for oral mucositis in bone marrow transplant patients* [chlorhexidine gluconate; alcohol 11.6%] 0.12%

Peridin-C *tablets* OTC *vitamin C supplement with bioflavonoids* [ascorbic acid; hesperidin] 200•200 mg

perifosine *investigational (orphan) antineoplastic for neuroblastoma*

Periguard *ointment* OTC *moisturizer; emollient* ② Procardia

perilla (Perilla frutescens) *plant medicinal herb for asthma, inducing sweating, nausea, gastrointestinal spasms, and sunstroke* ② Paral; Prelu; Prolia

perimetazine INN

perindopril USAN, INN, BAN *angiotensin-converting enzyme (ACE) inhibitor for hypertension*

perindopril erbumine USAN *angiotensin-converting enzyme (ACE) inhibitor for hypertension and stable coronary artery disease (CAD)* 2, 4, 8 mg oral

perindoprilat INN, BAN

PerioChip *biodegradable polymer implant* ℞ *antimicrobial adjunct to scaling and root planing procedures in periodontitis* [chlorhexidine gluconate] 2.5 mg

PerioGard *mouth rinse* ℞ *antimicrobial; gingivitis treatment* [chlorhexidine gluconate; alcohol 11.6%] 0.12%

PerioMed *oral rinse* ℞ *dental caries preventative* [stannous fluoride] 0.64% ② Paremyd; ProMod

Periostat *tablets* ℞ *antibiotic for periodontal disease* [doxycycline hyclate] 20 mg ② Pro-Stat

peripheral blood mononuclear cells *investigational (orphan) treatment for pancreatic cancer*

peripheral vasodilators *a class of cardiovascular drugs that cause dilation of the blood vessels*

Periploca sylvestris *medicinal herb* [see: gymnema]

perisoxal INN

peritoneal dialysis solution with 1.1% amino acids *nutritional supplement for continuous ambulatory peritoneal dialysis patients (orphan)*

periwinkle (Catharanthus roseus) *plant medicinal herb for cancer, diabetes, diarrhea, insect stings, nervousness, ocular inflammation, and ulcers; not generally regarded as safe and effective for ingestion because of toxicity*

Perlane subcu injectable gel in prefilled syringes ℞ *transparent dermal filler for deep wrinkles and facial folds* [hyaluronic acid] 20 mg/mL ⊠ Prelone; proline

Perlane-L subcu injectable gel in pre-filled syringes ℞ *transparent dermal filler for deep wrinkles and facial folds; local anesthetic* [hyaluronic acid; lidocaine] 20 mg/mL•0.3%

perlapine USAN, INN *hypnotic*

Perles (dosage form) *soft gelatin capsule*

Perloxx tablets ℞ *narcotic analgesic; antipyretic* [oxycodone HCl; acetaminophen] 2.5•300, 5•300, 7.5•300, 10•300 mg ⊠ Pyrlex

permanganic acid, potassium salt [see: potassium permanganate]

Permapen Isoject (unit dose syringe) for deep IM injection ℞ *natural penicillin antibiotic* [penicillin G benzathine] 1 200 000 U ⊠ prampine

Permax tablets (removed from the market in 2007 due to safety concerns) ℞ *dopamine agonist for Parkinson disease; also used for restless legs syndrome (RLS); investigational (orphan) for Tourette syndrome* [pergolide mesylate] 0.05, 0.25, 1 mg

permethrin USAN, INN, BAN *topical ectoparasiticide for scabies and lice; also used for papulopustular rosacea* 1%, 5% topical

Perna canaliculus natural remedy [see: New Zealand green-lipped mussel]

Pernox Scrub; Pernox Lathering Lotion OTC *antiseptic and keratolytic cleanser for acne* [sulfur; salicylic acid]

peroxide, dibenzoyl [see: benzoyl peroxide]

peroxisome proliferator–activated receptor (PPAR) agonists *a class of agents that increase insulin receptor sensitivity in type 2 diabetes; PPAR-alpha blockers are associated with lower triglyceride and higher HDL levels; PPAR-gamma blockers are associated with lower blood glucose levels*

Peroxyl mouth rinse, oral gel OTC *cleansing of oral wounds* [hydrogen peroxide] 1.5%

perphenazine USP, INN *conventional (typical) phenothiazine antipsychotic for schizophrenia and psychotic disorders; treatment for nausea and vomiting* 2, 4, 8, 16 mg oral

Persantine sugar-coated tablets ℞ *platelet aggregation inhibitor to prevent postoperative thromboembolic complications of cardiac valve replacement* [dipyridamole] 25, 50, 75 mg

Persantine IV injection (discontinued 2010) ℞ *diagnostic aid for coronary artery function* [dipyridamole] 10 mg

Persea americana; P. gratissima medicinal herb [see: avocado]

Persian bark; Persian berries medicinal herb [see: buckthorn]

Persian walnut medicinal herb [see: English walnut]

persic oil NF *vehicle*

persilic acid INN

pertussis immune globulin USP *passive immunizing agent*

pertussis immune human globulin [now: pertussis immune globulin]

pertussis vaccine USP *active immunizing agent*

pertussis vaccine, acellular [see: diphtheria & tetanus toxoids & acellular pertussis (DTaP) vaccine, adsorbed]

pertussis vaccine, component (alternate name for acellular pertussis vaccine) [see: diphtheria & tetanus toxoids & acellular pertussis (DTaP) vaccine, adsorbed]

pertussis vaccine, whole-cell [see: diphtheria & tetanus toxoids & whole-cell pertussis (DTwP) vaccine, adsorbed]

pertussis vaccine adsorbed USP *active immunizing agent*

Peruvian balsam NF *topical protectant; rubefacient*

Peruvian balsam (Myroxylon balsamum; M. pereirae) oil *medicinal herb for edema, expelling worms, hemostasis, topical infections, and wound healing*

Peruvian bark; yellow Peruvian bark *medicinal herb* [see: quinine]

Peruvian ginseng *medicinal herb* [see: maca]

Petasites hybridus medicinal herb [see: butterbur]

pethidine INN, BAN *narcotic analgesic; also abused as a street drug* [also: meperidine HCl]

pethidine HCl [see: meperidine HCl]

PETN (pentaerythritol tetranitrate) [q.v.]

petrichloral INN

petrolatum USP *ointment base; emollient/protectant* [also: yellow petrolatum]

petrolatum, hydrophilic USP *absorbent ointment base; topical protectant*

petrolatum, liquid [see: mineral oil]

petrolatum, liquid emulsion [see: mineral oil emulsion]

petrolatum, white USP, JAN *oleaginous ointment base; topical protectant*

petrolatum gauze [see: gauze, petrolatum]

petroleum benzin [see: benzin, petroleum]

petroleum distillate inhalants *vapors from butane, toluene, acetone, benzene, gasoline, etc. which produce psychoactive effects, abused as street drugs* [see also: nitrous oxide; volatile nitrites]

petroleum jelly [see: petrolatum]

Petroselinum sativum medicinal herb [see: parsley]

Peumus boldus medicinal herb [see: boldo]

pexantel INN

Pexeva tablets ℞ *selective serotonin reuptake inhibitor (SSRI) for depression, obsessive-compulsive disorder, and panic disorder* [paroxetine mesylate] 10, 20, 30, 40 mg

pexiganan acetate USAN *broad-spectrum antibiotic*

PFA (phosphonoformic acid) [see: foscarnet sodium]

Pfaffia paniculata medicinal herb [see: suma]

Pfeiffer's Cold Sore lotion OTC *skin protectant; mild anesthetic; antipruritic; counterirritant; antiseptic* [gum benzoin; camphor; menthol; eucalyptol; alcohol 85%] 7% • ⓘ • ⓘ • ⓘ

Pfizerpen powder for injection ℞ *natural penicillin antibiotic* [penicillin G potassium] 5, 20 million U

PFL (Platinol, fluorouracil, leucovorin [rescue]) *chemotherapy protocol for head, neck, and gastric cancer*

PG (paregoric) [q.v.]

PG (prostaglandin) [q.v.]

PGA (pteroylglutamic acid) [see: folic acid]

PGE₁ (prostaglandin E₁) [now: alprostadil]

PGE₂ (prostaglandin E₂) [now: dinoprostone]

PGF₂α (prostaglandin F₂α) [see: dinoprost]

PGF₂α (prostaglandin F₂α) THAM [see: dinoprost tromethamine]

PGI₂ (prostaglandin I₂) [now: epoprostenol]

PGX (prostaglandin X) [now: epoprostenol]

PGxTest: Warfarin *genetic test for professional use* ℞ *measures levels of the VKORC1 and CYP2C9 genes to help determine the appropriate dosing regimen*

Phaenicia sericata natural treatment [see: maggots]

Phanatuss DM Cough syrup (discontinued 2007) OTC *antitussive; expectorant* [dextromethorphan hydrobromide; guaifenesin] 20 • 200 mg/10 mL

phanchinone [see: phanquinone; phanquone]

phanquinone INN [also: phanquone]

phanquone BAN [also: phanquinone] ⓘ phenacaine

pharmaceutical glaze [see: glaze, pharmaceutical]

Pharmaflur; Pharmaflur df; Pharmaflur 1.1 chewable tablets ℞ *dental caries preventative* [sodium fluoride] 2.2 mg; 2.2 mg; 1.1 mg

Pharmalgen subcu or IM injection ℞ *venom sensitivity testing (subcu); venom desensitization therapy (IM)* [extracts of honeybee, yellow jacket, yellow hornet, white-faced hornet, mixed vespid, and wasp venom]

Pharmia regina natural treatment [see: maggots]

Phazyme tablets, softgels, oral drops OTC *antiflatulent* [simethicone] 60 mg; 180 mg; 40 mg/0.6 mL

Phazyme 95 tablets OTC *antiflatulent* [simethicone] 95 mg

Phazyme Quick Dissolve chewable tablets OTC *antiflatulent* [simethicone] 125 mg

phebutazine [see: febuverine]

phebutyrazine [see: febuverine]

phemfilcon A USAN *hydrophilic contact lens material*

Phenabid extended-release tablets ℞ *decongestant; antihistamine* [phenylephrine HCl; chlorpheniramine maleate] 20•8 mg

Phenabid DM timed-release caplets ℞ *antitussive; antihistamine; decongestant* [dextromethorphan hydrobromide; chlorpheniramine maleate; phenylephrine HCl] 30•8•20 mg

phenacaine INN [also: phenacaine HCl] 🔲 phanquone

phenacaine HCl USP [also: phenacaine]

phenacemide USP, INN, BAN *anticonvulsant*

phenacetin USP, INN *(withdrawn from market)*

phenacon [see: fenaclon]

phenactropinium chloride INN, BAN

phenacyl 4-morpholineacetate [see: mobecarb]

N-phenacylhomatropinium chloride [see: phenactropinium chloride]

phenacylpivalate [see: pibecarb]

phenadoxone INN, BAN

Phenadoz suppositories ℞ *antihistamine; sedative; antiemetic; motion sickness relief* [promethazine HCl] 12.5, 25 mg

phenaglycodol INN

phenamazoline INN

phenamazoline HCl [see: phenamazoline]

phenampromide INN

Phenapap tablets (discontinued 2007) OTC *decongestant; analgesic; antipyretic* [pseudoephedrine HCl; acetaminophen] 30•325 mg

phenaphthazine *pH indicator*

phenarbutal [see: phetharbital]

phenarsone sulfoxylate INN

Phenaseptic throat spray OTC *antipruritic/counterirritant; mild local anesthetic* [phenol] 1.4%

PhenaVent dual-release capsules ℞ *decongestant; expectorant* [phenylephrine HCl (extended release); guaifenesin (immediate release)] 15•600 mg

PhenaVent D film-coated extended-release caplets ℞ *decongestant; expectorant* [phenylephrine HCl; guaifenesin] 40•1200 mg

PhenaVent LA dual-release capsules ℞ *decongestant; expectorant* [phenylephrine HCl (extended release); guaifenesin (immediate release)] 30•400 mg

PhenaVent LA film-coated caplets (discontinued 2007) ℞ *decongestant; expectorant* [phenylephrine HCl; guaifenesin] 30•600 mg

PhenaVent PED dual-release capsules (discontinued 2008) ℞ *decongestant; expectorant* [phenylephrine HCl (extended release); guaifenesin (immediate release)] 7.5•200 mg

phenazocine INN

phenazocine hydrobromide [see: phenazocine]

PhenazoForte Plus film-coated tablets ℞ *urinary analgesic; antispasmodic; sedative* [phenazopyridine HCl; hyoscyamine hydrobromide; butabarbital] 150•0.3•15 mg

phenazone INN, BAN *analgesic* [also: antipyrine]

phenazopyridine INN, BAN *urinary tract analgesic for relief of pain, burning, urgency, and frequency due to mucosal irritation from surgery, catheterization, endoscopic procedures, or trauma; adjunct to antibacterial agents for urinary tract infection (UTI)* [also: phenazopyridine HCl]

phenazopyridine HCl USAN, USP *urinary tract analgesic for relief of pain, burning, urgency, and frequency due to mucosal irritation from surgery, catheterization, endoscopic procedures, or trauma; adjunct to antibacterial agents for urinary tract infection (UTI)* [also: phenazopyridine] 100, 200 mg oral

Phenazopyridine Plus tablets ℞ *urinary analgesic; antispasmodic; sedative* [phenazopyridine HCl; hyoscyamine hydrobromide; butabarbital] 150•0.3•15 mg

phenbenicillin BAN [also: fenbenicillin]

phenbutazone sodium glycerate USAN *anti-inflammatory*

phenbutrazate BAN [also: fenbutrazate]

Phencarb GG syrup ℞ *antitussive; decongestant; expectorant* [carbetapentane citrate; phenylephrine HCl; guaifenesin] 20•10•100 mg/5 mL

phencarbamide USAN *anticholinergic* [also: fencarbamide]

phencyclidine INN *anesthetic* [also: phencyclidine HCl]

phencyclidine HCl USAN *anesthetic* [also: phencyclidine]

phendimetrazine INN *CNS stimulant; anorexiant* [also: phendimetrazine tartrate]

phendimetrazine tartrate USP *CNS stimulant; anorexiant* [also: phendimetrazine] 35, 105 mg oral

phenelzine INN, BAN *antidepressant; MAO inhibitor* [also: phenelzine sulfate]

phenelzine sulfate USP *MAO inhibitor for atypical, nonendogenous, or neurotic depression; also used for bulimia, post-traumatic stress disorder (PTSD), chronic migraine, and social anxiety disorder (SAD)* [also: phenelzine] 15 mg oral

phenemal [see: phenobarbital]

Phenerbel-S tablets (discontinued 2008) ℞ *GI/GU anticholinergic/antispasmodic; sedative; analgesic* [belladonna alkaloids; phenobarbital; ergotamine tartrate] 0.2•40•0.6 mg

Phenergan tablets, suppositories, injection ℞ *antihistamine; sedative; antiemetic; motion sickness relief* [promethazine HCl] 12.5, 25, 50 mg; 12.5, 25 mg; 25, 50 mg/mL

Phenergan VC syrup (discontinued 2007) ℞ *decongestant; antihistamine* [phenylephrine HCl; promethazine HCl; alcohol 7%] 5•6.25 mg/5 mL

pheneridine INN

phenethanol [see: phenylethyl alcohol]

phenethazine [see: fenethazine]

phenethicillin potassium USP [also: pheneticillin]

phenethyl alcohol BAN *antimicrobial agent* [also: phenylethyl alcohol]

N-phenethylanthranilic acid [see: enfenamic acid]

phenethylazocine bromide [see: phenazocine hydrobromide]

phenethylhydrazine sulfate [see: phenelzine sulfate]

pheneticillin INN [also: phenethicillin potassium]

pheneticillin potassium [see: phenethicillin potassium]

phenetsal [see: acetaminosalol]

pheneturide INN, BAN [also: acetylpheneturide]

Phenex-1 powder OTC *formula for infants with phenylketonuria*

Phenex-2 powder OTC *enteral nutritional therapy for phenylketonuria (PKU)*

Phenflu G tablets OTC *antitussive; decongestant; expectorant; analgesic; antipyretic* [dextromethorphan hydrobromide; phenylephrine HCl; guaifenesin; acetaminophen] 30•15•600•500 mg

phenformin INN, BAN *biguanide antidiabetic that decreases hepatic glucose production and increases cellular response to insulin* [also: phenformin HCl]

phenformin HCl USP *biguanide antidiabetic that decreases hepatic glucose production and increases cellular response to insulin (removed from the market by the FDA in 1977)* [also: phenformin]

phenglutarimide INN, BAN

phenicarbazide INN

phenidiemal [see: phetharbital]

phenindamine INN *nonselective piperidine antihistamine* [also: phenindamine tartrate]

phenindamine tartrate USAN *nonselective piperidine antihistamine for allergic rhinitis* [also: phenindamine]

phenindione USP, INN *anticoagulant*

pheniodol sodium INN [also: iodoalphionic acid]

pheniprazine INN, BAN

pheniprazine HCl [see: pheniprazine]

pheniramine INN [also: pheniramine maleate] ☒ fenharmane

pheniramine maleate USAN *antihistamine* [also: pheniramine]

pheniramine maleate & naphazoline HCl *topical ophthalmic antihistamine and decongestant* 0.3%•0.025% eye drops

phenisonone hydrobromide

phenmetraline HCl [see: phenmetrazine HCl]

phenmetrazine INN, BAN *anorexiant; CNS stimulant; also abused as a street drug* [also: phenmetrazine HCl]

phenmetrazine HCl USP *anorexiant; CNS stimulant; also abused as a street drug* [also: phenmetrazine]

phenobamate [see: febarbamate]

phenobarbital USP, INN, JAN *anticonvulsant; hypnotic; sedative; also abused as a street drug* [also: phenobarbitone] 15, 30, 60, 100 mg oral; 15, 20 mg/5 mL oral ☒ vinbarbital

phenobarbital & belladonna alkaloids *gastrointestinal anticholinergic/antispasmodic; sedative* 16.2•0.13 mg oral

phenobarbital sodium USP, INN, JAN *anticonvulsant; hypnotic; sedative; also abused as a street drug* 30, 60, 65, 130 mg/mL injection ☒ vinbarbital sodium

phenobarbitone BAN *anticonvulsant; hypnotic; sedative; also abused as a street drug* [also: phenobarbital] ☒ vinbarbitone

phenobutiodil INN

phenododecinium bromide [see: domiphen bromide]

phenol USP *topical antiseptic/antipruritic; local anesthetic; preservative* ☒ fennel; vanilla

phenol, liquefied USP *topical antipruritic*

phenol, sodium salt [see: phenolate sodium]

phenol red [see: phenolsulfonphthalein]

phenolate sodium USAN *disinfectant*

Phenolated Calamine lotion OTC *poison ivy treatment* [calamine; zinc oxide; phenol] 8%•8%•1%

phenolphthalein USP, INN *stimulant laxative* banned in all OTC laxatives in 1998

phenolphthalein, white [see: phenolphthalein]

phenolphthalein, yellow USP *stimulant laxative* banned in all OTC laxatives in 1998

phenolsulfonphthalein USP

phenolsulphonate sodium USP

phenomorphan INN, BAN

phenomycilline [see: penicillin V]

phenoperidine INN, BAN

phenopryldiasulfone sodium [see: solasulfone]

Phenoptin *investigational (orphan) treatment for mild to moderate phenylketonuria* [phenylalanine ammonia lyase (PAL)]

phenosulfophthalein [see: phenolsulfonphthalein]

phenothiazine NF, INN *antipsychotic* ☒ fenethazine

phenothiazines *a class of dopamine receptor antagonists with antipsychotic, hypotensive, antiemetic, antispasmodic, and antihistaminic activity*

phenothrin INN, BAN

phenoxazoline HCl [see: fenoxazoline HCl]

phenoxybenzamine INN *antihypertensive* [also: phenoxybenzamine HCl]

phenoxybenzamine HCl USP *antihypertensive; pheochromocytomic agent* [also: phenoxybenzamine]

phenoxymethylpenicillin INN *natural penicillin antibiotic* [also: penicillin V]

phenoxypropazine BAN [also: fenoxy-propazine]

phenoxypropylpenicillin [see: propicillin]

phenozolone [see: fenozolone]

phenprobamate INN, BAN

phenprocoumon USAN, USP, INN *anticoagulant*

phenprocumone [see: phenprocoumon]

phenpromethadrine [see: phenpromethamine]

phenpromethamine INN

phenpropamine citrate [see: alverine citrate]

phensuximide USP, INN, BAN *succinimide anticonvulsant*

phentermine USAN, INN *anorexiant; CNS stimulant; an adrenergic isomer of amphetamine*

phentermine HCl USP *anorexiant; CNS stimulant; an adrenergic isomer of amphetamine* 8, 15, 18.75, 30, 37.5 mg oral

phenthiazine [see: phenothiazine]

phentolamine INN, BAN *antihypertensive; pheochromocytomic agent* [also: phentolamine HCl]

phentolamine HCl USP *antihypertensive; pheochromocytomic agent* [also: phentolamine]

phentolamine mesilate INN, JAN *antiadrenergic; antihypertensive; pheochromocytomic agent* [also: phentolamine mesylate]

phentolamine mesylate USP *alpha-adrenergic blocker; antihypertensive for pheochromocytoma; reverses soft-tissue anesthesia following oral surgery* [also: phentolamine mesilate] 5 mg injection

phentolamine methanesulfonate [now: phentolamine mesylate]

Phentrol 2; Phentrol 4; Phentrol 5 capsules ℞ *anorexiant; CNS stimulant* [phentermine HCl] 30 mg ☒ fenoterol

phentydrone

Phenydex oral liquid (discontinued 2007) ℞ *antitussive; antihistamine; sleep aid; decongestant; expectorant*

[dextromethorphan hydrobromide; pyrilamine maleate; phenylephrine HCl; guaifenesin] 20•25•10•200 mg/5 mL

Phenydex Pediatric oral liquid (discontinued 2007) ℞ *antitussive; decongestant; expectorant; for children 2–12 years* [dextromethorphan hydrobromide; phenylephrine HCl; guaifenesin] 5•2.5•50 mg/5 mL

phenyl aminosalicylate USAN, BAN *antibacterial; tuberculostatic* [also: fenamisal]

Phenyl Chlor-Tan Pediatric oral suspension ℞ *decongestant; antihistamine* [phenylephrine tannate; chlorpheniramine tannate] 5•4.5 mg/5 mL

phenyl salicylate NF *analgesic; not generally regarded as safe and effective as an antidiarrheal*

phenylalanine (L-phenylalanine) USAN, USP, INN *essential amino acid; symbols: Phe, F*

phenylalanine ammonia lyase (PAL) *investigational (orphan) treatment for mild to moderate phenylketonuria*

phenylalanine mustard (PAM) [see: melphalan]

L-phenylalanine mustard (L-PAM) [see: melphalan]

Phenylase *investigational (orphan) for hyperphenylalaninemia* [phenylalanine ammonia lyase (PAL)]

phenylazo diamino pyridine HCl [see: phenazopyridine HCl]

phenylbenzyl atropine [see: xenytropium bromide]

phenylbutazone USP, INN *antirheumatic; anti-inflammatory; antipyretic; analgesic*

phenylbutylpiperadines *a class of dopamine receptor antagonists with conventional (typical) antipsychotic activity* [also called: butyrophenones]

phenylbutyrate sodium [see: sodium phenylbutyrate]

2-phenylbutyrylurea [see: phenetu-ride; acetylpheneturide]

phenylcarbinol [see: benzyl alcohol]

phenylcinchoninic acid [now: cinchophen]

α-phenyl-p-cresol carbamate [see: diphenan]

phenylcyclohexyl piperidine (PCP) [see: PCP; phencyclidine HCl]

2-phenylcyclopentylamine HCl [see: cypenamine HCl]

phenyldimazone [see: normethadone]

phenylephrine (PE) INN, BAN *nasal decongestant; ocular vasoconstrictor; vasopressor for hypotensive or cardiac shock* [also: phenylephrine HCl]

phenylephrine bitartrate *bronchodilator; vasoconstrictor*

Phenylephrine CM extended-release caplets ℞ *decongestant; antihistamine; anticholinergic to dry mucosal secretions* [phenylephrine HCl; chlorpheniramine maleate; methscopolamine nitrate] 40•8•2.5 mg

Phenylephrine Complex oral liquid ℞ *decongestant; antihistamine; antitussive* [phenylephrine HCl; brompheniramine maleate; dextromethorphan hydrobromide] 7.5•4•15 mg/5 mL

phenylephrine HCl USP *nasal decongestant; ocular/otic vasoconstrictor; vasopressor for hypotensive or cardiac shock; investigational (orphan) treatment for fecal incontinence due to ileal pouch anal anastomosis* [also: phenylephrine] 0.25%, 0.5%, 1% nose drops or spray; 2.5%, 10% eye drops; 1% injection

phenylephrine HCl & brompheniramine maleate *decongestant; antihistamine* 7.5•6, 15•12 mg oral

phenylephrine HCl & chlorpheniramine maleate *decongestant; antihistamine* 20•4 mg oral; 12.5•4 mg/5 mL oral; 3.5•1 mg/mL oral

phenylephrine HCl & codeine phosphate & promethazine HCl *decongestant; narcotic antitussive; antihistamine* 5•10•6.25 mg/5 mL oral

phenylephrine HCl & dihydrocodeine bitartrate & brompheniramine maleate *decongestant; narcotic analgesic and antitussive; antihistamine* 7.5•3•4• mg oral

phenylephrine HCl & guaifenesin *decongestant; expectorant* 15•600, 40•600, 25•900, 30•900, 30•1200 mg oral; 5•200 mg/5 mL oral

phenylephrine HCl & promethazine HCl *decongestant; antihistamine* 5•5, 5•6.25 mg/5 mL oral

phenylephrine tannate *nasal decongestant*

phenylephrine tannate & chlorpheniramine tannate & pyrilamine tannate *decongestant; antihistamine* 5•2•12.5 mg/5 mL oral

phenylephrine tannate & brompheniramine tannate *decongestant; antihistamine* 20•12 mg/5 mL oral

phenylephrine tannate & dexchlorpheniramine tannate & dextromethorphan tannate *decongestant; antihistamine; antitussive* 20•2•30 mg/5 mL oral

phenylephrine tannate & pyrilamine tannate & dextromethorphan tannate *decongestant; antihistamine; sleep aid; antitussive* 15.5•15.5•25 mg/5 mL oral

phenylethanol [see: phenylethyl alcohol]

phenylethyl alcohol USP *antimicrobial agent; preservative* [also: phenethyl alcohol]

phenylethylmalonylurea [see: phenobarbital]

Phenyl-Free oral liquid, powder for oral solution OTC *special diet for infants with phenylketonuria (PKU)*

Phenylgesic tablets (discontinued 2007) OTC *antihistamine; sleep aid; analgesic; antipyretic* [phenyltoloxamine citrate; acetaminophen] 30•325 mg

Phenylhistine DH oral liquid ℞ *narcotic antitussive; antihistamine; decongestant* [codeine phosphate; chlorpheniramine maleate; pseudoephedrine HCl] 10•2•30 mg/5 mL

phenylindanedione [see: phenindione]

phenylmercuric acetate NF *antimicrobial agent; preservative*

phenylmercuric borate INN

phenylmercuric chloride NF

phenylmercuric nitrate NF *antimicrobial agent; preservative; topical antiseptic*

phenylone [see: antipyrine]

phenylpropanolamine (PPA) INN, BAN *vasoconstrictor; nasal decongestant; nonprescription diet aid (banned in all OTC products in 2001)* [also: phenylpropanolamine HCl]

phenylpropanolamine HCl USP *vasoconstrictor; nasal decongestant; nonprescription diet aid* [also: phenylpropanolamine] PPA was banned in all OTC products in 2001

phenylpropanolamine polistirex USAN *adrenergic; vasoconstrictor (banned in all OTC products in 2001)*

1-phenylsemicarbazide [see: phenicarbazide]

Phenyl-T oral suspension (discontinued 2009) ℞ *nasal decongestant* [phenylephrine tannate] 7.5 mg/5 mL

phenylthilone [see: phenythilone]

phenyltoloxamine INN *antihistamine; sleep aid*

phenyltoloxamine citrate *antihistamine; sleep aid*

Phenyltoloxamine PE CPM oral liquid ℞ *antihistamine; sleep aid; decongestant* [phenyltoloxamine citrate; phenylephrine HCl; chlorpheniramine maleate] 7.5•5•2.5 mg/5 mL

phenyltriazines *a class of anticonvulsants*

phenyracillin INN

phenyramidol HCl USAN *analgesic; skeletal muscle relaxant* [also: fenyramidol]

Phenytek extended-release capsules ℞ *once-daily hydantoin anticonvulsant* [phenytoin sodium] 200, 300 mg

phenythilone INN ② fenethylline

phenytoin USAN, USP, INN, BAN *hydantoin anticonvulsant* 125 mg/5 mL oral ② Vantin

phenytoin redox [see: redox-phenytoin]

phenytoin sodium USP *hydantoin anticonvulsant* 30, 100, 200, 300 mg oral; 50 mg/mL injection

phetharbital INN

phezathion [see: fezatione]

Phicon cream OTC *anesthetic; emollient* [pramoxine HCl; vitamins A and E] 0.5%•7500 IU•2000 IU

Phicon F cream OTC *local anesthetic; antifungal* [pramoxine HCl; undecylenic acid] 0.05%•8%

Phillips' caplets OTC *antacid; magnesium supplement* [magnesium (as magnesium oxide)] 500 mg (829 mg) ② Folpace

Phillips' Chewable tablets OTC *antacid* [magnesium hydroxide] 311 mg

Phillips' Liqui-Gels OTC *laxative; stool softener* [docusate sodium] 100 mg

Phillips' Milk of Magnesia; Concentrated Phillips' Milk of Magnesia oral liquid OTC *antacid; saline laxative* [magnesium hydroxide] 400 mg/5 mL; 800 mg/5 mL

pHisoDerm; pHisoDerm for Baby topical liquid OTC *soap-free therapeutic skin cleanser*

pHisoDerm Cleansing Bar OTC *therapeutic skin cleanser*

pHisoHex topical liquid ℞ *bacteriostatic skin cleanser* [hexachlorophene] 3%

P-Hist syrup ℞ *antitussive; antihistamine; sleep aid; decongestant* [dextromethorphan hydrobromide; pyrilamine maleate; dexchlorpheniramine maleate; phenylephrine HCl] 5•5•1.25•5 mg/5 mL

P-Hist DM oral drops ℞ *antitussive; antihistamine; decongestant* [dextromethorphan hydrobromide; brompheniramine maleate; pseudoephedrine HCl] 5•1•12 mg/mL

Phlemex-PE; Phlemex Forte extended-release tablets ℞ *antitussive; decongestant; expectorant* [dextromethorphan hydrobromide; phenylephrine HCl; guaifenesin] 20•20•800 mg; 30•30•1200 mg

phloropropiophenone [see: flopropione]

pholcodine INN
pholedrine INN, BAN
pholescutol [see: folescutol]
Phoradendron flavescens; P. sero-tinum; P. tomentosum medicinal herb
[see: mistletoe]
PhosChol softgels, oral liquid concentrate OTC *natural lipotropic supplement* [phosphatidylcholine] 565, 900 mg; 3 g/5 mL
phoscolic acid [see: foscolic acid]
Phos-Flur oral rinse R *dental caries preventative* [acidulated phosphate fluoride] 0.44 mg/mL
PhosLo capsules, gelcaps R *calcium supplement; buffering agent for hyper-phosphatemia in end-stage renal disease (orphan)* [calcium (as acetate)] 169 mg (667 mg) ② Feosol; VazoI; VSL
PhosLo tablets (discontinued 2008) R *calcium supplement; buffering agent for hyperphosphatemia in end-stage renal disease (orphan)* [calcium (as acetate)] 169 mg ② Feosol; VazoI; VSL
Phoslyra oral solution R *calcium supplement; buffering agent for hyperphos-phatemia in end-stage renal disease (orphan)* [calcium (as acetate)] 169 mg/5 mL (667 mg/5 mL)
Phos-NaK powder for oral solution OTC *electrolyte supplement* [phosphorus; potassium; sodium] 250•280• 160 mg/pkt.
Phospha 250 Neutral film-coated caplets R *urinary acidifier; phosphorus supplement* [monobasic sodium phosphate; monobasic potassium phosphate; dibasic sodium phosphate] 130•155•852 mg (250 mg P)
Phosphasal tablets R *urinary antibiotic; antiseptic; analgesic; antispasmodic* [methenamine; sodium phosphate; phenyl salicylate; methylene blue; hyoscyamine sulfate] 81.6• 40.8•36.2•10.8•0.12 mg ② fosfosal
phosphate salt of tricyclic nucleoside [now: triciribine phosphate]
phosphatidylcholine (PC) [see: lecithin]

phosphatidylserine (PS) *natural agent to improve neural function, maintain brain cell membrane integrity, and protect the brain against age-related functional deterioration*
phosphinic acid [see: hypophosphorous acid]
2,2'-phosphinicodilactic acid (PDLA) [see: foscolic acid]
Phosphocol P 32 suspension for intra-cavitary instillation, interstitial injection (discontinued 2010) R *radiopharmaceutical antineoplastic* [chromic phosphate P 32] 10, 15 mCi
phosphocysteamine *investigational (orphan) for cystinosis*
phosphodiesterase III (PDE III) inhibitors *a class of platelet aggregation inhibitors*
Phospholine Iodide powder for eye drops R *antiglaucoma agent; irreversible cholinesterase inhibitor miotic* [echothiophate iodide] 0.125%
phosphonoformic acid (PFA) [see: foscarnet sodium]
phosphonomethoxypropyladenine (PMPA) [see: tenofovir]
phosphorated carbohydrate solution (hyperosmolar solution with phosphoric acid) *antiemetic for nausea associated with influenza, morning sickness, motion sickness, inhalation anesthesia, or food and drink indiscretions*
phosphoric acid NF *solvent; acidifying agent*
phosphoric acid, aluminum salt [see: aluminum phosphate gel]
phosphoric acid, calcium salt [see: calcium phosphate, dibasic]
phosphoric acid, chromium salt [see: chromic phosphate Cr 51 & P 32]
phosphoric acid, diammonium salt [see: ammonium phosphate]
phosphoric acid, dipotassium salt [see: potassium phosphate, dibasic]
phosphoric acid, disodium salt heptahydrate [see: sodium phosphate, dibasic]

phosphoric acid, disodium salt hydrate [see: sodium phosphate, dibasic]

phosphoric acid, magnesium salt [see: magnesium phosphate]

phosphoric acid, monopotassium salt [see: potassium phosphate, monobasic]

phosphoric acid, monosodium salt dihydrate [see: sodium phosphate, monobasic]

phosphoric acid, monosodium salt monohydrate [see: sodium phosphate, monobasic]

phosphorofluoridic acid, disodium salt [see: sodium monofluorophosphate]

phosphorothiolate antisense oligodeoxynucleotide, TGF(β)2-specific *investigational (orphan) for malignant glioma*

phosphorothiolate oligonucleotide *investigational (orphan) for amyotrophic lateral sclerosis (ALS)*

phosphorus *element (P); electrolyte; urinary acidifier*

Phospho-soda [see: Fleet Phospho-soda]

phosphothiamine [see: monophosphothiamine]

Photofrin PDT powder for IV injection ℞ *laser light–activated antineoplastic for photodynamic therapy (PDT) of esophageal (orphan) and non–small cell lung cancers (NSCLC); used for ablation of high-grade dysplasia in Barrett esophagus patients; investigational (orphan) for bladder cancer* [porfimer sodium] 75 mg

phoxim INN, BAN

Phrenilin tablets (discontinued 2011) ℞ *barbiturate sedative; analgesic; antipyretic* [butalbital; acetaminophen] 50•325 mg

Phrenilin Forte capsules ℞ *barbiturate sedative; analgesic; antipyretic* [butalbital; acetaminophen] 50•650 mg

Phrenilin with Caffeine and Codeine capsules ℞ *barbiturate sedative; narcotic antitussive; analgesic;* *antipyretic* [butalbital; codeine phosphate; acetaminophen; caffeine] 50•30•325•40 mg

phthalofyne USAN *veterinary anthelmintic* [also: ftalofyne]

phthalylsulfacetamide NF

phthalylsulfamethizole INN

phthalylsulfathiazole USP, INN

phylcardin [see: aminophylline]

phyllindon [see: aminophylline]

phylloquinone [see: phytonadione]

Phylorinol mouthwash/gargle OTC *oral antiseptic; antipruritic/counterirritant; mild local anesthetic* [phenol] 0.6%

Phylorinol topical liquid OTC *antipruritic/counterirritant; mild local anesthetic; antiseptic; astringent; oral deodorant* [phenol; boric acid; strong iodine solution; chlorophyllin copper complex] 0.6%•?•?•?

physic root *medicinal herb* [see: Culver root]

physiological irrigating solution *sterile irrigant for general washing and rinsing; not for injection*

Physiolyte topical liquid ℞ *sterile irrigant for general washing and rinsing* [physiological irrigating solution]

PhysioSol topical liquid ℞ *sterile irrigant* [physiological irrigating solution]

physostigmine USP, BAN *reversible cholinesterase inhibitor miotic for glaucoma*

physostigmine salicylate USP *cholinergic to reverse anticholinergic overdose; investigational (orphan) for Friedreich and other inherited ataxias; also used for delirium tremens and Alzheimer disease* 1 mg/mL injection

physostigmine sulfate USP *ophthalmic cholinergic for glaucoma; miotic*

phytate persodium USAN *pharmaceutic aid*

phytate sodium USAN *calcium chelating agent*

phytic acid [see: fytic acid]

Phytolacca americana; P. decandra; P. rigida *medicinal herb* [see: pokeweed]

phytomenadione (vitamin K$_1$) INN, BAN *fat-soluble vitamin; prothrombogenic* [also: phytonadione]

phytonadiol sodium diphosphate INN

phytonadione (vitamin K₁) USP, JAN *fat-soluble vitamin; prothrombogenic* [also: phytomenadione] 0.1 mg oral; 2 mg/mL injection

phytosterols *a class of natural, plant-based extracts that are used to lower cholesterol*

pibecarb INN

piberaline INN ⑨ piperylone

piboserod HCl USAN, BAN *selective serotonin 5-HT₄ receptor antagonist for irritable bowel syndrome*

pibrozelesin hydrobromide USAN *antineoplastic*

picafibrate INN

picartamide INN

Picea excelsa; P. mariana medicinal herb [see: spruce tree]

picenadol INN *analgesic* [also: picenadol HCl]

picenadol HCl USAN *analgesic* [also: picenadol]

picilorex INN

pick purse; pickpocket *medicinal herb* [see: shepherd's purse]

piclamilast USAN *phosphodiesterase type IV inhibitor for asthma*

piclonidine INN

piclopastine INN

picloxydine INN, BAN

picobenzide INN

picodralazine INN

picolamine INN

piconol INN

picoperine INN

picoplatin *investigational (Phase III) antineoplastic for small cell lung cancer*

picoprazole INN

picotrin INN *keratolytic* [also: picotrin diolamine]

picotrin diolamine USAN *keratolytic* [also: picotrin]

Picrasma excelsa medicinal herb [see: quassia]

picric acid [see: trinitrophenol]

picrotoxin NF

picumast INN, BAN

picumeterol INN, BAN *bronchodilator* [also: picumeterol fumarate]

picumeterol fumarate USAN *bronchodilator* [also: picumeterol]

pidolacetamol INN

pidolic acid INN

pifarnine USAN, INN *gastric antiulcerative*

pifenate INN, BAN

pifexole INN ⑨ pivoxil

piflutixol INN

pifoxime INN

pigeonberry *medicinal herb* [see: pokeweed]

piketoprofen INN

pildralazine INN

pilewort (Erechtites hieracifolia) *plant medicinal herb used as an astringent and emetic*

Pilocar eye drops (discontinued 2009) ℞ *antiglaucoma agent; direct-acting miotic* [pilocarpine HCl] 1%, 2%, 3%, 4%, 6%

pilocarpine USP, BAN *antiglaucoma agent; ophthalmic cholinergic*

pilocarpine HCl USP *ophthalmic cholinergic; antiglaucoma; miotic; treatment of xerostomia and keratoconjunctivitis sicca due to radiotherapy or Sjögren syndrome (orphan); also for dry mouth* 0.5%, 1%, 2%, 4%, 6%, 8% eye drops; 5, 7.5 mg oral

pilocarpine nitrate USP *ophthalmic cholinergic; antiglaucoma; miotic*

Pilopine HS ophthalmic gel ℞ *antiglaucoma agent; direct-acting miotic* [pilocarpine HCl] 4%

Piloptic-½; Piloptic-1; Piloptic-2; Piloptic-3; Piloptic-4; Piloptic-6 eye drops ℞ *antiglaucoma agent; direct-acting miotic* [pilocarpine HCl] 0.5%; 1%; 2%; 3%; 4%; 6%

Pilopto-Carpine eye drops ℞ *antiglaucoma agent; direct-acting miotic* [pilocarpine HCl] 4%

Pilostat eye drops ℞ *antiglaucoma agent; direct-acting miotic* [pilocarpine HCl] 0.5%, 1%, 2%, 3%, 4%, 6%

Pilpak (trademarked packaging form) *patient compliance package*

Pima syrup ℞ *expectorant* [potassium iodide] 325 mg/5 mL

pimagedine HCl USAN *advanced glycosylation inhibitor for type 1 diabetes*

Pimalev tablets ℞ *narcotic analgesic; antipyretic* [oxycodone HCl; acetaminophen] 2.5•300, 5•300, 7.5• 300, 10•300 mg

pimaricin JAN *ophthalmic antibacterial/ antifungal antibiotic* [also: natamycin]

pimavanserin *investigational (Phase III) treatment for Parkinson disease–related psychosis*

pimeclone INN

pimecrolimus USAN, INN *calcineurin inhibitor; immunomodulator for atopic dermatitis*

pimefylline INN ▨ bamifylline

pimelautide INN

Pimenta dioica; P. officinalis medicinal herb [see: allspice]

pimetacin INN

pimethixene INN

pimetine INN *antihyperlipoproteinemic* [also: pimetine HCl]

pimetine HCl USAN *antihyperlipoproteinemic* [also: pimetine]

pimetixene [see: pimethixene]

pimetremide INN

pimeverine [see: pimetremide]

piminodine INN [also: piminodine esylate]

piminodine esylate NF [also: piminodine]

piminodine ethanesulfonate [see: piminodine esylate]

pimobendan USAN, INN *cardiotonic*

pimonidazole INN, BAN

pimozide USAN, USP, INN, BAN, JAN *antispasmodic/antidyskinetic for Tourette syndrome*

pimpernel; small pimpernel *medicinal herb* [see: burnet]

pimpernel, blue *medicinal herb* [see: skullcap]

pimpernel, water *medicinal herb* [see: brooklime]

Pimpinella anisum medicinal herb [see: anise]

Pimpinella magna; P. saxifrage medicinal herb [see: burnet]

pinacidil USAN, INN *antihypertensive (approved in 1989, but not marketed by the manufacturer)*

pinadoline USAN, INN *analgesic* ▨ binedaline

pinafide INN

pinaverium bromide INN *GI antispasmodic*

pinazepam INN

pincainide INN

pindolol USAN, USP, INN, BAN *betablocker for hypertension; also used for fibromyalgia* 5, 10 mg oral

pine, Norway *medicinal herb* [see: spruce]

pine, prince's *medicinal herb* [see: pipsissewa]

pine bark extract *natural free radical scavenger for inflammatory collagen disease and peripheral vascular disease; contains 80%–85% procyanidolic oligomers (PCOs)*

pine needle oil NF

pine tar USP

pineapple (*Ananas comosus*) *fruit medicinal herb for constipation, jaundice, soft tissue inflammation, and topical wound debridement*

Pink Bismuth *oral liquid* OTC *antidiarrheal; antinauseant* [bismuth subsalicylate] 130, 262 mg/15 mL

pinolcaine INN

pinoxepin INN *antipsychotic* [also: pinoxepin HCl] ▨ benaxibine

pinoxepin HCl USAN *antipsychotic* [also: pinoxepin]

Pin-Rid *oral liquid (discontinued 2010)* OTC *anthelmintic for ascariasis (roundworm) and enterobiasis (pinworm)* [pyrantel (as pamoate)] 50 mg/mL

Pin-Rid *softgels* OTC *anthelmintic for ascariasis (roundworm) and enterobiasis (pinworm)* [pyrantel (as pamoate)] 62.5 mg

Pinus palustris natural remedy [see: turpentine]

Pinus strobus medicinal herb [see: white pine]

Pin-X *oral liquid, chewable tablets* OTC *anthelmintic for ascariasis (roundworm)*

and enterobiasis (pinworm) [pyrantel (as pamoate)] 50 mg/mL; 250 mg ⑨ Pain-X

pioglitazone INN *thiazolidinedione (TZD) antidiabetic and peroxisome proliferator–activated receptor–gamma (PPARγ) agonist that increases cellular response to insulin without increasing insulin secretion* [also: pioglitazone HCl]

pioglitazone HCl USAN *thiazolidinedione (TZD) antidiabetic and peroxisome proliferator–activated receptor–gamma (PPARγ) agonist that increases cellular response to insulin without increasing insulin secretion* [also: pioglitazone]

pioglitazone HCl & metformin HCl *combination thiazolidinedione (TZD)/ peroxisome proliferator–activated receptor–gamma (PPARγ) agonist and biguanide antidiabetic that increases cellular response to insulin and decreases hepatic production of glucose* 15•500, 15•850 mg oral

pipacycline INN

pipamazine INN

pipamperone USAN, INN *antipsychotic*

pipaneperone [see: pipamperone]

pipazetate INN *antitussive* [also: pipazethate]

pipazethate USAN *antitussive* [also: pipazetate]

pipe plant; Dutchman's pipe; Indian pipe *medicinal herb* [see: fit root]

pipebuzone INN

pipecuronium bromide USAN, INN, BAN *nondepolarizing neuromuscular blocking agent; muscle relaxant; adjunct to general anesthesia*

pipemidic acid INN

pipenzolate bromide INN

pipenzolate methylbromide [see: pipenzolate bromide]

pipenzolone bromide [see: pipenzolate bromide]

pipequaline INN

Piper cubeba medicinal herb [see: cubeb]

Piper methysticum medicinal herb [see: kava kava]

piperacetazine USAN, USP, INN *antipsychotic*

piperacillin INN, BAN *extended-spectrum penicillin antibiotic* [also: piperacillin sodium]

piperacillin sodium USAN, USP, JAN *extended-spectrum penicillin antibiotic* [also: piperacillin] 2, 3, 4, 40 g injection

piperacillin sodium & tazobactam sodium *extended-spectrum penicillin antibiotic plus synergist* 2•0.25, 3• 0.375, 4•0.5, 36•4.5 g/vial injection

piperamide INN *anthelmintic* [also: piperamide maleate]

piperamide maleate USAN *anthelmintic* [also: piperamide]

piperamine [see: bamipine]

piperazine USP *anthelmintic for enterobiasis (pinworm) and ascariasis (roundworm)*

piperazine calcium edetate INN *anthelmintic* [also: piperazine edetate calcium]

piperazine citrate USP *anthelmintic* 250 mg oral; 500 mg/mL oral

piperazine citrate hydrate [see: piperazine citrate]

piperazine edetate calcium USAN *anthelmintic* [also: piperazine calcium edetate]

piperazine estrone sulfate [now: estropipate]

piperazine hexahydrate [see: piperazine citrate]

piperazine phosphate

piperazine phosphate monohydrate [see: piperazine phosphate]

piperazine theophylline ethanoate [see: acefylline piperazine]

piperidine phosphate

piperidines *a class of antihistamines*

piperidolate INN [also: piperidolate HCl]

piperidolate HCl USP [also: piperidolate]

piperilate [see: pipethanate]

piperine USP *natural pepper extract that increases the absorption of various natural remedies*

piperocaine INN [also: piperocaine HCl]

piperocaine HCl USP [also: pipero-
caine]
piperonyl butoxide *pediculicide for lice*
piperoxan INN
piperphenidol HCl
piperylone INN 🔢 piberaline
pipethanate INN
pipobroman USAN, USP, INN *alkylating
antineoplastic*
pipoctanone INN
pipofezine INN
piposulfan USAN, INN *antineoplastic*
pipotiazine INN *phenothiazine antipsychotic* [also: pipotiazine palmitate]
pipotiazine palmitate USAN *phenothiazine antipsychotic* [also: pipotiazine]
pipoxizine INN
pipoxolan INN *muscle relaxant* [also:
pipoxolan HCl]
pipoxolan HCl USAN *muscle relaxant*
[also: pipoxolan]
pipradimadol INN
pipradrol INN [also: pipradrol HCl]
pipradrol HCl NF [also: pipradrol]
pipramadol INN
pipratecol INN
piprinhydrinate INN, BAN
piprocurarium iodide INN
piprofurol INN
piprozolin USAN, INN *choleretic*
pipsissewa (*Chimaphila umbellata*)
plant *medicinal herb used as an astringent, diaphoretic, and diuretic*
piquindone INN *antipsychotic* [also:
piquindone HCl]
piquindone HCl USAN *antipsychotic*
[also: piquindone]
piquizil INN *bronchodilator* [also: piquizil HCl] 🔢 Paxil
piquizil HCl USAN *bronchodilator* [also:
piquizil]
piracetam USAN, INN, BAN *cognition
adjuvant; investigational (orphan) for
myoclonus*
pirandamine INN *antidepressant* [also:
pirandamine HCl]
pirandamine HCl USAN *antidepressant*
[also: pirandamine]
pirarubicin INN
piraxelate INN

pirazmonam INN *antimicrobial* [also:
pirazmonam sodium]
pirazmonam sodium USAN *antimicrobial* [also: pirazmonam]
pirazofurin INN *antineoplastic* [also:
pyrazofurin]
pirazolac USAN, INN, BAN *antirheumatic*
pirbenicillin INN *antibacterial* [also:
pirbenicillin sodium]
pirbenicillin sodium USAN *antibacterial* [also: pirbenicillin]
pirbuterol INN *sympathomimetic bronchodilator* [also: pirbuterol acetate]
pirbuterol acetate USAN *sympathomimetic bronchodilator for asthma and
bronchospasm* [also: pirbuterol]
pirbuterol HCl USAN *bronchodilator*
pirdonium bromide INN
pirenoxine INN
pirenperone USAN, INN, BAN *tranquilizer*
pirenzepine INN, BAN *tricyclic benzodiazepine for peptic ulcers* [also: pirenzepine HCl] 🔢 Principen
pirenzepine HCl USAN, JAN *tricyclic
benzodiazepine for peptic ulcers* [also:
pirenzepine]
pirepolol INN
piretanide USAN, INN *diuretic*
pirfenidone USAN, INN *anti-inflammatory; investigational (NDA filed,
orphan) TGF-beta inhibitor for idiopathic pulmonary fibrosis (IPF)*
piribedil INN 🔢 Prepidil
piribenzyl methylsulfate [see: bevonium metilsulfate]
piridicillin INN *antibacterial* [also: piridicillin sodium]
piridicillin sodium USAN *antibacterial*
[also: piridicillin]
piridocaine INN 🔢 paridocaine
piridocaine HCl [see: piridocaine]
piridoxilate INN, BAN
piridronate sodium USAN *calcium regulator*
piridronic acid INN
pirifibrate INN
pirinidazole INN
pirinitramide [see: piritramide]
pirinixic acid INN

pirinixil INN
piriprost USAN *antiasthmatic*
piriprost potassium USAN *antiasthmatic*
piriqualone INN
pirisudanol INN
piritramide INN, BAN
piritrexim INN *antiproliferative agent* [also: piritrexim isethionate]
piritrexim isethionate USAN *investigational (orphan) antiproliferative for* Pneumocystis, Toxoplasma gondii, *and* Mycobacterium avium-intracellulare *infections* [also: piritrexim]
pirlimycin HCl USAN *antibacterial*
pirlindole INN
pirmagrel USAN, INN *thromboxane synthetase inhibitor*
pirmenol INN *antiarrhythmic* [also: pirmenol HCl]
pirmenol HCl USAN *antiarrhythmic* [also: pirmenol]
pirnabin INN *antiglaucoma agent* [also: pirnabine]
pirnabine USAN *antiglaucoma agent* [also: pirnabin]
piroctone USAN, INN *antiseborrheic*
piroctone olamine USAN *antiseborrheic*
pirodavir USAN, INN, BAN *antiviral*
pirogliride INN *antidiabetic* [also: pirogliride tartrate]
pirogliride tartrate USAN *antidiabetic* [also: pirogliride]
piroheptine INN
pirolate USAN, INN *antiasthmatic* ☒ Prialt
pirolazamide USAN, INN *antiarrhythmic*
piromidic acid INN
piroxantrone INN *antineoplastic* [also: piroxantrone HCl]
piroxantrone HCl USAN *antineoplastic* [also: piroxantrone]
piroxicam USAN, USP, INN, BAN, JAN *analgesic; nonsteroidal anti-inflammatory drug (NSAID) for osteoarthritis and rheumatoid arthritis* 10, 20 mg oral
piroxicam β-cyclodextrin [see: piroxicam betadex]
piroxicam betadex USAN *analgesic; nonsteroidal anti-inflammatory drug (NSAID) for osteoarthritis and rheumatoid arthritis*

piroxicam cinnamate USAN *anti-inflammatory*
piroxicam olamine USAN *analgesic; anti-inflammatory*
piroxicillin INN
piroximone USAN, INN, BAN *cardiotonic* ☒ pyroxamine
pirozadil INN
pirprofen USAN, INN, BAN *anti-inflammatory*
pirquinozol USAN, INN *antiallergic* ☒ parconazole
pirralkonium bromide INN
pirroksan [now: proroxan HCl]
pirsidomine USAN, INN *vasodilator*
pirtenidine INN *treatment for gingivitis* [also: pirtenidine HCl]
pirtenidine HCl USAN *treatment for gingivitis* [also: pirtenidine]
pistachio *medicinal herb* [see: witch hazel]
pitavastatin calcium *HMG-CoA reductase inhibitor for hyperlipidemia and mixed dyslipidemia* (base=96%)
pitch tree, Canada; hemlock pitch tree *medicinal herb* [see: hemlock]
pitcher plant (Sarracenia purpurea) root *medicinal herb used as an astringent, diuretic, and stimulant*
pitenodil INN
Pitocin IV, IM injection ℞ *oxytocic for induction of labor, postpartum bleeding, and incomplete abortion* [oxytocin] 10 U/mL
pitofenone INN
pitrakinra *investigational oral leukotriene inhibitor for asthma*
Pitressin Synthetic IM or subcu injection ℞ *pituitary antidiuretic hormone for diabetes insipidus or prevention of abdominal distention* [vasopressin] 20 U/mL
pituitary, anterior
pituitary, posterior USP *antidiuretic hormone for postoperative ileus and surgical hemostasis*
pituxate INN
pivalate USAN, INN, BAN *combining name for radicals or groups*

pivampicillin INN *aminopenicillin antibiotic* [also: pivampicillin HCl]

pivampicillin HCl USAN *aminopenicillin antibiotic* [also: pivampicillin]

pivampicillin pamoate USAN *antibacterial*

pivampicillin probenate USAN *antibacterial*

pivenfrine INN

pivmecillinam INN, BAN *aminopenicillin antibiotic* [also: amdinocillin pivoxil; pivmecillinam HCl]

pivmecillinam HCl JAN *aminopenicillin antibiotic* [also: amdinocillin pivoxil; pivmecillinam]

pivopril USAN *antihypertensive*

pivoxazepam INN

pivoxetil USAN, INN *combining name for radicals or groups*

pivoxil USAN, INN *combining name for radicals or groups* ② pifexole

pivsulbactam BAN *beta-lactamase inhibitor; penicillin/cephalosporin synergist* [also: sulbactam pivoxil]

pix pini [see: pine tar]

pixantrone *investigational (NDA filed) treatment for relapsed, aggressive non-Hodgkin lymphoma*

Pixuvri *investigational (NDA filed) treatment for relapsed, aggressive non-Hodgkin lymphoma* [pixantrone]

pizotifen INN, BAN *anabolic; antidepressant; serotonin inhibitor (migraine specific)* [also: pizotyline]

pizotyline USAN *anabolic; antidepressant; serotonin inhibitor (migraine specific)* [also: pizotifen]

placebo *an inert substance with no therapeutic value* [also: obecalp]

placebo effect [L. I will please] *a perceived therapeutic effect from an inert substance* [compare to: nocebo effect]

plafibride INN

plague vaccine USP *active bacterin for plague* (Yersinia pestis)

Plan B tablets (in packs of 2) OTC ≥ 18 years; Ⅸ ≤ 17 years *emergency progestin-only postcoital contraceptive* [levonorgestrel] 0.75 mg

Plan B One Step tablets OTC ≥ 17 years; Ⅸ ≤ 16 years *emergency progestin-only postcoital contraceptive* [levonorgestrel] 1.5 mg

planadalin [see: carbromal]

Plantago lanceolata; P. major **and other species** *medicinal herb* [see: plantain]

Plantago ovata **(psyllium)** *medicinal herb* [see: plantain]

plantago seed USP *laxative*

plantain (*Plantago lanceolata; P. major* **and other species**) leaves and seeds *medicinal herb for bed-wetting, bladder infections, blood poisoning, constipation, diarrhea, diverticulitis, edema, hyperlipidemia, kidney disorders, neuralgia, snake bites, sores, and topical inflammation*

Plaquase powder for injection *investigational (orphan) for Peyronie disease* [collagenase]

Plaquenil film-coated tablets (discontinued 2008) Ⅸ *antimalarial; antirheumatic; lupus erythematosus suppressant* [hydroxychloroquine sulfate] 200 mg

Plaretase 8000 tablets (discontinued 2009) Ⅸ *porcine-derived digestive enzymes* [pancrelipase (lipase; protease; amylase)] 8000•30 000•30 000 USP units

Plasbumin-5; Plasbumin-20; Plasbumin-25 IV infusion Ⅸ *blood volume expander for shock, burns, and hypoproteinemia* [human albumin] 5%; 20%; 25%

plasma, antihemophilic human USP

plasma concentrate factor IX [see: factor IX complex]

plasma expanders *a class of therapeutic blood modifiers used to increase the volume of circulating blood* [also called: blood volume expanders]

plasma protein fraction USP *blood volume supporter/expander for shock due to burns, trauma, and surgery*

plasma protein fraction, human [now: plasma protein fraction]

plasma protein fractions *a class of therapeutic blood modifiers used to regulate the volume of circulating blood*

plasma thromboplastin component (PTC) [see: factor IX]

Plasma-Lyte A pH 7.4; Plasma-Lyte R; Plasma-Lyte 148 IV infusion ℞ *intravenous electrolyte therapy* [combined electrolyte solution]

Plasma-Lyte M (R; 56; 148) and 5% Dextrose IV infusion ℞ *intravenous nutritional/electrolyte therapy* [combined electrolyte solution; dextrose]

Plasmanate IV infusion ℞ *blood volume expander for shock due to burns, trauma, and surgery* [plasma protein fraction] 5%

Plasma-Plex IV infusion ℞ *blood volume expander for shock due to burns, trauma, and surgery* [plasma protein fraction] 5%

Plasmatein IV infusion (discontinued 2011) ℞ *blood volume expander for shock due to burns, trauma, and surgery* [plasma protein fraction] 5%

plasmid DNA vector *investigational (orphan) genetic therapy for cystic fibrosis*

plasmin BAN [also: fibrinolysin, human]

Plateau Cap (trademarked dosage form) *controlled-release capsule*

platelet cofactor II [see: factor IX]

platelet concentrate USP *platelet replenisher*

platinum *element (Pt)* ⍰ plutonium

cis-**platinum** [now: cisplatin]

cis-**platinum II** [now: cisplatin]

platinum diamminodichloride [see: cisplatin]

plaunotol INN

plauracin USAN, INN *veterinary growth stimulant*

Plavix film-coated tablets ℞ *platelet aggregation inhibitor for stroke, myocardial infarction, peripheral artery disease, and acute coronary syndrome; also used before coronary stent implantation surgery* [clopidogrel (as bisulfate)] 75, 300 mg

Plax mouthwash/gargle OTC *oral antiseptic* [sodium pyrophosphate; alcohol 8.7%]

pleconaril USAN *viral replication inhibitor*

PledgaClin pledgets ℞ *antibiotic for acne and rosacea* [clindamycin; alcohol 50%] 1%

Plegisol solution ℞ *cardioplegic solution* [calcium chloride; magnesium chloride; potassium chloride; sodium chloride] 17.6•325.3•119.3•643 mg/100 mL

Plenaxis powder for IM injection (discontinued 2009) ℞ *GnRH antagonist to suppress LH and FSH, leading to the cessation of testosterone production (medical castration, androgen ablation); treatment for prostate cancer* [abarelix] 100 mg/vial

Plendil extended-release tablets (discontinued 2008) ℞ *antihypertensive; calcium channel blocker* [felodipine] 2.5, 5, 10 mg

plerixafor *CXCR-4 chemokine receptor blocker used to mobilize stem cells for autologous stem cell transplants in patients with non-Hodgkin lymphoma and multiple myeloma*

Pletal tablets ℞ *platelet aggregation inhibitor and vasodilator for intermittent claudication* [cilostazol] 50 mg

pleurisy root (*Asclepias tuberosa*) *medicinal herb for asthma, bronchitis, dysentery, emphysema, fever, pleurisy, and pneumonia*

pleuromulin INN

Plexion topical liquid, cleansing cloths ℞ *antibiotic and keratolytic for acne* [sulfacetamide sodium; sulfur] 10%•5%

Plexion SCT cream ℞ *antibiotic and keratolytic for acne* [sulfacetamide sodium; sulfur] 10%•5%

Plexion TS topical suspension ℞ *antibiotic and keratolytic for acne* [sulfacetamide sodium; sulfur] 10%•5%

Pliagel solution OTC *surfactant cleaning solution for soft contact lenses*

Pliaglis cream ℞ *anesthetic* [lidocaine; tetracaine] 7%•7%

plicamycin USAN, USP, INN *antibiotic antineoplastic for malignant testicular tumors*

plitidepsin *investigational (orphan) antineoplastic for multiple myeloma*

plomestane USAN *antineoplastic; aromatase inhibitor*

plum *(Prunus americana; P. domestica; P. spinosa)* fruit and bark *medicinal herb used as an anthelmintic, astringent, and laxative*

plutonium *element (Pu)* ⊠ platinum

PLX (PLacental eXpanded) stem cells *mesenchymal-like adherent stromal cells (ASC) derived from full-term placenta; investigational (Phase II/III) treatment for critical limb ischemia (CLI); investigational (Phase II) for intermittent claudication (IC); investigational (orphan) for thromboangiitis obliterans (Buerger disease)*

pMDI (dosage form) *pressurized metered-dose inhaler*

PMMA (polymethylmethacrylate) [q.v.]

PMPA (phosphonomethoxypropyladenine) [see: tenofovir]

PMPA prodrug [see: tenofovir disoproxil fumarate]

pneumococcal polysaccharide vaccine [see: pneumococcal vaccine, polyvalent]

pneumococcal vaccine, 7-valent (PCV7) *active bacterin for pneumococcal pneumonia; polysaccharide isolates of seven strains of* Streptococcus pneumoniae: *4, 6B, 9V, 14, 18C, 19F, and 23F*

pneumococcal vaccine, 13-valent (PCV13) *active bacterin for pneumococcal pneumonia; polysaccharide isolates of thirteen strains of* Streptococcus pneumoniae: *1, 3, 4, 5, 6A, 6B, 7F, 9V, 14, 18C, 19A, 19F, and 23F*

pneumococcal vaccine, polyvalent *active bacterin for pneumococcal pneumonia (polysaccharide isolates of 23 strains of* Streptococcus pneumoniae)

Pneumopent *for inhalation investigational (orphan) prophylaxis of* Pneu- mocystis *pneumonia (PCP)* [pentamidine isethionate]

Pneumotussin caplets (discontinued 2007) ℞ *narcotic antitussive; expectorant* [hydrocodone bitartrate; guaifenesin] 2.5•300 mg ⊠ niometacin

Pneumotussin 2.5 Cough syrup (discontinued 2011) ℞ *narcotic antitussive; expectorant* [hydrocodone bitartrate; guaifenesin] 2.5•200 mg/5 mL

Pneumovax 23 subcu or IM injection ℞ *active immunization against 23 strains of* Streptococcus pneumoniae [pneumococcal vaccine, polyvalent] 25 mcg of each strain per 0.5 mL dose

PNV-DHA softgels ℞ *vitamin/calcium/iron/nutritional supplement* [multiple vitamins; calcium; iron; folate; docosahexaenoic acid (DHA)] ±•75•27•1.4•250 mg

PNV-Iron tablets ℞ *vitamin/mineral/calcium/iron supplement* [multiple vitamins & minerals; calcium; iron; folic acid; L-methylfolate calcium; biotin] ±•200•29•0.4•1•0.03 mg

pobilukast edamine USAN *antiasthmatic*

POC (procarbazine, Oncovin, CCNU) *chemotherapy protocol for pediatric brain tumors*

Pockethaler (trademarked delivery form) *nasal inhalation aerosol*

pod pepper *medicinal herb* [see: cayenne]

podilfen INN

Podocon-25 topical liquid ℞ *keratolytic for genital warts* [podophyllum resin] 25%

podofilox USAN *topical antimitotic for genital warts* [also: podophyllotoxin] 0.5% topical

Podofin topical liquid ℞ *keratolytic for genital warts* [podophyllum resin] 25%

podophyllin [see: podophyllum resin]

podophyllotoxin BAN *topical antimitotic* [also: podofilox]

podophyllotoxins *a class of mitotic-inhibiting antineoplastics derived from podophyllotoxin*

podophyllum USP *caustic; cytotoxic agent for genital warts*

Podophyllum peltatum *medicinal herb*
[see: mandrake]

podophyllum resin USP *caustic; cytotoxic agent for genital warts*

poinsettia *(Euphorbia pulcherrima; E. poinsettia; Poinsettia pulcherrima)* plant and sap *medicinal herb for fever, pain relief, stimulating lactation, toothache, and warts; also used as an antibacterial and depilatory* ② boneset; Panacet

Point-Two oral rinse ℞ *dental caries preventative* [sodium fluoride; alcohol 6%] 0.2%

poison, dog *medicinal herb* [see: dog poison]

poison ash *medicinal herb* [see: fringe tree]

poison flag *medicinal herb* [see: blue flag]

poison hemlock *(Conium maculatum)* plant *medicinal herb that has been used for analgesia and sedation and as a method of execution; it is extremely poisonous*

poison ivy extract, alum precipitated USAN *ivy poisoning counteractant*

poison oak *(Tocicodendron diversilobum)* extract *medicinal herb used in homeopathic remedies for osteoarthritis*

poison oak extract USAN *antiallergic*

poke root *(Phytolacca decandra) medicinal herb* [see: pokeweed]

pokeweed *(Phytolacca americana; P. decandra; P. rigida)* root and young shoots *medicinal herb for arthritis, blood cleansing, bowel evacuation, dysmenorrhea, mucous membrane inflammation and discharge, mumps, pain, rheumatism, ringworm, scabies, syphilis, and tonsillitis; not generally regarded as safe and effective*

polacrilex [see: nicotine polacrilex]

polacrilin USAN, INN *pharmaceutic aid*

polacrilin potassium USAN, NF *tablet disintegrant*

Polaramine Expectorant pediatric oral liquid (discontinued 2007) ℞ *decongestant; antihistamine; expectorant* [pseudoephedrine sulfate; dexchlorpheniramine maleate; guaifenesin; alcohol 7.2%] 20•2•100 mg/5 mL

poldine methylsulfate USAN, USP *anticholinergic* [also: poldine metilsulfate]

poldine metilsulfate INN *anticholinergic* [also: poldine methylsulfate]

polecat weed *medicinal herb* [see: skunk cabbage]

Polibar, Liquid; Liquid Polibar Plus oral/rectal suspension ℞ *radiopaque contrast agent* [barium sulfate] 100%; 105%

policapram USAN, INN *tablet binder*

policosanol *natural supplement from sugar cane plants; enhanced extract of octacosanol (q.v.) used for hypercholesterolemia; therapeutic effects are similar to statin drugs but without side effects such as liver dysfunction and muscle atrophy*

policresulen INN

polidexide sulfate INN

polidocanol INN, JAN *polyethylene glycol monododecyl ether*

polifeprosan INN *pharmaceutic aid; implantable, biodegradable drug carrier* [also: polifeprosan 20]

polifeprosan 20 USAN *pharmaceutic aid; implantable, biodegradable drug carrier* [also: polifeprosan]

poligeenan USAN, INN *dispersing agent*

poliglecaprone 25 USAN *absorbable surgical suture material*

poliglecaprone 90 USAN *absorbable surgical suture coating*

poliglusam USAN *antihemorrhagic*

polignate sodium USAN *pepsin enzyme inhibitor*

polihexanide INN [also: polyhexanide]

poliomyelitis vaccine [now: poliovirus vaccine, inactivated]

poliovirus vaccine, enhanced inactivated (eIPV) *active immunizing agent for poliomyelitis*

poliovirus vaccine, inactivated (IPV) USP *active immunizing agent for poliomyelitis*

poliovirus vaccine, live oral (OPV) USP *active immunizing agent for poliomyelitis*

polipropene 25 USAN *tablet excipient*
polisaponin INN
politef INN *prosthetic aid* [also: polytef]
polixetonium chloride USAN, INN
  preservative
Polocaine injection, dental injection
  ℞ *local anesthetic* [mepivacaine HCl]
  1%, 2%; 3% ▢ Bellacane
Polocaine MPF injection ℞ *local
  anesthetic* [mepivacaine HCl] 1%,
  1.5%, 2%
Polocaine with Levonordefrin dental injection (discontinued 2009) ℞
  local anesthetic; vasoconstrictor [mepi-
  vacaine HCl; levonordefrin] 2%•
  1:20 000
polonium *element (Po)*
poloxalene USAN, INN, BAN *surfactant*
poloxamer USAN, NF, INN, BAN *ointment and suppository base; tablet binder*
poloxamer 124 USAN *surfactant; emulsifier; solubilizer; stabilizer*
poloxamer 188 USAN *surfactant; emulsifier; solubilizer; investigational (Phase
  III, orphan) for sickle cell crisis; investigational (orphan) for severe burns and
  vasospasm following cerebral aneurysm
  repair*
poloxamer 237 USAN *surfactant; emulsifier; solubilizer; stabilizer*
poloxamer 331 *investigational (orphan)
  for toxoplasmosis of AIDS*
poloxamer 338 USAN *surfactant; emulsifier; solubilizer; stabilizer*
poloxamer 407 USAN *surfactant; emulsifier; solubilizer; stabilizer*
Poly Hist DHC oral liquid ℞ *narcotic
  antitussive; antihistamine; sleep aid;
  decongestant* [dihydrocodeine bitartrate; pyrilamine maleate; phenylephrine HCl] 7.5•7.5•5 mg/5 mL
Poly Hist DM oral liquid ℞ *antitussive;
  antihistamine; sleep aid; decongestant*
  [dextromethorphan hydrobromide;
  pyrilamine maleate; phenylephrine
  HCl] 15•12.5•7.5 mg/5 mL
Poly Hist HC oral liquid (discontinued
  2009) ℞ *narcotic antitussive; antihistamine; sleep aid; decongestant* [hydro-
  codone bitartrate; pyrilamine male-

ate; phenylephrine HCl] 3.5•12.5•
  7.5 mg/5 mL
Poly Hist NC oral liquid ℞ *narcotic
  antitussive; decongestant; antihistamine*
  [codeine phosphate; pseudoephedrine HCl; triprolidine HCl] 10•15•
  1.25 mg/5 mL
poly I: poly C12U *investigational (Phase
  III, orphan) RNA synthesis inhibitor
  and immunomodulator for AIDS, renal
  cell carcinoma, metastatic melanoma,
  and chronic fatigue syndrome*
Poly Tan D oral suspension (discontinued 2011) ℞ *decongestant; antihistamine; sleep aid* [phenylephrine tannate; dexbrompheniramine tannate;
  pyrilamine maleate] 25•4•3.5 mg/5
  mL
Poly Tan DM oral suspension ℞ *antitussive; antihistamine; sleep aid; decongestant* [dextromethorphan tannate;
  dexbrompheniramine tannate; pyrilamine maleate; phenylephrine tan-
  nate] 30•4•3.5•25 mg/5 mL
polyamine-methylene resin
polyanhydroglucose [see: dextran]
polyanhydroglucuronic acid [see:
  dextran]
polybenzarsol INN
polybutester USAN *surgical suture
  material*
polybutilate USAN *surgical suture coating*
polycarbokane [see: polycarbophil]
polycarbophil USP, INN, BAN *bulk laxative; antidiarrheal*
Polycitra syrup (discontinued 2008)
  ℞ *urinary alkalinizing agent* [potas-
  sium citrate; sodium citrate; citric
  acid] 550•500•334 mg/5 mL
Polycitra-K oral solution, crystals for
  oral solution (discontinued 2008) ℞
  urinary alkalizing agent [potassium
  citrate; citric acid] 1100•334 mg/5
  mL; 3300•1002 mg/pkt.
Polycitra-LC solution (discontinued
  2008) ℞ *urinary alkalizing agent*
  [potassium citrate; sodium citrate;
  citric acid] 550•500•334 mg/5 mL
**polycosanol & acetic acid & anti-
  pyrine & benzocaine** *analgesic;*

anesthetic 0.01%•0.01%•5.4%•1.4% otic drops

Polycose oral liquid, powder for oral liquid OTC *carbohydrate caloric supplement* [glucose polymers]

polydextrose USAN *food additive*

polydimethylsiloxane *surgical aid (retinal tamponade) for retinal detachment*

Polydine ointment, scrub, solution OTC *broad-spectrum antimicrobial* [povidone-iodine] ⑫ Paladin

polydioxanone USAN *absorbable surgical suture material*

polyelectrolyte 211 [see: sodium alginate]

polyenes *a class of antifungals produced by a species of* Streptomyces *that damage fungal cell membranes*

polyestradiol phosphate INN, BAN *estrogen; hormonal antineoplastic*

polyetadene INN *antacid* [also: polyethadene]

polyethadene USAN *antacid* [also: polyetadene]

polyethylene excipient NF *stiffening agent*

polyethylene glycol (PEG) NF *moisturizer/lubricant; ointment and suppository base; solvent*

polyethylene glycol *n* (*n* refers to the molecular weight: 300, 1000, etc.)

polyethylene glycol *n* **dioleate** (*n* refers to the molecular weight: 300, 1000, etc.)

polyethylene glycol 8 monostearate [see: polyoxyl 8 stearate]

polyethylene glycol 1000 monocetyl ether [see: cetomacrogol 1000]

polyethylene glycol 1540 NF

polyethylene glycol 3350 *laxative; bowel evacuant* 255, 527 g oral

polyethylene glycol 3350 & potassium chloride & sodium bicarbonate & sodium chloride *hyperosmotic laxative; pre-procedure bowel evacuant* 420•1.48•5.72•11.2 g/bottle

polyethylene glycol 3350 & potassium chloride & sodium bicarbonate & sodium chloride & sodium sulfate *hyperosmotic laxative;*

pre-procedure bowel evacuant 236• 2.97•6.74•5.86•22.74, 240•2.98• 6.72•5.84•22.73 g/bottle

polyethylene glycol 4000 USP [also: macrogol 4000]

polyethylene glycol 6000 USP

polyethylene glycol–electrolyte solution (PEG-ES) *pre-procedure bowel evacuant* [contains polyethylene glycol 3350, potassium chloride, sodium bicarbonate, and sodium chloride] 60, 105 g/L

polyethylene glycol monoleyl ether [see: polyoxyl 10 oleyl ether]

polyethylene glycol monomethyl ether NF *excipient*

polyethylene glycol monostearate [see: polyoxyl 40 & 50 stearate]

polyethylene glycol–superoxide dismutase (PEG-SOD) [see: pegorgotein]

polyethylene oxide NF *suspending and viscosity agent; tablet binder*

polyferose USAN *hematinic*

Polygala senega medicinal herb [see: senega]

Polygam S/D freeze-dried powder for IV infusion (discontinued 2008) ℞ *passive immunizing agent for HIV, idiopathic thrombocytopenic purpura, and B-cell chronic lymphocytic leukemia* [immune globulin (IGIV), solvent/detergent treated] 90% (2.5, 5, 10 g/dose)

polygeline INN, BAN

polyglactin 370 USAN *absorbable surgical suture coating*

polyglactin 910 USAN *absorbable surgical suture material*

polyglycolic acid USAN, INN *surgical suture material*

polyglyconate USAN, BAN *absorbable surgical suture material*

Polygonatum multiflorum; P. odoratum medicinal herb [see: Solomon's seal]

Polygonum aviculare; P. hydropiper; P. persicaria; P. punctatum medicinal herb [see: knotweed]

Polygonum bistorta medicinal herb [see: bistort]

Polygonum multiflorum medicinal herb [see: fo-ti; ho-shou-wu]

polyhexanide BAN [also: polihexanide]

Polyhist PD oral suspension ℞ *decongestant; antihistamine; sleep aid* [phenylephrine HCl; chlorpheniramine maleate; pyrilamine maleate] 7.5•2• 12.5 mg/5 mL

Poly-Histine elixir ℞ *antihistamine for allergic and vasomotor rhinitis, allergic conjunctivitis, and mild urticaria; sleep aid* [pheniramine maleate; pyrilamine maleate; phenyltoloxamine citrate] 4•4•4 mg/5 mL

poly-ICLC *investigational (orphan) agent for orthopoxvirus infections and primary brain tumors* [polyinosinic-polycytidilic acid]

polyinosinic-polycytidilic acid *investigational (orphan) agent for orthopoxvirus infections and primary brain tumors*

Poly-Iron capsules OTC *iron supplement* [iron (as polysaccharide-iron complex)] 150 mg

poly-L-lactic acid *synthetic polymer for the correction of facial lipoatrophy due to HIV infections*

polyloxyl 8 stearate USAN *surfactant*

polymacon USAN *hydrophilic contact lens material*

polymanoacetate [now: acemannan]

polymeric oxygen [see: oxygen, polymeric]

polymetaphosphate P 32 USAN *radioactive agent*

polymethyl methacrylate (PMMA) *rigid hydrophobic polymer used for hard contact lenses*

polymixin E [see: colistin sulfate]

polymonine

polymyxin BAN *bactericidal antibiotic* [also: polymyxin B sulfate; polymyxin B]

polymyxin B INN *bactericidal antibiotic* [also: polymyxin B sulfate; polymyxin]

polymyxin B sulfate USP *bactericidal antibiotic* [also: polymyxin B; polymyxin] 500 000 U/vial injection

polymyxin B sulfate & bacitracin zinc *topical antibiotic* 10 000•500 U/g ophthalmic

polymyxin B sulfate & bacitracin zinc & neomycin sulfate *topical antibiotic* 10 000 U•400 U•5 mg per g ophthalmic

polymyxin B sulfate & gramicidin & neomycin sulfate *topical antibiotic* 10 000 U•0.025 mg•1.75 mg per mL eye drops

polymyxin B sulfate & neomycin *antibiotic* 200 000 U•40 mg per mL intravesical solution

polymyxin B sulfate & neomycin sulfate & dexamethasone *topical ophthalmic antibiotic and corticosteroidal anti-inflammatory* 10 000 U/mL• 0.35%•0.1% eye drops

polymyxin B sulfate & neomycin sulfate & hydrocortisone *topical ophthalmic/otic antibiotic and corticosteroidal anti-inflammatory* 10 000 U/mL•0.35%•1% eye drops; 10 000 U/mL•5 mg/mL•1% ear drops

polymyxin B sulfate & trimethoprim sulfate *topical ophthalmic antibiotic* 10 000 U•1 mg per mL eye drops

polymyxin B₁ [see: polymyxin B]

polymyxin B₂ [see: polymyxin B]

polymyxin B₃ [see: polymyxin B]

polymyxin E [see: colistin sulfate]

polynoxylin INN, BAN

polyolprepolymer *topical base for gels and creams*

polyoxyethylene 20 sorbitan monolaurate [see: polysorbate 20]

polyoxyethylene 20 sorbitan monooleate [see: polysorbate 80]

polyoxyethylene 20 sorbitan monopalmitate [see: polysorbate 40]

polyoxyethylene 20 sorbitan monostearate [see: polysorbate 60]

polyoxyethylene 20 sorbitan trioleate [see: polysorbate 85]

polyoxyethylene 20 sorbitan tristearate [see: polysorbate 65]

polyoxyethylene 50 stearate [now: polyoxyl 50 stearate]

polyoxyethylene glycol 1000 mono-cetyl ether [see: cetomacrogol 1000]

polyoxyethylene nonyl phenol *surfactant/wetting agent*

polyoxyl 10 oleyl ether NF *surfactant*

polyoxyl 20 cetostearyl ether NF *surfactant*

polyoxyl 35 castor oil NF *emulsifying agent; surfactant*

polyoxyl 40 hydrogenated castor oil NF *emulsifying agent; surfactant*

polyoxyl 40 stearate USAN, NF *surfactant*

polyoxyl 50 stearate NF *surfactant; emulsifying agent*

polyoxypropylene 15 stearyl ether USAN *solvent*

polyphosphoric acid, sodium salt [see: sodium polyphosphate]

Polypodium vulgare *medicinal herb* [see: female fern]

Poly-Pred eye drop suspension ℞ *corticosteroidal anti-inflammatory; antibiotic* [prednisolone acetate; neomycin sulfate; polymyxin B sulfate] 0.5%•0.35%•10 000 U per mL

polypropylene glycol NF

polyribonucleotide [see: poly I: poly C12U]

polysaccharide-iron complex *hematinic; iron supplement* 150 mg Fe oral

Polysorb Hydrate cream (discontinued 2009) OTC *moisturizer; emollient*

polysorbate 20 USAN, NF, INN *surfactant/wetting agent*

polysorbate 40 USAN, NF, INN *surfactant*

polysorbate 60 USAN, NF, INN *surfactant*

polysorbate 65 USAN, INN *surfactant*

polysorbate 80 USAN, NF, INN *surfactant/wetting agent; viscosity-increasing agent*

polysorbate 85 USAN, INN *surfactant*

Polysporin ointment OTC *antibiotic* [polymyxin B sulfate; bacitracin zinc] 10 000•500 U/g

Polysporin topical powder (discontinued 2008) OTC *antibiotic* [polymyxin

B sulfate; bacitracin zinc] 10 000•500 U/g

Polytabs-F pediatric chewable tablets (discontinued 2008) ℞ *vitamin supplement; dental caries preventative* [multiple vitamins; fluoride; folic acid] $\pm$•1•0.3 mg

Polytar shampoo OTC *antiseborrheic; antipsoriatic; antipruritic; antibacterial* [coal tar (solution includes pine tar and juniper tar)] 0.5% (4.5%)

Polytar soap (discontinued 2008) OTC *antiseborrheic; antipsoriatic; antipruritic; antibacterial* [coal tar (solution includes pine tar and juniper tar)] 0.5% (2.5%)

polytef USAN *prosthetic aid* [also: politef]

polytetrafluoroethylene (PTFE) [see: polytef]

polythiazide USAN, USP, INN *diuretic; antihypertensive*

Poly-Tussin AC oral liquid ℞ *narcotic antitussive; decongestant; antihistamine* [codeine phosphate; phenylephrine HCl; brompheniramine maleate] 10•7.5•4 mg/5 mL

Poly-Tussin DHC oral liquid ℞ *narcotic antitussive; antihistamine; decongestant* [dihydrocodeine bitartrate; brompheniramine maleate; phenylephrine HCl] 3•4•7.5 mg/5 mL

Poly-Tussin EX oral liquid ℞ *narcotic antitussive; decongestant; expectorant* [dihydrocodeine bitartrate; phenylephrine HCl; guaifenesin] 7.5•7.5•50 mg/5 mL

Poly-Tussin HD syrup (discontinued 2009) ℞ *narcotic antitussive; antihistamine; decongestant* [hydrocodone bitartrate; chlorpheniramine maleate; phenylephrine HCl] 6•2•5 mg/5 mL

Poly-Tussin XP oral liquid ℞ *narcotic antitussive; decongestant; expectorant* [hydrocodone bitartrate; phenylephrine HCl; guaifenesin] 5•10•200 mg/5 mL

polyurethane foam USAN *internal bone splint*

polyvalent Crotaline antivenin [see: antivenin (Crotalidae) polyvalent]

polyvalent gas gangrene antitoxin [see: gas gangrene antitoxin, pentavalent]

Poly-Vent DM caplets OTC *antitussive; decongestant; expectorant* [dextromethorphan hydrobromide; pseudoephedrine HCl; guaifenesin] 15•45•400 mg

Poly-Vent Plus caplets OTC *decongestant; expectorant; analgesic; antipyretic* [pseudoephedrine HCl; guaifenesin; acetaminophen] 45•200•500 mg

polyvidone INN *dispersing, suspending and viscosity-increasing agent* [also: povidone]

Poly-Vi-Flor chewable tablets (discontinued 2008) ℞ *vitamin supplement; dental caries preventative* [multiple vitamins; sodium fluoride; folic acid] ±• 0.25•0.3, ±•0.5•0.3, ±•1•0.3 mg

Poly-Vi-Flor oral drops (discontinued 2008) ℞ *vitamin supplement; dental caries preventative* [multiple vitamins; sodium fluoride] ±•0.25, ±•0.5 mg/mL

Poly-Vi-Flor with Iron chewable tablets (discontinued 2008) ℞ *vitamin/ iron supplement; dental caries preventative* [multiple vitamins & minerals; sodium fluoride; iron; folic acid] ±• 0.25•12•0.3, ±•0.5•12•0.3, ±•1• 12•0.3 mg

Poly-Vi-Flor with Iron oral drops (discontinued 2008) ℞ *vitamin/iron supplement; dental caries preventative* [multiple vitamins & minerals; sodium fluoride; iron] ±•0.25•10, ±•0.5•10 mg/mL

polyvinyl acetate phthalate NF *coating agent*

polyvinyl alcohol (PVA) USP *ophthalmic moisturizer; viscosity-increasing agent*

polyvinyl chloride, radiopaque *oral radiopaque contrast medium for severe constipation*

polyvinylpyrrolidone (PVP) [now: povidone]

Poly-Vi-Sol chewable tablets (discontinued 2008) OTC *vitamin supplement*

[multiple vitamins; folic acid] ±•0.3 mg

Poly-Vi-Sol oral drops (discontinued 2008) OTC *vitamin supplement* [multiple vitamins]

Poly-Vi-Sol with Iron chewable tablets (discontinued 2008) OTC *vitamin/iron supplement* [multiple vitamins; iron; folic acid] ±•12•0.3 mg

Poly-Vi-Sol with Iron oral drops (discontinued 2008) OTC *vitamin/iron supplement* [multiple vitamins; iron] ±•10 mg/mL

Poly-Vitamin oral drops OTC *vitamin supplement* [multiple vitamins]

Polyvitamin Fluoride chewable tablets (discontinued 2008) ℞ *vitamin supplement; dental caries preventative* [multiple vitamins; fluoride; folic acid] ±•0.5•0.3, ±•1•0.3 mg

Polyvitamin Fluoride with Iron chewable tablets (discontinued 2008) ℞ *vitamin/iron supplement; dental caries preventative* [multiple vitamins & minerals; fluoride; iron; folic acid] ± •1•12•0.3 mg

PolyVitamin with Fluoride oral drops ℞ *vitamin supplement; dental caries preventative* [multiple vitamins; fluoride] ±•0.25, ±•0.5 mg/mL (note: one of two products with the same name)

PolyVitamin with Fluoride oral drops ℞ *vitamin/iron supplement; dental caries preventative* [multiple vitamins; iron (as ferrous sulfate); fluoride] ±•10•0.25, ±•10•0.5 mg/mL (note: one of two products with the same name)

Poly-Vitamin with Iron oral drops (discontinued 2008) OTC *vitamin/iron supplement* [multiple vitamins; iron] ±•10 mg/mL

Polyvitamin with Iron and Fluoride oral drops (discontinued 2008) ℞ *vitamin/iron supplement; dental caries preventative* [multiple vitamins; iron; fluoride] ±•10•0.25 mg/mL

Polyvitamins with Fluoride and Iron chewable tablets (discontinued

2007) ℞ *vitamin/iron supplement; dental caries preventative* [multiple vitamins; fluoride; iron; folic acid] ± •0.5•12•0.3 mg

pomegranate *(Punica granatum)* seeds and fruit rind *medicinal herb used as an anthelmintic and astringent*

ponalrestat USAN, INN, BAN *aldose reductase inhibitor*

ponfibrate INN ⧉ binifibrate

Ponstel capsules ℞ *analgesic; nonsteroidal anti-inflammatory drug (NSAID) for mild to moderate pain and primary dysmenorrhea* [mefenamic acid] 250 mg

Pontocaine cream (discontinued 2007) OTC *anesthetic* [tetracaine HCl] 1% ⧉ pentaquine

Pontocaine ointment (discontinued 2007) OTC *anesthetic; antipruritic; counterirritant* [tetracaine; menthol] 0.5%•0.5% ⧉ pentaquine

Pontocaine HCl injection, powder for injection ℞ *local anesthetic for spinal anesthesia* [tetracaine HCl] 0.2%, 0.3%, 1%; 20 mg

Pontocaine HCl oral solution (discontinued 2007) ℞ *mucous membrane anesthetic to abolish laryngeal and esophageal reflex* [tetracaine HCl; chlorobutanol] 2%•0.4%

poplar *(Populus tremuloides)* bark and buds *medicinal herb used as an antiperiodic, balsamic, febrifuge, and stomachic*

poplar, balsam *medicinal herb* [see: balm of Gilead]

poplar, black *medicinal herb* [see: black poplar]

Po-Pon-S sugar-coated tablets (discontinued 2008) OTC *vitamin/mineral supplement* [multiple vitamins & minerals]

Populus balsamifera; P. candicans medicinal herb [see: balm of Gilead]

Populus nigra; P. tremula medicinal herb [see: black poplar]

Populus tremuloides medicinal herb [see: poplar]

poractant alfa BAN *porcine lung extract containing 90% phospholipids for emergency rescue and treatment of respiratory distress syndrome (RDS) in premature infants* (orphan)

porcine islet preparation, encapsulated *investigational* (orphan) *antidiabetic for type 1 patients on immunosuppression*

porfimer sodium USAN, INN *laser light–activated antineoplastic for photodynamic therapy (PDT) of esophageal* (orphan) *and non–small cell lung cancers; used for ablation of high-grade dysplasia in Barrett esophagus patients* (orphan); *investigational* (orphan) *for bladder cancer*

porfiromycin USAN, INN, BAN *antibacterial; investigational* (Phase III, orphan) *antineoplastic for head, neck, and cervical cancers*

Porites spp. natural material [see: coral]

porofocon A USAN *hydrophobic contact lens material* ⧉ parvaquone

porofocon B USAN *hydrophobic contact lens material*

porphobilinogen deaminase, erythropoietic form, recombinant human *investigational* (orphan) *for prophylaxis of acute attacks of intermittent porphyria*

porphobilinogen deaminase, recombinant human *investigational* (orphan) *for treatment of acute attacks of intermittent porphyria*

Porphozyme *investigational* (orphan) *treatment for acute attacks of intermittent porphyria* [porphobilinogen deaminase, recombinant human]

Portagen powder OTC *enteral nutritional therapy* [lactose-free formula]

Portia film-coated tablets (in packs of 21 or 28) ℞ *monophasic oral contraceptive; emergency postcoital contraceptive* [levonorgestrel; ethinyl estradiol] 0.15 mg•30 mcg

posaconazole USAN *broad-spectrum triazole antifungal for the treatment of oropharyngeal candidiasis and prophylaxis of serious invasive fungal infec-*

*tions in immunocompromised patients;
investigational (orphan) for zygomycosis*
posatirelin INN
posedrine [see: benzchlorpropamid]
poskine INN, BAN
Posoril *investigational (orphan) broad-spectrum triazole antifungal for zygomycosis* [posaconazole]
posterior pituitary [see: pituitary, posterior]
Posture tablets OTC *calcium supplement* [calcium (as tribasic calcium phosphate)] 600 mg (1540 mg)
Posture-D film-coated tablets (discontinued 2008) OTC *dietary supplement* [calcium (as phosphate, tribasic); vitamin D] 600 mg•125 IU
Potaba tablets, capsules, Envules (powder for oral solution) ℞ *water-soluble vitamin; "possibly effective" for scleroderma and other skin diseases and Peyronie disease* [aminobenzoate potassium] 500 mg; 500 mg; 2 g
Potasalan oral liquid ℞ *electrolyte replenisher* [potassium (as chloride); alcohol 4%] 20 mEq/15 mL
potash, sulfurated USP *source of sulfides*
potassic saline, lactated NF
potassium *element (K)*
potassium acetate USP *electrolyte replenisher* (10.2 mEq K/g) 2, 4 mEq/mL injection
potassium acid phosphate *urinary acidifier*
potassium alpha-phenoxyethyl penicillin [see: phenethicillin potassium]
potassium alum [see: alum, potassium]
potassium aminobenzoate [see: aminobenzoate potassium]
potassium aspartate [see: L-aspartate potassium]
potassium aspartate & magnesium aspartate USAN *nutrient* 90 mg K• 90 mg Mg oral
potassium benzoate NF *preservative*
potassium benzyl penicillin [see: penicillin G potassium]
potassium bicarbonate USP *pH buffer; electrolyte replacement*
potassium bitartrate USAN

potassium borate *pH buffer*
potassium canrenoate JAN *aldosterone antagonist* [also: canrenoate potassium; canrenoic acid]
potassium carbonate USP *alkalizing agent*
potassium chloride (KCl) USP *electrolyte replenisher* (13.4 mEq K/g) 8, 10, 20 mEq oral; 20, 40 mEq/15 mL oral; 20 mEq/pkt oral; 2, 10, 20, 30, 40, 60, 90 mEq/mL injection
potassium chloride K 42 USAN *radioactive agent*
potassium chloride & sodium bicarbonate & sodium chloride & polyethylene glycol 3350 *hyperosmotic laxative; pre-procedure bowel evacuant* 1.48•5.72•11.2•420 g/bottle
potassium chloride & sodium bicarbonate & sodium chloride & sodium sulfate & polyethylene glycol 3350 *hyperosmotic laxative; pre-procedure bowel evacuant* 2.97• 6.74•5.86•22.74•236, 2.98•6.72• 5.84•22.73•240 g/bottle
potassium citrate USP *electrolyte replacement; urinary alkalizer for nephrolithiasis and hypocitruria prevention (orphan)* 5, 10 mEq oral
potassium citrate & citric acid *investigational (orphan) agent for the dissolution and control of uric acid and cysteine calculi in the urinary tract*
potassium clavulanate & amoxicillin [see: amoxicillin]
potassium clavulanate & ticarcillin [see: ticarcillin disodium]
potassium dichloroisocyanurate [see: troclosene potassium]
potassium gamma hydroxybutyrate (KGHB) [see: gamma hydroxybutyrate (GHB)]
potassium glucaldrate USAN, INN *antacid*
potassium gluconate USP *electrolyte replenisher* 500, 595 mg oral; 20 mEq/15 mL oral
potassium guaiacolsulfonate USP *expectorant* [also: sulfogaiacol]

potassium hydroxide (KOH) NF *alkalizing agent*

potassium hydroxymethoxyben-zenesulfonate hemihydrate [see: potassium guaiacolsulfonate]

potassium iodate *thyroid saturation agent to block the uptake of radioactive iodine after a nuclear accident or attack*

potassium iodide USP *antifungal; expectorant; dietary iodine supplement; thyroid agent; thyroid saturation agent to block the uptake of radioactive iodine after a nuclear accident or attack (orphan)* 1 g/mL oral

potassium mercuric iodide NF

potassium metabisulfite NF *antioxidant*

potassium metaphosphate NF *buffering agent*

potassium nitrate *tooth desensitizer*

potassium nitrazepate INN

potassium para-aminobenzoate (PAB) [see: aminobenzoate potassium]

potassium penicillin G [see: penicillin G potassium]

potassium permanganate USP *topical anti-infective*

potassium phosphate, dibasic (K_2HPO_4) USP *calcium regulator; phosphorus replacement; pH buffer* (11.5 mEq K/g)

potassium phosphate, monobasic (KH_2PO_4) NF *pH buffer; phosphorus replacement* (7.3 mEq K/g)

potassium sodium tartrate USP *laxative*

potassium sorbate NF *antimicrobial/ antiseptic*

potassium tetraborate *pH buffer*

potassium thiocyanate NF

potassium-sparing diuretics *a class of diuretic agents that interfere with sodium reabsorption, thus decreasing potassium secretion*

potato, wild; wild sweet potato vine *medicinal herb* [see: wild jalap]

Potentilla anserina; P. canadensis; P. reptans medicinal herb [see: cinquefoil]

Potentilla tormentilla medicinal herb [see: tormentil]

Potiga tablets ℞ *adjunctive treatment of partial-onset epilepsy in adults* [ezogabine] 50, 200, 300, 400 mg

Povidine ointment, scrub, solution OTC *broad-spectrum antimicrobial* [povidone-iodine] 10%, 5%, 10%

povidone USAN, USP *dispersing, suspending, and viscosity-increasing agent* [also: polyvidone]

povidone I 125 USAN *radioactive agent*

povidone I 131 USAN *radioactive agent*

povidone-iodine USP, BAN *broad-spectrum antimicrobial* 10% topical

powdered cellulose [see: cellulose, powdered]

powdered ipecac [see: ipecac, powdered]

powdered opium [see: opium, powdered]

PowerMate tablets (discontinued 2008) OTC *vitamin/mineral supplement* [multiple vitamins & minerals] ⑦ buramate

PowerSleep tablets OTC *vitamin/mineral supplement; sleep aid* [multiple vitamins & minerals; 5-hydroxytryptophan; L-glutamine; melatonin; valerian] ≛•250•25•0.25•75 mg

PowerVites tablets OTC *vitamin/mineral supplement* [multiple vitamins & minerals; folic acid; biotin] ≛•150• 25 mcg

PPA (phenylpropanolamine) [q.v.]

PPAR (peroxisome proliferator–activated receptor) agonists *a class of agents that increase insulin receptor sensitivity in type 2 diabetes; PPARα agonists are associated with lower triglyceride and higher HDL levels; PPARγ agonists are associated with lower blood glucose levels*

PPD (purified protein derivative [of tuberculin]) [see: tuberculin]

PPG-15 stearyl ether [now: polyoxypropylene 15 stearyl ether]

PPIs (proton pump inhibitors) [q.v.]

PR cream OTC *moisturizer; emollient* [cyclomethicone; dimethicone]

PR Natal 400; PR Natal 430 film-coated tablets + softgels ℞ *prenatal*

vitamin/mineral/calcium/iron/omega-3 supplement [multiple vitamins & minerals; calcium; iron; folic acid + docosahexaenoic acid (DHA)] ☒•200•29•1 mg (tablets) + 400 mg (softgels); ☒•200•29•1 mg (tablets) + 430 mg (softgels) ⑨ Prenatal; pyrantel

PR Natal 400ec; PR Natal 430ec film-coated tablets + enteric-coated softgels ℞ *prenatal vitamin/mineral/calcium/iron/omega-3 supplement* [multiple vitamins & minerals; calcium; iron; folic acid + docosahexaenoic acid (DHA)] ☒•200•29•1 mg (tablets) + 400 mg (softgels); ☒•200•29•1 mg (tablets) + 430 mg (softgels)

PR-1 vaccine *investigational (orphan) antineoplastic for myelodysplastic syndromes and acute or chronic myelogenous leukemia*

PR-122 (redox-phenytoin) *investigational (orphan) emergency rescue for grand mal status epilepticus*

PR-225 (redox-acyclovir) *investigational (orphan) treatment for AIDS-related herpes simplex infections*

PR-239 (redox penicillin G) *investigational (orphan) treatment for AIDS-related neurosyphilis*

PR-320 (molecusol & carbamazepine) *investigational (orphan) emergency rescue for grand mal status epilepticus*

practolol USAN, INN *antiadrenergic (beta-blocker)*

Pradaxa capsules ℞ *anticoagulant for the prevention of stroke, deep vein thrombosis (DVT), or other venous thromboembolism (VTE) following total hip or total knee replacement surgery* [dabigatran etexilate] 75, 150 mg (110 mg available in Europe)

prajmalium bitartrate INN, BAN

pralatrexate *folic acid antagonist; antineoplastic for peripheral T-cell lymphoma*

pralidoxime chloride USAN, USP *cholinesterase reactivator for organophosphate poisoning and anticholinesterase overdose*

pralidoxime iodide USAN, INN *cholinesterase reactivator*

pralidoxime mesylate USAN *cholinesterase reactivator*

pralmorelin dihydrochloride USAN *growth hormone secretagogue*

PramCort cream ℞ *corticosteroidal anti-inflammatory; local anesthetic* [hydrocortisone acetate; pramoxine] 1%•1%

PrameGel gel OTC *anesthetic; antipruritic; counterirritant* [pramoxine HCl; menthol] 1%•0.5%

Pram-HCA anorectal cream ℞ *corticosteroidal anti-inflammatory; local anesthetic* [hydrocortisone acetate; pramoxine] 2.35%•1%

Pramilet FA Filmtabs (film-coated tablets) (discontinued 2008) ℞ *prenatal vitamin/mineral/calcium/iron supplement* [multiple vitamins & minerals; calcium; iron; folic acid] ☒•250•40•1 mg

pramipexole USAN, INN *dopamine agonist for Parkinson disease*

pramipexole dihydrochloride USAN *dopamine agonist for idiopathic Parkinson disease; treatment for primary restless legs syndrome (RLS)* 0.125, 0.25, 0.5, 0.75, 1, 1.5 mg oral

pramiracetam INN *cognition adjuvant* [also: pramiracetam HCl]

pramiracetam HCl USAN *cognition adjuvant* [also: pramiracetam]

pramiracetam sulfate USAN *cognition adjuvant; investigational (orphan) to manage cognitive dysfunction and enhance antidepressant activity*

pramiverine INN, BAN

pramlintide USAN *antidiabetic for types 1 and 2 diabetes; synthetic amylin analogue that slows gastric emptying and decreases hepatic glucose production*

pramlintide acetate USAN *antidiabetic for types 1 and 2 diabetes; synthetic amylin analogue that slows gastric emptying and decreases hepatic glucose production*

pramocaine INN *topical anesthetic*
[also: pramoxine HCl; pramoxine] ⧄
primaquine

pramocaine HCl [see: pramoxine HCl]

Pramosone cream, lotion, ointment
℞ *corticosteroidal anti-inflammatory;
local anesthetic* [hydrocortisone acetate; pramoxine] 1%•1%, 2.5%•1%;
2.5%•1%; 2.5%•1% ⧄ primycin;
promazine

Pramosone E cream ℞ *corticosteroidal
anti-inflammatory; local anesthetic*
[hydrocortisone acetate; pramoxine]
2.5%•1% ⧄ primycin; promazine

pramoxine BAN *topical anesthetic* [also:
pramoxine HCl; pramocaine]

Pramoxine HC anorectal aerosol
foam, cream (discontinued 2007) ℞
*corticosteroidal anti-inflammatory; local
anesthetic* [hydrocortisone acetate;
pramoxine HCl] 1%•1%; 2.5%•1%

pramoxine HCl USP *topical anesthetic*
[also: pramocaine; pramoxine]

**pramoxine HCl & hydrocortisone
acetate** *local anesthetic; corticosteroidal
anti-inflammatory* 1%•2.5% topical

prampine INN, BAN ⧄ Permapen

PrandiMet tablets ℞ *combination antidiabetic for type 2 diabetes that stimulates the release of insulin from the
pancreas, decreases hepatic glucose production, and increases cellular response
to insulin* [repaglinide; metformin]
1•500, 2•500 mg

Prandin tablets ℞ *meglitinide antidiabetic for type 2 diabetes that stimulates
the release of insulin from the pancreas*
[repaglinide] 0.5, 1, 2 mg

pranidipine INN

pranlukast INN, BAN *antiasthmatic*

pranolium chloride USAN, INN *antiarrhythmic*

pranoprofen INN

pranosal INN

praseodymium *element* (Pr)

prasterone INN *synthetic dehydroepiandrosterone (DHEA); investigational
(NDA filed) agent to increase bone
density in patients with systemic lupus*
erythematosus (SLE) *on corticosteroid
therapy*

prasugrel HCl *oral adenosine phosphate
inhibitor to block platelet aggregation in
patients with acute coronary syndrome*
(ACS) (base=92%)

Pravachol tablets ℞ *HMG-CoA
reductase inhibitor for hyperlipidemia,
hypertriglyceridemia, atherosclerosis,
coronary procedures, and recurrent
myocardial infarctions* [pravastatin
sodium] 10, 20, 40, 80 mg

pravadoline INN *analgesic* [also: pravadoline maleate]

pravadoline maleate USAN *analgesic*
[also: pravadoline]

pravastatin INN, BAN *HMG-CoA
reductase inhibitor for hyperlipidemia,
atherosclerosis, coronary procedures,
and recurrent myocardial infarctions*
[also: pravastatin sodium]

pravastatin sodium USAN, JAN *HMG-CoA reductase inhibitor for hyperlipidemia, atherosclerosis, coronary procedures, and recurrent myocardial infarctions* [also: pravastatin] 10, 20, 40,
80 mg oral

Prax lotion, cream OTC *anesthetic* [pramoxine HCl] 1%

praxadine INN

prazarelix acetate USAN *gonadotropinreleasing hormone (GnRH) antagonist
for uterine fibroids, endometriosis, and
prostate cancer*

prazepam USAN, USP, INN *sedative;
anxiolytic*

prazepine INN ⧄ prozapine

praziquantel USAN, USP, INN, BAN *anthelmintic for schistosomiasis (liver
flukes); investigational (orphan) for
neurocysticercosis*

prazitone INN, BAN

prazocillin INN

prazosin INN, BAN *antihypertensive;
alpha₁ blocker* [also: prazosin HCl]

prazosin HCl USAN, USP, JAN *antihypertensive; alpha₁ blocker* [also: prazosin] 1, 2, 5 mg oral

Pre-Attain oral liquid OTC *enteral nutritional therapy* [lactose-free formula]

prebiotics *a class of natural foods, such as inulin and other fructo-oligosaccharides (FOS), that enhances or supports the growth of probiotic (beneficial) bacteria in the digestive system, thereby suppressing the growth of harmful bacteria* [compare to: probiotics]

PreCare chewable tablets ℞ *prenatal vitamin/mineral/calcium/iron supplement* [multiple vitamins & minerals; calcium; iron (as ferrous fumarate); folic acid] ≐•250•40•1 mg

PreCare Conceive film-coated tablets ℞ *pre-conception vitamin/mineral/calcium/iron supplement* [multiple vitamins & minerals; calcium; iron; folic acid] ≐•200•30•1 mg

PreCare Premier film-coated caplets ℞ *prenatal vitamin/mineral/calcium/iron supplement; stool softener* [multiple vitamins & minerals; calcium; iron (as sumalate); folic acid; docusate sodium] ≐•250•30•1•50 mg

PreCare Prenatal film-coated caplet ℞ *prenatal vitamin/mineral/calcium/iron supplement* [multiple vitamins & minerals; calcium; iron (as ferrous fumarate); folic acid] ≐•250•40•1 mg

precatory bean (Abrus precatorius) plant *medicinal herb for eye inflammation, hastening labor, and stimulating abortion; not generally regarded as safe and effective as it is highly toxic and ingestion may be fatal*

Precedex IV infusion ℞ *sedative for intubated and ventilated patients in an intensive care setting; premedication to anesthesia; also used for postanesthetic shivering* [dexmedetomidine (as HCl)] 100 mcg/mL

precipitated calcium carbonate JAN *antacid; dietary calcium supplement* [also: calcium carbonate]

precipitated chalk [see: calcium carbonate]

precipitated sulfur [see: sulfur, precipitated]

Precision High Nitrogen Diet powder OTC *enteral nutritional therapy* [lactose-free formula]

Precision LR Diet powder OTC *enteral nutritional therapy* [lactose-free formula]

preclamol INN

Precose tablets ℞ *antidiabetic agent for type 2 diabetes; alpha-glucosidase inhibitor that delays the digestion of dietary carbohydrates* [acarbose] 25, 50, 100 mg

Pred Mild; Pred Forte eye drop suspension ℞ *corticosteroidal anti-inflammatory* [prednisolone acetate] 0.12%; 1%

Predcor-50 IM injection (discontinued 2008) ℞ *corticosteroid; anti-inflammatory* [prednisolone acetate] 50 mg/mL

Pred-G eye drop suspension ℞ *corticosteroidal anti-inflammatory; antibiotic* [prednisolone acetate; gentamicin sulfate] 1%•0.3%

Pred-G ophthalmic ointment ℞ *corticosteroidal anti-inflammatory; antibiotic* [prednisolone acetate; gentamicin sulfate; chlorobutanol] 0.6%•0.3%•0.5%

prednazate USAN, INN *anti-inflammatory*

prednazoline INN

prednicarbate USAN, INN *corticosteroid; anti-inflammatory* 0.1% topical

Prednicen-M tablets (discontinued 2008) ℞ *corticosteroid; anti-inflammatory; immunosuppressant* [prednisone] 5 mg

prednimustine USAN, INN *investigational (orphan) antineoplastic for malignant non-Hodgkin lymphomas*

Prednisol eye drops (discontinued 2010) ℞ *corticosteroidal anti-inflammatory* [prednisolone (as sodium phosphate)] 1%

Prednisol TBA intra-articular, intralesional, or soft tissue injection (discontinued 2008) ℞ *corticosteroid; anti-inflammatory* [prednisolone tebutate] 20 mg/mL

prednisolamate INN, BAN

prednisolone USP, INN *corticosteroidal anti-inflammatory* 5 mg oral; 15 mg/5 mL oral

prednisolone acetate USP, BAN *corticosteroidal anti-inflammatory* (base= 90%) 1% eye drops

prednisolone hemisuccinate USP *corticosteroidal anti-inflammatory*

prednisolone sodium phosphate USP *corticosteroidal anti-inflammatory* (base=74%) 5, 10, 15, 20, 25 mg/5 mL oral; 1% eye drops

prednisolone sodium succinate USP *corticosteroidal anti-inflammatory*

prednisolone steaglate INN, BAN *corticosteroidal anti-inflammatory*

prednisolone tebutate USP *corticosteroidal anti-inflammatory*

prednisone USP, INN *corticosteroidal anti-inflammatory; immunosuppressant* 1, 2.5, 5, 10, 20, 50 mg oral; 1, 5 mg/mL oral

prednival USAN *corticosteroidal anti-inflammatory*

prednylidene INN, BAN

prefenamate INN

PreferaOB tablets ℞ *prenatal vitamin/ mineral/iron supplement* [multiple vitamins & minerals; folic acid; iron] ±•1•² mg

Prefest tablets (in packs of 30) ℞ *hormone replacement therapy for postmenopausal symptoms* [estradiol; norgestimate] 1•0 mg × 3 days; 1•0.09 mg × 3 days; repeat without interruption

Prefill (delivery form) *prefilled applicator* ℞ Bravelle

Preflex Daily Cleaner Especially for Sensitive Eyes solution OTC *surfactant cleaning solution for soft contact lenses*

pregabalin USAN *gabamimetic anticonvulsant for partial-onset seizures; agent for the management of neuropathic pain from diabetic peripheral neuropathy (DPN), postherpetic neuralgia (PHN), and fibromyalgia; investigational (NDA filed) for generalized anxiety disorder*

pregelatinized starch [see: starch, pregelatinized]

Pregestimil powder OTC *hypoallergenic infant food for severe malabsorption*

disorders [enzymatically hydrolyzed protein formula]

pregnandiol JAN

pregneninolone [see: ethisterone]

pregnenolone INN *natural hormone precursor* [also: pregnenolone succinate]

pregnenolone succinate USAN *hormone precursor* [also: pregnenolone]

Pregnosis slide test for home use OTC *in vitro diagnostic aid; urine pregnancy test* [latex agglutination test]

Pregnyl powder for IM injection ℞ *a human-derived hormone used for prepubertal cryptorchidism or hypogonadism and to induce ovulation in anovulatory women* [chorionic gonadotropin] 1000 U/mL ⊡ proguanil

Prehist sustained-release capsules ℞ *decongestant; antihistamine* [phenylephrine HCl; chlorpheniramine maleate] 20•8 mg

Pre-Hist-D sustained-release tablets ℞ *decongestant; antihistamine; anticholinergic to dry mucosal secretions* [phenylephrine HCl; chlorpheniramine maleate; methscopolamine nitrate] 20•8•2.5 mg

preladenant *investigational (Phase III) treatment for Parkinson disease*

Prelief tablets OTC *calcium/phosphorus supplement* [calcium; phosphorus] 65•50 mg

Prelone syrup ℞ *corticosteroid; anti-inflammatory* [prednisolone; alcohol 5%] 15 mg/5 mL ⊡ Perlane; proline

Prelu-2 timed-release capsules ℞ *CNS stimulant; anorexiant* [phendimetrazine tartrate] 105 mg ⊡ Paral; perilla; Prolia

premafloxacin USAN, INN *veterinary antibacterial*

Premarin tablets ℞ *a mixture of equine estrogens for the prevention and treatment of postmenopausal symptoms; palliative therapy for prostate and breast cancer* [conjugated estrogens] 0.3, 0.45, 0.625, 0.9, 1.25 mg ⊡ Primorine

Premarin Intravenous IV or IM injection ℞ *a mixture of equine estrogens for the treatment of abnormal uter-*

ine bleeding due to hormonal imbalance [conjugated estrogens] 25 mg/vial

Premarin Vaginal cream ℞ *a mixture of equine estrogens for postmenopausal atrophic vaginitis and dyspareunia* [conjugated estrogens] 0.625 mg/g

premazepam INN, BAN ② bromazepam

Premesis Rx film-coated tablets (discontinued 2011) ℞ *prenatal vitamin/ calcium supplement* [vitamins B_6 and B_{12}; calcium (as carbonate); folic acid] 75•0.012•200•1 mg

Premphase tablets (in packs of 28) ℞ *a mixture of equine and synthetic hormones; hormone replacement therapy for postmenopausal symptoms* [conjugated estrogens; medroxyprogesterone acetate]
Phase 1 (14 days): 0.625•0 mg;
Phase 2 (14 days): 0.625•5 mg

Prempro tablets (in packs of 28) ℞ *a mixture of equine and synthetic hormones; hormone replacement therapy for postmenopausal symptoms* [conjugated estrogens; medroxyprogesterone acetate] 0.3•1.5, 0.45•1.5, 0.625•2.5, 0.625•5 mg

Prēmsyn PMS caplets OTC *analgesic; antipyretic; diuretic; antihistamine; sleep aid* [acetaminophen; pamabrom; pyrilamine maleate] 500•25•15 mg

PrenaFirst film-coated tablets ℞ *prenatal vitamin/mineral/calcium/iron supplement* [multiple vitamins & minerals; calcium; iron (as ferrous fumarate); folic acid] ±•200•17•1 mg

Prenaissance softgels ℞ *prenatal vitamin/calcium/iron/omega-3 supplement; stool softener* [multiple vitamins; calcium; iron (as ferrous fumarate); folic acid; DHA; docusate sodium] ±• 160•29•1.25•325•55 mg

prenalterol INN, BAN *adrenergic* [also: prenalterol HCl]

prenalterol HCl USAN *adrenergic* [also: prenalterol]

Prenatabs CBF film-coated tablets ℞ *prenatal vitamin/mineral/calcium/iron supplement* [multiple vitamins & minerals; calcium; iron (as carbonyl); folic acid] ±•200•50•1 mg

Prenatabs FA tablets ℞ *prenatal vitamin/mineral/calcium/iron supplement* [multiple vitamins & minerals; calcium; iron (as ferrous fumarate); folic acid] ±•200•29•1 mg

Prenatabs OBN film-coated tablets ℞ *prenatal vitamin/mineral/calcium/iron supplement* [multiple vitamins & minerals; calcium; iron (as ferrous fumarate); folic acid] ±•200•29•1 mg

Prenatabs RX film-coated tablets ℞ *prenatal vitamin/mineral/calcium/iron supplement* [multiple vitamins & minerals; calcium; iron (as carbonyl); folic acid; biotin] ±•200•29•1• 0.03 mg

Prenatal tablets OTC *prenatal vitamin/ mineral/calcium/iron supplement* [multiple vitamins & minerals; calcium; iron (as ferrous fumarate); folic acid] ±•200•27•0.8 mg ② PR Natal; pyrantel

Prenatal 19 chewable tablets ℞ *prenatal vitamin/mineral/calcium/iron supplement* [multiple vitamins & minerals; calcium; iron (as ferrous fumarate); folic acid] ±•200•29•1 mg ② PR Natal; pyrantel

Prenatal 19 tablets ℞ *prenatal vitamin/ mineral/calcium/iron supplement; stool softener* [multiple vitamins & minerals; calcium; iron (as ferrous fumarate); folic acid; docusate sodium] ± •200•29•1•50 mg ② PR Natal; pyrantel

Prenatal AD film-coated tablets ℞ *prenatal vitamin/mineral/calcium/iron supplement* [multiple vitamins & minerals; calcium; iron (as carbonyl); folic acid] ±•200•90•1 mg

Prenatal-H capsules (discontinued 2009) ℞ *prenatal vitamin/mineral/iron supplement* [multiple vitamins & minerals; iron (as ferrous fumarate); folic acid] ±•106.5•1 mg ② PR Natal; pyrantel

Prenatal H.P. tablets (discontinued 2008) ℞ *prenatal vitamin/calcium/iron*

supplement [multiple vitamins; calcium; iron; folic acid] ± • 50 • 30 • 0.8 mg

Prenatal Maternal tablets (discontinued 2008) ℞ *prenatal vitamin/mineral/calcium/iron supplement* [multiple vitamins & minerals; calcium; iron; folic acid; biotin] ± • 250 • 60 • 1 • 0.03 mg

Prenatal MR 90 film-coated tablets (discontinued 2009) ℞ *prenatal vitamin/mineral/calcium/iron supplement; stool softener* [multiple vitamins and minerals; calcium; iron (as ferrous fumarate); folic acid; dosusate sodium] ± • 250 • 90 • 1 • 50 mg

Prenatal MTR with Selenium film-coated caplets ℞ *prenatal vitamin/mineral/calcium/iron supplement* [multiple vitamins and minerals; calcium; iron (as ferrous fumarate); folic acid; biotin] ± • 200 • 27 • 1 • 0.03 mg

Prenatal PC 40 film-coated caplets (discontinued 2008) ℞ *prenatal vitamin/mineral/calcium/iron supplement* [multiple vitamins and minerals; calcium; iron; folic acid] ± • 250 • 40 • 1 mg

Prenatal Plus tablets (discontinued 2008) ℞ *prenatal vitamin/calcium/iron supplement* [multiple vitamins; calcium; iron; folic acid] ± • 200 • 65 • 1 mg ⍰ Par-Natal Plus

Prenatal Plus Improved tablets (discontinued 2007) ℞ *prenatal vitamin/calcium/iron supplement* [multiple vitamins; calcium; iron; folic acid] ± • 200 • 65 • 1 mg ⍰ Par-Natal Plus

Prenatal Plus Iron tablets ℞ *prenatal vitamin/calcium/iron supplement* [multiple vitamins; calcium; iron; folic acid] ± • 200 • 27 • 1 mg ⍰ Par-Natal Plus

Prenatal Rx 1 tablets (discontinued 2009) ℞ *prenatal vitamin/mineral/calcium/iron supplement* [multiple vitamins and minerals; calcium; iron (as ferrous fumarate); folic acid; biotin] ± • 200 • 60 • 1 • 0.03 mg

Prenatal Rx with Betacarotene tablets (discontinued 2008) ℞ *prenatal vitamin/calcium/iron supplement* [mul-

tiple vitamins; calcium; iron; folic acid; biotin] ± • 200 • 60 • 1 • 0.03 mg

Prenatal-S tablets OTC *prenatal vitamin/calcium/iron supplement* [multiple vitamins; calcium; iron (as ferrous fumarate); folic acid] ± • 200 • 27 • 0.8 mg

Prenatal-U capsules ℞ *prenatal vitamin/mineral/iron supplement* [multiple vitamins & minerals; iron (as ferrous fumarate); folic acid] ± • 106.5 • 1 mg ⍰ PR Natal; pyrantel

Prenatal with Folic Acid tablets (discontinued 2008) OTC *prenatal vitamin/calcium/iron supplement* [multiple vitamins; calcium; iron; folic acid] ± • 200 • 60 • 0.8 mg

Prenatal Z Advanced Formula film-coated tablets (discontinued 2009) ℞ *prenatal vitamin/mineral/calcium/iron supplement* [multiple vitamins and minerals; calcium; iron (as ferrous fumarate); folic acid; hydrogenated oil] ± • 200 • 65 • 1 mg

Prenatal-1 + Iron tablets (discontinued 2008) ℞ *prenatal vitamin/calcium/iron supplement* [multiple vitamins; calcium; iron; folic acid] ± • 200 • 65 • 1 mg

Prenate Advance; Prenate Elite delayed-release film-coated tablets ℞ *prenatal vitamin/calcium/iron supplement* [multiple vitamins; calcium; iron; folic acid] ± • 200 • 90 • 1 mg; ± • 120 • 27 • 1 mg

Prenate DHA softgel ℞ *prenatal vitamin/calcium/iron/omega-3 supplement* [multiple vitamins; calcium; iron (as ferrous fumarate); folic acid; L-methylfolate; docosahexaenoic acid (DHA)] ± • 150 • 27 • 0.4 • 0.6 • 300 mg

PreNate Plus tablets ℞ *prenatal vitamin/mineral/calcium/iron supplement* [multiple vitamins & minerals; calcium; iron; folic acid] ± • 200 • 27 • 1 mg

Prenavite tablets OTC *prenatal vitamin/mineral/calcium/iron supplement* [multiple vitamins and minerals; calcium; iron (as ferrous fumarate); folic acid] ± • 200 • 28 • 0.8 mg

PreNexa capsules ℞ *once-daily prenatal vitamin/mineral/calcium/iron/omega-3 supplement; stool softener* [multiple vitamins and minerals; calcium (as tribasic calcium phosphate); iron (as ferrous fumarate); folic acid; docosahexaenoic acid; docusate sodium] ± •160•30•1.2•265•55 mg

prenisteine INN

prenoverine INN

prenoxdiazine INN

prenylamine USAN, INN *coronary vasodilator*

Preparation H anorectal cream OTC *local anesthetic and astringent for temporary relief of hemorrhoidal symptoms* [pramoxine HCl; phenylephrine HCl; petrolatum; glycerin] 1%•0.25%•15%•14.4%

Preparation H anorectal ointment OTC *emollient and astringent for temporary relief of hemorrhoidal symptoms* [shark liver oil; phenylephrine HCl] 3%•0.25%

Preparation H cleansing tissues OTC *moisturizer and cleanser for external rectal/vaginal areas* [propylene glycol]

Preparation H rectal suppositories OTC *emollient for temporary relief of hemorrhoidal symptoms* [shark liver oil] 3%

Preparation H Cooling Gel OTC *emollient and astringent for temporary relief of hemorrhoidal symptoms* [phenylephrine HCl; hamamelis water (witch hazel); alcohol 7.5%] 0.25%•50%

prepared chalk [see: calcium carbonate]

Prepcat oral suspension ℞ *radiopaque contrast medium for gastrointestinal imaging* [barium sulfate] 1.5%

Pre-Pen solution for dermal scratch test ℞ *diagnostic aid for penicillin hypersensitivity* [benzylpenicilloyl polylysine] 0.25 mL ② propane

Pre-Pen/MDM solution for dermal scratch test *investigational (orphan) agent for penicillin hypersensitivity assessment* [benzylpenicillin]

Prepidil gel ℞ *prostaglandin for cervical ripening at term* [dinoprostone] 0.5 mg ② piribedil

PreserVision Lutein softgel OTC *vitamin/mineral supplement* [vitamins C and E; multiple minerals; lutein] 226 mg•200 IU• ± •5 mg

Prestara *investigational (NDA filed) agent to increase bone density in patients with systemic lupus erythematosus (SLE) on corticosteroid therapy* [prasterone]

pretamazium iodide INN, BAN

prethcamide

prethrombin [see: prothrombin complex, activated]

pretiadil INN

Pretty Feet & Hands cream OTC *moisturizer; emollient*

Pretz solution OTC *nasal moisturizer* [sodium chloride (saline solution)] 0.6% ② protease

Pretz Irrigating solution OTC *for postoperative irrigation* [sodium chloride (saline solution); glycerin; eriodictyon] 0.75%

Pretz Moisturizing nose drops OTC *nasal moisturizer* [sodium chloride (saline solution); glycerin; eriodictyon] 0.75%

Prevacid delayed-release enteric-coated granules in capsules ℞ *proton pump inhibitor for gastric and duodenal ulcers, erosive esophagitis, gastroesophageal reflux disease (GERD), and other gastroesophageal disorders* [lansoprazole] 15, 30 mg

Prevacid delayed-release enteric-coated granules for oral suspension ℞ *proton pump inhibitor for gastric and duodenal ulcers, erosive esophagitis, gastroesophageal reflux disease (GERD), and other gastroesophageal disorders* [lansoprazole] 15, 30 mg

Prevacid 24HR delayed-release enteric-coated granules in capsules OTC *proton pump inhibitor for frequent heartburn* [lansoprazole] 15 mg

Prevacid I.V. powder for infusion (discontinued 2010) ℞ *proton pump inhib-*

itor for erosive esophagitis in hospitalized patients [lansoprazole] 30 mg/vial

Prevacid NapraPAC 375 tablets + capsules in 7-day dose packs (discontinued 2010) ℞ *nonsteroidal antiinflammatory; proton pump inhibitor; treatment for gastric and duodenal ulcers* [naproxen (tablets); lansoprazole (capsules)] 375•15

Prevacid SoluTab (delayed-release enteric-coated granules in orally disintegrating tablets) ℞ *proton pump inhibitor for gastric and duodenal ulcers, erosive esophagitis, gastroesophageal reflux disease (GERD), and other gastroesophageal disorders* [lansoprazole] 15, 30 mg

Prevalite powder for oral suspension ℞ *cholesterol-lowering antihyperlipidemic; treatment for pruritus due to partial biliary obstruction; also used for diarrhea and as an antidote to* Clostridium difficile *and digitalis toxicity* [cholestyramine resin] 4 g/dose

Prevelle Silk subcu injection in prefilled syringes ℞ *dermal filler for deep wrinkles and facial folds; topical anesthetic* [hyaluronic acid; lidocaine]

Preven kit (4 film-coated tablets + a pregnancy test) (discontinued 2008) ℞ (available OTC *from pharmacists in some states*) *emergency postcoital contraceptive* [levonorgestrel; ethinyl estradiol] 0.25•0.05 mg ② paraffin; Privine; Profen

PreviDent dental gel for self-application ℞ *caries preventative* [fluoride (as sodium fluoride)] 0.5% (1.1%)

PreviDent 5000 Plus dental cream for self-application ℞ *caries preventative* [fluoride (as sodium fluoride)] 0.5% (1.1%)

PreviDent Rinse oral solution ("swish and spit") ℞ *dental caries preventative* [sodium fluoride] 0.2%

Previfem tablets (in packs of 28) ℞ *monophasic oral contraceptive* [norgestimate; ethinyl estradiol] 0.25 mg• 35 mcg × 21 days; counters × 7 days

Prevnar IM injection ℞ *active immunization against seven strains of* Streptococcus pneumoniae *in infants and toddlers; investigational (Phase III) for adults over 50 years* [pneumococcal vaccine, 7-valent] 16 mcg total (2–4 mcg of each strain) per 0.5 mL dose

Prevnar 13 IM injection in prefilled syringes ℞ *active immunization against 13 strains of* Streptococcus pneumoniae *in infants and toddlers; investigational for use in adults* [pneumococcal vaccine, 13-valent] 30.8 mcg total (2.2–4.4 mcg of each strain) per 0.5 mL dose

Prevpac three-drug daily pack ℞ *triple therapy for* H. pylori: *an antisecretory and two antibiotics* [lansoprazole (capsules); clarithromycin (tablets); amoxicillin (capsules)] 2 × 30 mg; 2 × 500 mg; 4 × 500 mg

PreVue B. *burgdorferi* **Antibody Detection Assay** reagent kit for professional use ℞ *in vitro diagnostic aid for Lyme disease*

prezatide copper acetate USAN, INN *immunomodulator; investigational (Phase II) wound-healing gel for venous leg ulcers*

Prezista film-coated tablets ℞ *antiretroviral for HIV-1 infections* [darunavir (as ethanolate)] 75, 150, 400, 600 mg

Prialt intrathecal infusion ℞ *calcium-channel blocker; non-narcotic analgesic for intractable pain of cancer or AIDS* [ziconotide acetate] 25, 100 mcg/mL ② pirolate

pribecaine INN

prickly ash (*Xanthoxylum americanum; X. fraxineum*) bark *medicinal herb for fever, mouth sores, poor circulation, ulcers, and wounds*

prickly juniper (*Juniperus oxycedrus*) *medicinal herb* [see: juniper]

prickly pear *medicinal herb* [see: nopal]

pride of China (*Melia azedarach*) root bark and fruit *medicinal herb used as an anthelmintic, astringent, bit-*

ter tonic, emetic, emmenagogue, and purgative

pride weed medicinal herb [see: fleabane; horseweed]

pridefine INN antidepressant [also: pridefine HCl] ⑨ proadifen

pridefine HCl USAN antidepressant [also: pridefine]

prideperone INN

pridinol INN

priest's crown medicinal herb [see: dandelion]

prifelone USAN, INN dermatologic anti-inflammatory ⑨ Prophyllin

prifinium bromide INN

Priftin film-coated tablets ℞ antibacterial for tuberculosis (orphan); investigational (orphan) for AIDS-related Mycobacterium avium complex [rifapentine] 150 mg

prifuroline INN

Priligy ⒠ tablets (available in Finland and Sweden) investigational (NDA filed) selective serotonin reuptake inhibitor (SSRI) for moderate to severe premature ejaculation (PE) [dapoxetine]

priliximab USAN, INN monoclonal antibody for organ transplants and autoimmune lymphoproliferative diseases; investigational (orphan) for multiple sclerosis

prilocaine USAN, INN, BAN topical/local anesthetic

prilocaine HCl USAN, USP topical/local anesthetic [also: propitocaine HCl] 4% injection

prilocaine HCl & epinephrine bitartrate local anesthetic; vasoconstrictor 4%•0.005 mg/mL injection

prilocaine & lidocaine local anesthetic 2.5%•2.5% topical

Prilosec delayed-release enteric-coated granules in capsules, delayed-release granules for oral suspension ℞ proton pump inhibitor for gastric and duodenal ulcers, erosive esophagitis, GERD, and other gastroesophageal disorders [omeprazole] 10, 20, 40 mg; 2.5, 10 mg/pkt

Prilosec OTC delayed-release tablets OTC proton pump inhibitor for acid

indigestion and heartburn [omeprazole (as magnesium)] 20 mg

Prilovix investigational platelet aggregation inhibitor plus a proton pump inhibitor to reduce gastric side effects [clopidogrel; omeprazole] 75•20 mg

PrimaCare AM softgels + PM caplets (discontinued 2011) ℞ prenatal vitamin/mineral/calcium/iron/omega-3 supplement [DHA; EPA; ALA; calcium + multiple vitamins & minerals; calcium; iron (as ferrous asparto glycinate); folic acid; biotin] 260•40•40•150 mg (softgels) + ±•250•30•1•0.035 mg (caplets)

PrimaCare Advantage AM softgels + PM caplets ℞ prenatal vitamin/mineral/calcium/iron/omega-3 supplement [DHA; EPA; ALA + multiple vitamins & minerals; calcium; iron (as ferrous asparto glycinate); folic acid; biotin] 400•175•175 mg (softgels) + ±•250•30•1•0.035 mg (caplets)

PrimaCare ONE capsules ℞ prenatal vitamin/calcium/iron/omega-3 supplement [multiple vitamins; calcium; iron (as carbonyl and ferrous asparto glycinate); folic acid; DHA; EPA; ALA; hydrogenated oil] ±•150•27•1•260•40•30 mg

primachine phosphate [see: primaquine phosphate]

Primacor IV infusion (discontinued 2008) ℞ vasodilator for congestive heart failure [milrinone lactate] 0.2 mg/mL

primaperone INN

primaquine INN antimalarial [also: primaquine phosphate] ⑨ pramocaine

primaquine phosphate USP used to treat malarial symptoms and prevent relapse; investigational (orphan) treatment adjunct to Pneumocystis pneumonia (PCP) infection [also: primaquine] 26.3 mg oral

primaquine phosphate & clindamycin HCl investigational (orphan) for AIDS-associated Pneumocystis pneumonia (PCP)

Primatene Asthma tablets OTC bronchodilator; decongestant; expectorant

[ephedrine HCl; guaifenesin] 12.5•
200 mg

Primatene Mist inhalation aerosol
OTC *sympathomimetic bronchodilator
and vasopressor for bronchial asthma*
[epinephrine] 0.22 mg/spray

Primaxin I.M. powder for injection
R *carbapenem antibiotic* [imipenem;
cilastatin sodium] 500•500 mg

Primaxin I.V. powder for injection R
carbapenem antibiotic [imipenem; cilastatin sodium] 250•250, 500•500 mg

primidolol USAN, INN *antihypertensive;
antianginal; antiarrhythmic*

primidone USP, INN, BAN *anticonvulsant for grand mal, psychomotor, and
focal epileptic seizures; also used for
essential tremor and benign familial
tremor* 50, 250 mg oral

Primlev caplets R *narcotic analgesic;
antipyretic* [oxycodone HCl; aspirin]
5•300, 7.5•300, 10•300 mg

Primorine (trademarked ingredient)
*antioxidant; a proprietary blend of the
nutritional supplements aminobenzoic
acid, vitamin E, and alpha lipoic acid
(ALA); also known as* **Benzamine** ⦾
Premarin

Primsol oral solution R *antibiotic for
otitis media in children and urinary
tract infections in adults* [trimetho-
prim HCl] 50 mg/5 mL

primycin INN ⦾ Pramosone; promazine; puromycin

prince's pine *medicinal herb* [see: pip-
sissewa]

Principen capsules, powder for oral
suspension R *aminopenicillin antibiotic* [ampicillin] 250, 500 mg; 125,
250 mg/5 mL ⦾ pirenzepine

Prinivil tablets R *antihypertensive;
angiotensin-converting enzyme (ACE)
inhibitor; adjunctive treatment for congestive heart failure (CHF)* [lisinopril]
10, 20 mg

prinodolol [see: pindolol]

prinomastat USAN *matrix metallopro-
tease inhibitor*

prinomide INN *antirheumatic* [also: prinomide tromethamine]

prinomide tromethamine USAN *antirheumatic* [also: prinomide]

prinoxodan USAN, INN *cardiotonic*

Prinzide tablets R *combination angiotensin-converting enzyme (ACE) inhibitor and diuretic for hypertension* [lisino-
pril; hydrochlorothiazide] 10•12.5,
20•12.5, 20•25 mg

pristinamycin INN, BAN

Pristiq tablets R *once-daily selective
serotonin and norepinephrine reuptake
inhibitor (SSNRI) for major depressive
disorder (MDD); investigational (NDA
filed) for postmenopausal vasomotor
symptoms; investigational (Phase III)
for fibromyalgia and diabetic peripheral
neuropathy* [desvenlafaxine (as succinate)] 50, 100 mg

privet, Egyptian *medicinal herb* [see:
henna (*Lawsonia*)]

Privigen IM injection R *passive immunizing agent for primary (inherited)
immunodeficiency disorders and immune
thrombocytopenic purpura (ITP); also
used for Guillain-Barré syndrome,
myasthenia gravis, and multiple sclerosis* [immune globulin (IGIV)] 10%
(5, 10, 20 g/dose) ⦾ Brevicon

Privine nasal spray, nose drops OTC
nasal decongestant [naphazoline HCl]
0.05% ⦾ paraffin; Preven; Profen

prizidilol INN, BAN *antihypertensive*
[also: prizidilol HCl]

prizidilol HCl USAN *antihypertensive*
[also: prizidilol]

Pro Fem cream OTC *natural progesterone from soy; hormone replacement
therapy; postmenopausal osteoporosis
preventative* [progesterone USP (in a
liposomal base)] 2.5%

Pro Skin capsules (discontinued 2008)
OTC *vitamin/zinc supplement* [vitamins
A, B_5, C, and E; zinc] 6250 IU•10
mg•100 mg•100 IU•10 mg

proadifen INN *non-specific synergist*
[also: proadifen HCl] ⦾ pridefine

proadifen HCl USAN *non-specific synergist* [also: proadifen]

ProAir HFA inhalation aerosol with a
CFC-free propellant R *sympathomi-

metic bronchodilator [albuterol] 90 mcg/dose

ProAmatine tablets ℞ *vasopressor for orthostatic hypotension (orphan); also used for urinary incontinence* [midodrine HCl] 2.5, 5, 10 mg

proanthocyanidins *natural free radical scavenger found in grape seed extract and pine bark extract* [also: procyanidolic oligomers (PCOs); procyanidins]

Pro-Banthīne tablets (discontinued 2010) ℞ *GI anticholinergic/antispasmodic; adjunctive treatment for peptic ulcers* [propantheline bromide] 7.5, 15 mg

probarbital sodium NF, INN

Probax gel OTC *relief from minor oral irritations* [propolis] 2%

Probec-T tablets (discontinued 2008) OTC *vitamin supplement* [multiple B vitamins; vitamin C] ± • 600 mg

probenecid USP, INN, BAN *uricosuric for gout* 500 mg oral

probenecid & colchicine *treatment for frequent, recurrent attacks of gouty arthritis* [500 • 0.5 mg oral]

probicromil calcium USAN *prophylactic antiallergic* [also: ambicromil]

Pro-Bionate capsules, powder (discontinued 2008) OTC *natural intestinal bacteria; probiotic; dietary supplement; fever blister treatment; not generally regarded as safe and effective as an antidiarrheal* [*Lactobacillus acidophilus*] 2 billion CFU; 2 billion CFU/g

Probiotic Formula capsules OTC *natural intestinal bacteria; probiotic; dietary supplement* [*Lactobacillus acidophilus; L. casei; L. plantarum; L. salavarius; Bifidobacterium lactis*] 2 billion CFU of each

probiotics *a class of natural bacteria, such as* Lactobacillus acidophilus, *that favorably alter the microflora balance in the digestive system; an abundance of probiotic bacteria inhibit the growth of harmful bacteria and promote good digestion* [compare to: prebiotics]

probucol USAN, USP, INN *antihyperlipidemic*

probutate USAN *combining name for radicals or groups* [also: buteprate]

procainamide INN *antiarrhythmic* [also: procainamide HCl]

procainamide HCl USP *antiarrhythmic* [also: procainamide] 100, 500 mg/mL injection

procaine INN *injectable local anesthetic* [also: procaine borate] ⑨ Paracaine; Puregon; pyrrocaine

procaine borate NF *injectable local anesthetic* [also: procaine]

procaine HCl USP *injectable local anesthetic; sometimes used as a treatment for the overall effects of aging such as alopecia, arthritis, cerebral atherosclerosis, hypertension, progressive dementia, and sexual dysfunction* 1%, 2% ⑨ pyrrocaine HCl

procaine penicillin BAN *bactericidal antibiotic* [also: penicillin G procaine]

Pro-Cal tablets OTC *vitamin/mineral/ calcium supplement* [vitamins C and D; calcium; magnesium; potassium] 30 mg • 400 IU • 750 mg • 160 mg • 580 mg

ProcalAmine IV infusion ℞ *peripheral parenteral nutrition* [multiple essential and nonessential amino acids; electrolytes]

Procanbid film-coated extended-release tablets (discontinued 2010) ℞ *twice-daily antiarrhythmic* [procainamide HCl] 500, 1000 mg

procarbazine INN *antineoplastic* [also: procarbazine HCl]

procarbazine HCl USAN, USP *antineoplastic for Hodgkin disease; investigational (orphan) for malignant glioma; also used for other lymphomas, melanoma, brain tumors, and lung cancer* [also: procarbazine]

Procardia capsules ℞ *calcium channel blocker; vasodilator for angina with or without vasospasm; also used for anal fissures and Raynaud phenomenon* [nifedipine] 10, 20 mg ⑨ Periguard

Procardia XL film-coated sustained-release tablets ℞ *coronary vasodilator for angina with or without vasospasm;*

calcium channel blocker for hypertension; also used for anal fissures and Raynaud phenomenon [nifedipine] 30, 60, 90 mg ⊡ Periguard

procaterol INN, BAN *bronchodilator* [also: procaterol HCl]

procaterol HCl USAN *bronchodilator* [also: procaterol]

ProCentra oral liquid ℞ *amphetamine; CNS stimulant* [dextroamphetamine sulfate] 5 mg/5 mL

Prochieve vaginal gel in prefilled applicators (discontinued 2011) ℞ *natural progestin; hormone replacement for secondary amenorrhea; hormone supplementation for assisted reproductive technology (ART) treatments* [progesterone] 4%, 8% (45, 90 mg)

prochlorperazine USP, INN *conventional (typical) phenothiazine antipsychotic for schizophrenia; anxiolytic; antiemetic for nausea and vomiting; also used for acute treatment of migraine headaches* 2.5, 5, 25 mg suppositories; 5 mg/mL injection

prochlorperazine bimaleate *conventional (typical) phenothiazine antipsychotic for schizophrenia; anxiolytic; antiemetic for nausea and vomiting; also used for acute treatment of migraine headaches*

prochlorperazine edisylate USP *conventional (typical) phenothiazine antipsychotic for schizophrenia; anxiolytic; antiemetic for nausea and vomiting; also used for acute treatment of migraine headaches* 5 mg/mL injection

prochlorperazine ethanedisulfonate [see: prochlorperazine edisylate]

prochlorperazine maleate USP *conventional (typical) phenothiazine antipsychotic for schizophrenia; anxiolytic; antiemetic for nausea and vomiting; also used for acute treatment of migraine headaches* 5, 10, 25 mg oral

prochlorperazine mesylate *conventional (typical) phenothiazine antipsychotic for schizophrenia; anxiolytic; antiemetic for nausea and vomiting;*

also used for acute treatment of migraine headaches

procinolol INN

procinonide USAN, INN *adrenocortical steroid*

Pro-Clear capsules ℞ *narcotic antitussive; expectorant* [codeine phosphate; guaifenesin] 9•200 mg ⊡ PruClair

proclonol USAN, INN *anthelmintic; antifungal*

procodazole INN

ProCoMycin ointment OTC *antibiotic; anesthetic* [polymyxin B sulfate; neomycin sulfate; bacitracin; lidocaine] 10 000 U•3.5 mg•500 U•40 mg per g

proconvertin [see: factor VII]

ProCort anorectal cream ℞ *corticosteroidal anti-inflammatory; local anesthetic* [hydrocortisone acetate; pramoxine] 1.85%•1.15% (note: one of two products with the same name)

Procort cream, spray OTC *corticosteroidal anti-inflammatory* [hydrocortisone] 1% (note: one of two products with the same name)

Procrit IV or subcu injection ℞ *hematopoietic to stimulate RBC production for anemia of chronic renal failure, HIV, and chemotherapy (orphan) and to reduce the need for blood transfusions in surgery* [epoetin alfa] 2000, 3000, 4000, 10 000, 20 000, 40 000 U/mL

Proctocort anorectal cream, suppositories ℞ *corticosteroidal anti-inflammatory* [hydrocortisone] 1%; 30 mg

ProctoCream-HC 2.5% anorectal cream ℞ *corticosteroidal anti-inflammatory* [hydrocortisone acetate] 2.5%

ProctoFoam anorectal aerosol foam OTC *anesthetic* [pramoxine HCl] 1%

Proctofoam HC anorectal aerosol foam ℞ *corticosteroidal anti-inflammatory; anesthetic* [hydrocortisone acetate; pramoxine HCl] 1%•1%

Pro-Cute lotion OTC *moisturizer; emollient*

procyanidolic oligomers (PCOs) *natural free radical scavenger found in grape seed extract and pine bark extract* [also: proanthocyanidins; procyanidins]

ProCycle Gold tablets OTC *vitamin/ mineral supplement* [multiple vitamins & minerals; folic acid; biotin] ≜•200•100 mcg

procyclidine HCl USP *anticholinergic; antiparkinsonian; skeletal muscle relaxant* [also: procyclidine]

procymate INN

Procysteine *investigational (orphan) immunomodulator for adult respiratory distress syndrome and amyotrophic lateral sclerosis* [oxothiazolidine carboxylate]

prodeconium bromide INN

Proderm aerosol spray OTC *wound treatment for decubitus ulcers* [castor oil; Peruvian balsam] 650•72.5 mg/ 0.82 mL

prodilidine INN *analgesic* [also: prodilidine HCl]

prodilidine HCl USAN *analgesic* [also: prodilidine]

prodipine INN

Prodium tablets OTC *urinary tract analgesic for relief of pain, burning, urgency, and frequency due to mucosal irritation from surgery, catheterization, endoscopic procedures, or trauma; adjunct to antibacterial agents for urinary tract infection* [phenazopyridine HCl] 95 mg ⊡ Perdiem

prodolic acid USAN, INN *anti-inflammatory*

Prodose AAD (adaptive aerosol delivery) (trademarked delivery device) *oral inhalation solution dispenser*

Prodrin tablets ℞ *cerebral vasoconstrictor and analgesic for migraine and tension headaches* [isometheptene mucate; acetaminophen; caffeine] 130•500•20 mg

pro-drugs *a class of agents which metabolize into a therapeutic or more potent form in the body*

profadol INN *analgesic* [also: profadol HCl]

profadol HCl USAN *analgesic* [also: profadol]

Profasi powder for IM injection (discontinued 2011) ℞ *a human-derived hormone used for prepubertal cryptorchidism or hypogonadism and to induce ovulation in anovulatory women* [chorionic gonadotropin] 500, 1000 U/mL

Pro-Fast HS capsules ℞ *anorexiant; CNS stimulant* [phentermine HCl] 18.75 mg

Pro-Fast SA tablets (discontinued 2009) ℞ *anorexiant; CNS stimulant* [phentermine HCl] 8 mg

Pro-Fast SR capsules (discontinued 2009) ℞ *anorexiant; CNS stimulant* [phentermine HCl] 37.5 mg

Profen II; Profen Forte extended-release tablets (discontinued 2007) ℞ *decongestant; expectorant* [pseudoephedrine HCl; guaifenesin] 45•800 mg; 90•800 mg ⊡ paraffin; Preven; Privine

Profen II DM extended-release caplets (discontinued 2007) ℞ *antitussive; decongestant; expectorant* [dextromethorphan hydrobromide; pseudoephedrine HCl; guaifenesin] 30• 45•800 mg

Profen Forte DM sustained-release caplets (discontinued 2007) ℞ *antitussive; decongestant; expectorant* [dextromethorphan hydrobromide; pseudoephedrine HCl; guaifenesin] 60•90•800 mg ⊡ Parafon Forte

profenamine INN *antiparkinsonian* [also: ethopropazine HCl; ethopropazine]

profenamine HCl [see: ethopropazine HCl]

profexalone INN

Profiber oral liquid OTC *enteral nutritional therapy* [lactose-free formula]

Profilnine SD powder for IV infusion ℞ *systemic hemostatic; antihemophilic for factor IX deficiency (hemophilia B; Christmas disease) (orphan)* [factor IX complex (factors II, IX, and X), human, solvent/detergent treated] (actual number of units is indicated on the vial)

proflavine INN [also: proflavine dihydrochloride]

proflavine dihydrochloride NF [also: proflavine]

proflavine sulfate NF

proflazepam INN

ProFree/GP Weekly Enzymatic Cleaner tablets (discontinued 2010) OTC *enzymatic cleaner for rigid gas permeable contact lenses* [papain]

progabide USAN, INN *anticonvulsant; muscle relaxant*

Progestasert IUD (discontinued 2009) Ŗ *intrauterine contraceptive* [progesterone] 38 mg

progesterone USP, INN *natural progestin; intrauterine contraceptive; hormone replacement for secondary amenorrhea; hormone supplementation for assisted reproductive technology (ART) treatments; investigational (orphan) for in vitro fertilization and embryo transfer* 50 mg/mL injection

progestins *a class of sex hormones that cause a sloughing of the endometrial lining; also used as a hormonal antineoplastic*

proglumetacin INN

proglumide USAN, INN, BAN, JAN *anticholinergic*

Proglycem capsules, oral suspension Ŗ *glucose-elevating agent for hyperinsulinemia due to pancreatic cancer* [diazoxide] 50 mg; 50 mg/mL

Prograf capsules, IV infusion Ŗ *immunosuppressant for liver, kidney, and heart transplants (orphan); investigational (orphan) for graft-versus-host disease* [tacrolimus] 0.5, 1, 5 mg; 5 mg/mL

proguanil INN, BAN *antimalarial; dihydrofolate reductase inhibitor* [also: chloroguanide HCl]

proguanil HCl [see: chloroguanide HCl]

ProHance injection Ŗ *paramagnetic contrast agent for head and neck imaging and to enhance MRIs of the brain, spine, and other CNS tissue* [gadoteridol] 279.3 mg/mL

proheptazine INN

Prohist CF oral liquid Ŗ *antitussive; antihistamine* [chlophedianol HCl; triprolidine HCl] 25•2.5 mg/5 mL

Prohist DM oral drops Ŗ *antitussive; antihistamine; decongestant; for children 2–11 years* [dextromethorphan hydrobromide; brompheniramine maleate; pseudoephedrine HCl] 5•1•12 mg/mL

proinsulin human USAN *antidiabetic*

Prolastin powder for IV infusion Ŗ *enzyme replacement therapy for hereditary alpha$_1$-proteinase inhibitor deficiency, which leads to progressive panacinar emphysema (orphan)* [alpha$_1$-proteinase inhibitor] ≥ 20 mg/mL (500, 1000 mg/vial)

Proleukin powder for IV infusion Ŗ *antineoplastic for metastatic melanoma and renal cell carcinoma (orphan); investigational (orphan) for immunodeficiency diseases, acute myelogenous leukemia (AML), and non-Hodgkin lymphoma* [aldesleukin] 18 million IU/mL

Prolex DH oral liquid Ŗ *narcotic antitussive; expectorant* [hydrocodone bitartrate; potassium guaiacolsulfonate] 4.5•300 mg/5 mL

Prolex DM; Prolex DMX oral liquid Ŗ *antitussive; expectorant* [dextromethorphan hydrobromide; potassium guaiacolsulfonate] 15•300 mg/5 mL; 15•100 mg/5 mL

Prolia subcu injection Ŗ *twice-yearly injection to increase bone density and treat osteoporosis in postmenopausal women and men receiving androgen ablation therapy for prostate cancer* [denosumab] 60 mg ⑫ Paral; perilla; Prelu

proligestone INN

proline (L-proline) USAN, USP, INN *nonessential amino acid; symbols: Pro, P* ⑫ Perlane; Prelone

prolintane INN *antidepressant* [also: prolintane HCl]

prolintane HCl USAN *antidepressant* [also: prolintane]

prolonium iodide INN

Proloprim tablets ℞ *anti-infective; antibacterial* [trimethoprim] 100, 200 mg

ProMACE (prednisone, methotrexate, Adriamycin, cyclophosphamide, etoposide) [with leucovorin rescue] *chemotherapy protocol for non-Hodgkin lymphoma*

ProMACE/cytaBOM (ProMACE [above], cytarabine, bleomycin, Oncovin, mitoxantrone) [with Bactrim antibiotic] *chemotherapy protocol for non-Hodgkin lymphoma*

ProMACE/MOPP (full course of ProMACE, followed by MOPP) *chemotherapy protocol for non-Hodgkin lymphoma*

Promacet tablets ℞ *barbiturate sedative; analgesic; antipyretic* [butalbital; acetaminophen] 50•650 mg

Promacta film-coated tablets ℞ *hematopoietic; once-daily thrombopoietin (TPO) receptor agonist to increase platelet counts in idiopathic thrombocytopenic purpura (ITP)* [eltrombopag] 25, 50 mg

promazine INN *phenothiazine antipsychotic* [also: promazine HCl] ⑨ bromazine; Pramosone; primycin

promazine HCl USP *phenothiazine antipsychotic* [also: promazine]

Promega Pearls (softgels) (discontinued 2008) OTC *dietary supplement* [multiple vitamins & minerals; omega-3 fatty acids (eicosapentaenoic acid and docosahexaenoic acid)] ±• 600 mg (168 mg EPA; 72 mg DHA), ±•1000 mg (280 mg EPA; 120 mg DHA)

promegestone INN

promelase INN

promestriene INN

Prometh VC Plain syrup ℞ *decongestant; antihistamine* [phenylephrine HCl; promethazine HCl; alcohol 7%] 5•6.25 mg/5 mL

Prometh VC with Codeine syrup (discontinued 2007) ℞ *narcotic antitussive; antihistamine; decongestant* [codeine phosphate; promethazine

HCl; phenylephrine HCl; alcohol 7%] 10•6.25•5 mg/5 mL

Prometh with Codeine syrup (discontinued 2007) ℞ *narcotic antitussive; antihistamine* [codeine phosphate; promethazine HCl; alcohol 7%] 10•6.25 mg/5 mL

Prometh with Dextromethorphan syrup (discontinued 2007) ℞ *antitussive; antihistamine* [dextromethorphan hydrobromide; promethazine HCl; alcohol 7%] 15•6.25 mg/5 mL

promethazine INN *phenothiazine antihistamine; antiemetic; antidopaminergic; motion sickness relief* [also: promethazine HCl] ⑨ paramethasone; perimetazine

promethazine HCl USP *phenothiazine antihistamine; antiemetic; antidopaminergic; motion sickness relief* [also: promethazine] 12.5, 25, 50 mg oral; 6.25 mg/5 mL oral; 12.5, 25, 50 mg suppositories; 25, 50 mg/mL injection

promethazine HCl & codeine phosphate *antihistamine; narcotic antitussive* 6.25•10 mg/5 mL oral

promethazine HCl & dextromethorphan hydrobromide *antihistamine; antitussive* 6.25•15 mg/5 mL oral

promethazine HCl & meperidine HCl *narcotic analgesic; sedative* 25• 50 mg oral

promethazine HCl & phenylephrine HCl *antihistamine; decongestant* 5•5, 6.25•5 mg/5 mL oral

promethazine HCl & phenylephrine HCl & codeine phosphate *antihistamine; decongestant; narcotic antitussive* 6.25•5•10 mg/5 mL oral

promethazine teoclate INN *phenothiazine antihistamine*

Promethazine VC syrup ℞ *decongestant; antihistamine* [phenylephrine HCl; promethazine HCl] 5•6.25 mg/5 mL

Promethazine VC with Codeine syrup (discontinued 2007) ℞ *narcotic antitussive; antihistamine; decongestant* [codeine phosphate; promethazine

HCl; phenylephrine HCl; alcohol 7%] 10•6.25•5 mg/5 mL

Promethazine with Dextromethor-phan Cough syrup ℞ *antitussive; antihistamine* [dextromethorphan hydrobromide; promethazine HCl; alcohol 7%] 15•6.25 mg/5 mL

Promethegan suppositories ℞ *antihistamine; sedative; antiemetic; motion sickness relief* [promethazine HCl] 12.5, 25, 50 mg

promethestrol [see: methestrol]

promethium *element (Pm)*

Prometrium softgels ℞ *natural progestin for secondary amenorrhea and to prevent endometrial hyperplasia* [progesterone, micronized] 100, 200 mg

Promit IV injection ℞ *monovalent hapten for prevention of dextran-induced anaphylactic reactions; investigational (orphan) for cystic fibrosis* [dextran 1] 150 mg/mL

ProMod powder (discontinued 2008) OTC *oral protein supplement* [D-whey protein concentrate; soy lecithin] ⊉ Paremyd; PerioMed

promolate INN

promoxolane INN

prompt insulin zinc [see: insulin zinc, prompt]

Promycin *investigational (Phase III, orphan) antineoplastic for head, neck, and cervical cancers* [porfiromycin]

Pronemia Hematinic capsules (discontinued 2008) ℞ *hematinic* [iron (ferrous fumarate); vitamin B_{12}; vitamin C; intrinsic factor concentrate; folic acid] 115•0.015•150•75•1 mg

Pronestyl tablets (discontinued 2008) ℞ *antiarrhythmic* [procainamide HCl] 375, 500 mg

pronetalol INN [also: pronethalol]

pronethalol BAN [also: pronetalol]

Pronto shampoo OTC *pediculicide for lice* [pyrethrins; piperonyl butoxide] 0.33%•4%

Propac powder OTC *oral protein supplement* [whey protein; lactose]

Propacet 100 film-coated tablets (discontinued 2010) ℞ *narcotic analgesic; antipyretic; all products containing propoxyphene were withdrawn from the market in 2010 due to safety concerns* [propoxyphene napsylate; acetaminophen] 100•650 mg

propacetamol INN

propafenone INN, BAN *antiarrhythmic* [also: propafenone HCl]

propafenone HCl USAN *antiarrhythmic* [also: propafenone] 150, 225, 300, 325, 425 mg oral

propamidine INN, BAN

propamidine isethionate *investigational (orphan) eye drops for Acanthamoeba keratitis*

propaminodiphen [see: pramiverine]

propane NF *aerosol propellant* ⊉ Pre-Pen

1,2-propanediol [see: propylene glycol]

propanidid USAN, INN *intravenous anesthetic*

propanocaine INN

propanoic acid, sodium salt hydrate [see: sodium propionate]

2-propanol [see: isopropyl alcohol]

2-propanone [see: acetone]

propantheline bromide USP, INN *GI anticholinergic/antispasmodic; adjunctive treatment for peptic ulcers* 15 mg oral

PROPApH Acne cream OTC *keratolytic for acne* [salicylic acid] 2%

PROPApH Astringent Cleanser topical liquid OTC *keratolytic for acne* [salicylic acid; alcohol] 2%•55%

PROPApH Cleansing; PROPApH Cleansing for Sensitive Skin; PROPApH Cleansing Maximum Strength pads OTC *keratolytic for acne* [salicylic acid] 0.5%; 0.5%; 2%

PROPApH Cleansing for Normal/Combination Skin lotion OTC *keratolytic for acne* [salicylic acid] 0.5%

PROPApH Cleansing for Oily Skin lotion OTC *keratolytic for acne* [salicylic acid] 0.6%

PROPApH Foaming Face Wash topical liquid ℞ *keratolytic cleanser for acne* [salicylic acid] 2%

PROPApH Peel-Off Acne Mask OTC *keratolytic for acne* [salicylic acid] 2%

proparacaine HCl USP *topical ophthalmic anesthetic* [also: proxymetacaine] 0.5% eye drops

proparacaine HCl & fluorescein sodium *topical ophthalmic anesthetic; corneal disclosing agent* 0.5%•0.25% eye drops

propatyl nitrate USAN *coronary vasodilator* [also: propatylnitrate]

propatylnitrate INN *coronary vasodilator* [also: propatyl nitrate]

propazolamide INN

Propecia film-coated tablets ℞ *androgen hormone inhibitor for androgenic alopecia in men* [finasteride] 1 mg

1-propene homopolymer [see: polipropene 25]

propenidazole INN ② parbendazole

propentofylline INN

p-**propenylanisole** [see: anethole]

propenzolate HCl USAN *anticholinergic* [also: oxyclipine]

propericiazine [see: periciazine]

properidine INN, BAN

propetamide INN

propetandrol INN

prophenamine HCl [see: ethopropazine HCl]

Pro-Phree powder OTC *supplement to breast milk* [protein-free formula with vitamins & minerals]

Prophyllin ointment OTC *antifungal; vulnerary; wound deodorant* [sodium propionate; chlorophyll derivatives] 5%•0.0125% ② prifelone

propicillin INN, BAN

propikacin USAN, INN *antibacterial*

Propimex-1 powder OTC *formula for infants with propionic or methylmalonicacidemia*

Propimex-2 powder OTC *enteral nutritional therapy for propionic or methylmalonic acidemia*

Propine eye drops (discontinued 2009) ℞ *antiglaucoma agent* [dipivefrin HCl] 0.1% ② Pre-Pen

propinetidine INN

propiodal [see: prolonium iodide]

propiolactone (β-propiolactone) USAN, INN *disinfectant*

propiomazine USAN, INN *preanesthetic sedative*

propiomazine HCl USP *sedative; analgesic adjunct*

propionic acid NF *antimicrobial; acidifying agent*

propionyl erythromycin lauryl sulfate [see: erythromycin estolate]

propipocaine INN

propiram INN, BAN *narcotic agonist-antagonist analgesic* [also: propiram fumarate]

propiram fumarate USAN *narcotic agonist-antagonist analgesic* [also: propiram]

propisergide INN

propitocaine HCl JAN *topical/local anesthetic* [also: prilocaine HCl]

propiverine INN

propizepine INN

Proplex T powder for IV infusion (discontinued 2009) ℞ *systemic hemostatic; antihemophilic to correct factor VII, factor VIII (hemophilia A), and factor IX (hemophilia B; Christmas disease) deficiencies* [factor IX complex (factors II, VII, IX, and X), human, heat treated] (actual number of units is indicated on the vial)

propofol USAN, INN, BAN *rapid-acting general anesthetic* 1% injection

propolis *natural resin collected from the buds of certain trees by bees and used as an antibiotic, anti-inflammatory, antioxidant, antineoplastic, fungicide, immune system stimulant, and vulnerary*

propoxate INN

propoxycaine INN *local anesthetic* [also: propoxycaine HCl]

propoxycaine HCl USP *local anesthetic* [also: propoxycaine]

propoxyphene HCl USAN, USP *narcotic analgesic for mild to moderate pain; withdrawn from the market in 2010 due to safety concerns* [also: dextropropoxyphene HCl] 65 mg oral

propoxyphene napsylate USAN, USP *narcotic analgesic for mild to moderate pain; withdrawn from the market in 2010 due to safety concerns*

propoxyphene napsylate & aceta-minophen *narcotic analgesic combination; withdrawn from the market in 2010 due to safety concerns* 100•500, 100•650 mg oral

propranolol INN, BAN *antiadrenergic (beta-blocker); antianginal; antiarrhythmic; antihypertensive* [also: propranolol HCl]

propranolol HCl USAN, USP *antiadrenergic (beta-blocker); antianginal; antiarrhythmic; antihypertensive; also used for traumatic brain injury* [also: propranolol] 10, 20, 40, 60, 80, 120, 160 mg oral; 4, 8 mg/mL oral; 1 mg/mL injection

propranolol HCl & hydrochlorothiazide *combination beta-blocker and diuretic for hypertension* 40•25, 80•25 mg oral

Propranolol Intensol oral solution (discontinued 2010) ℞ *beta-blocker; antianginal; antiarrhythmic; antihypertensive* [propranolol HCl] 80 mg/mL

propyl p-aminobenzoate [see: risocaine]

propyl docetrizoate INN, BAN

propyl gallate NF *antioxidant*

propyl p-hydroxybenzoate [see: propylparaben]

propyl p-hydroxybenzoate, sodium salt [see: propylparaben sodium]

N-propylajmalinium tartrate [see: prajmalinum bitartrate]

propylene carbonate NF *gelling agent*

propylene glycol USP *humectant; solvent; moisturizer/lubricant; suspending and viscosity-increasing agent*

propylene glycol alginate NF *suspending agent; viscosity-increasing agent*

propylene glycol diacetate NF *solvent*

propylene glycol ether of methylcellulose [see: hydroxypropyl methylcellulose]

propylene glycol monostearate NF *emulsifying agent*

propylhexedrine USP, INN, BAN *vasoconstrictor; nasal decongestant*

propyliodone USP, INN *radiopaque contrast medium (56.7% iodine)*

propylorvinol [see: etorphine]

propylparaben USAN, NF *antifungal agent; preservative*

propylparaben sodium USAN, NF *antimicrobial preservative*

2-propylpentanoic acid [see: valproic acid]

propylthiouracil (PTU) USP, INN *thyroid inhibitor for Graves disease* 50 mg oral

2-propylvaleramide [see: valpromide]

propylvaleric acid [see: valproic acid]

propyperone INN

propyphenazone INN, BAN

propyromazine bromide INN

Pro-Q foam OTC *skin protectant* [dimethicone; glycerin; parabens

ProQuad powder for subcu injection ℞ *measles, mumps, rubella, and varicella vaccine* [measles, mumps, rubella, and varicella virus vaccine, live attenuated] 0.5 mL/dose

proquamezine BAN [also: aminopromazine]

proquazone USAN, INN *anti-inflammatory*

Proquin XR film-coated extended-release tablets ℞ *broad-spectrum fluoroquinolone antibiotic* [ciprofloxacin (as HCl)] 500 mg

proquinolate USAN, INN *coccidiostat for poultry*

Pro-Red syrup (discontinued 2009) ℞ *narcotic antitussive; antihistamine; sleep aid; decongestant* [hydrocodone bitartrate; pyrilamine maleate; phenylephrine HCl] 2•8.38•5 mg/5 mL

Pro-Red AC syrup ℞ *narcotic antitussive; antihistamine; sleep aid; decongestant* [codeine phosphate; pyrilamine maleate; phenylephrine HCl] 9•8.33•5 mg/5 mL

prorenoate potassium USAN, INN *aldosterone antagonist*

proroxan INN *antiadrenergic (alpha-blocker)* [also: proroxan HCl]

proroxan HCl USAN *antiadrenergic (alpha-blocker)* [also: proroxan]

Proscar film-coated tablets ℞ *androgen hormone inhibitor for benign prostatic* *hyperplasia (BPH); investigational for aggressive prostate tumors* [finasteride] 5 mg

proscillaridin USAN, INN *cardiotonic*

proscillaridin A [see: proscillaridin]

Prosed/DS sugar-coated tablets ℞ *urinary antibiotic; antiseptic; analgesic; antispasmodic* [methenamine; phenyl salicylate; methylene blue; benzoic acid; hyoscyamine sulfate] 81.6•36.2•10.8•9•0.12 mg

ProSight Lutein capsules OTC *vitamin/mineral supplement* [vitamins C and E; multiple minerals; lutein] 60 mg•30 IU•≜•6 mg

ProSobee oral liquid, powder for oral liquid OTC *hypoallergenic infant food* [soy protein formula]

ProSobee LIPIL oral liquid, powder for oral liquid OTC *hypoallergenic infant food fortified with omega-3 fatty acids* [soy protein formula]

ProSom tablets (discontinued 2007) ℞ *benzodiazepine sedative and hypnotic* [estazolam] 1, 2 mg

prospidium chloride INN

prostacyclin [now: epoprostenol]

prostaglandin agonists *a class of antiglaucoma agents that reduce intraocular pressure (IOP) by increasing the outflow of aqueous humor*

prostaglandin E$_1$ (PGE$_1$) [now: alprostadil]

prostaglandin E$_1$ enol ester *investigational (orphan) for advanced chronic critical limb ischemia*

prostaglandin E$_2$ (PGE$_2$) [see: dinoprostone]

prostaglandin F$_{2\alpha}$ (PGF$_{2\alpha}$) [see: dinoprost]

prostaglandin I$_2$ (PGI$_2$) [now: epoprostenol]

prostaglandin X (PGX) [now: epoprostenol]

prostaglandins *a class of agents that stimulate uterine contractions, used for abortions, cervical ripening, and postpartum hemorrhage*

prostalene USAN, INN *prostaglandin*

ProstaScint IV infusion ℞ *radiodiagnostic imaging agent for new or recurrent prostate cancer and its metastases* [capromab pendetide, radiolabeled with indium In 111] 0.5 mg

Pro-Stat 64; Pro-Stat 101 oral liquid OTC *enteral nutritional therapy* [collagen hydrolysate formula] 887 mL and 30 mL single serving ⑦ Periostat

Prosteon tablets OTC *vitamin/mineral/calcium supplement* [cholecalciferol (vitamin D$_3$); vitamin K; multiple minerals] 500 IU•25 mcg•≜

Prostigmin subcu or IM injection (discontinued 2009) ℞ *muscle stimulant for myasthenia gravis; urinary stimulant for postsurgical urinary retention; antidote to neuromuscular blockers* [neostigmine methylsulfate] 1:1000 (1 mg/mL), 1:2000 (0.5 mg/mL), 1:4000 (0.25 mg/mL); 1:400 (2.5 mg/mL) is available in Canada

Prostigmin tablets ℞ *muscle stimulant for myasthenia gravis* [neostigmine bromide] 15 mg

Prostin E2 vaginal suppository ℞ *prostaglandin-type abortifacient* [dinoprostone] 20 mg ⑦ perastine; prazitone

Prostin VR Pediatric IV injection ℞ *vasodilator; platelet aggregation inhibitor* [alprostadil] 500 mcg/mL

prosulpride INN

prosultiamine INN

ProSure oral liquid OTC *enteral nutritional therapy for cancer patients* 8 oz.

protactinium *element (Pa)*

protamine sulfate USP, INN *antidote to heparin overdose* [also: protamine sulphate] 10 mg/mL IV infusion

protamine sulphate BAN *antidote to heparin overdose* [also: protamine sulfate]

protamine zinc insulin (PZI) INN *antidiabetic* [also: insulin, protamine zinc; insulin zinc protamine]

protargin, mild [see: silver protein, mild]

protease *digestive enzyme (digests protein)* [100 IU/mg in pancrelipase; 25 IU/mg in pancreatin]

protease inhibitors *a class of antivirals that block HIV replication*

proteasome inhibitors *a class of antineoplastics*

ProTech First Aid Stik topical liquid OTC *analgesic; antiseptic* [lidocaine; povidone-iodine] 2.5% • 10%

Protectol Medicated topical powder OTC *antifungal* [calcium undecylenate] 15%

Protegra softgels OTC *vitamin/mineral supplement* [vitamins A, C, and E; multiple minerals; grapeseed extract] 5000 IU • 250 mg • 60 IU • 50 mg

Protegra Cardio softgels OTC *vitamin/mineral/EFA supplement* [multiple vitamins & minerals; omega-3 fatty acids (eicosapentaenoic acid and docosahexaenoic acid)] $\pm$ • 250 mg (45 mg EPA; 30 mg DHA)

protein C concentrate (human) *thrombolytic; replacement therapy for severe congenital protein C deficiency in children and adults to prevent or treat thrombosis, pulmonary emboli, and purpura fulminans (orphan)*

protein hydrolysate USP *fluid and nutrient replenisher*

α_1-**proteinase inhibitor** [see: alpha$_1$-proteinase inhibitor]

Protenate IV infusion $\mathbb{R}$ *blood volume expander for shock due to burns, trauma, and surgery* [plasma protein fraction] 5%

proterguride INN

protheobromine INN

prothionamide BAN [also: protionamide]

prothipendyl INN

prothipendyl HCl [see: prothipendyl]

prothixene INN

prothrombin complex, activated BAN

ProTime test kit for home use OTC *in vitro diagnostic aid for the management of anticoagulation therapy*

protiofate INN

protionamide INN [also: prothionamide]

protirelin USAN, INN, BAN *prothyrotropin; diagnostic aid for thyroid function;* *investigational (orphan) for infant respiratory distress syndrome of prematurity and amyotrophic lateral sclerosis*

protizinic acid INN

protokylol HCl

proton pump inhibitors (PPIs) *a class of gastric antisecretory agents that inhibit the ATPase "proton pump" within the gastric parietal cell* [also called: ATPase inhibitors; substituted benzimidazoles]

Protonix delayed-release tablets, enteric-coated delayed-release granules for oral suspension $\mathbb{R}$ *proton pump inhibitor for erosive esophagitis associated with gastroesophageal reflux disease (GERD) and Zollinger-Ellison syndrome* [pantoprazole (as sodium)] 20, 40 mg; 40 mg/pkt

Protonix I.V. powder for infusion $\mathbb{R}$ *proton pump inhibitor for erosive esophagitis associated with gastroesophageal reflux disease (GERD) and Zollinger-Ellison syndrome* [pantoprazole (as sodium)] 40 mg/vial

Protopam Chloride powder for IV injection $\mathbb{R}$ *antidote to organophosphate poisoning and anticholinesterase overdose* [pralidoxime chloride] 1 g

Protopic ointment $\mathbb{R}$ *treatment for moderate to severe atopic dermatitis; also used for vitiligo and psoriasis* [tacrolimus] 0.03%, 0.1%

Protostat tablets $\mathbb{R}$ *antibiotic; antiprotozoal; amebicide* [metronidazole] 250, 500 mg

protoveratrine A

Protox *investigational (orphan) for toxoplasmosis of AIDS* [poloxamer 331]

protriptyline INN *tricyclic antidepressant* [also: protriptyline HCl]

protriptyline HCl USAN, USP *tricyclic antidepressant* [also: protriptyline] 5, 10 mg oral

prourokinase [see: saruplase]

Provenge suspension for IV infusion $\mathbb{R}$ *autologous cellular immunotherapy antineoplastic (theraccine) for metastatic castrate-resistant (hormone-refractory) prostate cancer (CRPC)* [sipuleucel-T] 50 million autologous CD54 cells/dose

Proventil inhalation aerosol (discontinued 2008) ℞ *sympathomimetic bronchodilator* [albuterol] 90 mcg/dose

Proventil solution for inhalation ℞ *sympathomimetic bronchodilator* [albuterol sulfate] 0.5% (5 mg/mL)

Proventil tablets, syrup (discontinued 2010) ℞ *sympathomimetic bronchodilator* [albuterol sulfate] 2, 4 mg; 4 mg; 2 mg/5 mL

Proventil HFA inhalation aerosol with a CFC-free propellant ℞ *sympathomimetic bronchodilator* [albuterol] 90 mcg/dose

Provera tablets ℞ *synthetic progestin for secondary amenorrhea, abnormal uterine bleeding, and endometrial hyperplasia* [medroxyprogesterone acetate] 2.5, 5, 10 mg

Provigil caplets ℞ *analeptic for excessive daytime sleepiness due to narcolepsy (orphan), obstructive sleep apnea, or shift work sleep disorder (SWSD); also used for fatigue associated with multiple sclerosis* [modafinil] 100, 200 mg ⊠ Pravachol

Proviron *brand name for mesterolone, an androgen abused with anabolic steroid street drugs*

ProVisc prefilled syringes ℞ *cohesive viscoelastic agent for ophthalmic surgery* [hyaluronate sodium] 10 mg/mL

provitamin A [see: beta carotene]

Provocholine powder for inhalation solution ℞ *bronchoconstrictor for in vivo pulmonary function challenge test* [methacholine chloride] 100 mg/5 mL

proxazole USAN, INN *smooth muscle relaxant; analgesic; anti-inflammatory*

proxazole citrate USAN *smooth muscle relaxant; analgesic; anti-inflammatory*

proxetil INN *combining name for radicals or groups*

proxibarbal INN

proxibutene INN

proxicromil USAN, INN *antiallergic*

proxifezone INN

proxorphan INN *analgesic; antitussive* [also: proxorphan tartrate]

proxorphan tartrate USAN *analgesic; antitussive* [also: proxorphan]

proxymetacaine INN, BAN *topical ophthalmic anesthetic* [also: proparacaine HCl]

proxymetacaine HCl [see: proparacaine HCl]

proxyphylline INN, BAN

Prozac Pulvules (capsules), oral solution ℞ *selective serotonin reuptake inhibitor (SSRI) for major depressive disorder, obsessive-compulsive disorder, bulimia nervosa, premenstrual dysphoric disorder, and panic disorder; investigational (orphan) for autism and body dysmorphic disorder* [fluoxetine HCl] 10, 20, 40 mg; 20 mg/5 mL

Prozac tablets (discontinued 2008) ℞ *selective serotonin reuptake inhibitor (SSRI) for major depressive disorder (MDD), obsessive-compulsive disorder (OCD), bulimia nervosa, premenstrual dysphoric disorder (PMDD), and panic disorder; investigational (orphan) for autism* [fluoxetine HCl] 10 mg

Prozac Weekly enteric-coated delayed-release pellets in capsules ℞ *selective serotonin reuptake inhibitor (SSRI) for major depressive disorder (MDD), obsessive-compulsive disorder (OCD), and bulimia nervosa; once-weekly dosing for maintenance* [fluoxetine HCl] 90 mg

prozapine INN ⊠ prazepine

Prozine-50 IM injection ℞ *conventional (typical) antipsychotic* [promazine HCl] 50 mg/mL

prucalopride HCl USAN *prokinetic agent for severe constipation*

prucalopride succinate USAN *prokinetic agent for severe constipation*

PruClair cream ℞ *antipruritic; moisturizer; emollient* [Butyrospermum parkii; glyceryl; PEG] ⊠ Pro-Clear

Prudoxin cream ℞ *antihistamine; antipruritic* [doxepin HCl] 5% ⊠ pyridoxine

prulifloxacin *investigational (Phase III) oral antibiotic for traveler's diarrhea*

PruMyx cream ℞ *moisturizer; emollient*

Prunella vulgaris *medicinal herb* [see: woundwort]

Prunus africana *medicinal herb* [see: pygeum]

Prunus americana; P. domestica; P. spinosa *medicinal herb* [see: plum]

Prunus amygdalus *medicinal herb* [see: almond]

Prunus armeniaca *medicinal herb* [see: apricot]

Prunus persica *medicinal herb* [see: peach]

Prunus serotina *medicinal herb* [see: wild black cherry]

Prunus virginiana *medicinal herb* [see: wild cherry]

PSE (pseudoephedrine HCl) [q.v.]

PSE 120/MSC 2.5 sustained-release tablets ℞ *decongestant; anticholinergic to dry mucosal secretions* [pseudoephedrine HCl; methscopolamine nitrate] 120•2.5 mg

PSE 15/CPM 2 chewable tablets ℞ *decongestant; antihistamine* [pseudoephedrine HCl; chlorpheniramine maleate] 15•2 mg

PSE Brom DM syrup ℞ *antitussive; antihistamine; decongestant* [dextromethorphan hydrobromide; brompheniramine maleate; pseudoephedrine HCl] 30•4•60 mg/5 mL

PSE CPM chewable tablets ℞ *decongestant; antihistamine* [pseudoephedrine HCl; chlorpheniramine maleate] 15•2 mg

PSE-BPM oral liquid ℞ *decongestant; antihistamine* [pseudoephedrine HCl; brompheniramine maleate] 60•4 mg/5 mL

Pseudo Carb Pediatric oral liquid ℞ *decongestant; antihistamine* [pseudoephedrine HCl; carbinoxamine maleate] 12.5•2 mg/5 mL

Pseudo CM TR timed-release tablets (discontinued 2007) ℞ *decongestant; antihistamine; anticholinergic to dry mucosal secretions* [pseudoephedrine HCl; chlorpheniramine maleate; methscopolamine nitrate] 120•8•2.5 mg

Pseudo Cough oral liquid OTC *antitussive; decongestant; expectorant* [dextromethorphan hydrobromide; pseudoephedrine HCl; guaifenesin] 15•32•175 mg/5 mL

Pseudo-Carb DM Pediatric oral liquid ℞ *antitussive; antihistamine; decongestant; for adults and children ≥ 18 months* [dextromethorphan hydrobromide; carbinoxamine maleate; pseudoephedrine HCl] 15•3•12.5 mg/5 mL

pseudoephedrine INN, BAN *vasoconstrictor; nasal decongestant* [also: pseudoephedrine HCl]

pseudoephedrine HCl USAN, USP *vasoconstrictor; nasal decongestant* [also: pseudoephedrine] 30, 60, 120 mg oral; 30 mg/5 mL oral

pseudoephedrine HCl & brompheniramine maleate *decongestant; antihistamine* 7.5•1, 60•4 mg/5 mL oral

pseudoephedrine HCl & brompheniramine maleate & hydrocodone bitartrate *decongestant; antihistamine; narcotic antitussive* 30•3•2.5 mg/5 mL oral

pseudoephedrine HCl & carbinoxamine maleate & hydrocodone bitartrate *nasal decongestant; antihistamine; antitussive* 30•2•5 mg/5 mL oral

pseudoephedrine HCl & chlorpheniramine maleate *decongestant; antihistamine* 100•12, 120•8, 120•12 mg oral

pseudoephedrine HCl & chlorpheniramine maleate & dextromethorphan hydrobromide *decongestant; antihistamine; antitussive* 30•4•30 mg oral

pseudoephedrine HCl & dextromethorphan hydrobromide & guaifenesin *decongestant; antitussive; expectorant* 90•60•800 mg oral

pseudoephedrine HCl & fexofenadine HCl *decongestant and antihista-*

mine combination for *allergic rhinitis* 120•60, 240•180 mg oral

pseudoephedrine HCl & guaifenesin *decongestant; expectorant* 45•800, 48•595, 50•1200, 60•500, 85•795, 90•800 mg oral

pseudoephedrine HCl & triprolidine HCl *decongestant; antihistamine* 60•2.5 mg/10 mL oral

pseudoephedrine polistirex USAN *nasal decongestant*

pseudoephedrine sulfate USAN, USP *bronchodilator; nasal decongestant*

pseudoephedrine sulfate & desloratadine *decongestant; antihistamine* 240•5 mg oral

pseudoephedrine tannate *bronchodilator; nasal decongestant*

pseudoephedrine tannate & chlorpheniramine tannate *decongestant; antihistamine*

Pseudomonas aeruginosa **purified extract** *investigational (orphan) agent to increase platelet count in immune thrombocytopenic purpura*

Pseudomonas **immune globulin** [see: mucoid exopolysaccharide *Pseudomonas* hyperimmune globulin]

pseudomonic acid A [see: mupirocin]

Pseudovent dual-release capsules (discontinued 2008) ℞ *decongestant; expectorant* [pseudoephedrine HCl (extended release); guaifenesin (immediate release)] 120•250 mg

Pseudovent-PED dual-release capsules ℞ *decongestant; expectorant* [pseudoephedrine HCl (extended release); guaifenesin (immediate release)] 60•300 mg

psilocin *a hallucinogenic street drug closely related to psilocybin* ⃞ Salacyn; Selsun; xylazine

psilocybin BAN *a hallucinogenic street drug derived from the* Psilocybe mexicana *mushroom* [also: psilocybine] ⃞ Soluspan

psilocybine INN *a hallucinogenic street drug derived from the* Psilocybe mexicana *mushroom* [also: psilocybin] ⃞ Soluspan

psoralens *a class of oral or topical skin photosensitizing agents used with ultraviolet A light (320–400 nm wavelength) for the treatment of severe recalcitrant psoriasis*

Psor-a-set bar OTC *keratolytic skin cleanser* [salicylic acid] 2%

Psorcon E cream, ointment ℞ *corticosteroidal anti-inflammatory* [diflorasone diacetate] 0.05%

Psorent topical liquid OTC *antipsoriatic; antiseptic* [coal tar] 2.3%

Psoriatec cream (discontinued 2009) ℞ (available OTC in Canada as **Micanol**) *antipsoriatic* [anthralin] 1% ⃞ Zyrtec

psyllium *(Plantago ovata) medicinal herb* [see: plantain]

psyllium husk USP *bulk laxative* ⃞ Sulmasque

psyllium hydrocolloid *bulk laxative*

psyllium hydrophilic mucilloid *bulk laxative*

psyllium seed [see: plantago seed]

P-Tann D oral suspension (discontinued 2008) ℞ *decongestant; antihistamine* [phenylephrine tannate; chlorpheniramine tannate] 10•8 mg/5 mL

PTC (plasma thromboplastin component) [see: factor IX]

P.T.E.-4 IV injection (discontinued 2010) ℞ *intravenous nutritional therapy* [multiple trace elements (metals)]

P.T.E.-5 IV injection (discontinued 2008) ℞ *intravenous nutritional therapy* [multiple trace elements (metals)]

pterins *a class of investigational antineoplastics*

pteroyldiglutamic acid (PDGA)

pteroylglutamic acid (PGA) [see: folic acid]

P-Tex oral suspension ℞ *antihistamine* [brompheniramine tannate] 10 mg/5 mL

PTFE (polytetrafluoroethylene) [see: polytef]

PTU (propylthiouracil) [q.v.]

Pt/VM (Platinol, VM-26) *chemotherapy protocol for pediatric neuroblastoma*

ptyalagogues *a class of agents that stimulate the secretion of saliva* [also called: sialagogues]

puccoon, yellow *medicinal herb* [see: goldenseal]

Pueraria lobata; P. thunbergiana *medicinal herb* [see: kudzu]

puffball *medicinal herb* [see: dandelion]

Pulexn DM syrup (discontinued 2007) ℞ *antitussive; expectorant* [dextromethorphan hydrobromide; guaifenesin] 20•200 mg/10 mL

Pulmicort Flexhaler (dry powder in a metered-dose inhaler) ℞ *corticosteroidal anti-inflammatory for chronic asthma* [budesonide] 80, 160 mcg/dose

Pulmicort Respules (single-dose ampule for inhalation) ℞ *corticosteroidal anti-inflammatory for chronic asthma in children* [budesonide] 0.25, 0.5, 1 mg

Pulmicort Turbuhaler (dry powder in a metered-dose inhaler) (discontinued 2009) ℞ *corticosteroidal anti-inflammatory for chronic asthma* [budesonide] 160 mcg/dose

Pulmocare ready-to-use oral liquid OTC *enteral nutritional therapy for pulmonary problems* [lactose-free formula] 240 mL, 1 L

PulmoLAR *investigational (orphan) for pulmonary arterial hypertension (PAH)* [2-methoxyestradiol]

Pulmonaria officinalis *medicinal herb* [see: lungwort]

pulmonary surfactant replacement, porcine [now: poractant alfa]

Pulmozyme solution for inhalation ℞ *mucolytic to reduce viscoelasticity of sputum in cystic fibrosis patients (orphan)* [dornase alfa] 1 mg/mL

pulse VAC (vincristine, Adriamycin, cyclophosphamide) *chemotherapy protocol for sarcomas* [also: VAC; VAC pulse]

PulsePak (trademarked packaging form) *one-week dosage pack*

Pulvule (trademarked dosage form) *bullet-shaped capsule*

Pulzium *investigational (NDA filed) antiarrhythmic for atrial fibrillation* [tedisamil]

pumice USP *dental abrasive*

pumitepa INN

Punctum Plug ℞ *blocks the puncta and canaliculus to eliminate tear loss in keratitis sicca* [silicone plug]

Punica granatum *medicinal herb* [see: pomegranate]

Puralube ophthalmic ointment (discontinued 2010) OTC *ocular moisturizer/lubricant* [white petrolatum; mineral oil]

Puralube Tears eye drops OTC *moisturizer/lubricant* [polyvinyl alcohol; polyethylene glycol 400] 1%•1%

Pure C 500 tablets OTC *vitamin supplement* [vitamin C] 500 mg

purgatives *a class of agents that cause vigorous evacuation of the bowels by increasing bulk, stimulating peristaltic action, etc.* [also called: cathartics]

Purge oral liquid (discontinued 2009) OTC *stimulant laxative* [castor oil] 95% ▢ borage

Puricase *investigational (Phase III, orphan) uricase enzyme for hyperuricemia due to severe gout* [pegloticase]

purified cotton [see: cotton, purified]

purified protein derivative (PPD) of tuberculin [see: tuberculin]

purified rayon [see: rayon, purified]

purified siliceous earth [see: siliceous earth, purified]

purified water [see: water, purified]

H-purin-6-amine [see: adenine]

Purinethol tablets ℞ *antimetabolite antineoplastic for acute lymphocytic, lymphoblastic, myelogenous, and myelomonocytic leukemias* [mercaptopurine] 50 mg ▢ PR Natal; Prenatal; pyrantel

puromycin USAN, INN *antineoplastic; antiprotozoal (Trypanosoma)* ▢ primycin

puromycin HCl USAN *antineoplastic; antiprotozoal (Trypanosoma)*

purple angelica *medicinal herb* [see: angelica]

purple boneset *medicinal herb* [see: boneset]

purple cone flower *medicinal herb* [see: echinacea]

purple leptandra *medicinal herb* [see: Culver root]

Purpose Alpha Hydroxy Moisture lotion, cream OTC *moisturizer; emollient; exfoliant* [glycolic acid] 8%

Purpose Dry Skin cream OTC *moisturizer; emollient*

Purpose Soap bar OTC *therapeutic skin cleanser*

purshiana bark *medicinal herb* [see: cascara sagrada]

purslain, water *medicinal herb* [see: brooklime]

purvain *medicinal herb* [see: blue vervain]

pussywillow *medicinal herb* [see: willow]

PUVA *an acronym for psoralens (P) and ultraviolet A (UVA) light, used as a treatment for severe recalcitrant psoriasis* [see: psoralens; methoxsalen]

PVA (polyvinyl alcohol) [q.v.]

PVA (prednisone, vincristine, asparaginase) *chemotherapy protocol for acute lymphocytic leukemia (ALL)*

PVB (Platinol, vinblastine, bleomycin) *chemotherapy protocol for testicular cancer and adenocarcinoma*

PVC (polyvinyl chloride) [see: polyvinyl chloride, radiopaque]

PVDA (prednisone, vincristine, daunorubicin, asparaginase) [with Bactrim antibiotic] *chemotherapy protocol for acute lymphocytic leukemia (ALL)*

PVP (polyvinylpyrrolidone) [now: povidone]

PVS Basics ℞ *hydrophobic contact lens material* [paflufocon E]

P-V-Tussin caplets (discontinued 2009) ℞ *narcotic antitussive; antihistamine* [hydrocodone bitartrate; pseudoephedrine HCl] 5•60 mg

P-V-Tussin syrup (discontinued 2009) ℞ *narcotic antitussive; antihistamine; decongestant* [hydrocodone bitartrate; chlorpheniramine maleate; pseudo-

ephedrine HCl; alcohol 5%] 2.5•2•30 mg/5 mL

Pycnanthemum virginianum *medicinal herb* [see: wild hyssop]

Pycnogenol OTC *natural free radical scavenger* [pine bark extract]

pygeum *(Prunus africana; Pygeum africanum)* bark *medicinal herb for prostate gland enlargement and urinary disorders* ℞ PCM

Pylera capsules ℞ *triple therapy for the eradication of H. pylori infections* [bismuth subcitrate potassium; metronidazole; tetracycline HCl] 140•125•125 mg

Pylori-Check test kit for professional use ℞ *in vivo diagnostic aid for H. pylori in the breath*

Pyloriset reagent kit for professional use ℞ *in vitro diagnostic aid for GI disorders*

pyrabrom USAN *antihistamine*

pyradone [see: aminopyrine]

Pyramax *investigational artemisinin-based therapy for malaria; effective against both Plasmodium falciparum and P. vivax* [pyronaridine artesunate]

pyrantel INN *anthelmintic for ascariasis (roundworm) and enterobiasis (pinworm)* [also: pyrantel pamoate] ℞ PR Natal; Prenatal

pyrantel pamoate USAN, USP *anthelmintic for ascariasis (roundworm) and enterobiasis (pinworm)* (base=34.7%) [also: pyrantel]

pyrantel tartrate USAN *anthelmintic*

pyrathiazine HCl [see: parathiazine]

pyrazinamide (PZA) USP, INN, BAN *bactericidal; primary tuberculostatic* 500 mg oral

pyrazinecarboxamide [see: pyrazinamide]

pyrazofurin USAN *antineoplastic* [also: pirazofurin]

pyrazoline [see: antipyrine]

pyrazolopyrimidines *a class of sedative/hypnotics with rapid onset and short duration of action, used in the short-term treatment of insomnia*

pyrbenzindole [see: benzindopyrine HCl]

pyrbuterol HCl [see: pirbuterol HCl]

Pyrelle H.B. caplets (discontinued 2011) ℞ *urinary analgesic; antispasmodic; sedative* [phenazopyridine HCl; hyoscyamine hydrobromide; butabarbital] 150•0.3•15 mg

pyrethrins *a class of natural pesticides derived from pyrethrum flowers, especially* Chrysanthemum cinerariaefolium *and* C. coccineum

Pyrethrum parthenium medicinal herb [see: feverfew]

pyricarbate INN [also: pyridinol carbamate]

Pyrichlor PE oral liquid ℞ *decongestant; antihistamine; sleep aid* [phenylephrine HCl; chlorpheniramine maleate; pyrilamine maleate] 10•2•10 mg/10 mL

pyridarone INN

4-pyridinamine [see: fampridine]

2-pyridine aldoxime methylchloride (2-PAM) [see: pralidoxime chloride]

3-pyridine carboxamide [see: niacinamide; nicotinamide]

3-pyridinecarboxylic acid [see: niacin]

4-pyridinecarboxylic acid hydrazide [see: isoniazid]

3-pyridinecarboxylic acid methyl ester [see: methyl nicotinate]

3-pyridinemethanol [see: nicotinyl alcohol]

2-pyridinemethanol [see: piconol]

3-pyridinemethanol tartrate [see: nicotinyl tartrate]

pyridinol carbamate JAN [also: pyricarbate]

Pyridium tablets ℞ *urinary tract analgesic for relief of pain, burning, urgency, and frequency due to mucosal irritation from surgery, catheterization, endoscopic procedures, or trauma; adjunct to antibacterial agents for urinary tract infection* [phenazopyridine HCl] 100, 200 mg ℞ Baridium; Perdiem; Prodium

Pyridium Plus tablets ℞ *urinary analgesic; antispasmodic; sedative* [phenazo-

pyridine HCl; hyoscyamine hydrobromide; butabarbital] 150•0.3•15 mg

pyridofylline INN

pyridostigmine bromide USP, INN *anticholinesterase muscle stimulant for myasthenia gravis; antidote to muscle relaxants* 60 mg oral

pyridoxal-5'-phosphate [see: pyridoxine HCl]

pyridoxamine [see: pyridoxine HCl]

pyridoxine (vitamin B₆) INN *water-soluble vitamin; enzyme cofactor* [also: pyridoxine HCl] ℞ Prudoxin

pyridoxine HCl (vitamin B₆) USP *water-soluble vitamin; enzyme cofactor; treatment for vitamin B₆ deficiency; also used for hydrazine poisoning, premenstrual syndrome (PMS), oxalate kidney stones, pregnancy-related nausea and vomiting, and carpal tunnel syndrome* [also: pyridoxine] 50, 100, 250, 500 mg oral; 100 mg/mL injection

β-pyridylcarbinol [see: nicotinyl alcohol]

pyridylmethanol *me+* [see: nicotinyl alcohol]

Pyril DM oral suspension ℞ *antitussive; decongestant; antihistamine; sleep aid* [dextromethorphan hydrobromide; phenylephrine HCl; pyrilamine maleate] 15•5•16 mg/5 mL

pyrilamine maleate USP *anticholinergic; nonselective ethylenediamine antihistamine; sleep aid* [also: mepyramine]

pyrilamine tannate USP *anticholinergic; nonselective ethylenediamine antihistamine; sleep aid* [also: mepyramine]

pyrilamine tannate & dextromethorphan tannate & phenylephrine tannate *antihistamine; sleep aid; antitussive; decongestant* 15.5•25•15.5 mg/5 mL oral

pyrilamine tannate & phenylephrine tannate & chlorpheniramine tannate *antihistamine; decongestant* 12.5•5•2 mg/5 mL oral

pyrimethamine USP, INN *folic acid antagonist for malaria suppression and transmission control; toxoplasmosis treatment adjunct*

pyrimethamine & sulfadiazine *treatment for* Toxoplasma gondii *encephalitis (orphan)*

pyrimidinedione [see: uracil]

pyrimitate INN, BAN

pyrinoline USAN, INN *antiarrhythmic*

Pyrinyl Plus shampoo OTC *pediculicide for lice* [pyrethrins; piperonyl butoxide] 0.33%•4%

pyrithen [see: chlorothen citrate]

pyrithione sodium USAN *topical antimicrobial*

pyrithione zinc USAN, INN, BAN *topical antibacterial; antifungal; antiseborrheic*

pyrithyldione INN

pyritidium bromide INN

pyritinol INN, BAN

Pyrlex oral suspension (discontinued 2009) ℞ *antihistamine; sleep aid* [pyrilamine tannate] 12 mg/5 mL ⊡ Perloxx

Pyrlex CB oral suspension ℞ *antitussive; antihistamine; sleep aid* [carbetapentane tannate; pyrilamine tannate] 22.5•12 mg/5 mL

pyrodifenium bromide [see: prifinium bromide]

pyrogallic acid [see: pyrogallol]

pyrogallol NF ⊡ pargolol

pyronaridine artesunate *investigational artemisinin-based therapy for malaria; effective against both* Plasmodium falciparum *and* P. vivax

pyrophendane INN

pyrophenindane [see: pyrophendane]

pyrovalerone INN *CNS stimulant* [also: pyrovalerone HCl]

pyrovalerone HCl USAN *CNS stimulant* [also: pyrovalerone]

pyroxamine INN *antihistamine* [also: pyroxamine maleate] ⊡ piroximone

pyroxamine maleate USAN *antihistamine* [also: pyroxamine]

pyroxylin USP, INN *pharmaceutic necessity for collodion* ⊡ perhexiline

pyrrobutamine phosphate USP

pyrrocaine USAN, INN *local anesthetic* ⊡ Paracaine; procaine

pyrrocaine HCl NF ⊡ procaine HCl

pyrrolifene INN *analgesic* [also: pyrroliphene HCl]

pyrrolifene HCl [see: pyrroliphene HCl]

pyrroliphene HCl USAN *analgesic* [also: pyrrolifene]

pyrrolnitrin USAN, INN *antifungal*

pyrroxane [now: proroxan HCl]

Pyrroxate caplets OTC *decongestant; antihistamine; analgesic; antipyretic* [phenylephrine HCl; chlorpheniramine maleate; acetaminophen] 10•4•650 mg ⊡ Percocet

Pyrus malus medicinal herb [see: apple]

pyruvate *investigational (orphan) for interstitial lung disease*

pyrvinium chloride INN

pyrvinium embonate [see: pyrvinium pamoate]

pyrvinium pamoate USP *anthelmintic* [also: viprynium embonate]

pytamine INN

PYtest reagent kit for professional use ℞ *in vitro diagnostic aid for* H. pylori *in the breath* [carbon C 14 urea] 1 mCi

PYY (peptide YY) [q.v.]

PZA (pyrazinamide) [q.v.]

PZI (protamine zinc insulin) [q.v.]

Qdall sustained-release capsules (discontinued 2007) ℞ *decongestant; antihistamine* [pseudoephedrine HCl; chlorpheniramine maleate] 100•12 mg

Qdall AR dual-release capsules ℞ *antihistamine* [chlorpheniramine maleate] 12 mg (2 mg immediate release; 10 mg sustained release)

Q-dryl oral liquid OTC *antihistamine; antitussive; sleep aid* [diphenhydramine HCl] 12.5 mg/5 mL

Qnaze HFA CFC-free metered-dose inhaler *investigational (Phase III) dry-formulation corticosteroidal anti-inflammatory for seasonal or perennial rhinitis* [beclomethasone dipropionate]

Qnexa controlled release *investigational (NDA filed) combination therapy for weight loss* [phentermine HCl; topiramate]

Q-Pap tablets OTC *analgesic; antipyretic* [acetaminophen] 325, 500 mg ☒ cubeb

Q-Pap, Children's oral liquid, oral suspension, elixir OTC *analgesic; antipyretic* [acetaminophen] 160 mg/5 mL

Q-Pap Infant Drops (discontinued 2011) OTC *analgesic; antipyretic* [acetaminophen] 100 mg/mL

Q-Tapp elixir OTC *decongestant; antihistamine* [pseudoephedrine HCl; brompheniramine maleate] 30•2 mg/10 mL ☒ Cotab; CTAB; K-Tab

Q-Tapp DM Cold & Cough elixir OTC *antitussive; antihistamine; decongestant* [dextromethorphan hydrobromide; brompheniramine maleate; pseudoephedrine HCl] 10•2•30 mg/10 mL

Q-Tussin CF oral liquid (discontinued 2009) OTC *antitussive; decongestant; expectorant* [dextromethorphan hydrobromide; phenylephrine HCl; guaifenesin] 10•5•100 mg/5 mL

Quad Tann caplets (discontinued 2007) ℞ *antitussive; antihistamine; decongestant* [carbetapentane tannate; chlorpheniramine tannate; phenylephrine tannate; ephedrine tannate] 60•5•10•10 mg ☒ codeine; Kadian

Quad Tann Pediatric oral suspension (discontinued 2008) ℞ *antitussive; antihistamine; decongestant* [carbetapentane tannate; chlorpheniramine tannate; phenylephrine tannate; ephedrine tannate] 30•4•5•5 mg/5 mL

quadazocine INN, BAN *opioid antagonist* [also: quadazocine mesylate]

quadazocine mesylate USAN *opioid antagonist* [also: quadazocine]

Quadra-Hist D; Quadra-Hist D Ped extended-release capsules (discontinued 2007) ℞ *decongestant; antihistamine; sleep aid* [pseudoephedrine HCl; phenyltoloxamine citrate; pyrilamine maleate; pheniramine maleate] 80•16•16•16 mg; 40•8•8•8 mg

Quadramet IV injection ℞ *radiopharmaceutical for treatment of bone pain from osteoblastic metastatic tumors* [samarium Sm 153 lexidronam] 1850 MBq/mL (50 mCi/mL)

Quadrapax elixir ℞ *GI/GU anticholinergic/antispasmodic; sedative* [atropine sulfate; scopolamine hydrobromide; hyoscyamine sulfate; phenobarbital] 0.0194•0.0065•0.1037•16.2 mg/5 mL

quadrosilan INN

Quad-Tuss Tannate Pediatric oral suspension ℞ *antitussive; antihistamine; decongestant* [carbetapentane tannate; chlorpheniramine tannate; phenylephrine tannate; ephedrine tannate] 30•4•5•5 mg/5 mL

quaking aspen *medicinal herb* [see: poplar]

Qualaquin capsules ℞ *antimalarial for chloroquine-resistant falciparum malaria; also used for nocturnal leg cramps* [quinine sulfate] 324 mg

Qual-Tussin oral drops (discontinued 2008) ℞ *decongestant; antihistamine; expectorant; for children 2–24 months* [phenylephrine HCl; chlorpheniramine maleate; guaifenesin] 2•1•20 mg/mL

Qual-Tussin syrup (discontinued 2007) ℞ *antitussive; antihistamine; decongestant; expectorant* [dextromethorphan hydrobromide; chlorpheniramine maleate; phenylephrine HCl; guaifenesin] 15•4•20•200 mg/10 mL

Qual-Tussin DC syrup (discontinued 2007) ℞ *narcotic antitussive; decongestant; expectorant* [hydrocodone bitartrate; phenylephrine HCl; guaifenesin] 2.5•7.5•50 mg/5 mL

Quantaffirm reagent kit for professional use ℞ *in vitro diagnostic aid for mononucleosis*

Quasense film-coated tablets (in packs of 91) ℞ *extended-cycle (3 months) monophasic oral contraceptive* [levonorgestrel; ethinyl estradiol] 0.15 mg• 30 mcg × 84 days; counters × 7 days

quassia (Picrasma excelsa; Quassia amara) bark *medicinal herb used as an anthelmintic, antimalarial, appetizer, digestive aid, febrifuge, insecticide, pediculicide, and tonic*

quatacaine INN ⧉ ketocaine

quaternium-18 bentonite [see: bentoquatam]

quazepam USAN, INN *benzodiazepine sedative and hypnotic*

quazinone USAN, INN *cardiotonic*

quazodine USAN, INN *cardiotonic; bronchodilator*

quazolast USAN, INN *antiasthmatic; mediator release inhibitor*

Queen Anne's lace *medicinal herb* [see: carrot]

queen of the meadow (Eupatorium purpureum) leaves *medicinal herb for bursitis, gallstones, kidney infections and stones, neuralgias, rheumatism, ringworm, urinary disorders, and water retention* [also see: boneset; meadowsweet]

Quelicin IV or IM injection ℞ *neuromuscular blocker* [succinylcholine chloride] 20, 100 mg/mL ⧉ Cleocin

quercetin *natural flavonoid used to protect capillary walls; antioxidant; active flavonol of rutin* 50, 250 mg oral

Quercus alba *medicinal herb* [see: white oak]

Questran; Questran Light powder for oral suspension ℞ *cholesterol-lowering antihyperlipidemic; treatment for pruritus due to partial biliary obstruction; also used for diarrhea and as an antidote to* Clostridium difficile *and digitalis toxicity* [cholestyramine resin] 4 g/dose

quetiapine fumarate USAN *novel (atypical) dibenzothiazepine antipsy-* chotic for schizophrenia and both manic and depressive episodes of a bipolar disorder; also used for obsessive-compulsive disorder; investigational (NDA filed) for generalized anxiety disorder (base=87%)

Quibron; Quibron-300 capsules (discontinued 2007) ℞ *antiasthmatic; bronchodilator; expectorant* [theophylline; guaifenesin] 150•90 mg; 300• 180 mg

Quick Care solutions (discontinued 2010) OTC *two-step chemical disinfecting system for soft contact lenses* [hydrogen peroxide–based]

Quick Melts Children's Non-Aspirin, Quick Melts Jr. Strength Non-Aspirin orally disintegrating tablets OTC *analgesic; antipyretic* [acetaminophen] 80 mg; 160 mg

Quicklets (trademarked dosage form) *quickly dissolving tablets*

Quickscreen test kit for home use OTC *in vitro diagnostic aid for detection of multiple illicit drugs in the urine*

quick-set *medicinal herb* [see: hawthorn]

QuickVue H. pylori gII test kit for professional use ℞ *in vitro diagnostic aid for* H. pylori *in serum or plasma*

QuickVue Influenza Test for professional use ℞ *in vitro diagnostic aid for detection of influenza* A and B *from nasal excretions*

QuickVue Pregnancy Test cassettes for professional use ℞ *in vitro diagnostic aid; urine pregnancy test*

quifenadine INN

quiflapon sodium USAN *leukotriene biosynthesis inhibitor for asthma and inflammatory bowel disease*

quillaia (Quillaja saponaria) bark *medicinal herb for bronchitis and cough; also used topically for dandruff and scalp itchiness*

quillifoline INN

quilostigmine USAN *cholinesterase inhibitor for Alzheimer disease*

quinacainol INN

quinacillin INN, BAN

quinacrine HCl USP *antimalarial; anthelmintic for giardiasis and cestodiasis (tapeworm); investigational (orphan) to prevent the recurrence of pneumothorax in high-risk patients* [also: mepacrine]

quinalbarbitone sodium BAN *hypnotic; sedative* [also: secobarbital sodium]

quinaldine blue USAN *obstetric diagnostic aid*

quinambicide [see: clioquinol]

quinapril INN, BAN *angiotensin-converting enzyme (ACE) inhibitor for hypertension; adjunctive treatment for congestive heart failure (CHF)* [also: quinapril HCl]

quinapril HCl USAN *angiotensin-converting enzyme (ACE) inhibitor for hypertension; adjunctive treatment for congestive heart failure (CHF)* [also: quinapril] 5, 10, 20, 40 mg

quinapril HCl & hydrochlorothiazide *combination angiotensin-converting enzyme (ACE) inhibitor and diuretic for hypertension* 10•12.5, 20•12.5, 20•25 mg oral

quinaprilat USAN, INN *antihypertensive; angiotensin-converting enzyme (ACE) inhibitor*

Quinaretic film-coated tablets ℞ *combination angiotensin-converting enzyme (ACE) inhibitor and diuretic for hypertension* [quinapril HCl; hydrochlorothiazide] 20•12.5, 20•25 mg

quinazosin INN *antihypertensive* [also: quinazosin HCl]

quinazosin HCl USAN *antihypertensive* [also: quinazosin]

quinbolone USAN, INN *anabolic*

quincarbate INN

quindecamine INN *antibacterial* [also: quindecamine acetate]

quindecamine acetate USAN *antibacterial* [also: quindecamine]

quindonium bromide USAN, INN *antiarrhythmic*

quindoxin INN, BAN

quinelorane INN *antihypertensive; antiparkinsonian* [also: quinelorane HCl]

quinelorane HCl USAN *antihypertensive; antiparkinsonian* [also: quinelorane]

quinestradol INN, BAN

quinestrol USAN, USP, INN, BAN *estrogen replacement therapy for postmenopausal disorders*

quinetalate INN *smooth muscle relaxant* [also: quinetolate]

quinethazone USP, INN *diuretic; antihypertensive*

quinetolate USAN *smooth muscle relaxant* [also: quinetalate]

quinezamide INN

quinfamide USAN, INN *antiamebic*

quingestanol INN *progestin* [also: quingestanol acetate]

quingestanol acetate USAN *progestin* [also: quingestanol]

quingestrone USAN, INN *progestin*

quinidine NF, BAN *antiarrhythmic*

quinidine gluconate USP *antiarrhythmic; antimalarial* (base=62%) 324 mg oral; 80 mg/mL injection

quinidine sulfate USP *antiarrhythmic* (base=83%) 100, 200, 300 mg oral

quinine (Cinchona calisaya; C. ledgeriana; C. succirubra) NF, BAN bark *medicinal herb for cancer, fever, hemorrhoids, indigestion, inducing abortion, jaundice, malaria, mouth and throat diseases, parasites, stimulation of hair growth, and varicose veins*

quinine ascorbate USAN *smoking deterrent*

quinine biascorbate [now: quinine ascorbate]

quinine bisulfate NF

quinine dihydrochloride NF *antiinfective for pernicious malaria*

quinine ethylcarbonate NF

quinine glycerophosphate NF

quinine HCl NF

quinine hydrobromide NF

quinine hypophosphite NF

quinine monohydrobromide [see: quinine hydrobromide]

quinine monohydrochloride [see: quinine HCl]

quinine monosalicylate [see: quinine salicylate]

quinine phosphate NF

quinine phosphinate [see: quinine hypophosphite]

quinine salicylate NF

quinine sulfate USP *cinchona alkaloid; antimalarial for chloroquine-resistant falciparum malaria (orphan); also used for nocturnal leg cramps* 200, 260, 325 mg oral

quinine sulfate dihydrate [see: quinine sulfate]

quinine tannate USP

quinisocaine INN [also: dimethisoquin HCl; dimethisoquin] ⊡ guanisoquine

quinocide INN

8-quinolinol [see: oxyquinoline]

8-quinolinol benzoate [see: benzoxiquine]

quinolizidines *a class of antibiotics based on the quinolizidine (norlupinane) structure* [also called: norlupinanes]

quinolones [see: fluoroquinolones]

quinoxyl [see: chiniofon]

quinpirole INN *antihypertensive* [also: quinpirole HCl]

quinpirole HCl USAN *antihypertensive* [also: quinpirole]

quinprenaline INN *bronchodilator* [also: quinterenol sulfate]

quinprenaline sulfate [see: quinterenol sulfate]

Quinsana Plus powder OTC *antifungal* [tolnaftate] 1%

quinsy berry *medicinal herb* [see: currant]

Quintabs tablets OTC *vitamin supplement* [multiple vitamins; folic acid; biotin] ≛•400•30 mcg

Quintabs-M tablets OTC *vitamin/mineral/calcium/iron supplement* [multiple vitamins & minerals; calcium (as ascorbate and carbonate); iron (as ferrous fumarate); folic acid] ≛•30•10•0.4 mg

quinterenol sulfate USAN *bronchodilator* [also: quinprenaline]

quintiofos INN, BAN

3-quinuclidinol benzoate [see: benzoclidine]

quinuclium bromide USAN, INN *antihypertensive*

quinupramine INN

quinupristin USAN, INN *streptogramin antibiotic; bacteriostatic to gram-positive infections*

quipazine INN *antidepressant; oxytocic* [also: quipazine maleate] ⊡ Cubicin

quipazine maleate USAN *antidepressant; oxytocic* [also: quipazine]

quisultazine INN

quisultidine [see: quisultazine]

Quixin eye drops ℞ *fluoroquinolone antibiotic for bacterial conjunctivitis* [levofloxacin] 0.5%

Qutenza transdermal patch ℞ *counterirritant; topical analgesic for the management of neuropathic pain due to postherpetic neuralgia (orphan); investigational (orphan) for erythromelalgia and painful HIV-related neuropathy* [capsaicin] 8%

QV-Allergy syrup ℞ *decongestant; antihistamine; anticholinergic to dry mucosal secretions* [phenylephrine HCl; chlorpheniramine maleate; methscopolamine nitrate] 10•2•0.625 mg/5 mL

Qvar pressurized metered-dose inhaler (pMDI) with a CFC-free propellant ℞ *antiasthmatic* [beclomethasone dipropionate] 40, 80 mcg/puff

R & D Calcium Carbonate/600 *investigational (orphan) agent for hyperphosphatemia of end-stage renal disease* [calcium carbonate]

RA Lotion OTC *antiseptic, antifungal, and keratolytic for acne* [resorcinol; alcohol] 3%•43%

RabAvert IM injection ℞ *rabies vaccine for pre-exposure vaccination or post-exposure prophylaxis* [rabies vaccine, chick embryo cell] ≥ 2.5 IU/mL

rabeprazole INN *proton pump inhibitor for duodenal ulcers, erosive or ulcerative gastroesophageal reflux disease (GERD), and other gastroesophageal disorders* [also: rabeprazole sodium]

rabeprazole sodium USAN *proton pump inhibitor for duodenal ulcers, erosive or ulcerative gastroesophageal reflux disease (GERD), H. pylori infection, and other gastroesophageal disorders* [also: rabeprazole]

rabies immune globulin (RIG) USP *passive immunizing agent for use after rabies exposure*

rabies vaccine USP *rabies vaccine for pre-exposure vaccination or post-exposure prophylaxis; the virus is grown in either human diploid cells or chick embryo cells*

rabies vaccine, adsorbed (RVA) [see: rabies vaccine]

rabies vaccine, DCO (diploid cell origin) [see: rabies vaccine]

rabies vaccine, HDCV (human diploid cell vaccine) [see: rabies vaccine]

race ginger *medicinal herb* [see: ginger]

racefemine INN

racefenicol INN *antibacterial* [also: racephenicol]

racemethadol [see: dimepheptanol]

racemethionine USAN, USP *urinary acidifier to control ammonia production* [also: methionine (the DL- form)]

racemethorphan INN, BAN

racemetirosine INN

racemic [def.] *A chemical compound with equal parts of (+) (formerly d- or dextro-) and (−) (formerly l- or levo-) enantiomers. Designated by the prefix (±) (formerly dl-).* [see also: isomer; enantiomer]

racemic amphetamine phosphate

racemic amphetamine sulfate [see: amphetamine sulfate]

racemic calcium pantothenate [see: calcium pantothenate, racemic]

racemoramide INN, BAN

racemorphan INN

racephedrine HCl USAN

racephenicol USAN *antibacterial* [also: racefenicol]

racepinefrine INN *sympathomimetic bronchodilator* [also: racepinephrine]

racepinephrine USP *sympathomimetic bronchodilator* [also: racepinefrine]

racepinephrine HCl USP *sympathomimetic bronchodilator*

raclopride INN, BAN

raclopride C 11 USAN *radiopharmaceutical*

racoonberry *medicinal herb* [see: mandrake]

ractopamine INN *veterinary growth stimulant* [also: ractopamine HCl]

ractopamine HCl USAN *veterinary growth stimulant* [also: ractopamine]

RadiaPlexRx gel ℞ *moisturizer; emollient*

Radiesse subcu implant in prefilled syringes ℞ *collagen production stimulant for HIV-related facial lipoatrophy and moderate to severe facial wrinkles and folds* [calcium hydroxylapatite] 0.3, 1.3 mL/syringe

radio-chromated serum albumin [see: albumin, chromated]

Radiogardase capsules ℞ *chelating agent for internal contamination with radioactive or nonradioactive cesium and/or thallium (orphan)* [ferric hexacyanoferrate (insoluble Prussian blue)] 500 mg

radio-iodinated I 125 serum albumin [see: albumin, iodinated]

radio-iodinated I 131 serum albumin [see: albumin, iodinated]

radiomerisoprol ^{197}Hg [see: merisoprol Hg 197]

radioselenomethionine ^{75}Se [see: selenomethionine Se 75]

radiotolpovidone I 131 INN *hypoalbuminemia test; radioactive agent* [also: tolpovidone I 131]

radish (Raphanus sativus) *root medicinal herb used as an antispasmodic, astringent, cholagogue, and diuretic*

radium *element (Ra)* ② rhodium

radium-233 chloride *investigational (Phase III) radiotherapeutic agent for advanced prostate cancer with bone metastases*

radon *element (Rn)*

rafoxanide USAN, INN *anthelmintic*

ragged cup (Silphium perfoliatum) *root and gum medicinal herb used as an antispasmodic, diaphoretic, and stimulant*

Ragus *tablets* OTC *vitamin/mineral/calcium/iron/amino acid supplement* [multiple vitamins & minerals; calcium (as dicalcium phosphate); iron (as ferrous gluconate); multiple amino acids] ≐•193•6.67• ≐ mg

ragwort *medicinal herb* [see: life root]

ralitoline USAN, INN *anticonvulsant*

Ralivia ER *controlled-release tablets (discontinued 2007)* ℞ *once-daily opioid analgesic for moderate to severe pain* [tramadol HCl] 100, 200, 300 mg

Ralix *extended-release tablets* ℞ *decongestant; antihistamine; anticholinergic to dry mucosal secretions* [phenylephrine HCl; chlorpheniramine maleate; methscopolamine nitrate] 40•8•2.5 mg ② RuLox

raloxifene INN *antiestrogen; selective estrogen receptor modulator (SERM) for the prevention for postmenopausal osteoporosis* [also: raloxifene HCl]

raloxifene HCl USAN *selective estrogen receptor modulator (SERM) for the prevention and treatment of postmeno-* pausal osteoporosis; hormone antagonist for breast cancer (orphan); also used for uterine leiomyomas, pubertal gynecomastia, and prostate cancer [also: raloxifene]

raltegravir (RGV) *integrase inhibitor; antiretroviral for drug-resistant HIV-1 infection*

raltegravir potassium *integrase inhibitor; oral antiretroviral for drug-resistant HIV-1 infection (base=92%)*

raltitrexed USAN *antimetabolite antineoplastic; thymidylate synthase inhibitor*

raluridine USAN *antiviral*

rambufaside [see: meproscillarin]

ramciclane INN

ramelteon *melatonin MT$_1$ and MT$_2$ receptor agonist; hypnotic for insomnia due to difficulty with sleep onset*

ramifenazone INN

ramipril USAN, INN, BAN *antihypertensive; angiotensin-converting enzyme (ACE) inhibitor; treatment for myocardial infarction (MI), congestive heart failure (CHF), and stroke* 1.25, 2.5, 5, 10 mg oral

ramiprilat INN

ramixotidine INN

ramnodigin INN

ramoplanin USAN, INN *broad-spectrum glycolipodepsipeptide antibiotic*

Ranamine *(trademarked ingredient) a proprietary blend of vitamins B$_6$, B$_{12}$, and folic acid* ② RenAmin

Ranexa *film-coated extended-release tablets* ℞ *antianginal for chronic stable angina, ventricular arrhythmias, atrial fibrillation, and bradycardia* [ranolazine (as HCl)] 500, 1000 mg ② Renax

ranibizumab *vascular endothelial growth factor (VEGF-A) inhibitor for neovascular (wet) age-related macular degeneration (AMD) and macular edema; investigational for diabetic retinopathy*

Raniclor *chewable tablets* ℞ *second-generation cephalosporin antibiotic* [cefaclor] 125, 187, 250, 375 mg

ranimustine INN

ranimycin USAN, INN *antibacterial*

ranitidine USAN, INN, BAN *histamine H$_2$ antagonist for gastric ulcers* 75, 150, 300 mg oral; 25 mg/mL injection

ranitidine bismuth citrate USAN *histamine H$_2$ antagonist for gastric ulcers with H. pylori infection* [also: ranitidine bismutrex]

ranitidine bismutrex BAN *histamine H$_2$ antagonist for gastric ulcers with H. pylori infection* [also: ranitidine bismuth citrate]

ranitidine HCl USP, JAN *histamine H$_2$ antagonist for gastric ulcers* 75, 150, 300 mg oral; 15 mg/mL oral

ranolazine INN *antianginal* [also: ranolazine HCl]

ranolazine HCl USAN *antianginal for chronic stable angina, ventricular arrhythmias, atrial fibrillation, and bradycardia* [also: ranolazine]

ranpirnase USAN, INN *investigational (Phase III) antineoplastic for unresectable malignant mesothelioma (UMM)*

Ranunculus acris; R. bulbosus; R. scleratus medicinal herb [see: buttercup]

rapacuronium bromide USAN *neuromuscular blocker; adjunct to general anesthesia*

Rapaflo capsules ℞ *alpha$_{1a}$ blocker for benign prostatic hyperplasia (BPH)* [silodosin] 4, 8 mg

Rapamune tablets, oral solution ℞ *immunosuppressant for renal transplantation; investigational (Phase III) for liver transplantation; also used for psoriasis* [sirolimus] 0.5, 1, 2 mg; 1 mg/mL

rapamycin [now: sirolimus]

Raphanus sativus medicinal herb [see: radish]

Rapid Anthrax Test reagents for use with **LightCycler** assay device ℞ *diagnostic aid for anthrax DNA in human and environmental samples* [polymerase chain reaction (PCR) test]

Rapid B-12 Energy sublingual spray OTC *vitamin B$_{12}$ supplement* [cyanocobalamin] 200 mcg/spray

RapidVue test kit for home use OTC *in vitro diagnostic aid; urine pregnancy test*

Rapimelt (trademarked dosage form) *orally disintegrating tablets*

Rapirun H. pylori Antibody Detection Kit test kit for professional use ℞ *in vitro diagnostic aid for the detection of anti-H. pylori IgG antibodies in urine*

RapiTabs (trademarked dosage form) *orally disintegrating tablets*

Raptiva powder for subcu injection (withdrawn from the market in 2009 due to safety concerns) ℞ *immunosuppressant for plaque psoriasis* [efalizumab] 125 mg/dose

rasagiline INN *monoamine oxidase B (MAO-B) inhibitor for Parkinson disease*

rasagiline mesylate USAN *monoamine oxidase B (MAO-B) inhibitor for Parkinson disease*

rasburicase USAN, INN *antimetabolite antineoplastic for leukemia, lymphoma, and solid tumor malignancies (orphan)*

raspberry, ground *medicinal herb* [see: goldenseal]

raspberry, red; wild red raspberry *medicinal herb* [see: red raspberry]

raspberry [syrup] USP

rathyronine INN

rattleroot *medicinal herb* [see: black cohosh]

rattlesnake antivenin [see: antivenin (Crotalidae) polyvalent]

rattlesnake root *medicinal herb* [see: birthroot; black cohosh; senega]

rattleweed *medicinal herb* [see: black cohosh]

rauwolfia serpentina USP *antihypertensive; peripheral antiadrenergic; antipsychotic*

rauwolfia serpentina & bendroflumethiazide *combination peripheral antiadrenergic and diuretic for hypertension* 50•4 mg oral

Rauzide tablets (discontinued 2007) ℞ *antihypertensive; diuretic* [bendroflumethiazide; rauwolfia serpentina] 4•50 mg

raxibacumab *investigational (NDA filed) treatment for inhalational anthrax poisoning*

rayon, purified USAN, USP *surgical aid*

Razadyne film-coated tablets, oral drops ℞ *acetylcholinesterase inhibitor to increase cognition in Alzheimer disease* [galantamine hydrobromide] 4, 8, 12 mg; 4 mg/mL

Razadyne ER extended-release pellets in capsules ℞ *acetylcholinesterase inhibitor to increase cognition in Alzheimer disease* [galantamine hydrobromide] 8, 16, 24 mg

razinodil INN

razobazam INN

razoxane INN, BAN

⁸⁶Rb [see: rubidium chloride Rb 86]

rCD4 (recombinant CD4) [see: CD4, recombinant soluble human]

RCF oral liquid OTC *hypoallergenic infant formula* [soy protein formula, carbohydrate free]

RE Benzoyl Perozide cream ℞ *keratolytic for acne* [benzoyl peroxide] 3.5%, 5.5%, 8.5%

RE Chlordiazepoxide/Clidinium capsules ℞ *anxiolytic; GI anticholinergic* [chlordiazepoxide HCl; clidinium bromide] 5•2.5 mg

RE DCP oral drops (discontinued 2011) ℞ *antitussive; antihistamine; decongestant; for children 2–12 years* [dextromethorphan hydrobromide; chlorpheniramine maleate; phenylephrine HCl] 2.75•0.75•1.75 mg/mL

RE MultiVit with Fluoride chewable tablets ℞ *vitamin supplement; dental caries preventative* [multiple vitamins; fluoride] ≟•0.25, ≟•0.5, ≟•1 mg

RE-U40 topical aerosol foam ℞ *moisturizer; emollient; keratolytic* [urea] 40%

RE Urea 50 topical solution ℞ *moisturizer; emollient; keratolytic* [urea] 50%

RE2+30 syrup ℞ *antihistamine; decongestant* [chlorpheniramine maleate; pseudoephedrine HCl] 2•30 mg/5 mL

Reabilan; Reabilan HN ready-to-use oral liquid OTC *enteral nutritional therapy* [lactose-free formula]

reactrol [see: clemizole HCl]

Readi-Cat oral suspension ℞ *radiopaque contrast medium for gastrointestinal imaging* [barium sulfate] 2.1%

Readi-Cat; Readi-Cat 2 oral/rectal suspension ℞ *radiopaque contrast medium for gastrointestinal imaging* [barium sulfate] 1.3%; 2%

RealTime CT/NG Assay for professional use ℞ *in vitro diagnostic aid for detection of* Chlamydia trachomatis *and* Neisseria gonorrhoeae *from urine, female vaginal/endocervical swabs, or male urethral swabs* polymerase chain reaction (PCR) assay

rebamipide INN

Rebetol capsules, oral solution ℞ *antiviral for chronic hepatitis C infections (orphan) and clinically stable HIV disease; also used for viral hemorrhagic fevers* [ribavirin] 200 mg; 40 mg/mL

Rebetron capsules + subcu or IM injection (discontinued 2009) ℞ *combination treatment for chronic hepatitis C* [Rebetol (ribavirin capsules); Intron A (interferon alfa-2b injection)] 200 mg•3 million IU

Rebif prefilled syringes for subcu injection ℞ *immunomodulator for relapsing remitting multiple sclerosis (orphan); investigational (orphan) for malignant melanoma, metastatic renal cell carcinoma, T-cell lymphoma, and Kaposi sarcoma* [interferon beta-1a] 8.8, 22, 44 mcg (2.4, 6, 12 MIU)

reboxetine INN *fast-acting selective norepinephrine reuptake inhibitor for depression*

reboxetine mesilate INN, BAN *fast-acting selective norepinephrine reuptake inhibitor for depression* (base=76.5%) [also: reboxetine mesylate]

reboxetine mesylate USAN *fast-acting selective norepinephrine reuptake inhibitor for depression* (base=76.5%) [also: reboxetine mesilate]

recainam INN, BAN *antiarrhythmic* [also: recainam HCl]

recainam HCl USAN *antiarrhythmic* [also: recainam]

recainam tosylate USAN *antiarrhythmic*

Recal D chewable wafers ℞ *vitamin/ mineral/calcium supplement* [multiple vitamins & minerals; calcium (as citrate); folic acid] ±•282•1 mg

recanescin [see: deserpidine]

Recentin *investigational (Phase III) antineoplastic for metastatic colorectal cancer*

Receptin *investigational (Phase II, orphan) antiviral for AIDS* [CD4, recombinant soluble human]

Reclast IV infusion ℞ *single-dose bisphosphonate bone resorption inhibitor for Paget disease of the bone; annual or biannual treatment for male, postmenopausal, or glucocorticoid-induced osteoporosis* [zoledronic acid] 5 mg

reclazepam USAN, INN *sedative*

Reclipsen tablets (in packs of 28) ℞ *monophasic oral contraceptive* [desogestrel; ethinyl estradiol] 0.15 mg• 30 mcg × 21 days; counters × 7 days

Reclomide tablets (discontinued 2007) ℞ *antiemetic for chemotherapy and postoperative nausea and vomiting; GI stimulant for diabetic gastroparesis and gastroesophageal reflux* [metoclopramide (as HCl)] 10 mg

Recombigen HIV-1 LA Test reagent kit for professional use (discontinued 2008) ℞ *in vitro diagnostic aid for HIV-1 antibodies in blood, serum, or plasma* [latex agglutination test]

recombinant factor VIII [see: antihemophilic factor, recombinant]

recombinant human activated protein C (rhAPC) [see: drotrecogan alfa]

recombinant human deoxyribonuclease (rhDNase) [see: dornase alfa]

recombinant human growth hormone (rhGH) [see: somatropin]

recombinant soluble human CD4 (rCD4) [see: CD4, recombinant soluble human]

recombinant tissue plasminogen activator (rtPA; rt-PA) [see: alteplase]

Recombinate powder for IV injection ℞ *systemic hemostatic; antihemophilic for the prevention and control of bleeding in classical hemophilia (hemophilia A) and von Willebrand disease (orphan)* [antihemophilic factor concentrate, recombinant] 250, 500, 1000 IU

Recombivax HB adult IM injection, pediatric/adolescent IM injection, dialysis formulation ℞ *active immunizing agent for hepatitis B and D* [hepatitis B virus vaccine, inactvated, recombinant] 10 mcg/mL; 5 mcg/0.5 mL; 40 mcg/mL

Recomparin *investigational synthetic heparin*

Recothrom powder for solution ℞ *topical hemostat for surgery* [thrombin, recombinant] 1000 U/mL (5000, 20 000 U/vial)

Rectacort rectal suppositories ℞ *corticosteroidal anti-inflammatory* [hydrocortisone acetate] 10%

Rectagene rectal suppositories OTC *temporary relief of hemorrhoidal symptoms* [live yeast cell derivative; shark liver oil] 2000 SRF U/oz.

Rectagene Medicated Rectal Balm ointment OTC *temporary relief of hemorrhoidal symptoms* [shark liver oil; phenyl mercuric nitrate; live yeast cell derivative] 3%•1:10 000•66.67 U/g

Rectiv intra-anal ointment ℞ *coronary vasodilator; emergency antianginal* [nitroglycerin] 0.4%

Rectolax suppositories OTC *stimulant laxative* [bisacodyl] 10 mg

red bay; red laurel *medicinal herb* [see: magnolia]

red bearberry *medicinal herb* [see: uva ursi]

red blood cells [see: blood cells, red]

red bush tea (*Aspalathus contaminata; A. linearis; Borbonia pinifolia*) leaves and stems *medicinal herb used as a free radical scavenger; investigational antineoplastic; investigational for preventing brain damage caused by aging*

red clover (*Trifolium pratense*) flower *medicinal herb for blood cleansing, bronchitis, cancer, clearing toxins, nervous disorders, and spasms*

Red Cross Toothache topical liquid OTC *oral analgesic* [eugenol] 85%

red currant *(Ribes rubrum) medicinal herb* [see: currant]

red elm *medicinal herb* [see: slippery elm]

red ferric oxide [see: ferric oxide, red]

red ink berries; red ink plant *medicinal herb* [see: pokeweed]

red laurel; red bay *medicinal herb* [see: magnolia]

red legs *medicinal herb* [see: bistort]

red mulberry *(Morus rubra) medicinal herb* [see: mulberry]

red oak *(Quercus rubra) medicinal herb* [see: white oak]

red paint root *medicinal herb* [see: bloodroot]

red pepper; African red pepper; American red pepper *medicinal herb* [see: cayenne]

red pimpernel *(Anagallis arvensis)* plant *medicinal herb used as a cholagogue, diaphoretic, diuretic, expectorant, nervine, purgative, and stimulant*

red puccoon *medicinal herb* [see: bloodroot]

red raspberry *(Rubus idaeus; R. strigosus)* leaves *medicinal herb for childbirth afterpains, diarrhea and other bowel disorders, fever, flu, morning sickness, menstrual disorders, mouth sores, nausea, and vomiting*

red root *medicinal herb* [see: bloodroot; danshen; New Jersey tea]

red sarsaparilla *medicinal herb* [see: sarsaparilla]

Red Throat Spray; Green Throat Spray OTC *mild mucous membrane anesthetic; antipruritic; counterirritant* [phenol] 1.4%

red veterinarian petrolatum (RVP) [see: petrolatum]

red weed *medicinal herb* [see: pokeweed]

redberry *medicinal herb* [see: ginseng]

Redi Vial (trademarked delivery form) *dual-compartment vial*

Rediject (trademarked delivery form) *prefilled disposable syringe*

Redipak (trademarked delivery form) *unit dose or unit-of-issue package*

RediTabs (trademarked dosage form) *rapidly disintegrating tablets*

Reditux IV infusion ℞ *monoclonal antibody for non-Hodgkin B-cell lymphoma and rheumatoid arthritis* [rituximab (biosimilar)] 10 mg/mL

redmond clay (montmorillonite) *natural remedy for bug bites and stings and other skin problems*

Redness Reliever eye drops (discontinued 2010) OTC *decongestant; vasoconstrictor* [tetrahydrozoline HCl] 0.05%

Redur-PCM oral suspension (discontinued 2009) ℞ *decongestant; antihistamine; anticholinergic to dry mucosal secretions* [phenylephrine tannate; chlorpheniramine tannate; methscopolamine nitrate] 10•2•1.5 mg/5 mL

Redutemp tablets (discontinued 2008) OTC *analgesic; antipyretic* [acetaminophen] 500 mg

Reese's Pinworm caplets, oral suspension OTC *anthelmintic for ascariasis (roundworm) and enterobiasis (pinworm)* [pyrantel (as pamoate)] 62.5 mg; 50 mg/mL

ReFacto powder for IV injection ℞ *short-term anticoagulant for prophylaxis of spontaneous bleeding and for surgical procedures (orphan)* [antihemophilic factor, recombinant] 250, 500, 1000, 2000 IU

Refensen Plus Severe Strength Cough & Cold Medicine caplets (discontinued 2007) OTC *decongestant; expectorant* [pseudoephedrine HCl; guaifenesin] 60•400 mg

Refludan powder for IV injection ℞ *anticoagulant for heparin-associated thrombocytopenia (orphan)* [lepirudin] 50 mg ⑫ rofelodine

Refresh Classic eye drops OTC *moisturizer/lubricant* [polyvinyl alcohol] 1.4%

Refresh Dry Eye Therapy eye drops OTC *moisturizer/lubricant* [glycerin; polysorbate 80] 1%•1%

Refresh Eye Itch Relief eye drops OTC *antihistamine and mast cell stabilizer for allergic conjunctivitis* [ketotifen fumarate] 0.025%

Refresh Lacri-Lube; Refresh P.M.
ophthalmic ointment OTC *ocular
moisturizer/lubricant* [white petrolatum; mineral oil; lanolin]

Refresh Liquigel eye drops OTC *moisturizer/lubricant* [carboxymethylcellulose] 1%

Refresh Plus; Refresh Tears eye
drops OTC *moisturizer/lubricant* [carboxymethylcellulose] 0.5%

Refresh Redness Relief eye drops OTC
decongestant; vasoconstrictor; moisturizer; lubricant [phenylephrine HCl;
polyvinyl alcohol] 0.12%•1.4%

refrigerants *a class of agents that lower
abnormal body heat (a term used in
folk medicine)*

regadenoson *selective adenosine* A_{2A}
*receptor agonist; coronary vasodilator to
induce pharmacological stress for myocardial perfusion imaging*

Rēgain snack bar OTC *enteral nutritional
therapy for impaired renal function*
[multiple essential amino acids] ②
Rogaine

Regenecare gel OTC *anesthetic* [lidocaine] 2%

Reglan tablets, IV infusion ℞ *antiemetic for chemotherapy and postoperative nausea and vomiting; GI stimulant
for diabetic gastroparesis, gastroesophageal reflux, small bowel intubation, and
radiological examination of the intestine;
also used for hiccups* [metoclopramide
(as HCl)] 5, 10 mg; 5 mg/mL

regorafenib *investigational (Phase III)
antineoplastic for bowel cancer*

regramostim USAN, INN *antineutropenic; hematopoietic stimulant; biologic
response modifier; bone marrow stimulant*

Regranex gel ℞ *recombinant platelet-derived growth factor B for diabetic foot
and leg ulcers* [becaplermin] 0.01%

Regroton tablets (discontinued 2007)
℞ *antihypertensive; diuretic* [chlorthalidone; reserpine] 50•0.25 mg

regulator, female *medicinal herb* [see:
life root]

Regulax SS capsules (discontinued
2008) OTC *laxative; stool softener* [docusate sodium] 100 mg

Reguloid powder OTC *bulk laxative* [psyllium hydrophilic mucilloid] 3.4 g/tsp.

Rehydralyte oral solution OTC *electrolyte replacement* [sodium, potassium,
and chloride electrolytes]

reishi mushrooms body and stem
*medicinal herb for AIDS, allergies,
fatigue, heart problems, and insomnia*

Rejuvenex cream OTC *antioxidant,
moisturizer, and sunscreen for the face*

Rejuvex caplets OTC *natural/herbal
supplement for the relief or postmenopausal symptoms* [multiple vitamins
and minerals; phytoestrogens]

Rekinla *investigational (NDA filed)
CNS depressant for fibromyalgia*
[sodium oxybate]

Relacon-DM NR oral liquid (discontinued 2007) ℞ *antitussive; decongestant; expectorant* [dextromethorphan
hydrobromide; pseudoephedrine HCl;
guaifenesin] 15•32•200 mg/5 mL

Relacon-HC; Relacon-HC NR oral
liquid (discontinued 2009) ℞ *narcotic antitussive; antihistamine; decongestant* [hydrocodone bitartrate;
chlorpheniramine maleate; phenylephrine HCl] 3.5•2.5•10 mg/5 mL;
3.5•2.5•8 mg/5 mL

Relagesic oral liquid ℞ *analgesic; antipyretic; antihistamine; sleep aid* [acetaminophen; phenyltoloxamine citrate] 160•5 mg/5 mL

Relagesic tablets (discontinued 2007)
℞ *analgesic; antipyretic; antihistamine;
sleep aid* [acetaminophen; phenyltoloxamine citrate] 650•50 mg

Relahist-DM oral drops (discontinued
2010) ℞ *antitussive; antihistamine;
decongestant; for children 2–12 years*
[dextromethorphan hydrobromide;
chlorpheniramine maleate; phenylephrine HCl] 3•1•2 mg/mL

Relamine tablets ℞ *nutritional supplement for osteoarthritis* [glucosamine;
chondroitin; Primorine (q.v.)] 400•
300•425 mg

Relasin DM oral liquid OTC *antitussive; decongestant; expectorant* [dextromethorphan hydrobromide; pseudoephedrine HCl; guaifenesin] 15•32•175 mg/5 mL

Relasin-HC oral liquid (discontinued 2009) ℞ *narcotic antitussive; antihistamine; decongestant* [hydrocodone bitartrate; chlorpheniramine maleate; phenylephrine HCl] 3.25•2.5•8 mg/5 mL

relaxin, recombinant human *investigational (orphan) for progressive systemic sclerosis; investigational (Phase III) for acute heart failure*

Relcof CPM extended-release caplets ℞ *antihistamine; anticholinergic to dry mucosal secretions* [chlorpheniramine maleate; methscopolamine nitrate] 8•2.5 mg

Relcof DN PE extended-release caplets in a "day and night" package ℞ *decongestant; antihistamine; anticholinergic to dry mucosal secretions* [day: **Relcof PE** (q.v.); night: **Relcof CPM** (q.v.)]

Relcof DN PSE extended-release caplets in a "day and night" package ℞ *decongestant; antihistamine; anticholinergic to dry mucosal secretions* [day: **Relcof PSE** (q.v.); night: **Relcof CPM** (q.v.)]

Relcof PE extended-release caplets ℞ *decongestant; antihistamine; anticholinergic to dry mucosal secretions* [phenylephrine HCl; chlorpheniramine maleate; methscopolamine nitrate] 20•8•2.5 mg

Relcof PSE extended-release caplets ℞ *decongestant; antihistamine; anticholinergic to dry mucosal secretions* [pseudoephedrine HCl; chlorpheniramine maleate; methscopolamine nitrate] 120•8•2.5 mg

Release-Tabs (dosage form) *timed-release tablets*

Relenza Rotadisks (powder for oral inhalation, for use with a **Diskhaler** device) ℞ *antiviral for the prophylaxis and treatment of acute influenza A and B virus infections; also used for H1N1 swine flu* [zanamivir] 5 mg

Relhist chewable tablets ℞ *decongestant; antihistamine* [phenylephrine tannate; brompheniramine tannate] 15•6 mg

Reli On Ketone Test Strips reagent strips for home use OTC *in vitro diagnostic aid for acetone (ketones) in the urine*

Reliable Gentle Laxative delayed-release enteric-coated tablets, suppositories OTC *stimulant laxative* [bisacodyl] 5 mg; 10 mg

Relief eye drops (discontinued 2010) OTC *decongestant* [phenylephrine HCl] 0.12%

Relistor subcu injection ℞ *opioid receptor antagonist for opioid-induced constipation (orphan); investigational (NDA filed) for postoperative ileus* [methylnaltrexone bromide] 12 mg/0.6 mL vial

relomycin USAN, INN *antibacterial*

Relora tablets, capsules OTC *dietary supplement to relieve stress and anxiety by reducing cortisol levels and increasing DHEA levels; adjunct to weight reduction* [Magnolia officinalis extract; Phellodendron amurense extract] 250 mg

Reloxin (available in 23 countries) *investigational (NDA filed) neurotoxin complex for cosmetic wrinkle treatments* [botulinum toxin]

Relpax film-coated tablets ℞ *vascular serotonin 5-HT$_{1B/1D/1F}$ receptor agonist for the acute treatment of migraine* [eletriptan (as hydrobromide)] 20, 40 mg

Reluri extended-release caplets ℞ *decongestant; expectorant* [phenylephrine HCl; guaifenesin] 30•1200 mg

remacemide INN *neuroprotective anticonvulsant* [also: remacemide HCl]

remacemide HCl USAN *neuroprotective anticonvulsant; investigational (orphan) for Huntington disease* [also: remacemide]

Reme Hist DM oral liquid ℞ *antitussive; antihistamine; sleep aid; decongestant* [dextromethorphan hydrobromide; pyrilamine maleate; phenylephrine HCl] 15•12.5•7.5 mg/5 mL

Remedy topical solution OTC *antiseptic* [benzalkonium chloride] 0.12%

Remedy Calazime topical paste OTC *astringent; mild anesthetic; antipruritic; counterirritant* [zinc oxide; menthol] 20%•0.2%

Remeron film-coated tablets ℞ *tetracyclic antidepressant* [mirtazapine] 15, 30, 45 mg

Remeron SolTabs (orally disintegrating tablets) ℞ *tetracyclic antidepressant* [mirtazapine] 15, 30, 45 mg

Remicade powder for IV infusion ℞ *anti-inflammatory for severe and fistulizing Crohn disease (orphan), ulcerative colitis, rheumatoid and psoriatic arthritis, ankylosing spondylitis, and plaque psoriasis; also used for juvenile arthritis* [infliximab] 100 mg

Remifemin Menopause tablets OTC *natural remedy for postmenopausal symptoms* [black cohosh (standardized extract)] 20 mg (1 mg triterpene glycosides)

remifentanil INN, BAN *short-acting narcotic analgesic for general anesthesia* [also: remifentanil HCl]

remifentanil HCl USAN *short-acting narcotic analgesic for general anesthesia* [also: remifentanil]

remikiren INN

remiprostol USAN, INN *antiulcerative*

Remitogen *investigational (orphan) agent for non-Hodgkin B-cell lymphoma* [monoclonal antibody 1D10, humanized]

Remodulin continuous subcu or IV infusion ℞ *peripheral vasodilator for pulmonary arterial hypertension (PAH; orphan)* [treprostinil sodium] 1, 2.5, 5, 10 mg/mL

remoxipride USAN, INN, BAN *antipsychotic*

remoxipride HCl USAN *antipsychotic*

Remoxy gelcaps *investigational (NDA filed) abuse-resistant form of* **OxyContin** [oxycodone]

Remular-S tablets ℞ *skeletal muscle relaxant* [chlorzoxazone] 250 mg

Remura eye drops *long-acting nonsteroidal anti-inflammatory drug (NSAID); investigational (Phase III) treatment for dry eye syndrome* [bromfenac sodium]

Renacidin powder for solution (discontinued 2010) ℞ *bladder and catheter irrigant for apatite or struvite calculi (orphan)* [citric acid; D-gluconic acid lactone; magnesium hydroxycarbonate] 6.602•0.198•3.177 g/100 mL

Renacidin Irrigation solution ℞ *bladder and catheter irrigant for apatite or struvite calculi (orphan)* [citric acid; glucono-delta-lactone; magnesium carbonate]

ReNaf chewable tablets ℞ *dental caries preventative* [fluoride] 0.25, 0.5, 1 mg

Renagel film-coated tablets ℞ *phosphate-binding polymer for hyperphosphatemia in dialysis patients with chronic kidney disease (CKD); also used for hyperuricemia in dialysis patients* [sevelamer (as HCl)] 400, 800 mg

Renal Caps softgels ℞ *vitamin supplement* [multiple B vitamins; vitamin C; folic acid; biotin] ≚•60•1•0.15 mg

RenAmin IV infusion ℞ *nutritional therapy for renal failure* [multiple essential and nonessential amino acids; electrolytes] ② Ranamine

renanolone INN

RenaPlex tablets OTC *vitamin supplement* [multiple B vitamins; vitamin C; folic acid; biotin] ≚•60•0.8•0.3 mg

Renatabs caplets ℞ *vitamin supplement* [multiple vitamins; folic acid; biotin] ≚•1•0.3 mg

Renatabs with Iron film-coated caplets ℞ *hematinic* [iron (as elemental iron and carbonyl iron); multiple B vitamins; vitamin C; folic acid; biotin] 100•≚•60•1•0.3 mg

Rena-Vite tablets OTC *vitamin supplement* [multiple B vitamins; vitamin C; folic acid; biotin] ≚•60•0.8•0.3 mg

Rena-Vite Rx tablets ℞ *vitamin supplement* [multiple B vitamins; vitamin C; folic acid; biotin] ≚•60•1•0.3 mg

Renax; Renax 5.5 film-coated caplets ℞ *nutritional therapy for azotemia (uremia)* [multiple vitamins & minerals; folic acid; biotin; hydrogenated oil] ≐•2.5•0.3 mg; ≐•5.5•0.3 mg ⊡ Ranexa

Renese-R tablets (discontinued 2007) ℞ *antihypertensive; diuretic* [polythiazide; reserpine] 2•0.25 mg

renin inhibitors *a class of antihypertensives that reduce the amount of serum angiotensin II by blocking the action of renin, an enzyme required to create its precursor, angiotensin I* [compare to: angiotensin-converting enzyme inhibitors; angiotensin II receptor antagonists]

rennet, cheese *medicinal herb* [see: bedstraw]

Reno-30 intracavitary instillation (discontinued 2010) ℞ *radiopaque contrast medium for urological imaging* [diatrizoate meglumine (46.67% iodine)] 300 mg/mL (141 mg/mL)

Reno-60; Reno-Dip injection (discontinued 2010) ℞ *radiopaque contrast medium* [diatrizoate meglumine (46.67% iodine)] 600 mg/mL (282 mg/mL); 300 mg/mL (141 mg/mL)

RenoCal-76 injection ℞ *radiopaque contrast medium* [diatrizoate meglumine; diatrizoate sodium (48.7% total iodine)] 660•100 mg/mL (370 mg/mL)

Renografin-60 injection ℞ *radiopaque contrast medium* [diatrizoate meglumine; diatrizoate sodium (48.75% total iodine)] 520•80 mg/mL (292.5 mg/mL)

Renoquid tablets ℞ *broad-spectrum bacteriostatic* [sulfacytine] 250 mg

Renova cream ℞ *retinoid for photodamage, fine wrinkles, mottled hyperpigmentation, and roughness of facial skin* [tretinoin] 0.02%, 0.05%

rentiapril INN

ReNu solution OTC *rinsing/storage solution for soft contact lenses* [sodium chloride (preserved saline solution)]

ReNu Effervescent Enzymatic Cleaner; ReNu Thermal Enzymatic Cleaner tablets (discontinued 2010) OTC *enzymatic cleaner for soft contact lenses* [subtilisin]

ReNu Multi-Purpose solution (discontinued 2010) OTC *chemical disinfecting solution for soft contact lenses* [polyaminopropyl biguanide; EDTA] 0.00005%•0.01%

Renvela film-coated tablets, powder for oral suspension ℞ *phosphate-binding polymer for hyperphosphatemia in dialysis patients with chronic kidney disease (CKD); also used for hyperuricemia in dialysis patients* [sevelamer (as carbonate)] 800 mg; 0.8, 2.4 g/packet

renytoline INN *anti-inflammatory* [also: paranyline HCl]

renytoline HCl [see: paranyline HCl]

renzapride INN, BAN

ReoPro IV injection ℞ *platelet aggregation inhibitor for PTCA and acute arterial occlusive disorders* [abciximab] 2 mg/mL

repaglinide USAN *meglitinide antidiabetic for type 2 diabetes that stimulates the release of insulin from the pancreas* 0.5, 1, 2 mg oral

Repan tablets ℞ *barbiturate sedative; analgesic; antipyretic* [butalbital; acetaminophen; caffeine] 50•325•40 mg ⊡ Riopan

Repan CF caplets ℞ *barbiturate sedative; analgesic; antipyretic* [butalbital; acetaminophen] 50•650 mg

reparixin *investigational (orphan) to prevent delayed graft function of solid organ transplants*

Repetab (trademarked dosage form) *extended-release tablet* ⊡ Ribatab; Robitab

repirinast USAN, INN *antiallergic; antiasthmatic*

Replagal *investigational (NDA filed, orphan) enzyme replacement therapy for Fabry disease* [agalsidase alfa]

Replens vaginal gel OTC *moisturizer/lubricant* [glycerin; mineral oil]

Replete ready-to-use oral liquid OTC *enteral nutritional therapy* [lactose-free formula]

Repliva 21/7 film-coated tablets (in packs of 28) (discontinued 2011) ℞ *hematinic* [iron (as ferrous fumarate, ferrous aspartoglycinate, and elemental iron); vitamin B$_{12}$; vitamin C; folic acid] 151•0.01•200•1 mg × 21 days; counters × 7 days

rEPO (recombinant erythropoietin) [see: epoetin alfa; epoetin beta]

repository corticotropin [see: corticotropin, repository]

Reprexain film-coated tablets ℞ *narcotic analgesic; antipyretic* [hydrocodone bitartrate; ibuprofen] 2.5•200, 5•200, 10•200 mg

repromicin USAN, INN *antibacterial*

Repronex powder or pellet for IM or subcu injection ℞ *gonadotropin; follicle-stimulating hormone (FSH) and luteinizing hormone (LH) for the induction of ovulation in women and spermatogenesis in men; adjunct to assisted reproductive technologies (ART)* [menotropins] 75, 150 FSH units + 75, 150 LH units

reproterol INN, BAN *bronchodilator* [also: reproterol HCl]

reproterol HCl USAN *bronchodilator* [also: reproterol]

Requip film-coated tablets ℞ *dopamine agonist for idiopathic Parkinson disease; treatment for primary restless legs syndrome (RLS)* [ropinirole (as HCl)] 0.25, 0.5, 1, 2, 3, 4, 5 mg

Requip CR (controlled release) *investigational (NDA filed) dopamine agonist for restless legs syndrome (RLS)* [ropinirole HCl]

Requip XL film-coated extended-release caplets ℞ *once-daily dopamine agonist for idiopathic Parkinson disease* [ropinirole (as HCl)] 2, 4, 6, 8, 12 mg

rescimetol INN

rescinnamine NF, INN, BAN *antihypertensive; rauwolfia derivative*

Rescon caplets ℞ *decongestant; antihistamine; anticholinergic to dry mucosal secretions* [phenylephrine HCl; chlorpheniramine maleate; methscopolamine nitrate] 40•12•1.25 mg ② risocaine

Rescon Jr. sustained-release caplets ℞ *decongestant; antihistamine* [phenylephrine HCl; dexchlorpheniramine maleate] 20•3 mg

Rescon-DM oral liquid OTC *antitussive; antihistamine; decongestant* [dextromethorphan hydrobromide; chlorpheniramine maleate; pseudoephedrine HCl] 10•2•30 mg/5 mL

Rescon-GG oral liquid OTC *decongestant; expectorant* [phenylephrine HCl; guaifenesin] 10•200 mg/10 mL

Rescon-MX caplets ℞ *decongestant; antihistamine* [phenylephrine HCl; dexchlorpheniramine maleate] 40•6 mg

Rescriptor caplets ℞ *antiretroviral for HIV-1 infection* [delavirdine mesylate] 100, 200 mg

Rescue Pak (trademarked delivery form) *unit dose package*

Resectisol solution (discontinued 2008) ℞ *genitourinary irrigant* [mannitol] 5 g/100 mL

reserpine USP, INN *antihypertensive; peripheral antiadrenergic; rauwolfia derivative* 0.1, 0.25 mg oral

resibufogenin [see: bufogenin]

resiniferatoxin (RTX) *investigational (orphan) neuronal desensitizing agent for intractable pain at end-stage disease*

resocortol butyrate USAN *topical anti-inflammatory*

Resol oral solution OTC *electrolyte replacement* [sodium, potassium, chloride, calcium, magnesium, and phosphate electrolytes] ② rose oil

Resolve/GP solution OTC *cleaning solution for hard or rigid gas permeable contact lenses*

resorantel INN

resorcin [see: resorcinol]

resorcin acetate [see: resorcinol monoacetate]

resorcin brown NF

resorcinol USP *keratolytic; antifungal*

resorcinol monoacetate USP *antiseborrheic; keratolytic*

ReSource; ReSource Plus; ReSource Diabetic; ReSource Just for Kids ready-to-use oral liquid in **Tetra Brik** packs OTC *enteral nutritional therapy* [lactose-free formula] 237 mL/pack

ReSource Arginaid powder for oral liquid OTC *arginine-rich enteral nutritional therapy to speed recovery of pressure ulcers, burns, or surgery*

ReSource Fruit Beverage ready-to-use oral liquid OTC *enteral nutritional therapy* [whey protein formula] 237 mL/pkt.

Respa A.R. tablets ℞ *decongestant; antihistamine; anticholinergic to dry mucosal secretions* [pseudoephedrine HCl; chlorpheniramine maleate; belladonna alkaloids (atropine, hyoscyamine, scopolamine)] 90•8• 0.024 mg

Respa C&C caplets ℞ *decongestant; antihistamine; sleep aid; antitussive; analgesic; antipyretic* [phenylephrine HCl; diphenhydramine HCl; dextromethorphan hydrobromide; acetaminophen] 18•37.5•30•575 mg

Respa-1st sustained-release tablets ℞ *decongestant; expectorant* [pseudoephedrine HCl; guaifenesin] 58•600 mg

Respa-DM sustained-release tablets ℞ *antitussive; expectorant* [dextromethorphan hydrobromide; guaifenesin] 28•600 mg

Respahist sustained-release capsules ℞ *decongestant; antihistamine* [pseudoephedrine HCl; brompheniramine maleate] 60•6 mg

Respahist-II extended-release caplets ℞ *decongestant; antihistamine* [phenylephrine HCl; brompheniramine maleate] 19•6 mg

Respaire-60 SR extended-release capsules ℞ *decongestant; expectorant* [pseudoephedrine HCl; guaifenesin] 60•200 mg

Respaire-120 SR dual-release capsules ℞ *decongestant; expectorant* [pseudo-

ephedrine HCl (extended release); guaifenesin (immediate release)] 120•250 mg

Respalor ready-to-use oral liquid OTC *enteral nutritional therapy for pulmonary problems*

Respa-SA caplets ℞ *decongestant; antihistamine; sleep aid* [pseudoephedrine HCl; diphenhydramine HCl] 58• 37.5 mg

Resperal syrup ℞ *antitussive; antihistamine; sleep aid; decongestant* [dextromethorphan hydrobromide; pyrilamine maleate; dexchlorpheniramine maleate; phenylephrine HCl] 5•5• 1.25•5 mg/5 mL

RespiGam IV infusion (discontinued 2009) ℞ *preventative for respiratory syncytial virus (RSV) infections in high-risk infants (orphan)* [respiratory syncytial virus immune globulin (RSV-IG)] 50 mg/mL (2500 mg/dose)

Respihaler (trademarked delivery form) *oral inhalation aerosol*

RespiPak (trademarked packaging form) *tablets in daily compliance packaging*

Respiracult-Strep culture paddles for professional use ℞ *in vitro diagnostic test for Group A streptococci from throat and nasopharyngeal sources*

respiratory syncytial virus immune globulin (RSV-IG) *preventative for respiratory syncytial virus (RSV) infections in high-risk infants (orphan); investigational (orphan) treatment for RSV*

Respirgard II (trademarked delivery device) *nebulizer*

Respi-Tann chewable tablets, oral suspension ℞ *antitussive; decongestant* [carbetapentane tannate; pseudoephedrine tannate] 25•75 mg; 25• 75 mg/5 mL

Respi-Tann G oral suspension (discontinued 2009) ℞ *antitussive; expectorant* [carbetapentane citrate; guaifenesin] 7.5•200 mg/5 mL

Respi-Tann Pd oral suspension ℞ *antitussive; decongestant* [carbetapentane tannate; pseudoephedrine tannate] 15•60 mg/5 mL

Respules (trademarked delivery form) *single-dose ampule for inhalation*

Restasis eye drop emulsion ℞ *immunomodulator and anti-inflammatory to increase tear production in patients with Sjögren keratoconjunctivitis sicca (orphan)* [cyclosporine] 0.05%

restoratives *a class of agents that promote a restoration of strength and vigor (a term used in folk medicine)*

Restore-X powder for oral solution OTC *vitamin/mineral/amino acid supplement* [multiple vitamins & minerals; multiple amino acids; folic acid] ≛•≛•400 mcg

Restoril capsules ℞ *benzodiazepine sedative and hypnotic* [temazepam] 7.5, 15, 22.5, 30 mg

Restylane subcu injection in prefilled syringes ℞ *transparent dermal filler for deep wrinkles and facial folds* [hyaluronic acid] 20 mg/mL

Restylane-L subcu injectable gel in prefilled syringes ℞ *transparent dermal filler for deep wrinkles and facial folds; local anesthetic* [hyaluronic acid; lidocaine] 20 mg/mL•0.3%

Re-Tann oral suspension ℞ *antitussive; decongestant* [carbetapentane tannate; pseudoephedrine tannate] 25•75 mg/5 mL 🔄 R-Tanna; rutin; Ry-Tann

retapamulin *topical pleuromutilin antibiotic for impetigo caused by* Staphylococcus aureus *and* Streptococcus pyogenes *infections*

Retavase powder for IV infusion ℞ *thrombolytic; tissue plasminogen activator (tPA) for acute myocardial infarction* [reteplase] 18.8 mg (10.8 IU)

retelliptine INN

reteplase USAN, INN *thrombolytic; tissue plasminogen activator (tPA) for acute myocardial infarction*

retigabine INN *potassium channel opener for adjunctive treatment of partial-onset epilepsy in adults* [also: ezogabine]

Retin-A cream, gel ℞ *keratolytic for acne* [tretinoin] 0.025%, 0.05%,

0.1% (0.01% available in Canada); 0.01%, 0.025%, 0.1% 🔄 R-Tanna; rutin; Ry-Tann

Retin-A Micro gel ℞ *keratolytic for acne* [tretinoin] 0.04%, 0.1%

retinoic acid (all-*trans*-retinoic acid) [see: tretinoin]

9-*cis*-retinoic acid [see: alitretinoin]

13-*cis*-retinoic acid [see: isotretinoin]

retinoids *a class of antineoplastics chemically related to vitamin A*

Retinol cream OTC *moisturizer; emollient* [vitamin A] 100 000 IU

retinol INN, BAN *vitamin A₁*

Retinol-A cream OTC *moisturizer; emollient* [vitamin A palmitate] 10 000 IU/g

Retisert ocular implant ℞ *corticosteroidal anti-inflammatory for uveitis (orphan)* [fluocinolone acetonide] 0.59 mg

R-etodolac *investigational (orphan) treatment for chronic lymphocytic leukemia*

Retrovir film-coated tablets, capsules, syrup, IV injection ℞ *antiretroviral for AIDS and AIDS-related complex (orphan), HIV-1 infection, and the prevention of maternal-fetal HIV-1 transmission* [zidovudine] 300 mg; 100 mg; 50 mg/5 mL; 10 mg/mL

retroviral vector gamma-c cDNA [see: gamma-c cDNA, retroviral vector]

retroviral vector glucocerebrosidase (GC) [see: glucocerebrosidase, recombinant retroviral vector]

Revatio film-coated tablets, IV injection ℞ *selective vasodilator for pulmonary arterial hypertension (PAH)* [sildenafil citrate] 20 mg

Reveal Rapid HIV-1 Antibody Test kit for professional use ℞ *in vitro diagnostic aid for HIV-1 in blood*

revenast INN

reverse transcriptase (RT) inhibitors *a class of antiretroviral drugs that inhibit the activity of reverse transcriptase in viral cells, preventing cell replication; subdivided into nucleoside (purine- or pyrimidine-based) and non-*

nucleoside types [reverse transcriptase is also known as DNA polymerase]

reversible proton pump inhibitors [see: proton pump inhibitors]

Reversol IV or IM injection ℞ *short-acting muscle stimulant; diagnostic aid for myasthenia gravis; antidote to curare* [edrophonium chloride] 10 mg/mL

Revex IV, IM, or subcu injection (discontinued 2008) ℞ *narcotic antagonist; antidote to opioid overdose; postanesthesia "stir-up"* [nalmefene] 0.1 mg/mL (postop), 1 mg/mL (antidote)

Rēv-Eyes powder for eye drops (discontinued 2009) ℞ *miotic to reverse iatrogenic mydriasis* [dapiprazole HCl] 0.5% ☒ Rivasa

ReVia film-coated tablets ℞ *narcotic antagonist for opiate dependence or overdose (orphan) and alcoholism; also used for pruritus and irritable bowel syndrome* [naltrexone HCl] 50 mg

reviparin sodium *investigational (orphan) for deep vein thrombosis (DVT) in pediatric or pregnant patients*

Revlimid capsules ℞ *immunomodulator for multiple myeloma and transfusion-dependent anemia in patients with myelodysplastic syndrome (orphan)* [lenalidomide] 5, 10, 15, 25 mg

Revonto powder for IV injection ℞ *skeletal muscle relaxant* [dantrolene sodium] 20 mg/vial (0.32 mg/mL)

revospirone INN, BAN

Rexin-G IV injection *investigational (NDA filed, orphan) tumor-targeted gene therapy for pancreatic cancer* [Mx-dnG1 retroviral vector]

Reyataz capsules ℞ *antiretroviral for HIV-1 infection* [atazanavir (as sulfate)] 100, 150, 200, 300 mg

Rezamid lotion OTC *antiseptic and keratolytic for acne* [sulfur; resorcinol; alcohol] 5%•2%•28%

Rezipas *investigational (orphan) for ulcerative colitis* [aminosalicylic acid]

Rezira oral liquid ℞ *narcotic antitussive; decongestant* [hydrocodone bitartrate; pseudoephedrine HCl] 5•60 mg/5 mL

Rezonic *investigational (NDA filed) NK-1 receptor antagonist for the prevention of chemotherapy-induced nausea and vomiting* [casopitant]

ReZyst IM chewable tablets OTC *natural intestinal bacteria; probiotic; dietary supplement* [Lactobacillus sp.; Bifidobacterium sp.] 150 mg

rGCR (recombinant glucocerebrosidase) [see: glucocerebrosidase, recombinant retroviral vector]

rG-CSF (recombinant granulocyte colony-stimulating factor) [see: lenograstim]

R-Gel (discontinued 2010) OTC *counterirritant; analgesic for muscle and joint pain* [capsaicin] 0.025%

R-Gen elixir ℞ *expectorant* [iodinated glycerol] 60 mg/5 mL ☒ Rēgain; Rogaine

R-Gene 10 IV injection ℞ *diagnostic aid for pituitary (growth hormone) function* [arginine HCl] 10% (950 mOsmol/L) ☒ Rēgain; Rogaine

RGG0853, E1A lipid complex *investigational (orphan) for advanced ovarian cancer*

rGM-CSF; rhGM-CSF; rhuGM-CSF (granulocyte-macrophage colony-stimulating factor) [q.v.]

RGV (raltegravir) [q.v.]

Rhamnus cathartica; R. frangula *medicinal herb* [see: buckthorn]

Rhamnus purshiana *medicinal herb* [see: cascara sagrada]

rhAPC (recombinant human activated protein C) [see: drotrecogan alfa]

(rhATIII) recombinant human antithrombin III) [see: antithrombin III]

rhDNase (recombinant human deoxyribonuclease) [see: dornase alfa]

rhenium *element (Re)*

Rheomacrodex IV infusion ℞ *plasma volume expander for shock due to hemorrhage, burns, or surgery* [dextran 40] 10%

rheotran (45) [see: dextran 45]

rhetinic acid [see: enoxolone]

Rheum palmatum *medicinal herb* [see: rhubarb]

Rheumatex slide tests for professional use ℞ *in vitro diagnostic aid for rheumatoid factor in the blood*

rheumatism root *medicinal herb* [see: twin leaf; wild yam]

rheumatism weed *medicinal herb* [see: pipsissewa]

Rheumaton slide tests for professional use ℞ *in vitro diagnostic aid for rheumatoid factor in serum or synovial fluid*

Rheumatrex Dose Pack (tablets) ℞ *antimetabolite antineoplastic for leukemia; systemic antipsoriatic; antirheumatic for adult and juvenile rheumatoid arthritis (orphan)* [methotrexate] 2.5 mg

rhFSH (recombinant human follicle-stimulating hormone) [see: menotropins]

rhGAA (recombinant human glucosidase-alpha acid) [see: alglucosidase alfa]

rhGH (recombinant human growth hormone) [see: somatropin]

rhIGF-1 (recombinant human insulin-like growth factor-1) [now: mecasermin]

rhIL-1R; rhu IL-1R (recombinant human interleukin-1 receptor) [see: interleukin-1 receptor]

rhIL-11 (recombinant human interleukin-11) [see: oprelvekin]

rhIL-12 (recombinant human interleukin-12) [see: interleukin-12]

Rhinabid extended-release capsules (discontinued 2007) ℞ *decongestant; antihistamine* [phenylephrine HCl; brompheniramine maleate] 15•12 mg

Rhinabid PD extended-release pediatric capsules (discontinued 2007) ℞ *decongestant; antihistamine* [phenylephrine HCl; brompheniramine maleate] 7.5•6 mg

Rhinacon A extended-release caplets ℞ *decongestant; antihistamine; sleep aid* [phenylephrine HCl; chlorpheniramine maleate; phenyltoloxamine citrate] 20•4•40 mg

Rhinall nasal spray, nose drops OTC *decongestant* [phenylephrine HCl] 0.25% ② ronnel

Rhinaris nasal solution, nasal gel OTC *nasal moisturizer* [sodium chloride (saline solution)] 0.2%

Rhinaris Lubricating Mist nasal spray, nasal gel OTC *nasal moisturizer* [polyethylene glycol; propylene glycol] 15%•5%; 15%•20%

Rhinatate Pediatric oral suspension (discontinued 2007) ℞ *decongestant; antihistamine; sleep aid* [phenylephrine tannate; chlorpheniramine tannate; pyrilamine tannate] 5•2•12.5 mg/5 mL

Rhinatate-NF Pediatric oral suspension (discontinued 2007) ℞ *decongestant; antihistamine* [phenylephrine tannate; chlorpheniramine tannate] 5•4.5 mg/5 mL

Rhinocort Aqua nasal spray in a metered-dose pump ℞ *corticosteroidal anti-inflammatory for seasonal or perennial allergic rhinitis* [budesonide] 32 mcg/dose

Rh$_O$(D) immune globulin USP *passive immunizing agent for antenatal or postpartum prophylaxis of Rh hemolytic disease of the newborn; treatment for immune thrombocytopenic purpura (orphan)* [also see: globulin, immune]

Rh$_O$(D) immune human globulin [now: Rh$_O$(D) immune globulin]

rhodine [see: aspirin]

rhodium *element (Rh)* ② radium

RhoGAM Ultra Filtered Plus IM injection in prefilled syringes ℞ *immunizing agent for antenatal or postpartum prophylaxis of Rh hemolytic disease of the newborn* [Rh$_O$(D) immune globulin] 300 mcg (1500 IU)

Rhophylac IV or IM injection in prefilled syringes ℞ *immunizing agent for antenatal or postpartum prophylaxis of Rh hemolytic disease of the newborn; treatment for immune thrombocytopenic purpura (orphan)* [Rh$_O$(D) immune globulin] 300 mcg (1500 IU)

rHSA (recombinant human serum albumin) [see: albumin, human]

rhubarb *(Rheum palmatum)* root *medicinal herb for colon and liver disorders*

Rhucin *investigational (NDA filed) agent to prevent acute attacks of angioedema in adolescents or adults with hereditary angioedema (HAE)* [C1-inhibitor, human]

rHuIFN-beta; rIFN-beta (recombinant [human] interferon beta) [see: interferon beta-1b, recombinant]

rhuMAb-E25 (monoclonal antibody E25, recombinant human) [now: omalizumab]

rhuMAb-VEGF (monoclonal antibody to vascular endothelial growth factor, recombinant human) [now: bevacizumab]

Rhus glabra medicinal herb [see: sumach]

RiaSTAP powder for injection ℞ *systemic hemostatic to control bleeding in fibrinogen-deficient patients (orphan)* [fibrinogen, human] 1 g/vial

Riba 3.0 SIA reagent kit for professional use ℞ *in vitro diagnostic aid for hepatitis C* [strip immunoblot assay (SIA)]

ribaminol USAN, INN *memory adjuvant*

RibaPak film-coated caplets (in 14 packs) (discontinued 2011) ℞ *antiviral for chronic hepatitis C infections (orphan) and clinically stable HIV disease; also used for viral hemorrhagic fevers* [ribavirin] 400 mg × 14, 600 mg × 14, 400 mg × 7 + 600 mg × 7

Ribasphere pellet-filled capsules, film-coated caplets ℞ *antiviral for chronic hepatitis C infections (orphan) and clinically stable HIV disease; also used for viral hemorrhagic fevers* [ribavirin] 200 mg; 200, 400, 600 mg

Ribatab film-coated caplets (discontinued 2011) ℞ *antiviral for chronic hepatitis C infections (orphan) and clinically stable HIV disease; also used for viral hemorrhagic fevers* [ribavirin] 400, 600 mg ⊡ Repetab; Robitab

ribavirin USP, INN *nucleoside antiviral for severe lower respiratory tract infections, chronic hepatitis C infections (orphan), and stable HIV disease; investigational (orphan) for hemorrhagic fever with renal syndrome* [also: tribavirin] 200 mg oral

Ribes nigrum; R. rubrum medicinal herb [see: currant]

ribgrass; ribwort *medicinal herb* [see: plantain]

riboflavin (vitamin B₂) USP, INN *water-soluble vitamin; enzyme cofactor* 50, 100 mg oral

riboflavin 5′-phosphate sodium USP *vitamin*

riboflavine [see: riboflavin]

riboprine USAN, INN *antineoplastic*

ribostamycin INN, BAN

riboxamide [see: tiazofurin]

ricainide [see: indecainide HCl]

rice bran oil (gamma oryzanol) extract *medicinal herb used as a hypolipidemic and to treat gastrointestinal and menopausal symptoms*

richweed *medicinal herb* [see: black cohosh; stone root]

Ricola Herb Throat Drops lozenges OTC *mild anesthetic; antipruritic; counterirritant* [menthol] 1.1 mg

RID shampoo + gel OTC *pediculicide for lice* [pyrethrins; piperonyl butoxide] 0.33%•4%

RID Pure Alternative gel OTC *pediculicide for lice* [dimethicone] 100%

ridaforolimus *investigational (NDA filed) angiogenesis inhibitor antineoplastic for bone and cartilage sarcoma*

Rid-A-Pain oral gel OTC *mucous membrane anesthetic* [benzocaine] 10% ⊡ riodipine

Rid-A-Pain-HP cream OTC *counterirritant; analgesic for muscle and joint pain* [capsaicin] 0.075%

Ridaura capsules ℞ *antirheumatic* [auranofin] 3 mg

ridazolol INN

Ridenol elixir (discontinued 2008) OTC *analgesic; antipyretic* [acetaminophen] 80 mg/5 mL

ridogrel USAN, INN, BAN *thromboxane synthetase inhibitor*

rifabutin USAN, INN *antiviral; antibacterial; for prevention of* Mycobacterium avium *complex (MAC) in advanced HIV patients (orphan)*

Rifadin capsules, powder for IV injection ℞ *tuberculostatic (orphan)* [rifampin] 150, 300 mg; 600 mg

rifalazil USAN *rifampin derivative; investigational (orphan) for pulmonary tuberculosis*

Rifamate capsules ℞ *tuberculostatic* [rifampin; isoniazid] 300●150 mg

rifametane USAN, INN *antibacterial*

rifamexil USAN *antibacterial*

rifamide USAN, INN *antibacterial*

rifampicin INN, BAN, JAN *antibacterial* [also: rifampin]

rifampin USAN, USP *antibacterial; antituberculosis agent (orphan)* [also: rifampicin] 150, 300 mg oral; 600 mg injection

rifampin & isoniazid & pyrazinamide *short-course treatment of tuberculosis (orphan)*

rifamycin INN, BAN

rifamycin diethylamide [see: rifamide]

rifamycin M-14 [see: rifamide]

rifapentine USAN, INN, BAN *antibacterial for tuberculosis (orphan); investigational (orphan) for AIDS-related* Mycobacterium avium *complex (MAC)*

Rifater tablets ℞ *short-course treatment for tuberculosis (orphan)* [rifampin; isoniazid; pyrazinamide] 120●50●300 mg

rifaximin USAN, INN *broad-spectrum rifamycin antibiotic for traveler's diarrhea and hepatic encephalopathy (orphan); also used for irritable bowel syndrome (IBS)*

rIFN-A (recombinant interferon alfa) [see: interferon alfa-2a, recombinant]

rIFN-α2 (recombinant interferon alfa-2) [see: interferon alfa-2b, recombinant]

rIFN-beta; rHuIFN-beta (recombinant [human] interferon beta) [see: interferon beta-1a, recombinant]

rifomycin [see: rifamycin]

RIG (rabies immune globulin) [q.v.]

rilapine INN

rilmazafone INN

rilmenidine INN

rilonacept *immunosuppressant; interleukin-1 (IL-1) blocker for cryopyrin-associated periodic syndromes (CAPS), including familial cold autoinflammatory syndrome (FCAS) and Muckle-Wells syndrome (MWS); investigational (Phase II) for chronic gout* [also known as: IL-1 Trap]

rilopirox INN

rilozarone INN

rilpivirine HCl *oral non-nucleoside reverse transcriptase inhibitor (NNRTI) for HIV-1 infection* (base=91%)

Rilutek film-coated caplets ℞ *neuroprotective agent for amyotrophic lateral sclerosis (ALS) (orphan); investigational (orphan) for Huntington disease* [riluzole] 50 mg

riluzole USAN, INN *neuroprotective agent for amyotrophic lateral sclerosis (ALS) (orphan); investigational (orphan) for Huntington disease*

rimabotulinumtoxin B *neurotoxin complex derived from* Clostridium botulinum, *type B; symptomatic treatment of cervical dystonia (orphan)*

Rimactane capsules ℞ *tuberculostatic* [rifampin] 300 mg

rimantadine INN *antiviral for the prophylaxis and treatment of influenza A infection* [also: rimantadine HCl]

rimantadine HCl USAN *antiviral for the prophylaxis and treatment of influenza A infection* [also: rimantadine] 100 mg oral

rimazolium metilsulfate INN

rimcazole INN *antipsychotic* [also: rimcazole HCl]

rimcazole HCl USAN *antipsychotic* [also: rimcazole]

rimexolone USAN, INN, BAN *topical ophthalmic corticosteroidal anti-inflammatory*

rimiterol INN *bronchodilator* [also: rimiterol hydrobromide]

rimiterol hydrobromide USAN *bronchodilator* [also: rimiterol]

rimonabant *investigational (NDA filed) selective cannabinoid CB$_1$ blocker for smoking cessation, weight loss, increasing HDL, increasing insulin sensitivity, and decreasing C-reactive protein (CRP)*

rimoprogin INN

Rimso-50 solution for bladder instillation R *anti-inflammatory for symptomatic relief of interstitial cystitis* [dimethyl sulfoxide (DMSO)] 50% ℞ RMS

Rindal HD Plus syrup (discontinued 2009) R *narcotic antitussive; antihistamine; decongestant* [hydrocodone bitartrate; chlorpheniramine maleate; phenylephrine HCl] 3.5•2•7.5 mg/5 mL

Rindal HPD syrup (discontinued 2009) R *narcotic antitussive; antihistamine; sleep aid; decongestant* [hydrocodone bitartrate; diphenhydramine HCl; phenylephrine HCl] 2•12.5•7.5 mg/5 mL

Ringer injection USP *fluid and electrolyte replenisher* [also: compound solution of sodium chloride] 500, 1000 mL

Ringer injection, lactated USP *fluid and electrolyte replenisher; systemic alkalizer* [also: compound solution of sodium lactate] 250, 500, 1000 mL

Ringer irrigation USP *irrigation solution* 1000 mL

Ringer irrigation, lactated *irrigation solution* 300 mL

Ringer solution [now: Ringer irrigation]

Rinnovi Nail System topical stick R *moisturizer; emollient; keratolytic* [urea] 50%

riodipine INN ℞ Rid-A-Pain

Riomet oral liquid R *biguanide antidiabetic that decreases hepatic glucose production and increases cellular response to insulin* [metformin HCl] 500 mg/5 mL

Riopan oral suspension OTC *antacid* [magaldrate] 540 mg/5 mL ℞ Repan

Riopan Plus chewable tablets, oral suspension OTC *antacid; antiflatulent*

[magaldrate; simethicone] 480•20, 1080•20 mg; 540•40, 1080•40 mg/5 mL

rioprostil USAN, INN *gastric antisecretory*

ripazepam USAN, INN *minor tranquilizer*

ripple grass *medicinal herb* [see: plantain]

Riquent *investigational (NDA filed, orphan) immunosuppressant for lupus-associated nephritis* [abetimus sodium]

risedronate sodium USAN *bisphosphonate bone resorption inhibitor for Paget disease and corticosteroid-induced or age-related osteoporosis in men and women*

rismorelin porcine USAN *growth stimulant for growth hormone deficiencies*

risocaine USAN, INN *local anesthetic* ℞ Rescon

risotilide HCl USAN *antiarrhythmic*

Risperdal tablets, M-Tabs (orally disintegrating tablets), oral drops R *novel (atypical) benzisoxazole antipsychotic for schizophrenia, manic episodes of a bipolar disorder, pediatric behavioral problems, and autism; also used for obsessive-compulsive disorder (OCD) and Tourette syndrome* [risperidone] 0.25, 0.5, 1, 2, 3, 4 mg; 0.5, 1, 2, 3, 4 mg; 1 mg/mL

Risperdal Consta powder for long-acting injection R *novel (atypical) benzisoxazole antipsychotic for schizophrenia and bipolar disorder* [risperidone (encapsulated in polymer microspheres)] 12.5, 25, 37.5, 50 mg

risperidone USAN, INN, BAN *novel (atypical) benzisoxazole antipsychotic for schizophrenia, manic episodes of a bipolar disorder, pediatric behavioral problems, and autism; also used for obsessive-compulsive disorder (OCD) and Tourette syndrome* 0.25, 0.5, 1, 2, 3, 4 mg oral; 1 mg/mL oral

ristianol INN, BAN *immunoregulator* [also: ristianol phosphate]

ristianol phosphate USAN *immunoregulator* [also: ristianol]

ristocetin USP, INN, BAN

Ritalin tablets R *CNS stimulant for attention-deficit/hyperactivity disorder*

(ADHD) and narcolepsy; also abused as a street drug [methylphenidate HCl] 5, 10, 20 mg

Ritalin LA dual-release capsules (50% immediate release, 50% delayed release) ℞ CNS stimulant for attention-deficit/hyperactivity disorder (ADHD) [methylphenidate HCl] 10, 20, 30, 40 mg

Ritalin SR sustained-release tablets ℞ CNS stimulant for attention-deficit/hyperactivity disorder (ADHD) and narcolepsy [methylphenidate HCl] 20 mg

ritanserin USAN, INN, BAN serotonin S_2 antagonist for various psychiatric illnesses and substance abuse

ritiometan INN

ritodrine USAN, INN smooth muscle relaxant

ritodrine HCl USAN, USP smooth muscle relaxant; uterine relaxant to arrest preterm labor

ritolukast USAN, INN antiasthmatic; leukotriene antagonist

ritonavir USAN, INN antiretroviral protease inhibitor for HIV infection 100 mg oral

ritropirronium bromide INN

ritrosulfan INN

Rituxan IV infusion ℞ monoclonal antibody for chronic lymphocytic leukemia (orphan), non-Hodgkin lymphoma (orphan), rheumatoid arthritis, microscopic polyangiitis, and granulomatosis; investigational (orphan) for ITP; investigational for vasculitis; also used for macroglobulinemia [rituximab] 10 mg/mL (100, 500 mg/vial)

rituximab USAN monoclonal antibody for chronic lymphocytic leukemia (orphan), non-Hodgkin lymphoma (orphan), rheumatoid arthritis, microscopic polyangiitis, and granulomatosis; investigational (orphan) for ITP; investigational for vasculitis; also used for macroglobulinemia

rivaroxaban factor Xa coagulation inhibitor; once-daily oral antithrombotic for the prevention of deep vein thrombosis (DVT) following knee or hip replacement surgery; investigational

(NDA filed) for venous thromboembolism (VTE) and stroke prevention

rivastigmine USAN acetylcholinesterase inhibitor to increase cognition in Alzheimer and Parkinson disease

rivastigmine tartrate acetylcholinesterase inhibitor to increase cognition in Alzheimer and Parkinson disease 1.5, 3, 4.5, 6 mg oral

rivoglitazone USAN antidiabetic for type 2 diabetes

Rizaben investigational (orphan) for malignant glioma [tranilast]

rizatriptan benzoate USAN vascular serotonin 5-$HT_{1B/1D}$ receptor agonist for the acute treatment of migraine

rizatriptan sulfate USAN vascular serotonin 5-$HT_{1B/1D}$ receptor agonist for the acute treatment of migraine

rizolipase INN

r-metHuLeptin [see: metreleptin]

RMP-7 (receptor-mediated permeabilizer) [see: lobradimil]

RMS suppositories ℞ narcotic analgesic [morphine sulfate] 5, 10, 20, 30 mg

rNPA (recombinant novel plasminogen activator) [see: novel plasminogen activator]

rob elder medicinal herb [see: elderberry]

Robafen CF oral liquid OTC antitussive; decongestant; expectorant [dextromethorphan hydrobromide; pseudoephedrine HCl; guaifenesin] 10•30•100 mg/5 mL

Robafen DM; Robafen DM Max oral liquid OTC antitussive; expectorant [dextromethorphan hydrobromide; guaifenesin] 10•100 mg/5 mL; 10•200 mg/5 mL

Robafen PE oral liquid (discontinued 2007) OTC decongestant; expectorant [pseudoephedrine HCl; guaifenesin] 60•200 mg/10 mL

RoBathol Bath Oil OTC bath emollient

Robaxin tablets, IV or IM injection ℞ skeletal muscle relaxant [methocarbamol] 500, 750 mg; 100 mg/mL

robenidine INN coccidiostat for poultry [also: robenidine HCl]

robenidine HCl USAN *coccidiostat for poultry* [also: robenidine]

Robicap (trademarked dosage form) *capsule*

Robinul tablets, IV or IM injection ℞ GI *anticholinergic/antispasmodic/antisecretory; adjunctive treatment for peptic ulcers* [glycopyrrolate] 1 mg; 0.2 mg/5 mL

Robinul Forte tablets ℞ GI *antispasmodic; anticholinergic; peptic ulcer treatment adjunct; antisecretory* [glycopyrrolate] 2 mg

Robitab (trademarked dosage form) *tablet* ⃞ Repetab; Ribatab

Robitussin oral liquid OTC *expectorant* [guaifenesin] 100 mg/5 mL

Robitussin Children's Cough & Cold CF oral liquid ℞ *antitussive; decongestant; expectorant* [dextromethorphan hydrobromide; phenylephrine HCl; guaifenesin] 5•2.5•50 mg/5 mL

Robitussin Cold, Cold & Congestion caplets OTC *antitussive; decongestant; expectorant* [dextromethorphan hydrobromide; pseudoephedrine HCl; guaifenesin] 10•30•200 mg

Robitussin Cough oral liquid OTC *antitussive* [dextromethorphan hydrobromide; alcohol 1.4%] 15 mg/5 mL

Robitussin Cough, Cold & Flu Nighttime syrup OTC *antitussive; antihistamine; decongestant; analgesic; antipyretic* [dextromethorphan hydrobromide; chlorpheniramine maleate; phenylephrine HCl; acetaminophen] 10•2•5•320 mg/10 mL

Robitussin Cough & Allergy oral liquid (discontinued 2010) OTC *antitussive; antihistamine; decongestant* [dextromethorphan hydrobromide; brompheniramine maleate; phenylephrine HCl] 10•2•5 mg/5 mL

Robitussin Cough & Cold D oral liquid OTC *antitussive; decongestant; expectorant* [dextromethorphan hydrobromide; pseudoephedrine HCl; guaifenesin] 30•60•400 mg/10 mL

Robitussin Cough & Congestion oral liquid OTC *antitussive; expectorant* [dextromethorphan hydrobromide; guaifenesin] 10•200 mg/5 mL

Robitussin Cough Drops (lozenges) OTC *mild anesthetic; antipruritic; counterirritant* [menthol] 7.4, 10 mg

Robitussin Cough Sugar-Free DM oral liquid OTC *antitussive; expectorant* [dextromethorphan hydrobromide; guaifenesin] 10•100 mg/5 mL

Robitussin CoughGels liquid-filled gelcaps OTC *antitussive* [dextromethorphan hydrobromide] 15 mg

Robitussin Liquid Center Cough Drops (lozenges) OTC *mild anesthetic; antipruritic; counterirritant* [menthol] 10 mg

Robitussin PE Head and Chest Congestion oral liquid OTC *decongestant; expectorant* [phenylephrine HCl; guaifenesin] 10•200 mg/10 mL

Robitussin Pediatric Cough oral liquid OTC *antitussive* [dextromethorphan hydrobromide] 7.5 mg/5 mL

Robitussin Pediatric Cough & Cold Long-Acting oral liquid OTC *antitussive; antihistamine; for adults and children* ≥ 6 *years* [dextromethorphan hydrobromide; chlorpheniramine maleate] 15•2 mg/10 mL

Robitussin Pediatric Cough & Cold Nighttime oral liquid (discontinued 2010) OTC *antitussive; antihistamine; decongestant; for adults and children* ≥ 6 *years* [dextromethorphan hydrobromide; chlorpheniramine maleate; phenylephrine HCl] 10•2•5 mg/10 mL

Robitussin Pediatric Cough/Cold CF oral drops OTC *antitussive; decongestant; expectorant; for children 2–5 years* [dextromethorphan hydrobromide; phenylephrine HCl; guaifenesin] 2•1•40 mg/mL

Robitussin-DM oral liquid OTC *antitussive; expectorant* [dextromethorphan hydrobromide; guaifenesin] 10•100 mg/5 mL

Rocaltrol capsules, oral solution ℞ *vitamin D therapy for hypoparathyroidism and hypocalcemia due to chronic renal dialysis; also used to decrease the severity of psoriatic lesions* [calcitriol] 0.25, 0.5 mcg; 1 mcg/mL

rocastine INN *antihistamine* [also: rocastine HCl]

rocastine HCl USAN *antihistamine* [also: rocastine]

Rocephin powder or frozen premix for IV or IM injection ℞ *third-generation cephalosporin antibiotic* [ceftriaxone sodium] 0.5, 1, 2 g

rochelle salt [see: potassium sodium tartrate]

rociverine INN

rock brake; rock polypod *medicinal herb* [see: female fern]

rock elm *medicinal herb* [see: slippery elm]

rock parsley *medicinal herb* [see: parsley]

rock rose *(Helianthemum canadense)* plant *medicinal herb used as an astringent and tonic*

Rocky Mountain grape *medicinal herb* [see: Oregon grape]

Rocky Mountain spotted fever vaccine USP

rocuronium bromide USAN, INN, BAN *nondepolarizing neuromuscular blocking agent; muscle relaxant; adjunct to general anesthesia* 10 mg/mL injection

rodocaine USAN, INN *local anesthetic*

rodorubicin INN

rofelodine INN ⑨ Refludan

Roferon-A subcu or IM injection in prefilled syringes (discontinued 2009) ℞ *immunostimulant for hairy cell leukemia, hepatitis C, Kaposi sarcoma (orphan), and chronic myelogenous leukemia (orphan); investigational (orphan) for malignant melanoma and esophageal, renal, colorectal, and other cancers* [interferon alfa-2a] 3, 6, 9 million IU

roflumilast *once-daily oral phosphodiesterase 4 (PDE-4) inhibitor for chronic obstructive pulmonary disease (COPD)*

roflurane USAN, INN *inhalation anesthetic*

Rogaine; Rogaine for Men; Rogaine for Women topical solution OTC *hair growth stimulant* [minoxidil] 2%; 2%, 5%; 2% ⑨ Rēgain

Rogaine Men's Extra Strength topical foam OTC *hair growth stimulant* [minoxidil] 5%

rogletimide USAN, INN, BAN *antineoplastic; aromatase inhibitor*

Rohypnol (banned in the U.S.) ℞ *sedative and hypnotic; smuggled into the U.S. as a street drug, commonly called "roofies" or "the date rape drug"* [flunitrazepam]

rokitamycin INN

Rolaids; Calcium Rich Rolaids chewable tablets OTC *antacid* [magnesium hydroxide; calcium carbonate] 110•550, 135•675 mg; 80•412 mg

Rolaids Multi-Symptom chewable tablets OTC *antacid; antiflatulent* [magnesium hydroxide; calcium carbonate; simethicone] 135•675•60 mg

Rolaids Plus Gas Relief chewable tablets OTC *antacid; antiflatulent* [calcium carbonate; simethicone] 1177•80 mg

Rolaids Softchews OTC *antacid; calcium supplement* [calcium (as carbonate)] 471 mg (1177 mg)

roletamide USAN, INN *hypnotic*

rolgamidine USAN, INN, BAN *antidiarrheal*

rolicton [see: amisometradine]

rolicyclidine INN

rolicypram BAN *antidepressant* [also: rolicyprine]

rolicyprine USAN, INN *antidepressant* [also: rolicypram]

rolipram USAN, INN *tranquilizer*

rolitetracycline USAN, USP, INN *antibacterial*

rolitetracycline nitrate USAN *antibacterial*

rolodine USAN, INN *skeletal muscle relaxant*

rolofylline *investigational (Phase III) agent for acute heart failure*

rolziracetam INN, BAN

Roman camomile *medicinal herb* [see: chamomile]

Roman laurel *medicinal herb* [see: laurel]

romazarit USAN, INN, BAN *anti-inflammatory; antirheumatic*

Romazicon IV injection ℞ *benzodiazepine antagonist to reverse anesthesia or treat overdose; also used for hepatic encephalopathy* [flumazenil] 0.1 mg/mL

rometin [see: clioquinol]

romidepsin *histone deacetylase (HDAC) inhibitor for cutaneous T-cell lymphoma*

romifenone INN

romifidine INN

Romilar AC oral liquid (discontinued 2007) ℞ *narcotic antitussive; expectorant* [codeine phosphate; guaifenesin] 20•200 mg/10 mL

romiplostim *hematopoietic; oral thrombopoietin (TPO) receptor agonist to increase platelet production in immune thrombocytopenic purpura (ITP)*

romurtide INN

ronactolol INN

Rondamine-DM syrup (discontinued 2007) ℞ *antitussive; antihistamine; decongestant* [dextromethorphan hydrobromide; brompheniramine maleate; pseudoephedrine HCl] 15•4•60 mg/5 mL

Rondec oral drops (discontinued 2011) ℞ *decongestant; antihistamine; drops for children 6–24 months* [phenylephrine HCl; chlorpheniramine maleate] 3.5•1 mg/mL

Rondec syrup (discontinued 2009) ℞ *decongestant; antihistamine; drops for children 6–24 months* [phenylephrine HCl; chlorpheniramine maleate] 12.5•4 mg/5 mL

Rondec tablets (discontinued 2007) ℞ *decongestant; antihistamine* [pseudoephedrine HCl; carbinoxamine maleate] 60•4 mg

Rondec-DM oral drops (discontinued 2010) ℞ *antitussive; antihistamine; decongestant; for children 6–24 months* [dextromethorphan hydrobromide; carbinoxamine maleate; phenylephrine HCl] 3•1•3.5 mg/mL

Rondec-DM syrup (discontinued 2007) ℞ *antitussive; antihistamine; decongestant* [dextromethorphan hydrobromide; chlorpheniramine maleate; phenylephrine HCl] 15•4•12.5 mg/5 mL

Rondec-TR timed-release tablets (discontinued 2007) ℞ *decongestant; antihistamine* [pseudoephedrine HCl; carbinoxamine maleate] 120•8 mg

Rondex oral drops (discontinued 2011) ℞ *decongestant; antihistamine; for children 6–24 months* [phenylephrine HCl; chlorpheniramine maleate] 3.5•1 mg/mL

Rondex-DM oral drops ℞ *antitussive; antihistamine; decongestant; for children 6–24 months* [dextromethorphan hydrobromide; carbinoxamine maleate; phenylephrine HCl] 3•1•3.5 mg/mL

ronidazole USAN, INN *antiprotozoal*

ronifibrate INN

ronipamil INN

ronnel USAN *systemic insecticide* [also: fenclofos; fenchlorphos] ② Rhinall

ropinirole INN, BAN *dopamine agonist for idiopathic Parkinson disease; treatment for primary restless legs syndrome (RLS)* [also: ropinirole HCl]

ropinirole HCl USAN *dopamine agonist for idiopathic Parkinson disease; treatment for primary restless legs syndrome (RLS)* [also: ropinirole] 0.25, 0.5, 1, 2, 3, 4, 5 mg

ropitoin INN *antiarrhythmic* [also: ropitoin HCl]

ropitoin HCl USAN *antiarrhythmic* [also: ropitoin]

ropivacaine INN *long-acting injectable local anesthetic*

ropivacaine HCl *long-acting local or regional anesthetic for surgery; epidural block for cesarean section*

ropizine USAN, INN *anticonvulsant*

roquinimex USAN, INN *investigational (orphan) bone marrow transplant adjunct for leukemia*

Rosa acicularis; R. canina; R. rugosa **and other species** *medicinal herb* [see: rose]

Rosac cream ℞ *antibiotic and keratolytic for acne* [sulfacetamide sodium; sulfur] 10%•5%

Rosac Wash emulsion ℞ *antibiotic and keratolytic for acne* [sulfacetamide sodium; sulfur] 10%•1%

Rosaderm wash ℞ *antibiotic and keratolytic for acne* [sulfacetamide sodium; sulfur] 10%•5%

rosamicin [now: rosaramicin]

rosamicin butyrate [now: rosaramicin butyrate]

rosamicin propionate [now: rosaramicin propionate]

rosamicin sodium phosphate [now: rosaramicin sodium phosphate]

rosamicin stearate [now: rosaramicin stearate]

Rosanil cleanser ℞ *antibiotic and keratolytic for acne* [sulfacetamide sodium; sulfur] 10%•5%

rosaprostol INN

rosaramicin USAN, INN *antibacterial*

rosaramicin butyrate USAN *antibacterial*

rosaramicin propionate USAN *antibacterial*

rosaramicin sodium phosphate USAN *antibacterial*

rosaramicin stearate USAN *antibacterial*

rosary pea *medicinal herb* [see: precatory bean]

rose (*Rosa acicularis; R. canina; R. rugosa* **and other species**) *flowers and hips medicinal herb for blood cleansing, cancer, colds, flu, infections, and sore throat; also used as a diuretic, mild laxative, and source of vitamin C*

rose, sun *medicinal herb* [see: rock rose]

rose bengal *diagnostic aid for corneal or conjunctival injury and pathology* 1.3 mg/strip

rose bengal sodium (^{131}I) INN *hepatic function test; radioactive agent* [also: rose bengal sodium I 131]

rose bengal sodium I 125 USAN *radioactive agent*

rose bengal sodium I 131 USAN, USP *hepatic function test; radioactive agent* [also: rose bengal sodium (^{131}I)]

rose laurel *medicinal herb* [see: mountain laurel]

rose oil NF *perfume* ② Resol

rose petal aqueous infusion *ocular emollient*

rose water, stronger NF *perfume*

rose water ointment USP *emollient; ointment base*

rosemary (*Rosmarinus officinalis*) leaves *medicinal herb for flatulence, gastrointestinal spasm, halitosis, heart tonic, inducing diaphoresis, migraine headache, promoting menstrual flow, stimulating abortion, and stomach disorders*

Rosets ophthalmic strips (discontinued 2010) OTC *diagnostic aid for corneal or conjunctival injury and pathology* [rose bengal] 1.3 mg

rosiglitazone maleate USAN *thiazolidinedione (TZD) antidiabetic and peroxisome proliferator–activated receptor–gamma (PPARγ) agonist that increases cellular response to insulin without increasing insulin secretion*

rosin USP

rosoxacin USAN, INN *antibacterial* [also: acrosoxacin]

rostaporfin USAN *photosensitizer; investigational (orphan) to prevent access graft disease in hemodialysis patients*

rosterolone INN

Rosula soap, gel ℞ *antibiotic and keratolytic for acne and rosacea* [sulfacetamide sodium; sulfur; urea] 10%•5%•10% ② Resol

Rosula Aqueous Cleanser topical liquid (discontinued 2009) ℞ *antibiotic and keratolytic for acne and rosacea* [sulfacetamide sodium; sulfur; urea] 10%•5%•10%

Rosula Clarifying Wash topical liquid ℞ *antibiotic and keratolytic for acne and rosacea* [sulfacetamide sodium; sulfur; urea] 10%•4%•10%

Rosula Foam ℞ *antibiotic and keratolytic for acne and rosacea* [sulfacetamide sodium; sulfur] 10%•4%

Rosula NS cleansing pads ℞ *antibiotic for acne and rosacea* [sulfacetamide sodium; urea] 10%•10%

rosuvastatin calcium USAN *HMG-CoA reductase inhibitor for hypercholesterolemia, mixed dyslipidemia, and hypertriglyceridemia; reduces atheroma (plaque build-up) in arteries and serum C-reactive protein (CRP) levels to prevent stroke and myocardial infarction* 5, 10, 20, 40 mg oral

rosuvastatin zinc *investigational (NDA filed) HMG-CoA reductase inhibitor for hypercholesterolemia, mixed dyslipidemia, and hypertriglyceridemia; new salt form of rosuvastatin* 5, 10, 20, 40 mg oral

Rotacaps (trademarked dosage form) *encapsulated powder for inhalation*

Rotadisk (trademarked dosage form) *powder for inhalation* [used in a **Diskhaler** delivery device]

rotamicillin INN

Rotarix powder for oral suspension ℞ *immunization against rotavirus G1, G3, G4, and G9 gastroenteritis in infants 6–24 weeks* [rotavirus vaccine, live attenuated] 1 mL/dose

RotaTeq oral suspension in single-dose tubes ℞ *live oral immunization against rotavirus G1, G2, G3, and G4 gastroenteritis in infants 6–32 weeks* [rotavirus vaccine, live pentavalent] 2 mL/tube

rotavirus vaccine *live oral immunization against rotavirus gastroenteritis in infants 6–32 weeks*

rotigotine *dopamine D_2 agonist for early-stage Parkinson disease*

rotoxamine USAN, INN *antihistamine*

rotoxamine tartrate NF

rotraxate INN

round-leaved plantain *medicinal herb* [see: plantain]

Rovamycine *macrolide antibiotic; investigational (orphan) treatment for chronic cryptosporidiosis in immunocompromised patients* [spiramycin]

rovelizumab USAN, INN *immunomodulator; cell adhesion inhibitor*

Rowasa suppositories (discontinued 2008) ℞ *anti-inflammatory for active ulcerative colitis, proctosigmoiditis, and proctitis* [mesalamine (5-aminosalicylic acid)] 500 mg

Rowasa; sfRowasa enema (note: "sf"=sulfite free) ℞ *anti-inflammatory for active ulcerative colitis, proctosigmoiditis, and proctitis* [mesalamine (5-aminosalicylic acid)] 4 g/60 mL

roxadimate USAN, INN *sunscreen*

Roxanol; Roxanol T; Roxanol 100 oral concentrate ℞ *narcotic analgesic* [morphine sulfate] 20 mg/mL; 20 mg/mL; 100 mg/5 mL

roxarsone USAN, INN *antibacterial*

roxatidine INN, BAN *histamine H_2 antagonist for gastric and duodenal ulcers* [also: roxatidine acetate HCl]

roxatidine acetate HCl USAN *histamine H_2 antagonist for gastric and duodenal ulcers* [also: roxatidine]

roxibolone INN

Roxicet tablets, oral solution ℞ *narcotic analgesic; antipyretic* [oxycodone HCl; acetaminophen] 5•325 mg; 5•325 mg/5 mL

Roxicet 5/500 caplets ℞ *narcotic analgesic; antipyretic* [oxycodone HCl; acetaminophen] 5•500 mg

Roxicodone tablets, oral solution, Intensol (concentrated oral solution) ℞ *narcotic analgesic* [oxycodone HCl] 5, 15, 30 mg; 5 mg/5 mL; 20 mg/mL

roxifiban acetate USAN *antithrombotic; fibrinogen receptor antagonist*

Roxilox capsules ℞ *narcotic analgesic; antipyretic* [oxycodone HCl; acetaminophen] 5•500 mg

roxindole INN

Roxiprin tablets ℞ *narcotic analgesic; antipyretic* [oxycodone HCl; oxycodone terephthalate; aspirin] 4.5•0.38•325 mg

roxithromycin USAN, INN *macrolide antibiotic*

roxolonium metilsulfate INN

roxoperone INN

royal jelly *natural remedy for improving fertility and increasing longevity*

Rozerem film-coated tablets ℞ *hypnotic for insomnia due to difficulty with sleep onset* [ramelteon] 8 mg

rPA; r-PA (recombinant plasminogen activator) *more properly called "recombinant tissue plasminogen activator" (rtPA)* [see: alteplase; anistreplase; lanoteplase; monteplase; reteplase; saruplase; tenecteplase]

R/S lotion OTC *antiseptic, antifungal, and keratolytic for acne* [sulfur; resorcinol; alcohol] 5%•2%•28%

rSP-C lung surfactant *investigational (orphan) for adult respiratory distress syndrome (ARDS)*

RSV-IG (respiratory syncytial virus immune globulin) [q.v.]

RT (reverse transcriptase) inhibitors [q.v.]

R-Tanna caplets ℞ *decongestant; antihistamine* [phenylephrine tannate; chlorpheniramine tannate] 25•9 mg ☑ Re-Tann; rutin; Ry-Tann

R-Tanna 12 oral suspension ℞ *decongestant; antihistamine; sleep aid* [phenylephrine tannate; pyrilamine tannate] 5•30 mg/5 mL ☑ Re-Tann; rutin; Ry-Tann

R-Tanna S Pediatric oral suspension (discontinued 2007) ℞ *decongestant; antihistamine* [phenylephrine tannate; chlorpheniramine tannate] 5•4.5 mg/5 mL

rtPA; rt-PA (recombinant tissue plasminogen activator) [see: alteplase; anistreplase; lanoteplase; monteplase; reteplase; saruplase; tenecteplase]

Rubazyme reagent kit for professional use ℞ *in vitro diagnostic aid for rubella virus IgG antibodies in serum* [enzyme immunoassay (EIA)]

rubbing alcohol [see: alcohol, rubbing]

rubbing isopropyl alcohol [see: isopropyl alcohol, rubbing]

rubefacients *a class of gentle local irritants that redden the skin by producing active or passive hyperemia*

rubella & mumps virus vaccine, live *active immunizing agent for rubella and mumps*

rubella virus vaccine, live USP *active immunizing agent for rubella*

rubeola vaccine [see: measles virus vaccine, live]

rubidium *element (Rb)*

rubidium chloride Rb 82 USAN *radioactive diagnostic aid for cardiac disease*

rubidium chloride Rb 86 USAN *radioactive agent*

rubidomycin [now: daunorubicin]

rubitecan USAN *topoisomerase I inhibitor; investigational (Phase III, orphan) for pediatric HIV/AIDS infections*

Rubus fructicosus; R. villosus *medicinal herb* [see: blackberry]

Rubus idaeus; R. strigosus *medicinal herb* [see: red raspberry]

rue (*Ruta bracteosa; R. graveolens; R. montana*) *plant medicinal herb for cramps, hypertension, hysteria, muscle strains, neuralgia, nervous disorders, sciatica, stimulation of abortion and menstruation, tendon strains, and trauma*

rufinamide USAN, INN *triazole anticonvulsant; adjunctive therapy for Lennox-Gastaut syndrome (orphan)*

rufloxacin INN

rufocromomycin INN, BAN *antineoplastic* [also: streptonigrin]

Ru-lets M 500 film-coated tablets (discontinued 2008) OTC *vitamin/mineral supplement* [multiple vitamins & minerals]

RuLox oral suspension OTC *antacid; antiflatulent* [aluminum hydroxide; magnesium hydroxide; simethicone] 200•200•20 mg/5 mL ☑ Ralix

RuLox Plus chewable tablets OTC *antacid; antiflatulent* [aluminum hydroxide; magnesium hydroxide; simethicone] 200•200•25 mg

RuLox Plus oral suspension (discontinued 2010) OTC *antacid; antiflatulent* [aluminum hydroxide; magnesium hydroxide; simethicone] 500•450•40 mg/5 mL

rum cherry *medicinal herb* [see: wild black cherry]

Rumex acetosa medicinal herb [see: sorrel]

Rumex crispus medicinal herb [see: yellow dock]

Rumex hymenosepalus medicinal herb [see: canaigre]

ruplizumab USAN *treatment for immune thrombocytopenic purpura and systemic lupus erythematosus (SLE) (orphan); investigational (orphan) for hemophilia A and B and to prevent rejection of pancreatic islet cell and solid organ transplants*

Ruscus aculeatus medicinal herb [see: butcher's broom]

rush, sweet *medicinal herb* [see: calamus]

Ruta bracteosa; R. graveolens; R. montana medicinal herb [see: rue]

rutamycin USAN, INN *antifungal*

ruthenium *element (Ru)*

rutin NF *a bioflavonoid (q.v.)* [also: rutoside] ☒ Re-Tann; R-Tanna; Ry-Tann

Rutiplen C capsules OTC *vitamin C supplement with multiple bioflavonoids* [vitamins C and E; citrus bioflavonoids; rutin] 600 mg•25 IU•100 mg•50 mg

rutoside INN [also: rutin]

ruvazone INN

ruxoltinib *investigational (NDA filed) antineoplastic for myelofibrosis*

RVA (rabies vaccine, adsorbed) [see: rabies vaccine]

RVP (red veterinarian petrolatum) [see: petrolatum]

Rx Support Heartburn & Acid Reflux tablets OTC *vitamin/calcium supplement* [vitamins B_6, B_{12}, and D; calcium; folic acid] 10 mg•200 mcg•1000 U•≚•400 mcg

Rx Support Heartburn & Acid Reflux Plus Aloe tablets OTC *vitamin/calcium supplement* [vitamins B_6, B_{12}, and D; calcium; folic acid; aloe vera powder] 10 mg•200 mcg•1000 U•≚•400 mcg•100 mg

RxPak; ℞Pak (trademarked packaging form) *prescription package*

Rybix ODT (orally disintegrating tablets) ℞ *opioid analgesic for moderate to severe chronic pain* [tramadol HCl] 50 mg

Ryna-12 caplets ℞ *decongestant; antihistamine; sleep aid* [phenylephrine tannate; pyrilamine tannate] 25•60 mg

Ryna-12 S oral suspension ℞ *decongestant; antihistamine; sleep aid* [phenylephrine tannate; pyrilamine tannate] 5•30 mg/5 mL

Ryna-12X tablets, oral suspension ℞ *decongestant; antihistamine; sleep aid; expectorant* [phenylephrine tannate; pyrilamine tannate; guaifenesin] 25•60•200 mg; 5•30•100 mg/5 mL ☒ Ranexa; Renax

Rynatan caplets ℞ *decongestant; antihistamine* [phenylephrine tannate; chlorpheniramine tannate] 25•9 mg

Rynatan Pediatric chewable tablets, oral suspension ℞ *decongestant; antihistamine* [phenylephrine tannate; chlorpheniramine tannate] 5•4.5 mg; 5•4.5 mg/5 mL

Rynatuss caplets ℞ *antitussive; antihistamine; decongestant* [carbetapentane tannate; chlorpheniramine tannate; phenylephrine tannate; ephedrine tannate] 60•5•10•10 mg

Rynatuss Pediatric oral suspension ℞ *antitussive; antihistamine; decongestant* [carbetapentane tannate; chlorpheniramine tannate; phenylephrine tannate; ephedrine tannate] 30•4•5•5 mg/5 mL

Rynesa 12S oral suspension ℞ *decongestant; antihistamine; sleep aid* [phenylephrine tannate; pyrilamine tannate] 5•30 mg/5 mL

Rynex PE oral liquid ℞ *decongestant; antihistamine* [phenylephrine HCl; brompheniramine maleate] 2.5•1 mg/5 mL

Ryneze extended-release tablets (discontinued 2007) ℞ *antihistamine; anticholinergic to dry mucosal secretions* [chlorpheniramine maleate; methscopolamine nitrate] 8•2.5 mg

Ryneze oral liquid ℞ *antihistamine; anticholinergic to dry mucosal secretions* [chlorpheniramine maleate; scopolamine] 4•1.25 mg/5 mL
RY-T-12 oral suspension ℞ *decongestant; antihistamine; sleep aid* [phenylephrine tannate; pyrilamine tannate] 5•30 mg/5 mL
Ry-Tann caplets ℞ *decongestant; antihistamine* [phenylephrine tannate; chlorpheniramine tannate] 25•9 mg
🔲 Re-Tann; R-Tanna; rutin

Rythmol film-coated tablets ℞ *antiarrhythmic* [propafenone HCl] 150, 225 mg
Rythmol SR extended-release capsules ℞ *antiarrhythmic* [propafenone HCl] 225, 325, 425 mg
Ryzolt controlled-release tablets ℞ *once-daily opioid analgesic for moderate to severe pain; also used for premature ejaculation* [tramadol HCl] 100, 200, 300 mg

S

S-2 solution for inhalation OTC *sympathomimetic bronchodilator and vasopressor for bronchial asthma* [epinephrine (as racepinephrine chloride)] 1.125%
^{35}S [see: sodium sulfate S 35]
SA (salicylic acid) [q.v.]
SA (serum albumin) [see: albumin, human]
SA 6% cream, lotion ℞ *keratolytic* [salicylic acid] 6%
Sabatia angularis medicinal herb [see: American centaury]
sabcomeline HCl USAN *muscarinic receptor agonist for Alzheimer disease*
sabeluzole USAN, INN, BAN *anticonvulsant; antihypoxic*
Sabin vaccine [see: poliovirus vaccine, live oral]
Sabril film-coated tablets, powder for oral solution ℞ *anticonvulsant for infantile spasms (orphan) and complex partial seizures; investigational (Phase II) treatment for cocaine and methamphetamine addictions* [vigabatrin] 500 mg; 500 mg/packet
saccharated ferric oxide JAN *hematinic for iron-deficiency anemia in patients with chronic kidney disease* [also: iron sucrose]
saccharated iron; saccharated iron oxide [see: iron sucrose; saccharated ferric oxide]

saccharin NF *flavoring agent*
saccharin calcium USP *non-nutritive sweetener*
saccharin sodium USP *non-nutritive sweetener*
Saccharomyces boulardii; Saccharomyces boulardii lyo natural intestinal bacteria; probiotic; dietary supplement
sacred bark medicinal herb [see: cascara sagrada]
sacrosidase USAN *enzyme replacement therapy for congenital sucrase-isomaltase deficiency (orphan)*
S-adenosyl-L-methionine (SAMe) *natural amino acid derivative used to treat depression and protect the liver from toxic overload; regenerates liver function and restores hepatic glutathione levels when taken with B vitamins; investigational (orphan) for AIDS-related myelopathy*
Saf-Clens spray OTC *wound cleanser*
Safe Tussin CD oral liquid OTC *antitussive; decongestant* [dextromethorphan hydrobromide; phenylephrine HCl] 15•2.5 mg/5 mL
Safe Tussin DM oral liquid OTC *antitussive; expectorant* [dextromethorphan hydrobromide; guaifenesin] 15•100 mg/5 mL
safflower (*Carthamus tinctorius*) flowers *medicinal herb for delirium,*

digestive disorders, fever, gout, inducing sweating, jaundice, liver disorders, lowering cholesterol, promoting expectoration, uric acid build-up, and urinary disorders

safflower oil USP *oleaginous vehicle; essential fatty acid supplement*

saffron (Crocus sativus) *flowers medicinal herb for fever, gout, inducing sweating, measles, rheumatism, scarlet fever, and sedation; also used as an aphrodisiac and expectorant* ☒ Zofran; Zophren

saffron, American; bastard saffron *medicinal herb* [see: safflower]

safingol USAN *antipsoriatic; antineoplastic adjunct*

safingol HCl USAN *antipsoriatic; antineoplastic adjunct*

Saflutan eye drops *investigational (NDA filed) prostaglandin analogue for glaucoma* [tafluprost]

safrole USP

Safyral film-coated tablets (in packs of 28) ℞ *monophasic oral contraceptive; iron supplement* [drospirenone; ethinyl estradiol; folic acid (as levomefolate calcium)] 3•0.03•0.451 mg × 21 days; 0•0•0.451 mg × 7 days

sagackhomi *medicinal herb* [see: uva ursi]

sage (Salvia lavandulaefolia; S. lyrata; S. officinalis) leaves *medicinal herb for cough, diarrhea, dysmenorrhea, fever, gastritis, gum and mouth sores, memory improvement, nausea, nervous disorders, and sore throat*

SAHA (suberoylanilide hydroxamic acid) [see: vorinostat]

sailor's tobacco *medicinal herb* [see: mugwort]

St. Benedict thistle *medicinal herb* [see: blessed thistle]

St. James weed; St. James wort *medicinal herb* [see: shepherd's purse]

St. John's wort (Hypericum perforatum) plant *medicinal herb for AIDS, antiviral therapy, anxiety, bronchitis, cancer, childbirth afterpains, depression, gastritis, insomnia, and skin disorders*

St. Joseph Adult Chewable Aspirin chewable tablets OTC *analgesic; antipyretic; anti-inflammatory* [aspirin] 81 mg

St. Josephwort *medicinal herb* [see: basil]

Saizen powder for subcu or IM injection ℞ *growth hormone for children and adults with congenital or endogenous growth hormone deficiency (GHD), short bowel syndrome, or AIDS-wasting syndrome; for children with Turner syndrome, Prader-Willi syndrome, or renal-induced growth failure* [somatropin] 5, 8.8 mg (15, 26.4 IU) per vial ☒ Susano; Zosyn

Saizen click.easy prefilled cartridge for subcu injection, used with a **cool.click** (needle-free injector) or **one.click** (disposable needle injector) pen ℞ *growth hormone for children and adults with congenital or endogenous growth hormone deficiency (GHD), short bowel syndrome, or AIDS-wasting syndrome; for children with Turner syndrome, Prader-Willi syndrome, or renal-induced growth failure* [somatropin] 8.8 mg (26.4 IU) per cartridge

SalAc topical liquid (discontinued 2011) OTC *keratolytic cleanser for acne* [salicylic acid] 2% ☒ Soyalac

salacetamide INN ☒ cilostamide

salacetin [see: aspirin]

Sal-Acid plaster (discontinued 2010) OTC *keratolytic* [salicylic acid in a collodion-like vehicle] 40%

Salactic Film topical liquid OTC *keratolytic* [salicylic acid in a collodion-like vehicle] 17%

Salacyn cream, lotion ℞ *keratolytic* [salicylic acid] 6% ☒ psilocin; Selsun; xylazine

salafibrate INN

Salagen film-coated tablets ℞ *treatment of xerostomia and keratoconjunctivitis sicca due to radiotherapy or Sjögren syndrome (orphan); also for dry mouth* [pilocarpine HCl] 5, 7.5 mg ☒ silicon; Solaquin; Xylocaine

salantel USAN, INN *veterinary anthelmintic* ☒ zilantel

salazodine INN

salazosulfadimidine INN [also: salazo-sulphadimidine]

salazosulfamide INN

salazosulfapyridine JAN *broad-spectrum bacteriostatic; anti-inflammatory for ulcerative colitis; antirheumatic* [also: sulfasalazine; sulphasalazine]

salazosulfathiazole INN

salazosulphadimidine BAN [also: salazosulfadimidine]

salbutamol INN, BAN *sympathomimetic bronchodilator* [also: albuterol]

salbutamol sulfate JAN *sympathomimetic bronchodilator* [also: albuterol sulfate]

salcatonin BAN *synthetic analogue of calcitonin (salmon); calcium regulator* [also: calcitonin salmon (synthesis)]

salcetogen [see: aspirin]

Sal-Clens Acne Cleanser gel OTC *keratolytic for acne* [salicylic acid] 2%

salcolex USAN, INN *analgesic; anti-inflammatory; antipyretic*

Salese lozenges OTC *mucous membrane moisturizer for dry mouth* [eucalyptus oil; wintergreen oil; zinc] ⚇ Cialis; Silace; xylose

Salese with Xylitol lozenges OTC *mucous membrane moisturizer for dry mouth* [eucalyptus oil; wintergreen oil; zinc; xylitol]

SalEst test kit for professional use ℞ *in vitro diagnostic aid for estriol levels in saliva, used to predict spontaneous preterm labor and delivery*

saletamide INN *analgesic* [also: salethamide maleate]

saletamide maleate [see: salethamide maleate]

salethamide maleate USAN *analgesic* [also: saletamide]

saletin [see: aspirin]

Saleto tablets OTC *analgesic; antipyretic; anti-inflammatory* [acetaminophen; aspirin; salicylamide; caffeine] 115•210•65•16 mg

Salex cream, lotion, shampoo ℞ *keratolytic for acne* [salicylic acid] 6% ⚇ Celexa; Cylex; Xolox

Salflex film-coated tablets OTC *analgesic; antipyretic; anti-inflammatory; antirheumatic* [salsalate] 500, 750 mg ⚇ Sulfolax

salfluverine INN

salicain [now: salicyl alcohol]

salicin USP ⚇ psilocin; Selsun

salicin willow *medicinal herb* [see: willow]

salicyl alcohol USAN *local anesthetic*

salicylamide USP *analgesic*

salicylanilide NF

salicylate meglumine USAN *antirheumatic; analgesic*

salicylates *a class of drugs that have analgesic, antipyretic, and anti-inflammatory effects*

salicylazosulfapyridine [now: sulfasalazine]

salicylic acid (SA) USP *keratolytic; antiseborrheic; antipsoriatic* 6%, 26% topical

salicylic acid, bimolecular ester [see: salsalate]

salicylic acid acetate [see: aspirin]

Salicylic Acid and Sulfur Soap bar OTC *antiseptic and keratolytic cleanser for acne* [salicylic acid; precipitated sulfur] 3%•10%

Salicylic Acid Cleansing bar OTC *medicated cleanser for acne* [salicylic acid] 2%

salicylic acid dihydrogen phosphate [see: fosfosal]

Salicylic Acid Shampoo ℞ *medicated shampoo for seborrhea* [salicylic acid] 6%

salicylsalicylic acid [see: salsalate]

saligenin [now: salicyl alcohol]

saligenol [now: salicyl alcohol]

salinazid INN, BAN

saline, lactated potassic [see: potassic saline, lactated]

saline laxatives *a subclass of laxatives that work by attracting and retaining water in the intestines to increase intraluminal pressure and cholecystokinin release* [see also: laxatives]

saline solution (SS) [also: normal saline]

SalineX nasal mist, nose drops OTC *nasal moisturizer* [sodium chloride (saline solution)] 0.4%

saliniazid [see: salinazid]

salinomycin INN, BAN *investigational antineoplastic for breast cancer stem cells*

Saliva Substitute oral solution OTC *saliva substitute*

saliva substitutes *a class of oral moisturizers used to relieve dry mouth and throat (xerostomia) due to Sjögren syndrome, Bell palsy, surgery or radiation near the salivary glands, HIV/AIDS, lupus, diabetes, aging, or various medications*

Salivart throat spray OTC *saliva substitute*

SalivaSure lozenges OTC *saliva substitute*

Salix alba; S. caprea; S. nigra; S. purpurea medicinal herb [see: willow]

Salkera topical foam ℞ *keratolytic* [salicylic acid] 6% ⧉ Xalkori

salmaterol [see: salmeterol]

salmefamol INN, BAN

salmeterol USAN, INN, BAN *long-acting beta$_2$ agonist (LABA); sympathomimetic bronchodilator for asthma and bronchospasm, and for the long-term treatment of COPD*

salmeterol xinafoate USAN *long-acting beta$_2$ agonist (LABA); sympathomimetic bronchodilator for asthma and bronchospasm, and for the long-term treatment of COPD* (base=69%)

salmisteine INN

salmon calcitonin [see: salcatonin]

Salmonella typhi **vaccine** [see: typhoid vaccine]

salmotin [see: adicillin]

salnacedin USAN *topical anti-inflammatory*

Sal-Oil-T hair dressing ℞ *antipsoriatic; antiseborrheic; keratolytic* [coal tar; salicylic acid] 10%•6%

salol [see: phenyl salicylate]

Salonpas patch OTC *analgesic; mild anesthetic; counterirritant* [methyl salicylate; menthol] 10%•3%

Sal-Plant gel OTC *keratolytic* [salicylic acid in a collodion-like vehicle] 17%

salprotoside INN

salsalate USAN, USP, INN, BAN *analgesic; antipyretic; anti-inflammatory; antirheumatic; investigational for heart disease and type 2 diabetes* 500, 750 mg oral

Salsitab film-coated tablets ℞ *analgesic; antipyretic; anti-inflammatory; antirheumatic* [salsalate] 500, 750 mg

salt [def.] *The inactive part of a compound, made by combining an acid with an alkali. In naproxen sodium, for example, the base is naproxen (an acid) and the salt is sodium (from sodium hydroxide, an alkali).* [compare to: base]

Sal-Tropine tablets ℞ *GI/GU antispasmodic; antiparkinsonian; anticholinergic "drying agent" for the respiratory tract; antidote to insecticide poisoning* [atropine sulfate] 0.4 mg ⧉ sulotroban

Saluron tablets (discontinued 2008) ℞ *diuretic; antihypertensive* [hydroflumethiazide] 50 mg

Salutensin; Salutensin-Demi tablets (discontinued 2007) ℞ *antihypertensive* [hydroflumethiazide; reserpine] 50•0.125 mg; 25•0.125 mg

saluzide [see: opiniazide]

salvarsan [see: arsphenamine]

Salvax topical foam ℞ *keratolytic* [salicylic acid] 6%

Salvax Duo topical foam ℞ *keratolytic and moisturizer/emollient* [salicylic acid; urea] 6%•40%

salverine INN

Salvia lavandulaefolia; S. lyrata; S. officinalis medicinal herb [see: sage]

Salvia miltiorrhiza medicinal herb [see: danshen]

samarium *element (Sm)*

samarium Sm 153 EDTMP (ethylenediaminetetramethylenephosphoric acid) [see: samarium Sm 153 lexidronam]

samarium Sm 153 lexidronam USAN *radiopharmaceutical for treatment of bone pain from osteoblastic metastatic tumors*

Sambucus canadensis; S. ebulus; S. nigra; S. racemosa medicinal herb [see: elder flower; elderberry]

SAMe (*S*-adenosyl-L-methionine) [q.v.]

Samsca tablets ℞ *selective vasopressin receptor antagonist for heart failure and hyponatremia* [tolvaptan] 15, 30 mg

Sanchi ginseng (*Panax pseudoginseng*) *medicinal herb* [see: ginseng]

Sanctura film-coated tablets ℞ *urinary antispasmodic for overactive bladder with urinary frequency, urgency, and incontinence* [trospium chloride] 20 mg

Sanctura XR extended-release capsules ℞ *urinary antispasmodic for overactive bladder with urinary frequency, urgency, and incontinence* [trospium chloride] 60 mg

Sancuso transdermal patch ℞ *antiemetic to prevent chemotherapy-induced nausea and vomiting (CINV)* [granisetron (as HCl)] 3.1 mg/day

sancycline USAN, INN *antibacterial*

sandalwood (*Santalum album*) oil *medicinal herb for headache, stomach ache, and urogenital disorders; also used topically as an antiseptic and astringent*

Sandimmune gelcaps, oral solution, IV injection ℞ *immunosuppressant for allogenic kidney, liver, and heart transplants (orphan)* [cyclosporine] 25, 100 mg; 100 mg/mL; 50 mg/mL ☒ xinidamine

SandoPak (trademarked packaging form) *unit dose blister package*

Sandostatin subcu or IV injection ℞ *gastric antisecretory for acromegaly and severe diarrhea due to VIPomas and other tumors (orphan)* [octreotide acetate] 0.05, 0.1, 0.2, 0.5, 1 mg/mL

Sandostatin LAR Depot suspension for monthly IM injection ℞ *gastric antisecretory for acromegaly and severe diarrhea due to VIPomas and other tumors (orphan)* [octreotide] 10, 20, 30 mg/5 mL

sanfetrinem INN, BAN *antibacterial* [also: sanfetrinem sodium]

sanfetrinem cilexetil USAN *antibacterial*

sanfetrinem sodium USAN *antibacterial* [also: sanfetrinem]

Sanguinaria canadensis *medicinal herb* [see: bloodroot]

sanguinarine chloride [now: sanguinarium chloride]

sanguinarium chloride USAN, INN *antifungal; antimicrobial; anti-inflammatory*

sanicle (*Sanicula europea*; *S. marilandica*) root *medicinal herb used as an astringent, expectorant, discutient, depurative, nervine, and vulnerary* ☒ Xenical

Sani-Pak (trademarked packaging form) *sanitary dispensing box* ☒ Cinobac

Sani-Supp suppositories OTC *hyperosmolar laxative* [glycerin]

Santalum album *medicinal herb* [see: sandalwood]

santonin NF

Santyl ointment ℞ *enzyme for wound débridement* [collagenase] 250 U/g

Sanvar *antineoplastic; synthetic octapeptide analogue of somatostatin; investigational (Phase III, orphan) treatment for acute esophageal variceal bleeding secondary to portal hypertension; investigational (orphan) for acromegaly and carcinoid tumors* [vapreotide acetate]

sapacitabine *investigational (Phase III, orphan) antineoplastic for acute myeloid leukemia (AML), myelodysplastic syndromes, bone marrow stem cell disorder, and lung cancer*

saperconazole USAN, INN, BAN *antifungal*

Saphris sublingual tablets ℞ *novel (atypical) antipsychotic for schizophrenia and manic episodes of a bipolar disorder* [asenapine] 5, 10 mg ☒ sfRowasa

Saponaria officinalis *medicinal herb* [see: soapwort]

saprisartan INN, BAN *angiotensin receptor blocker (ARB) for hypertension* [also: saprisartan potassium]

saprisartan potassium USAN *angiotensin receptor blocker (ARB) for hypertension* [also: saprisartan]

sapropterin INN

sapropterin dihydrochloride oral *phenylalanine hydroxylase (PAH)* *enzyme for mild to moderate phenylke-tonuria (PKU)*

saquinavir USAN, INN, BAN *antiretroviral protease inhibitor for HIV infection* [also: saquinavir mesylate]

saquinavir mesylate USAN *oral antiretroviral protease inhibitor for HIV infection* [also: saquinavir]

Sarafem tablets, Pulvules (capsules) ℞ *selective serotonin reuptake inhibitor (SSRI) for premenstrual dysphoric disorder (PMDD)* [fluoxetine HCl] 10, 15, 20 mg; 10, 20 mg

sarafloxacin INN, BAN *anti-infective; DNA gyrase inhibitor* [also: sarafloxacin HCl]

sarafloxacin HCl USAN *anti-infective; DNA gyrase inhibitor* [also: sarafloxacin]

saralasin INN *antihypertensive* [also: saralasin acetate]

saralasin acetate USAN *antihypertensive* [also: saralasin]

Saratoga ointment OTC *astringent; antiseptic; wound protectant* [zinc oxide; boric acid; eucalyptol]

sarcolysin INN

L-sarcolysin [see: melphalan]

Sardo Bath & Shower oil OTC *bath emollient*

Sardoettes towelettes OTC *moisturizer; emollient*

sargramostim USAN, INN, BAN *hematopoietic stimulant for graft delay (orphan) and bone marrow transplant in patients with acute lymphoblastic leukemia (ALL), Hodgkin disease, or non-Hodgkin lymphoma (NHL)*

sarmazenil INN

sarmoxicillin USAN, INN *antibacterial*

Sarmustine *investigational (orphan) for malignant glioma* [2-chloroethyl-3-sarcosinamide-1-nitrosourea]

Sarna Anti-Itch foam, lotion OTC *mild anesthetic; antipruritic; counterirritant* [camphor; menthol] 0.5%•0.5%

Sarna Sensitive wash OTC *disinfectant/antiseptic* [triclosan] 0.2%

Sarna Sensitive Anti-Itch lotion OTC *anesthetic* [pramoxine HCl] 1%

Sarna Ultra cream OTC *anesthetic; antipruritic; counterirritant; emollient* [pramoxine HCl; menthol; petrolatum] 1%•0.5%•30%

saroten [see: amitriptyline]

Sarothamnus scoparius *medicinal herb* [see: broom]

sarpicillin USAN, INN *antibacterial*

Sarracenia purpurea *medicinal herb* [see: pitcher plant]

sarsaparilla (*Smilax* spp.) root *medicinal herb for blood cleansing (binding and expulsion of endotoxins), joint aches including arthritis and rheumatism, hormonal disorders, skin diseases including leprosy and psoriasis, and syphilis*

sarsasapogenin *investigational (orphan) agent for amyotrophic lateral sclerosis (ALS)*

saruplase INN *prourokinase (pro-UK)*

sassafras (*Sassafras albidum; S. officinale*) root and bark *medicinal herb for acne, blood cleansing, insect bites and stings, obesity, psoriasis, skin diseases, and water retention; not generally regarded as safe and effective and banned by the FDA as a carcinogen with other serious side effects*

sassafras, swamp *medicinal herb* [see: magnolia]

SAStid Soap bar OTC *antiseptic and keratolytic cleanser for acne* [sulfur; salicylic acid] 5%•3%

saterinone INN

satinflower *medicinal herb* [see: chickweed]

satoribine [now: isatoribine]

satranidazole INN

satraplatin USAN *investigational (Phase III) antineoplastic for hormone-refractory prostate cancer*

satumomab INN, BAN *radiodiagnostic monoclonal antibody for ovarian and colorectal carcinoma* [also: indium In 111 satumomab pendetide]

satumomab pendetide [see: indium In 111 satumomab pendetide]

Satureja hortensis *medicinal herb* [see: summer savory]

Satureja montana; S. obovata medicinal herb [see: winter savory]

Savella film-coated tablets ℞ *selective serotonin and norepinephrine reuptake inhibitor (SNRI) antidepressant for fibromyalgia syndrome* [milnacipran HCl] 12.5, 25, 50, 100 mg

savory *medicinal herb* [see: summer savory; winter savory]

savoxepin INN

saw palmetto *(Serenoa repens; S. serrulata) berries medicinal herb for benign prostatic hypertrophy (BPH) and genitourinary, glandular, and reproductive disorders; also used to enlarge breasts, increase sperm production, promote weight gain, and enhance sexual vigor*

saxagliptin HCl *dipeptidyl peptidase-4 (DPP-4) inhibitor; oral antidiabetic that enhances the function of the body's incretin system to increase insulin production in the pancreas and reduce glucose production in the liver* (base= 89.6%)

saxifrage, burnet; European burnet saxifrage; small burnet saxifrage; small saxifrage *medicinal herb* [see: burnet]

saxifrax *medicinal herb* [see: sassafras]

SB-408075 *investigational (orphan) agent for pancreatic cancer*

SBR-Lipocream OTC *emollient for dry skin* [oil-in-water emulsion] 70% oil•30% water

SC (succinylcholine) [see: succinylcholine chlorine]

scabicides *a class of agents effective against scabies*

scabwort *medicinal herb* [see: elecampane]

Scadan scalp lotion OTC *antiseptic; antiseborrheic* [myristyltrimethylammonium bromide; stearyl dimethyl benzyl ammonium chloride] 1%•0.1%

S-Caine Peel cream ℞ *anesthetic* [lidocaine; tetracaine] 7%•7%

Scalacort; Scalacort DK (defense kit) lotion ℞ *corticosteroidal anti-inflammatory for scalp dermatoses;* the "kit" includes a salicylic acid and sulfur shampoo [hydrocortisone] 2%

Scalpicin topical liquid OTC *antiseborrheic* [salicylic acid] 3%

scaly dragon's claw *medicinal herb* [see: coral root]

scammony, wild *medicinal herb* [see: wild jalap]

scandium *element* (Sc)

Scandonest dental injection ℞ *local anesthetic* [mepivacaine HCl] 3%

Scandonest L dental injection ℞ *local anesthetic; vasoconstrictor* [mepivacaine HCl; levonordefrin] 2%• 1:20 000

Scanlux-300; Scanlux-370 injection ℞ *radiopaque contrast medium* [iopamidol (49% iodine)] 61% (300 mg/mL); 76% (370 mg/mL)

Scar Cream OTC *to reduce the appearance of surgical scars; sunscreens* [octinoxate; octisalate] 7.5%•5%

scarlet bergamot *medicinal herb* [see: Oswego tea]

scarlet berry *medicinal herb* [see: bittersweet nightshade]

scarlet fever streptococcus toxin

scarlet red NF *promotes wound healing*

Scarlet Red Ointment Dressings medication-impregnated gauze ℞ *wound dressing; vulnerary* [scarlet red] 5%

scarlet sumach *medicinal herb* [see: sumach]

SCCS (simethicone-coated cellulose suspension) [see: SonoRx]

sCD4-PE40 [see: alvircept sudotox]

SCE-A (synthetic conjugated estrogens A) [see: estrogens A, synthetic conjugated]

SCE-B (synthetic conjugated estrogens B) [see: estrogens B, synthetic conjugated]

Sceletium tortuosum medicinal herb [see: kanna]

SCF (stem cell factor) [see: methionyl stem cell factor]

SCH-58500 *investigational (orphan) gene therapy for ovarian tumors*

SCH-530348 *investigational (Phase III) oral thrombin receptor antagonist for the prevention and treatment of atherosclerotic events in high-risk patients*

Schamberg lotion OTC *mild anesthetic; antipruritic; counterirritant; astringent; emollient* [menthol; phenol; zinc oxide] 0.25%•1.5%•8.25%

Schick test [see: diphtheria toxin for Schick test]

Schick test control USP *dermal reactivity indicator*

Schirmer Tear Test ophthalmic strips ℞ *diagnostic tear flow test aid*

schizandra *(Schisandra arisanensis; S. chinensis; S. rubriflora; S. sphenanthera)* berries *medicinal herb for cough, gastrointestinal disorders, increasing energy and mental alertness, nervous disorders, respiratory illnesses, and stress; also used as a liver protectant*

SCIG, IGSC (subcutaneous immune globulin) [see: globulin, immune]

Sclerex tablets OTC *vitamin/mineral/calcium/iron supplement* [multiple vitamins & minerals; calcium; iron (as ferrous gluconate); folic acid] ± • 8.33•3.33•0.033 mg

Scleromate IV injection ℞ *sclerosing agent for varicose veins* [morrhuate sodium] 50 mg/mL

Sclerosol aerosol ℞ *treatment for malignant pleural effusion and pneumothorax via intrapleural thoracoscopy administration (orphan)* [talc, sterile]

scoke *medicinal herb* [see: pokeweed]

Scopace tablets ℞ *anticholinergic CNS depressant for postencephalitic parkinsonism and other spasticities; motion sickness preventative; GI antispasmodic/ antiemetic* [scopolamine hydrobromide] 0.4 mg

scopafungin USAN *antibacterial; antifungal*

Scope mouthwash OTC *oral antiseptic* [cetylpyridinium chloride]

scopolamine *oral/transdermal motion sickness preventative; post-surgical antiemetic*

scopolamine hydrobromide USP *anticholinergic CNS depressant for postencephalic parkinsonism and other spasticities, delirium tremens and other maniacal states, and general sedation; motion sickness preventative; GI antispasmodic/ antiemetic; cycloplegic; mydriatic* [also: hyoscine hydrobromide] 0.3, 0.4, 0.86, 1 mg/mL injection

scopolamine methyl nitrate [see: methscopolamine nitrate]

scopolamine methylbromide [see: methscopolamine bromide]

Scott's Emulsion (discontinued 2008) OTC *vitamin supplement* [vitamins A and D] 1250•100 IU/5 mL

Scot-Tussin Allergy Relief Formula Clear oral liquid OTC *antihistamine; sleep aid* [diphenhydramine HCl] 12.5 mg/5 mL

Scot-Tussin DM oral liquid OTC *antitussive; antihistamine* [dextromethorphan hydrobromide; chlorpheniramine maleate] 15•2 mg/5 mL

Scot-Tussin DM Cough Chasers lozenges OTC *antitussive* [dextromethorphan hydrobromide] 5 mg

Scot-Tussin Expectorant oral liquid OTC *expectorant* [guaifenesin] 100 mg/5 mL

Scot-Tussin Original 5-Action Cold Formula syrup, oral liquid OTC *decongestant; antihistamine; analgesic* [phenylephrine HCl; pheniramine maleate; sodium citrate; sodium salicylate; caffeine citrate] 4.2•13.3• 83.3•83.3•25 mg

Scot-Tussin Senior Clear oral liquid OTC *antitussive; expectorant* [dextromethorphan hydrobromide; guaifenesin] 15•200 mg/5 mL

sCR1 (soluble complement receptor 1) [see: complement receptor type I, soluble recombinant human]

scrofula plant *medicinal herb* [see: figwort]

Scrophularia nodosa *medicinal herb* [see: figwort]

scullcap *medicinal herb* [see: skullcap]

Sculptra dermal injection ℞ *synthetic polymer for the correction of facial lipoatrophy due to HIV infections* [poly-L-lactic acid]

scuroforme [see: butyl aminobenzoate]

Scutellaria lateriflora medicinal herb [see: skullcap]

Scytera topical foam OTC *antipsoriatic; antipruritic; emollient* [coal tar] 2% ⃞ Cytra; Zetar

SD (streptodornase) [q.v.]

SE 10-5 SS cream ℞ *antibiotic and keratolytic for acne* [sulfacetamide sodium; sulfur] 10%•5%

SE BPO soap, topical wipes OTC *keratolytic for acne* [benzoyl peroxide] 7%; 3%, 6%, 9%

^{75}Se [see: selenomethionine Se 75]

sea girdles *medicinal herb* [see: kelp (*Laminaria*)]

Seale's Lotion Modified (discontinued 2009) OTC *antiseptic and keratolytic for acne* [sulfur] 6.4%

sealroot; sealwort *medicinal herb* [see: Solomon's seal]

Sea-Omega 30 softgels OTC *dietary supplement* [omega-3 fatty acids (eicosapentaenoic acid and docosahexaenoic acid)] 360 mg (216 mg EPA; 144 mg DHA) ⃞ Zomig

Sea-Omega 50 softgels OTC *dietary supplement* [omega-3 fatty acids (eicosapentaenoic acid and docosahexaenoic acid)] 500 mg (300 mg EPA; 200 mg DHA) ⃞ Zomig

Sea-Omega 70 softgels OTC *dietary supplement* [omega-3 fatty acids (eicosapentaenoic acid and docosahexaenoic acid); vitamin E] 700 mg•15 IU (400 mg EPA; 200 mg DHA) ⃞ Zomig

Seasonale film-coated tablets (in packs of 91) ℞ *extended-cycle (3 months) monophasic oral contraceptive* [levonorgestrel; ethinyl estradiol] 0.15 mg•30 mcg × 84 days; counters × 7 days

Seasonique film-coated tablets (in packs of 91) ℞ *extended-cycle (3 months) biphasic oral contraceptive* [levonorgestrel; ethinyl estradiol]

Phase 1 (84 days): 0.15 mg•30 mcg; Phase 2 (7 days): 0•10 mcg

seawrack *medicinal herb* [see: kelp (*Fucus*)]

Seba-Nil Cleansing Mask scrub OTC *abrasive cleanser for acne*

Seba-Nil Oily Skin Cleanser topical liquid OTC *cleanser for acne* [alcohol; acetone]

Sebasorb lotion OTC *keratolytic for acne* [salicylic acid; attapulgite] 2%•10%

Sebex shampoo OTC *antiseborrheic; keratolytic; antiseptic* [sulfur; salicylic acid] 2%•2%

Sebex-T shampoo OTC *antiseborrheic; antipsoriatic; keratolytic; antiseptic* [sulfur; salicylic acid; coal tar] 2%•2%•5%

Seb-Prev lotion ℞ *antibiotic for acne* [sulfacetamide sodium] 10%

Seb-Prev Wash (soap) ℞ *antibiotic; antiseborrheic* [sulfacetamide sodium] 10%

Sebulex with Conditioners shampoo OTC *antiseborrheic; keratolytic; antiseptic* [sulfur; salicylic acid] 2%•2%

secalciferol USAN, INN, BAN *calcium regulator; investigational (orphan) for familial hypophosphatemic rickets*

secbutabarbital sodium INN *sedative; hypnotic* [also: butabarbital sodium]

secbutobarbitone BAN *sedative; hypnotic* [also: butabarbital]

seclazone USAN, INN *anti-inflammatory; uricosuric* ⃞ cyclizine

secnidazole INN, BAN

secobarbital USP, INN *hypnotic; sedative*

secobarbital sodium USP, JAN *hypnotic; sedative; also abused as a street drug* [also: quinalbarbitone sodium] 100 mg oral; 50 mg/mL injection

Seconal Sodium Pulvules (capsules) ℞ *sedative; hypnotic; also abused as a street drug* [secobarbital sodium] 100 mg

secoverine INN

Secran oral liquid (discontinued 2008) OTC *vitamin supplement* [vitamins B$_1$, B$_3$, and B$_{12}$; alcohol 17%] 10 mg•10 mg•25 mcg per 5 mL

SecreFlo powder for IV injection (discontinued 2008) ℞ *diagnostic aid for pancreatic function* [secretin] 16 mcg/vial

secretin INN, BAN *diagnostic aid for pancreatic function*

secretin, synthetic human; secretin, synthetic porcine *investigational (orphan) diagnostic aid for pancreatic function*

secretory leukocyte protease inhibitor, recombinant *investigational (orphan) for bronchopulmonary dysplasia*

Sectral capsules ℞ *antihypertensive (beta-blocker); antiarrhythmic for premature ventricular contractions (PVCs); also used for ventricular tachycardia* [acebutolol HCl] 200, 400 mg

Secule (trademarked delivery form) *single-dose vial* ⊡ squill

securinine INN

sedaform [see: chlorobutanol]

Sedapap caplets ℞ *barbiturate sedative; analgesic; antipyretic* [butalbital; acetaminophen] 50•650 mg

sedatine [see: antipyrine]

sedatives *a class of soothing agents that reduce excitement, nervousness, distress, or irritation* [also called: calmatives]

sedecamycin USAN, INN *veterinary antibacterial*

sedeval [see: barbital]

sedge, sweet *medicinal herb* [see: calamus]

Se-Donna PB HYOS elixir ℞ *GI/GU anticholinergic/antispasmodic; sedative* [atropine sulfate; scopolamine hydrobromide; hyoscyamine sulfate; phenobarbital] 0.0194•0.0065•0.1037•16.2 mg/5 mL

sedoxantrone trihydrochloride [now: ledoxantrone trihydrochloride]

seganserin INN, BAN

seglitide INN *antidiabetic* [also: seglitide acetate]

seglitide acetate USAN *antidiabetic* [also: seglitide]

selamectin USAN, INN *veterinary antiparasitic*

selective estrogen receptor modulators (SERMs) *a class of osteoporosis prevention agents that reduce bone resorption and decrease overall bone turnover in postmenopausal women*

selective serotonin 5-HT₃ (hydroxytryptamine) blockers *a class of antiemetic and antinauseant agents used primarily after emetogenic cancer chemotherapy* [also called: 5-HT₃ receptor antagonists]

selective serotonin and norepinephrine reuptake inhibitors (SSNRIs) *a class of oral antidepressants that inhibit neuronal uptake of the CNS neurotransmitters serotonin (5-HT) and norepinephrine*

selective serotonin reuptake inhibitors (SSRIs) *a class of oral antidepressants that inhibit neuronal uptake of the CNS neurotransmitter serotonin (5-HT)*

Select-OB caplets ℞ *prenatal vitamin/mineral/iron supplement* [multiple vitamins and minerals; iron (as polysaccharide iron complex); hydrogenated oil] ≠•29•1 mg

selegiline INN, BAN *monoamine oxidase inhibitor (MAOI); dopaminergic for Parkinson disease (PD); transdermal treatment for major depressive disorder (MDD)* [also: selegiline HCl]

selegiline HCl USAN *monoamine oxidase inhibitor (MAOI); dopaminergic for Parkinson disease (orphan)* [also: selegiline] 5 mg oral

selenious acid USP *dietary selenium supplement; additive to IV solutions for total parenteral nutrition (61% elemental selenium)* 65.4 mcg/mL (40 mcg/mL Se) injection

selenium *element (Se)*

selenium dioxide, monohydrated [see: selenious acid]

selenium sulfide USP *antiseborrheic; antipsoriatic; antifungal for tinea versicolor* 1%, 2.25%, 2.5% topical

selenomethionine (⁷⁵Se) INN *pancreas function test; radioactive agent* [also: selenomethionine Se 75]

658   selenomethionine Se 75

selenomethionine Se 75 USAN, USP *pancreas function test; radioactive agent* [also: selenomethionine (^{75}Se)]

Selenos shampoo ℞ *antiseborrheic; dandruff treatment* [selenium sulfide] 2.25% ⑤ "cillins"

Sele-Pak IV injection (discontinued 2010) ℞ *selenium supplement* [selenious acid (61% elemental selenium)] 65.4 mcg/mL (40 mcg Se/mL)

Selepen IV injection (discontinued 2010) ℞ *selenium supplement* [selenious acid (61% elemental selenium)] 65.4 mcg/mL (40 mcg Se/mL)

Selfemra capsules ℞ *selective serotonin reuptake inhibitor (SSRI) for premenstrual dysphoric disorder (PMDD)* [fluoxetine HCl] 10, 20 mg

selfotel USAN NMDA (N-methyl-D-aspartate) *antagonist for treatment of stroke-induced impairment*

selprazine INN

Selsun lotion ℞ *antiseborrheic; antipsoriatic; antifungal for tinea versicolor* [selenium sulfide] 2.5% ⑤ psilocin; Salacyn

Selsun Blue Medicated Treatment lotion/shampoo OTC *antiseborrheic; dandruff treatment* [selenium sulfide] 1%

Selzentry film-coated tablets ℞ *twice-daily antiretroviral for early-stage HIV-1 infections* [maraviroc] 150, 300 mg

semagacestat *investigational (Phase III) oral gamma secretase inhibitor to block the production of amyloid beta plaque in the brain for Alzheimer disease*

sematilide INN *antiarrhythmic* [also: sematilide HCl]

sematilide HCl USAN *antiarrhythmic* [also: sematilide]

semduramicin USAN, INN *coccidiostat*

semduramicin sodium USAN *coccidiostat*

Semicid vaginal suppositories OTC *spermicidal contraceptive* [nonoxynol 9] 100 mg

semisodium valproate BAN *anticonvulsant for complex partial seizures and simple or complex absence seizures; treatment for manic episodes of a bipolar disorder; migraine headache prophylaxis* [also: divalproex sodium; valproate semisodium]

semparatide acetate USAN *parathyroid hormone analogue to enhance fracture healing*

Semprex-D capsules ℞ *decongestant; antihistamine* [pseudoephedrine HCl; acrivastine] 60•8 mg

semustine USAN, INN *antineoplastic*

senecio, golden *medicinal herb* [see: life root]

Senecio aureus; S. jacoboea; S. vulgaris *medicinal herb* [see: life root]

senega (Polygala senega) root *medicinal herb used as an antitussive for asthma, chronic bronchitis, croup, lung congestion, and pneumonia* ⑤ Cena-K; zinc

Senexon tablets, oral liquid OTC *stimulant laxative* [sennosides] 8.6 mg; 8.8 mg/5 mL

Senilezol elixir (discontinued 2008) ℞ *vitamin/iron supplement* [multiple B vitamins; iron (as ferric pyrophosphate); alcohol 15%] ±•1 mg/5 mL

senna USP *stimulant laxative* 176 mg/5 mL oral

Senna syrup OTC *stimulant laxative* [sennosides] 8.8 mg/5 mL

senna (Cassia acutifolia; C. angustifolia; C. senna) leaves *medicinal herb for bowel evacuation before gastrointestinal procedures, constipation, edema, and expelling worms*

Senna Concentrate tablets (discontinued 2010) OTC *stimulant laxative* [sennosides] 8.6 mg

Senna Plus tablets OTC *stimulant laxative; stool softener* [sennosides; docusate sodium] 8.6•50 mg

Senna Prompt capsules OTC *stimulant and bulk laxative combination* [sennosides; psyllium] 9•500 mg

Senna Smooth tablets OTC *stimulant laxative* [sennosides] 15 mg

Senna-Gen tablets OTC *stimulant laxative* [sennosides] 8.6 mg ⑤ Sinequan; Zincon

Senna-S tablets OTC *stimulant laxative; stool softener* [sennosides; docusate sodium] 8.6•50 mg ☒ Zencia

sennosides USP *stimulant laxative*

Senokot tablets, granules, syrup OTC *stimulant laxative* [sennosides] 8.6 mg; 15 mg/5 mL; 8.8 mg/5 mL ☒ Cyanokit

Senokot-S tablets OTC *stimulant laxative; stool softener* [sennosides; docusate sodium] 8.6•50 mg

SenokotXtra tablets OTC *stimulant laxative* [sennosides] 17 mg

Sensability kit OTC *breast self-examination aid*

Sensi-Care Moisturizing Body Cream OTC *emollient/protectant* [dimethicone; petrolatum] 1%•30%

Sensipar film-coated tablets ℞ *treatment for hypercalcemia due to parathyroid carcinoma (orphan), primary hyperparathyroidism, or secondary hyperparathyroidism (SHPT) due to chronic kidney disease* [cinacalcet (as HCl)] 30, 60, 90 mg

Sensitive Eyes; Sensitive Eyes Plus solution OTC *rinsing/storage solution for soft contact lenses* [sodium chloride (preserved saline solution)]

Sensitive Eyes Daily Cleaner; Sensitive Eyes Saline/Cleaning Solution OTC *surfactant cleaning solution for soft contact lenses*

Sensitive Eyes Drops OTC *rewetting solution for soft contact lenses*

Sensitivity Protection Crest toothpaste OTC *tooth desensitizer; dental caries preventative* [potassium nitrate; sodium fluoride]

Sensodyne Cool Gel; Sensodyne iso-active Multi Action; Sensodyne iso-active Whitening toothpaste OTC *tooth desensitizer; dental caries preventative* [potassium nitrate; sodium fluoride] 5%•0.15%

Sensodyne Fresh Mint toothpaste OTC *tooth desensitizer; dental caries preventative* [potassium nitrate; sodium monofluorophosphate]

Sensodyne-SC toothpaste OTC *tooth desensitizer* [strontium chloride hexahydrate] 10%

SensoGARD oral gel OTC *mucous membrane anesthetic* [benzocaine] 20%

Sensorcaine injection ℞ *local anesthetic* [bupivacaine HCl] 0.25%, 0.5%

Sensorcaine injection ℞ *local anesthetic* [bupivacaine HCl; epinephrine] 0.25%•1:200 000; 0.5%•1:200 000

Sensorcaine MPF injection ℞ *local anesthetic* [bupivacaine HCl] 0.25%, 0.5%, 0.75%

Sensorcaine MPF injection ℞ *local anesthetic* [bupivacaine HCl; epinephrine] 0.25%•1:200 000, 0.5%• 1:200 000, 0.75%•1:200 000

Sensorcaine MPF Spinal injection ℞ *local anesthetic* [bupivacaine HCl] 0.75%

Sentinel test kit for professional use ℞ *urine test for HIV-1 antibodies*

sepazonium chloride USAN, INN *topical anti-infective*

seperidol HCl USAN *antipsychotic* [also: clofl);

Sensodyne [also: clofluperol]

Seprafilm hydrated gel film ℞ *to reduce the incidence, extent, and severity of postoperative adhesions* [hyaluronate sodium; carboxymethylcellulose]

seprilose USAN *antirheumatic*

seproxetine HCl USAN *antidepressant*

Septocaine intraoral injection (discontinued 2009) ℞ *local anesthetic for dentistry* [articaine HCl; epinephrine] 4%•1:100 000

septomonab [see: nebacumab]

Septopal polymethyl methacrylate (PMMA) beads on surgical wire *investigational (orphan) agent for chronic osteomyelitis* [gentamicin sulfate]

Septra oral suspension (discontinued 2010) ℞ *broad-spectrum sulfonamide antibiotic* [sulfamethoxazole; trimethoprim] 200•40 mg/5 mL

Septra; Septra DS tablets ℞ *broad-spectrum sulfonamide antibiotic* [sulfamethoxazole; trimethoprim] 400•80 mg; 800•160 mg

Septra IV infusion (discontinued 2007) ℞ *broad-spectrum sulfonamide antibiotic* [sulfamethoxazole; trimethoprim] 400•80 mg/5 mL

Sequels (trademarked dosage form) *sustained-release capsule or tablet* ⊡ Cyclessa

sequential AC/paclitaxel (Adriamycin, cyclophosphamide; paclitaxel) *chemotherapy protocol for breast cancer*

sequential DOX (doxorubicin) → CMF (cyclophosphamide, methotrexate, fluorouracil) *chemotherapy protocol for breast cancer*

sequential epirubicin + paclitaxel + cyclophosphamide, dose dense [with filgrastim hematopoietic and mesna rescue] *chemotherapy protocol for breast cancer*

sequifenadine INN

seractide INN *adrenocorticotropic hormone* [also: seractide acetate]

seractide acetate USAN *adrenocorticotropic hormone* [also: seractide]

Serada *investigational (Phase III) for moderate to severe postmenopausal hot flashes* [gabapentin]

Seradex-LA extended-release caplets ℞ *decongestant; antihistamine* [phenylephrine HCl; brompheniramine maleate] 19•6 mg

Ser-Ap-Es tablets (discontinued 2007) ℞ *antihypertensive; vasodilator; diuretic* [hydrochlorothiazide; reserpine; hydralazine HCl] 15•0.1•25 mg ⊡ Surpass

seratrodast USAN, INN *anti-inflammatory; antiasthmatic; thromboxane receptor antagonist*

Serax capsules, tablets (discontinued 2009) ℞ *benzodiazepine anxiolytic; sedative; alcohol withdrawal aid* [oxazepam] 10, 15, 30 mg; 15 mg

serazapine HCl USAN *anxiolytic*

Serc tablets ℞ *vasodilator; treatment for vertigo due to Meniere syndrome* [betahistine HCl] 24 mg

Serdolect Ⓔ (available in Europe) *investigational (NDA filed) novel*

(atypical) antipsychotic; neuroleptic [sertindole]

Sereine solution OTC *cleaning solution for hard contact lenses* (note: multiple products with the same name) ⊡ Ceron

Sereine solution OTC *wetting solution for hard contact lenses* (note: multiple products with the same name) ⊡ Ceron

Sereine solution OTC *wetting/soaking solution for hard contact lenses* (note: multiple products with the same name) ⊡ Ceron

Serenoa repens; S. serrulata medicinal herb [see: saw palmetto]

Serevent Diskus oral inhalation powder ℞ *twice-daily sympathomimetic bronchodilator for asthma, bronchospasm, and chronic obstructive pulmonary disease (COPD)* [salmeterol (as xinafoate)] 50 mcg/dose

serfibrate INN

sergolexole INN *antimigraine* [also: sergolexole maleate]

sergolexole maleate USAN *antimigraine* [also: sergolexole]

serine (L-serine) USAN, USP, INN *nonessential amino acid; symbols: Ser, S* ⊡ Ceron

L-serine diazoacetate [see: azaserine]

L-serine & L-leucine & L-tyrosine *investigational (orphan) for hepatocellular carcinoma*

84-L-serineplasminogen activator [see: monteplase]

sermetacin USAN, INN *anti-inflammatory*

sermorelin INN, BAN *diagnostic aid for pituitary function; treatment for growth hormone deficiency, anovulation, and AIDS-related weight loss* [also: sermorelin acetate]

sermorelin acetate USAN *diagnostic aid for pituitary function; treatment for growth hormone deficiency (orphan), anovulation (orphan), and AIDS-related weight loss (orphan)* [also: sermorelin]

SERMs (selective estrogen receptor modulators) [q.v.]

SeroJet (trademarked delivery device) *needle-free subcutaneous injector for Serostim*

Seromycin Pulvules (capsules) ℞ *tuberculostatic* [cycloserine] 250 mg ② cyromazine

Serophene tablets ℞ *ovulation stimulant* [clomiphene citrate] 50 mg

Seroquel film-coated tablets ℞ *novel (atypical) antipsychotic for schizophrenia and both manic and depressive episodes of a bipolar disorder; also used for obsessive-compulsive disorder (OCD)* [quetiapine (as fumarate)] 25, 50, 100, 200, 300, 400 mg

Seroquel XR extended-release film-coated caplets ℞ *novel (atypical) antipsychotic for schizophrenia and both manic and depressive episodes of a bipolar disorder; also used for obsessive-compulsive disorder (OCD); investigational (NDA filed) for generalized anxiety disorder* [quetiapine] 50, 150, 200, 300, 400 mg

Serostim powder for subcu injection ℞ *growth hormone for children and adults with congenital or endogenous growth hormone deficiency (GHD), short bowel syndrome, or AIDS-wasting syndrome; for children with Turner syndrome, Prader-Willi syndrome, or renal-induced growth failure* [somatropin] 4, 5, 6, 8.8 mg (12, 15, 18, 26.4 IU) per vial

Serostim prefilled one.click auto-injector syringe (discontinued 2008) ℞ *growth hormone for children and adults with congenital or endogenous growth hormone deficiency (GHD), short bowel syndrome, or AIDS-wasting syndrome; for children with Turner syndrome, Prader-Willi syndrome, or renal-induced growth failure* [somatropin] 8.8 mg (26.4 IU) per syringe

Serostim LQ subcu injection cartridges (discontinued 2008) ℞ *growth hormone for children and adults with congenital or endogenous growth hormone deficiency (GHD), short bowel syndrome, or AIDS-wasting syndrome; for*

children with Turner syndrome, Prader-Willi syndrome, or renal-induced growth failure [somatropin] 6 mg (18 IU) per 0.5 mL cartridge

serotonin (5-hydroxytriptamine$_1$; 5-HT$_1$) [see: selective serotonin reuptake inhibitors; vascular serotonin receptor antagonists]

SERPACWA (Skin Exposure Reduction Paste Against Chemical Warfare Agents) cream ℞ *to delay absorption of chemical warfare agents through the skin when applied before exposure; used in conjunction with MOPP (Mission Oriented Protective Posture) gear* [polytef; perfluoroalkylpolyether]

serrapeptase INN

Serratia marcescens **extract (polyribosomes)** *investigational (orphan) for primary brain malignancies*

sertaconazole INN *topical antifungal*

sertaconazole nitrate *topical antifungal*

sertindole USAN, INN *investigational (NDA filed) novel (atypical) antipsychotic; neuroleptic*

Sertoli cells, porcine *investigational (orphan) intracerebral implant for stage 4 and 5 Parkinson disease (for co-implantation with fetal neural cells)*

sertraline INN, BAN *selective serotonin reuptake inhibitor (SSRI) for depression, obsessive-compulsive disorder (OCD), panic disorder, post-traumatic stress disorder (PTSD), premenstrual dysphoric disorder (PMDD), and social anxiety disorder (SAD)* [also: sertraline HCl]

sertraline HCl USAN *selective serotonin reuptake inhibitor (SSRI) for depression, obsessive-compulsive disorder (OCD), panic disorder, post-traumatic stress disorder (PTSD), premenstrual dysphoric disorder (PMDD), and social anxiety disorder (SAD)* [also: sertraline] 25, 50, 100 mg; 20 mg/mL oral

serum albumin (SA) [see: albumin, human]

serum albumin, iodinated (^{125}I) human [see: albumin, iodinated I 125 serum]

serum albumin, iodinated (^{131}I) human [see: albumin, iodinated I 131 serum]

serum fibrinogen (SF) [see: fibrinogen, human]

serum globulin (SG) [see: globulin, immune]

serum gonadotrophin [see: gonadotrophin, serum]

serum gonadotropin [see: gonadotrophin, serum]

serum prothrombin conversion accelerator (SPCA) factor [see: factor VII]

Serutan granules OTC *bulk laxative* [psyllium] 2.5 g/tsp. ⊘ Soriatane

Servira extended-release tablets ℞ *GI/GU anticholinergic/antispasmodic; sedative* [atropine sulfate; scopolamine hydrobromide; hyoscyamine hydrobromide; phenobarbital] 0.0582•0.0195•0.3111•48.6 mg

sesame oil NF *solvent; oleaginous vehicle*

Sesame Street Complete chewable tablets (discontinued 2008) OTC *vitamin/mineral/calcium/iron supplement* [multiple vitamins & minerals; calcium; iron; folic acid; biotin] ±•80•10•0.2•0.015 mg

Sesame Street Plus Iron chewable tablets (discontinued 2008) OTC *vitamin/iron supplement* [multiple vitamins; iron; folic acid] ±•10•0.2 mg

sestamibi (scan) [see: technetium Tc 99m sestamibi]

setastine INN

setazindol INN

setiptiline INN

setoperone USAN, INN *antipsychotic*

setwall *medicinal herb* [see: valerian]

sevelamer carbonate *phosphate-binding polymer for hyperphosphatemia in dialysis patients with chronic kidney disease (CKD); also used for hyperuricemia in dialysis patients*

sevelamer HCl USAN *phosphate-binding polymer for hyperphosphatemia in dialysis patients with chronic kidney disease (CKD); also used for hyperuricemia in dialysis patients*

7 + 3 protocol (cytarabine, daunorubicin) *chemotherapy protocol for acute myelocytic leukemia (AML)*

7 + 3 protocol (cytarabine, idarubicin) *chemotherapy protocol for acute myelocytic leukemia (AML)*

7 + 3 protocol (cytarabine, mitoxantrone) *chemotherapy protocol for acute myelocytic leukemia (AML)*

7 + 3 + 7 protocol (cytarabine, daunorubicin, etoposide) *chemotherapy protocol for acute myelocytic leukemia (AML)*

seven barks *medicinal herb* [see: hydrangea]

17 alpha-hydroxyprogesterone caproate *synthetic progesterone; hormone therapy to prevent preterm birth in women with a history of spontaneous preterm delivery*

Severe Congestion Tussin softgels OTC *decongestant; expectorant* [pseudoephedrine HCl; guaifenesin] 30•200 mg

sevirumab USAN, INN *antiviral*

sevitropium mesilate INN

sevoflurane USAN, INN *inhalation general anesthetic*

sevopramide INN ⊘ cefpiramide

sezolamide HCl USAN *carbonic anhydrase inhibitor*

SF (serum fibrinogen) [see: fibrinogen, human]

SF 1.1% dental gel ℞ *dental caries preventative* [fluoride (as sodium fluoride)] 0.5% (1.1%)

SF 5000 Plus toothpaste ℞ *dental caries preventative* [fluoride (as sodium fluoride)] 0.5% (1.1%)

SFC lotion (discontinued 2010) OTC *soap-free therapeutic skin cleanser*

sfericase INN ⊘ Zephrex; Zovirax

sfRowasa "sulfite free" enema ℞ *anti-inflammatory for active ulcerative colitis, proctosigmoiditis, and proctitis* [mesalamine (5-aminosalicylic acid)] 4 g/60 mL ⊘ Saphris

SG (serum globulin) [see: globulin, immune]

SG (soluble gelatin) [see: gelatin]

SGLT-2 (sodium-glucose transporter 2) inhibitors *a class of investigational (NDA filed) antidiabetic agents that lower blood glucose by causing increased secretion of glucose by the kidneys*

shamrock, Indian *medicinal herb* [see: birthroot]

shamrock, water *medicinal herb* [see: buckbean]

shark cartilage (derived from *Sphyrna lewini*, *Squalus acanthias*, and other species) *natural remedy for cancer* [also: squalamine]

shark liver oil *emollient/protectant*

shavegrass *medicinal herb* [see: horsetail]

shea butter (*Butyrospermum parkii*) *emollient*

sheep laurel *medicinal herb* [see: mountain laurel]

Sheik Elite *premedicated condom* OTC *spermicidal/barrier contraceptive* [nonoxynol 9] 8%

shell flower *medicinal herb* [see: turtle-bloom]

shellac NF *tablet coating agent* ☒ Cholac

Shellgel *intraocular injection* ℞ *viscoelastic agent for ophthalmic surgery* [hyaluronate sodium] 12 mg/mL

Shepard's Cream Lotion; Shepard's Skin Cream OTC *moisturizer; emollient*

shepherd's club *medicinal herb* [see: mullein]

shepherd's heart *medicinal herb* [see: shepherd's purse]

shepherd's purse (*Capsella bursa-pastoris*) *plant medicinal herb for bleeding, ear disease, hypertension, painful menstruation, and urinary bleeding*

shigoka *medicinal herb* [see: eleuthero]

shiitake mushrooms (*Lentinula edodes*; *Tricholomopsis edodes*) *stem and cap medicinal herb for boosting the immune system, cancer, lowering cholesterol, and viral illnesses*

Shohl solution, modified (sodium citrate & citric acid) *urinary alkalizer; compounding agent*

short chain fatty acids *investigational (orphan) for left-sided ulcerative colitis and chronic radiation proctitis*

short-leaved buchu *medicinal herb* [see: buchu]

Shur-Clens *solution* OTC *wound cleanser* [poloxamer 188] 20%

Shur-Seal *vaginal gel* OTC *spermicidal contraceptive (for use with a diaphragm)* [nonoxynol 9] 2%

siagoside INN

sialagogues *a class of agents that stimulate the secretion of saliva* [also called: ptyalagogues]

Sibelium *investigational (orphan) vasodilator for alternating hemiplegia* [flunarizine HCl]

sibenadet HCl USAN *treatment for chronic obstructive pulmonary disease (COPD)*

Siberian ginseng (*Acanthopanax senticosus*; *Eleutherococcus senticosus*) *an older (and incorrect) name for eleuthero; "Siberian ginseng" is not in the ginseng family* [now: eleuthero; compare to: ginseng]

sibopirdine USAN *cognition enhancer for Alzheimer disease; nootropic*

sibrafiban USAN *platelet inhibitor; fibrinogen receptor antagonist; glycoprotein IIb/IIIa receptor antagonist*

sibutramine INN, BAN *anorexiant for the treatment of obesity; monoamine reuptake inhibitor antidepressant* [also: sibutramine HCl]

sibutramine HCl USAN *anorexiant for the treatment of obesity; monoamine reuptake inhibitor antidepressant* [also: sibutramine]

siccanin INN ☒ zocainone

Sickledex *test kit for professional use* ℞ *in vitro diagnostic aid for hemoglobin S (sickle cell)*

sicklewort *medicinal herb* [see: woundwort]

side-flowering skullcap *medicinal herb* [see: skullcap]

SigPak *(trademarked packaging form) unit-of-use package*

Sigtab tablets OTC *vitamin supplement* [multiple vitamins; folic acid] ≛•400 mcg

Sigtab-M tablets (discontinued 2008) OTC *vitamin/mineral/calcium/iron supplement* [multiple vitamins & minerals; calcium; iron; folic acid; biotin] ≛•200•18•0.4•0.045 mg

siguazodan INN, BAN

Silace syrup, oral liquid OTC *laxative; stool softener* [docusate sodium] 60 mg/15 mL; 10 mg/mL ⧉ Cialis; Salese; xylose

Siladryl oral liquid OTC *antihistamine; sleep aid* [diphenhydramine HCl] 12.5 mg/5 mL

Silafed syrup OTC *decongestant; antihistamine* [pseudoephedrine HCl; triprolidine HCl] 30•1.25 mg/5 mL

silafilcon A USAN *hydrophilic contact lens material* ⧉ xylofilcon A

silafocon A USAN *hydrophobic contact lens material*

silandrone USAN, INN *androgen*

Silapap, Children's oral liquid, elixir OTC *analgesic; antipyretic* [acetaminophen] 160 mg/5 mL

Silapap, Infant's oral drops (discontinued 2011) OTC *analgesic; antipyretic* [acetaminophen] 100 mg/mL

Sildec oral drops ℞ *decongestant; antihistamine; for children 1–24 months* [pseudoephedrine HCl; carbinoxamine maleate] 15•1 mg/mL

Sildec syrup ℞ *decongestant; antihistamine* [pseudoephedrine HCl; brompheniramine maleate] 45•4 mg/5 mL

Sildec-DM oral drops (discontinued 2007) ℞ *antitussive; antihistamine; decongestant; for children 1–24 months* [dextromethorphan hydrobromide; carbinoxamine maleate; pseudoephedrine HCl] 4•1•15 mg/mL

Sildec-DM syrup ℞ *antitussive; antihistamine; decongestant* [dextromethorphan hydrobromide; brompheniramine maleate; pseudoephedrine HCl] 15•4•45 mg/5 mL

sildenafil citrate USAN *phosphodiesterase type 5 (PDE-5) inhibitor; selective vasodilator for erectile dysfunction (ED) and pulmonary arterial hypertension (PAH); also used for antidepressant- or antipsychotic-induced sexual dysfunction*

Silenor tablets ℞ *low-dose tricyclic antidepressant for the treatment of chronic insomnia* [doxepin HCl] 3, 6 mg

Silfedrine, Children's oral liquid (discontinued 2011) OTC *nasal decongestant* [pseudoephedrine HCl] 30 mg/5 mL

silibinin INN

silica, dental-type NF *pharmaceutic aid*

silica gel [now: silicon dioxide]

siliceous earth, purified NF *filtering medium*

silicic acid, magnesium salt [see: magnesium trisilicate]

silicon *element (Si)* ⧉ silicone; Solaquin; Xylocaine

silicon dioxide NF *dispersing and suspending agent*

silicon dioxide, colloidal NF *suspending agent; tablet and capsule diluent*

silicone ⧉ silicon; Solaquin; Xylocaine

Silicone No. 2 ointment OTC *skin protectant* [silicone; hydrophobic starch derivative] 10%•≛

silicone oil [see: polydimethylsiloxane]

silicristin INN

silidianin INN

silkweed *medicinal herb* [see: milkweed; pleurisy root]

silky swallow wort; Virginia silk *medicinal herb* [see: milkweed]

silodosin *alpha$_{1a}$ blocker for benign prostatic hyperplasia (BPH)*

silodrate USAN *antacid* [also: simaldrate]

Silphen DM syrup OTC *antitussive* [dextromethorphan hydrobromide; alcohol 5%] 10 mg/5 mL

Silphium perfoliatum *medicinal herb* [see: ragged cup]

Sil-Tex oral liquid ℞ *decongestant; expectorant* [phenylephrine HCl; guaifenesin] 7.5•100 mg/5 mL

Siltussin DAS oral liquid OTC *expectorant* [guaifenesin] 100 mg/5 mL

Siltussin DM oral liquid OTC *antitussive; expectorant* [dextromethorphan hydrobromide; guaifenesin] 10•100 mg/5 mL

Siltussin SA oral liquid OTC *expectorant* [guaifenesin] 100 mg/5 mL

Silvadene cream ℞ *broad-spectrum bactericidal for adjunctive burn treatment* [silver sulfadiazine] 10 mg/g

silver *element (Ag); antiseptic; broad-spectrum antimicrobial*

silver nitrate USP *ophthalmic neonatal anti-infective; strong caustic* 10%, 25%, 50%, 75% topical

silver nitrate, toughened USP *caustic*

silver protein, mild NF *ophthalmic antiseptic; ophthalmic surgical aid*

silver sulfadiazine (SSD) USAN, USP *broad-spectrum bactericidal; adjunct to burn therapy* [also: sulfadiazine silver]

silver sulfadiazine & cerium nitrate *investigational (orphan) for life-threatening burns*

silverweed; silver cinquefoil *medicinal herb* [see: cinquefoil]

Silybum marianum *medicinal herb* [see: milk thistle]

Simaal Gel 2 oral liquid (discontinued 2007) OTC *antacid; antiflatulent* [aluminum hydroxide; magnesium hydroxide; simethicone] 500•400•40 mg/5 mL

simaldrate INN *antacid* [also: silodrate]

Simcor film-coated, extended-release tablets ℞ *combination treatment for hypercholesterolemia and hypertriglyceridemia: HMG-CoA reductase inhibitor to lower LDL and total cholesterol plus niacin to raise HDL and lower triglycerides* [simvastatin; niacin] 20•500, 20•750, 40•500, 40•1000 mg

simethicone USAN, USP *antiflatulent; adjunct to gastrointestinal imaging* 80 mg oral; 40 mg/0.6 mL oral

simethicone-coated cellulose suspension (SCCS) [see: SonoRx]

simetride INN

simfibrate INN

Similac Advance with Iron ready-to-use oral liquid, powder for oral liquid OTC *infant formula fortified with omega-3 fatty acids*

Similac Human Milk Fortifier powder OTC *supplement to breast milk* 900 mg/pkt.

Similac Low Iron oral liquid, powder for oral liquid OTC *total or supplementary infant feeding*

Similac PM 60/40 Low-Iron oral liquid OTC *formula for infants predisposed to hypocalcemia* [whey formula with lowered mineral levels]

Similac with Iron oral liquid, powder for oral liquid OTC *total or supplementary infant feeding*

simple syrup [see: syrup]

Simpler's joy *medicinal herb* [see: blue vervain]

Simplet tablets (discontinued 2007) OTC *decongestant; antihistamine; analgesic; antipyretic* [pseudoephedrine HCl; chlorpheniramine maleate; acetaminophen] 60•4•650 mg

Simply Cough oral liquid OTC *antitussive* [dextromethorphan hydrobromide] 5 mg/5 mL

Simply Saline nasal spray OTC *nasal moisturizer* [sodium chloride (saline solution)]

Simply Sleep tablets OTC *antihistamine; sleep aid* [diphenhydramine HCl] 25 mg

Simply Stuffy oral liquid (discontinued 2009) OTC *nasal decongestant* [pseudoephedrine HCl] 15 mg/5 mL

Simply Stuffy tablets OTC *nasal decongestant* [pseudoephedrine HCl] 30 mg

Simponi prefilled autoinjector for subcu injections ℞ *once-monthly treatment for rheumatoid arthritis, psoriatic arthritis, and ankylosing spondylitis* [golimumab] 50 mg

Simron Plus capsules (discontinued 2008) OTC *vitamin/iron supplement* [multiple vitamins; ferrous gluconate; folic acid] ±•10•0.1 mg

simtrazene USAN, INN *antineoplastic*

Simuc extended-release tablets (discontinued 2008) ℞ *decongestant; expec-*

torant [phenylephrine HCl; guaifenesin] 25•900 mg ② sumach; Zomig

Simuc-GP extended-release tablets ℞ *decongestant; expectorant* [phenylephrine HCl; guaifenesin] 25•1200 mg ② sumach; Zomig

Simuc-HD elixir ℞ *narcotic antitussive; decongestant; expectorant* [hydrocodone bitartrate; phenylephrine HCl; guaifenesin] 2.5•10•225 mg/5 mL ② sumach; Zomig

Simulect powder for IV infusion ℞ *immunosuppressant; IL-2 receptor antagonist for the prevention of acute rejection of renal transplants (orphan)* [basiliximab] 20 mg

simvastatin USAN, INN, BAN *HMG-CoA reductase inhibitor for hyperlipidemia, hypertriglyceridemia, and coronary heart disease (CHD)* 5, 10, 20, 40, 80 mg oral

Sina-12X caplets, pediatric oral suspension ℞ *decongestant; expectorant* [phenylephrine tannate; guaifenesin] 25•200 mg; 5•100 mg/5 mL ② Xanax

Sinadrin PE caplets OTC *decongestant; antihistamine; analgesic; antipyretic* [phenylephrine HCl; dexbrompheniramine maleate; acetaminophen] 10•2•650 mg

Sinapis alba medicinal herb [see: mustard]

sinapultide USAN *pulmonary surfactant for respiratory distress syndrome*

sincalide USAN, INN *choleretic; diagnostic aid for gallbladder function*

sinecatechins *a class of natural polyphenolic antioxidants; topical treatment for external genital and perianal warts (condyloma acuminatum) in immunocompromised adults* [also known as: kunecatechins]

sinefungin USAN, INN *antifungal*

Sinemet 10-100; Sinemet 25-100; Sinemet 25-250 tablets ℞ *dopamine precursor for Parkinson disease; decarboxylase inhibitor (levodopa potentiator)* [levodopa; carbidopa] 100•10 mg; 100•25 mg; 250•25 mg

Sinemet CR sustained-release tablets ℞ *dopamine precursor for Parkinson*

disease; decarboxylase inhibitor (levodopa potentiator) [levodopa; carbidopa] 100•25, 200•50 mg

Sine-Off Cough/Cold; Sine-Off Multi Symptom Relief tablets OTC *antitussive; decongestant; expectorant; analgesic; antipyretic* [dextromethorphan hydrobromide; phenylephrine HCl; guaifenesin; acetaminophen] 15•5•200•325 mg

Sine-Off Non-Drowsy tablets OTC *decongestant; analgesic; antipyretic* [phenylephrine HCl; acetaminophen] 5•500 mg

Sine-Off Sinus/Cold caplets OTC *decongestant; antihistamine; analgesic; antipyretic* [phenylephrine HCl; chlorpheniramine maleate; acetaminophen] 5•2•500 mg

Sinequan capsules, concentrate for oral solution ℞ *tricyclic antidepressant; anxiolytic* [doxepin HCl] 10, 25, 50, 75, 100, 150 mg; 10 mg/mL ② Zincon

Sinex [also see: DayQuil Sinex; NyQuil Sinex]

Sinex 12-Hour Long Acting; Sinex 12-Hour Ultra Fine Mist for Sinus Relief nasal spray OTC *nasal decongestant* [oxymetazoline HCl] 0.05%

Sinex Ultra Fine Mist nasal spray OTC *decongestant* [phenylephrine HCl] 0.5%

SingleJect (trademarked delivery form) *prefilled syringe*

Singlet for Adults tablets (discontinued 2007) OTC *decongestant; antihistamine; analgesic; antipyretic* [pseudoephedrine HCl; chlorpheniramine maleate; acetaminophen] 60•4•650 mg

Singulair film-coated tablets, chewable tablets, granules for oral solution ℞ *leukotriene receptor antagonist (LTRA) for allergic rhinitis, exercise-induced bronchoconstriction (EIB), and the prophylaxis and chronic treatment of asthma* [montelukast (as sodium)] 10 mg; 4, 5 mg; 4 mg/pkt.

Sinografin intracavitary instillation ℞ *radiopaque contrast medium for gyne-*

cological imaging [diatrizoate meglumine; iodipamide meglumine (47.8% total iodine)] 727•268 mg/mL (380 mg/mL)

sinorphan [now: ecadotril]

sintropium bromide INN 🔢 xenytropium bromide

Sinuhist tablets ℞ *decongestant; antihistamine* [phenylephrine HCl; brompheniramine maleate] 45•6 mg 🔢 Sonahist

Sinus Relief caplets (discontinued 2007) OTC *decongestant; analgesic; antipyretic* [pseudoephedrine HCl; acetaminophen] 30•500 mg

Sinustop capsules OTC *nasal decongestant* [pseudoephedrine HCl] 60 mg

Sinutab Non-Drying capsules OTC *decongestant; expectorant* [phenylephrine HCl; guaifenesin] 5•200 mg

Sinutab Sinus caplets OTC *decongestant; analgesic; antipyretic* [phenylephrine HCl; acetaminophen] 5•325 mg

Sinutab Sinus Allergy caplets (discontinued 2009) OTC *decongestant; antihistamine; analgesic; antipyretic* [pseudoephedrine HCl; chlorpheniramine maleate; acetaminophen] 30• 2•500 mg

SINUtuss DM caplets ℞ *antitussive; decongestant; expectorant* [dextromethorphan hydrobromide; phenylephrine HCl; guaifenesin] 30•15•600 mg

SINUvent PE extended-release caplets ℞ *decongestant; expectorant* [phenylephrine HCl; guaifenesin] 15•600 mg

siplizumab *investigational (orphan) monoclonal antibody for T-cell lymphomas*

sipuleucel-T *recombinant fusion protein of prostatic acid phosphatase linked to granulocyte-macrophage colony-stimulating factor (GM-CSF); autologous cellular immunotherapy antineoplastic (theraccine) for metastatic hormone-refractory prostate cancer*

sirolimus USAN *immunosuppressant for renal transplantation; investigational (Phase III) for liver transplantation; also used for psoriasis*

sisomicin USAN, INN *antibacterial* [also: sissomicin]

sisomicin sulfate USAN, USP *antibacterial*

sissomicin BAN *antibacterial* [also: sisomicin]

sitafloxacin USAN, INN *antibacterial; DNA-gyrase inhibitor*

sitagliptin phosphate *dipeptidyl peptidase-4 (DPP-4) inhibitor; oral antidiabetic that enhances the function of the body's incretin system to increase insulin production in the pancreas and reduce glucose production in the liver*

sitalidone INN

sitaxsentan sodium *endothelin receptor antagonist (ERA) vasodilator; investigational (NDA filed, orphan) once-daily oral antihypertensive for pulmonary arterial hypertension (PAH)*

sitofibrate INN

sitogluside USAN, INN *antiprostatic hypertrophy*

sitosterols NF

Sitrex extended-release caplets ℞ *decongestant; expectorant* [phenylephrine HCl; guaifenesin] 20•1200 mg 🔢 storax

Sitrex PD oral liquid ℞ *decongestant; expectorant* [phenylephrine HCl; guaifenesin] 7.5•75 mg/5 mL

Sitzmarks capsules ℞ *radiopaque contrast medium for severe constipation* [polyvinyl chloride, radiopaque] 24 rings/capsule

666 Cold Preparation oral liquid (discontinued 2007) OTC *antitussive; decongestant; analgesic; antipyretic* [dextromethorphan hydrobromide; pseudoephedrine HCl; acetaminophen] 10•30•325 mg/15 mL

sizofiran INN

SK (streptokinase) [q.v.]

Skeeter Stik topical liquid OTC *anesthetic; antipruritic; counterirritant* [lidocaine; menthol] 4%•1%

Skelaxin tablets ℞ *skeletal muscle relaxant* [metaxalone] 800 mg

Skelid tablets ℞ *bisphosphonate bone resorption inhibitor for Paget disease;*

also used for osteoporosis [tiludronate (as disodium)] 200 mg

SK&F 110679 *investigational (orphan) long-term treatment for children with growth failure due to lack of endogenous growth hormone*

skin respiratory factor (SRF) *claimed to promote wound healing*

Skin Shield topical liquid OTC *skin protectant; local anesthetic* [dyclonine HCl; benzethonium chloride] 0.75%•0.2%

skullcap (Scutellaria lateriflora) plant *medicinal herb for convulsions, epilepsy, fever, hypertension, infertility, insomnia, nervous disorders, rabies, and restlessness*

skunk cabbage (Symplocarpus foetidus) root *medicinal herb used as an antispasmodic, diuretic, emetic, expectorant, pectoral, stimulant, and sudorific*

skunk weed *medicinal herb* [see: skunk cabbage]

SL (sodium lactate) [q.v.]

Sleepinal capsules, soft gels OTC *antihistamine; sleep aid* [diphenhydramine HCl] 50 mg

Sleepwell 2-nite tablets OTC *antihistamine; sleep aid* [diphenhydramine HCl] 25 mg

Slidecase (packaging form) *patient compliance package for oral contraceptives*

slippery elm (Ulmus fulva; U. rubra) inner bark *medicinal herb for asthma, blackened or bruised eyes, boils, bronchitis, burns, cold sores, colitis, cough, diaper rash, diarrhea, indigestion, lung disorders, sore throat, and urinary tract inflammation*

slippery root *medicinal herb* [see: comfrey]

Slo-bid Gyrocaps (extended-release capsules) (discontinued 2008) ℞ *antiasthmatic; bronchodilator* [theophylline] 50, 75, 100, 125, 200, 300 mg

Slocaps (trademarked dosage form) *sustained-release capsules*

Slo-Niacin controlled-release tablets OTC *vitamin B_3 supplement; peripheral vasodilator; antihyperlipidemic* [niacin] 250, 500, 750 mg

Slo-phyllin tablets, syrup (discontinued 2008) ℞ *antiasthmatic; bronchodilator* [theophylline] 100, 200 mg; 80 mg/15 mL ⑨ sulfalene

Slo-Salt-K slow-release tablets OTC *electrolyte replacement; dehydration preventative* [sodium chloride; potassium chloride] 410•150 mg

slow channel blockers *a class of coronary vasodilators that inhibit cardiac muscle contraction and slow cardiac electrical conduction velocity* [also called: calcium channel blockers; calcium antagonists]

Slow Fe slow-release tablets OTC *iron supplement* [iron (as ferrous sulfate)] 45 mg (142 mg)

Slow Fe with Folic Acid slow-release tablets OTC *vitamin/iron supplement* [ferrous sulfate; folic acid] 50•0.4 mg

Slow-Mag enteric-coated delayed-release tablets OTC *magnesium supplement* [magnesium (as chloride); calcium] 143•238 mg

Slow-Mag enteric-coated tablets OTC *magnesium supplement* [magnesium chloride hexahydrate] 64 mg Mg

Slow-Mag with Calcium delayed-release tablets OTC *calcium/magnesium supplement* [calcium (as carbonate); magnesium (as chloride)] 113•64 mg

Slow-Release Iron extended-release tablets OTC *iron supplement* [iron (as ferrous sulfate, dried)] 50 mg (160 mg)

small burnet saxifrage *medicinal herb* [see: burnet]

small pimpernel *medicinal herb* [see: burnet]

small saxifrage *medicinal herb* [see: burnet]

smallpox vaccine USP *active immunizing agent*

SMART anti-tac; humanized anti-tac [now: daclizumab]

SmartMist (trademarked delivery device) *hand-held inhalation device*

smartweed; water smartweed *medicinal herb* [see: knotweed]

SMF (streptozocin, mitomycin, fluorouracil) *chemotherapy protocol for pancreatic cancer*

Smilax **spp.** *medicinal herb* [see: sarsaparilla]

smooth sumach *medicinal herb* [see: sumach]

SMX; SMZ (sulfamethoxazole) [q.v.]

SMZ-TMP (sulfamethoxazole & trimethoprim) [q.v.]

SN (streptonigrin) [q.v.]

snake bite *medicinal herb* [see: birthroot]

snake head *medicinal herb* [see: turtlebloom]

snake lily *medicinal herb* [see: blue flag]

snake weed *medicinal herb* [see: bistort; plantain]

snakebite antivenin [see: antivenin, Crotalidae & Micrurus fulvius]

snakeroot *medicinal herb* [see: echinacea]

snakeroot, black *medicinal herb* [see: black cohosh; sanicle]

snapping hazel *medicinal herb* [see: witch hazel]

SnapTab (trademarked dosage form) *scored tablet*

SnET2 (tin ethyl etiopurpurin) [see: rostaporfin]

Snooze Fast tablets OTC *antihistamine; sleep aid* [diphenhydramine HCl] 50 mg

Sno-Strips ophthalmic strips (discontinued 2009) OTC *diagnostic tear flow test aid*

snout, swine *medicinal herb* [see: dandelion]

snowball, wild *medicinal herb* [see: New Jersey tea]

snowdrop tree; snowflower *medicinal herb* [see: fringe tree]

soap, green USP *detergent*

soapwort (*Saponaria officinalis*) *plant and roots medicinal herb for acne, boils, eczema, poison ivy rash and psoriasis; also used in skin disinfectants and soaps* ⦾ Supprette

Sochlor eye drops OTC *corneal edema-reducing agent* [sodium chloride (hypertonic saline solution)] 5% ⦾ Ceclor; Zyclara

SOD (superoxide dismutase) [see: orgotein]

soda lime NF *carbon dioxide absorbent*

SodiPhluor oral drops ℞ *dental caries preventative* [sodium fluoride] 0.5 mg/mL

sodium *element (Na)*

sodium acetate USP *dialysis aid; electrolyte replenisher; pH buffer* 2, 4 mEq/mL (16.4%, 32.8%) injection

sodium acetate trihydrate [see: sodium acetate]

sodium acetrizoate INN, BAN [also: acetrizoate sodium]

sodium acetylsalicylate *analgesic*

sodium acid phosphate *urinary acidifier*

sodium alginate NF *suspending agent*

sodium aluminosilicate *investigational (orphan) for chronic hepatic encephalopathy*

sodium amidotrizoate INN *oral/rectal/parenteral radiopaque contrast medium (59.87% iodine)* [also: diatrizoate sodium; sodium diatrizoate]

sodium aminobenzoate [see: aminobenzoate sodium]

sodium amylopectin sulfate [see: sodium amylosulfate]

sodium amylosulfate USAN *enzyme inhibitor*

sodium anoxynaphthonate BAN *blood volume and cardiac output test* [also: anazolene sodium]

sodium antimony gluconate [see: sodium stibogluconate]

sodium antimonylgluconate BAN

sodium apolate INN, BAN *anticoagulant* [also: lyapolate sodium]

sodium arsenate, exsiccated NF

sodium arsenate As 74 USAN *radioactive agent*

sodium ascorbate (vitamin C) USP, INN *water-soluble vitamin; antiscorbutic*

sodium aurothiomalate INN *antirheumatic* [also: gold sodium thiomalate]

sodium aurotiosulfate INN [also: gold sodium thiosulfate]

sodium azodisalicylate [now: olsalazine sodium]

sodium benzoate USAN, NF, JAN *adjunctive therapy (rescue agent) to prevent and treat hyperammonemia due to urea cycle enzymopathy; antifungal agent; preservative*

sodium benzoate & caffeine *analeptic for respiratory depression due to an overdose of CNS depressants* 250 mg/mL injection

sodium benzoate & sodium phenylacetate *adjunctive therapy (rescue agent) to prevent and treat hyperammonemia due to urea cycle enzymopathy (orphan)*

sodium benzyl penicillin [see: penicillin G sodium]

sodium bicarbonate USP *electrolyte replenisher; systemic alkalizer; antacid* 325, 600, 650 mg oral; 0.5, 0.6, 0.9, 1 mEq/mL (4.2%, 5%, 7.5%, 8.4%) injection

sodium bicarbonate & sodium chloride & polyethylene glycol 3350 & potassium chloride *hyperosmotic laxative; pre-procedure bowel evacuant* 5.72•11.2•420•1.48 g/bottle

sodium bicarbonate & sodium chloride & sodium sulfate & polyethylene glycol 3350 & potassium chloride *hyperosmotic laxative; pre-procedure bowel evacuant* 6.74•5.86• 22.74•236•2.97, 6.72•5.84•22.73• 240•2.98 g/bottle

sodium biphosphate *urinary acidifier; pH buffer*

sodium bisulfite NF *antioxidant*

sodium bitionolate INN *topical anti-infective* [also: bithionolate sodium]

sodium borate NF *alkalizing agent; antipruritic; bacteriostatic agent in cold creams, eye washes, and mouth rinses*

sodium borocaptate (^{10}B) INN *antineoplastic; radioactive agent* [also: borocaptate sodium B 10]

sodium cacodylate NF

sodium calcium edetate INN *heavy metal chelating agent* [also: edetate calcium disodium; sodium calciumedetate; calcium disodium edetate]

sodium calciumedetate BAN *heavy metal chelating agent* [also: edetate calcium disodium; sodium calcium edetate; calcium disodium edetate]

sodium caprylate *antifungal*

sodium carbonate NF *alkalizing agent*

sodium chloride (NaCl) USP *ophthalmic hypertonic; electrolyte replacement; abortifacient* [sterile isotonic solution] 650, 1000 mg oral; 0.45%, 0.9%, 3%, 5%, 14.6%, 23.4% injection/diluent

0.45% sodium chloride (½ normal saline; ½ NS) *electrolyte replacement*

0.9% sodium chloride (normal saline; NS) *electrolyte replacement* [also: saline solution]

sodium chloride, compound solution of INN *fluid and electrolyte replenisher* [also: Ringer's injection]

sodium chloride Na 22 USAN *radioactive agent*

sodium chloride & polyethylene glycol 3350 & potassium chloride & sodium bicarbonate *hyperosmotic laxative; pre-procedure bowel evacuant* 11.2•420•1.48•5.72 g/bottle

sodium chloride & sodium sulfate & polyethylene glycol 3350 & potassium chloride & sodium bicarbonate *hyperosmotic laxative; pre-procedure bowel evacuant* 5.86• 22.74•236•2.97•6.74, 5.84•22.73• 240•2.98•6.72 g/bottle

sodium chondroitin sulfate [see: chondroitin sulfate sodium]

sodium chromate (^{51}Cr) INN *blood volume test; radioactive agent* [also: sodium chromate Cr 51]

sodium chromate Cr 51 USAN *blood volume test; radioactive agent* [also: sodium chromate (^{51}Cr)]

sodium citrate USP *systemic alkalizer; pH buffer; antacid; investigational (orphan) adjunct to leukapheresis procedures*

sodium citrate & citric acid *urinary alkalinizing agent* 500•334 mg/5 mL oral

sodium colistin methanesulfonate [see: colistimethate sodium]

sodium copper chlorophyllin [see: chlorophyllin copper complex]

sodium cromoglycate [see: cromolyn sodium]

sodium cyclamate NF, INN

sodium cyclohexanesulfamate [see: sodium cyclamate]

sodium dehydroacetate NF *antimicrobial preservative*

sodium dehydrocholate INN [also: dehydrocholate sodium]

sodium denyl [see: phenytoin sodium]

sodium diatrizoate BAN *oral/rectal/parenteral radiopaque contrast medium (59.87% iodine)* [also: diatrizoate sodium; sodium amidotrizoate]

sodium dibunate INN, BAN

sodium dichloroacetate (sodium DCA) USAN *pyruvate dehydrogenase activator; investigational (orphan) for severe head trauma, lactic acidosis, homozygous familial hypercholesterolemia, and monochloroacetic acid poisoning*

sodium diethyldithiocarbamate [see: ditiocarb sodium]

sodium diiodomethanesulfonate [see: dimethiodal sodium]

sodium dioctyl sulfosuccinate INN *stool softener; surfactant* [also: docusate sodium]

sodium diphenylhydantoin [see: phenytoin sodium]

sodium diprotrizoate INN, BAN [also: diprotrizoate sodium]

Sodium Edecrin [see: Edecrin Sodium]

sodium edetate [see: edetate sodium]

sodium estrone sulfate *estrogen replacement therapy for postmenopausal disorders* 0.625, 1.25, 2.5, 5 mg oral

sodium etasulfate INN *detergent* [also: sodium ethasulfate]

sodium ethasulfate USAN *detergent* [also: sodium etasulfate]

sodium feredetate INN [also: sodium ironedetate]

sodium ferric gluconate *hematinic for iron deficiency due to chronic hemodial-*ysis with epoetin therapy 62.5 mg/5 mL injection

sodium fluoride USP *fluoride replacement therapy; dental caries preventative* (45% fluoride) 1.1, 2.2 mg oral; 0.125, 0.25, 0.5 mg/mL oral

sodium fluoride F 18 USP 10–200 mCi/mL injection

sodium fluoride & phosphoric acid USP *dental caries preventative*

sodium formaldehyde sulfoxylate NF *preservative*

sodium gamma hydroxybutyrate (NaGHB) [see: gamma hydroxybutyrate (GHB); sodium oxybate]

sodium gammahydroxyburate [see: sodium oxybate]

sodium gentisate INN

sodium glucaspaldrate INN, BAN

sodium gluconate USP *electrolyte replenisher*

sodium glucosulfone USP

sodium glutamate

sodium glycerophosphate NF

sodium glycocholate [see: bile salts]

sodium gualenate INN [also: azulene sulfonate sodium]

sodium hyaluronate [see: hyaluronate sodium]

sodium hydroxide NF *alkalizing agent*

sodium hydroxybenzenesulfonate [see: phenolsulphonate sodium]

sodium 4-hydroxybutyrate [see: sodium oxybate]

sodium hypochlorite USP, JAN *disinfectant; bleach; used for utensils and equipment*

sodium hypochlorite, diluted NF [also: antiformin, dental]

sodium hypophosphite NF

sodium iodide USP *dietary iodine supplement; additive to IV solutions for total parenteral nutrition (85% elemental iodine)*

sodium iodide (^{123}I) JAN *thyroid function test; radioactive agent* [also: sodium iodide I 123]

sodium iodide (^{125}I) INN *thyroid function test; radioactive agent* [also: sodium iodide I 125]

sodium iodide (¹³¹I) JAN *radioactive antineoplastic for thyroid carcinoma; thyroid inhibitor for hyperthyroidism* [also: sodium iodide I 131]

sodium iodide I 123 USP *diagnostic aid for thyroid function; radioactive agent* [also: sodium iodide (¹²³I)] 3.7, 7.4 MBq oral

sodium iodide I 125 USAN, USP *thyroid function test; radioactive agent* [also: sodium iodide (¹²⁵I)]

sodium iodide I 131 USAN, USP, INN *radioactive antineoplastic for thyroid carcinoma; thyroid inhibitor for hyperthyroidism* [also: sodium iodide (¹³¹I)] 0.75–100, 3.5–150 mCi oral

sodium iodohippurate (¹³¹I) INN, JAN *renal function test; radioactive agent* [also: iodohippurate sodium I 131]

sodium iodomethanesulfonate [see: methiodal sodium]

sodium iopodate JAN *oral radiopaque contrast medium for cholecystography (61.4% iodine)* [also: ipodate sodium; sodium ipodate]

sodium iotalamate (¹²⁵I) INN *radioactive agent* [also: iothalamate sodium I 125]

sodium iotalamate (¹³¹I) INN *radioactive agent* [also: iothalamate sodium I 131]

sodium iothalamate BAN *parenteral radiopaque contrast medium (59.9% iodine)* [also: iothalamate sodium]

sodium ioxaglate BAN *radiopaque contrast medium* [also: ioxaglate sodium]

sodium ipodate INN, BAN *oral radiopaque contrast medium for cholecystography (61.4% iodine)* [also: ipodate sodium; sodium iopodate]

sodium ironedetate BAN [also: sodium feredetate]

sodium lactate (SL) USP *electrolyte replenisher* 167 mEq/L (1/6 molar) injection

sodium lactate, compound solution of INN *electrolyte and fluid replenisher; systemic alkalizer* [also: Ringer's injection, lactated]

sodium lauryl sulfate NF *surfactant/ wetting agent* [also: laurilsulfate]

sodium lignosulfonate [see: polignate sodium]

sodium metabisulfite NF *antioxidant*

sodium metrizoate INN *radiopaque contrast medium* [also: metrizoate sodium]

sodium monododecyl sulfate [see: sodium lauryl sulfate]

sodium monofluorophosphate USP *dental caries preventative*

sodium monomercaptoundecahy-dro-closo-dodecaborate *investigational (orphan) for boron neutron capture therapy (BNCT) for glioblastoma multiforme*

sodium morrhuate INN *sclerosing agent* [also: morrhuate sodium]

sodium nitrite USP *adjunct to cyanide detoxification; also used for hydrogen sulfide poisoning* 30 mg/mL injection

sodium nitrite & sodium thiosulfate & amyl nitrite [inhalant] *emergency treatment of cyanide poisoning (orphan)* 300 mg•12.5 g•0.3 mL kit

sodium nitroferricyanide [see: sodium nitroprusside]

sodium nitroferricyanide dihydrate [see: sodium nitroprusside]

sodium nitroprusside USP *emergency antihypertensive; vasodilator; investigational (orphan) for the prevention and treatment of cerebral vasospasm following subarachnoid hemorrhage* 50 mg/ dose injection

sodium noramidopyrine methane-sulfonate [see: dipyrone]

sodium oxybate USAN *adjunct to anesthesia; CNS depressant for narcolepsy (orphan), cataplexy, sleep paralysis, and hypnagogic hallucinations; investigational (Phase III) for fibromyalgia; also used for fatigue* [also known as: gamma hydroxybutyrate (GHB)]

sodium oxychlorosene [see: oxychlorosene sodium]

sodium paratoluenesulfan chloramide [see: chloramine-T]

sodium PCA; Na PCA (sodium pyrrolidone carboxylic acid) [q.v.]

sodium penicillin G [see: penicillin G sodium]

sodium pentosan polysulfate [see: pentosan polysulfate sodium]

sodium perborate *topical antiseptic/ germicidal*

sodium perborate monohydrate USAN *topical antiseptic/germicidal*

sodium pertechnetate Tc 99m USAN, USP *radioactive agent*

sodium phenolate [see: phenolate sodium]

sodium phenylacetate USAN *adjunctive therapy (rescue agent) to prevent and treat hyperammonemia due to urea cycle enzymopathy*

sodium phenylacetate & sodium benzoate *adjunctive therapy (rescue agent) to prevent and treat hyperammonemia due to urea cycle enzymopathy (orphan)*

sodium phenylbutyrate USAN *antihyperammonemic for urea cycle disorders (orphan); investigational (orphan) for malignant glioma and various sickling disorders and spinal muscular atrophy*

sodium phosphate (^{32}P) INN *antineoplastic; antipolycythemic; neoplasm test* [also: sodium phosphate P 32]

sodium phosphate, dibasic (Na_2HPO_4) USP *saline laxative; phosphorus replacement; calcium regulator; pH buffer*

sodium phosphate, monobasic (NaH_2PO_4) USP *saline laxative; calcium regulator; phosphorus replacement; pH buffer*

sodium phosphate P 32 USAN, USP *antipolycythemic; radiopharmaceutical antineoplastic for various leukemias and skeletal metastases* [also: sodium phosphate (^{32}P)] 0.67 mCi/mL

sodium picofosfate INN

sodium picosulfate INN

sodium polyphosphate USAN *pharmaceutic aid*

sodium polystyrene sulfonate USP *potassium-removing ion-exchange resin for hyperkalemia* 15, 454 g oral or rectal

sodium propionate NF *preservative; antifungal*

sodium propionate hydrate [see: sodium propionate]

sodium 2-propylvalerate [see: valproate sodium]

sodium psylliate NF

sodium pyrophosphate USAN *pharmaceutic aid*

sodium pyrrolidone carboxylic acid (sodium PCA; Na PCA) *natural skin moisturizing factor; humectant*

sodium pyruvate *investigational (orphan) for cystic fibrosis*

sodium radiochromate [see: sodium chromate Cr 51]

sodium rhodanate [see: thiocyanate sodium]

sodium salicylate (SS) USP *analgesic; antipyretic; anti-inflammatory; antirheumatic* 325, 650 mg oral

sodium starch glycolate NF *tablet excipient*

sodium stearate NF *emulsifying and stiffening agent*

sodium stearyl fumarate NF *tablet and capsule lubricant*

sodium stibocaptate INN [also: stibocaptate]

sodium stibogluconate INN, BAN *investigational antiparasitic for leishmaniasis and trypanosomiasis*

Sodium Sulamyd eye drops, ophthalmic ointment ℞ *antibiotic* [sulfacetamide sodium] 10%, 30%; 10%

sodium sulfacetamide [see: sulfacetamide sodium]

sodium sulfate USP *calcium regulator*

sodium sulfate & polyethylene glycol 3350 & potassium chloride & sodium bicarbonate & sodium chloride *hyperosmotic laxative; preprocedure bowel evacuant* 22.74•236•2.97•6.74•5.86, 22.73•240•2.98•6.72•5.84 g/bottle

sodium sulfate S 35 USAN *radioactive agent*

sodium sulfocyanate [see: thiocyanate sodium]

sodium taurocholate [see: bile salts]

sodium tetradecyl (STD) sulfate
INN *sclerosing agent for varicose veins*

sodium thiomalate, gold [see: gold sodium thiomalate]

sodium thiosalicylate *analgesic; antipyretic; anti-inflammatory; antirheumatic* 50 mg/mL injection

sodium thiosulfate USP *antidote to cyanide poisoning; antiseptic; antifungal; also used for cisplatin-induced nephrotoxicity in adults; investigational (orphan) for platinum-induced ototoxicity in children* 10%, 25% (100, 250 mg/mL) injection

sodium thiosulfate, gold [see: gold sodium thiosulfate]

sodium thiosulfate & hydroxocobalamin *investigational (orphan) for severe acute cyanide poisoning*

sodium thiosulfate pentahydrate [see: sodium thiosulfate]

sodium thiosulfate & sodium nitrite & amyl nitrite [inhalant] *emergency treatment of cyanide poisoning (orphan)* 12.5 g•300 mg•0.3 mL kit

sodium timerfonate INN *topical antiinfective* [also: thimerfonate sodium]

sodium trimetaphosphate USAN *pharmaceutic aid*

sodium tyropanoate INN *oral radioopaque contrast medium for cholecystography (57.4% iodine)* [also: tyropanoate sodium]

sodium valproate [see: valproate sodium]

Sodol Compound tablets ℞ *skeletal muscle relaxant; analgesic; antipyretic* [carisoprodol; aspirin] 200•325 mg

sofalcone INN

Sof-lax softgels OTC *laxative; stool softener* [docusate sodium] 100 mg ⊘ ZFlex

Soft Mate Comfort Drops for Sensitive Eyes OTC *rewetting solution for soft contact lenses*

Soft Mate Consept solution + aerosol spray OTC *two-step chemical disinfecting system for soft contact lenses* [hydrogen peroxide–based]

Soft Mate Disinfecting for Sensitive Eyes solution OTC *chemical disinfecting solution for soft contact lenses* [EDTA; chlorhexidine gluconate] 0.1%•0.005%

Soft Mate Hands Off Daily Cleaner solution OTC *surfactant cleaning solution for soft contact lenses*

soft pine *medicinal herb* [see: white pine]

Soft Sense lotion OTC *moisturizer; emollient*

Softabs (trademarked dosage form) *chewable tablets*

softgels (dosage form) *soft gelatin capsules*

SoftWear solution OTC *rinsing/storage solution for soft contact lenses* [sodium chloride (preserved saline solution)]

Sojourn liquid for vaporization ℞ *inhalation general anesthetic* [sevoflurane]

Solagé topical solution ℞ *depigmenting agent for solar lentigines* [mequinol; tretinoin; alcohol 77.8%] 2%•0.01%

solanezumab *investigational (Phase III) monoclonal antibody to amyloid beta plaque in the brain for Alzheimer disease*

Solanum dulcamara *medicinal herb* [see: bittersweet nightshade]

solapsone BAN [also: solasulfone]

Solaquin cream OTC *hyperpigmentation bleaching agent* [hydroquinone in a sunscreen base] 2% ⊘ silicon; Xylocaine

Solaquin Forte cream, gel ℞ *hyperpigmentation bleaching agent* [hydroquinone (in a sunscreen base)] 4%

Solaraze gel ℞ *anti-inflammatory for actinic keratosis (AK)* [diclofenac sodium] 3%

Solarcaine aerosol spray, lotion OTC *anesthetic; disinfectant/antiseptic* [benzocaine; triclosan] 20%•0.13%

Solarcaine Aloe Extra Burn Relief cream, gel, topical spray OTC *anesthetic* [lidocaine] 0.5%

Solarcaine Medicated First Aid Spray OTC *anesthetic; disinfectant/antiseptic* [benzocaine; triclosan] 20%•0.13%

solasulfone INN [also: solapsone]

soldier's woundwort *medicinal herb*
[see: yarrow]

Solfoton tablets, capsules ℞ *long-acting barbiturate sedative, hypnotic, and anticonvulsant* [phenobarbital] 16 mg

Solganal IM injection (discontinued 2009) ℞ *antirheumatic* [aurothioglucose] 50 mg/mL

Solia tablets (in packs of 28) ℞ *monophasic oral contraceptive* [desogestrel; ethinyl estradiol] 0.15 mg•30 mcg × 21 days; counters × 7 days

Solidago nemoralis; S. odora; S. virgaurea medicinal herb [see: goldenrod]

solifenacin succinate *selective muscarinic* M_3 *receptor antagonist; urinary antispasmodic for overactive bladder with urinary incontinence, urgency, and frequency*

Soliris IV infusion ℞ *monoclonal antibody; antihemolytic for paroxysmal nocturnal hemoglobinuria (PNH; orphan); investigational (orphan) for idiopathic membranous glomerular nephropathy* [eculizumab] 10 mg/mL (300 mg/vial)

Solodyn film-coated extended-release tablets ℞ *tetracycline antibiotic for severe acne* [minocycline (as HCl)] 45, 55, 65, 80, 90, 105, 115, 135 mg

Solomon's seal *(Polygonatum multiflorum; P. odoratum) root medicinal herb used as an astringent, demulcent, emetic, and expectorant*

SoloStar (trademarked insulin delivery device) *prefilled subcu injector for* **Lantus**

Solotuss oral suspension (discontinued 2009) ℞ *antitussive* [carbetapentane tannate] 30 mg/5 mL

solpecainol INN

SolTabs (trademarked dosage form) *orally disintegrating tablets*

Soltamox oral solution (discontinued 2010) ℞ *antiestrogen antineoplastic for the treatment of breast cancer and the reduction of breast cancer incidence in high-risk women* [tamoxifen citrate] 10 mg/5 mL

Soltice Quick-Rub ointment OTC *analgesic; counterirritant* [menthol; camphor] 5.1%•5.1%

soluble ferric pyrophosphate [see: ferric pyrophosphate, soluble]

soluble gelatin (SG) [see: gelatin]

Soluble T4 *investigational (orphan) treatment for AIDS* [CD4 human truncated 369 AA polypeptide]

Soluclenz gel ℞ *keratolytic for acne* [benzoyl peroxide] 5%

Solu-Cortef powder for IV or IM injection ℞ *corticosteroid; antiinflammatory* [hydrocortisone sodium succinate] 100, 250, 500, 1000 mg

Solu-Medrol powder for IV or IM injection ℞ *corticosteroid; anti-inflammatory; immunosuppressant* [methylprednisolone sodium succinate] 40, 125, 500, 1000, 2000 mg/vial

Solumol ointment OTC *nontherapeutic base for compounding various dermatological preparations*

Soluspan (trademarked dosage form) *injectable suspension* 🄿 psilocybin

Soluvite C.T. pediatric chewable tablets (discontinued 2008) ℞ *vitamin supplement; dental caries preventative* [multiple vitamins; fluoride; folic acid] ±•1•0.3 mg

Solvent-G topical liquid OTC *nontherapeutic base for compounding various dermatological preparations*

Solvet (trademarked dosage form) *soluble tablet*

solypertine INN *antiadrenergic* [also: solypertine tartrate]

solypertine tartrate USAN *antiadrenergic* [also: solypertine]

Soma tablets ℞ *skeletal muscle relaxant* [carisoprodol] 250, 350 mg

Soma Compound tablets (discontinued 2008) ℞ *skeletal muscle relaxant; analgesic; antipyretic* [carisoprodol; aspirin] 200•325 mg

Soma Compound with Codeine tablets (discontinued 2008) ℞ *skeletal muscle relaxant; narcotic antitussive; analgesic; antipyretic* [carisopro-

dol; aspirin; codeine phosphate]
200•325•16 mg

somagrebove USAN *veterinary galactopoietic agent*

somalapor USAN, INN, BAN *porcine growth hormone*

somantadine INN *antiviral* [also: somantadine HCl]

somantadine HCl USAN *antiviral* [also: somantadine]

SomatoKine *investigational (orphan) treatment for growth hormone insensitivity syndrome (Laron syndrome) and extreme insulin-resistance syndromes (type A, type B, Rabson-Mendenhall syndrome, leprechaunism)* [mecasermin rinfabate]

somatomedin-C [see: mecasermin]

somatorelin INN *growth hormone-releasing factor (GH-RF)*

somatostatin (SS) INN, BAN *growth hormone-release inhibiting factor; investigational (orphan) for cutaneous gastrointestinal fistulas and bleeding esophageal varices*

somatostatin analogue, multi-ligand *investigational (orphan) for functional gastroenteropancreatic neuroendocrine tumors (insulinoma, gastrinoma, somatostatinoma, GRFoma, VIPoma, and glucagonoma)*

SomatoTher *investigational (orphan) radiotherapeutic agent for somatostatin receptor–positive neuroendocrine tumors* [indium In 111 pentetreotide]

somatotropin, human [see: somatropin]

Somatrel *investigational (orphan) diagnostic aid for pituitary release of growth hormone* [NG-29 (code name — generic name not yet assigned)]

somatrem USAN, INN, BAN *growth hormone for congenital growth failure due to lack of endogenous growth hormone (orphan); investigational (orphan) for short stature due to Turner syndrome*

somatropin USAN, INN, BAN, JAN *growth hormone for children and adults with congenital or endogenous growth hormone deficiency (GHD), short bowel syndrome, or AIDS-wasting syndrome; for children with Turner syndrome, Prader-Willi syndrome, or renal-induced growth failure* [also: human growth hormone]

somatropin & glutamine *investigational (orphan) for GI malabsorption due to short bowel syndrome*

Somatuline Depot subcu injection in prefilled syringes ℞ *reduces endogenous growth hormone (GH) and insulin growth factor-1 (IGF-1) levels to treat acromegaly (orphan)* [lanreotide (as acetate)] 60, 90, 120 mg

Somavert subcu injection ℞ *growth hormone receptor antagonist for acromegaly (orphan)* [pegvisomant] 10, 15, 20 mg/dose

somavubove USAN, INN *veterinary galactopoietic agent*

somenopor USAN *porcine growth hormone*

sometribove USAN, INN, BAN *veterinary growth stimulant*

sometripor USAN, INN, BAN *veterinary growth stimulant*

somfasepor USAN *veterinary growth stimulant*

somidobove USAN, INN *synthetic bovine growth hormone*

Sominex tablets, caplets OTC *antihistamine; sleep aid* [diphenhydramine HCl] 25 mg; 50 mg

Sominex Pain Relief tablets OTC *antihistamine; sleep aid; analgesic; antipyretic* [diphenhydramine HCl; acetaminophen] 25•500 mg

Somnote capsules ℞ *nonbarbiturate sedative and hypnotic; also abused as a street drug* [chloral hydrate] 500 mg

Sonahist oral drops ℞ *decongestant; antihistamine; for children 2–12 years* [phenylephrine HCl; chlorpheniramine maleate] 2•1 mg/mL ⊘ Sinuhist

Sonahist DM oral drops ℞ *antitussive; antihistamine; decongestant; for children 2–12 years* [dextromethorphan hydrobromide; chlorpheniramine maleate; phenylephrine HCl] 3•1•2 mg/mL

Sonata capsules ℞ *rapid-onset, short-duration hypnotic for the short-term treatment of insomnia* [zaleplon] 5, 10 mg

sonepiprazole mesylate USAN *dopamine D_4 antagonist; antipsychotic*

SonoRx oral suspension (discontinued 2010) ℞ *ultrasound imaging agent to reduce gas shadowing* [simethicone-coated cellulose] 7.5 mg/mL

Soothaderm lotion OTC *anesthetic; antihistamine; emollient* [pyrilamine maleate; benzocaine; zinc oxide] 2.07•2.08•41.35 mg/mL

Soothe eye drops OTC *moisturizer/lubricant* [polysorbate 80] 0.4%

Soothe & Cool cream OTC *diaper rash treatment* [zinc oxide; dimethicone] 5%•5%

Soothe XP eye drops OTC *moisturizer/lubricant* [mineral oil; light mineral oil] 4.5%•1%

sopecainol [see: solpecainol]

sopitazine INN

sopromidine INN

soproxil USAN *combining name for radicals or groups* [also: disoproxil]

soquinolol INN

sorafenib tosylate *multikinase inhibitor; antineoplastic for advanced renal cell carcinoma (orphan) and hepatocellular carcinoma* (base=73%)

sorb apple *medicinal herb* [see: mountain ash]

sorbic acid NF *antimicrobial agent; preservative*

sorbide nitrate [see: isosorbide dinitrate]

sorbimacrogol laurate 300 [see: polysorbate 20]

sorbimacrogol oleate 300 [see: polysorbate 80]

sorbimacrogol palmitate 300 [see: polysorbate 40]

sorbimacrogol stearate [see: polysorbate 60]

sorbimacrogol tristearate 300 [see: polysorbate 65]

sorbinicate INN

sorbinil USAN, INN, BAN *aldose reductase enzyme inhibitor*

sorbitan laurate INN *surfactant* [also: sorbitan monolaurate]

sorbitan monolaurate USAN, NF *surfactant* [also: sorbitan laurate]

sorbitan monooleate USAN, NF *surfactant* [also: sorbitan oleate]

sorbitan monopalmitate USAN, NF *surfactant* [also: sorbitan palmitate]

sorbitan monostearate USAN, NF *surfactant* [also: sorbitan stearate]

sorbitan oleate INN *surfactant* [also: sorbitan monooleate]

sorbitan palmitate INN *surfactant* [also: sorbitan monopalmitate]

sorbitan sesquioleate USAN, INN *surfactant*

sorbitan stearate INN *surfactant* [also: sorbitan monostearate]

sorbitan trioleate USAN, INN *surfactant*

sorbitan tristearate USAN, INN *surfactant*

sorbitol NF *flavoring agent; tablet excipient; urologic irrigant* 3%, 3.3% solution

sorbitol solution (D-sorbitol) USP *flavoring agent; urologic irrigant* 70% solution

Sorbsan pads OTC *absorbent dressing for wet wounds* [calcium alginate fiber]

Sorbus americana; S. aucuparia *medicinal herb* [see: mountain ash]

Sorbutuss NR oral liquid OTC *antitussive; expectorant; demulcent* [dextromethorphan hydrobromide; guaifenesin; potassium citrate] 15•150•127.5 mg/5 mL

Soriatane capsules ℞ *systemic antipsoriatic* [acitretin] 10, 17.5, 22.5, 25 mg ☑ Serutan

Soriatane CK ("convenience kit") capsules + topical foam (discontinued 2010) ℞ *antipsoriatic (capsules); emollient/protectant (foam)* [acitretin (capsules)] 10 mg

Sorilux aerosol foam ℞ *antipsoriatic* [calcipotriene] 0.005%

sorivudine USAN, INN, BAN *investigational (NDA filed) antiviral for herpes* *zoster (orphan) and varicella zoster infections in immunocompromised patients*

sornidipine INN

sorrel (*Rumex acetosa*) plant *medicinal herb used as an antiscorbutic, astringent, diuretic, laxative, refrigerant, and vermifuge* ⑨ Xiral

sorrel, common; mountain sorrel; white sorrel *medicinal herb* [see: wood sorrel]

sorrel, Jamaica *medicinal herb* [see: hibiscus]

sotalol INN, BAN *antiarrhythmic; antiadrenergic (beta-blocker)* [also: sotalol HCl]

sotalol HCl USAN *antiarrhythmic (beta-blocker) for ventricular arrhythmias (orphan)* [also: sotalol] 80, 120, 160, 240 mg oral; 15 mg/mL injection

Sotalol HCl AF tablets ℞ *antiarrhythmic (beta-blocker) for atrial fibrillation or atrial flutter* [sotalol HCl] 80, 120, 160 mg

soterenol INN *adrenergic; bronchodilator* [also: soterenol HCl] ⑨ cioteronel; citronella; SteriNail

soterenol HCl USAN *adrenergic; bronchodilator* [also: soterenol]

Sotradecol IV injection ℞ *sclerosing agent for varicose veins* [sodium tetradecyl sulfate] 10, 30 mg/mL

Sotret softgels ℞ *keratolytic for severe recalcitrant cystic acne* [isotretinoin] 10, 20, 30, 40 mg

sour dock *medicinal herb* [see: yellow dock]

sourberry; sowberry *medicinal herb* [see: barberry]

sourgrass *medicinal herb* [see: sorrel]

Southern ginseng *medicinal herb* [see: jiaogulan]

Soviet gramicidin [see: gramicidin S]

sowberry; sourberry *medicinal herb* [see: barberry]

soy; soya; soybean (*Glycine max*) *medicinal herb and food crop; isoflavone compounds provide phytoestrogens to alleviate menopausal symptoms, including osteoporosis, and provide antineoplastic, cardiovascular, and gastrointestinal benefits*

Soyalac; I-Soyalac oral liquid, powder for oral liquid OTC *hypoallergenic infant food* [soy protein formula] ⑨ SalAc

soybean oil USP *pharmaceutic necessity*

spaglumic acid INN

Span C tablets OTC *vitamin C supplement with bioflavonoids* [ascorbic acid and rose hips; citrus bioflavonoids] 200•300 mg

Spancap No. 1 sustained-release capsules ℞ *CNS stimulant* [dextroamphetamine sulfate] 15 mg

Spancaps (dosage form) *timed-release capsules*

Spanidin *investigational (orphan) immunosuppressant for acute renal graft rejection* [gusperimus]

Spanish chestnut *medicinal herb* [see: horse chestnut]

Spanish pepper *medicinal herb* [see: cayenne]

Spansule (trademarked dosage form) *sustained-release capsule*

sparfloxacin (SPFX) USAN, INN, BAN *broad-spectrum fluoroquinolone antibiotic* ⑨ ciprofloxacin

sparfosate sodium USAN *antineoplastic* [also: sparfosic acid]

sparfosic acid INN *antineoplastic* [also: sparfosate sodium]

Sparkles effervescent granules OTC *antacid; antiflatulent; aid in endoscopic examination* [sodium bicarbonate; citric acid; simethicone] 2000• 1500• 2̲ mg/dose

sparsomycin USAN, INN *antineoplastic*

Spartaject (trademarked delivery device) *investigational (Phase II/III) intravenous injector*

Spartaject Busulfan *investigational (orphan) alkylating antineoplastic for neoplastic meningitis and primary brain malignancies* [busulfan]

sparteine INN *oxytocic* [also: sparteine sulfate]

sparteine sulfate USAN *oxytocic* [also: sparteine]

Spasmolin tablets ℞ *GI antispasmodic; anticholinergic; sedative* [atropine sulfate; scopolamine hydrobromide; hyoscyamine hydrobromide; phenobarbital] 0.0194•0.0065•0.1037•16.2 mg

SPCA (serum prothrombin conversion accelerator) factor [see: factor VII]

spearmint NF

spearmint *(Mentha spicata)* leaves *medicinal herb for colds, colic, flu, gas, nausea, and vomiting*

spearmint oil NF

Spec-T lozenges OTC *mucous membrane anesthetic* [benzocaine] 10 mg

Spectazole cream ℞ *antifungal* [econazole nitrate] 1%

spectinomycin INN *antibiotic* [also: spectinomycin HCl]

spectinomycin HCl USAN, USP *antibiotic for gonorrhea* [also: spectinomycin]

Spectracef film-coated tablets ℞ *broad-spectrum cephalosporin antibiotic* [cefditoren pivoxil] 200, 400 mg

Spectro-Jel topical liquid OTC *soap-free therapeutic skin cleanser*

speedwell *(Veronica officinalis)* flowering plant *medicinal herb used as a diuretic, expectorant, and stomachic*

speedwell, tall *medicinal herb* [see: Culver root]

spenbolic [see: methandriol]

spermaceti, synthetic [see: cetyl esters wax]

spermicides *a class of topical contraceptive agents that kill sperm*

SPFX (sparfloxacin) [q.v.]

Spherulin intradermal injection (discontinued 2010) ℞ *diagnostic aid for coccidioidomycosis* [coccidioidin] 1:100, 1:10

spiceberry *medicinal herb* [see: wintergreen]

spiclamine INN

spiclomazine INN

spicy wintergreen *medicinal herb* [see: wintergreen]

spider bite antivenin [see: antivenin (Latrodectus mactans)]

spignet *medicinal herb* [see: spikenard]

spikenard *(Aralia racemosa)* root *medicinal herb for asthma, childbirth, cough, and rheumatism*

spindle tree *medicinal herb* [see: wahoo]

spinosad *topical pediculicide for lice*

spiperone USAN, INN *antipsychotic*

spiradoline INN *analgesic* [also: spiradoline mesylate]

spiradoline mesylate USAN *analgesic* [also: spiradoline]

spiramide INN

spiramycin USAN, INN, BAN *macrolide antibiotic; investigational (orphan) treatment for chronic cryptosporidiosis in immunocompromised patients* [also: acetylspiramycin]

spirapril INN, BAN *antihypertensive; angiotensin-converting enzyme (ACE) inhibitor* [also: spirapril HCl]

spirapril HCl USAN *antihypertensive; angiotensin-converting enzyme (ACE) inhibitor* [also: spirapril]

spiraprilat USAN, INN *antihypertensive; angiotensin-converting enzyme (ACE) inhibitor*

spirazine INN 🄯 Sprayzoin

spirazine HCl [see: spirazine]

spirendolol INN

spirgetine INN

spirilene INN, BAN

spirit of nitrous ether [see: ethyl nitrite]

Spiriva powder in capsules for inhalation (used with **HandiHaler** device) ℞ *once-daily bronchodilator for emphysema and chronic obstructive pulmonary disease (COPD)* [tiotropium (as bromide)] 18 mcg/dose

spirobarbital sodium

spirofylline INN

spirogermanium INN, BAN *antineoplastic* [also: spirogermanium HCl]

spirogermanium HCl USAN *antineoplastic* [also: spirogermanium]

spirohydantoin mustard [now: spiromustine]

spiromustine USAN, INN *antineoplastic*

spironolactone USP, INN, BAN, JAN *aldosterone antagonist; antihypertensive; potassium-sparing diuretic for essential hypertension, hypokalemia, congestive heart failure, severe heart failure, cirrhosis of the liver, and*

*nephrotic syndrome; also used for
female hirsutism* 25, 50, 100 mg oral

spiroplatin USAN, INN, BAN *antineoplastic*

spirorenone INN

spirotriazine HCl [see: spirazine]

spiroxamide [see: spiroxatrine]

spiroxasone USAN, INN *diuretic*

spiroxatrine INN

spiroxepin INN

spirulina *(Spirulina pratensis)* plant
*medicinal herb for chronic disease,
enhancing antibody production, lowering
serum lipids and triglycerides, and reducing gastric secretory activity; also used
as a blood builder and food supplement*

spizofurone INN

spoonwood *medicinal herb* [see: linden
tree]

Sporanox capsules, PulsePak ℞ *systemic triazole antifungal* [itraconazole]
100 mg; 100 mg × 28

Sporanox IV infusion (discontinued
2007) ℞ *systemic triazole antifungal*
[itraconazole] 10 mg/mL

Sporanox oral solution ("swish and
swallow") ℞ *antifungal for esophageal
and oropharyngeal candidiasis* [itraco-
nazole] 10 mg/mL

Sporidin-G *investigational (orphan)
treatment of cryptosporidiosis-induced
diarrhea in immunocompromised patients*
[*Cryptosporidium parvum* bovine
colostrum IgG concentrate]

Sports Spray OTC *analgesic; mild anesthetic; antipruritic; counterirritant;
antiseptic* [methyl salicylate; menthol; camphor; alcohol 58%] 3.5%•
10%•5%

Sportscreme OTC *analgesic* [trolamine
salicylate] 10%

Sportscreme Ice gel OTC *analgesic;
mild anesthetic; antipruritic; counterirritant* [trolamine; menthol] ≟•2%

spotted alder *medicinal herb* [see:
witch hazel]

spotted comfrey *medicinal herb* [see:
lungwort]

spotted cranesbill *medicinal herb* [see:
alum root]

spotted geranium *medicinal herb* [see:
alum root]

**spotted hemlock; spotted cowbane;
spotted parsley** *medicinal herb* [see:
poison hemlock]

spotted lungwort *medicinal herb* [see:
lungwort]

spotted thistle *medicinal herb* [see:
blessed thistle]

spp. plural of *species*

**SPPG (sulfated polysaccharide pep-
tidoglycan)** [see: tecogalan sodium]

Sprayzoin spray OTC *skin protectant;
antiseptic* [benzoin; ethyl alcohol] ℞
spirazine

spring wintergreen *medicinal herb*
[see: wintergreen]

Sprinkle Caps (trademarked dosage
form) *powder*

Sprintec tablets (in packs of 28) ℞
monophasic oral contraceptive [norges-
timate; ethinyl estradiol] 0.25 mg•
35 mcg × 21 days; counters × 7 days

Sprix nasal spray ℞ *nonsteroidal anti-
inflammatory drug (NSAID) for moderate to moderately severe pain*
[ketorolac tromethamine] 15.75 mg/
spray ℞ Suprax; Zyprexa

sprodiamide USAN *heart and CNS
imaging aid for MRI*

spruce *(Picea excelsa; P. mariana)*
young shoots *medicinal herb used as a
calmative, diaphoretic, expectorant, and
pectoral*

spruce, Norway *medicinal herb* [see:
spruce]

spruce, weeping *medicinal herb* [see:
hemlock]

Sprycel film-coated tablets ℞ *antineoplastic for chronic myeloid leukemia
(CML) and acute lymphoblastic leukemia in patients expressing the Philadelphia chromosome (Ph+ ALL)* [dasa-
tinib] 20, 50, 70, 80, 100, 140 mg

SPS oral or rectal suspension ℞ *potassium-removing agent for hyperkalemia*
[sodium polystyrene sulfonate] 15 g/
60 mL

spurge laurel; spurge olive *medicinal
herb* [see: mezereon]

squalamine lactate *natural remedy; shark cartilage derivative; investigational (orphan) angiogenesis inhibitor for ovarian cancer* [also: shark cartilage]

squalane NF *oleaginous vehicle*

square, carpenter's *medicinal herb* [see: figwort]

squaw balm; squaw mint *medicinal herb* [see: pennyroyal]

squaw root *medicinal herb* [see: black cohosh; blue cohosh]

squaw tea *medicinal herb* [see: ephedra]

squaw vine (Mitchella repens) *plant medicinal herb for easing childbirth, lactation, and menstruation and for uterine disorders*

squaw weed *medicinal herb* [see: life root]

squawberry *medicinal herb* [see: squaw vine]

squill (Urginea indica; U. maritima; U. scilla) *bulb medicinal herb for edema and inducing emesis and expectoration; also used as a rat poison* ② Secule

squirrel pea, ground *medicinal herb* [see: twin leaf]

⁸⁵Sr [see: strontium chloride Sr 85]

⁸⁵Sr [see: strontium nitrate Sr 85]

⁸⁵Sr [see: strontium Sr 85]

SRF (skin respiratory factor) [q.v.]

Sronyx film-coated tablets (in packs of 28) ℞ *monophasic oral contraceptive* [levonorgestrel; ethinyl estradiol] 0.1 mg•20 mcg × 21 days; counters × 7 days

SS (saline solution)

SS (sodium salicylate) [q.v.]

SS (somatostatin) [q.v.]

SSD (silver sulfadiazine) [q.v.]

SSD; SSD AF cream ℞ *broad-spectrum bactericidal for adjunctive burn treatment* [silver sulfadiazine] 10 mg/g

SSKI oral solution ℞ *expectorant* [potassium iodide] 1 g/mL

SSNRIs (selective serotonin and norepinephrine reuptake inhibitors) [q.v.]

SSRIs (selective serotonin reuptake inhibitors) [q.v.]

SSS 10-4 topical foam ℞ *antibiotic and keratolytic for acne* [sulfacetamide sodium; sulfur] 10%•4%

S.S.S. Tonic oral liquid OTC *vitamin/iron supplement* [multiple B vitamins; iron (as ferric ammonium citrate); alcohol 12%] ±•11.1 mg/5 mL

S.S.S. Tonic tablets OTC *vitamin/mineral/calcium/iron supplement* [multiple vitamins & minerals; calcium (as di- and tricalcium phosphate); iron (as ferrous fumarate); folic acid] ±• 100•27•0.2 mg

S.T. 37 topical solution OTC *antiseptic* [hexylresorcinol] 0.1%

S-T Cort lotion ℞ *corticosteroidal anti-inflammatory* [hydrocortisone] 0.5% ② Cetacort

S-T Forte 2 oral liquid (discontinued 2007) ℞ *narcotic antitussive; antihistamine* [hydrocodone bitartrate; chlorpheniramine maleate] 2.5•2 mg/5 mL

ST1-RTA immunotoxin (SR 44163) *investigational (orphan) for graft vs. host disease and B-chronic lymphocytic leukemia*

Staarvisc intraocular injection ℞ *viscoelastic agent for ophthalmic surgery* [hyaluronate sodium]

stable factor [see: factor VII]

Staccato (trademarked delivery device) *investigational (NDA filed) single-dose oral inhaler, currently being tested with* **loxapine** *for acute agitation associated with schizophrenia*

Stachys officinalis *medicinal herb* [see: betony]

Stadol IV or IM injection (discontinued 2011) ℞ *narcotic agonist-antagonist analgesic* [butorphanol tartrate] 1, 2 mg/mL ② cetiedil

staff vine *medicinal herb* [see: bittersweet nightshade]

Staflex caplets ℞ *analgesic; antipyretic; antihistamine; sleep aid* [acetaminophen; phenyltoloxamine citrate] 500•55 mg

Stagesic capsules ℞ *narcotic analgesic; antipyretic* [hydrocodone bitartrate; acetaminophen] 5•500 mg

staggerweed *medicinal herb* [see: turkey corn]

staghorn *medicinal herb* [see: club moss]

Stahist sustained-release tablets ℞ *decongestant; antihistamine; anticholinergic to dry mucosal secretions* [phenylephrine HCl; pseudoephedrine HCl; chlorpheniramine maleate; hyoscyamine sulfate; atropine sulfate; scopolamine hydrobromide] 25•40•8•0.19•0.04•0.01 mg

Stalevo 50; Stalevo 75; Stalevo 100; Stalevo 125; Stalevo 150; Stalevo 200 film-coated tablets ℞ *multi-modal treatment for Parkinson disease: dopamine precursor + decarboxylase inhibitor (levodopa potentiator) + COMT (catechol-O-methyltransferase) inhibitor* [levodopa; carbidopa; entacapone] 50•12.5•200 mg; 75•18.75•200 mg; 100•25•200 mg; 125•31.25•200 mg; 150•37.5•200 mg; 200•50•200 mg

stallimycin INN *antibacterial* [also: stallimycin HCl]

stallimycin HCl USAN *antibacterial* [also: stallimycin]

Stamoist E caplets ℞ *decongestant; expectorant* [pseudoephedrine HCl; guaifenesin] 45•600 mg

Stanback Headache Powder OTC *analgesic; antipyretic; anti-inflammatory* [aspirin; caffeine] 845•65 mg/pkt.

standard VAC *chemotherapy protocol for sarcomas* [see: VAC standard]

Stanford V (mechlorethamine, doxorubicin, vinblastine, vincristine, bleomycin, etoposide, prednisone) [with Bactrim, ketoconazole, and acyclovir] *chemotherapy protocol for Hodgkin lymphoma*

stannous chloride USAN *pharmaceutic aid*

stannous fluoride USP *dental caries preventative* 0.4%, 0.63% topical oral

stannous pyrophosphate USAN *skeletal imaging aid*

stannous sulfur colloid USAN *bone, liver and spleen imaging aid*

stannsoporfin USAN *bilirubin inhibitor*

stanolone BAN *anabolic steroid; investigational (orphan) for AIDS-wasting syndrome* [also: androstanolone]

stanozolol USAN, USP, INN, BAN *androgen; anabolic steroid for hereditary angioedema*

StaphAseptic gel OTC *anesthetic; antiseptic* [lidocaine HCl; benzethonium chloride] 2.5%•0.2%

Staphylococcus aureus **immune globulin, human** *investigational (orphan) prophylaxis against S. aureus infections in low birthweight neonates*

Staphylococcus aureus **vaccine, pentavalent** *investigational multi-component active bacterin against methicillin-resistant S. aureus (MRSA)*

star anise (*Illicium anisatum; I. verum*) seeds *medicinal herb used as a carminative, stimulant, and stomachic; also added to other herbal medications to improve digestibility and taste*

star chickweed; starweed *medicinal herb* [see: chickweed]

star grass (*Aletris farinosa*) root and rhizome *medicinal herb for diarrhea, dysmenorrhea and menstrual discomfort, gas and colonic cramps, and rheumatism*

star root *medicinal herb* [see: star grass]

starch NF *dusting powder; pharmaceutic aid*

starch, pregelatinized NF *tablet excipient*

starch, topical USP *dusting powder*

starch carboxymethyl ether, sodium salt [see: sodium starch glycolate]

starch glycerite NF

starch 2-hydroxyethyl ether [see: hetastarch; pentastarch]

Starlix tablets ℞ *meglitinide antidiabetic for type 2 diabetes that stimulates the release of insulin from the pancreas* [nateglinide] 60, 120 mg ⊘ Citralax

Star-Otic ear drops OTC *antibacterial; antifungal; antiseptic; astringent* [acetic acid; aluminum acetate; boric acid]

Starvisc [see: Staarvisc]

starwort; mealy starwort *medicinal herb* [see: chickweed; star grass]

Stat-Crit electrode device for professional use ℞ *in vitro diagnostic aid for hemoglobin/hematocrit measurement*

STATdose (trademarked delivery form) *prefilled syringes for self-administration*

"statins" *brief term for a class of antihyperlipidemics that include atorvastatin, cerivastatin, fluvastatin, lovastatin, pitavastatin, pravastatin, rosuvastatin, and simvastatin* [properly called: HMG-CoA reductase inhibitors]

statolon USAN *antiviral* [also: vistatolon]

Stat-Pak (trademarked packaging form) *unit-dose package*

Statuss Green oral liquid (discontinued 2009) ℞ *narcotic antitussive; antihistamine; sleep aid; decongestant* [hydrocodone bitartrate; chlorpheniramine maleate; pyrilamine maleate; phenylephrine HCl; pseudoephedrine HCl] 2.5•2•3.3•5•3.3 mg/5 mL

staunch, blood *medicinal herb* [see: fleabane; horseweed]

stavudine USAN, INN *nucleoside reverse transcriptase inhibitor (NRTI); antiretroviral for HIV-1 infection* 15, 20, 30, 40 mg oral; 1 mg/mL oral

stavudine & lamivudine *combination nucleoside reverse transcriptase inhibitor (NRTI) for HIV and AIDS* 30•150, 40•150 mg oral

stavudine & nevirapine & lamivudine *combination nucleoside reverse transcriptase inhibitor (NRTI) and non-nucleoside reverse transcriptase inhibitor (NNRTI) for HIV and AIDS* 6•50•30, 12•100•60, 30•200•150, 40•200•150 mg oral

Stavzor delayed-release softgels ℞ *anticonvulsant for complex partial seizures and simple or complex absence seizures; treatment for manic episodes of a bipolar disorder; migraine prophylactic* [valproic acid] 125, 250, 500 mg

Staxyn orally disintegrating tablets ℞ *selective vasodilator for erectile dysfunction (ED)* [vardenafil (as HCl)] 10 mg ⊘ Cytoxan

Stay Awake tablets OTC *CNS stimulant; analeptic* [caffeine] 200 mg

Stay-Wet 3; Stay-Wet 4 solution (discontinued 2010) OTC *disinfecting/wetting/soaking solution for rigid gas permeable contact lenses*

STD (sodium tetradecyl sulfate) [q.v.]

steaglate INN *combining name for radicals or groups*

stearethate 40 [see: polyoxyl 40 stearate]

stearic acid NF *emulsion adjunct; tablet and capsule lubricant* ⊘ citric acid

stearyl alcohol NF *emulsion adjunct*

stearyl dimethyl benzyl ammonium chloride

stearylsulfamide INN

Stedesa *investigational (NDA filed) once-daily adjunctive therapy for partial-onset seizures in adults* [eslicarbazepine acetate] 800, 1200 mg

steffimycin USAN, INN *antibacterial; antiviral*

Stelara subcu injection ℞ *immunomodulator for moderate to severe plaque psoriasis* [ustekinumab] 90 mg/mL

Stellaria media *medicinal herb* [see: chickweed]

stem and progenitor cells derived from ex vivo allogenic umbilical cord blood *investigational (orphan) hematopoietic support for patients on high-dose therapy for hematologic malignancies*

stem cells, T-cell depleted, derived from peripheral blood stem cells *investigational (orphan) for chronic granulomatous disease*

StemEx *investigational (orphan) hematopoietic support for patients on high-dose therapy for hematologic malignancies* [stem and progenitor cells derived from ex vivo allogenic umbilical cord blood]

stenbolone INN *anabolic steroid; also abused as a street drug* [also: stenbolone acetate]

stenbolone acetate USAN *anabolic steroid; also abused as a street drug* [also: stenbolone]

Stenorol *investigational (orphan) antiprotozoal for scleroderma* [halofuginone hydrobromide]

stepronin INN

Sterapred; Sterapred DS tablets, Unipak (dispensing pack) (discontinued 2010) ℞ *corticosteroid; anti-inflammatory* [prednisone] 5 mg; 10 mg

Sterculia tragacantha; S. urens; S. villosa medicinal herb [see: karaya gum]

stercuronium iodide INN

Sterecyt *investigational (orphan) antineoplastic for malignant non-Hodgkin lymphomas* [prednimustine]

Steri-Dose (trademarked delivery form) *prefilled disposable syringe*

SteriLid foaming eye wash OTC *extraocular irrigating solution*

SteriNail topical solution (discontinued 2008) OTC *antifungal* [undecylenic acid; tolnaftate] 🗇 cioteronel; citronella; soterenol

Steritalc *investigational (orphan) treatment for malignant pleural effusion and pneumothorax* [talc, sterile]

Steri-Vial (trademarked delivery form) *ampule*

Sterules (trademarked dosage form) *solution for nebulization*

stevaladil INN

stevia *(Stevia rebaudiana) leaves medicinal herb used as a non-caloric sugar substitute; also used for diabetes, food cravings, hypertension, obesity, and tobacco cravings*

stibamine glucoside INN, BAN

stibocaptate BAN [also: sodium stibocaptate]

stibophen NF

stibosamine INN

stickwort; sticklewort *medicinal herb* [see: agrimony]

stigmata maidis (corn silk) *medicinal herb* [see: Indian corn]

stilbamidine isethionate [see: stilbamidine isetionate]

stilbamidine isetionate INN

stilbazium iodide USAN, INN *anthelmintic*

stilbestroform [see: diethylstilbestrol]

stilbestrol [see: diethylstilbestrol]

stilbestronate [see: diethylstilbestrol dipropionate]

stilboestroform [see: diethylstilbestrol]

stilboestrol BAN *estrogen* [also: diethylstilbestrol]

stilboestrol DP [see: diethylstilbestrol dipropionate]

stillingia (Stillingia ligustina) root *medicinal herb for acne, eczema, and other skin disorders, blood cleansing, liver disorders, respiratory illnesses, and syphilis*

stilonium iodide USAN, INN *antispasmodic*

stilronate [see: diethylstilbestrol dipropionate]

Stimate metered-dose nasal spray ℞ *posterior pituitary hormone for hemophilia A and von Willebrand disease (orphan)* [desmopressin acetate] 150 mcg (600 IU)/dose

stimulant laxatives *a subclass of laxatives that work by direct action on the intestinal mucosa and nerve plexus to increase peristaltic action* [see also: laxatives]

stimulants *a class of agents that excite the activity of physiological processes*

Stimuvax *investigational (Phase III) antineoplastic vaccine against MUC-1 for the treatment of non–small cell lung cancer* [BLP-25 liposome vaccine]

Sting-Eze topical solution concentrate OTC *anesthetic; antihistamine; antipruritic; antiseptic* [benzocaine; diphenhydramine HCl; camphor; phenol; eucalyptol]

stinging nettle *medicinal herb* [see: nettle]

Sting-Kill swabs, wipes OTC *anesthetic; antipruritic; counterirritant* [benzocaine; menthol; isopropyl alcohol 15%] 20%•1%

stingless nettle *medicinal herb* [see: blind nettle]

stinking nightshade *medicinal herb* [see: henbane]

stirimazole INN, BAN

stiripentol USAN, INN *anticonvulsant*

stirocainide INN

stirofos USAN *veterinary insecticide*

stitchwort *medicinal herb* [see: chickweed]

stomachics *a class of agents that promote the functional activity of the stomach*

stone root (Collinsonia canadensis) roots and leaves *medicinal herb used as a diuretic and vulnerary*

Stool Softener capsules OTC *laxative; stool softener* [docusate sodium] 100, 250 mg

Stool Softener; Stool Softener DC capsules OTC *laxative; stool softener* [docusate calcium] 240 mg

stool-softening laxatives *a subclass of laxatives that work by increasing the amount of fat and water in the stool to ease its movement through the intestines* [see also: laxatives]

Stop gel ℞ *dental caries preventative* [stannous fluoride] 0.4%

storax (Liquidambar orientalis; L. styraciflua) USP leaves and gum *medicinal herb for diarrhea, inducing expectoration, parasitic infections, promoting sweating and diuresis, skin sores and wounds, and sore throat* ② Sitrex

Storz-Sulf eye drops (discontinued 2010) ℞ *antibiotic* [sulfacetamide sodium] 10%

stramonium [see: jimsonweed]

Strattera capsules ℞ *non-stimulant treatment for attention-deficit/hyperactivity disorder (ADHD); also used for nocturnal enuresis; investigational (orphan) for Tourette syndrome* [atomoxetine (as HCl)] 10, 18, 25, 40, 60, 80, 100 mg

strawberry (Fragaria vesca) leaves *medicinal herb for blood cleansing, diarrhea, eczema, intestinal disorders, preventing miscarriage, and stomach cleansing*

strawberry bush; strawberry tree *medicinal herb* [see: wahoo]

Strep Detect slide tests for professional use ℞ *in vitro diagnostic aid for streptococcal antigens in throat swabs*

Streptase powder for IV or intracoronary infusion ℞ *thrombolytic enzyme for lysis of thrombi and catheter clearance* [streptokinase] 250 000, 750 000, 1 500 000 IU

streptococcus immune globulin, group B *investigational (orphan) for neonatal group B streptococcal infection*

Streptococcus thermophilus *natural intestinal bacteria; probiotic; dietary supplement* [see also: lactic acid bacteria]

streptodornase (SD) INN, BAN

streptoduocin USP

streptogramins *a class of antibiotics, isolated from Streptomyces pristinaespirales, used for gram-positive infections*

streptokinase (SK) INN *thrombolytic enzymes for myocardial infarction, thrombosis or embolism*

streptomycin INN, BAN *aminoglycoside antibiotic; primary tuberculostatic* [also: streptomycin sulfate]

streptomycin sulfate USP *aminoglycoside antibiotic; primary tuberculostatic* [also: streptomycin] 1 g injection

Streptonase-B test kit for professional use ℞ *in vitro diagnostic test for DNAse-B streptococcal antigens in serum*

streptoniazid INN *antibacterial* [also: streptonicozid]

streptonicozid USAN *antibacterial* [also: streptoniazid]

streptonigrin (SN) USAN *antineoplastic* [also: rufocromomycin]

streptovarycin INN

streptozocin USAN, INN *nitrosourea-type alkylating antineoplastic for metastatic islet cell carcinoma of the pancreas*

streptozotocin [see: streptozocin]

Streptozyme slide tests for professional use ℞ *in vitro diagnostic test for streptococcal extracellular antigens in blood, plasma, and serum*

Stress 600 with Zinc tablets (discontinued 2008) OTC *vitamin/mineral sup-*

plement [multiple vitamins & minerals; folic acid; biotin] ± • 400 • 45 mcg

Stress B Complex tablets (discontinued 2008) OTC *vitamin/mineral supplement* [multiple vitamins & minerals; folic acid; biotin] ± • 400 • 45 mcg

Stress B Complex with Vitamin C timed-release tablets (discontinued 2008) OTC *vitamin/mineral supplement* [multiple B vitamins; vitamin C; zinc] ± • 300 • 15 mg

Stress Formula; Stress Formula Vitamins capsules, tablets OTC *vitamin supplement* [multiple vitamins; folic acid; biotin] ± • 400 • 45 mcg

Stress Formula 600 tablets (discontinued 2008) OTC *vitamin supplement* [multiple vitamins; folic acid; biotin] ± • 400 • 45 mcg

Stress Formula with Iron film-coated tablets (discontinued 2008) OTC *vitamin/iron supplement* [multiple B vitamins; vitamins C and E; iron (as ferrous fumarate); folic acid; biotin] ± • 500 mg • 30 IU • 27 mg • 0.4 mg • 45 mcg

Stress Formula with Zinc tablets OTC *vitamin/iron supplement* [multiple B vitamins; vitamins C and E; multiple minerals; folic acid; biotin] ± • 500 mg • 30 IU • ± • 0.4 mg • 45 mcg

Stress with Iron tablets OTC *vitamin/iron supplement* [multiple vitamins; iron (as ferrous fumarate); folic acid; biotin] ± • 18 • 0.4 • 45 mg

Stresstabs tablets (discontinued 2008) OTC *vitamin supplement* [multiple vitamins; folic acid; biotin] ± • 400 • 45 mcg

Stresstabs + Iron film-coated tablets (discontinued 2008) OTC *vitamin/iron supplement* [multiple B vitamins; vitamins C and E; iron (as ferrous fumarate); folic acid; biotin] ± • 500 mg • 30 IU • 18 mg • 0.4 mg • 45 mcg

Stresstabs + Zinc film-coated tablets OTC *vitamin/mineral supplement* [multiple vitamins & minerals; folic acid; biotin] ± • 400 • 45 mcg

Stresstein powder for oral solution OTC *enteral nutritional therapy for moderate to severe stress or trauma* [multiple branched chain amino acids]

Striant mucoadhesive buccal tablets ℞ *androgen for hypogonadism or testosterone deficiency in men; hormone replacement therapy (HRT) for postandropausal symptoms* [testosterone] 30 mg

Stri-Dex pads OTC *keratolytic cleanser for acne* [salicylic acid; alcohol] 0.5% • 28%, 2% • 44%, 2% • 54%

Stri-Dex Cleansing bar OTC *disinfectant/antiseptic; medicated cleanser for acne* [triclosan] 1%

Stri-Dex Clear gel OTC *keratolytic for acne* [salicylic acid; alcohol] 2% • 9.3%

Stri-Dex Face Wash solution OTC *disinfectant/antiseptic; medicated cleanser for acne* [triclosan] 1%

strinoline INN

striped alder *medicinal herb* [see: winterberry; witch hazel]

Stromectol tablets ℞ *anthelmintic for strongyloidiasis and onchocerciasis; also used to prevent the transmission of scabies to healthcare workers* [ivermectin] 3 mg

strong ammonia solution [see: ammonia solution, strong]

Strong Iodine oral solution, tincture ℞ *treatment for hyperthyroidism* [iodine; potassium iodide] 5% • 10%

Strong Start chewable tablets ℞ *vitamin/mineral/calcium/iron supplement* [multiple vitamins & minerals; calcium; iron; folic acid] ± • 200 • 29 • 1 mg

Strong Start tablets ℞ *vitamin/mineral/calcium/iron supplement* [multiple vitamins & minerals; calcium (as carbonate); iron (as ferrous fumarate); folic acid] ± • 250 • 35 • 1 mg

stronger rose water [see: rose water, stronger]

strontium *element (Sr)*

strontium chloride *topical anti-irritant*

strontium chloride Sr 85 USAN *radioactive agent*

strontium chloride Sr 89 USAN *radioactive agent; analgesic for metastatic bone pain*

strontium nitrate Sr 85 USAN *radioactive agent*

strontium salicylate NF

strontium Sr 85 USP

Strovite tablets ℞ *vitamin supplement* [multiple B vitamins; vitamin C; folic acid] ≛•500•0.5 mg

Strovite Advance caplets ℞ *vitamin/mineral supplement* [multiple vitamins & minerals; folic acid; biotin; alpha-lipoic acid; lutein] ≛•1•0.1• 15•5 mg

Strovite Forte syrup ℞ *vitamin/mineral/iron supplement* [multiple vitamins & minerals; iron (as ferrous gluconate); folic acid] ≛•10•1 mg/15 mL

Strovite Forte; Strovite Plus caplets ℞ *vitamin/mineral/iron supplement* [multiple vitamins & minerals; iron (as ferrous fumarate); folic acid; biotin] ≛•10•1•0.15 mg; ≛•27•0.8• 0.15 mg

Strovite One caplets ℞ *vitamin/mineral supplement* [multiple vitamins & minerals; folic acid; biotin] ≛•1•0.1 mg

structum *natural remedy* [see: chondroitin sulfate]

strychnine NF *an extremely poisonous CNS stimulant; occasionally abused as a street drug in combination with LSD*

strychnine glycerophosphate NF

strychnine nitrate NF

strychnine phosphate NF

strychnine sulfate NF

strychnine valerate NF

Stuart Formula tablets (discontinued 2008) OTC *vitamin/mineral/iron supplement* [multiple vitamins & minerals; iron; folic acid] ≛•18•0.1 mg

Stuart Prenatal tablets OTC *prenatal vitamin/mineral/calcium/iron supplement* [multiple vitamins and minerals; calcium; iron (as ferrous fumarate); folic acid] ≛•200•28•0.8 mg

StuartNatal Plus 3 tablets (discontinued 2008) ℞ *vitamin/calcium/iron supplement* [multiple vitamins; calcium; iron; folic acid] ≛•200•28•1 mg

stugeron [see: cinnarizine]

stutgin [see: cinnarizine]

Stye ophthalmic ointment OTC *emollient* [white petrolatum; mineral oil] 58%•32%

styptics *a class of hemostatic agents that stop bleeding of the skin by astringent action* [see also: astringents; hemostatics]

Stypto-Caine topical solution OTC *styptic to the stop bleeding of minor cuts* [aluminum chloride; tetracaine HCl; oxyquinoline sulfate] 250•2.5•1 mg/g

styramate INN

styronate resins

subathizone INN ⍰ sopitazine

subendazole INN

suberoylanilide hydroxamic acid (SAHA) [see: vorinostat]

Sublimaze IV or IM injection (discontinued 2011) ℞ *narcotic analgesic for breakthrough pain in cancer patients; adjunct to anesthesia* [fentanyl citrate] 50 mcg/mL

sublimed sulfur [see: sulfur, sublimed]

Sublingual B Total drops (discontinued 2008) OTC *vitamin supplement* [multiple B vitamins; vitamin C] ≛ •60 mg/mL

Suboxone sublingual tablets, sublingual film ℞ *narcotic agonist-antagonist analgesic for outpatient maintenance of opiate dependence (orphan)* [buprenorphine (as HCl); naloxone (as HCl)] 2•0.5, 8•2 mg

substance F [see: demecolcine]

substituted benzimidazoles *a class of gastric antisecretory agents that inhibit the ATPase "proton pump" within the gastric parietal cell* [also called: proton pump inhibitors; ATPase inhibitors]

Subutex sublingual tablets ℞ *narcotic agonist-antagonist analgesic for inpatient treatment of opiate dependence (orphan)* [buprenorphine HCl] 2, 8 mg

Suby G solution; Suby solution G (citric acid, magnesium oxide,

sodium carbonate) *urologic irrigant to dissolve phosphatic calculi*

succimer USAN, INN, BAN *heavy metal chelating agent for lead poisoning (orphan); investigational (orphan) for mercury poisoning and cysteine kidney stones*

succinchlorimide NF

succinimides *a class of anticonvulsants*

succinylcholine chloride USP *neuromuscular blocker; muscle relaxant; anesthesia adjunct* [also: suxamethonium chloride] 20 mg/mL injection

succinyldapsone [see: succisulfone]

succinylsulfathiazole USP

succisulfone INN

succory *medicinal herb* [see: chicory]

Succus Cineraria Maritima *eye drops (discontinued 2009)* ℞ *natural treatment for optic opacity caused by cataract* [senecio compositae; hamamelis water (witch hazel); boric acid]

suclofenide INN, BAN

Sucraid *oral solution* ℞ *enzyme replacement therapy for congenital sucrase-isomaltase deficiency (orphan)* [sacrosidase] 8500 IU/mL

sucralfate USAN, INN, BAN *cytoprotective agent for gastric ulcers; investigational (orphan) for oral mucositis and stomatitis following cancer radiation or chemotherapy* 1 g oral; 1 g/10 mL oral

sucralose BAN

sucralox INN, BAN

Sucrets *throat spray* OTC *antipruritic/counterirritant; mild local anesthetic* [dyclonine HCl] 0.1%

Sucrets Children's Formula; Sucrets Maximum Strength Sore Throat *lozenges* OTC *mucous membrane anesthetic* [dyclonine HCl] 1.2 mg; 3 mg

Sucrets Complete *lozenges* OTC *mucous membrane anesthetic* [dyclonine HCl; menthol] 3•6 mg

Sucrets Defense Kid's Formula *lozenges* OTC *vitamin/mineral supplement* [vitamin C; zinc; glutathione] 3.9•0.93•20 mg

Sucrets DM Cough Formula; Sucrets DM Cough Suppressant

lozenges OTC *antitussive* [dextromethorphan hydrobromide] 10 mg

Sucrets Herbal *lozenges* OTC *mild anesthetic; antipruritic; counterirritant* [menthol; pectin] 50•60 mg

Sucrets Original Formula Sore Throat (Cherry) *lozenges* OTC *mucous membrane anesthetic* [dyclonine HCl] 2 mg

Sucrets Original Formula Sore Throat (Mint) *lozenges* OTC *antiseptic* [hexylresorcinol] 2.4 mg

sucrose NF *flavoring agent; tablet excipient* ② Xigris

sucrose octaacetate NF *alcohol denaturant*

sucrosofate potassium USAN *antiulcerative*

Sudafed *tablets* OTC *nasal decongestant* [pseudoephedrine HCl] 30, 60 mg

Sudafed, Children's *chewable tablets (discontinued 2009)* OTC *nasal decongestant* [pseudoephedrine HCl] 15 mg

Sudafed, Children's Non-Drowsy *oral liquid* OTC *nasal decongestant* [pseudoephedrine HCl] 15 mg/5 mL

Sudafed Children's Non-Drowsy Cold & Cough *oral liquid (discontinued 2009)* OTC *antitussive; decongestant* [dextromethorphan hydrobromide; pseudoephedrine HCl] 5•15 mg/5 mL

Sudafed Non-Drowsy *tablets (discontinued 2009)* OTC *nasal decongestant* [pseudoephedrine HCl] 30 mg

Sudafed Non-Drowsy 12 Hour Long Acting *extended-release caplets* OTC *nasal decongestant* [pseudoephedrine HCl] 120 mg

Sudafed Non-Drowsy 24 Hour Long Acting *dual-release tablets* OTC *nasal decongestant* [pseudoephedrine HCl] 240 mg (60 mg immediate release, 180 mg extended release)

Sudafed PE *tablets* OTC *nasal decongestant* [phenylephrine HCl] 10 mg

Sudafed PE Day & Night *caplets* OTC *decongestant; antihistamine/sleep aid added* PM [phenylephrine HCl;

diphenhydramine HCl added PM] 10 mg AM; 10•25 mg PM

Sudafed PE Multi-Symptom Cold and Cough caplets OTC *antitussive; decongestant; expectorant; analgesic; antipyretic* [dextromethorphan hydrobromide; phenylephrine HCl; guaifenesin; acetaminophen] 10•5•100•325 mg

Sudafed PE Multi-Symptom Severe Cold caplets OTC *decongestant; antihistamine; sleep aid; analgesic; antipyretic* [phenylephrine HCl; diphenhydramine HCl; acetaminophen] 5•12.5•325 mg

Sudafed PE Nighttime Cold caplets OTC *decongestant; antihistamine; sleep aid; analgesic; antipyretic* [phenylephrine HCl; diphenhydramine HCl; acetaminophen] 5•25•325 mg

Sudafed PE Nighttime Nasal Decongestant tablets OTC *decongestant; antihistamine; sleep aid* [phenylephrine HCl; diphenhydramine HCl] 10•25 mg

Sudafed PE Non-Drying Sinus caplets OTC *decongestant; expectorant* [phenylephrine HCl; guaifenesin] 5•200 mg

Sudafed PE Quick-Dissolve orally disintegrating film (discontinued 2009) OTC *nasal decongestant* [phenylephrine HCl] 10 mg

Sudafed PE Sinus & Allergy tablets OTC *decongestant; antihistamine* [phenylephrine HCl; chlorpheniramine maleate] 10•4 mg

Sudafed PE Sinus Headache caplets OTC *decongestant; analgesic; antipyretic* [phenylephrine HCl; acetaminophen] 5•325 mg

Sudafed Sinus & Allergy tablets (discontinued 2009) OTC *decongestant; antihistamine* [pseudoephedrine HCl; chlorpheniramine maleate] 60•4 mg

Sudafed Sinus & Cold Non-Drowsy Liqui-Caps (liquid-filled gelcaps) (discontinued 2009) OTC *decongestant; analgesic; antipyretic* [pseudo-

ephedrine HCl; acetaminophen] 30•325 mg

Sudafed Sinus Nighttime Plus Pain Relief caplets (discontinued 2009) OTC *decongestant; antihistamine; sleep aid; analgesic; antipyretic* [pseudoephedrine HCl; diphenhydramine HCl; acetaminophen] 30•25•500 mg

SudaHist extended-release caplets ℞ *decongestant; antihistamine* [pseudoephedrine HCl; chlorpheniramine maleate] 120•12 mg

Sudal-12 chewable tablets, extended-release oral suspension (discontinued 2007) ℞ *decongestant; antihistamine* [pseudoephedrine polistirex; chlorpheniramine polistirex] 30•4 mg; 30•6 mg/5 mL ☑ Xodol

Sudal-12 Tannate chewable tablets ℞ *decongestant; antihistamine* [pseudoephedrine HCl; chlorpheniramine maleate] 30•4 mg

Sudal-DM sustained-release tablets (discontinued 2007) ℞ *antitussive; expectorant* [dextromethorphan hydrobromide; guaifenesin] 30•500 mg

SudaTex G tablets OTC *decongestant; expectorant* [pseudoephedrine HCl; guaifenesin] 40•400 mg

Sudatuss-2 DF oral liquid (discontinued 2007) ℞ *narcotic antitussive; decongestant; expectorant* [codeine phosphate; pseudoephedrine HCl; guaifenesin; alcohol 1.4%] 10•30•100 mg/5 mL

Sudex dual-release caplets (discontinued 2009) ℞ *decongestant; expectorant* [phenylephrine HCl; guaifenesin] 20•600 mg (5•200 mg immediate release; 15•400 mg extended release) ☑ Cedax; ciadox; Cidex; Z-Dex

sudexanox INN

sudismase INN

Sudodrin tablets (discontinued 2007) OTC *nasal decongestant* [pseudoephedrine HCl] 30 mg

SudoGest Non-Drowsy tablets ℞ *decongestant* [pseudoephedrine HCl] 30 mg

SudoGest Sinus tablets (discontinued 2007) OTC *decongestant; analgesic; antipyretic* [pseudoephedrine HCl; acetaminophen] 30•500 mg

SudoGest Sinus & Allergy tablets OTC *decongestant; antihistamine* [pseudoephedrine HCl; chlorpheniramine maleate] 60•4 mg

sudorifics *a class of agents that promote profuse perspiration* [also called: diaphoretics]

sudoxicam USAN, INN *anti-inflammatory*

Sufenta IV injection or infusion ℞ *narcotic analgesic for general or epidural anesthesia* [sufentanil citrate] 50 mcg/mL

sufentanil USAN, INN, BAN *narcotic analgesic*

sufentanil citrate USAN *narcotic analgesic for general or epidural anesthesia* 50 mcg/mL

sufosfamide INN

sufotidine USAN, INN, BAN *antagonist to histamine H_2 receptors*

sugammadex *investigational (NDA filed) selective relaxation binding agent (SRBA) to reverse the effects of strong muscle relaxants, used for postanesthesia "stir-up"*

sugar, compressible NF *flavoring agent; tablet excipient*

sugar, confectioner's NF *flavoring agent; tablet excipient*

sugar, invert (50% dextrose & 50% fructose) USP *fluid and nutrient replenisher; caloric replacement*

sugar spheres NF *solid carrier vehicle*

sulamserod HCl USAN *selective 5-HT_4 receptor antagonist; antiarrhythmic; treatment for urge incontinence*

Sulamyd [see: Sodium Sulamyd]

Sular extended-release film-coated tablets ℞ *calcium channel blocker for hypertension* [nisoldipine] 8.5, 17, 25.5, 34 mg ⚠ celery; Xolair

sulazepam USAN, INN *minor tranquilizer* ⚠ zolazepam

sulbactam INN, BAN *beta-lactamase inhibitor; penicillin/cephalosporin synergist*

sulbactam benzathine USAN *beta-lactamase inhibitor; penicillin/cephalosporin synergist*

sulbactam pivoxil USAN *beta-lactamase inhibitor; penicillin/cephalosporin synergist* [also: pivsulbactam]

sulbactam sodium USAN, USP *beta-lactamase inhibitor; penicillin/cephalosporin synergist*

sulbenicillin INN

sulbenox USAN, INN *veterinary growth stimulant*

sulbentine INN

sulbutiamine INN [also: bisibutiamine]

sulclamide INN

sulconazole INN, BAN *antifungal* [also: sulconazole nitrate]

sulconazole nitrate USAN, USP *topical antifungal* [also: sulconazole]

sulergine [see: disulergine]

sulesomab USAN *monoclonal antibody; diagnostic aid for infectious lesions* [also: technetium Tc 99m sulesomab]

Sulf-10 eye drops ℞ *antibiotic* [sulfacetamide sodium] 10%

sulfabenz USAN, INN *antibacterial; coccidiostat for poultry*

sulfabenzamide USAN, USP, INN *bacteriostatic antibiotic*

sulfabromomethazine sodium NF

sulfacarbamide INN [also: sulphaurea]

sulfacecole INN

sulfacetamide USP, INN *bacteriostatic antibiotic*

sulfacetamide sodium USP *bacteriostatic antibiotic* 10% eye drops; 10% topical

sulfacetamide sodium & sulfur *antibiotic and keratolytic for acne* 8%•4%, 9%•4%, 10%•4%, 10%•5% topical

Sulfacet-R lotion ℞ *antibiotic and keratolytic for acne* [sulfacetamide sodium; sulfur] 10%•5%

sulfachlorpyridazine INN

sulfachrysoidine INN

sulfacitine INN *antibacterial* [also: sulfacytine]

SulfaCleanse 8/4 soap ℞ *antibiotic and keratolytic for acne* [sulfacetamide sodium; sulfur] 8%•4%

sulfaclomide INN

sulfaclorazole INN

sulfaclozine INN

sulfacombin [see: sulfadiazine]

sulfacytine USAN *broad-spectrum bacteriostatic* [also: sulfacitine]

sulfadiasulfone sodium INN *antibacterial; leprostatic* [also: acetosulfone sodium]

sulfadiazine USP, INN, JAN *broad-spectrum sulfonamide bacteriostatic* [also: sulphadiazine] 500 mg oral

sulfadiazine & pyrimethamine *oral* Toxoplasma gondii *encephalitis treatment (orphan)*

sulfadiazine silver JAN *broad-spectrum bactericidal; adjunct to burn therapy* [also: silver sulfadiazine]

sulfadiazine sodium USP, INN *antibacterial* [also: sulphadiazine sodium]

sulfadicramide INN

sulfadicrolamide [see: sulfadicramide]

sulfadimethoxine NF [also: sulphadimethoxine]

sulfadimidine INN, BAN *antibacterial* [also: sulfamethazine]

sulfadoxine USAN, USP *bacteriostatic; antimalarial adjunct*

sulfaethidole NF, INN [also: sulphaethidole]

sulfafurazole INN *broad-spectrum sulfonamide bacteriostatic* [also: sulfisoxazole; sulphafurazole]

sulfaguanidine NF, INN

sulfaguanole INN

sulfaisodimidine [see: sulfisomidine]

sulfalene USAN, INN *antibacterial* [also: sulfametopyrazine] ⊡ Slo-phyllin

sulfaloxic acid INN [also: sulphaloxic acid]

sulfamates *a class of broad-spectrum anticonvulsants*

sulfamazone INN

sulfamerazine USP, INN *broad-spectrum bacteriostatic*

sulfamerazine sodium NF, INN

sulfameter USAN *antibacterial* [also: sulfametoxydiazine; sulfamethoxydiazine]

sulfamethazine USP *broad-spectrum bacteriostatic* [also: sulfadimidine]

sulfamethizole USP, INN, JAN *broad-spectrum sulfonamide bacteriostatic* [also: sulphamethizole]

sulfamethoxazole (SMX; SMZ) USAN, USP, INN, JAN *broad-spectrum sulfonamide antibiotic* [also: sulphamethoxazole; acetylsulfamethoxazole; sulfamethoxazole sodium]

sulfamethoxazole sodium JAN *broad-spectrum sulfonamide antibiotic* [also: sulfamethoxazole; sulphamethoxazole; acetylsulfamethoxazole]

sulfamethoxazole & trimethoprim *broad-spectrum sulfonamide antibiotic* 400•80, 800•160 mg oral; 200•40 mg/5 mL oral; 80•16 mg/mL injection

sulfamethoxydiazine BAN *antibacterial* [also: sulfameter; sulfametoxydiazine]

sulfamethoxypyridazine USP, INN [also: sulphamethoxypyridazine]

sulfamethoxypyridazine acetyl

sulfametin [see: sulfameter]

sulfametomidine INN

sulfametopyrazine BAN *antibacterial* [also: sulfalene]

sulfametoxydiazine INN *antibacterial* [also: sulfameter; sulfamethoxydiazine]

sulfametrole INN, BAN

sulfamidothiodiazol [see: glybuzole]

sulfamonomethoxine USAN, INN, BAN *antibacterial*

sulfamoxole USAN, INN *antibacterial* [also: sulphamoxole]

p-**sulfamoylbenzoic acid** [see: carzenide]

4′-sulfamoylsuccinanilic acid [see: sulfasuccinamide]

Sulfamylon cream ℞ *broad-spectrum bacteriostatic for second- and third-degree burns* [mafenide (as acetate)] 85 mg/g

Sulfamylon powder for topical solution ℞ *broad-spectrum bacteriostatic to prevent meshed autograft loss on second- and third-degree burns (orphan)* [mafenide (as acetate)] 5%

sulfanilamide NF, INN *broad-spectrum sulfonamide antibiotic* 15% topical

sulfanilanilide [see: sulfabenz]

sulfanilate zinc USAN *antibacterial*

N-sulfanilylacetamide [see: sulfacetamide]

N-sulfanilylacetamide monosodium salt monohydrate [see: sulfacetamide sodium]

N-p-sulfanilylphenylglycine sodium [see: acediasulfone sodium]

N-sulfanilylstearamide [see: stearylsulfamide]

4'-sulfanilylsuccinanilic acid [see: succisulfone]

sulfanilylurea [see: sulfacarbamide]

sulfanitran USAN, INN, BAN *antibacterial; coccidiostat for poultry*

sulfaperin INN

sulfaphenazole INN [also: sulphaphenazole]

sulfaphtalythiazol [see: phthalylsulfathiazole]

sulfaproxyline INN [also: sulphaproxyline]

sulfapyrazole INN, BAN *antibacterial* [also: sulfazamet]

sulfapyridine USAN, INN *investigational (orphan) dermatitis herpetiformis suppressant* [also: sulphapyridine]

sulfapyridine sodium NF

sulfaquinoxaline INN, BAN

sulfarsphenamine NF, INN

sulfasalazine USAN, USP, INN *broad-spectrum bacteriostatic; anti-inflammatory for ulcerative colitis, rheumatoid arthritis (RA), and juvenile rheumatoid arthritis (JRA); also used for ankylosing spondylitis, Crohn disease, and regional enteritis* [also: sulphasalazine; salazosulfapyridine] 500 mg oral

sulfasomizole USAN, INN *antibacterial* [also: sulphasomizole]

sulfasoxizole & erythromycin ethylsuccinate *antibiotic combination for acute otitis media in children* 600•200 mg oral

sulfastearyl [see: stearylsulfamide]

sulfasuccinamide INN

sulfasymazine INN

sulfated polysaccharide peptidoglycan (SPPG) [see: tecogalan sodium]

sulfathiazole USP, INN *bacteriostatic antibiotic* [also: sulphathiazole]

sulfathiazole sodium NF

sulfathiocarbamide [see: sulfathiourea]

sulfathiourea INN

sulfatolamide INN

Sulfatrim oral suspension ℞ *broad-spectrum sulfonamide antibiotic* [sulfamethoxazole; trimethoprim] 200•40 mg/5 mL

sulfatroxazole INN

sulfatrozole INN

sulfazamet USAN *antibacterial* [also: sulfapyrazole]

sulfinalol INN *antihypertensive* [also: sulfinalol HCl]

sulfinalol HCl USAN *antihypertensive* [also: sulfinalol]

sulfinpyrazone USP, INN *uricosuric for gout* [also: sulphinpyrazone] 100, 200 mg oral

sulfiram INN [also: monosulfiram]

sulfisomidine [also: sulphasomidine]

sulfisoxazole USP, JAN *broad-spectrum sulfonamide antibiotic* [also: sulfafurazole; sulphafurazole]

sulfisoxazole acetyl USP *broad-spectrum sulfonamide antibiotic*

sulfisoxazole diolamine USAN, USP *broad-spectrum sulfonamide antibiotic*

Sulfoam shampoo OTC *antiseborrheic; keratolytic; antiseptic* [sulfur] 2%

sulfobenzylpenicillin [see: sulbenicillin]

sulfobromophthalein sodium USP *hepatic function test*

sulfobromphthalein sodium [see: sulfobromophthalein sodium]

sulfocon B USAN *hydrophobic contact lens material*

sulfogaiacol INN *expectorant* [also: potassium guaiacolsulfonate]

Sulfolax soft gels OTC *laxative; stool softener* [docusate calcium] 240 mg ⑨ Salflex

sulfomyxin USAN, INN *antibacterial* [also: sulphomyxin sodium]

sulfonal [see: sulfonmethane]

sulfonamides *a class of broad-spectrum bacteriostatic antibiotics effective against both gram-positive and gram-negative organisms*

sulfonated hydrogenated castor oil [see: hydroxystearin sulfate]

sulfonethylmethane NF

sulfonmethane NF

sulfonterol INN *bronchodilator* [also: sulfonterol HCl]

sulfonterol HCl USAN *bronchodilator* [also: sulfonterol]

sulfonylureas *a class of antidiabetic agents that stimulate insulin production in the pancreas*

Sulforcin lotion OTC *antiseptic and keratolytic for acne* [sulfur; resorcinol; alcohol] 5%•2%•11.65%

sulforidazine INN

sulfosalicylic acid

sulfoxone sodium USP *antibacterial; leprostatic* [also: aldesulfone sodium]

Sulfoxyl Regular lotion ℞ *antiseptic and keratolytic for acne* [benzoyl peroxide; sulfur] 5%•2%

Sulfoxyl Strong lotion (discontinued 2010) ℞ *antiseptic and keratolytic for acne* [benzoyl peroxide; sulfur] 10%•5%

sulfur *element (S)* [see: sulfur, precipitated; sulfur, sublimed]

sulfur, precipitated USP *scabicide; topical antibacterial; topical exfoliant*

sulfur, sublimed USP *scabicide; topical antibacterial; topical exfoliant*

sulfur dioxide NF *antioxidant*

sulfur hexafluoride (SF₆) USAN *ultrasound imaging agent*

Sulfur Soap bar OTC *antiseptic and keratolytic cleanser for acne* [precipitated sulfur] 10%

sulfur & sulfacetamide sodium *keratolytic and antibiotic for acne* 4%•8%, 4%•9%, 4%•10%, 5%•10% topical

sulfurated lime solution [see: lime, sulfurated]

sulfurated potash [see: potash, sulfurated]

sulfuric acid NF *acidifying agent*

sulfuric acid, aluminum ammonium salt, dodecahydrate [see: alum, ammonium]

sulfuric acid, aluminum potassium salt, dodecahydrate [see: alum, potassium]

sulfuric acid, aluminum salt, hydrate [see: aluminum sulfate]

sulfuric acid, barium salt [see: barium sulfate]

sulfuric acid, calcium salt [see: calcium sulfate]

sulfuric acid, copper salt pentahydrate [see: cupric sulfate]

sulfuric acid, disodium salt decahydrate [see: sodium sulfate]

sulfuric acid, magnesium salt [see: magnesium sulfate]

sulfuric acid, manganese salt [see: manganese sulfate]

sulfuric acid, zinc salt hydrate [see: zinc sulfate]

sulfurous acid, monosodium salt [see: sodium bisulfite]

sulglicotide INN [also: sulglycotide]

sulglycotide BAN [also: sulglicotide]

sulicrinat INN

sulindac USAN, USP, INN, BAN *nonsteroidal anti-inflammatory drug (NSAID) for osteoarthritis, rheumatoid arthritis, ankylosing spondylitis, acute bursitis/tendinitis, and other inflammatory conditions* 150, 200 mg oral

sulisatin INN ② Celestone

sulisobenzone USAN, INN *ultraviolet screen*

sulmarin USAN, INN *hemostatic*

Sulmasque mask OTC *antiseptic and keratolytic for acne* [sulfur] 6.4% ② psyllium husk

sulmazole INN

sulmepride INN

sulnidazole USAN, INN *antiprotozoal (Trichomonas)*

sulocarbilate INN

suloctidil USAN, INN, BAN *peripheral vasodilator*

sulodexide INN *glycosaminoglycan*

sulofenur USAN, INN *antineoplastic*

sulopenem USAN, INN *antibacterial*

sulosemide INN

sulotroban USAN, INN, BAN *treatment for glomerulonephritis* ② Sal-Tropine

suloxifen INN *bronchodilator* [also: suloxifen oxalate]

suloxifen oxalate USAN *bronchodilator* [also: suloxifen]

sulphabutin [see: busulfan]

sulphadiazine BAN *broad-spectrum bacteriostatic* [also: sulfadiazine]

sulphadiazine sodium BAN *antibacterial* [also: sulfadiazine sodium]

sulphadimethoxine BAN [also: sulfadimethoxine]

sulphaethidole BAN [also: sulfaethidole]

sulphafurazole BAN *broad-spectrum sulfonamide bacteriostatic* [also: sulfisoxazole; sulfafurazole]

sulphaloxic acid BAN [also: sulfaloxic acid]

sulphamethizole BAN *broad-spectrum sulfonamide bacteriostatic* [also: sulfamethizole]

sulphamethoxazole BAN *broad-spectrum sulfonamide bacteriostatic* [also: sulfamethoxazole; acetylsulfamethoxazole; sulfamethoxazole sodium]

sulphamethoxypyridazine BAN [also: sulfamethoxypyridazine]

sulphamoxole BAN *antibacterial* [also: sulfamoxole]

sulphan blue BAN *lymphangiography aid* [also: isosulfan blue]

sulphaphenazole BAN [also: sulfaphenazole]

sulphaproxyline BAN [also: sulfaproxyline]

sulphapyridine BAN *dermatitis herpetiformis suppressant* [also: sulfapyridine]

sulphasalazine BAN *broad-spectrum bacteriostatic; antirheumatic; antiinflammatory for ulcerative colitis* [also: sulfasalazine; salazosulfapyridine]

sulphasomidine BAN [also: sulfisomidine]

sulphasomizole BAN *antibacterial* [also: sulfasomizole]

sulphathiazole BAN *antibacterial* [also: sulfathiazole]

sulphaurea BAN [also: sulfacarbamide]

sulphinpyrazone BAN *uricosuric for gout* [also: sulfinpyrazone]

sulphocarbolate sodium [see: phenolsulphonate sodium]

Sulpho-Lac cream, soap OTC *antiseptic and keratolytic for acne* [sulfur] 5% ⑨ Salofalk

Sulpho-Lac Acne Medication cream OTC *antiseptic and keratolytic for acne* [sulfur; zinc sulfate] 5%•27%

sulphomyxin sodium BAN *antibacterial* [also: sulfomyxin]

sulphonal [see: sulfonmethane]

sulpiride USAN, INN *antidepressant*

sulprosal INN

sulprostone USAN, INN *prostaglandin*

sultamicillin USAN, INN, BAN *antibacterial*

sulthiame USAN *anticonvulsant* [also: sultiame]

sultiame INN *anticonvulsant* [also: sulthiame]

sultopride INN

sultosilic acid INN

sultroponium INN

sulukast USAN, INN *antiasthmatic; leukotriene antagonist*

sulverapride INN

SulZee Wash (discontinued 2010) ℞ *antibiotic and keratolytic for acne* [sulfacetamide sodium; sulfur] 10%•1%

suma *(Pfaffia paniculata)* bark and root *medicinal herb for circulatory disorders, chronic disease, fatigue, hormone regulation, immune system stimulation, lowering cholesterol levels, and stress; also used as a tonic*

Sumacal powder OTC *carbohydrate caloric supplement* [glucose polymers]

sumacetamol INN, BAN

sumach *(Rhus glabra)* bark, leaves, and berries *medicinal herb used as an antiseptic, astringent, diaphoretic, diuretic, emmenagogue, febrifuge, and refrigerant* ⑨ Simuc; Zomig

sumarotene USAN, INN *keratolytic*

sumatriptan INN, BAN *vascular serotonin 5-HT$_1$ receptor agonist for the acute treatment of migraine headaches* [also: sumatriptan succinate] 25, 50, 100 mg oral; 5, 20 mg nasal spray

sumatriptan succinate USAN *vascular serotonin 5-HT₁ receptor agonist for the acute treatment of migraine and cluster headaches* (base=71.4%) [also: sumatriptan] 25, 50, 100 mg oral; 4, 6 mg/0.5 mL injection

Sumavel DosePro subcu injection in a prefilled self-injector ℞ *vascular serotonin receptor agonist for the acute treatment of migraine and cluster headaches* [sumatriptan (as succinate)] 6 mg/0.5 mL dose

Sumaxin medicated pads ℞ *antibiotic and keratolytic for acne* [sulfacetamide sodium; sulfur] 10%•4% 🔲 ciamexon

Sumaxin TS topical suspension ℞ *antibiotic and keratolytic for acne* [sulfacetamide sodium; sulfur] 8%•4%

Sumaxin Wash topical liquid ℞ *antibiotic and keratolytic for acne* [sulfacetamide sodium; sulfur] 9%•4%

sumetizide INN

summer savory (*Calamintha hortensis; Satureja hortensis*) leaves and stems *medicinal herb for diarrhea, nausea, promoting expectoration, relieving gas and flatulence, and stimulation of menstruation; also used as an aphrodisiac*

Summer's Eve Anti-Itch vaginal gel (discontinued 2009) OTC *anesthetic* [pramoxine HCl] 1%

Summer's Eve Disposable Douche vaginal solution OTC *antifungal; cleanser and deodorizer; acidity modifier* [sodium benzoate; citric acid]

Summer's Eve Disposable Douche; Summer's Eve Disposable Douche Extra Cleansing vaginal solution OTC *acidity modifier; cleanser and deodorizer* [vinegar (acetic acid)]

Summer's Eve Feminine Bath topical liquid OTC *external perivaginal cleanser*

Summer's Eve Feminine Powder OTC *vaginal moisture absorbent; antiseptic* [cornstarch; benzethonium chloride]

Summer's Eve Feminine Wash topical liquid, wipes OTC *external perivaginal cleanser*

Summer's Eve Medicated Disposable Douche vaginal solution OTC *antiseptic/germicidal cleanser and deodorizer* [povidone-iodine] 0.3%

Summer's Eve Post-Menstrual Disposable Douche vaginal solution OTC *cleanser and deodorizer; acidity modifier* [monosodium phosphate; disodium phosphate]

Summit Extra Strength coated caplets OTC *analgesic; antipyretic; antiinflammatory* [acetaminophen; aspirin; caffeine] 250•250•65 mg

Sumycin syrup ℞ *broad-spectrum antibiotic* [tetracycline HCl] 125 mg/5 mL

Sumycin '250'; Sumycin '500' capsules, tablets ℞ *broad-spectrum antibiotic* [tetracycline HCl] 250 mg; 500 mg

sun rose *medicinal herb* [see: rock rose]

sunagrel INN

suncillin INN *antibacterial* [also: suncillin sodium]

suncillin sodium USAN *antibacterial* [also: suncillin]

sunepitron HCl USAN *anxiolytic; antidepressant*

sunitinib malate *receptor tyrosine kinase (RTK) inhibitor antineoplastic for gastrointestinal stromal tumor (GIST), metastatic renal cell carcinoma, and pancreatic neuroendocrine tumors*

SunKist Multivitamins Complete, Children's chewable tablets (discontinued 2008) OTC *vitamin/mineral/iron supplement* [multiple vitamins & minerals; iron; folic acid; biotin] ≚•18 mg•400 mcg•40 mcg

SunKist Multivitamins + Extra C chewable tablets (discontinued 2008) OTC *vitamin supplement* [multiple vitamins; folic acid] ≚•0.3 mg

SunKist Vitamin C chewable tablets OTC *vitamin C supplement* [ascorbic acid and sodium ascorbate] 60, 250, 500 mg

Sunnie tablets OTC *vitamin/mineral/herb supplement* [multiple B vitamins and minerals; vitamin C; folic acid; bio-

tin; gingko biloba; St. John's wort] ±
•125•0.1•0.0125•2.5•225 mg

SunVite tablets OTC *vitamin/mineral/
calcium/iron supplement* [multiple
vitamins & minerals; calcium (as
carbonate and dicalcium phosphate);
iron (as ferrous fumarate); folic acid;
biotin] ± •162•18•0.4•0.03 mg

Supartz intra-articular injection in
prefilled syringes ℞ *viscoelastic lubricant and "shock absorber" for osteoarthritis and TMJ syndrome* [hyaluro-
nate sodium] 25 mg/2.5 mL

Super 2 Daily softgels OTC *vitamin/
mineral supplement* [multiple vitamins & minerals; fish oil concentrate; lecithin; phosphatidyl choline;
bioflavonoids; lutein] ± •385•30•
25•12.5•0.025 mg

Super CalciCaps tablets (discontinued 2008) OTC *calcium supplement*
[calcium (as dibasic calcium phosphate, gluconate, and carbonate);
vitamin D] 400 mg•133 IU

Super CalciCaps M-Z tablets (discontinued 2008) OTC *vitamin/mineral
supplement* [vitamins A and D; multiple minerals] 1667 mg•133 IU• ±

Super Calcium '1200' softgels (discontinued 2008) OTC *calcium supplement*
[calcium; vitamin D] 600 mg•200 IU

Super Carnosine capsules OTC *anti-
aging supplement; glycation inhibitor*
[carnosine] 500 mg

Super D Perles (capsules) (discontinued 2008) OTC *vitamin supplement*
[vitamins A and D] 10 000•400 IU

Super Flavons; Super Flavons-300
tablets (discontinued 2007) OTC *dietary supplement* [mixed bioflavonoids]
300 mg

Super Hi Potency tablets (discontinued 2008) OTC *vitamin/mineral supplement* [multiple vitamins & minerals; folic acid; biotin] ± •0.4 mg•
0.075 mg

Super Ivy-Dry lotion OTC *poison ivy
treatment* [zinc acetate; benzyl alcohol; isopropanol] 2%•10%•35%

Super MiraForte with Chrysin capsules OTC *natural supplement to
increase free testosterone levels in men*
[chrysin; muira puama; maca; nettle;
ginger; piperine; zinc] 375•212.5•
80•70.5•12.5•3.75•3.75 mg

Super Quints-50 tablets OTC *vitamin
supplement* [multiple B vitamins;
folic acid; biotin] ± •400•50 mcg

Super Strength Vitamin D 2000 tablets OTC *vitamin D supplement* [chole-
calciferol (vitamin D_3)] 2000 IU

Superdophilus powder OTC *natural
intestinal bacteria; probiotic; dietary
supplement; fever blister treatment; not
generally regarded as safe and effective
as an antidiarrheal* [Lactobacillus acidophilus DDS-1] 2 billion CFU/g

SuperEPA 1200 softgels (discontinued 2008) OTC *dietary supplement*
[omega-3 fatty acids (eicosapentaenoic acid and docosahexaenoic acid)]
1200 mg (360 mg EPA; 240 mg DHA)

SuperEPA 2000 softgels OTC *dietary
supplement* [omega-3 fatty acids (eicosapentaenoic acid and docosahexaenoic acid); vitamin E] 1000 mg•20
IU (500 mg EPA; 310 mg DHA)

superoxide dismutase (SOD) [see:
orgotein]

Superplex-T tablets OTC *vitamin supplement* [multiple B vitamins; vitamin C] ± •500 mg

Supervent *investigational (orphan) surfactant for cystic fibrosis* [tyloxapol]

supidimide INN

Suplena ready-to-use oral liquid OTC
*enteral nutritional therapy for renal
failure* [milk-based formula] 240 mL

Supprelin LA once-yearly subcu
implant ℞ *gonadotropin suppressant
for the treatment of central precocious
puberty (orphan)* [histrelin acetate]
50 mg

Supprette (trademarked dosage form)
suppository ⑨ soapwort

Suprane liquid for vaporization ℞
inhalation general anesthetic [desflu-
rane] ⑨ Syprine

Suprax chewable tablets, film-coated tablets ℞ *third-generation cephalosporin antibiotic* [cefixime] 100, 150, 200 mg; 400 mg ⊡ Sprix; Zyprexa

Suprax powder for oral suspension ℞ *third-generation cephalosporin antibiotic* [cefixime] 100, 200 mg/5 mL ⊡ Sprix; Zyprexa

Suprenza orally disintegrating tablets ℞ *anorexiant; CNS stimulant* [phentermine HCl] 15, 30 mg

Suprep oral solution ℞ *pre-procedure bowel evacuant* [sodium sulfate; potassium sulfate; magnesium sulfate] 17.5•3.13•1.6 g ⊡ X-Prep

suproclone USAN, INN *sedative*

suprofen USAN, INN, BAN *ocular non-steroidal anti-inflammatory drug (NSAID); antimiotic*

Supule (trademarked dosage form) *suppository*

suramin hexasodium USAN *investigational (NDA filed, orphan) growth factor antagonist for prostate cancer*

suramin sodium USP, BAN *antiparasitic for African trypanosomiasis and onchocerciasis*

Surbex Filmtabs (film-coated tablets) (discontinued 2008) OTC *vitamin supplement* [multiple B vitamins] ⊡ Cerebyx

Surbex 750 with Iron Filmtabs (film-coated tablets) (discontinued 2008) OTC *vitamin/iron supplement* [multiple B vitamins; vitamins C and E; iron (as ferrous sulfate); folic acid] ±• 750 mg•30 IU•27 mg•0.4 mg

Surbex 750 with Zinc Filmtabs (film-coated tablets) OTC *vitamin/zinc supplement* [multiple vitamins; zinc sulfate; folic acid] ±•22.5•0.4 mg

Surbex-C Filmtabs (film-coated tablets) OTC *vitamin supplement* [multiple B vitamins; vitamin C] ±•225 mg ⊡ Cerebyx

Surbex-T Filmtabs (film-coated tablets) (discontinued 2010) OTC *vitamin supplement* [multiple B vitamins; vitamin C] ±•450 mg

Surbu-Gen-T film-coated tablets (discontinued 2008) OTC *vitamin supplement* [multiple B vitamins; vitamin C] ±•500 mg

Sure Cell Chlamydia Test reagent kit for professional use ℞ *in vitro diagnostic aid for* Chlamydia trachomatis [monoclonal antibody-based enzyme-linked immunosorbent assay]

Sure Cell Herpes (HSV) Test reagent kit for professional use ℞ *in vitro diagnostic aid for herpes simplex virus in genital, rectal, oral, or dermal swabs* [monoclonal antibody-based enzyme-linked immunosorbent assay (ELISA)]

Sure Cell Pregnancy test kit for professional use ℞ *in vitro diagnostic aid; urine pregnancy test* [monoclonal/polyclonal antibody ELISA test]

Sure Cell Streptococci test kit for professional use ℞ *in vitro diagnostic aid for Group A streptococcal antigens in blood and throat swabs* [enzyme-linked immunosorbent assay (ELISA)]

SureLac chewable tablets OTC *digestive aid for lactose intolerance* [lactase enzyme] 3000 U

surface active extract of saline lavage of bovine lungs [see: beractant]

surfactant, human amniotic fluid derived *investigational (orphan) agent for the prevention and treatment of respiratory distress syndrome (RDS) in premature infants*

surfactant laxatives *a subclass of laxatives that work by increasing the amount of fat and water in the stool to ease its movement through the intestines* [more commonly called stool softeners]

surfactant TA [see: beractant]

surfactant TA, modified bovine lung surfactant extract [see: beractant]

Surfak Stool Softener softgels OTC *laxative; stool softener* [docusate calcium] 240 mg

Surfaxin *investigational (NDA filed, orphan) KL4 pulmonary surfactant for acute respiratory distress syndrome*

(ARDS) and meconium aspiration syndrome (MAS) [lucinactant]

surfilcon A USAN *hydrophilic contact lens material*

Surfol Post-Immersion Bath Oil OTC *bath emollient*

surfomer USAN, INN *hypolipidemic*

Surgel vaginal gel OTC *moisturizer/ lubricant* [propylene glycol; glycerin] ⊡ Seroquel

surgibone USAN *internal bone splint*

surgical catgut [see: suture, absorbable surgical]

surgical gut [see: suture, absorbable surgical]

Surgicel strips, Nu-knit pads ℞ *topical hemostat for surgery* [cellulose, oxidized]

Surgilube topical jelly OTC *broad-spectrum antimicrobial; germicidal* [chlorhexidine gluconate]

suricainide INN *antiarrhythmic* [also: suricainide maleate]

suricainide maleate USAN, INN *antiarrhythmic* [also: suricainide]

suriclone INN, BAN

Surinam wood *medicinal herb* [see: quassia]

suritozole USAN, INN *antidepressant*

Surmontil capsules ℞ *tricyclic antidepressant* [trimipramine maleate] 25, 50, 100 mg

suronacrine INN *cholinesterase inhibitor* [also: suronacrine maleate]

suronacrine maleate USAN *cholinesterase inhibitor* [also: suronacrine]

Surpass chewing gum OTC *antacid; calcium supplement* [calcium (as carbonate)] 120, 180 mg (300, 450 mg) ⊡ Ser-Ap-Es

Survanta suspension for intratracheal instillation ℞ *pulmonary surfactant for neonatal respiratory distress syndrome or respiratory failure (orphan)* [beractant] 25 mg/mL

Susano elixir (discontinued 2008) ℞ *GI/GU anticholinergic/antispasmodic; sedative* [atropine sulfate; scopolamine hydrobromide; hyoscyamine hydrobromide; phenobarbital]

0.0194•0.0065•0.1037•16.2 mg/5 mL ⊡ Saizen; Zosyn

Sustacal powder OTC *enteral nutritional therapy* [milk-based formula]

Sustacal pudding OTC *enteral nutritional therapy* [milk-based formula]

Sustacal ready-to-use oral liquid OTC *enteral nutritional therapy* [lactose-free formula]

Sustacal Basic; Sustacal Plus ready-to-use oral liquid OTC *enteral nutritional therapy* [lactose-free formula]

Sustagen powder OTC *enteral nutritional therapy* [milk-based formula] ⊡ Cystagon

Sustain tablets ℞ *electrolyte replacement; dehydration preventative* [sodium chloride; potassium chloride; calcium carbonate] 220•15•18 mg ⊡ cystine; Systane

Sustenna (extended-release injectable doseform of **Invega**) [q.v.]

Sustiva capsules, film-coated caplets ℞ *antiretroviral for HIV-1 infection* [efavirenz] 50, 200 mg; 600 mg

Sutent capsules ℞ *antineoplastic for gastrointestinal stromal tumor (GIST), metastatic renal cell carcinoma, and pancreatic neuroendocrine tumors; investigational (Phase III) for lung, breast, and colorectal cancers* [sunitinib malate] 12.5, 25, 50 mg

sutilains USAN, USP, INN, BAN *topical proteolytic enzymes for necrotic tissue debridement*

sutoprofen [see: suprofen]

suture, absorbable surgical USP *surgical aid*

suture, nonabsorbable surgical USP *surgical aid*

Su-Tuss DM oral liquid (discontinued 2009) ℞ *antitussive; expectorant* [dextromethorphan hydrobromide; guaifenesin; alcohol 5%] 20•200 mg/5 mL

Su-Tuss HD elixir ℞ *narcotic antitussive; decongestant; expectorant* [hydrocodone bitartrate; pseudoephedrine HCl; guaifenesin] 2.5•30•100 mg/5 mL

suxamethone [see: succinylcholine chloride]

suxamethonium chloride INN, BAN *neuromuscular blocking agent* [also: succinylcholine chloride]

suxemerid INN *antitussive* [also: suxemerid sulfate]

suxemerid sulfate USAN *antitussive* [also: suxemerid]

suxethonium chloride INN

suxibuzone INN

swallow wort, orange *medicinal herb* [see: pleurisy root]

swallow wort, silky *medicinal herb* [see: milkweed]

swamp cabbage *medicinal herb* [see: skunk cabbage]

swamp laurel; swamp sassafras *medicinal herb* [see: magnolia]

Sween Cream OTC *moisturizer; emollient* [vitamins A and D]

sweet, mountain *medicinal herb* [see: New Jersey tea]

sweet, winter *medicinal herb* [see: marjoram]

sweet anise; sweet chervil *medicinal herb* [see: sweet cicely]

sweet balm *medicinal herb* [see: lemon balm]

sweet basil *medicinal herb* [see: basil]

sweet bay *medicinal herb* [see: laurel]

sweet birch *medicinal herb* [see: birch]

sweet birch oil [see: methyl salicylate]

sweet cicely (Osmorhiza longistylis) *root medicinal herb used as a carminative, expectorant, and stomachic*

sweet clover *medicinal herb* [see: melilot]

sweet dock *medicinal herb* [see: bistort]

sweet elder *medicinal herb* [see: elderberry]

sweet elm *medicinal herb* [see: slippery elm]

sweet fennel *medicinal herb* [see: fennel]

sweet flag *medicinal herb* [see: calamus]

sweet grass *medicinal herb* [see: calamus]

sweet leaf *medicinal herb* [see: stevia]

sweet magnolia *medicinal herb* [see: magnolia]

sweet marjoram *medicinal herb* [see: marjoram]

sweet myrtle *medicinal herb* [see: calamus]

sweet orange peel tincture [see: orange peel tincture, sweet]

sweet potato vine, wild *medicinal herb* [see: wild jalap]

sweet root *medicinal herb* [see: calamus]

sweet rush *medicinal herb* [see: calamus]

sweet sedge *medicinal herb* [see: calamus]

sweet spirit of nitre [see: ethyl nitrite]

sweet vernal grass (Anthoxanthum odoratum) *natural flavoring banned by the FDA as it is not generally regarded as safe and effective*

sweet violet *medicinal herb* [see: violet]

sweet water lily; sweet-scented water lily *medicinal herb* [see: white pond lily]

sweet weed *medicinal herb* [see: marsh mallow]

sweet woodruff (Asperula odorata; Galium odoratum) *plant medicinal herb for diuresis, inducing expectoration, liver disorders, promoting wound healing, relieving gastrointestinal spasms, and sedation*

sweet wormwood (Artemisia annua) *plant medicinal herb for malaria*

sweet-scented pond lily; sweet-scented water lily *medicinal herb* [see: white pond lily]

sweetwood *medicinal herb* [see: licorice]

Swim-Ear ear drops (discontinued 2008) OTC *antiseptic* [isopropyl alcohol] 95% ☑ Zemaira; Zymar

swine snout *medicinal herb* [see: dandelion]

Syeda film-coated tablets (in packs of 28) ℞ *monophasic oral contraceptive* [drospirenone; ethinyl estradiol] 3 mg•30 mcg × 21 days; counters × 7 days

Sylatron powder for subcu injection ℞ *immunomodulator for malignant melanoma; also used for chronic myelogenous leukemia and renal cell carcinoma* [peginterferon alfa-2b] 40, 60, 120 mcg/0.1 mL

Syllact powder OTC *bulk laxative* [psyllium husks] 3.3 g/tsp.

Symax Duotab dual-release caplets (33% immediate release, 67% extended-release) ℞ *GI/GU antispasmodic; antiparkinsonian; anticholinergic "drying agent" for allergic rhinitis and hyperhidrosis* [hyoscyamine sulfate] 0.375 mg

Symax FasTab (orally disintegrating tablets) ℞ *GI/GU antispasmodic; antiparkinsonian; anticholinergic "drying agent" for allergic rhinitis and hyperhidrosis* [hyoscyamine sulfate] 0.125 mg

Symax-SL sublingual tablets ℞ *GI/GU antispasmodic; antiparkinsonian; anticholinergic "drying agent" for allergic rhinitis and hyperhidrosis* [hyoscyamine sulfate] 0.125 mg

Symax-SR sustained-release caplets ℞ *GI/GU antispasmodic; antiparkinsonian; anticholinergic "drying agent" for allergic rhinitis and hyperhidrosis* [hyoscyamine sulfate] 0.375 mg

Symbicort inhalation aerosol in a metered-dose inhaler ℞ *corticosteroidal anti-inflammatory and bronchodilator combination for chronic asthma, chronic obstructive pulmonary disease (COPD), bronchitis, and emphysema* [budesonide; formoterol fumarate] 80•4.5, 160•4.5 mcg/dose

Symbyax capsules ℞ *combination antipsychotic plus selective serotonin reuptake inhibitor (SSRI) for treatment-resistant depression (TRD) and depressive episodes of a bipolar disorder* [olanzapine; fluoxetine (as HCl)] 3•25, 6•25, 6•50, 12•25, 12•50 mg

symclosene USAN, INN *topical anti-infective*

symetine INN *antiamebic* [also: symetine HCl]

symetine HCl USAN *antiamebic* [also: symetine]

SymlinPen 60; SymlinPen 120 self-injectors prefilled with **Symlin** ℞ *antidiabetic for types 1 and 2 diabetes; synthetic amylin analogue that slows gastric emptying and decreases hepatic glucose production* [pramlintide acetate] 15, 30, 45, 60 mcg/dose; 60, 120 mcg/dose

Symmetrel tablets, syrup ℞ *antiviral for influenza A infections; dopaminergic antiparkinson agent* [amantadine HCl] 100 mg; 50 mg/5 mL ⊉ cimaterol

SymPak AM+PM tablets in a 14-day pack ℞ *decongestant; expectorant added* AM; *antihistamine and anticholinergic to dry mucosal secretions added* PM [phenylephrine HCl; guaifenesin added AM; chlorpheniramine maleate, methscopolamine nitrate added PM] 15•600 mg AM; 25•8•2.5 mg PM

SymPak II AM+PM tablets in a 14-day pack ℞ *decongestant; antihistamine; anticholinergic to dry mucosal secretions added* PM [pseudoephrine HCl, brompheniramine maleate AM; phenylephrine HCl, chlorpheniramine maleate, methscopolamine nitrate PM] 45•6 mg AM; 25•8•2.5 mg PM

SymPak PDX AM+PM tablets in a 14-day pack ℞ *antihistamine; anticholinergic to dry mucosal secretions; decongestant added* AM [chlorpheniramine maleate; methscopolamine nitrate; phenylephrine HCl added AM] 2•1.5•10 mg AM; 2•1.5 mg PM

sympatholytics *a class of cardiovascular drugs that block the passage of impulses through the sympathetic nervous system* [also called: antiadrenergics]

sympathomimetics *a class of bronchodilators that relax the bronchial muscles, reducing bronchospasm; a class of cardiac agents that increase myocardial contractility, causing a vasopressor effect to counteract shock (inadequate tissue perfusion)* [also called: adrenergic agonists]

Symphytum officinale; S. tuberosum medicinal herb [see: comfrey]

Symplocarpus foetidus medicinal herb [see: skunk cabbage]

Synacort cream ℞ *corticosteroidal anti-inflammatory* [hydrocortisone] 1%, 2.5%

Synagis IM injection ℞ *monoclonal antibody for prophylaxis of respiratory syncytial virus (RSV) in infants* [palivizumab] 100 mg/mL ☑ Xanax

Synalar cream, ointment, topical solution ℞ *corticosteroidal anti-inflammatory* [fluocinolone acetonide] 0.01, 0.25%; 0.025%; 0.01%

Synalgos-DC capsules ℞ *narcotic analgesic; antipyretic* [dihydrocodeine bitartrate; aspirin; caffeine] 16•356.4•30 mg

Synarel nasal spray ℞ *gonadotropin-releasing hormone for central precocious puberty (orphan) and endometriosis* [nafarelin acetate] 2 mg/mL (200 mcg/spray)

SynBiotics-3 capsules OTC *natural intestinal bacteria; probiotic; dietary supplement* [*Bifidobacterium longum; Lactobacillus rhamnosus* A; *L. plantarum; Saccharomyces boulardii*] 4.5 billion CFU total

Syncria *investigational (Phase III) glucagon-like peptide-1 (GLP-1) for type 2 diabetes* [albiglutide]

Synemol cream ℞ *corticosteroidal anti-inflammatory* [fluocinolone acetonide] 0.025%

Synera transdermal patch ℞ *local anesthetic* [lidocaine; tetracaine] 70•70 mg

Synercid powder for IV infusion ℞ *semi-synthetic streptogramin antibiotic for life-threatening infections* [quinupristin; dalfopristin] 150•350 mg/10 mL

synestrin [see: diethylstilbestrol]

synnematin B [see: adicillin]

Synophylate-GG syrup (discontinued 2007) ℞ *antiasthmatic; bronchodilator; expectorant* [theophylline; guaifenesin; alcohol 10%] 150•100 mg/15 mL

Synsorb Pk *investigational (Phase III, orphan) E. coli neutralizer for traveler's diarrhea and hemolytic uremic syndrome*

Syntest D.S.; Syntest H.S. film-coated caplets (discontinued 2008) ℞ *estrogen/androgen hormone replacement for postmenopausal symptoms* [esterified estrogens; methyltestosterone] 1.25•2.5 mg; 0.625•1.25 mg

synthestrin [see: diethylstilbestrol]

synthetic conjugated estrogens [see: estrogens, synthetic conjugated (A and B)]

synthetic lung surfactant [see: colfosceril palmitate]

synthetic monosaccharides *a class of investigational synthetic carbohydrates with immunomodulatory and anti-inflammatory effects being evaluated for the treatment of rheumatic arthritis*

synthetic paraffin [see: paraffin, synthetic]

synthetic spermaceti [now: cetyl esters wax]

synthoestrin [see: diethylstilbestrol]

Synthroid tablets, powder for injection ℞ *synthetic thyroid hormone (T_4 fraction only)* [levothyroxine sodium] 25, 50, 75, 88, 100, 112, 125, 137, 150, 175, 200, 300 mcg; 200, 500 mcg

synvinolin [now: simvastatin]

Synvisc; Synvisc-One intra-articular injection in prefilled syringes ℞ *viscoelastic lubricant and "shock absorber" for osteoarthritis and TMJ syndrome* [hylan G-F 20] 8 mg/mL

Syprine capsules ℞ *copper chelating agent for Wilson disease (orphan)* [trientine HCl] 250 mg ☑ Suprane

syrosingopine NF, INN, BAN

syrup NF *flavoring agent*

syrupus cerasi [see: cherry juice]

Syrvite oral liquid (discontinued 2008) OTC *vitamin supplement* [multiple vitamins]

Systane eye drops OTC *moisturizer/lubricant* [polyethylene glycol 400; polypropylene glycol] 0.4%•0.3% ☑ cystine; Sustain

Systane Balance eye drops OTC *moisturizer/lubricant* [propylene glycol] 0.6%

Systane Nighttime eye drops OTC *moisturizer/lubricant* [petrolatum; mineral oil] 94%•3%

Syzygium aromaticum medicinal herb [see: cloves]

Syzygium claviflorum medicinal herb for *diarrhea and bleeding disorders*

(S)-zopiclone [see: esopiclone]

T₃ (liothyronine sodium) [q.v.]

T₄ (levothyroxine sodium) [q.v.]

T4 endonuclease V (T4N5), lipo-some encapsulated *investigational (orphan) for prevent cutaneous neoplasms in xeroderma pigmentosum*

Tab-A-Vite + Iron; Tab-A-Vite Women's tablets OTC *vitamin/iron supplement* [multiple vitamins; iron (as ferrous fumarate); folic acid] ≛•18•0.4 mg

Tab-A-Vite Maximum tablets OTC *vitamin/mineral/calcium/iron supplement* [multiple vitamins & minerals; calcium; iron; folic acid] ≛•162•18•0.4 mg

Tab-A-Vite with Beta-Carotene; Tab-A-Vite Essential with Beta-Carotene tablets OTC *vitamin supplement* [multiple vitamins; folic acid] ≛•400 mcg

Tabebuia avellanedae; T. impetiginosa medicinal herb [see: pau d'arco]

Tabernanthe iboga street drug [see: iboga]

tabilautide INN

Tabloid (trademarked dosage form) *tablet with raised lettering*

Tabloid tablets ℞ *antimetabolite antineoplastic for acute nonlymphocytic leukemias (ANLL); also used for psoriasis, ulcerative colitis, and Crohn disease* [thioguanine] 40 mg

Tabules (dosage form) *tablets*

Tac-3 IM, intra-articular, intrabursal, intradermal injection (discontinued 2008) ℞ *corticosteroid; anti-inflammatory* [triamcinolone acetonide] 3 mg/mL

Tac-40 suspension for injection (discontinued 2008) ℞ *corticosteroid; anti-inflammatory* [triamcinolone acetonide] 40 mg/mL

TachoSil 4.8 cm × 4.8 cm, 4.8 cm × 9.5 cm dressings ℞ *premedicated dressings used to control bleeding during cardiovascular surgery* [fibrin sealant, human; thrombin, human] 5.5 mg•2 IU per cm² ⑨ Taxol; Tygacil

taclamine INN *minor tranquilizer* [also: taclamine HCl]

taclamine HCl USAN *minor tranquilizer* [also: taclamine]

Taclonex ointment ℞ *antipsoriatic; steroidal anti-inflammatory for plaque psoriasis* [calcipotriene; betamethasone dipropionate] 0.005%•0.064%

Taclonex Scalp topical suspension ℞ *antipsoriatic; steroidal anti-inflammatory for plaque psoriasis* [calcipotriene; betamethasone dipropionate] 0.005%•0.064%

tacmahac *medicinal herb* [see: balm of Gilead]

tacrine INN, BAN *reversible cholinesterase inhibitor; cognition adjuvant for Alzheimer dementia* [also: tacrine HCl]

tacrine HCl USAN *reversible cholinesterase inhibitor; cognition adjuvant for mild-to-moderate Alzheimer dementia* [also: tacrine]

tacrolimus USAN, INN *topical treatment for moderate to severe atopic dermatitis; systemic immunosuppressant for liver, kidney, and heart transplants (orphan); investigational (orphan) for graft-versus-host disease* 0.5, 1, 5 mg oral

TAD (thioguanine, ara-C, daunorubicin) *chemotherapy protocol for acute myelocytic leukemia (AML)* [also known as: DAT; DCT]

tadalafil *phosphodiesterase type 5 (PDE-5) inhibitor; selective vasodilator for erectile dysfunction (ED) and pulmonary arterial hypertension (PAH; orphan)*

taeniacides *a class of agents that destroy tapeworms* [see also: anthelmintics; vermicides; vermifuges]

tafamidis meglumine *investigational (Phase III) disease-modifying agent for transthyretin amyloid polyneuropathy (ATTR-PN), a rare neurodegenerative disease*

tafluprost *investigational (NDA filed) prostaglandin analogue for glaucoma*

Tagamet film-coated tablets ℞ *hista-mine H₂ antagonist for gastric and duo-denal ulcers and gastric hypersecretory conditions* [cimetidine] 400, 800 mg

Tagamet HB 200 film-coated tablets OTC *histamine H₂ antagonist for epi-sodic heartburn and acid indigestion* [cimetidine] 200 mg

taglutimide INN

taheebo *medicinal herb* [see: pau d'arco]

tail, colt's; cow's tail; horse tail; mare's tail *medicinal herb* [see: flea-bane; horseweed]

tail, lion's *medicinal herb* [see: mother-wort]

tailed cubebs; tailed pepper *medici-nal herb* [see: cubeb]

TAK-603 *investigational (orphan) for Crohn disease*

Talacen caplets (discontinued 2010) ℞ *narcotic agonist-antagonist analgesic; antipyretic* [pentazocine (as HCl); acetaminophen] 25•650 mg ☒ tylosin

talampicillin INN *antibacterial* [also: talampicillin HCl]

talampicillin HCl USAN *antibacterial* [also: talampicillin]

talastine INN

talbutal USP, INN *barbiturate sedative; hypnotic*

talc USP, JAN *dusting powder; tablet and capsule lubricant*

talc, sterile aerosol *treatment for malig-nant pleural effusion and pneumothorax via intrapleural thoracoscopy adminis-tration (orphan)*

taleranol USAN, INN *gonadotropin enzyme inhibitor*

taliglucerase alfa *investigational (Phase III, orphan) recombinant glucocerebro-sidase (GCD) for Gaucher disease*

talinolol INN

talipexole INN

talisomycin USAN, INN *antineoplastic*

tall speedwell *medicinal herb* [see: Cul-ver root]

tall veronica *medicinal herb* [see: Cul-ver root]

tallimustine INN *antineoplastic*

tallow shrub *medicinal herb* [see: bay-berry]

tallysomycin A [now: talisomycin]

talmetacin USAN, INN *analgesic; anti-inflammatory; antipyretic*

talmetoprim INN

talnetant HCl USAN *NK₃ receptor antagonist for urinary frequency, urgency, and incontinence*

talniflumate USAN, INN *anti-inflamma-tory; analgesic*

talopram INN *catecholamine potentiator* [also: talopram HCl]

talopram HCl USAN *catecholamine potentiator* [also: talopram]

talosalate USAN, INN *analgesic; anti-inflammatory*

taloximine INN, BAN

talsaclidine INN

talsaclidine fumarate USAN *musca-rinic M₁ agonist for Alzheimer disease*

talsupram INN

taltibride [see: metibride]

taltrimide INN

taludipine [see: teludipine]

taludipine HCl [see: teludipine HCl]

Talwin IV, IM, or subcu injection, Carpuject (prefilled syringes) ℞ *nar-cotic agonist-antagonist analgesic for moderate to severe pain; adjunct to surgical anesthesia; also abused as a street drug* [pentazocine lactate] 30 mg/mL; 60 mg

Talwin Compound caplets (discon-tinued 2010) ℞ *narcotic agonist-antagonist analgesic; antipyretic; also abused as a street drug* [pentazocine HCl; aspirin] 12.5•325 mg

Talwin NX tablets (discontinued 2010) ℞ *narcotic agonist-antagonist analgesic; also abused as a street drug* [pentazocine HCl; naloxone HCl] 50•0.5 mg

tamarind (*Tamarindus indica*) fruit and leaves *medicinal herb used as an anthelmintic, laxative, and refrigerant*

tamatinib fosdium *investigational (Phase III) treatment for autoimmune disorders, including rheumatoid arthritis*

(RA) and idiopathic thrombocytopenic purpura (ITP)

Tambocor tablets ℞ *antiarrhythmic* [flecainide acetate] 50, 100, 150 mg

tameridone USAN, INN, BAN *veterinary sedative*

tameticillin INN

tametraline INN *antidepressant* [also: tametraline HCl]

tametraline HCl USAN *antidepressant* [also: tametraline]

Tamiflu capsules, powder for oral suspension ℞ *antiviral for the prophylaxis and treatment of influenza A and B infections; also used for the prophylaxis and treatment of H1N1 influenza A (swine flu; Mexican pandemic flu) infections* [oseltamivir (as phosphate)] 30, 45, 75 mg; 12 mg/mL

tamitinol INN

tamoxifen INN, BAN *antiestrogen antineoplastic for breast cancer* [also: tamoxifen citrate]

tamoxifen citrate USAN, USP, JAN *antiestrogen antineoplastic for the treatment of breast cancer and the reduction of breast cancer incidence in high-risk women* (base=65.8%) [also: tamoxifen] 10, 20 mg oral

tamoxifen + epirubicin *chemotherapy protocol for breast cancer*

tampramine INN *antidepressant* [also: tampramine fumarate]

tampramine fumarate USAN *antidepressant* [also: tampramine]

Tamp-R-Tel (trademarked packaging form) *tamper-evident cartridge-needle unit*

tamsulosin INN *alpha$_1$-adrenergic blocker for benign prostatic hyperplasia (BPH)* [also: tamsulosin HCl]

tamsulosin HCl USAN, JAN *alpha$_1$-adrenergic blocker for benign prostatic hyperplasia (BPH); also used as adjunctive therapy for ureteral stones* [also: tamsulosin] 0.4 mg oral

Tanabid SR tablets ℞ *antihistamine; decongestant* [brompheniramine maleate; phenylephrine HCl] 6•30 mg

Tanac gel OTC *oral anesthetic; vulnerary* [dyclonine HCl; allantoin] 1%•0.5%

Tanac topical liquid OTC *mucous membrane anesthetic; antiseptic* [benzocaine; benzalkonium chloride] 10%•0.12%

Tanac Dual Core stick OTC *mucous membrane anesthetic; antiseptic; astringent* [benzocaine; benzalkonium chloride; tannic acid] 7.5%•0.12%•6%

Tanacetum parthenium medicinal herb [see: feverfew]

Tanacetum vulgare medicinal herb [see: tansy]

TanaCof A12 oral suspension (discontinued 2007) ℞ *decongestant; antihistamine; sleep aid* [phenylephrine tannate; chlorpheniramine tannate; pyrilamine tannate] 30•12•75 mg/ 30 mL

TanaCof-DM oral suspension (discontinued 2007) ℞ *antitussive; antihistamine; decongestant* [dextromethorphan tannate; dexchlorpheniramine tannate; pseudoephedrine tannate] 50•5•150 mg/10 mL

Tanafed DMX oral suspension (discontinued 2007) ℞ *antitussive; antihistamine; decongestant* [dextromethorphan tannate; dexchlorpheniramine tannate; pseudoephedrine tannate] 50•5•150 mg/10 mL

Tanafed DP oral suspension (discontinued 2007) ℞ *decongestant; antihistamine* [pseudoephedrine tannate; dexchlorpheniramine tannate] 150• 9 mg/10 mL

TanaHist-D Pediatric oral drops ℞ *antihistamine; decongestant* [chlorpheniramine tannate; phenylephrine tannate] 2•6 mg/mL

TanaHist-PD oral suspension ℞ *antihistamine* [chlorpheniramine tannate] 2 mg/mL

Tanate DMP-DEX oral liquid (discontinued 2007) ℞ *antitussive; antihistamine; decongestant* [dextromethorphan tannate; dexchlorpheniramine tannate; pseudoephedrine tannate] 50•5•150 mg/10 mL

Tanavan oral suspension (discontinued 2007) ℞ *decongestant; antihistamine; sleep aid* [phenylephrine tannate; pyrilamine tannate] 12.5•30 mg/5 mL

tandamine INN *antidepressant* [also: tandamine HCl]

tandamine HCl USAN *antidepressant* [also: tandamine]

Tandem capsules ℞ *hematinic* [iron (as ferrous fumarate and polysaccharide-iron complex)] 106 mg

Tandem DHA capsules ℞ *prenatal vitamin/iron/omega-3 supplement* [vitamins B_6 & C; iron (as ferrous sulfate and carbonyl); folic acid; docosahexaenoic acid (DHA); eicosapentaenoic acid (EPA)] 25•20•30•1•215•53.5 mg

Tandem F capsules (discontinued 2008) ℞ *hematinic* [iron (as ferrous fumarate and polysaccharide-iron complex); folic acid] 106•1 mg

Tandem OB capsules ℞ *prenatal vitamin/mineral/iron supplement* [multiple vitamins & minerals; iron; folic acid] ±•277•1 mg

Tandem Plus capsules ℞ *vitamin/mineral/iron supplement* [multiple vitamins & minerals; iron; folic acid] ±•106•1 mg

tandospirone INN, BAN *anxiolytic* [also: tandospirone citrate]

tandospirone citrate USAN *anxiolytic* [also: tandospirone]

TanDur DM oral suspension (discontinued 2009) ℞ *antitussive; antihistamine; decongestant* [dextromethorphan tannate; dexchlorpheniramine tannate; pseudoephedrine tannate] 27.5•3•50 mg/5 mL

tanezumab INN *monoclonal antibody; nerve growth factor inhibitor; investigational (Phase III) for osteoarthritis; investigational (Phase II) for endometriosis and cancer pain*

taniplon INN

Tannate 12 S oral suspension (discontinued 2009) ℞ *antitussive; antihistamine* [carbetapentane tannate; chlorpheniramine tannate] 30•4 mg/5 mL

Tannate-12D S oral suspension (discontinued 2010) ℞ *antitussive; antihistamine; sleep aid; decongestant* [carbetapentane tannate; pyrilamine tannate; phenylephrine tannate] 30•30•5 mg/5 mL

Tannate DMP-DEX oral suspension (discontinued 2009) ℞ *antitussive; antihistamine; decongestant* [dextromethorphan tannate; dexchlorpheniramine tannate; pseudoephedrine tannate] 25•2.5•75 mg/5 mL

Tannate Pediatric oral suspension ℞ *antihistamine; decongestant* [chlorpheniramine tannate; phenylephrine tannate] 4.5•5 mg/5 mL

Tannate-V-DM oral suspension (discontinued 2009) ℞ *antitussive; antihistamine; sleep aid; decongestant* [dextromethorphan tannate; pyrilamine tannate; phenylephrine tannate] 25•30•12.5 mg/5 mL

tannic acid USP, JAN *astringent; topical mucosal protectant*

tannic acid acetate [see: acetyltannic acid]

Tannic-12 caplets ℞ *antitussive; antihistamine* [carbetapentane tannate; chlorpheniramine tannate] 60•5 mg

Tannic-12 oral suspension (discontinued 2007) ℞ *antitussive; antihistamine; decongestant* [carbetapentane tannate; chlorpheniramine tannate; phenylephrine tannate] 30•4•5 mg/5 mL

Tannic-12 S oral suspension ℞ *antitussive; antihistamine* [carbetapentane tannate; chlorpheniramine tannate] 30•4 mg/5 mL ☒ TNKase; tonics

Tannihist-12 D oral suspension ℞ *antitussive; antihistamine; sleep aid; decongestant* [carbetapentane tannate; pyrilamine tannate; phenylephrine tannate] 30•30•5 mg/5 mL

tannin [see: tannic acid]

tannyl acetate [see: acetyltannic acid]

tansy *(Chrysanthemum vulgare; Tanacetum vulgare)* leaves and seeds *medicinal herb for inducing diaphoresis,* promoting wound healing, relieving spasms, stimulating menstruation, and treating worm infections

tantalum *element (Ta)*

Tantum *investigational (orphan) radioprotectant for oral mucosa following radiation therapy for head and neck cancer* [benzydamine HCl]

taoryi edisylate [see: caramiphen edisylate]

Tapanol tablets, caplets, gelcaps (discontinued 2007) OTC *analgesic; antipyretic* [acetaminophen] 325, 500 mg; 500 mg; 500 mg

Tapazole tablets R̥ *thyroid inhibitor for hyperthyroidism* [methimazole] 5, 10 mg

tape, adhesive USP *surgical aid*

tapentadol HCl *central analgesic for moderate to severe pain*

TaperPak (trademarked packaging form) *corticosteroid packaging to taper off the dosage*

taprostene INN

tar [see: coal tar]

tarweed *medicinal herb* [see: yerba santa]

Tarabine PFS subcu, intrathecal, or IV injection R̥ *antimetabolite antineoplastic for various leukemias* [cytarabine] 20 mg/mL

taranabant *investigational (Phase III) selective cannabinoid CB₁ blocker for weight loss*

Taraphilic ointment OTC *antipsoriatic; antiseborrheic* [coal tar] 1%

Taraxacum officinale *medicinal herb* [see: dandelion]

Tarceva film-coated tablets R̥ *antineoplastic for advanced or metastatic non–small cell lung cancer (NSCLC) and pancreatic cancer; investigational (orphan) for malignant gliomas* [erlotinib (as HCl)] 25, 100, 150 mg

tarenflurbil *investigational (Phase III) amyloid-beta-42–blocking agent to delay the progression of mild Alzheimer disease*

targeted monoclonal antibody vehicles (T-MAVs) *a class of agents that deliver a cytotoxic drug or radioactivity directly to the targeted tissue, usually a*

cancerous tumor; T-MAVs are not therapeutic per se, but transport the therapeutic agent (effector molecule) to a specific site [also see: antibody-drug conjugate (ADC)]

Targretin capsules, gel R̥ *synthetic retinoid analogue antineoplastic for cutaneous T-cell lymphoma (orphan);* [bexarotene] 75 mg; 1%

Tarka film-coated dual-release tablets R̥ *once-daily combination angiotensin-converting enzyme (ACE) inhibitor and calcium channel blocker for hypertension* [trandolapril (immediate release); verapamil HCl (extended release)] 1•240, 2•180, 2•240, 4•240 mg ⓩ Tri-K

Tarlene hair lotion OTC *antiseborrheic; antipsoriatic; keratolytic* [salicylic acid; coal tar] 2.5%•2% ⓩ triolein

Taron-Crystals powder for oral solution R̥ *urinary alkalizing agent* [potassium citrate; citric acid] 3300•1002 mg/pkt.

tarragon (Artemisia dracunculus) flowering plant *medicinal herb used as a diuretic, emmenagogue, hypnotic, and stomachic* ⓩ Torecan; Treagan; Trocaine

Tarsum shampoo OTC *antipsoriatic; antiseborrheic; keratolytic* [coal tar; salicylic acid] 10%•5%

tartar emetic [see: antimony potassium tartrate]

tartaric acid NF *buffering agent*

Tasigna capsules R̥ *antineoplastic for Philadelphia chromosome–positive chronic myeloid leukemia (CML)* [nilotinib (as HCl)] 150, 200 mg

tasimelteon *investigational (Phase III) melatonin agonist to treat insomnia and circadian rhythm sleep disorders; investigational (orphan) for circadian rhythm sleep disorders in blind people with no light perception*

tasisulam *investigational (Phase III) antineoplastic for soft-tissue sarcoma, leukemia, and breast, ovarian, renal, and non–small cell lung cancers*

Tasmar film-coated tablets ℞ *COMT (catechol-O-methyltransferase) inhibitor for Parkinson disease* [tolcapone] 100, 200 mg

tasocitinib *investigational (Phase III) janus-associated kinase (JAK) inhibitor for rheumatoid arthritis*

tasosartan USAN, INN *angiotensin receptor blocker (ARB) for hypertension*

taspoglutide *investigational (Phase III) glucagon-like peptide-1 (GLP-1) for type 2 diabetes*

tasuldine INN

taurine INN [also: aminoethylsulfonic acid]

taurocholate sodium [see: sodium taurocholate]

taurolidine INN, BAN *antitoxin*

tauromustine INN *antineoplastic* ⊘ trimustine

tauroselcholic acid INN, BAN

taurultam INN, BAN

Tavist Allergy tablets OTC *antihistamine for allergic rhinitis and urticaria* [clemastine fumarate] 1.34 mg

Tavist Allergy/Sinus/Headache caplets (discontinued 2007) OTC *decongestant; antihistamine; analgesic; antipyretic* [pseudoephedrine HCl; clemastine fumarate; acetaminophen] 30•0.335•500 mg

Tavist ND tablets (discontinued 2008) OTC *nonsedating antihistamine for allergic rhinitis; also used for chronic idiopathic urticaria* [loratadine] 10 mg

Tavist Sinus caplets (discontinued 2007) OTC *decongestant; analgesic; antipyretic* [pseudoephedrine HCl; acetaminophen] 30•500 mg

Tavocept *investigational (Phase III) neuroprotectant for paclitaxel and cisplatin therapy for non–small cell lung cancer*

taxanes; taxoids *a class of antineoplastics that inhibits cancer cell mitosis by disrupting the cells' microtubular network*

Taxol IV infusion (discontinued 2010) ℞ *antineoplastic for AIDS-related Kaposi sarcoma (orphan), breast and ovarian cancers, and non–small cell lung cancer (NSCLC)* [paclitaxel] 6 mg/mL ⊘ TachoSil; Tygacil

Taxoprexin *investigational (orphan) taxane for hormone-refractory prostate cancer* [docosahexaenoic acid (DHA); paclitaxel]

Taxotere IV infusion ℞ *antineoplastic for advanced or metastatic breast, prostate, stomach, head, neck, and non–small cell lung cancer (NSCLC); also used for ovarian, esophageal, and other cancers; analogue to paclitaxel* [docetaxel] 20, 80 mg/vial

Taxus bacatta **and other species** *medicinal herb* [see: yew]

tazadolene INN *analgesic* [also: tazadolene succinate]

tazadolene succinate USAN *analgesic* [also: tazadolene]

tazanolast INN

tazarotene USAN, INN *retinoid prodrug; topical keratolytic for acne and psoriasis; adjuvant treatment for facial wrinkles, hyper- and hypopigmentation, and benign lentigines; investigational (NDA filed) for acute acne*

tazasubrate INN, BAN

tazeprofen INN

Tazicef powder or frozen premix for IV or IM injection ℞ *third-generation cephalosporin antibiotic* [ceftazidime] 1, 2, 6 g

Tazidime powder for IV or IM injection ℞ *third-generation cephalosporin antibiotic* [ceftazidime] 1, 2, 6 g ⊘ Tusso-DM

tazifylline INN *antihistamine* [also: tazifylline HCl]

tazifylline HCl USAN *antihistamine* [also: tazifylline]

taziprinone INN

tazobactam USAN, INN, BAN *beta-lactamase inhibitor; penicillin synergist*

tazobactam sodium USAN *beta-lactamase inhibitor; penicillin synergist*

tazofelone USAN

tazolol INN *cardiotonic* [also: tazolol HCl]

tazolol HCl USAN *cardiotonic* [also: tazolol]

tazomeline citrate USAN *cholinergic agonist for Alzheimer disease*

Tazorac cream, gel ℞ *retinoid pro-drug; keratolytic for acne and psoriasis* [tazarotene] 0.05%, 0.1%

Taztia XT extended-release capsules ℞ *antihypertensive; calcium channel blocker* [diltiazem HCl] 120, 180, 240, 300, 360 mg

TBZ (thiabendazole) [q.v.]

3TC [now: lamivudine]

99mTc [see: macrosalb (99mTc)]

99mTc [see: sodium pertechnetate Tc 99m]

99mTc [see: technetium Tc 99m albumin]

99mTc [see: technetium Tc 99m albumin aggregated]

99mTc [see: technetium Tc 99m albumin colloid]

99mTc [see: technetium Tc 99m albumin microaggregated]

99mTc [see: technetium Tc 99m antimony trisulfide colloid]

99mTc [see: technetium Tc 99m biciromab]

99mTc [see: technetium Tc 99m bicisate]

99mTc [see: technetium Tc 99m disofenin]

99mTc [see: technetium Tc 99m etidronate]

99mTc [see: technetium Tc 99m exametazine]

99mTc [see: technetium Tc 99m ferpentetate]

99mTc [see: technetium Tc 99m furifosmin]

99mTc [see: technetium Tc 99m gluceptate]

99mTc [see: technetium Tc 99m lidofenin]

99mTc [see: technetium Tc 99m mebrofenin]

99mTc [see: technetium Tc 99m medronate]

99mTc [see: technetium Tc 99m medronate disodium]

99mTc [see: technetium Tc 99m mertiatide]

99mTc [see: technetium Tc 99m oxidronate]

99mTc [see: technetium Tc 99m pentetate]

99mTc [see: technetium Tc 99m pentetate calcium trisodium]

99mTc [see: technetium Tc 99m (pyro- & trimeta-) phosphates]

99mTc [see: technetium Tc 99m pyrophosphate]

99mTc [see: technetium Tc 99m red blood cells]

99mTc [see: technetium Tc 99m sestamibi]

99mTc [see: technetium Tc 99m siboroxime]

99mTc [see: technetium Tc 99m succimer]

99mTc [see: technetium Tc 99m sulfur colloid]

99mTc [see: technetium Tc 99m teboroxime]

99mTc [see: technetium Tc 99m tetrofosmin]

99mTc [see: technetium Tc 99m tiatide]

TCC (trichlorocarbanilide) [see: triclocarban]

T-cell depleted stem cells derived from peripheral blood stem cells *investigational (orphan) for chronic granulomatous disease*

T-cell receptor (TCR) ligand, recombinant *investigational (orphan) for multiple sclerosis*

TCF (Taxol, cisplatin, fluorouracil) *chemotherapy protocol for esophageal cancer*

TCI Ovulation Tester test kit for home use OTC *in vitro diagnostic aid to predict ovulation time from a saliva sample*

TCR (T-cell receptor) ligand [q.v.]

TD; Td (tetanus & diphtheria [toxoids]) the designation TD (or DT) denotes the pediatric vaccine; Td denotes the adult vaccine [see: diphtheria & tetanus toxoids, adsorbed]

Tdap (tetanus, diphtheria, acellular pertussis) vaccine Tdap (tetanus predominant) is the booster vaccine used in adults and children ≥ 10 years; compare to Dtap [see: diphtheria & tetanus toxoids & acellular pertussis (DTaP; Dtap; Tdap) vaccine]

T-DM1 ("targeted DM1") *investigational (NDA filed) antineoplastic for breast cancer that uses* **Herceptin** (trastuzumab) *as a targeted monoclonal antibody vehicle (T-MAV; q.v.) to deliver* **DM1** (maytansine) *to HER-2–positive breast cancer tumors*

tea, Canada; mountain tea; redberry tea *medicinal herb* [see: wintergreen]

tea tree oil *(Melaleuca alternifolia) medicinal herb for acne, boils, burns, Candida infections, cold sores, joint pain, skin disorders, staphylococcal and streptococcal infections, and sunburn; also used as a douche for trichomonal cervicitis and vaginal candidiasis*

TEAB (tetraethylammonium bromide) [see: tetrylammonium bromide]

teaberry oil [see: methyl salicylate]

TEAC (tetraethylammonium chloride) [q.v.]

teamster's tea *medicinal herb* [see: ephedra]

TearGard eye drops (discontinued 2010) OTC *moisturizer/lubricant* [hydroxyethylcellulose] ⊡ terguride

Teargen eye drops (discontinued 2010) OTC *moisturizer/lubricant* [polyvinyl alcohol] ⊡ tarragon; Torecan; Treagan; Trocaine; Trugene

Tearisol eye drops OTC *moisturizer/lubricant* [hydroxypropyl methylcellulose] 0.5% ⊡ Terazol

Tears Again gel OTC *ophthalmic moisturizer/lubricant* [hydroxypropyl methylcellulose] 0.7% ⊡ triaziquone

Tears Naturale; Tears Naturale II; Tears Naturale Free eye drops OTC *moisturizer/lubricant* [hydroxypropyl methylcellulose] 0.3%

Tears Naturale Forte eye drops OTC *moisturizer/lubricant* [hydroxypropyl methylcellulose; glycerin] 0.3%•0.2%

Tears Plus eye drops OTC *moisturizer/lubricant* [polyvinyl alcohol] 1.4%

Tears Renewed eye drops (discontinued 2010) OTC *moisturizer/lubricant* [hydroxypropyl methylcellulose] 0.3%

Tears Renewed ophthalmic ointment (discontinued 2010) OTC *ocular moisturizer/lubricant* [white petrolatum; mineral oil]

TearSaver Punctum Plugs ℞ *blocks the puncta and canaliculus to eliminate tear loss in keratitis sicca* [silicone plug]

Tebamide suppositories, pediatric suppositories (removed from the market in 2007 due to lack of efficacy) ℞ *anticholinergic; post-surgical antiemetic; local anesthetic* [trimethobenzamide HCl; benzocaine] 200 mg•2%; 100 mg•2%

tebatizole INN

tebethion [see: thioacetazone; thiacetazone]

tebufelone USAN, INN *analgesic; anti-inflammatory*

tebuquine USAN, INN *antimalarial* ⊡ Topicaine

tebutate USAN, INN *combining name for radicals or groups*

teceleukin USAN, INN, BAN *immunostimulant; investigational (orphan) for metastatic renal cell carcinoma and metastatic malignant melanoma*

technetium *element (Tc)*

technetium (⁹⁹ᵐTc) dimercaptosuccinic acid JAN *diagnostic aid for renal function testing* [also: technetium Tc 99m succimer]

technetium (⁹⁹ᵐTc) human serum albumin JAN *radioactive agent*

technetium (⁹⁹ᵐTc) labeled macroaggregated human albumin JAN [also: macrosalb (⁹⁹ᵐTc)]

technetium (⁹⁹ᵐTc) methylenediphosphonate JAN *radioactive diagnostic aid for skeletal imaging* [also: technetium Tc 99m medronate]

technetium (⁹⁹ᵐTc) phytate JAN *radioactive agent*

technetium Tc 99m albumin USP *radioactive agent*

technetium Tc 99m albumin aggregated USAN, USP *radioactive diagnostic aid for lung imaging*

technetium Tc 99m albumin colloid USAN, USP *radioactive agent*

technetium Tc 99m albumin microaggregated USAN *radioactive agent*

technetium Tc 99m antimony trisulfide colloid USAN *radioactive agent*

technetium Tc 99m apcitide *radiopharmaceutical diagnostic aid for acute venous thrombosis*

technetium Tc 99m arcitumomab USAN *radiopharmaceutical diagnostic aid for recurrent or metastatic thyroid and colorectal cancers*

technetium Tc 99m bectumomab *monoclonal antibody IgG$_{2a}$ to B cell, murine; investigational (Phase III, orphan) diagnostic aid for non-Hodgkin B-cell lymphoma, AIDS-related lymphomas, and other acute and chronic B-cell leukemias* [also: bectumomab]

technetium Tc 99m biciromab *radioactive diagnostic aid for deep vein thrombosis*

technetium Tc 99m bicisate USAN, INN, BAN *radioactive diagnostic aid for brain imaging*

technetium Tc 99m disofenin USP *radioactive diagnostic aid for hepatobiliary function testing*

technetium Tc 99m DMSA (dimercaptosuccinic acid) [see: technetium Tc 99m succimer]

technetium Tc 99m DTPA (diethylenetriaminepentaacetic acid) [see: technetium Tc 99m pentetate]

technetium Tc 99m etidronate USP *radioactive agent*

technetium Tc 99m exametazine USAN *radioactive agent*

technetium Tc 99m ferpentetate USP *radioactive agent*

technetium Tc 99m furifosmin USAN, INN *radioactive agent; diagnostic aid for cardiac disease*

technetium Tc 99m gluceptate USP *radioactive agent*

technetium Tc 99m HSA (human serum albumin) [see: technetium Tc 99m albumin]

technetium Tc 99m iron ascorbate pentetic acid complex [now: technetium Tc 99m ferpentetate]

technetium Tc 99m lidofenin USAN, USP *radioactive agent*

technetium Tc 99m MAA (microaggregated albumin) [see: technetium Tc 99m albumin aggregated]

technetium Tc 99m MDP (methylenediphosphonate) [see: technetium Tc 99m medronate]

technetium Tc 99m mebrofenin USAN, USP *radioactive hepatobiliary imaging agent for cholescintigraphy 100 mCi in 45 mg injection*

technetium Tc 99m medronate USP *radioactive diagnostic aid for skeletal imaging* [also: technetium (^{99m}Tc) methylenediphosphonate]

technetium Tc 99m medronate disodium USAN *radioactive agent*

technetium Tc 99m mertiatide USAN *radioactive diagnostic aid for renal function testing*

technetium Tc 99m oxidronate USP *radioactive diagnostic aid for skeletal imaging*

technetium Tc 99m pentetate USP *radioactive agent* [also: human serum albumin diethylenetriaminepentaacetic acid technetium (^{99m}Tc)]

technetium Tc 99m pentetate calcium trisodium USAN *radioactive agent*

technetium Tc 99m pentetate sodium [now: technetium Tc 99m pentetate]

technetium Tc 99m pterotetramide *investigational (orphan) radiodiagnostic aid for ovarian carcinoma*

technetium Tc 99m (pyro- and trimeta-) phosphates USP *radioactive agent*

technetium Tc 99m pyrophosphate USP, JAN *radioactive agent*

technetium Tc 99m red blood cells USAN *radioactive agent*

technetium Tc 99m rh-Annexin V
*investigational (orphan) radiodiagnostic
aid to assess the rejection status of heart
and lung transplants*

technetium Tc 99m sestamibi USAN,
INN, BAN *radioactive/radiopaque diagnostic aid for cardiac perfusion imaging
and mammography* 5 mL injection

technetium Tc 99m siboroxime
USAN, INN *radiodiagnostic aid for brain
imaging*

**technetium Tc 99m sodium glu-
ceptate** [now: technetium Tc 99m
gluceptate]

technetium Tc 99m succimer USP
*radiodiagnostic aid for renal function
testing* [also: technetium (⁹⁹ᵐTc)
dimercaptosuccinic acid]

technetium Tc 99m sulesomab
*radiodiagnostic monoclonal antibody for
infectious lesions* [also: sulesomab]

**technetium Tc 99m sulfur colloid
(TSC)** USAN, USP *radioactive agent*

technetium Tc 99m teboroxime
USAN, INN, BAN *radioactive/radi-
opaque diagnostic aid for cardiac perfusion imaging*

technetium Tc 99m tetrofosmin
*radioactive agent for cardiovascular
imaging*

technetium Tc 99m tiatide BAN

**technetium Tc 99m TSC (techne-
tium sulfur colloid)** [see: technetium Tc 99m sulfur colloid]

**technetium Tc 99m-labeled CEA
scan** [see: arcitumomab]

Techni-Care surgical scrub ℞ *broad-
spectrum microbicide* [chloroxylenol]
3%

Technosphere (trademarked delivery
device) *investigational (NDA filed)
oral inhalation device for* **Afrezza**

teclothiazide INN, BAN

teclozan USAN, INN *antiamebic*

Tecnu Outdoor Skin Cleanser lotion
OTC *for the removal of toxic oils from
poison ivy, oak, or sumac; use before
or as soon as rash appears; can also be
used to clean clothing and equipment*

[deodorized mineral spirits; propylene glycol; fatty acid soap]

tecogalan sodium USAN *antiangiogenic
antineoplastic*

Teczem film-coated extended-release
tablets (discontinued 2007) ℞ *antihypertensive; angiotensin-converting
enzyme (ACE) inhibitor; calcium channel blocker* [diltiazem maleate; enalapril maleate] 180•5 mg

tedisamil INN *investigational (NDA filed)
antiarrhythmic for atrial fibrillation*

Tedrigen tablets (discontinued 2007)
OTC *antiasthmatic; bronchodilator;
decongestant; sedative* [theophylline;
ephedrine HCl; phenobarbital] 120•
22.5•7.5 mg

teduglutide *investigational (Phase III)
glucagon-like peptide 2 (GLP-2) analogue for short bowel syndrome*

tefazoline INN ⑫ tofisoline

tefenperate INN

Teflaro powder for IV infusion ℞ *broad-
spectrum cephalosporin antibiotic for
complicated skin and skin structure infections (cSSSI), methicillin-resistant S.
aureus (MRSA), and multidrug-resistant
Streptococcus pneumoniae (MDRSP)*
[ceftaroline fosamil] 400, 600 mg

tefludazine INN

teflurane USAN, INN *inhalation anesthetic*

teflutixol INN

tegafur USAN, INN, BAN *antineoplastic;
prodrug of fluorouracil*

tegaserod USAN *selective serotonin 5-
HT₄ receptor antagonist for irritable
bowel syndrome (IBS)*

tegaserod maleate *selective serotonin
5-HT₄ receptor antagonist for irritable
bowel syndrome (IBS) with chronic
constipation in women and chronic
idiopathic constipation in all patients*

Tegretol chewable tablets, caplets,
oral suspension ℞ *iminostilbene anticonvulsant; analgesic for trigeminal
neuralgia; also used for restless legs
syndrome (RLS), alcohol withdrawal,
and postherpetic neuralgia* [carbamaze-
pine] 100 mg; 200 mg; 100 mg/5 mL

Tegretol-XR extended-release film-coated tablets ℞ *twice-daily anticonvulsant; analgesic for trigeminal neuralgia; also used for restless legs syndrome (RLS), alcohol withdrawal, and postherpetic neuralgia* [carbamazepine] 100, 200, 400 mg

Tegrin-HC ointment OTC *corticosteroidal anti-inflammatory* [hydrocortisone] 1%

teholamine [see: aminophylline]

TEIB (triethyleneiminobenzoquinone) [see: triaziquone]

teicoplanin USAN, INN, BAN *glycopeptide antibiotic*

teicoplanin A$_{2-1}$, A$_{2-2}$, A$_{2-3}$, A$_{2-4}$, A$_{2-5}$, and A$_{3-1}$ *components of teicoplanin*

Tekamlo film-coated tablets ℞ *combination direct renin inhibitor and calcium channel blocker for hypertension* [aliskiren (as hemifumarate); amlodipine besylate] 150•5, 150•10, 300•5, 300•10 mg

Tekral caplets OTC *decongestant; antihistamine; sleep aid* [pseudoephedrine HCl; diphenhydramine HCl] 120•100 mg

Tekturna film-coated tablets ℞ *once-daily direct renin inhibitor for hypertension* [aliskiren (as hemifumarate)] 150, 300 mg

Tekturna HCT film-coated tablets ℞ *combination direct renin inhibitor and diuretic for hypertension* [aliskiren hemifumarate; hydrochlorothiazide] 150•12.5, 150•25, 300•12.5, 300•25 mg

Teladar cream (discontinued 2007) ℞ *corticosteroidal anti-inflammatory* [betamethasone dipropionate] 0.05%

telaprevir *oral hepatitis C virus (HCV) protease inhibitor for the treatment of HCV infections*

telavancin HCl *lipoglycopeptide antibiotic for drug-resistant gram-positive complicated skin and skin structure infections (cSSSI); semisynthetic derivative of vancomycin*

telbermin USAN *angiogenic growth factor; vascular endothelial growth factor,* recombinant human (rhVEGF); investigational (Phase II, orphan) for peripheral vascular disease and coronary artery disease

telbivudine *nucleoside reverse-transcriptase inhibitor (NRTI); oral antiviral for chronic hepatitis B virus (HBV) infection*

telcagepant *investigational (NDA filed) calcitonin gene-related peptide (CGRP) receptor antagonist for migraine headaches*

Telcyta *investigational (Phase III) antineoplastic for non–small cell lung cancers*

Tel-E-Amp (trademarked delivery form) *unit dose ampule*

Tel-E-Dose (trademarked packaging form) *unit dose package*

Tel-E-Ject (trademarked delivery form) *prefilled disposable syringe*

telenzepine INN

Tel-E-Pack (trademarked packaging form) *packaging system*

Tel-E-Vial (trademarked packaging form) *unit dose vial*

telinavir USAN *antiviral; HIV protease inhibitor*

telithromycin *broad-spectrum ketolide antibiotic for community-acquired pneumonia (CAP); approval to treat other types of respiratory tract infections was withdrawn by the FDA in 2007*

tellurium *element (Te)*

telmisartan USAN *angiotensin receptor blocker (ARB) for hypertension*

teloxantrone INN *antineoplastic* [also: teloxantrone HCl]

teloxantrone HCl USAN *antineoplastic* [also: teloxantrone]

teludipine INN, BAN *antihypertensive; calcium channel antagonist* [also: teludipine HCl]

teludipine HCl USAN *antihypertensive; calcium channel antagonist* [also: teludipine]

temafloxacin INN, BAN *antibacterial; microbial DNA topoisomerase inhibitor* [also: temafloxacin HCl]

temafloxacin HCl USAN *antibacterial; microbial DNA topoisomerase inhibitor* [also: temafloxacin]

temarotene INN

tematropium methylsulfate USAN *anticholinergic* [also: tematropium metilsulfate]

tematropium metilsulfate INN *anticholinergic* [also: tematropium methylsulfate]

temazepam USAN, INN *benzodiazepine sedative and hypnotic* 7.5, 15, 22.5, 30 mg oral

Tembid (trademarked dosage form) *sustained-action capsule*

temefos USAN, INN *veterinary ectoparasiticide*

temelastine USAN, INN, BAN *antihistamine*

temocapril HCl USAN *antihypertensive*

temocillin USAN, INN, BAN *antibacterial*

temocillin sodium *investigational (orphan) antibiotic for pulmonary* Burkholderia cepacia *infections*

Temodar capsules, powder for IV injection ℞ *alkylating antineoplastic for refractory anaplastic astrocytoma (AA), recurrent glioblastoma multiforme (GBM), and malignant glioma (orphan); investigational (NDA filed, orphan) for advanced metastatic melanoma* [temozolomide] 5, 20, 100, 140, 180, 250 mg; 100 mg/vial

temodox USAN, INN *veterinary growth stimulant*

temoporfin USAN, INN, BAN *photosensitizer for photodynamic cancer therapy; investigational (NDA filed, orphan) palliative treatment for head and neck cancer*

Temovate ointment, gel, cream, scalp application ℞ *corticosteroidal anti-inflammatory* [clobetasol propionate] 0.05%

Temovate Emollient cream ℞ *corticosteroidal anti-inflammatory* [clobetasol propionate in an emollient base] 0.05%

temozolomide INN, BAN *alkylating antineoplastic for refractory anaplastic astrocytoma (AA), recurrent glioblastoma multiforme (GBM), and malignant glioma (orphan); investigational (NDA filed, orphan) for advanced metastatic melanoma* 5, 20, 100, 140, 180, 250 mg oral

Temp Tab tablets OTC *electrolyte replacement* [sodium (as chloride), potassium (as chloride), and chloride (as sodium and potassium chloride) electrolytes] 180•15•287 mg

Tempo chewable tablets OTC *antacid; antiflatulent* [aluminum hydroxide; magnesium hydroxide; calcium carbonate; simethicone] 133•81•414•20 mg

Tempra 1 oral drops (discontinued 2008) OTC *analgesic; antipyretic* [acetaminophen] 100 mg/mL

Tempra 2 syrup (discontinued 2008) OTC *analgesic; antipyretic* [acetaminophen] 160 mg/5 mL

Tempra 3 chewable tablets (discontinued 2008) OTC *analgesic; antipyretic* [acetaminophen] 80, 160 mg

Tempra Quicklets (quickly dissolving tablets) (discontinued 2008) OTC *analgesic; antipyretic* [acetaminophen] 80, 160 mg

Tempule (trademarked dosage form) *timed-release capsule or tablet*

temsirolimus *antineoplastic for renal cell carcinoma (orphan); investigational (NDA filed) for mantle cell lymphoma; immunosuppressant*

temurtide USAN, INN, BAN *vaccine adjuvant*

10 Benzagel; 5 Benzagel gel ℞ *keratolytic for acne* [benzoyl peroxide] 10%; 5%

10% LMD IV injection ℞ *plasma volume expander for shock due to hemorrhage, burns, or surgery* [dextran 40] 10%

tenamfetamine INN

Tenar PSE oral liquid ℞ *decongestant; expectorant* [pseudoephedrine HCl; guaifenesin] 40•200 mg/5 mL

Tencon caplets ℞ *barbiturate sedative; analgesic; antipyretic* [butalbital; acetaminophen] 50•650 mg

tendamistat INN

tenecteplase USAN *genetically engineered mutation of tissue plasminogen activator (tPA); thrombolytic/fibrinolytic for acute myocardial infarction (AMI)*

Tenex tablets ℞ *antihypertensive; investigational (orphan) for fragile X syndrome* [guanfacine (as HCl)] 1, 2 mg

tenidap USAN, INN *anti-inflammatory for osteoarthritis and rheumatoid arthritis; cytokine inhibitor*

tenidap sodium USAN *anti-inflammatory for osteoarthritis and rheumatoid arthritis*

tenilapine INN

teniloxazine INN

tenilsetam INN

teniposide USAN, INN, BAN *antineoplastic for refractory childhood acute lymphoblastic leukemia (orphan); also used for adult acute lymphocytic leukemia and non-Hodgkin lymphoma*

Ten-K controlled-release tablets ℞ *electrolyte replenisher* [potassium (as chloride)] 10 mEq (750 mg)

tenoate INN *combining name for radicals or groups*

tenocyclidine INN

tenofovir USAN *nucleotide reverse transcriptase inhibitor (NRTI); antiviral for HIV-1 infection*

tenofovir disoproxil fumarate (tenofovir DF) *nucleotide reverse transcriptase inhibitor (NRTI); oral antiviral for HIV-1 and chronic hepatitis B virus (HBV) infections; investigational gel form for vaginal use to prevent HIV transmission to women during sex (base=82%)*

tenofovir disoproxil fumarate & efavirenz & emtricitabine *antiviral combination therapy for HIV infection in adults* 300•600•200 mg oral

tenonitrozole INN

Tenoretic 50; Tenoretic 100 tablets ℞ *combination beta-blocker and diuretic for hypertension* [atenolol; chlorthalidone] 50•25 mg; 100•25 mg

Tenormin IV injection (discontinued 2008) ℞ *antianginal; antihypertensive; beta-blocker* [atenolol] 5 mg/10 mL

Tenormin tablets ℞ *antianginal; antihypertensive; beta-blocker; treatment for acute myocardial infarction; also used to prevent migraine headaches* [atenolol] 25, 50, 100 mg

tenoxicam USAN, INN, BAN *anti-inflammatory*

Tensilon IV or IM injection (discontinued 2010) ℞ *short-acting muscle stimulant; diagnostic aid for myasthenia gravis; antidote to curare* [edrophonium chloride] 10 mg/mL ⓡ tinazoline; Tonsaline

Ten-Tab (trademarked dosage form) *controlled-release tablet*

tenylidone INN

teoclate INN *combining name for radicals or groups* [also: theoclate]

teopranitol INN

teoprolol INN

tepirindole INN

teplizumab *investigational (Phase II/III) to slow the progression of type 1 diabetes*

tepoxalin USAN, INN *antipsoriatic*

teprenone INN ⓡ tiopronin

teprosilate INN *combining name for radicals or groups*

teprotide USAN, INN *antihypertensive; angiotensin-converting enzyme (ACE) inhibitor*

Tera-Gel shampoo OTC *antiseborrheic; antipsoriatic; antipruritic; antibacterial* [coal tar] 0.5% ⓡ Trocal

Terak with Polymyxin B Sulfate ophthalmic ointment ℞ *antibiotic* [oxytetracycline HCl; polymyxin B sulfate] 5 mg•10 000 U per g

Terazol 3 vaginal suppositories, vaginal cream in prefilled applicator ℞ *antifungal* [terconazole] 80 mg; 0.8% ⓡ Tearisol

Terazol 7 vaginal cream in prefilled applicator ℞ *antifungal* [terconazole] 0.4% ⓡ Tearisol

terazosin INN, BAN *alpha$_1$ blocker for hypertension and benign prostatic hyperplasia (BPH)* [also: terazosin HCl]

terazosin HCl USAN *alpha$_1$ blocker for hypertension and benign prostatic* *hyperplasia (BPH)* [also: terazosin] 1, 2, 5, 10 mg oral

terbinafine USAN, INN, BAN *systemic allylamine antifungal* [also: terbinafine HCl]

terbinafine HCl JAN *allylamine antifungal* [also: terbinafine] 250 mg oral; 1% topical

Terbinex tablets ℞ *allylamine antifungal* [terbinafine (as HCl)] 250 mg

terbium *element (Tb)*

terbogrel USAN *platelet aggregation inhibitor*

terbucromil INN

terbufibrol INN

terbuficin INN

terbuprol INN

terbutaline INN, BAN *sympathomimetic bronchodilator for asthma and bronchospasm* [also: terbutaline sulfate]

terbutaline sulfate USAN, USP *sympathomimetic bronchodilator for asthma and bronchospasm; also used as a tocolytic to stop preterm labor* [also: terbutaline] 2.5, 5 mg oral; 1 mg/mL injection

terciprazine INN

terconazole USAN, INN, BAN *topical antifungal* 0.4%, 0.8%, 80 mg vaginal suppositories

terfenadine USAN, USP, INN, JAN *piperidine antihistamine*

terflavoxate INN

terfluranol INN

terguride INN *dopamine agonist* ☒ Tear-Gard

teriflunomide *investigational (Phase III) oral agent to reduce the relapse rate in multiple sclerosis patients*

teriparatide USAN, INN *human parathyroid hormone, recombinant; osteoporosis treatment that stimulates new bone formation (orphan); diagnostic aid for parathyroid-induced hypocalcemia (orphan); investigational (orphan) for hypoparathyroidism*

teriparatide acetate USAN, JAN *diagnostic aid for parathyroid-induced hypocalcemia (orphan)*

terizidone INN ☒ trazodone

terlakiren USAN *antihypertensive; renin inhibitor*

terlipressin INN, BAN *synthetic vasopressin derivative; investigational (NDA filed, orphan) hormone for bleeding esophageal varices and to improve renal function in patients with hepatorenal syndrome (HRS)*

ternidazole INN

Terocin lotion OTC *anesthetic; analgesic; antipruritic; counterirritant* [lidocaine; methyl salicylate; menthol; capsaicin] 2.5%•25%•10%•0.025% ☒ Trisan; tyrosine

terodiline INN, BAN, JAN *coronary vasodilator* [also: terodiline HCl]

terodiline HCl USAN *coronary vasodilator* [also: terodiline]

terofenamate INN

teroxalene INN *antischistosomal* [also: teroxalene HCl] ☒ trixolane

teroxalene HCl USAN *antischistosomal* [also: teroxalene]

teroxirone USAN, INN *antineoplastic*

terpin hydrate USP *expectorant* banned by the FDA in 1991

terpinol [see: terpin hydrate]

terrafungine [see: oxytetracycline]

Terramycin IM or IV injection (discontinued 2007) ℞ *broad-spectrum tetracycline antibiotic* [oxytetracycline; lidocaine] 100 mg•2%, 250 mg•2% per 2 mL dose ☒ Trimo-San

Terramycin with Polymyxin B ophthalmic ointment ℞ *ophthalmic antibiotic* [oxytetracycline HCl; polymyxin B sulfate] 5 mg•10 000 U per g

Terrell liquid for vaporization ℞ *inhalation general anesthetic* [isoflurane] ☒ Touro LA

Tersaseptic shampoo/cleanser OTC *soap-free therapeutic cleanser*

Tersi Foam topical foam OTC *antiseborrheic; dandruff treatment* [selenium sulfide] 2.5%

tertatolol INN, BAN

tertiary amyl alcohol [see: amylene hydrate]

***tert*-pentyl alcohol** [see: amylene hydrate]

tesamorelin acetate *growth hormone–releasing factor for HIV-associated lipodystrophy* (base–91%)

tesicam USAN, INN *anti-inflammatory*

tesimide USAN, INN *anti-inflammatory*

Teslac tablets (discontinued 2008) ℞ *adjunctive hormonal chemotherapy for advanced postmenopausal breast carcinoma* [testolactone] 50 mg

Teslascan IV injection (discontinued 2010) ℞ *radiopaque contrast agent to enhance MRIs of the liver* [mangafodipir trisodium] 37.9 mg/mL (50 mcmol/mL)

tesmilifene HCl USAN *antihistamine; chemopotentiator for adjunctive treatment of malignant tumors*

TESPA (triethylenethiophosphoramide) [see: thiotepa]

Tessalon Perles (capsules) ℞ *antitussive* [benzonatate] 100, 200 mg ⍰ tiosalan

Test Pack kit for professional use ℞ *in vitro diagnostic aid for Group A streptococcal antigens in throat swabs* [enzyme immunoassay]

Testim gel ℞ *androgen for hypogonadism or testosterone deficiency in men; hormone replacement therapy (HRT) for postandropausal symptoms* [testosterone; alcohol 74%] 1% (50 mg/pkt.)

testolactone USAN, USP, INN *aromatase inhibitor; antiandrogen antineoplastic for breast cancer*

Testopel pellets for subcu implantation ℞ *androgen for hypogonadism or testosterone deficiency in men; hormone replacement therapy (HRT) for postandropausal symptoms* [testosterone] 75 mg

testosterone USP, INN, BAN *natural androgen for hypogonadism or testosterone deficiency in men; hormone replacement therapy (HRT) for postandropausal symptoms; investigational (Phase II, orphan) for AIDS-wasting syndrome and delay of growth and puberty in boys*

Testosterone Aqueous IM injection ℞ *androgen for hypogonadism or testosterone deficiency in men, delayed puberty in boys, and androgen-responsive metastatic cancers in women; testosterone replacement therapy for postandropausal symptoms* [testosterone] 25, 50, 100 mg/mL

testosterone cyclopentanepropionate [see: testosterone cypionate]

testosterone cyclopentylpropionate [see: testosterone cypionate]

testosterone cypionate USP *parenteral natural androgen for hypogonadism or testosterone deficiency in men; hormone replacement therapy (HRT) for postandropausal symptoms; sometimes abused as a street drug* 100, 200 mg/mL (in oil) injection

testosterone enanthate USP *parenteral natural androgen for testosterone deficiency in men, delayed puberty in boys, and metastatic breast cancer in women; hormone replacement therapy (HRT) for postandropausal symptoms; sometimes abused as a street drug* 200 mg/mL (in oil) injection

testosterone heptanoate [see: testosterone enanthate]

testosterone ketolaurate USAN, INN *androgen*

testosterone 3-oxododecanoate [see: testosterone ketolaurate]

testosterone phenylacetate USAN *androgen*

testosterone propionate USP *parenteral androgen for hypogonadism or testosterone deficiency in men; hormone replacement therapy (HRT) for postandropausal symptoms; investigational (orphan) topical treatment for vulvar dystrophies* 100 mg/mL injection

testosterone undecanoate *investigational (Phase III) parenteral natural androgen for testosterone deficiency in men*

TestPack [see: Abbott TestPack]

Testred capsules ℞ *synthetic androgen for hypogonadism or testosterone deficiency in men, delayed puberty in boys, and metastatic breast cancer in women; hormone replacement therapy (HRT)* for postandropausal symptoms; also abused as a street drug [methyltestosterone] 10 mg

tetanus antitoxin USP *passive immunizing agent*

tetanus & gas gangrene antitoxins NF

tetanus & gas gangrene polyvalent antitoxin [see: tetanus & gas gangrene antitoxins]

tetanus immune globulin (TIG) USP *passive immunizing agent for postexposure tetanus prophylaxis in patients with incomplete or uncertain pre-exposure immunization with tetanus toxoids*

tetanus immune human globulin [now: tetanus immune globulin]

tetanus toxoid USP *active immunizing agent*

tetanus toxoid, adsorbed USP *active immunizing agent*

tetanus toxoid & diphtheria toxoid & acellular pertussis (TDaP; Tdap) vaccine *active immunizing agent for tetanus, diphtheria, and pertussis; vaccine booster for adolescents 10–18 years*

Tetcaine eye drops ℞ *topical anesthetic* [tetracaine HCl] 0.5%

tetiothalein sodium [see: iodophthalein sodium]

tetnicoran [see: nicofurate]

Tetra Brik packs (trademarked delivery form) *ready-to-use liquid containers*

tetrabarbital INN

tetrabenazine INN, BAN *selective dopamine depletor for chorea associated with Huntington disease (orphan)*

tetracaine USP, INN *topical/local anesthetic* [also: amethocaine]

tetracaine HCl USP, JAN *ophthalmological local anesthetic; injectable local anesthetic for spinal anesthesia* [also: amethocaine HCl] 0.5% eye drops; 1% injection

tetrachloroethylene USP

tetrachloromethane [see: carbon tetrachloride]

tetracosactide INN *adrenocorticotropic hormone* [also: cosyntropin; tetracosactrin]

tetracosactrin BAN *adrenocorticotropic hormone* [also: cosyntropin; tetracosactide]

tetracyclics *a class of antidepressants which enhance noradrenergic and serotonergic activity by blocking norepinephrine or serotonin uptake*

tetracycline USP, INN, BAN *bacteriostatic antibiotic; antirickettsial*

tetracycline HCl USP *bacteriostatic antibiotic; antirickettsial* 250, 500 mg oral

tetracycline phosphate complex USP, BAN *antibacterial*

tetracyclines *a class of bacteriostatic, antimicrobial antibiotics*

tetradecanoic acid, methylethyl ester [see: isopropyl myristate]

tetradonium bromide INN

tetraethylammonium bromide (TEAB) [see: tetrylammonium bromide]

tetraethylammonium chloride (TEAC)

tetraethylthiuram disulfide [see: disulfiram]

tetrafilcon A USAN *hydrophilic contact lens material*

Tetra-Formula lozenges OTC *antitussive; mucous membrane anesthetic* [dextromethorphan hydrobromide; benzocaine] 10•15 mg

tetraglycine hydroperiodide *source of iodine for disinfecting water*

tetrahydroacridinamine (THA) [see: tacrine HCl]

tetrahydroaminoacridine (THA) [see: tacrine HCl]

tetrahydrocannabinol (THC), delta-9 *a psychoactive derivative of the* Cannabis sativa *(marijuana) plant; approved in Canada as an analgesic for pain associated with cancer and multiple sclerosis* [also: dronabinol]

tetrahydrolipstatin [see: orlistat]

tetrahydrozoline BAN *vasoconstrictor; nasal decongestant; topical ophthalmic* *decongestant* [also: tetrhydrozoline HCl; tetryzoline]

tetrahydrozoline HCl USP *vasocon-strictor; nasal decongestant; topical oph-thalmic decongestant* [also: tetryzoline; tetrahydrozoline] 0.05% eye drops

tetraiodophenolphthalein sodium [see: iodophthalein sodium]

tetraiodothyroacetic acid *investiga-tional (orphan) for the suppression of thyroid-stimulating hormone (TSH) in patients with thyroid cancer*

tetrallobarbital [see: butalbital]

tetramal [see: tetrabarbital]

tetrameprozine [see: aminopromazine]

tetramethrin INN

tetramethylene dimethanesulfonate [see: busulfan]

tetramisole INN *anthelmintic* [also: tetramisole HCl]

tetramisole HCl USAN *anthelmintic* [also: tetramisole]

tetranitrol [see: erythrityl tetranitrate]

tetrantoin

TetraPaks (trademarked delivery form) *ready-to-use open system containers*

tetrasodium ethylenediaminetetra-acetate [see: edetate sodium]

tetrasodium pyrophosphate [see: sodium pyrophosphate]

tetrazepam INN

tetrazolast INN *antiallergic; antiasth-matic* [also: tetrazolast meglumine]

tetrazolast meglumine USAN *antial-lergic; antiasthmatic* [also: tetrazolast]

tetridamine INN *analgesic; anti-inflam-matory* [also: tetrydamine]

tetriprofen INN

Tetrix cream ℞ *nonsteroidal antipruri-tic, moisturizer, and emollient for hand eczema and dermatitis*

tetrofosmin USAN, INN, BAN *diagnostic aid*

tetronasin INN, BAN *veterinary growth promoter* [also: tetronasin sodium; tetronasin 5930]

tetronasin 5930 INN *veterinary growth promoter* [also: tetronasin sodium; tetronasin]

tetronasin sodium USAN *veterinary growth promoter* [also: tetronasin; tetronasin 5930]

tetroquinone USAN, INN *systemic kera-tolytic*

tetroxoprim USAN, INN *antibacterial*

tetrydamine USAN *analgesic; anti-inflammatory* [also: tetridamine]

tetrylammonium bromide INN

tetryzoline INN *vasoconstrictor; nasal decongestant; topical ocular decongest-ant* [also: tetrahydrozoline HCl; tet-rahydrozoline]

tetryzoline HCl [see: tetrahydrozoline HCl]

Tetterine ointment ℞ *antifungal for tinea pedis, tinea cruris, and tinea cor-poris* [miconazole nitrate] 2%

tetterwort *medicinal herb* [see: blood-root; celandine]

Teveten film-coated caplets ℞ *angio-tensin receptor blocker (ARB) for hypertension* [eprosartan mesylate] 400, 600 mg

Teveten HCT film-coated caplets ℞ *combination angiotensin receptor blocker (ARB) and diuretic for hypertension* [eprosartan mesylate; hydrochlorothi-azide] 600•12.5, 600•25 mg

Tev-Tropin powder for subcu injection ℞ *growth hormone for children and adults with congenital or endogenous growth hormone deficiency (GHD), short bowel syndrome, or AIDS-wast-ing syndrome; for children with Turner syndrome, Prader-Willi syndrome, or renal-induced growth failure* [somatro-pin] 5 mg (15 IU) per vial

Texacort topical solution ℞ *cortico-steroidal anti-inflammatory* [hydrocor-tisone] 2.5%

texacromil INN

tezacitabine USAN *antineoplastic for colon and rectal cancers; investigational (orphan) for adenocarcinoma of the esophagus and stomach*

6-TG (6-thioguanine) [see: thiogua-nine]

TG (thyroglobulin) [q.v.]

TG PSE/BRM/DM caplets ℞ *decongestant; antihistamine; antitussive* [pseudoephedrine HCl; brompheniramine hydrobromide; dextromethorphan hydrobromide] 40•4•20 mg

T-Gen suppositories, pediatric suppositories (removed from the market in 2007 due to lack of efficacy) ℞ *anticholinergic; post-surgical antiemetic; local anesthetic* [trimethobenzamide HCl; benzocaine] 200 mg•2%; 100 mg•2% ▣ Tigan

T-Gesic capsules ℞ *narcotic analgesic; antipyretic* [hydrocodone bitartrate; acetaminophen] 5•500 mg

αTGI (α-triglycidyl isocyanurate) [see: teroxirone]

TGO 30PSE/150GFN/15DM oral liquid ℞ *decongestant; expectorant; antitussive* [pseudoephedrine HCl; guaifenesin; dextromethorphan hydrobromide] 30•150•15 mg/5 mL

TGQ 15DM/5PEH/2CPM oral liquid ℞ *antitussive; decongestant; antihistamine* [dextromethorphan hydrobromide; phenylephrine HCl; chlorpheniramine maleate] 15•5•2 mg/5 mL

TGQ 30PSE/3BRM/15DM; TGQ 40PSE/4BRM/20DM; TGQ 50PSE/3BRM/30DM syrup ℞ *decongestant; antihistamine; antitussive* [pseudoephedrine HCl; brompheniramine hydrobromide; dextromethorphan hydrobromide] 30•3•15 mg/5 mL; 40•4•20 mg/5 mL; 50•3•30 mg/5 mL

TGQ 7.5PEH/4BRM/15DM oral liquid ℞ *decongestant; antihistamine; antitussive* [phenylephrine HCl; brompheniramine maleate; dextromethorphan hydrobromide] 7.5•4• 15 mg/5 mL

TH (theophylline) [q.v.]

TH (thyroid hormone) [see: levothyroxine sodium]

THA (tetrahydroaminoacridine or tetrahydroacridinamine) [see: tacrine HCl]

thalidomide USAN, INN, BAN *immunomodulator for erythema nodosum leprosum (ENL; orphan) and multiple myeloma (orphan); investigational (orphan) for aphthous ulcers, graft vs. host disease, AIDS-wasting syndrome, Crohn disease, mycobacterial infections, and various cancers*

Thalitone tablets ℞ *antihypertensive; diuretic for congestive heart failure, hepatic cirrhosis, and corticosteroid therapy* [chlorthalidone] 15 mg

thallium *element (Tl)* ▣ thulium

thallous chloride Tl 201 USAN, USP *radiopaque contrast medium; radioactive agent*

Thalomid capsules ℞ *immunomodulator for erythema nodosum leprosum (ENL; orphan) and multiple myeloma (orphan); investigational (orphan) for aphthous ulcers, graft vs. host disease, AIDS-wasting syndrome, Crohn disease, mycobacterial infections, and various cancers* [thalidomide] 50, 100, 200 mg

Tham IV infusion ℞ *systemic alkalizer; corrects acidosis associated with cardiac bypass surgery or cardiac arrest* [tromethamine] 18 g/500 mL (150 mEq/ 500 mL)

thaumatin BAN

THC (tetrahydrocannabinol) [q.v.]

THC (thiocarbanidin)

theanine (L-theanine) *natural extract of green tea that produces calming and relaxing effects without drowsiness; effective in controlling PMS symptoms; increases brain levels of the neurotransmitters GABA and dopamine, which increase alpha brain wave activity*

thebacon INN, BAN ▣ tebuquine; Topicaine

theine [see: caffeine]

Thelin *endothelin receptor antagonist (ERA) vasodilator; investigational (NDA filed) once-daily oral antihypertensive for pulmonary arterial hypertension (PAH)* [sitaxsentan sodium]

thenalidine INN ▣ tenylidone

thenium closilate INN *veterinary anthelmintic* [also: thenium closylate]

thenium closylate USAN *veterinary anthelmintic* [also: thenium closilate]

thenyldiamine INN

thenylpyramine HCl [see: methapyrilene HCl]

Theo-24 extended-release capsules ℞ *antiasthmatic; bronchodilator* [theophylline] 100, 200, 300, 400 mg

theobromine NF

theobromine calcium salicylate NF

theobromine sodium acetate NF

theobromine sodium salicylate NF

Theobromo cacao medicinal herb [see: cocoa]

Theochron extended-release tablets ℞ *antiasthmatic; bronchodilator* [theophylline] 100, 200, 300, 450 mg ⧅ tacrine

theoclate BAN *combining name for radicals or groups* [also: teoclate]

theodrenaline INN, BAN

Theodrine tablets (discontinued 2007) OTC *antiasthmatic; bronchodilator; decongestant* [theophylline; ephedrine HCl] 120•22.5 mg

theofibrate USAN *antihyperlipoproteinemic* [also: etofylline clofibrate]

Theolair tablets (discontinued 2008) ℞ *antiasthmatic; bronchodilator* [theophylline] 125 mg

Theolair-SR sustained-release tablets (discontinued 2008) ℞ *antiasthmatic; bronchodilator* [theophylline] 200, 250, 300, 500 mg

Theolate oral liquid (discontinued 2007) ℞ *antiasthmatic; bronchodilator; expectorant* [theophylline; guaifenesin] 150•90 mg/15 mL ⧅ Twilite

Theomax DF pediatric syrup (discontinued 2007) ℞ *antiasthmatic; bronchodilator; decongestant; antihistamine* [theophylline; ephedrine sulfate; hydroxyzine HCl; alcohol 5%] 97.5•18.75•7.5 mg/15 mL

theophyldine [see: aminophylline]

theophyllamine [see: aminophylline]

Theophyllin KI elixir (discontinued 2007) ℞ *antiasthmatic; bronchodilator; expectorant* [theophylline; potassium iodide] 80•130 mg/15 mL

theophylline (TH) USP, BAN *bronchodilator* 100, 125, 200, 300, 400, 450, 600 mg oral; 80 mg/15 mL oral; 0.8, 1.6, 2, 3.2, 4 mg/mL injection

theophylline aminoisobutanol [see: ambuphylline]

theophylline calcium salicylate *bronchodilator*

theophylline ethylenediamine [now: aminophylline]

theophylline monohydrate [see: theophylline]

theophylline olamine USP

theophylline sodium acetate NF

theophylline sodium glycinate USP *smooth muscle relaxant*

Thera caplets, tablets OTC *vitamin supplement* [multiple vitamins; folic acid; biotin] ±•400•30 mcg

Thera oral liquid OTC *vitamin supplement* [multiple vitamins]

Thera Hematinic tablets (discontinued 2008) OTC *vitamin/iron supplement* [multiple vitamins; iron (as ferrous fumarate); folic acid] ±•66.7•0.33 mg

Thera Multi-Vitamin oral liquid (discontinued 2008) OTC *vitamin supplement* [multiple vitamins]

Thera Tears Lubricant eye drops OTC *moisturizer/lubricant* [carboxymethylcellulose] 0.25%

Therabid tablets (discontinued 2008) OTC *vitamin supplement* [multiple vitamins]

theraccines *a class of vaccines with therapeutic action, usually used to help prevent the spread of cancer*

TheraCLEC-Total *investigational (orphan) digestive enzymes for pancreatic insufficiency* [pancrelipase (amylase; lipase; protease)]

TheraCys powder for intravesical instillation ℞ *antineoplastic for urinary bladder cancer* [BCG vaccine, live] 81 mg (1.8–19.2 × 10⁸ CFU)

TheraDerm lotion OTC *emollient/protectant* [castor oil; lanolin; mineral oil; PEG] ⧅ Triderm

TheraDerm transdermal patch *investigational (Phase II, orphan) for AIDS-wasting syndrome* [testosterone]

TheraFlu Cold & Cough powder for oral solution OTC *antitussive; antihistamine; decongestant* [dextromethorphan hydrobromide; pheniramine maleate; phenylephrine HCl] 20•20•20 mg/pkt.

TheraFlu Cold & Sore Throat powder for oral solution OTC *decongestant; antihistamine; analgesic; antipyretic* [phenylephrine HCl; pheniramine maleate; acetaminophen] 10•20•325 mg/pkt.

TheraFlu Daytime Severe Cold powder for oral solution (discontinued 2009) OTC *decongestant; analgesic; antipyretic* [phenylephrine HCl; acetaminophen] 10•650 mg/pkt.

TheraFlu Daytime Severe Cold & Cough caplets, powder for oral solution OTC *antitussive; decongestant; analgesic; antipyretic* [dextromethorphan hydrobromide; phenylephrine HCl; acetaminophen] 10•5•325 mg; 20•10•650 mg/pkt.

Theraflu Flu & Chest Congestion powder for oral solution OTC *expectorant; analgesic; antipyretic* [guaifenesin; acetaminophen] 400•1000 mg

TheraFlu Flu & Sore Throat powder for oral solution OTC *decongestant; antihistamine; analgesic; antipyretic* [phenylephrine HCl; pheniramine maleate; acetaminophen] 10•20•650 mg/pkt.

TheraFlu Nighttime Severe Cold caplets OTC *antitussive; decongestant; antihistamine; decongestant; analgesic; antipyretic* [dextromethorphan hydrobromide; chlorpheniramine maleate; phenylephrine HCl; acetaminophen] 10•2•5•325 mg

TheraFlu Nighttime Severe Cold powder for oral solution (discontinued 2009) OTC *decongestant; antihistamine; analgesic; antipyretic* [phenylephrine HCl; pheniramine maleate; acetaminophen] 10•20•650 mg/pkt.

TheraFlu Nighttime Severe Cough & Cold; TheraFlu Sugar-Free Nighttime Severe Cough & Cold powder for oral solution OTC *decongestant; antihistamine; sleep aid; analgesic; antipyretic* [phenylephrine HCl; diphenhydramine HCl; acetaminophen] 10•25•650 mg/pkt.

Theraflu Thin Strips Daytime Cough & Cold orally disintegrating film OTC *antitussive; decongestant* [dextromethorphan hydrobromide; phenylephrine HCl] 20•10 mg

TheraFlu Thin Strips Long Acting Cough orally disintegrating film OTC *antitussive* [dextromethorphan hydrobromide] 15 mg

Theraflu Thin Strips Nighttime Cold & Cough orally disintegrating film OTC *decongestant; antihistamine; sleep aid* [phenylephrine HCl; diphenhydramine HCl] 10•25 mg

TheraFlu Warming Relief Daytime Multi-Symptom Cold caplets OTC *antitussive; decongestant; analgesic; antipyretic* [dextromethorphan hydrobromide; phenylephrine HCl; acetaminophen] 10•5•325 mg

TheraFlu Warming Relief Flu & Sore Throat oral liquid OTC *decongestant; antihistamine; sleep aid; analgesic; antipyretic* [phenylephrine HCl; diphenhydramine HCl; acetaminophen; alcohol 10%] 1.67•4.16•108.3 mg/5 mL

Thera-Flur; Thera-Flur-N gel for self-application ℞ *dental caries preventative* [fluoride (as sodium fluoride)] 0.5% (1.1%)

Thera-Gesic cream OTC *analgesic; mild anesthetic; antipruritic; counterirritant* [methyl salicylate; menthol] 15%• ≟

Theragran caplets (discontinued 2008) OTC *vitamin supplement* [multiple vitamins; folic acid; biotin] ≟• 400•30 mcg

Theragran oral liquid (discontinued 2008) OTC *vitamin supplement* [multiple vitamins]

Theragran AntiOxidant softgels (discontinued 2008) OTC *vitamin/mineral supplement* [vitamins A, C, and E; multiple minerals] 5000 IU•250 mg•200 IU• ±

Theragran Stress Formula tablets (discontinued 2008) OTC *vitamin/iron supplement* [multiple B vitamins; vitamins C and E; iron (as ferrous fumarate); folic acid; biotin] ± •600 mg•30 IU•27 mg•0.4 mg•45 mcg

Theragyn *investigational (Phase III, orphan) adjunctive treatment for ovarian cancer* [monoclonal antibody to polymorphic epithelial mucin, murine]

Thera-Hist Cold & Allergy pediatric syrup (discontinued 2007) OTC *decongestant; antihistamine* [pseudoephedrine HCl; chlorpheniramine maleate] 30•2 mg/10 mL

Thera-Hist Cold & Cough syrup (discontinued 2007) OTC *antitussive; antihistamine; decongestant* [dextromethorphan hydrobromide; chlorpheniramine maleate; pseudoephedrine HCl] 10•2•30 mg/10 mL

Thera-Hist Expectorant Chest Congestion pediatric oral liquid (discontinued 2007) OTC *decongestant; expectorant* [pseudoephedrine HCl; guaifenesin] 15•50 mg/5 mL

Thera-Ject (trademarked delivery form) *prefilled disposable syringe*

Thera-M with Minerals tablets OTC *vitamin/mineral/calcium/iron supplement* [multiple vitamins & minerals; calcium (as tricalcium phosphate); iron (as ferrous fumarate); folic acid; biotin] ± •40•27•0.4•0.035 mg

Theramill Plus capsules OTC *vitamin/mineral/calcium/iron supplement* [multiple vitamins & minerals; calcium (as citrate malate, glycinate, and carbonate); iron (as glycine chelate); folic acid] ± •66.7•2.5•0.07 mg

TheraPatch Cold Sore transmucosal patch OTC *mucous membrane anesthetic; antipruritic; counterirritant; emollient* [lidocaine; camphor; aloe vera; eucalyptus oil] 4%•0.5%• ± • ±

TheraPatch Vapor Patch for Kids Cough Suppressant (discontinued 2007) OTC *mild anesthetic; antipruritic; counterirritant* [camphor; menthol] 4.7%•2.6%

Therapeutic tablets OTC *vitamin supplement* [multiple vitamins; folic acid; biotin] ± •400•30 mcg

Therapeutic B with C capsules OTC *vitamin supplement* [multiple B vitamins; vitamin C] ± •300 mg

Therapeutic Bath lotion, oil OTC *moisturizer; emollient*

Therapeutic Mineral Ice; Therapeutic Mineral Ice Exercise Formula gel OTC *mild anesthetic; antipruritic; counterirritant* [menthol] 2%; 4%

Therapeutic-H tablets (discontinued 2008) OTC *vitamin/iron supplement* [multiple vitamins; iron (as ferrous fumarate); folic acid] ± •66.7•0.33 mg

Therapeutic-M tablets (discontinued 2008) OTC *vitamin/mineral/iron supplement* [multiple vitamins & minerals; iron; folic acid; biotin] ± •27 mg•0.4 mg•30 mcg

Thera-Plus oral liquid OTC *vitamin supplement* [vitamins A, B₁, B₂, B₃, B₅, B₆, B₁₂, C, and D] 5000•10•10•100•21.4•4.1•0.005•200•400 mg

Therapy Ice gel OTC *mild anesthetic; antipruritic; counterirritant* [menthol] 2%

TheraTears gel OTC *ophthalmic moisturizer/lubricant* [carboxymethylcellulose sodium] 1%

Theravee tablets (discontinued 2008) OTC *vitamin supplement* [multiple vitamins; folic acid; biotin] ± •400• 15 mcg ⑨ Thrive

Theravee Hematinic tablets (discontinued 2008) OTC *vitamin/iron supplement* [multiple vitamins; iron (as ferrous fumarate); folic acid] ± •66.7• 0.33 mg

Theravee-M tablets (discontinued 2008) OTC *vitamin/mineral/iron supplement* [multiple vitamins & minerals; iron; folic acid; biotin] ± •27 mg•0.4 mg•15 mcg

Theravim tablets (discontinued 2008) OTC *vitamin supplement* [multiple vitamins; folic acid; biotin] ±•400•35 mcg

Theravim-M film-coated tablets OTC *vitamin/mineral/calcium/iron supplement* [multiple vitamins & minerals; calcium (as dicalcium phosphate); iron (as ferrous fumarate); folic acid; biotin] ±•40•27•0.4•0.03 mg

Theravite oral liquid OTC *vitamin supplement* [multiple vitamins]

Therems tablets (discontinued 2008) OTC *vitamin supplement* [multiple vitamins; folic acid; biotin] ±•400•15 mcg

Therems-H film-coated tablets OTC *vitamin/mineral/calcium supplement* [multiple vitamins & minerals; calcium; folic acid] ±•130•0.33 mg

Therems-M tablets OTC *vitamin/mineral/calcium supplement* [multiple vitamins & minerals; calcium; folic acid; biotin] ±•40•0.4•0.03 mg

Therevac-Plus disposable enema OTC *hyperosmotic laxative; stool softener; local anesthetic* [glycerin; docusate sodium; benzocaine] 275•283•20 mg

Therevac-SB disposable enema OTC *hyperosmotic laxative; stool softener* [glycerin; docusate sodium] 275•283 mg

Thermazene cream ℞ *broad-spectrum bactericidal for adjunctive burn treatment* [silver sulfadiazine] 10 mg/g ⊡ Trimo-San

ThermoDox IV injection *investigational (Phase III, orphan) antineoplastic for primary liver cancer* [doxorubicin HCl, liposome-encapsulated, heat-treated]

ThexForte caplets OTC *vitamin supplement* [multiple B vitamins; vitamin C] ±•500 mg

THF (thymic humoral factor) [q.v.]

thiabendazole (TBZ) USAN, USP *anthelmintic for strongyloidiasis (threadworm), larva migrans, and trichinosis* [also: tiabendazole]

thiabutazide [see: buthiazide]

thiacetarsamide sodium INN

thiacetazone BAN [also: thioacetazone]

thialbarbital INN [also: thialbarbitone]

thialbarbitone BAN [also: thialbarbital]

thialisobumal sodium [see: buthalital sodium]

thiamazole INN *thyroid inhibitor* [also: methimazole]

thiambutosine INN, BAN

Thiamilate enteric-coated tablets OTC *vitamin B_1 supplement* [thiamine HCl] 20 mg

thiamine (vitamin B_1) INN *water-soluble vitamin; enzyme cofactor* [also: thiamine HCl; compare: benfotiamine]

thiamine HCl (vitamin B_1) USP *water-soluble vitamin; enzyme cofactor* [also: thiamine; compare: benfotiamine] 25, 50, 100, 250 mg oral; 100 mg/mL injection

thiamine mononitrate USP *vitamin B_1; enzyme cofactor*

thiamine propyl disulfide [see: prosultiamine]

thiaminogen *medicinal herb* [see: rice bran oil]

thiamiprine USAN *antineoplastic* [also: tiamiprine] ⊡ timiperone

thiamphenicol USAN, INN, BAN *antibacterial*

thiamylal USP *barbiturate general anesthetic* ⊡ timolol

thiamylal sodium USP, JAN *barbiturate general anesthetic*

thiazesim HCl USAN *antidepressant* [also: tiazesim]

thiazides *a class of diuretic agents that increase urinary excretion of sodium and chloride in approximately equal amounts* ⊡ TZDs

thiazinamium chloride USAN *antiallergic*

thiazinamium metilsulfate INN

4-thiazolidinecarboxylic acid [see: timonacic]

thiazolidinediones (TZDs) *a class of antidiabetic agents that increase cellular response to insulin without increasing insulin secretion*

thiazolsulfone [see: thiazosulfone]

thiazosulfone INN
thiazothielite [see: antienite]
thiazothienol [see: antazonite]
thienamycins *a class of antibiotics*
thienobenzodiazepines *a class of novel (atypical) antipsychotic agents*
thiethylperazine USAN, INN *antiemetic; antidopaminergic*
thiethylperazine malate USP *antiemetic; antipsychotic*
thiethylperazine maleate USAN, USP *antiemetic for postoperative nausea and vomiting*
thihexinol methylbromide NF, INN
thimbleberry *medicinal herb* [see: blackberry]
thimerfonate sodium USAN *topical anti-infective* [also: sodium timerfonate]
thimerosal USP *topical anti-infective; preservative (49% mercury)* [also: thiomersal] 1:1000 topical
thioacetazone INN [also: thiacetazone]
thiocarbanidin (THC)
thiocarlide BAN [also: tiocarlide]
thiocolchicine glycoside [see: thiocolchicoside]
thiocolchicoside INN
thioctan; thioctacid; thioctic acid *natural antioxidant* [see: alpha lipoic acid]
thiocyanate sodium NF
thiodiglycol INN
thiodiphenylamine [see: phenothiazine]
thiofuradene INN
thioguanine (6-TG) USAN, USP *antimetabolite antineoplastic for acute non-lymphocytic leukemias (ANLL); also used for psoriasis, ulcerative colitis, and Crohn disease* [also: tioguanine]
thiohexallymal [see: thialbarbital]
thiohexamide INN
Thiola *sugar-coated tablets* R̥ *prevention of cystine nephrolithiasis in homozygous cystinuria (orphan)* [tiopronin] 100 mg
thiomebumal sodium [see: thiopental sodium]
thiomersal INN, BAN *topical anti-infective; preservative* [also: thimerosal]

thiomesterone BAN [also: tiomesterone]
thiomicid [see: thioacetazone; thiacetazone]
thioparamizone [see: thioacetazone; thiacetazone]
thiopental sodium USP, INN, JAN *barbiturate general anesthetic; anticonvulsant* [also: thiopentone sodium] 2%, 2.5% (20, 25 mg/mL) injection
thiopentone sodium BAN *general anesthetic; anticonvulsant* [also: thiopental sodium]
thiophanate BAN
thiophosphoramide [see: thiotepa]
Thioplex *powder for IV, intracavitary, or intravesical injection* R̥ *alkylating antineoplastic for lymphomas and carcinoma of the breast, ovary, or bladder* [thiotepa] 15 mg
thiopropazate INN [also: thiopropazate HCl]
thiopropazate HCl NF [also: thiopropazate]
thioproperazine INN, BAN *phenothiazine antipsychotic* [also: thioproperazine mesylate]
thioproperazine mesylate *phenothiazine antipsychotic* [also: thioproperazine]
thioproperazine methanesulfonate [see: thioproperazine mesylate]
thioridazine USAN, USP, INN *conventional (typical) phenothiazine antipsychotic for schizophrenia; sedative*
thioridazine HCl USP *conventional (typical) phenothiazine antipsychotic for schizophrenia; sedative* 10, 15, 25, 50, 100, 150, 200 mg oral
thiosalan USAN *disinfectant* [also: tiosalan] 2 Tessalon
thiosulfuric acid, disodium salt pentahydrate [see: sodium thiosulfate]
thiotepa USP, INN, BAN, JAN *alkylating antineoplastic for lymphomas and carcinoma of the breast, ovary, or bladder* 15, 30 mg injection
thiotetrabarbital INN
thiothixene USAN, USP, BAN *conventional (typical) thioxanthene antipsy-*

chotic for schizophrenia [also: tiotix-ene] 1, 2, 5, 10 mg oral

thiothixene HCl USAN, USP *conventional (typical) thioxanthene antipsychotic for schizophrenia*

thiouracil ⊠ Tearisol

thiourea *antioxidant*

thioxanthenes *a class of dopamine receptor antagonists with conventional (typical) antipsychotic activity*

thioxolone BAN [also: tioxolone]

thiphenamil HCl USAN *smooth muscle relaxant* [also: tifenamil]

thiphencillin potassium USAN *antibacterial* [also: tifencillin]

thiram USAN, INN *antifungal* ⊠ thorium; Triam

thistle, bitter; holy thistle; Saint Benedict thistle; spotted thistle *medicinal herb* [see: blessed thistle]

thistle, carline; ground thistle *medicinal herb* [see: carline thistle]

thonzonium bromide USAN, USP *detergent; surface-active agent* [also: tonzonium bromide]

thonzylamine HCl USAN, INN

Thorazine tablets, IV or IM injection, suppositories (discontinued 2008) ℞ *conventional antipsychotic for schizophrenia, manic episodes of a bipolar disorder, pediatric hyperactivity, and severe pediatric behavioral problems; treatment for acute intermittent porphyria, nausea/vomiting, and intractable hiccoughs* [chlorpromazine] 25, 50, 100, 200 mg; 25 mg/mL; 100 mg ⊠ Terocin; tyrosine

thorium *element (Th)* ⊠ thiram; Triam

thorn, Egyptian *medicinal herb* [see: acacia]

thorn-apple *medicinal herb* [see: hawthorn; jimsonweed]

thousand-leaf; thousand seal *medicinal herb* [see: yarrow]

thozalinone USAN *antidepressant* [also: tozalinone]

THQ (tetrahydroxybenzoquinone) [see: tetroquinone]

THR (trishydroxyethyl rutin) [see: troxerutin]

3 in 1 Toothache Relief topical liquid, gum, oral lotion/gel OTC *mucous membrane anesthetic* [benzocaine]

three-leaved nightshade *medicinal herb* [see: birthroot]

3TC [now: lamivudine]

threonine (L-threonine) USAN, USP, INN *essential amino acid; symbols: Thr, T; investigational (orphan) for familial spastic paraparesis and amyotrophic lateral sclerosis*

Threostat *investigational (orphan) for familial spastic paraparesis and amyotrophic lateral sclerosis* [L-threonine]

Thrive chewing gum OTC *smoking cessation aid for the relief of nicotine withdrawal symptoms* [nicotine polacrilex] 2, 4 mg ⊠ Theravee

Throat Discs lozenges OTC *analgesic; counterirritant* [capsicum; peppermint oil]

throatwort *medicinal herb* [see: figwort; foxglove]

Thrombate III powder for IV infusion ℞ *for thrombosis and pulmonary emboli due to congenital AT-III deficiency (orphan)* [antithrombin III, human] 500 IU

Thrombi-Gel 10; Thrombi-Gel 40; Thrombi-Gel 100 medicated pad ℞ *topical hemostat for wound management* [thrombin, bovine] 1000 U; 1000 U; 20 000 U

thrombin USP, INN *topical hemostat for surgery; trauma dressing for wound management*

thrombin receptor antagonist (TRA) *investigational (Phase III) antiplatelet agent*

Thrombinar powder (discontinued 2010) ℞ *topical hemostat for surgery* [thrombin] 1000, 5000, 50 000 U

Thrombin-JMI powder for solution ℞ *topical hemostat for surgery* [thrombin, bovine] 1000 U/mL (10 000, 20 000 U/vial)

thrombinogen (prothrombin)

Thrombi-Pad 3 × 3 medicated pad ℞ *topical hemostat for wound management* [thrombin, bovine] 200 U

Thrombogen powder (discontinued 2008) ℞ *topical hemostat for surgery* [thrombin] 1000, 5000, 10 000, 20 000 IU

thrombolytics *a class of enzymes that dissolve blood clots, used emergently to treat stroke, pulmonary embolus, and myocardial infarct*

thromboplastin USP

thrombopoietin, recombinant human *investigational (orphan) adjunct to hematopoietic stem cell transplantation*

Thrombostat powder (discontinued 2010) ℞ *topical hemostat for surgery* [thrombin] 5000, 10 000, 20 000 IU

throw-wort *medicinal herb* [see: motherwort]

thulium *element (Tm)* 🔲 thallium

thunder god vine (Tripterygium wilfordii) *plant medicinal herb for abscesses, autoimmune diseases, boils, fever, inflammation, tumors, and viruses; also used as an insecticide to kill maggots or larvae and as a rat and bird poison* [also: triptolide]

thymalfasin USAN *vaccine enhancer for hepatitis C, cancer, and infectious diseases; investigational (Phase III, orphan) for chronic active hepatitis B; investigational (orphan) for DiGeorge syndrome with immune defects and hepatocellular carcinoma*

thyme (Thymus serpyllum; T. vulgaris) *plant medicinal herb for acute bronchitis, colic, digestive disorders, gas, gout, headache, laryngitis, lung congestion, sciatica, and throat disorders*

thymidylate synthase (TS) inhibitors *a class of folate-based antineoplastics*

thymocartin INN

thymoctonan INN *antiviral*

Thymoglobulin powder for IV infusion ℞ *passive immunizing agent to prevent allograft rejection of renal transplants (orphan); investigational (orphan) for myelodysplastic syndrome (MDS); also used for other transplants and aplastic anemia* [antithymocyte globulin, rabbit] 25 mg

thymol NF *stabilizer; topical antiseptic*

thymol iodide NF

thymopentin USAN, INN, BAN *immunoregulator*

thymopoietin 32-36 [now: thymopentin]

thymosin alpha-1 [now: thymalfasin]

thymosin beta-4 *investigational (orphan) for epidermolysis bullosa*

thymostimulin INN *immunomodulator*

thymotrinan INN

thymoxamine BAN [also: moxisylyte]

thymoxamine HCl *investigational (orphan) to reverse phenylephrine-induced mydriasis in patients at risk for acute angle-closure glaucoma*

Thymus serpyllum; T. vulgaris *medicinal herb* [see: thyme]

Thyro-Block tablets (discontinued 2010) ℞ *thyroid saturation agent to block the uptake of radioactive iodine after a nuclear accident or attack* [potassium iodide] 130 mg

thyrocalcitonin [see: calcitonin]

Thyrogen powder for IM injection ℞ *recombinant human thyroid-stimulating hormone (rhTSH); diagnostic aid for thyroid cancer (orphan); adjunctive treatment for thyroid cancer (orphan)* [thyrotropin alfa] 1.1 mg 🔲 tarragon; Torecan; Treagan; Trocaine

thyroglobulin (TG) USAN, USP, INN *thyroid hormone for hypothyroidism or thyroid cancer*

thyroid USP *natural thyroid hormone (a 4:1 mixture of T_4 and T_3)* (Note: thyroid dosage is sometimes given in grains [gr.] and sometimes in milligrams [mg]. The exact equivalent is: 1 gr.=64.8 mg, but rounding to 65 mg is common.) 32.5, 65, 130, 195 mg oral 🔲 Triad

thyroid hormone (TH) [see: levothyroxine sodium]

thyroid-stimulating hormone (TSH) [see: thyrotropin]

Thyrolar tablets ℞ *synthetic thyroid hormone (a 4:1 mixture of T_4 and T_3)* [liotrix] 15, 30, 60, 120, 180 mg

thyromedan HCl USAN *thyromimetic* [also: tyromedan]

thyropropic acid INN

ThyroSafe tablets OTC *thyroid saturation agent to block the uptake of radioactive iodine after a nuclear accident or attack (orphan)* [potassium iodide] 65 mg

ThyroShield oral solution OTC *thyroid saturation agent to block the uptake of radioactive iodine after a nuclear accident or attack (orphan)* [potassium iodide] 65 mg/mL

Thyro-Tabs tablets ℞ *synthetic thyroid hormone (T_4 fraction only)* [levothyroxine sodium] 25, 50, 75, 88, 100, 112, 125, 150, 175, 200, 300 mcg

thyrotrophic hormone [see: thyrotrophin]

thyrotrophin INN *thyroid-stimulating hormone* [also: thyrotropin]

thyrotropin *thyroid-stimulating hormone; in vivo diagnostic aid for thyroid function* [also: thyrotrophin]

thyrotropin alfa USAN *recombinant human thyroid-stimulating hormone (rhTSH); diagnostic aid for thyroid cancer (orphan); adjunctive treatment for thyroid cancer (orphan)*

thyrotropin-releasing hormone (TRH) [see: protirelin]

thyroxine BAN *synthetic thyroid hormone (T_4 fraction only)* [also: levothyroxine sodium] 🔢 TriOxin

D-thyroxine [see: dextrothyroxine sodium]

L-thyroxine [see: levothyroxine sodium]

thyroxine I 125 USAN *radioactive agent* 🔢 TriOxin

thyroxine I 131 USAN *radioactive agent* 🔢 TriOxin

tiabendazole INN *anthelmintic* [also: thiabendazole]

tiacrilast USAN, INN *antiallergic*

tiacrilast sodium USAN *antiallergic*

tiadenol INN

tiafibrate INN

tiagabine INN *anticonvulsant; adjunctive treatment for partial seizures*

tiagabine HCl USAN *anticonvulsant; adjunctive treatment for partial seizures*

tiamenidine USAN, INN *antihypertensive*

tiamenidine HCl USAN, INN *antihypertensive*

tiametonium iodide INN

tiamiprine INN *antineoplastic* [also: thiamiprine]

tiamizide INN *diuretic; antihypertensive* [also: diapamide]

tiamulin USAN, INN *veterinary antibacterial*

tiamulin fumarate USAN *veterinary antibacterial*

tianafac INN

tianeptine INN

tiapamil INN, BAN *antagonist to calcium* [also: tiapamil HCl]

tiapamil HCl USAN *antagonist to calcium* [also: tiapamil]

tiapirinol INN

tiapride INN *investigational (orphan) for Tourette syndrome*

tiaprofenic acid INN *nonsteroidal antiinflammatory drug (NSAID)*

tiaprost INN

tiaramide INN, BAN *antiasthmatic* [also: tiaramide HCl]

tiaramide HCl USAN *antiasthmatic* [also: tiaramide]

Tiazac extended-release capsules ℞ *antihypertensive; antianginal; antiarrhythmic; calcium channel blocker* [diltiazem HCl] 120, 180, 240, 300, 360, 420 mg

tiazesim INN *antidepressant* [also: thiazesim HCl]

tiazesim HCl [see: thiazesim HCl]

tiazofurin USAN *investigational (Phase II/III, orphan) antineoplastic for chronic myelogenous leukemia* [also: tiazofurine]

tiazofurine INN *antineoplastic* [also: tiazofurin]

tiazuril USAN, INN *coccidiostat for poultry*

tibalosin INN

Tibamine LA sustained-release tablets (discontinued 2009) ℞ *decongestant; antihistamine* [pseudoephedrine HCl; chlorpheniramine maleate] 120•12 mg

tibenelast sodium USAN *antiasthmatic; bronchodilator*

tibenzate INN

tibezonium iodide INN

tibolone USAN, INN, BAN *synthetic steroid*

tibric acid USAN, INN *antihyperlipoproteinemic*

tibrofan USAN, INN *disinfectant*

ticabesone INN *corticosteroid; anti-inflammatory* [also: ticabesone propionate]

ticabesone propionate USAN *corticosteroid; anti-inflammatory* [also: ticabesone]

ticagrelor *reversible adenosine diphosphate (ADP) receptor antagonist; oral antiplatelet agent to prevent thrombotic events*

Ticar *powder for IV or IM injection (discontinued 2009)* R̶ *extended-spectrum penicillin antibiotic* [ticarcillin disodium] 3 g/vial

ticarbodine USAN, INN *anthelmintic*

ticarcillin INN *extended-spectrum penicillin antibiotic* [also: ticarcillin disodium]

ticarcillin cresyl sodium USAN *extended-spectrum penicillin antibiotic*

ticarcillin disodium USAN, USP *extended-spectrum penicillin antibiotic* [also: ticarcillin]

Tice BCG *powder for intravesical instillation* R̶ *antineoplastic for urinary bladder cancer* [BCG vaccine, live, Tice strain] 50 mg (1–8 × 10^8 CFU)

tickweed *medicinal herb* [see: pennyroyal]

ticlatone USAN, INN *antibacterial; antifungal*

Ticlid *film-coated tablets* R̶ *platelet aggregation inhibitor for stroke* [ticlopidine HCl] 250 mg

ticlopidine INN, BAN *platelet aggregation inhibitor* [also: ticlopidine HCl]

ticlopidine HCl USAN *platelet aggregation inhibitor for stroke* [also: ticlopidine] 250 mg oral

ticolubant USAN *leukotriene B₄ receptor antagonist for psoriasis*

ticrynafen USAN *diuretic; uricosuric; antihypertensive* [also: tienilic acid]

Tidefen DM *extended-release caplets* R̶ *antitussive; decongestant; expectorant* [dextromethorphan hydrobromide; pseudoephedrine HCl; guaifenesin] 60•90•800 mg

tidembersat USAN *antimigraine*

tidiacic INN

tiemonium iodide INN, BAN

tienilic acid INN *diuretic; uricosuric; antihypertensive* [also: ticrynafen]

tienocarbine INN

tienopramine INN

tienoxolol INN

tifacogin USAN *anticoagulant; lipoprotein-associated coagulation inhibitor (LACI); recombinant tissue factor pathway inhibitor*

tifemoxone INN

tifenamil INN *smooth muscle relaxant* [also: thiphenamil HCl]

tifenamil HCl [see: thiphenamil HCl]

tifencillin INN *antibacterial* [also: thiphencillin potassium]

tifencillin potassium [see: thiphencillin potassium]

tiflamizole INN

tiflorex INN

tifluadom INN

tiflucarbine INN

tiformin INN [also: tyformin]

tifurac INN *analgesic* [also: tifurac sodium]

tifurac sodium USAN *analgesic* [also: tifurac]

TIG (tetanus immune globulin) [q.v.]

Tigan *capsules, IM injection* R̶ *anticholinergic; post-surgical antiemetic* [trimethobenzamide HCl] 300 mg; 100 mg/mL

Tigan *suppositories, pediatric suppositories (removed from the market in 2007 due to lack of efficacy)* R̶ *anticholinergic; post-surgical antiemetic; local anesthetic* [trimethobenzamide HCl; benzocaine] 200 mg•2%; 100 mg•2%

tigecycline *broad-spectrum glycylcycline antibiotic for intra-abdominal and complicated skin structure infections,* *methicillin-resistant* Staphylococcus aureus *(MRSA), and community-acquired bacterial pneumonia (CABP)*

tigemonam INN *antimicrobial* [also: tigemonam dicholine]

tigemonam dicholine USAN *antimicrobial* [also: tigemonam]

Tiger Balm ointment OTC *mild anesthetic; antipruritic; counterirritant* [menthol; camphor] 8%•11%

tigestol USAN, INN *progestin*

tigloidine INN, BAN

tiglyl*pseudo*tropine [see: tigloidine]

tiglyltropeine [see: tropigline]

Tikosyn capsules ℞ *antiarrhythmic for the conversion of atrial fibrillation/atrial flutter* [dofetilide] 125, 250, 500 mcg ⃞ toquizine

tilactase INN *digestive enzyme*

Tilade oral inhalation aerosol (discontinued 2008) ℞ *respiratory antiinflammatory; mast cell stabilizer; antiasthmatic; bronchodilator* [nedocromil sodium] 1.75 mg/dose

tilbroquinol INN

tiletamine INN *anesthetic; anticonvulsant* [also: tiletamine HCl]

tiletamine HCl USAN *anesthetic; anticonvulsant* [also: tiletamine]

Tilia americana; T. cordata; T. europaea; T. platyphyllos medicinal herb [see: linden tree]

Tilia Fe tablets (in packs of 28) ℞ *triphasic oral contraceptive; iron supplement* [norethindrone acetate; ethinyl estradiol; ferrous fumarate]
Phase 1 (5 days): 1•0.02•75 mg;
Phase 2 (7 days): 1•0.03•75 mg;
Phase 3 (9 days): 1•0.035•75 mg;
Counters (7 days): 0•0•75 mg

tilidate HCl BAN *analgesic* [also: tilidine HCl; tilidine]

tilidine INN *analgesic* [also: tilidine HCl; tilidate HCl]

tilidine HCl USAN *analgesic* [also: tilidine; tilidate HCl]

tiliquinol INN

tilisolol INN

tilmicosin USAN, INN, BAN *veterinary antibacterial*

tilmicosin phosphate USAN *veterinary antibacterial*

tilomisole USAN, INN *immunoregulator*

tilorone INN *antiviral* [also: tilorone HCl]

tilorone HCl USAN *antiviral* [also: tilorone]

tilozepine INN

tilsuprost INN

Tiltab (trademarked dosage form) *film-coated tablets*

tiludronate disodium USAN *bisphosphonate bone resorption inhibitor for Paget disease; also used for osteoporosis* (base=83%)

tiludronic acid INN

timcodar dimesylate USAN *antineoplastic adjunct to prevent emergence of multidrug-resistant tumors*

Timecap (trademarked dosage form) *sustained-release capsule*

Timecelle (trademarked dosage form) *timed-release capsule*

timefurone USAN, INN *antiatherosclerotic*

timegadine INN

Time-Hist sustained-release capsules (discontinued 2007) ℞ *decongestant; antihistamine* [pseudoephedrine HCl; chlorpheniramine maleate] 120•8 mg

Time-Hist QD extended-release tablets ℞ *decongestant; antihistamine; anticholinergic to dry mucosal secretions* [pseudoephedrine HCl; chlorpheniramine maleate; methscopolamine bromide] 120•6•2.5 mg

timelotem INN

Timentin powder or frozen premix for IV infusion ℞ *extended-spectrum penicillin antibiotic plus synergist* [ticarcillin disodium; clavulanate potassium] 3•0.1 g

timepidium bromide INN

Time-Release Balanced B-50 timed-release tablets OTC *vitamin/mineral supplement* [multiple B vitamins and minerals; folic acid; biotin] ≚•400•50 mcg

Timespan (trademarked dosage form) *timed-release tablets*

Timesules (dosage form) *sustained-release capsules*

timiperone INN

timobesone INN *topical adrenocortical steroid* [also: timobesone acetate]

timobesone acetate USAN *topical adrenocortical steroid* [also: timobesone]

timofibrate INN

Timolide 10-25 tablets (discontinued 2009) ℞ *combination beta-blocker and diuretic for hypertension* [timolol maleate; hydrochlorothiazide] 10•25 mg

timolol USAN, INN, BAN *topical antiglaucoma agent (beta-blocker)*

timolol hemihydrate *topical antiglaucoma agent (beta-blocker)*

timolol maleate USAN, USP *antianginal; antihypertensive; antiadrenergic (beta-blocker); topical antiglaucoma agent; migraine prophylaxis* 5, 10, 20 mg oral; 0.25%, 0.5% eye drops

timolol maleate & dorzolamide HCl *combination beta-blocker and carbonic anhydrase inhibitor for glaucoma* 0.5%•2%

timonacic INN

timoprazole INN

Timoptic Ocumeter (eye drops), Ocu-dose (single-use eye drop dispenser) ℞ *antiglaucoma agent (beta-blocker)* [timolol maleate] 0.25%, 0.5%

Timoptic-XE gel-forming Ocumeter (eye drops) ℞ *once-daily antiglaucoma agent (beta-blocker)* [timolol maleate] 0.25%, 0.5%

tin *element (Sn)*

tin chloride dihydrate [see: stannous chloride]

tin ethyl etiopurpurin (SnET2) [see: rostaporfin]

tin fluoride [see: stannous fluoride]

tinabinol USAN, INN *antihypertensive*

Tinactin cream, powder, spray powder, spray liquid, topical solution OTC *antifungal* [tolnaftate] 1%

Tinactin for Jock Itch cream, spray powder OTC *antifungal* [tolnaftate] 1%

tinazoline INN ⚚ Tensilon; Tonsaline

TinBen tincture OTC *skin protectant; antiseptic* [benzoin; alcohol 75–83%]

Tincture of Green Soap topical liquid OTC *antiseptic cleanser* [green soap; alcohol 28–32%]

Tindamax film-coated tablets ℞ *antiprotozoal/amebicide for amebiasis (orphan), giardiasis (orphan), trichomoniasis, and bacterial vaginosis* [tinidazole] 250, 500 mg

Ting aerosol liquid OTC *antifungal* [tolnaftate] 1%

Ting aerosol powder OTC *antifungal for tinea pedis, tinea cruris, and tinea corporis* [miconazole nitrate] 2%

Ting cream OTC *antifungal* [tolnaftate] 1%

tinidazole USAN, INN *antiprotozoal/amebicide for amebiasis (orphan), giardiasis (orphan), trichomoniasis, and bacterial vaginosis* 250, 500 mg oral

tinisulpride INN

tinofedrine INN

tinoridine INN

Tinver lotion ℞ *antifungal; keratolytic; antipruritic; anesthetic* [sodium thiosulfate; salicylic acid; alcohol 10%] 25%•1%

tinzaparin sodium USAN, INN, BAN *a low molecular weight heparin–type anticoagulant and antithrombotic for the prevention and treatment of deep vein thrombosis (DVT)*

tiocarlide INN [also: thiocarlide]

tioclomarol INN

tioconazole USAN, USP, INN, BAN, JAN *topical antifungal*

tioctilate INN

tiodazosin USAN, INN *antihypertensive*

tiodonium chloride USAN, INN *antibacterial*

tiofacic [see: stepronin]

tioguanine INN *antineoplastic* [also: thioguanine]

tiomergine INN

tiomesterone INN [also: thiomesterone]

tioperidone INN *antipsychotic* [also: tioperidone HCl]

tioperidone HCl USAN *antipsychotic* [also: tioperidone]

tiopinac USAN, INN *anti-inflammatory; analgesic; antipyretic*

tiopronin INN *prevention of cystine nephrolithiasis in homozygous cystinuria (orphan)* ⊡ teprenone

tiopropamine INN

tiosalan INN *disinfectant* [also: thiosalan] ⊡ Tessalon

tiosinamine [see: allylthiourea]

tiospirone INN *antipsychotic* [also: tiospirone HCl] ⊡ tisopurine

tiospirone HCl USAN *antipsychotic* [also: tiospirone]

tiotidine USAN, INN *antagonist to histamine H₂ receptors*

tiotixene INN *conventional (typical) thioxanthene antipsychotic for schizophrenia* [also: thiothixene]

tiotropium bromide *long-acting anticholinergic bronchodilator for emphysema and chronic obstructive pulmonary disease (COPD) (base=80%)*

tioxacin INN

tioxamast INN

tioxaprofen INN

tioxidazole USAN, INN *anthelmintic*

tioxolone INN [also: thioxolone]

TIP (Taxol, isosfamide, Platinol) [with mesna rescue; with or without filgrastim hematopoietic] *chemotherapy protocol for head, neck, esophageal, and testicular cancers*

tipentosin INN, BAN *antihypertensive* [also: tipentosin HCl]

tipentosin HCl USAN *antihypertensive* [also: tipentosin]

tipepidine INN

tipetropium bromide INN

tipifarnib USAN *investigational (NDA filed, orphan) antineoplastic for acute myeloid leukemia (AML)*

tipindole INN

tipranavir disodium USAN *protease inhibitor; oral antiretroviral for HIV-1 infections*

tipredane USAN, INN, BAN *topical adrenocortical steroid*

tiprenolol INN *antiadrenergic (beta-blocker)* [also: tiprenolol HCl]

tiprenolol HCl USAN *antiadrenergic (beta-blocker)* [also: tiprenolol]

tiprinast INN *antiallergic* [also: tiprinast meglumine]

tiprinast meglumine USAN *antiallergic* [also: tiprinast]

tipropidil INN *vasodilator* [also: tipropidil HCl]

tipropidil HCl USAN *vasodilator* [also: tipropidil]

tiprostanide INN, BAN

tiprotimod INN

tiqueside USAN, INN *antihyperlipidemic*

tiquinamide INN *gastric anticholinergic* [also: tiquinamide HCl]

tiquinamide HCl USAN *gastric anticholinergic* [also: tiquinamide]

tiquizium bromide INN

tirapazamine USAN, INN *antineoplastic; investigational (Phase III, orphan) for head and neck cancers*

tiratricol INN *investigational (orphan) for suppression of thyroid-stimulating hormone (TSH) for thyroid cancer*

tirilazad INN, BAN *antioxidant; lipid peroxidation inhibitor; 21-aminosteroid (lazaroid)* [also: tirilizad mesylate]

tirilazad mesylate USAN *antioxidant; lipid peroxidation inhibitor; 21-aminosteroid (lazaroid)* [also: tirilizad]

tirofiban HCl USAN *glycoprotein (GP) IIb/IIIa receptor antagonist; platelet aggregation inhibitor for acute coronary syndrome, unstable angina, myocardial infarction, and cardiac surgery*

tiropramide INN

Tirosint capsules ℞ *synthetic thyroid hormone (T₄ fraction only)* [levothyroxine sodium] 13 mcg

tisilfocon A USAN *hydrophobic contact lens material*

Tisit lotion, gel, shampoo OTC *pediculicide for lice* [pyrethrins; piperonyl butoxide] 0.3%•2%; 0.3%•3%; 0.33%•4%

tisocromide INN

TiSol throat irrigation solution OTC *antiseptic; mild anesthetic; antipruritic; counterirritant* [benzyl alcohol; menthol] 1%•0.04% ⊡ Tussall

tisopurine INN ⊡ tiospirone

tisoquone INN ⊡ Tussigon

Tisseal topical liquid, powder for topical liquid ℞ *adjunct to hemostasis for cardiopulmonary surgery; adjunct to prevent leakage from colonic anastomoses during colostomies; the sealant and thrombin are mixed just before applying to the graft, and it "sets" in about 60 seconds* [fibrin sealant, human; thrombin, human] 96–125 mg/mL; 400–625 IU/mL ⧗ Tussall

tissue factor [see: thromboplastin]

tissue plasminogen activator (tPA; t-PA) [see: alteplase]

Tis-U-Sol solution ℞ *sterile irrigant for general washing and rinsing* [physiological irrigating solution]

TIT (Tarabine intrathecal) [with methotrexate and hydrocortisone] *chemotherapy protocol for pediatric acute lymphocytic leukemia (ALL); intrathecal (IT) administration*

Titan solution (discontinued 2010) OTC *cleaning solution for hard contact lenses*

titanium *element (Ti)*

titanium dioxide USP *topical protectant; astringent*

titanium oxide [see: titanium dioxide]

Titradose (trademarked dosage form) *scored tablet*

Titralac chewable tablets OTC *antacid* [calcium carbonate] 420, 750 mg

Titralac Plus chewable tablets, oral liquid OTC *antacid; antiflatulent* [calcium carbonate; simethicone] 420•21 mg; 500•20 mg/5 mL

tivanidazole INN

tivazine [see: piperazine citrate]

tivozanib *investigational (Phase III) antineoplastic for advanced kidney cancer*

tixadil INN

tixanox USAN *antiallergic* [also: tixanoxum]

tixanoxum INN *antiallergic* [also: tixanox]

tixocortol INN *topical anti-inflammatory* [also: tixocortol pivalate]

tixocortol pivalate USAN *topical anti-inflammatory* [also: tixocortol]

tizabrin INN

tizanidine INN, BAN *central alpha$_2$ agonist; skeletal muscle relaxant; antispasmodic* [also: tizanidine HCl]

tizanidine HCl USAN, JAN *central alpha$_2$ agonist; skeletal muscle relaxant; antispasmodic for multiple sclerosis and spinal cord injury (orphan)* (base= 87.3%) [also: tizanidine] 2.3, 4.6 mg (2, 4 mg base) oral

tizolemide INN

tizoprolic acid INN

TL 45% lotion ℞ *moisturizer; emollient; keratolytic* [urea] 45%

TL Icon capsules ℞ *hematinic* [iron; vitamin B$_{12}$; vitamin C; intrinsic factor; folic acid] 110•0.015•75•240•0.5 mg ⧗ tolycaine

^{201}Tl [see: thallous chloride Tl 201]

TL-DEX DM oral liquid ℞ *antitussive; decongestant; expectorant* [dextromethorphan hydrobromide; pseudoephedrine HCl; guaifenesin] 15•33•200 mg/5 mL

TL-Hist CM oral liquid ℞ *narcotic antitussive; antihistamine* [codeine phosphate; chlorpheniramine maleate] 10•2 mg/5 mL

TL-Hist DM oral liquid ℞ *antihistamine; decongestant; antitussive* [brompheniramine maleate; phenylephrine HCl; dextromethorphan hydrobromide] 4•7.5•15 mg/5 mL

T-lymphotrophic virus antigens [see: human T-lymphotropic virus type III (HTLV-III) gp-160 antigens]

T-MAVs (targeted monoclonal antibody vehicles) [q.v.]

TMB (trimedoxime bromide) [q.v.]

TMC125 *investigational (Phase III) non-nucleoside reverse transcriptase inhibitor (NNRTI) antiviral for HIV and AIDS in treatment-experienced patients*

TMG (trimethylglycine) [q.v.]

TMP (trimethoprim) [q.v.]

TMP-SMZ (trimethoprim & sulfamethoxazole) [q.v.]

TNF (tumor necrosis factor) [q.v.]

TNKase powder for IV injection ℞ *thrombolytic/fibrinolytic for the treatment*

of acute myocardial infarction (AMI) [tenecteplase] 50 mg/vial ② tonics

TNK·tPA *a genetically engineered mutation of tissue plasminogen activator (tPA); "TNK" refers to the three specific sites of genetic modification* [see: tenecteplase]

tobacco *dried leaves of the* Nicotiana tabacum *plant; sedative narcotic; emetic; diuretic; heart depressant; antispasmodic* [see also: nicotine]

tobacco, British *medicinal herb* [see: coltsfoot]

tobacco, Indian; wild tobacco *medicinal herb* [see: lobelia]

tobacco, sailor's *medicinal herb* [see: mugwort]

tobacco wood *medicinal herb* [see: witch hazel]

TOBI *solution for inhalation* ℞ *antibiotic for* Pseudomonas aeruginosa *lung infections in cystic fibrosis patients (orphan)* [tobramycin] 300 mg/5 mL

toborinone USAN *cardiotonic*

TobraDex *eye drop suspension* ℞ *corticosteroidal anti-inflammatory; antibiotic* [dexamethasone; tobramycin] 0.05%•0.3%, 0.1%•0.3%

TobraDex *ophthalmic ointment* ℞ *corticosteroidal anti-inflammatory; antibiotic* [dexamethasone; tobramycin; chlorobutanol] 0.1%•0.3%•0.5%

tobramycin USAN, USP, INN, BAN *aminoglycoside antibiotic; inhalant for* Pseudomonas aeruginosa *lung infections in cystic fibrosis patients (orphan)* 0.3% eye drops

tobramycin & dexamethasone *antibiotic; corticosteroidal anti-inflammatory* 0.3%•0.1% eye drops

Tobramycin in 0.9% Sodium Chloride *IV or IM injection* ℞ *aminoglycoside antibiotic* [tobramycin (as sulfate)] 0.8, 1.2 mg/mL (60, 80 mg/dose)

tobramycin sulfate USP *aminoglycoside antibiotic* 10, 40 mg/mL injection

Tobrex *Drop-Tainers (eye drops), ophthalmic ointment* ℞ *aminoglycoside antibiotic* [tobramycin] 0.3%; 3 mg/g

tobuterol INN

tocainide USAN, INN, BAN *antiarrhythmic*

tocainide HCl USP *antiarrhythmic*

tocamphyl USAN, INN *choleretic*

Tocicodendron diversilobum *medicinal herb* [see: poison oak]

tocilizumab *humanized monoclonal antibody to interleukin-6 receptors for moderate to severe rheumatoid arthritis*

tocladesine USAN *immunomodulator; antineoplastic*

tocofenoxate INN

tocofersolan INN *dietary vitamin E supplement* [also: tocophersolan]

tocofibrate INN

tocolytics *a class of drugs used to inhibit uterine contractions; often administered in an attempt to arrest preterm labor*

tocopherol, d-alpha [see: vitamin E]

tocopherol, dl-alpha [see: vitamin E]

tocopherols, mixed [see: vitamin E]

tocopherols excipient NF *antioxidant*

tocophersolan USAN *dietary vitamin E supplement; investigational (orphan) for vitamin E deficiency due to prolonged cholestatic hepatobiliary disease* [also: tocofersolan]

tocopheryl acetate, d-alpha [see: vitamin E]

tocopheryl acetate, dl-alpha [see: vitamin E]

tocopheryl acid succinate, d-alpha [see: vitamin E]

tocopheryl acid succinate, dl-alpha [see: vitamin E]

tocopheryl polyethylene glycol succinate (TPGS) [see: tocophersolan]

tocosol paclitaxel [see: paclitaxel tocosol]

Today *vaginal sponge* OTC *spermicidal/barrier contraceptive* [nonoxynol 9] 1 g

todralazine INN, BAN

tofacitinib *investigational (Phase III) janus-associated kinase (JAK) inhibitor for rheumatoid arthritis*

tofenacin INN *anticholinergic* [also: tofenacin HCl]

tofenacin HCl USAN *anticholinergic* [also: tofenacin]

tofesilate INN *combining name for radicals or groups*

tofetridine INN
tofisoline ⑨ tefazoline
tofisopam INN
Tofranil sugar-coated tablets ℞ tricyclic antidepressant; treatment for childhood enuresis [imipramine HCl] 10, 25, 50 mg
Tofranil-PM capsules ℞ tricyclic antidepressant [imipramine pamoate] 75, 100, 125, 150 mg
tolamolol USAN, INN vasodilator; antiarrhythmic; antiadrenergic (beta-blocker)
tolazamide USAN, USP, INN, BAN sulfonylurea antidiabetic that stimulates insulin secretion in the pancreas 100, 250, 500 mg oral
tolazoline INN antiadrenergic; peripheral vasodilator for hypertension [also: tolazoline HCl]
tolazoline HCl USP antiadrenergic; peripheral vasodilator for neonatal persistent pulmonary hypertension [also: tolazoline]
tolboxane INN
tolbutamide USP, INN, BAN sulfonylurea antidiabetic that stimulates insulin secretion in the pancreas 500 mg oral
tolbutamide sodium USP in vivo diagnostic aid for pancreatic islet cell adenoma
tolcapone USAN, INN COMT (catechol-O-methyltransferase) inhibitor for Parkinson disease
tolciclate USAN, INN antifungal
tolclotide [see: disulfamide]
toldimfos INN, BAN
Tolerex powder OTC enteral nutritional therapy [lactose-free formula]
tolfamide USAN, INN urease enzyme inhibitor
tolfenamic acid INN, BAN
Tolfrinic film-coated tablets (discontinued 2008) OTC vitamin/iron supplement [iron (as ferrous fumarate); vitamin B₁₂; vitamin C] 200•0.025•100 mg
tolgabide USAN, INN, BAN anticonvulsant
tolhexamide [see: glycyclamide]
tolimidone USAN, INN antiulcerative
tolindate USAN, INN antifungal

toliodium chloride USAN, INN veterinary food additive
toliprolol INN
tolmesoxide INN
tolmetin USAN, INN analgesic; nonsteroidal anti-inflammatory drug (NSAID) for osteoarthritis, rheumatoid arthritis, and juvenile rheumatoid arthritis
tolmetin sodium USAN, USP analgesic; nonsteroidal anti-inflammatory drug (NSAID) for osteoarthritis, rheumatoid arthritis, and juvenile rheumatoid arthritis 200, 400, 600 mg oral
tolnaftate USAN, USP, INN, BAN antifungal 1% topical
tolnapersine INN
tolnidamine INN
toloconium metilsulfate INN
tolofocon A USAN hydrophobic contact lens material
tolonidine INN
tolonium chloride INN blue dye used in histology; diagnostic aid for oral cancer
toloxatone INN
toloxichloral [see: toloxychlorinol]
toloxychlorinol INN
tolpadol INN
tolpentamide INN, BAN
tolperisone INN, BAN
tolpiprazole INN, BAN
tolpovidone I 131 USAN hypoalbuminemia test; radioactive agent [also: radiotolpovidone I 131]
tolpronine INN, BAN
tolpropamine INN, BAN
tolpyrramide USAN, INN antidiabetic
tolquinzole INN
tolrestat USAN, INN, BAN aldose reductase inhibitor
tolterodine USAN anticholinergic; muscarinic receptor antagonist for urinary frequency, urgency, and incontinence
tolterodine tartrate USAN anticholinergic; muscarinic receptor antagonist for urinary frequency, urgency, and incontinence
toltrazuril USAN, INN, BAN veterinary coccidiostat
tolu balsam USP pharmaceutic aid

p-**toluenesulfone dichloramine** [see: dichloramine T]

tolufazepam INN

toluidine blue O [see: tolonium chloride]

toluidine blue O chloride [see: tolonium chloride]

Tolu-Sed DM oral liquid (discontinued 2007) OTC *antitussive; expectorant* [dextromethorphan hydrobromide; guaifenesin; alcohol 10%] 10•100 mg/5 mL

tolvaptan *selective vasopressin V$_2$ receptor antagonist for heart failure and hyponatremia*

tolycaine INN, BAN ② TL Icon

tomelukast USAN, INN *antiasthmatic; leukotriene antagonist*

Tomocat concentrated rectal suspension ℞ *radiopaque contrast medium for gastrointestinal imaging* [barium sulfate] 5%

tomoglumide INN

tomoxetine INN *antidepressant* [also: tomoxetine HCl]

tomoxetine HCl USAN *antidepressant* [also: tomoxetine]

tomoxiprole INN

Tom's of Maine Natural Cough & Cold Rub Cough Suppressant vaporizing ointment (discontinued 2007) OTC *mild anesthetic; antipruritic; counterirritant* [menthol; camphor] 4.8%•2.6%

tonazocine INN *analgesic* [also: tonazocine mesylate]

tonazocine mesylate USAN *analgesic* [also: tonazocine]

tongue grass *medicinal herb* [see: chickweed]

tonics *a class of agents that restore normal tone to tissue and strengthen or invigorate organs (a term used in folk medicine)* ② Tannic; TNKase

tonka bean (*Dipteryx odorata; D. oppositifolia*) *fruit and seed medicinal herb for cramps, nausea, and schistosomiasis*

Tonopaque powder for oral/rectal suspension ℞ *radiopaque contrast medium*

for gastrointestinal imaging [barium sulfate] 95%

Tonsaline mouthwash OTC *oral antiseptic* [alcohol 4%] ② Tensilon; tinazoline

tonzonium bromide INN *detergent; surface-active agent* [also: thonzonium bromide]

tooth, lion's *medicinal herb* [see: dandelion]

Toothache oral gel OTC *mucous membrane anesthetic* [benzocaine]

toothache bush; toothache tree *medicinal herb* [see: prickly ash]

Topamax coated tablets, sprinkle caps ℞ *broad-spectrum sulfamate anticonvulsant for Lennox-Gastaut syndrome (orphan) and partial-onset and generalized tonic-clonic seizures; migraine headache preventative; also used for a variety of psychiatric disorders* [topiramate] 25, 50, 100, 200 mg; 15, 25 mg

Topic gel OTC *mild anesthetic; antipruritic; counterirritant; antiseptic* [benzyl alcohol; camphor; menthol; alcohol 30%] 5%•?•?

Topicaine gel OTC *anesthetic* [lidocaine HCl] 4%, 5% ② tebuquine

topical starch [see: starch, topical]

TopiCare (trademarked ingredient) cream, gel *nontherapeutic polyolprepolymer base for compounding various dermatological preparations*

Topicort ointment, cream, gel ℞ *corticosteroidal anti-inflammatory* [desoximetasone] 0.25%; 0.25%; 0.05%

Topicort LP cream ℞ *corticosteroidal anti-inflammatory* [desoximetasone] 0.05%

Topiragen tablets ℞ *broad-spectrum sulfamate anticonvulsant for Lennox-Gastaut syndrome (orphan) and partial-onset and generalized tonic-clonic seizures; migraine headache preventative; also used for a variety of psychiatric disorders* [topiramate] 25, 50, 100, 200 mg

topiramate USAN, INN, BAN *broad-spectrum sulfamate anticonvulsant for Lennox-Gastaut syndrome (orphan) and partial-onset and generalized tonic-*

clonic seizures; migraine headache preventative; also used for a variety of psychiatric disorders 15, 25, 50, 100, 200 mg oral

topo/CTX (topotecan, cyclophosphamide) [with mesna rescue and filgrastim hematopoietic] chemotherapy protocol for bone and soft tissue sarcomas [also known as: cyclophosphamide + topotecan]

topoisomerase I inhibitors a class of hormonal antineoplastics that prevent DNA replication of tumors by inhibiting the re-ligation of naturally occurring single-strand breaks

Toposar IV injection ℞ antineoplastic for testicular and small cell lung cancers (SCLC) [etoposide; alcohol 33.2%] 20 mg/mL

topotecan INN, BAN topoisomerase I inhibitor; antineoplastic for ovarian, cervical, and small cell lung cancers [also: topotecan HCl]

topotecan HCl USAN topoisomerase I inhibitor; antineoplastic for ovarian, cervical, and small cell lung cancers [also: topotecan] 1 mg/mL (1, 3, 4 mg/vial) injection

toprilidine INN

Toprol-XL film-coated extended-release tablets ℞ antihypertensive; long-term antianginal; beta-blocker [metoprolol succinate] 25, 50, 100, 200 mg

topterone USAN, INN antiandrogen

TOPV (trivalent oral poliovirus vaccine) [see: poliovirus vaccine, live oral]

toquizine USAN, INN anticholinergic ◫ Tikosyn

toralizumab investigational (orphan) for immune thrombocytopenic purpura

torasemide INN, BAN antihypertensive; loop diuretic [also: torsemide]

torbafylline INN

torcetrapib investigational cholesterol ester transfer protein (CETP) inhibitor to improve glycemic control in type 2 diabetes

Torecan IM injection (discontinued 2008) ℞ antiemetic for postoperative

nausea and vomiting [thiethylperazine maleate] 5 mg/mL ◫ tarragon; Treagan; Trocaine

toremifene INN, BAN antiestrogen; antineoplastic [also: toremifene citrate]

toremifene citrate USAN selective estrogen receptor modulator (SERM); antiestrogen antineoplastic for metastatic breast cancer in postmenopausal women (orphan); investigational (orphan) for desmoid tumors (base= 68%) [also: toremifene]

toripristone INN

Torisel IV infusion ℞ antineoplastic for renal cell carcinoma (orphan); investigational (NDA filed) for mantle cell lymphoma; immunosuppressant [temsirolimus] 25 mg/mL

tormentil (Potentilla tormentilla; Tormentilla erecta) root medicinal herb used as an antiphlogistic, antiseptic, astringent, and hemostatic

Tornalate solution for inhalation (discontinued 2008) ℞ sympathomimetic bronchodilator [bitolterol mesylate] 0.2%

torsemide USAN antihypertensive; loop diuretic for congestive heart failure, hepatic cirrhosis, and renal disease [also: torasemide] 5, 10, 20, 100 mg oral; 10 mg/mL injection

tosactide INN [also: octacosactrin]

tosifen USAN, INN antianginal

tosilate INN combining name for radicals or groups [also: tosylate]

tositumomab monoclonal antibody to non-Hodgkin lymphoma (orphan) [see also: iodine I 131 tositumomab]

tosufloxacin USAN, INN antibacterial

tosulur INN

tosylate USAN, BAN combining name for radicals or groups [also: tosilate]

tosylchloramide sodium INN [also: chloramine-T]

Total solution (discontinued 2010) OTC cleaning/soaking/wetting solution for hard contact lenses

Total B with C caplets, tablets OTC vitamin supplement [multiple B vitamins; vitamin C] ≛•300 mg

Total Formula; Total Formula-2 tablets OTC *vitamin/mineral/calcium/ iron supplement* [multiple vitamins & minerals; calcium (as carbonate, citrate, and phosphate); iron (as carbonyl iron); folic acid; biotin] ±• 100•20•0.4•0.3 mg

Total Formula-3 without Iron tablets (discontinued 2008) OTC *vitamin/mineral supplement* [multiple vitamins & minerals; folic acid; biotin] ±•0.4•0.3 mg

Totalday timed-release tablets OTC *vitamin/mineral/calcium/iron supplement* [multiple vitamins & minerals; calcium; iron; folic acid] ±•250• 18•1 mg

Totect powder for IV infusion ℞ *cytoprotectant for anthracycline extravasation during chemotherapy (orphan)* [dexrazoxane (as HCl)] 500 mg

touch-me-not; pale touch-me-not *medicinal herb* [see: celandine; jewelweed; eleuthero]

toughened silver nitrate [see: silver nitrate, toughened]

Touro Allergy tablets, sustained-release capsules ℞ *decongestant; antihistamine* [pseudoephedrine HCl; brompheniramine maleate] 45•6 mg; 60•5.75 mg

Touro CC sustained-release caplets (discontinued 2007) ℞ *antitussive; decongestant; expectorant* [dextromethorphan hydrobromide; pseudoephedrine HCl; guaifenesin] 30•60•575 mg

Touro CC-LD sustained-release caplets ℞ *antitussive; decongestant; expectorant* [dextromethorphan hydrobromide; pseudoephedrine HCl; guaifenesin] 30•25•575 mg

Touro DM sustained-release tablets ℞ *antitussive; expectorant* [dextromethorphan hydrobromide; guaifenesin] 30•575 mg

Touro HC extended-release caplets (discontinued 2007) ℞ *narcotic antitussive; expectorant* [hydrocodone bitartrate; guaifenesin] 5•575 mg

Touro LA sustained-release caplets ℞ *decongestant; expectorant* [pseudoephedrine HCl; guaifenesin] 120• 525 mg ⑨ Terrell

Tovalt ODT (orally disintegrating tablets) ℞ *imidazopyridine sedative and hypnotic for the short-term treatment of insomnia* [zolpidem tartrate] 5, 10 mg

Toviaz extended-release film-coated tablets ℞ *muscarinic receptor antagonist for overactive bladder* [fesoterodine fumarate] 4, 8 mg ⑨ Tyvaso

toxoids *a class of drugs used for active immunization that produce endogenous antibodies to toxins*

toywort *medicinal herb* [see: shepherd's purse]

tozalinone INN *antidepressant* [also: thozalinone]

tPA; t-PA (tissue plasminogen activator) [see: alteplase; anistreplase; lanoteplase; monteplase; reteplase; saruplase; tenecteplase]

TPGS (tocopheryl polyethylene glycol succinate) [see: tocophersolan]

T-Phyl timed-release tablets (discontinued 2008) ℞ *antiasthmatic; bronchodilator* [theophylline] 200 mg

TPM Test kit for professional use ℞ *in vitro diagnostic aid for* Toxoplasma gondii *antibodies in serum* [indirect hemagglutination test]

TPN Electrolytes; TPN Electrolytes II; TPN Electrolytes III IV admixture ℞ *intravenous electrolyte therapy* [combined electrolyte solution]

trabectedin *cytotoxic tetrahydroisoquinoline alkaloid; investigational (NDA filed, orphan) for soft tissue sarcoma and relapsed ovarian cancer; investigational (Phase III) for breast cancer; investigational (Phase II) for prostate cancer, advanced liposarcoma, and leiomyosarcoma*

traboxopine INN

tracazolate USAN, INN, BAN *sedative*

Trace Elements 4 Pediatric IV injection ℞ *intravenous nutritional therapy* [multiple trace elements (metals)]

Tracleer film-coated tablets ℞ *vasodilator for pulmonary arterial hypertension (orphan); also used to prevent digital ulcers in systemic sclerosis* [bosentan] 62.5, 125 mg

Tracrium IV infusion ℞ *nondepolarizing neuromuscular blocker; adjunct to anesthesia* [atracurium besylate] 10 mg/mL

Tradjenta film-coated tablets ℞ *antidiabetic for type 2 diabetes that enhances the function of the body's incretin system to increase insulin production in the pancreas and reduce glucose production in the liver* [linagliptin] 5 mg

trafermin USAN *fibroblast growth factor*

tragacanth NF *suspending agent*

tralonide USAN, INN *corticosteroid; anti-inflammatory*

tramadol INN *opioid analgesic for moderate to severe pain* [also: tramadol HCl]

Tramadol ER extended-release tablets ℞ *opioid analgesic for moderate to severe chronic pain* [tramadol HCl] 100, 200, 300 mg

tramadol HCl USAN *opioid analgesic for moderate to severe pain; also used for premature ejaculation; investigational (orphan) for HIV-associated neuropathy and postherpetic neuralgia; investigational (Phase III) for premature ejaculation* [also: tramadol] 50, 100, 200, 300 mg oral

tramadol HCl & acetaminophen *central analgesic for acute pain* 37.5• 325 mg oral

Tramadol ODT (orally disintegrating tablets) ℞ *opioid analgesic for moderate to severe chronic pain* [tramadol HCl] 50 mg

tramazoline INN *adrenergic* [also: tramazoline HCl]

tramazoline HCl USAN *adrenergic* [also: tramazoline]

tramiprosate *investigational (Phase III) amyloid-beta antagonist to reduce plaque formation in Alzheimer disease*

Trandate film-coated tablets ℞ *alpha- and beta-blocker; antihypertensive* [labetalol HCl] 100, 200, 300 mg

Trandate IV injection (discontinued 2011) ℞ *alpha- and beta-blocker; antihypertensive* [labetalol HCl] 5 mg/mL

trandolapril INN, BAN *antihypertensive; angiotensin-converting enzyme (ACE) inhibitor; treatment for congestive heart failure (CHF)* 1, 2, 4 mg oral

trandolapril & verapamil HCl *combination angiotensin-converting enzyme (ACE) inhibitor and calcium channel blocker for hypertension* 1•240, 2• 180, 2•240, 4•240 mg oral

trandolaprilat INN

tranexamic acid USAN, INN, BAN *systemic hemostatic for menorrhagia; also used as a surgical adjunct for patients with congenital coagulopathies (orphan); investigational (orphan) for hereditary angioneurotic edema; investigational to stop accident victims from bleeding to death* 100 mg/mL injection

tranilast USAN, INN *antiasthmatic; investigational (orphan) for malignant glioma*

trans AMCHA (*trans*-aminomethyl cyclohexanecarboxylic acid) [see: tranexamic acid]

transcainide USAN, INN *antiarrhythmic*

transclomiphene [now: zuclomiphene]

Transderm Scōp transdermal patch ℞ *motion sickness preventative; post-surgical antiemetic* [scopolamine] 1.5 mg (1 mg dose over 3 days)

transforming growth factor beta 2 *investigational (orphan) growth stimulator for full-thickness macular holes*

***trans*-π-oxocamphor** JAN *topical antipruritic; mild local anesthetic; counterirritant* [also: camphor]

***trans*-retinoic acid** [see: tretinoin]

Trans-Ver-Sal Adult-Patch; Trans-Ver-Sal Pedia-Patch; Trans-Ver-Sal Plantar-Patch patch OTC *keratolytic* [salicylic acid] 15%

trantelinium bromide INN

Tranxene T-tabs ("T"-imprinted tablets) ℞ *benzodiazepine anxiolytic; minor tranquilizer; alcohol withdrawal aid; anticonvulsant adjunct* [clorazepate dipotassium] 3.75, 7.5, 15 mg

Tranxene-SD; Tranxene-SD Half Strength extended-release tablets (discontinued 2009) ℞ *benzodiazepine anxiolytic; minor tranquilizer; alcohol withdrawal aid; anticonvulsant adjunct* [clorazepate dipotassium] 22.5 mg; 11.25 mg

tranylcypromine INN, BAN *antidepressant; MAO inhibitor* [also: tranylcypromine sulfate]

tranylcypromine sulfate USP *MAO inhibitor for major depression; also used for migraine prevention, social anxiety disorder (SAD), panic disorder, bipolar depression, and Alzheimer and Parkinson disease* [also: tranylcypromine] 10 mg oral

trapencaine INN

trapidil INN

trapymin [see: trapidil]

trastuzumab *monoclonal antibody to human epidermal growth factor receptor 2 (HER2) protein; antineoplastic for metastatic HER2-overexpressing breast and gastric cancers; investigational (orphan) for pancreatic cancer*

trastuzumab + anastrozole *chemotherapy protocol for breast cancer*

trastuzumab + docetaxel *chemotherapy protocol for breast cancer*

trastuzumab + gemcitabine *chemotherapy protocol for breast cancer*

trastuzumab + paclitaxel *chemotherapy protocol for breast cancer*

trastuzumab + vinorelbine *chemotherapy protocol for breast cancer*

Trasylol IV infusion ℞ *systemic hemostatic for coronary artery bypass graft (CABG) surgery (orphan)* [aprotinin] 10 000 KIU/mL (kallikrein inhibitor units)

TraumaCal ready-to-use oral liquid (discontinued 2009) OTC *enteral nutritional therapy for moderate to severe stress or trauma* [multiple branched chain amino acids]

Travasol 2.75% in 5% (10%, 25%) Dextrose; Travasol 4.25% in 5% (10%, 25%) Dextrose IV infusion ℞ *total parenteral nutrition; peripheral parenteral nutrition* [multiple essential and nonessential amino acids; dextrose]

Travasol 3.5% (5.5%, 8.5%) with Electrolytes IV infusion ℞ *total parenteral nutrition (all except 3.5%); peripheral parenteral nutrition (all)* [multiple essential and nonessential amino acids; electrolytes] ⧈ Triphasil

Travasol 5.5% (8.5%, 10%) IV infusion ℞ *total parenteral nutrition; peripheral parenteral nutrition* [multiple essential and nonessential amino acids] ⧈ Triphasil

Travasorb HN; Travasorb MCT; Travasorb STD powder OTC *enteral nutritional therapy* [lactose-free formula]

Travatan; Travatan Z Drop-Tainers (eye drops) ℞ *antihypertensive for glaucoma and ocular hypertension* [travoprost] 0.004%

Travelan caplets OTC *prophylaxis of traveler's diarrhea due to E. coli bacteria in food* [antienterotoxigenic *Escherichia coli* antibodies from bovine colostrum] 200 mg

traveler's joy *medicinal herb* [see: blue vervain; woodbine]

5% Travert and Electrolyte No. 2; 10% Travert and Electrolyte No. 2 IV infusion ℞ *intravenous nutritional/electrolyte therapy* [combined electrolyte solution; invert sugar (50% dextrose + 50% fructose)]

travoprost USAN *topical prostaglandin $F_{2\alpha}$ analogue; antihypertensive for glaucoma and ocular hypertension*

traxanox INN

traxoprodil mesylate USAN *selective NMDA receptor antagonist for traumatic brain injury*

Traypak (trademarked packaging form) *multivial carton*

trazitiline INN ⧈ trestolone

trazium esilate INN

trazodone INN *triazolopyridine antidepressant; serotonin uptake inhibitor; also used for aggressive behavior, alcoholism, panic disorder, agoraphobia,* *and cocaine withdrawal* [also: trazodone HCl] ⑨ terizidone

trazodone HCl USAN *triazolopyridine antidepressant; serotonin uptake inhibitor; also used for insomnia, prevention of migraine headaches, aggressive behavior, alcoholism, and cocaine withdrawal* [also: trazodone] 50, 100, 150, 300 mg oral

trazolopride INN

Treagan ear drops ℞ *anesthetic; analgesic* [benzocaine; antipyrine] 1.4%•5.4% ⑨ tarragon; Torecan; Trocaine

Treanda powder for IV infusion ℞ *alkylating antineoplastic for chronic lymphocytic leukemia (orphan) and non-Hodgkin lymphoma (orphan)* [bendamustine HCl] 25, 100 mg/vial

trebenzomine INN *antidepressant* [also: trebenzomine HCl]

trebenzomine HCl USAN *antidepressant* [also: trebenzomine]

trecadrine INN

Trecator film-coated tablets ℞ *tuberculostatic* [ethionamide] 250 mg

trecetilide fumarate USAN *antiarrhythmic*

trecovirsen sodium USAN *antisense antiviral for HIV and AIDS*

trefentanil HCl USAN *analgesic*

trefoil, bean; bitter trefoil; marsh trefoil *medicinal herb* [see: buckbean]

Trellium Plus tablets (discontinued 2009) ℞ *urinary analgesic; antispasmodic; sedative* [phenazopyridine HCl; hyoscyamine hydrobromide; butabarbital] 150•0.3•15 mg

treloxinate USAN, INN *antihyperlipoproteinemic*

Trelstar suspension for IM injection ℞ *gonadotropin-releasing hormone (GnRH) antineoplastic for palliative treatment of advanced prostate cancer; investigational (orphan) for palliative treatment of advanced ovarian cancer* [triptorelin pamoate] 3.75, 11.25, 22.5 mg

Trelstar Depot IM injection (once monthly) (discontinued 2010) ℞ *gonadotropin-releasing hormone (GnRH) antineoplastic for palliative*

treatment of advanced prostate cancer; investigational (orphan) for palliative treatment of advanced ovarian cancer [triptorelin pamoate] 3.75 mg

Trelstar LA IM injection (three-month depot) (discontinued 2010) ℞ *gonadotropin-releasing hormone (GnRH) antineoplastic for palliative treatment of advanced prostate cancer; investigational (orphan) for palliative treatment of advanced ovarian cancer* [triptorelin pamoate] 11.25 mg

tremacamra USAN *antiviral; inhibits viral attachment to host cells*

trembling poplar; trembling tree *medicinal herb* [see: poplar]

Trenadrol capsules OTC *precursor to the veterinary anabolic steroid* trenbolone; *also abused as a street drug* [17β-methoxy-trienbolone] 30 mg

trenbolone INN, BAN *veterinary anabolic steroid; also abused as a street drug* [also: trenbolone acetate]

trenbolone acetate USAN *veterinary anabolic steroid; also abused as a street drug* [also: trenbolone]

trenbolone hexahydrobenzylcarbonate *veterinary anabolic steroid; also abused as a street drug*

trengestone INN

trenizine INN

Trental film-coated controlled-release tablets ℞ *peripheral vasodilator to improve blood microcirculation in intermittent claudication* [pentoxifylline] 400 mg

treosulfan INN, BAN *investigational (orphan) for ovarian cancer*

trepibutone INN

trepipam INN *sedative* [also: trepipam maleate]

trepipam maleate USAN *sedative* [also: trepipam]

trepirium iodide INN

treprostinil sodium *prostacyclin analogue; peripheral vasodilator for pulmonary arterial hypertension (PAH; orphan)*

treptilamine INN

trequinsin INN

trestolone INN *antineoplastic; androgen* [also: trestolone acetate] ② trazitiline

trestolone acetate USAN *antineoplastic; androgen* [also: trestolone]

tretamine INN, BAN [also: triethylenemelamine]

trethinium tosilate INN

trethocanic acid INN

trethocanoic acid [see: trethocanic acid]

tretinoin USAN, USP, INN, BAN *first generation retinoid; topical keratolytic for acne; treatment for acute promyelocytic leukemia (APL; orphan); investigational (orphan) for other leukemias and ophthalmic squamous metaplasia* 0.01%, 0.025%, 0.0375%, 0.05%, 0.1% topical; 10 mg oral

Tretin-X cream, gel ℞ *keratolytic for acne* [tretinoin] 0.025%, 0.05%, 0.1%; 0.01%, 0.025%

tretoquinol INN

Trexall film-coated tablets ℞ *antimetabolite antineoplastic for leukemia; systemic antipsoriatic; antirheumatic for adult and juvenile rheumatoid arthritis* [methotrexate] 5, 7.5, 10, 15 mg ② Tricosal

Treximet tablets ℞ *combination 5-HT$_{1B/1D}$ agonist and nonsteroidal antiinflammatory drug (NSAID) for the acute treatment of migraine headaches* [sumatriptan; naproxen sodium] 85•500 mg

Trezix capsules ℞ *narcotic analgesic; antipyretic* [dihydrocodeine bitartrate; acetaminophen; caffeine] 16•356.4•30 mg

TRH (thyrotropin-releasing hormone) [see: protirelin]

TRI (triple reuptake inhibitor) [q.v.]

Tri Lo Sprintec tablets (in packs of 28) ℞ *triphasic oral contraceptive* [norgestimate; ethinyl estradiol] Phase 1 (7 days): 0.18 mg•25 mcg; Phase 2 (7 days): 0.215 mg•25 mcg; Phase 3 (7 days): 0.25 mg•25 mcg; Counters (7 days)

Tri Vit with Fluoride pediatric oral drops (discontinued 2007) ℞ *vitamin supplement; dental caries preventative* [vitamins A, C, and D; fluoride] 1500 IU•35 mg•400 IU•0.25 mg, 1500 IU•35 mg•400 IU•0.5 mg per mL

TRIAC (triiodothyroacetic acid) [q.v.]

Triacana *investigational (orphan) for suppression of thyroid-stimulating hormone (TSH) for thyroid cancer; used with levothyroxine sodium* [tiratricol]

Triacet cream ℞ *corticosteroidal antiinflammatory* [triamcinolone acetonide] 0.1% ② Trycet

triacetin USP, INN *antifungal*

triacetyloleandomycin BAN *macrolide antibiotic* [also: troleandomycin]

Triacin-C Cough syrup (discontinued 2007) ℞ *narcotic antitussive; antihistamine; decongestant* [codeine phosphate; triprolidine HCl; pseudoephedrine HCl; alcohol 4.3%] 20•2.5•60 mg/10 mL

triaconazole [now: terconazole]

Triacting oral liquid OTC *decongestant; expectorant; for children 2–12 years* [pseudoephedrine HCl; guaifenesin] 15•50 mg/5 mL

Triacting Cold & Allergy pediatric oral liquid (discontinued 2007) OTC *decongestant; antihistamine* [pseudoephedrine HCl; chlorpheniramine maleate] 30•2 mg/10 mL

Tri-Acting Cold & Allergy pediatric syrup (discontinued 2007) OTC *decongestant; antihistamine* [pseudoephedrine HCl; chlorpheniramine maleate] 30•2 mg/10 mL

Tri-Acting Cold & Cough syrup (discontinued 2007) OTC *antitussive; antihistamine; decongestant; for children 6–11 years* [dextromethorphan hydrobromide; chlorpheniramine maleate; pseudoephedrine HCl] 10•2•30 mg/10 mL

Triad capsules ℞ *barbiturate sedative; analgesic; antipyretic* [butalbital; acetaminophen; caffeine] 50•325•40 mg

triafungin USAN, INN *antifungal*

Trial AG (Anti-Gas) tablets OTC *antacid; antiflatulent* [aluminum hydroxide; magnesium hydroxide; simethicone] 200•200•25 mg

Trial Antacid tablets OTC *antacid; calcium supplement* [calcium (as carbonate)] 168 mg (420 mg)

Triam-A IM, intra-articular, intrabursal, intradermal injection (discontinued 2008) ℞ *corticosteroid; anti-inflammatory* [triamcinolone acetonide] 40 mg/mL

triamcinolone USP, INN, BAN, JAN *corticosteroid*

triamcinolone acetonide USP, JAN *topical corticosteroidal anti-inflammatory; oral inhalation aerosol for chronic asthma; nasal aerosol for allergic rhinitis* 0.025%, 0.1%, 0.5% topical; 10, 40 mg/mL injection; 55 mcg/dose nasal spray

triamcinolone acetonide sodium phosphate USAN *corticosteroidal anti-inflammatory*

triamcinolone benetonide INN *corticosteroidal anti-inflammatory*

triamcinolone diacetate USP, JAN *corticosteroidal anti-inflammatory*

triamcinolone furetonide INN *corticosteroidal anti-inflammatory*

triamcinolone hexacetonide USAN, USP, INN, BAN *corticosteroidal anti-inflammatory*

Triaminic Allerchews orally disintegrating tablets OTC *nonsedating antihistamine for allergic rhinitis* [loratadine] 10 mg

Triaminic Allergy Congestion Softchews (chewable tablets), pediatric oral liquid (discontinued 2009) OTC *nasal decongestant* [pseudoephedrine HCl] 15 mg; 15 mg/5 mL

Triaminic Chest & Nasal Congestion oral liquid OTC *decongestant; expectorant; for children 2–12 years* [phenylephrine HCl; guaifenesin] 2.5•50 mg/5 mL

Triaminic Children's Allergy orally disintegrating film OTC *antitussive; antihistamine; sleep aid* [diphenhydramine HCl] 12.5 mg

Triaminic Children's Thin Strips Daytime Cold & Cough orally disintegrating film OTC *antitussive; decongestant* [dextromethorphan hydrobromide; phenylephrine HCl] 5•2.5 mg

Triaminic Children's Thin Strips Night Time Cold & Cough orally disintegrating film OTC *decongestant; antihistamine; sleep aid* [phenylephrine HCl; diphenhydramine HCl] 5•12.5 mg

Triaminic Cold & Allergy oral liquid (discontinued 2011) OTC *decongestant; antihistamine; for children 6–11 years* [phenylephrine HCl; chlorpheniramine maleate] 5•2 mg/10 mL

Triaminic Cold & Cough Thin Strips orally disintegrating film OTC *antitussive; decongestant* [dextromethorphan; phenylephrine HCl] 5•2.5 mg

Triaminic Cough & Runny Nose chewable tablets OTC *antitussive; antihistamine* [dextromethorphan hydrobromide; chlorpheniramine maleate] 5•1 mg

Triaminic Cough & Runny Nose orally disintegrating film OTC *antitussive; antihistamine; sleep aid* [diphenhydramine HCl] 12.5 mg

Triaminic Cough & Sore Throat softchews, oral liquid OTC *antitussive; analgesic; antipyretic; for children 2–11 years* [dextromethorphan hydrobromide; acetaminophen] 5•160 mg; 5•160 mg/5 mL

Triaminic D Children's syrup OTC *antitussive; decongestant; antihistamine* [dextromethorphan hydrobromide; pseudoephedrine HCl; chlorpheniramine maleate] 7.5•15•1 mg/5 mL

Triaminic Daytime Cold & Cough pediatric oral liquid OTC *antitussive; decongestant; for children 2–11 years* [dextromethorphan; phenylephrine HCl] 5•2.5 mg

Triaminic Flu, Cough, & Fever oral liquid OTC *antitussive; antihistamine; analgesic; antipyretic; for children 6–11*

years [dextromethorphan hydrobromide; chlorpheniramine maleate; acetaminophen] 15•2•320 mg/10 mL

Triaminic Infant Decongestant Plus Cough Thin Strips orally disintegrating film OTC *antitussive; decongestant; for children 2–3 years* [dextromethorphan; phenylephrine HCl] 1.83•1.25 mg

Triaminic Infant Thin Strips (orally disintegrating film) (discontinued 2010) OTC *decongestant* [phenylephrine HCl] 1.25 mg

Triaminic Infant's Fever Reducer/ Pain Reliever oral drops (discontinued 2011) OTC *analgesic; antipyretic* [acetaminophen] 100 mg/mL

Triaminic Long Acting Cough oral liquid OTC *antitussive* [dextromethorphan hydrobromide] 7.5 mg/5 mL

Triaminic MultiSymptom orally disintegrating film OTC *antihistamine; sleep aid* [diphenhydramine HCl] 25 mg

Triaminic Night Time Cold & Cough oral liquid OTC *decongestant; antihistamine; sleep aid; for children 6– 11 years* [phenylephrine HCl; diphenhydramine HCl] 5•12.5 mg/10 mL

Triaminic Sore Throat Spray OTC *mild mucous membrane anesthetic; antipruritic; counterirritant* [phenol] 0.5%

Triaminic Thin Strips Cold orally disintegrating film OTC *decongestant* [phenylephrine HCl] 2.5 mg

Triaminic Thin Strips Long Acting Cough orally disintegrating film OTC *antitussive* [dextromethorphan hydrobromide] 7.5 mg

Triaminicin Cold, Allergy, Sinus Medicine tablets (discontinued 2007) OTC *decongestant; antihistamine; analgesic; antipyretic* [pseudoephedrine HCl; chlorpheniramine maleate; acetaminophen] 60•4•650 mg

Triamolone 40 IM injection ℞ *corticosteroid; anti-inflammatory* [triamcinolone diacetate] 40 mg/mL

Triamonide 40 IM, intra-articular, intrabursal, intradermal injection (discontinued 2008) ℞ *corticosteroid;*

anti-inflammatory [triamcinolone acetonide] 40 mg/mL

triampyzine INN *anticholinergic* [also: triampyzine sulfate]

triampyzine sulfate USAN *anticholinergic* [also: triampyzine]

triamterene USAN, USP, INN, BAN, JAN *antihypertensive; potassium-sparing diuretic for congestive heart failure, cirrhosis of the liver, nephrotic syndrome, idiopathic edema, and steroid-induced edema*

triamterene & hydrochlorothiazide *antihypertensive; potassium-sparing diuretic* 37.5•25 mg oral

Trianex ointment ℞ *corticosteroidal anti-inflammatory* [triamcinolone acetonide] 0.05%

trianisestrol [see: chlorotrianisene]

Triant-HC oral liquid (discontinued 2009) ℞ *narcotic antitussive; antihistamine; decongestant* [hydrocodone bitartrate; chlorpheniramine maleate; phenylephrine HCl] 1.67•2•5 mg/5 mL

Tri-A-Vite with FL oral drops ℞ *vitamin supplement; dental caries preventative* [vitamins A, C, and D; fluoride] 1500 IU•35 mg•400 IU•0.5 mg per mL

Triaz cleansing cloths ℞ *keratolytic for acne* [benzoyl peroxide] 3, 6%, 9%

Triaz lotion ℞ *keratolytic for acne* [benzoyl peroxide] 3%, 6%, 10%

triaziquone INN, BAN ⑨ Tears Again

triazolam USAN, USP, INN *benzodiazepine sedative and hypnotic* 0.125, 0.25 mg oral

Triban; Pediatric Triban suppositories (removed from the market in 2007 due to lack of efficacy) ℞ *anticholinergic; post-surgical antiemetic; local anesthetic* [trimethobenzamide HCl; benzocaine] 200 mg•2%; 100 mg•2%

tribasic calcium phosphate [see: calcium phosphate, tribasic]

tribavirin BAN *antiviral for severe lower respiratory tract infections* [also: ribavirin]

tribendilol INN

tribenoside USAN, INN *sclerosing agent*

Tribenzor tablets ℞ *combination calcium channel blocker, angiotensin receptor blocker (ARB), and diuretic for hypertension* [amlodipine (as besylate); olmesartan medoxomil; hydrochlorothiazide] 5•20•12.5, 5•40•12.5, 5•40•25, 10•40•12.5, 10•40•25 mg

Tri-Biozene ointment OTC *antibiotic; local anesthetic* [polymyxin B sulfate; neomycin sulfate; bacitracin zinc; pramoxine HCl] 10 000 U•3.5 mg• 500 U•10 mg per g ⑨ Trobicin

tribromoethanol NF

tribromomethane [see: bromoform]

tribromsalan USAN, INN *disinfectant*

tribuzone INN ⑨ Trobicin

tricalcium phosphate [see: calcium phosphate, tribasic]

tricarbocyanine dye [see: indocyanine green]

TriCardio B capsules OTC *vitamin B supplement* [vitamins B$_6$ and B$_{12}$; folic acid] 25•0.25•0.1 mg

tricetamide USAN *sedative*

Trichinella extract USP

Tri-Chlor topical liquid ℞ *cauterant; keratolytic* [trichloroacetic acid] 80% ⑨ Tracleer

trichlorethoxyphosphamide [see: defosfamide]

trichlorfon USP *veterinary anthelmintic; investigational (NDA filed) acetylcholinesterase inhibitor for Alzheimer dementia* [also: metrifonate; metriphonate]

trichlorisobutylalcohol [see: chlorobutanol]

trichlormethiazide USP, INN *diuretic; antihypertensive*

trichlormethine INN [also: trimustine]

trichloroacetic acid USP *strong keratolytic/cauterant*

trichlorocarbanilide (TCC) [see: triclocarban]

trichloroethylene NF, INN

trichlorofluoromethane [see: trichloromonofluoromethane]

trichlorofon [see: metrifonate]

trichloromonofluoromethane NF *aerosol propellant; topical anesthetic*

trichlorphon [see: metrifonate]

Tricholomopsis edodes medicinal herb [see: shiitake mushrooms]

trichorad [see: acinitrazole]

Trichosanthes kirilowii medicinal herb [see: Chinese cucumber]

Trichotine Douche solution OTC *antiseptic/germicidal; vaginal cleanser and deodorizer; acidity modifier* [sodium borate]

Trichotine Douche vaginal powder OTC *antiseptic/germicidal cleanser and deodorizer* [sodium perborate]

triciribine INN *antineoplastic* [also: triciribine phosphate]

triciribine phosphate USAN *antineoplastic* [also: triciribine]

tricitrates (sodium citrate, potassium citrate, and citric acid) USP *systemic alkalizer; urinary alkalizer; antiurolithic*

triclabendazole INN

triclacetamol INN

triclazate INN

triclobisonium chloride NF, INN

triclocarban USAN, INN *disinfectant; antiseptic*

triclodazol INN

triclofenate INN *combining name for radicals or groups*

triclofenol piperazine USAN, INN *anthelmintic*

triclofos INN *hypnotic; sedative* [also: triclofos sodium]

triclofos sodium USAN *hypnotic; sedative* [also: triclofos]

triclofylline INN

triclonide USAN, INN *anti-inflammatory*

triclosan USAN, INN, BAN *topical disinfectant/antiseptic*

Tricodene Cough and Cold oral liquid (discontinued 2007) ℞ *narcotic antitussive; antihistamine; sleep aid* [codeine phosphate; pyrilamine maleate] 16.4•25 mg/10 mL

Tricodene Sugar Free Cough & Cold oral liquid OTC *antitussive; antihistamine* [dextromethorphan hydrobromide; chlorpheniramine maleate] 10•2 mg/5 mL

Tricof syrup (discontinued 2007) ℞ *narcotic antitussive; antihistamine; decongestant* [dihydrocodeine bitartrate; chlorpheniramine maleate; pseudoephedrine HCl] 7.5•2•15 mg/5 mL

Tricof EXP syrup (discontinued 2007) ℞ *narcotic antitussive; decongestant; expectorant* [dihydrocodeine bitartrate; pseudoephedrine HCl; guaifenesin] 7.5•15•100 mg/5 mL

Tricof PD syrup (discontinued 2007) ℞ *narcotic antitussive; antihistamine; decongestant* [dihydrocodeine bitartrate; chlorpheniramine maleate; phenylephrine HCl] 3•2•7.5 mg/5 mL

TriCor tablets ℞ *antihyperlipidemic for primary hypercholesterolemia, hypertriglyceridemia, and mixed dyslipidemia; also used for hyperuricemia* [fenofibrate] 48, 145 mg

tricosactide INN

Tricosal film-coated tablets ℞ *analgesic; antipyretic; antirheumatic* [choline magnesium trisalicylate] 500, 750, 1000 mg ⍰ Trexall

tricyclamol chloride INN

Tri-Cyclen [see: Ortho Tri-Cyclen]

tricyclics *a class of antidepressants that inhibit reuptake of amines, norepinephrine, and serotonin*

Tridal syrup (discontinued 2007) ℞ *narcotic antitussive; decongestant; expectorant* [codeine phosphate; phenylephrine HCl; guaifenesin] 10•4•125 mg/5 mL

Tridal HD oral liquid (discontinued 2007) ℞ *narcotic antitussive; antihistamine; decongestant* [hydrocodone bitartrate; chlorpheniramine maleate; phenylephrine HCl] 4•4•15 mg/10 mL

Tridal HD Plus syrup (discontinued 2007) ℞ *narcotic antitussive; antihistamine; decongestant* [hydrocodone bitartrate; chlorpheniramine maleate; phenylephrine HCl] 7•4•15 mg/10 mL

Triderm cream ℞ *corticosteroidal anti-inflammatory* [triamcinolone acetonide] 0.1%

Tridesilon Otic [see: Otic Tridesilon]

tridihexethyl chloride USP *peptic ulcer treatment adjunct*

tridihexethyl iodide INN

tridolgosir HCl USAN *chemoprotectant for solid tumor chemotherapy*

Tridrate Bowel Cleansing System oral liquid + 3 tablets + suppository OTC *pre-procedure bowel evacuant* [magnesium citrate (solution); bisacodyl (tablets and suppository)] 19 g; 5 mg; 10 mg

trientine INN *copper chelating agent* [also: trientine HCl; trientine dihydrochloride]

trientine dihydrochloride BAN *copper chelating agent* [also: trientine HCl; trientine]

trientine HCl USAN, USP *copper chelating agent for Wilson disease (orphan)* [also: trientine; trientine dihydrochloride]

Triesence intravitreal injection ℞ *corticosteroidal anti-inflammatory for ophthalmic diseases and visualization during vitrectomy* [triamcinolone acetonide] 40 mg/mL

triest; triestrogen [see: estriol]

triethanolamine [now: trolamine]

triethyl citrate NF *plasticizer*

triethyleneiminobenzoquinone (TEIB) [see: triaziquone]

triethylenemelamine NF [also: tretamine]

triethylenethiophosphoramide (TSPA; TESPA) [see: thiotepa]

Tri-Fed X oral suspension (discontinued 2008) ℞ *antitussive; antihistamine; decongestant* [dextromethorphan tannate; dexchlorpheniramine tannate; pseudoephedrine tannate] 25•2.5•75 mg/5 mL

trifenagrel USAN, INN *antithrombotic*

trifezolac INN

triflocin USAN, INN *diuretic*

Tri-Flor-Vite with Fluoride pediatric oral drops (discontinued 2008) ℞

vitamin supplement; dental caries pre-ventative [vitamins A, C, and D; fluoride] 1500 IU•35 mg•400 IU•0.25 mg per mL

triflubazam USAN, INN *minor tranquilizer*

triflumidate USAN, INN *anti-inflammatory*

trifluomeprazine INN, BAN

trifluoperazine INN *conventional (typical) phenothiazine antipsychotic for schizophrenia; anxiolytic for nonpsychotic anxiety* [also: trifluoperazine HCl]

trifluoperazine HCl USP *conventional (typical) phenothiazine antipsychotic for schizophrenia; anxiolytic for nonpsychotic anxiety* [also: trifluoperazine] 1, 2, 5, 10 mg oral

trifluorothymidine [see: trifluridine]

trifluperidol USAN, INN *antipsychotic*

triflupromazine USP, INN *phenothiazine antipsychotic; antiemetic*

triflupromazine HCl USP *phenothiazine antipsychotic; antiemetic*

trifluridine USAN, INN *ophthalmic antiviral* 1% eye drops

triflusal INN

triflutate USAN, INN *combining name for radicals or groups*

Trifolium pratense medicinal herb [see: red clover]

trigevolol INN

Triglide tablets ℞ *antihyperlipidemic for primary hypercholesterolemia, hypertriglyceridemia, and mixed dyslipidemia; also used for hyperuricemia* [fenofibrate] 50, 160 mg

α-triglycidyl isocyanurate (αTGI) [see: teroxirone]

Trigofen DM oral drops ℞ *antitussive; antihistamine; decongestant; for children 6–12 years* [dextromethorphan hydrobromide; chlorpheniramine maleate; phenylephrine HCl] 3•1•2 mg/mL

Trigonella foenum-graecum medicinal herb [see: fenugreek]

TriHemic 600 film-coated tablets (discontinued 2008) ℞ *hematinic* [iron (as ferrous fumarate); vitamin

B$_{12}$; vitamin C; vitamin E; intrinsic factor concentrate; docusate sodium; folic acid] 115 mg•25 mcg•600 mg•30 IU•75 mg•50 mg•1 mg

Trihexy-2; Trihexy-5 tablets ℞ *anticholinergic; antiparkinsonian* [trihexyphenidyl HCl] 2 mg; 5 mg

trihexyphenidyl INN *anticholinergic; antiparkinsonian* [also: trihexyphenidyl HCl; benzhexol]

trihexyphenidyl HCl USP *anticholinergic; antiparkinsonian* [also: trihexyphenidyl; benzhexol] 2, 5 mg oral; 2 mg/5 mL oral

TriHIBit IM injection (discontinued 2010) ℞ *active immunizing agent for diphtheria, tetanus, pertussis, (DTP) and H. influenzae type b (HIB) infections* [diphtheria & tetanus toxoids & acellular pertussis (DTaP) vaccine; *Haemophilus influenzae* b conjugate vaccine] supplied as separate 0.5 mL vials of Tripedia (q.v.) and ActHib (q.v.)

Tri-Hydroserpine tablets (discontinued 2007) ℞ *antihypertensive; vasodilator; diuretic* [hydrochlorothiazide; reserpine; hydralazine HCl] 15•0.1•25 mg

3,5,3′-triiodothyroacetate *investigational (orphan) for thyroid carcinoma*

triiodothyroacetic acid (TRIAC) *thyroid hormone analogue*

triiodothyronine sodium, levo [see: liothyronine sodium]

Tri-K oral liquid ℞ *electrolyte replenisher* [potassium (as acetate, bicarbonate, and citrate)] 45 mEq/15 mL ⊘ Tarka

trikates USP *electrolyte replenisher*

Tri-Kort IM, intra-articular, intrabursal, or intradermal injection (discontinued 2008) ℞ *corticosteroid; anti-inflammatory* [triamcinolone acetonide] 40 mg/mL

TriLegest Fe tablets (in packs of 28) ℞ *triphasic oral contraceptive; iron supplement* [norethindrone acetate; ethinyl estradiol; ferrous fumarate] Phase 1 (5 days): 1•0.02•75 mg; Phase 2 (7 days): 1•0.03•75 mg;

Phase 3 (9 days): 1•0.035•75 mg;
Counters (7 days): 0•0•75 mg

Trileptal film-coated tablets, oral suspension ℞ *anticonvulsant for partial seizures in adults or children; also used for bipolar disorder and diabetic neuropathy* [oxcarbazepine] 150, 300, 600 mg; 300 mg/5 mL

triletide INN

Tri-Levlen film-coated tablets (in Slidecases of 28) (discontinued 2008) ℞ *triphasic oral contraceptive; emergency postcoital contraceptive* [levonorgestrel; ethinyl estradiol]
Phase 1 (6 days): 0.5 mg•30 mcg;
Phase 2 (5 days): 0.75 mg•40 mcg;
Phase 3 (10 days): 0.125 mg•30 mcg;
Counters (7 days)

Trilipix delayed-release capsules ℞ *PPARα agonist for primary hypercholesterolemia, hypertriglyceridemia, and mixed dyslipidemia* [fenofibrate (as fenofibric acid)] 45, 135 mg

trilithium citrate tetrahydrate [see: lithium citrate]

Trillium erectum; T. grandiflorum; T. pendulum medicinal herb [see: birthroot]

Trilog IM, intra-articular, intrabursal, intradermal injection (discontinued 2008) ℞ *corticosteroid; anti-inflammatory* [triamcinolone acetonide] 40 mg/mL

Tri-Lo-Sprintec film-coated tablets (in packs of 28) (discontinued 2010) ℞ *triphasic oral contraceptive* [norgestimate; ethinyl estradiol]
Phase 1 (7 days): 0.18 mg•25 mcg;
Phase 2 (7 days): 0.215 mg•25 mcg;
Phase 3 (7 days): 0.25 mg•25 mcg;
Counters (7 days)

trilostane USAN, INN, BAN *adrenocortical suppressant; antisteroidal antineoplastic*

Tri-Luma cream ℞ *short-term treatment for melasma of the face* [hydroquinone; fluocinolone acetonide; tretinoin] 4%•0.01%•0.05%

TriLyte powder for oral solution ℞ *pre-procedure bowel evacuant* [PEG 3350; sodium bicarbonate; sodium

chloride; potassium chloride] 420•5.72•11.2•1.48 g/4 L bottle

Trimagen film-coated tablets ℞ *hematinic* [iron; vitamin B$_{12}$; vitamin C (as calcium ascorbate and calcium threonate); desiccated stomach substance; succinic acid] 70•0.01•152•50•75 mg

Trimazide suppositories, pediatric suppositories (removed from the market in 2007 due to lack of efficacy) ℞ *anticholinergic; post-surgical antiemetic* [trimethobenzamide HCl] 200 mg; 100 mg

trimazosin INN, BAN *antihypertensive* [also: trimazosin HCl]

trimazosin HCl USAN *antihypertensive* [also: trimazosin]

trimebutine INN *GI antispasmodic*

trimecaine INN

trimedoxime bromide INN

trimegestone USAN *progestin for postmenopausal hormone deficiency*

trimeperidine INN, BAN

trimeprazine BAN *phenothiazine antihistamine; antipruritic* [also: trimeprazine tartrate; alimemazine; alimemazine tartrate]

trimeprazine tartrate USP *phenothiazine antihistamine; antipruritic* [also: alimemazine; trimeprazine; alimemazine tartrate]

trimeproprimine [see: trimipramine]

trimetamide INN

trimetaphan camsilate INN *antihypertensive* [also: trimethaphan camsylate; trimetaphan camsilate]

trimetaphan camsylate BAN *antihypertensive* [also: trimethaphan camsylate; trimetaphan camsilate]

trimetazidine INN, BAN

trimethadione USP, INN *oxazolidinedione anticonvulsant for absence (petit mal) seizures* [also: troxidone]

trimethamide [see: trimetamide]

trimethaphan camphorsulfonate [see: trimethaphan camsylate]

trimethaphan camsylate USP *emergency antihypertensive* [also: trimetaphan camsilate; trimetaphan camsylate]

trimethidinium methosulfate NF, INN

trimethobenzamide INN *anticholinergic; post-surgical antiemetic* [also: trimethobenzamide HCl]

trimethobenzamide HCl USP *anticholinergic; post-surgical antiemetic; suppositories removed from the market in 2007 due to lack of efficacy* [also: trimethobenzamide] 300 mg oral; 100 mg/mL injection

trimethoprim (TMP) USAN, USP, INN, BAN *antibacterial antibiotic* 100, 200 mg oral

trimethoprim & sulfamethoxazole *broad-spectrum sulfonamide antibiotic* 80•400, 160•800 mg oral; 40•200 mg/5 mL oral; 16•80 mg/mL injection

trimethoprim sulfate USAN *antibiotic*

trimethoprim sulfate & polymyxin B sulfate *topical ophthalmic antibiotic* 1 mg•10 000 U per mL eye drops

trimethoquinol [see: tretoquinol]

trimethylammonium chloride carbamate [see: bethanechol chloride]

3,3,5-trimethylcyclohexyl salicylate [see: homosalate]

trimethylene [see: cyclopropane]

trimethylglycine (TMG) *natural methylation agent used to prevent cardiovascular disease by lowering homocysteine levels, to boost neurological function by remyelinating nerve cells, and to slow cellular aging by protecting DNA; precursor to SAMe (q.v.)*

trimethyltetradecylammonium bromide [see: tetradonium bromide]

trimetozine USAN, INN *sedative*

trimetrexate USAN, INN, BAN *antimetabolic antineoplastic; systemic antiprotozoal*

trimetrexate glucuronate USAN *antiprotozoal for AIDS-related Pneumocystis pneumonia (PCP) (orphan); investigational (orphan) antineoplastic for multiple cancers*

trimexiline INN

trimipramine USAN, INN *tricyclic antidepressant*

trimipramine maleate USAN *tricyclic antidepressant*

trimolide [see: trimetozine]

trimopam maleate [now: trepipam maleate]

trimoprostil USAN, INN *gastric antisecretory*

Trimo-San vaginal jelly OTC *antiseptic; astringent* [oxyquinoline sulfate; boric acid; sodium borate] 0.025%•1%•0.7% ☒ Terramycin

Trimox chewable tablets, capsules, powder for oral suspension (discontinued 2008) ℞ *aminopenicillin antibiotic* [amoxicillin] 125, 250 mg; 250, 500 mg; 250 mg/5 mL ☒ Tyromex

Trimox powder for oral suspension ℞ *aminopenicillin antibiotic* [amoxicillin] 125 mg/5 mL ☒ Tyromex

trimoxamine INN *antihypertensive* [also: trimoxamine HCl]

trimoxamine HCl USAN *antihypertensive* [also: trimoxamine]

Trimpex tablets ℞ *anti-infective; antibacterial* [trimethoprim] 100 mg

trimustine BAN [also: trichlormethine] ☒ tauromustine

Trinam reservoir delivery device *investigational (Phase II, orphan) gene-based therapy for neointimal hyperplasia disease* [vascular endothelial growth factor 165, human (hVEGF165)]

Trinate film-coated tablets ℞ *prenatal vitamin/mineral/calcium/iron supplement* [multiple vitamins & minerals; calcium; iron (as ferrous fumarate); folic acid] ≛•200•28•1 mg

trinecol (pullus) USAN *collagen derivative for treatment of rheumatoid arthritis*

TriNessa tablets (in packs of 28) ℞ *triphasic oral contraceptive* [norgestimate; ethinyl estradiol]
Phase 1 (7 days): 0.18 mg•35 mcg;
Phase 2 (7 days): 0,215 mg•35 mcg;
Phase 3 (7 days): 0.25 mg•35 mcg;
Counters (7 days)

trinitrin [see: nitroglycerin]

trinitrophenol NF

Tri-Norinyl tablets (in Wallettes of 28) R̥ *triphasic oral contraceptive* [norethindrone; ethinyl estradiol]
Phase 1 (7 days): 0.5 mg•35 mcg;
Phase 2 (9 days): 1 mg•35 mcg;
Phase 3 (5 days): 0.5 mg•35 mcg;
Counters (7 days)

Trinsicon capsules (discontinued 2009) R̥ *hematinic* [iron (as ferrous fumarate); vitamin B_{12}; vitamin C; intrinsic factor concentrate; folic acid] 110•0.015•75•240•0.5 mg

2′,3′,5′-tri-o-acetyluridine *investigational (orphan) treatment for mitochondrial disease*

triolein I 125 USAN *radioactive agent* 🔲 Tarlene

triolein I 131 USAN *radioactive agent* 🔲 Tarlene

trional [see: sulfonethylmethane]

Trionate caplets R̥ *antitussive; antihistamine* [carbetapentane tannate; chlorpheniramine tannate] 60•5 mg

Triostat IV injection R̥ *synthetic thyroid hormone (T_3 fraction only) for myxedema coma or precoma (orphan)* [liothyronine sodium] 10 mcg/mL

Triotann Pediatric oral suspension R̥ *decongestant; antihistamine; sleep aid* [phenylephrine tannate; chlorpheniramine tannate; pyrilamine tannate] 5•2•12.5 mg/5 mL

Triotann-S Pediatric oral suspension (discontinued 2007) R̥ *decongestant; antihistamine; sleep aid* [phenylephrine tannate; chlorpheniramine tannate; pyrilamine tannate] 5•2•12.5 mg/5 mL

Tri-Otic ear drops (discontinued 2008) R̥ *corticosteroidal anti-inflammatory; anesthetic; antiseptic* [hydrocortisone; pramoxine HCl; chloroxylenol] 10•10•1 mg/mL

trioxifene INN *antiestrogen* [also: trioxifene mesylate]

trioxifene mesylate USAN *antiestrogen* [also: trioxifene]

TriOxin ear drops R̥ *corticosteroidal anti-inflammatory; anesthetic; antiseptic* [hydrocortisone; benzocaine; chloroxylenol] 10•15•1 mg/mL

trioxsalen USAN, USP *systemic psoralens for repigmentation of idiopathic vitiligo; also used to enhance pigmentation and increase tolerance to sunlight* [also: trioxsalen]

trioxyethylrutin [see: troxerutin]

trioxymethylene [see: paraformaldehyde]

trioxysalen INN *systemic psoralens for repigmentation of idiopathic vitiligo; also used to enhance pigmentation and increase tolerance to sunlight* [also: trioxsalen]

tripamide USAN, INN *antihypertensive; diuretic*

triparanol INN *(withdrawn from market)*

Tri-Pase 8; Tri-Pase 16 tablets R̥ *porcine-derived digestive enzymes* [pancrelipase (lipase; protease; amylase)] 8•30•30, 16•60•60 thousand USP units

Tripedia IM injection R̥ *active immunizing agent for diphtheria, tetanus, and pertussis; Dtap (diphtheria predominant) vaccine used in the initial immunization series of infants and children 6 weeks to 6 years* [diphtheria toxoid; tetanus toxoid; pertussis antigens] 6.7 LfU•5 LfU•46.8 mcg per 0.5 mL dose

tripelennamine INN *ethylenediamine antihistamine* [also: tripelennamine citrate]

tripelennamine citrate USP *ethylenediamine antihistamine* [also: tripelennamine]

tripelennamine HCl USP *ethylenediamine antihistamine*

Triphasil tablets (in packs of 21 or 28) R̥ *triphasic oral contraceptive; emergency postcoital contraceptive* [levonorgestrel; ethinyl estradiol] 🔲 Travasol
Phase 1 (6 days): 0.5 mg•30 mcg;
Phase 2 (5 days): 0.75 mg•40 mcg;
Phase 3 (10 days): 0.125 mg•30 mcg

Triple Antibiotic ointment OTC *antibiotic* [polymyxin B sulfate; neomycin sulfate; bacitracin] 5000 U•3.5 mg•400 U per g

Triple Cream OTC *moisturizer; emollient*

Triple Paste AF ointment (discontinued 2009) OTC *antifungal* [miconazole nitrate] 2%

triple reuptake inhibitors (TRIs) *a class of investigational oral antidepressants that inhibit neuronal uptake of the CNS neurotransmitters serotonin (5-HT), norepinephrine, and dopamine*

triple sulfa (sulfathiazole, sulfacetamide, and sulfabenzamide) [q.v.]

Triple Tannate Pediatric oral suspension ℞ *decongestant; antihistamine; sleep aid* [phenylephrine tannate; chlorpheniramine tannate; pyrilamine tannate] 5•2•12.5 mg/5 mL

Triple Vitamin ADC with Fluoride pediatric oral drops (discontinued 2008) ℞ *vitamin supplement; dental caries preventative* [vitamins A, C, and D; fluoride] 1500 IU•35 mg•400 IU•0.5 mg per mL

Triplex AD oral liquid (discontinued 2011) ℞ *decongestant; antihistamine; sleep aid* [phenylephrine HCl; chlorpheniramine maleate; pyrilamine maleate] 7.5•2•12.5 mg/5 mL

Triplex DM oral liquid ℞ *antitussive; antihistamine; sleep aid; decongestant* [dextromethorphan hydrobromide; pyrilamine maleate; phenylephrine HCl] 15•12.5•7.5 mg/5 mL

Tripohist D oral liquid ℞ *decongestant; antihistamine* [pseudoephedrine HCl; triprolidine HCl] 45•1.25 mg/5 mL

tripotassium citrate monohydrate [see: potassium citrate]

Tri-Previfem tablets (in packs of 28) ℞ *triphasic oral contraceptive* [norgestimate; ethinyl estradiol]
Phase 1 (7 days): 0.18 mg•35 mcg;
Phase 2 (7 days): 0.215 mg•35 mcg;
Phase 3 (7 days): 0.25 mg•35 mcg;
Counters (7 days)

triproamylin [see: pramlintide]

triprolidine INN *antihistamine* [also: triprolidine HCl]

triprolidine HCl USP *antihistamine* [also: triprolidine] 1.25 mg/5 mL oral

triprolidine HCl & pseudoephedrine HCl *antihistamine; decongestant* 2.5•60 mg/10 mL oral

Tripterygium wilfordii *medicinal herb* [see: thunder god vine]

Triptone long-acting caplets OTC *antinauseant; antiemetic; antivertigo; motion sickness preventative* [dimenhydrinate] 50 mg

triptorelin USAN, INN *gonadotropin-releasing hormone (GnRH) antineoplastic*

triptorelin pamoate *gonadotropin-releasing hormone (GnRH) antineoplastic for palliative treatment of advanced prostate cancer; investigational (orphan) for palliative treatment of advanced ovarian cancer*

trisaccharides A and B *investigational (orphan) for newborn hemolytic disease and ABO blood incompatibility of organ or bone marrow transplants*

Trisenox injection ℞ *antineoplastic for acute promyelocytic leukemia (orphan); investigational (orphan) for other leukemias, multiple myeloma, myelodysplastic syndromes, liver cancer, and malignant glioma* [arsenic trioxide] 10 mg/10 mL

trisodium calcium DTPA [see: pentetate calcium trisodium]

trisodium citrate [see: sodium citrate]

trisodium citrate dihydrate [see: sodium citrate]

trisodium hydrogen ethylenediaminetetraacetate [see: edetate trisodium]

trisodium zinc DTPA [see: pentetate zinc trisodium]

Trispec PSE oral liquid (discontinued 2007) ℞ *antitussive; decongestant; expectorant* [dextromethorphan hydrobromide; pseudoephedrine HCl; guaifenesin] 15•30•25 mg/5 mL

Tri-Sprintec tablets (in packs of 28) ℞ *triphasic oral contraceptive* [norgestimate; ethinyl estradiol]
Phase 1 (7 days): 0.18 mg•35 mcg;
Phase 2 (7 days): 0.215 mg•35 mcg;
Phase 3 (7 days): 0.25 mg•35 mcg;
Counters (7 days)

Tri-Statin II cream ℞ *corticosteroidal anti-inflammatory; antifungal* [triamcinolone acetonide; nystatin] 0.1% • 100 000 U per g

trisulfapyrimidines USP (a mixture of sulfadiazine, sulfamerazine, and sulfamethazine) *broad-spectrum bacteriostatic*

Tri-Super Flavons 1000 tablets OTC *dietary supplement* [mixed bioflavonoids] 1000 mg

Trital DM oral liquid ℞ *antitussive; antihistamine; decongestant* [dextromethorphan hydrobromide; chlorpheniramine maleate; phenylephrine HCl] 15 • 4 • 10 mg/5 mL

tritheon [see: acinitrazole]

tritiated water USAN *radioactive agent*

Triticum repens medicinal herb [see: couch grass]

tritiozine INN

tritoqualine INN

TriTuss syrup (discontinued 2011) ℞ *antitussive; decongestant; expectorant* [dextromethorphan hydrobromide; phenylephrine HCl; guaifenesin] 25 • 12.5 • 175 mg/5 mL

Trituss-A oral drops (discontinued 2007) ℞ *antitussive; antihistamine; decongestant; for children 3–24 months* [dextromethorphan hydrobromide; carbinoxamine maleate; phenylephrine HCl] 4 • 1 • 2 mg/mL

TriTuss-ER extended-release caplets ℞ *antitussive; decongestant; expectorant* [dextromethorphan hydrobromide; phenylephrine HCl; guaifenesin] 30 • 10 • 600 mg

Tritussin syrup (discontinued 2007) ℞ *narcotic antitussive; antihistamine; decongestant* [hydrocodone bitartrate; chlorpheniramine maleate; phenylephrine HCl] 10 • 4 • 10 mg/10 mL

Trivagizole 3 vaginal cream OTC *antifungal for yeast infections* [clotrimazole] 2%

trivalent oral poliovirus vaccine (TOPV) [see: poliovirus vaccine, live oral]

Trivaris gel suspension for ocular, IM, or intra-articular injection ℞ *corticosteroidal anti-inflammatory* [triamcinolone acetonide] 80 mg/mL

Tri-Vi-Flor pediatric chewable tablets, pediatric oral drops (discontinued 2008) ℞ *vitamin supplement; dental caries preventative* [vitamins A, C, and D; sodium fluoride] 2500 IU • 60 mg • 400 IU • 1 mg; 1500 IU • 35 mg • 400 IU • 0.25 mg, 1500 IU • 35 mg • 400 IU • 0.5 mg per mL

Tri-Vi-Flor with Iron pediatric oral drops ℞ *vitamin/iron supplement; dental caries preventative* [vitamins A, C, and D; iron; sodium fluoride] 1500 IU • 35 mg • 400 IU • 0.25 mg per mL

Tri-Vi-Sol oral drops OTC *vitamin supplement* [vitamins A, C, and D] 1500 IU • 35 mg • 400 IU per mL ⧈ Travasol

Tri-Vi-Sol with Iron oral drops OTC *vitamin/iron supplement* [vitamins A, C, and D; iron (as elemental iron and ferrous sulfate)] 1500 IU • 35 mg • 400 IU • 10 mg per mL

Tri-Vitamin oral drops OTC *vitamin supplement* [vitamins A, C, and D] 1500 IU • 35 mg • 400 IU per mL

Trivitamin Fluoride pediatric chewable tablets, pediatric oral drops (discontinued 2008) ℞ *vitamin supplement; dental caries preventative* [vitamins A, C, and D; fluoride] 2500 IU • 60 mg • 400 IU • 1 mg; 1500 IU • 35 mg • 400 IU • 0.25 mg, 1500 IU • 35 mg • 400 IU • 0.5 mg per mL

Tri-Vitamin with Fluoride pediatric oral drops (discontinued 2008) ℞ *vitamin supplement; dental caries preventative* [vitamins A, C, and D; fluoride] 1500 IU • 35 mg • 400 IU • 0.5 mg per mL

Trivora tablets (in packs of 28) ℞ *triphasic oral contraceptive* [levonorgestrel; ethinyl estradiol]
Phase 1 (6 days): 0.5 mg • 30 mcg;
Phase 2 (5 days): 0.75 mg • 40 mcg;
Phase 3 (10 days): 0.125 mg • 30 mcg;
Counters (7 days)

trixolane INN ② teroxalene
Trizivir film-coated caplets ℞ *antiretroviral nucleoside reverse transcriptase inhibitor (NRTI) for HIV infection* [abacavir sulfate; zidovudine; lamivudine] 300•300•150 mg
trizoxime INN
Trizyme (trademarked ingredient) *digestive enzymes* [amylolytic, proteolytic, and cellulolytic enzymes (amylase; protease; cellulase)]
Trizytek *investigational (NDA filed) non-porcine derived enzyme replacement therapy for patients with pancreatic insufficiency* [liprotamase]
Trobicin powder for IM injection (discontinued 2009) ℞ *antibiotic for gonorrhea* [spectinomycin HCl] 400 mg/mL ② Tri-Biozene
Trocaine lozenges OTC *mucous membrane anesthetic* [benzocaine] 10 mg ② tarragon; Torecan; Treagan
Trocal lozenges OTC *antitussive* [dextromethorphan hydrobromide] 7.5 mg
trocimine INN
troclosene potassium USAN, INN *topical anti-infective*
trofosfamide INN
troglitazone USAN, INN *thiazolidinedione (TZD) antidiabetic and peroxisome proliferator–activated receptor–gamma (PPARγ) agonist that increases cellular response to insulin without increasing insulin secretion*
trolamine USAN, NF *alkalizing agent; analgesic*
trolamine polypeptide oleate-condensate *cerumenolytic to emulsify and disperse ear wax*
trolamine salicylate *topical analgesic*
troleandomycin USAN, USP *macrolide antibiotic; investigational (orphan) for severe asthma* [also: triacetyloleandomycin]
trolnitrate INN
trolnitrate phosphate [see: trolnitrate]
tromantadine INN
trometamol INN, BAN *systemic alkalizer; corrects acidosis associated with*

cardiac bypass surgery or cardiac arrest [also: tromethamine]
tromethamine USAN, USP *systemic alkalizer; corrects acidosis associated with cardiac bypass surgery or cardiac arrest* [also: trometamol]
Tronolane anorectal cream OTC *local anesthetic; astringent; emollient* [pramoxine HCl; zinc oxide] 1%•5%
Tronolane rectal suppositories OTC *astringent* [phenylephrine HCl] 0.25%
Tronothane HCl cream OTC *anesthetic* [pramoxine HCl] 1% ② trientine HCl
tropabazate INN
Tropaeolum majus *medicinal herb* [see: Indian cress]
tropanserin INN, BAN *migraine-specific serotonin receptor antagonist* [also: tropanserin HCl]
tropanserin HCl USAN *migraine-specific serotonin receptor antagonist* [also: tropanserin]
tropapride INN
tropatepine INN
tropenziline bromide INN
TrophAmine 6%; TrophAmine 10% IV infusion ℞ *total parenteral nutrition; peripheral parenteral nutrition* [multiple essential and nonessential amino acids]
Trophite + Iron oral liquid (discontinued 2008) OTC *vitamin/iron supplement* [vitamin B₁; vitamin B₁₂; iron (as ferric pyrophosphate)] 30•0.075•60 mg/15 mL
trophosphamide [see: trofosfamide]
Tropicacyl eye drops ℞ *cycloplegic; mydriatic* [tropicamide] 0.5%, 1%
tropicamide USAN, USP, INN *ophthalmic anticholinergic; cycloplegic; short-acting mydriatic* 0.5%, 1% eye drops
tropigline INN, BAN
tropirine INN
tropisetron INN, BAN *antiemetic*
tropodifene INN
troquidazole INN
trospectomycin INN, BAN *broad-spectrum aminocyclitol antibiotic* [also: trospectomycin sulfate]

trospectomycin sulfate USAN *broad-spectrum aminocyclitol antibiotic* [also: trospectomycin]

trospium chloride INN *muscarinic receptor antagonist; urinary antispasmodic for overactive bladder with urinary frequency, urgency, and incontinence* 20 mg oral

trovafloxacin mesylate USAN *broad-spectrum fluoroquinolone antibiotic*

Trovan film-coated tablets (discontinued 2008) ℞ *broad-spectrum fluoroquinolone antibiotic* [trovafloxacin mesylate] 100, 200 mg

Trovan IV infusion (discontinued 2008) ℞ *broad-spectrum fluoroquinolone antibiotic* [alatrofloxacin mesylate] 5 mg/mL

Trovan/Zithromax Compliance Pak ℞ *single-dose antibiotic treatment for sexually transmitted diseases* [Trovan (trovafloxacin mesylate); Zithromax (azithromycin)] 100 mg tablet; 1 g pkt. of powder for oral suspension

TroVax *investigational (Phase III) immunotherapeutic for advanced or metastatic renal cell carcinoma (RCC)*

troxacitabine USAN, INN *antineoplastic for various leukemias and solid tumors; investigational (orphan) for acute myeloid leukemia*

Troxatyl *investigational (orphan) antineoplastic for acute myeloid leukemia* [troxacitabine]

troxerutin INN, BAN *vitamin P₄*

troxidone BAN *anticonvulsant* [also: trimethadione]

troxipide INN

troxolamide INN

troxonium tosilate INN [also: troxonium tosylate]

troxonium tosylate BAN [also: troxonium tosilate]

troxundate INN *combining name for radicals or groups*

troxypyrrolium tosilate INN [also: troxypyrrolium tosylate]

troxypyrrolium tosylate BAN [also: troxypyrrolium tosilate]

true ivy *medicinal herb* [see: English ivy]

T.R.U.E. Test patch ℞ *diagnostic aid for contact dermatitis* [skin test antigens (23 different) plus 1 negative control]

Trugene genetic testing system for professional use ℞ *in vitro diagnostic aid for HIV mutations that cause resistance to anti-AIDS drugs; used to determine which treatment regimen is most effective in individual patients* ☒ tarragon; Teargen; Torecan; Treagan; Trocaine

Trusopt eye drops ℞ *carbonic anhydrase inhibitor for glaucoma* [dorzolamide HCl] 2%

Truvada film-coated caplets ℞ *once-daily antiviral combination for HIV infections; approved to prevent HIV infection in sexually active gay men who test HIV negative at treatment initiation* [emtricitabine; tenofovir disoproxil fumarate] 200•300 mg

truxicurium iodide INN

truxipicurium iodide INN

Trycet film-coated caplets (discontinued 2010) ℞ *narcotic analgesic; antipyretic; all products containing propoxyphene were withdrawn from the market in 2010 due to safety concerns* [propoxyphene napsylate; acetaminophen] 100•325 mg ☒ Triacet

trypaflavine [see: acriflavine HCl]

trypan blue *surgical aid for staining the anterior capsule of the lens and other ophthalmic tissue during vitrectomy*

tryparsamide USP, INN

trypsin, crystallized USP *topical proteolytic enzyme; necrotic tissue debridement*

trypsin & chymotrypsin & papain *investigational (orphan) enzyme combination adjunct to chemotherapy for multiple myeloma*

tryptizol [see: amitriptyline]

tryptizol HCl [see: amitriptyline HCl]

tryptophan (L-tryptophan) USAN, USP, INN *essential amino acid; serotonin precursor banned by the FDA in 1997; returned to the market in 2008*

TSC (technetium sulfur colloid) [see: technetium Tc 99m sulfur colloid]

T/Scalp topical liquid OTC *corticoster-oidal anti-inflammatory* [hydrocorti-sone] 1%

TSH (thyroid-stimulating hormone) [see: thyrotropin]

TSPA (triethylenethiophosphor-amide) [see: thiotepa]

TST (tuberculin skin test) [see: tuberculin]

Tsuga canadensis *medicinal herb* [see: hemlock]

T-Tabs (trademarked dosage form) *tablets with a "T" imprint*

tuaminoheptane USP, INN *adrenergic; vasoconstrictor*

tuaminoheptane sulfate USP

tuberculin USP *tuberculosis skin test*

tuberculin, crude [see: tuberculin]

tuberculin, old (OT) [see: tuberculin]

tuberculin purified protein deriva-tive (PPD) [see: tuberculin]

tuberculosis vaccine [see: BCG vac-cine]

Tubersol intradermal injection ℞ *tuberculosis skin test* [tuberculin puri-fied protein derivative] 5 U/0.1 mL

Tubex (trademarked delivery device) *cartridge-needle unit*

tubocurarine chloride USP, INN, BAN *neuromuscular blocker; muscle relax-ant* 3 mg (20 U)/mL injection

tubocurarine chloride HCl pentahy-drate [see: tubocurarine chloride]

tubulozole INN *antineoplastic; micro-tubule inhibitor* [also: tubulozole HCl]

tubulozole HCl USAN, INN *antineo-plastic; microtubule inhibitor* [also: tubulozole]

tucaresol INN, BAN *immunopotentiator*

Tucks anorectal ointment OTC *cortico-steroidal anti-inflammatory* [hydrocor-tisone acetate] 1% (note: multiple products with the same name)

Tucks anorectal ointment OTC *local anesthetic; astringent* [pramoxine HCl; zinc oxide] 1%•12.5% (note: multi-ple products with the same name)

Tucks rectal suppositories OTC *emol-lient* [topical starch] 51%

Tucks; Tucks Take-Alongs cleansing pads OTC *moisturizer and cleanser for the perineal area; astringent* [witch hazel; glycerin] 50%•10%

Tucks Clear gel OTC *emollient; astrin-gent* [hamamelis water (witch hazel); glycerin] 50%•10%

tuclazepam INN

Tuinal Pulvules (capsules) ℞ *sedative; hypnotic; also abused as a street drug* [amobarbital sodium; secobarbital sodium] 50•50, 100•100 mg

tulobuterol INN, BAN, JAN [also: tulo-buterol HCl]

tulobuterol HCl JAN [also: tulobuterol]

tulopafant INN

tumeric root *medicinal herb* [see: gold-enseal]

tumor necrosis factor–binding pro-tein I and II *investigational (orphan) for symptomatic AIDS patients*

Tums chewable tablets (discontinued 2009) OTC *antacid; calcium supple-ment* [calcium (as carbonate)] 200 mg (500 mg)

Tums Calcium for Life Bone Health chewable tablets OTC *antacid; calcium supplement* [calcium (as carbonate)] 500 mg (1250 mg)

Tums Calcium for Life PMS; Tums E-X; Tums Kids; Tums Ultra chewable tablets OTC *antacid; calcium supplement* [calcium (as carbonate)] 300 mg (750 mg); 300 mg (750 mg); 300 mg (750 mg); 400 mg (1 g)

Tums Dual Action chewable tablets OTC *combination histamine H_2 antago-nist and antacid for acid indigestion and heartburn* [famotidine; calcium car-bonate; magnesium hydroxide] 10•800•165 mg

Tums Quick Pak oral powder OTC *antacid; calcium supplement* [calcium (as carbonate)] 400 mg (1 g)

Tums Smooth Dissolve (orally disin-tegrating tablets) OTC *antacid; cal-cium supplement* [calcium (as carbon-ate)] 300 mg (750 mg)

tung seed (*Aleurites cordata; A. moluccana***)** *seed and oil medicinal* herb for asthma, bowel evacuation, and tumors; not generally regarded as safe and effective as it is highly toxic

tungsten element (W)

Turbinaire (trademarked dosage form) nasal inhalation aerosol

Turbuhaler (trademarked delivery form) dry powder in a metered-dose inhaler

turkey corn (Corydalis formosa) root medicinal herb used as an antisyphilitic, bitter tonic, and diuretic

turkey pea; wild turkey pea medicinal herb [see: turkey corn]

turmeric (Curcuma domestica; C. longa) rhizomes medicinal herb for flatulence, hemorrhage, hepatitis and jaundice, topical analgesia, and ringworm

Turnera aphrodisiaca; T. diffusa; T. microphylla medicinal herb [see: damiana]

turosteride INN

turpentine (Pinus palustris) gum natural treatment for colds, cough, and toothache; also used topically as a counterirritant for muscle pain and rheumatic disorders

turtlebloom (Chelone glabra) leaves medicinal herb used as an anthelmintic, aperient, cholagogue, and detergent

Tusana-D oral liquid (discontinued 2009) ℞ narcotic antitussive; antihistamine; decongestant [hydrocodone bitartrate; chlorpheniramine maleate; phenylephrine HCl] 6•2•12 mg/5 mL

Tusdec-DM oral liquid ℞ antitussive; antihistamine; decongestant [dextromethorphan hydrobromide; brompheniramine maleate; phenylephrine HCl] 15•2•7.5 mg/5 mL

Tusdec-HC oral liquid (discontinued 2009) ℞ narcotic antitussive; decongestant [hydrocodone bitartrate; phenylephrine HCl] 3.75•7.5 mg/5 mL

Tusnel; Tusnel Pediatric oral liquid ℞ antitussive; decongestant; expectorant [dextromethorphan hydrobromide; pseudoephedrine HCl; guai-

fenesin] 15•30•200 mg/5 mL; 5•15•50 mg/5 mL

Tusnel C syrup ℞ narcotic antitussive; decongestant; expectorant [codeine phosphate; pseudoephedrine HCl; guaifenesin; alcohol 1.9%] 10•30•100 mg/5 mL

Tusnel-DM Pediatric oral liquid OTC antitussive; decongestant; expectorant [dextromethorphan hydrobromide; pseudoephedrine HCl; guaifenesin] 2.5•7.5•25 mg/5 mL

Tusnel-HC oral liquid (discontinued 2009) ℞ narcotic antitussive; antihistamine; decongestant [hydrocodone bitartrate; brompheniramine maleate; phenylephrine HCl] 2.5•4•7.5 mg/5 mL

Tussafed syrup (discontinued 2007) ℞ antitussive; antihistamine; decongestant [dextromethorphan hydrobromide; carbinoxamine maleate; pseudoephedrine HCl] 15•4•60 mg/5 mL

Tussafed Ex syrup (discontinued 2007) ℞ antitussive; decongestant; expectorant [dextromethorphan hydrobromide; phenylephrine HCl; guaifenesin] 30•10•200 mg/5 mL

Tussafed HC; Tussafed HCG syrup ℞ narcotic antitussive; decongestant; expectorant [hydrocodone bitartrate; phenylephrine HCl; guaifenesin] 2.5•7.5•50 mg/5 mL; 2.5•6•150 mg/5 mL

Tussafed LA sustained-release caplets (discontinued 2007) ℞ antitussive; decongestant; expectorant [dextromethorphan hydrobromide; pseudoephedrine HCl; guaifenesin] 30•60•600 mg

Tussall syrup ℞ antitussive; antihistamine; decongestant [dextromethorphan hydrobromide; dexbrompheniramine maleate; phenylephrine HCl] 20•2•10 mg/5 mL ▢ TiSol

Tussall-ER extended-release caplets ℞ antitussive; antihistamine; decongestant [dextromethorphan hydrobromide; dexbrompheniramine maleate; phenylephrine HCl] 30•6•20 mg

Tussbid extended-release capsules ℞ *decongestant; expectorant* [phenylephrine HCl; guaifenesin] 15•400 mg

Tussbid PD extended-release capsules ℞ *decongestant; expectorant* [phenylephrine HCl; guaifenesin] 7.5•200 mg

Tussend caplets (discontinued 2007) ℞ *narcotic antitussive; antihistamine; decongestant* [hydrocodone bitartrate; chlorpheniramine maleate; pseudoephedrine HCl] 5•4•60 mg

Tussend syrup (discontinued 2007) ℞ *narcotic antitussive; antihistamine; decongestant* [hydrocodone bitartrate; chlorpheniramine maleate; pseudoephedrine HCl; alcohol 5%] 5•4•60 mg/10 mL

Tussi-12 caplets ℞ *antitussive; antihistamine* [carbetapentane tannate; chlorpheniramine tannate] 60•5 mg

Tussi-12 D caplets ℞ *antitussive; decongestant; antihistamine; sleep aid* [carbetapentane tannate; phenylephrine tannate; pyrilamine tannate] 60•40•10 mg

Tussi-12 S oral suspension ℞ *antitussive; antihistamine* [carbetapentane tannate; chlorpheniramine tannate] 30•4 mg/5 mL

Tussi-12D S oral suspension ℞ *antitussive; antihistamine; sleep aid; decongestant* [carbetapentane tannate; pyrilamine tannate; phenylephrine tannate] 30•30•5 mg/5 mL

Tussi-bid sustained-release caplets ℞ *antitussive; expectorant* [dextromethorphan hydrobromide; guaifenesin] 60•1200 mg

TussiCaps Full Strength; TussiCaps Half Strength extended-release capsules ℞ *narcotic antitussive; antihistamine* [hydrocodone bitartrate; chlorpheniramine maleate] 10•8 mg; 5•4 mg

Tussiden DM oral liquid (discontinued 2009) ℞ *antitussive; expectorant* [dextromethorphan hydrobromide; guaifenesin] 10•100 mg/5 mL

Tussigon tablets ℞ *narcotic antitussive; anticholinergic* [hydrocodone bitartrate; homatropine methylbromide] 5•1.5 mg ☑ tisoquone

Tussilago farfara *medicinal herb* [see: coltsfoot]

TussiNATE syrup (discontinued 2007) ℞ *narcotic antitussive; antihistamine; sleep aid; decongestant* [hydrocodone bitartrate; diphenhydramine HCl; phenylephrine HCl] 7•25•10 mg/10 mL

Tussionex Pennkinetic extended-release oral suspension ℞ *narcotic antitussive; antihistamine* [hydrocodone polistirex; chlorpheniramine polistirex] 10•8 mg/5 mL

Tussi-Organidin DM NR oral liquid (discontinued 2010) ℞ *antitussive; expectorant* [dextromethorphan hydrobromide; guaifenesin] 10•300 mg/5 mL

Tussi-Organidin DM-S NR oral liquid with an oral syringe ℞ *antitussive; expectorant* [dextromethorphan hydrobromide; guaifenesin] 10•300 mg/5 mL

Tussi-Organidin NR; Tussi-Organidin-S NR oral liquid ("S" includes an oral syringe) ℞ *narcotic antitussive; expectorant* [codeine phosphate; guaifenesin] 10•300 mg/5 mL

Tussi-Pres; Tussi-Pres Pediatric oral liquid ℞ *antitussive; decongestant; expectorant* [dextromethorphan hydrobromide; phenylephrine HCl; guaifenesin] 15•5•200 mg/5 mL; 5•2.5•75 mg/5 mL

Tussirex oral liquid ℞ *narcotic antitussive; decongestant; antihistamine; expectorant; analgesic* [codeine phosphate; phenylephrine HCl; pheniramine maleate; sodium citrate; sodium salicylate; caffeine citrate] 10•4.17•13.33•83.3•83.33•25 mg/5 mL

Tussirex syrup (discontinued 2011) ℞ *narcotic antitussive; decongestant; antihistamine; expectorant; analgesic* [codeine phosphate; phenylephrine HCl; pheniramine maleate; sodium citrate; sodium salicylate; caffeine

citrate] 10•4.17•13.33•83.3•
83.33•25 mg/5 mL

Tussizone-12 RF caplets (discontinued 2009) ℞ *antitussive; antihistamine* [carbetapentane tannate; chlorpheniramine tannate] 60•5 mg

Tussizone-12 RF oral suspension ℞ *antitussive; antihistamine* [carbetapentane tannate; chlorpheniramine tannate] 30•4 mg/5 mL

Tusso-C syrup ℞ *narcotic antitussive; expectorant* [codeine phosphate; guaifenesin] 10•200 mg/5 mL

Tusso-DM dual-release caplets ℞ *antitussive; decongestant; expectorant* [dextromethorphan hydrobromide; phenylephrine HCl; guaifenesin] 23 mg (65% extended release)•9 mg (100% extended release)•600 mg (67% extended release) ⑤ Tazidime

Tusso-DMR capsules ℞ *antitussive; decongestant; expectorant* [dextromethorphan hydrobromide; phenylephrine HCl; guaifenesin] 14•7•288 mg

Tusso-HC caplets (discontinued 2011) ℞ *narcotic antitussive; expectorant* [hydrocodone bitartrate; guaifenesin] 10•1200 mg

Tusso-XR oral suspension ℞ *antitussive; decongestant; expectorant* [dextromethorphan hydrobromide; phenylephrine HCl; guaifenesin] 20•10•100 mg/5 mL

Tusso-ZMR capsules ℞ *antitussive; expectorant* [carbetapentane citrate; guaifenesin] 8•200 mg

Tusso-ZR syrup ℞ *antitussive; expectorant* [carbetapentane citrate; guaifenesin] 7.5•150 mg/5 mL

Tussplex syrup ℞ *narcotic antitussive; decongestant; antihistamine; sleep aid* [hydrocodone bitartrate; phenylephrine HCl; pyrilamine maleate] 6•5•12 mg/5 mL

Tusstat syrup ℞ *antihistamine; sleep aid* [diphenhydramine HCl; alcohol 5%] 12.5 mg/5 mL

Tustan 12S oral suspension ℞ *antitussive; antihistamine* [carbetapentane tannate; chlorpheniramine tannate] 30•4 mg/5 mL

tuvatidine INN

tuvirumab USAN, INN *investigational (orphan) prophylaxis of hepatitis B reinfection following liver transplants*

T-Vites tablets OTC *vitamin/mineral supplement* [multiple vitamins & minerals; folic acid; biotin] ±•400•30 mcg

12 Hour nasal spray OTC *nasal decongestant* [oxymetazoline HCl] 0.05%

Twelve Resin-K tablets OTC *vitamin B₁₂ supplement* [cyanocobalamin on resin] 1000 mcg

20/20 eye drops OTC *decongestant; vasoconstrictor; moisturizer/lubricant* [naphazoline HCl; glycerin] 0.012%•0.2%

Twice-A-Day 12-Hour nasal spray OTC *nasal decongestant* [oxymetazoline HCl] 0.05%

Twilite caplets OTC *antihistamine; sleep aid* [diphenhydramine HCl] 50 mg

twin leaf (Jeffersonia diphylla) root *medicinal herb used as an antirheumatic, antispasmodic, antisyphilitic, diuretic, emetic, and expectorant*

Twinject prefilled auto-injector (2 doses per unit) ℞ *vasopressor for shock; emergency treatment of anaphylaxis* [epinephrine] 1:1000 (0.15, 0.3 mg)

Twinrix IM injection in vials and prefilled syringes ℞ *immunizing agent for hepatitis A, B, and D in adults* [hepatitis A vaccine, inactivated; hepatitis B virus vaccine, recombinant] 720 EL.U.•20 mcg per mL

TwoCal HN ready-to-use oral liquid OTC *enteral nutritional therapy* [lactose-free formula]

Twynsta tablets ℞ *combination calcium channel blocker and angiotensin receptor blocker (ARB) for hypertension* [amlodipine (as besylate); telmisartan] 5•40, 5•80, 10•40, 10•80 mg

tybamate USAN, NF, INN, BAN *minor tranquilizer*

tyformin BAN [also: tiformin]

Tygacil powder for IV infusion ℞ *broad-spectrum antibiotic for intraabdominal and complicated skin struc-*

ture infections, methicillin-resistant Staphylococcus aureus (MRSA), and community-acquired bacterial pneumonia (CABP) [tigecycline] 50 mg/vial ⑨ TachoSil; Taxol

Tykerb film-coated tablets ℞ tyrosine kinase inhibitor; once-daily antineoplastic for advanced or metastatic HER2-positive breast cancer; investigational for kidney, head, neck, and colon cancers [lapatinib (as ditosylate)] 250 mg

tylcalsin [see: calcium acetylsalicylate]

tylemalum [see: carbubarb]

Tylenol tablets, caplets, oral liquid OTC analgesic; antipyretic [acetaminophen] 325 mg; 500 mg; 166.6 mg/5 mL

Tylenol, Children's oral suspension OTC analgesic; antipyretic [acetaminophen] 160 mg/5 mL

Tylenol 8 Hour extended-release caplets OTC analgesic; antipyretic [acetaminophen] 650 mg

Tylenol Allergy Multi-Symptom caplets, gelcaps OTC decongestant; antihistamine; analgesic; antipyretic [phenylephrine HCl; chlorpheniramine maleate; acetaminophen] 5•2•325 mg

Tylenol Allergy Multi-Symptom Convenience Pack caplets OTC decongestant; analgesic; antipyretic; antihistamine; sleep aid added PM [phenylephrine HCl; acetaminophen; chlorpheniramine maleate added AM; diphenhydramine HCl added PM] 5•325•2 mg AM; 5•325•25 mg PM

Tylenol Allergy Multi-Symptom Night-time caplets OTC decongestant; antihistamine; sleep aid; analgesic; antipyretic [phenylephrine HCl; diphenhydramine HCl; acetaminophen] 5•25•325 mg

Tylenol Arthritis Pain extended-release caplets, extended-release geltabs OTC analgesic; antipyretic [acetaminophen] 650 mg

Tylenol Chest Congestion caplets, oral liquid OTC expectorant; analgesic; antipyretic [guaifenesin; acetamino-phen] 200•325 mg; 400•1000 mg/30 mL

Tylenol Children's Meltaways orally disintegrating tablets OTC analgesic; antipyretic [acetaminophen] 80 mg

Tylenol Cold, Children's pediatric chewable tablets, oral liquid OTC decongestant; antihistamine; analgesic; antipyretic [pseudoephedrine HCl; chlorpheniramine maleate; acetaminophen] 7.5•0.5•80 mg; 15•1•160 mg/5 mL

Tylenol Cold Head Congestion Daytime gelcaps OTC antitussive; decongestant; analgesic; antipyretic [dextromethorphan hydrobromide; phenylephrine HCl; acetaminophen] 10•5•325 mg

Tylenol Cold Head Congestion Daytime Cool Burst; Tylenol Cold Multi-Symptom Daytime Cool Burst caplets OTC antitussive; decongestant; analgesic; antipyretic [dextromethorphan hydrobromide; phenylephrine HCl; acetaminophen] 10•5•325 mg

Tylenol Cold Head Congestion Nighttime Cool Burst; Tylenol Cold Multi-Symptom Nighttime Cool Burst caplets OTC antitussive; antihistamine; decongestant; analgesic; antipyretic [dextromethorphan hydrobromide; chlorpheniramine maleate; phenylephrine HCl; acetaminophen] 10•2•5•325 mg

Tylenol Cold Multi-Symptom Daytime Citrus Burst oral liquid OTC antitussive; decongestant; analgesic; antipyretic [dextromethorphan hydrobromide; phenylephrine HCl; acetaminophen] 20•10•650 mg/30 mL

Tylenol Cold Multi-Symptom Nighttime Cool Burst oral liquid OTC antitussive; antihistamine; sleep aid; decongestant; analgesic; antipyretic [dextromethorphan hydrobromide; doxylamine succinate; phenylephrine HCl; acetaminophen] 20•12.5•10•650 mg/30 mL

Tylenol Cold Severe Congestion caplets OTC *antitussive; decongestant; expectorant; analgesic; antipyretic* [dextromethorphan hydrobromide; pseudoephedrine HCl; guaifenesin; acetaminophen] 15•30•200•325 mg

Tylenol Cough & Sore Throat Daytime oral liquid OTC *antitussive; analgesic; antipyretic* [dextromethorphan hydrobromide; acetaminophen] 30•1000 mg/30 mL

Tylenol Cough & Sore Throat Nighttime oral liquid OTC *antitussive; antihistamine; sleep aid; analgesic; antipyretic* [dextromethorphan hydrobromide; doxylamine succinate; acetaminophen] 30•12.5•1000 mg/30 mL

Tylenol EZ Tabs tablets OTC *analgesic; antipyretic* [acetaminophen] 500 mg

Tylenol GoTabs chewable tablets OTC *analgesic; antipyretic* [acetaminophen] 500 mg

Tylenol Infants' Drops (discontinued 2011) OTC *analgesic; antipyretic* [acetaminophen] 100 mg/mL

Tylenol Infants' Drops Plus Cold (discontinued 2011) OTC *decongestant; analgesic; antipyretic* [phenylephrine HCl; acetaminophen] 2.5•160 mg/1.6 mL

Tylenol Jr. Meltaways orally disintegrating tablets OTC *analgesic; antipyretic* [acetaminophen] 160 mg

Tylenol Multi-Symptom Menstrual Relief, Women's caplets OTC *analgesic; antipyretic; diuretic* [acetaminophen; pamabrom] 500•25 mg

Tylenol No. 2, No. 3, and No. 4 [see: Tylenol with Codeine]

Tylenol Plus Children's Cold oral suspension OTC *decongestant; antihistamine; analgesic; antipyretic; for children 6–11 years* [phenylephrine HCl; chlorpheniramine maleate; acetaminophen] 5•2•320 mg/10 mL

Tylenol Plus Children's Cough & Runny Nose oral suspension OTC *antitussive; antihistamine; analgesic; antipyretic; for children 6–11 years* [dextromethorphan hydrobromide; chlorpheniramine maleate; acetaminophen] 10•2•320 mg/10 mL

Tylenol Plus Children's Cough & Sore Throat oral suspension OTC *antitussive; analgesic; antipyretic; for children 2–11 years* [dextromethorphan hydrobromide; acetaminophen] 5•160 mg/5 mL

Tylenol Plus Children's Flu; Tylenol Plus Children's Multi-Symptom Cold oral suspension OTC *antitussive; antihistamine; decongestant; analgesic; antipyretic; for children 6–11 years* [dextromethorphan hydrobromide; chlorpheniramine maleate; phenylephrine HCl; acetaminophen] 10•2•5•320 mg/10 mL

Tylenol Plus Infants' Cold & Cough Concentrated Drops (discontinued 2011) OTC *antitussive; decongestant; analgesic; antipyretic; for children 2–3 years* [dextromethorphan hydrobromide; phenylephrine HCl; acetaminophen] 5•2.5•160 mg/1.6 mL

Tylenol PM tablets, caplets, gelcaps OTC *analgesic; antipyretic; antihistamine; sleep aid* [acetaminophen; diphenhydramine HCl] 500•25 mg

Tylenol Rapid Release Gels OTC *analgesic; antipyretic* [acetaminophen] 500 mg

Tylenol Severe Allergy caplets OTC *antihistamine; sleep aid; analgesic; antipyretic* [diphenhydramine HCl; acetaminophen] 12.5•500 mg

Tylenol Sinus Congestion & Pain Nighttime caplets OTC *decongestant; antihistamine; analgesic; antipyretic* [phenylephrine HCl; chlorpheniramine maleate; acetaminophen] 5•2•325 mg

Tylenol Sinus Congestion & Pain Severe Daytime caplets OTC *decongestant; expectorant; analgesic; antipyretic* [phenylephrine HCl; guaifenesin; acetaminophen] 5•200•325 mg

Tylenol Sinus Non-Drowsy caplets, geltabs, gelcaps OTC *decongestant; analgesic; antipyretic* [pseudoephedrine HCl; acetaminophen] 30•500 mg

Tylenol Sinus Severe Congestion
caplets OTC *decongestant; expectorant; analgesic; antipyretic* [pseudoephedrine HCl; guaifenesin; acetaminophen] 30•200•325 mg

Tylenol Sore Throat Daytime oral liquid OTC *analgesic; antipyretic* [acetaminophen] 166.6 mg/5 mL

Tylenol Sore Throat Nighttime oral liquid OTC *antihistamine; sleep aid; analgesic; antipyretic* [diphenhydramine HCl; acetaminophen] 48•1000 mg/30 mL

Tylenol with Codeine elixir ℞ *narcotic antitussive; analgesic; antipyretic* [codeine phosphate; acetaminophen] 12•120 mg/5 mL

Tylenol with Codeine No. 2, No. 3, and No. 4 tablets ℞ *narcotic antitussive; analgesic; antipyretic; also abused as a street drug* [codeine phosphate; acetaminophen] 15•300 mg; 30•300 mg; 60•300 mg

Tylenol with Flavor Creator, Children's oral suspension OTC *analgesic; antipyretic* [acetaminophen] 160 mg/5 mL

tylosin INN, BAN ② Talacen

Tylox capsules ℞ *narcotic analgesic; antipyretic* [oxycodone HCl; acetaminophen] 5•500 mg ② Taloxa

tyloxapol USAN, USP, INN, BAN *detergent; wetting agent; cleaner/lubricant for artificial eyes; investigational (orphan) surfactant for cystic fibrosis*

Typhim Vi IM injection ℞ *typhoid vaccine for adults and children over 2 years* [typhoid vaccine (Ty2), Vi polysaccharide] 25 mcg/0.5 mL dose

typhoid vaccine USP *active bacterin for typhoid fever* (Salmonella typhi *Ty21a, attenuated*)

typhoid Vi capsular polysaccharide vaccine *active bacterin for typhoid fever* (Salmonella typhi *Ty2, inactivated*)

typhus vaccine USP

"typical" antipsychotics [see: conventional antipsychotics]

Tyrex-2 powder OTC *enteral nutritional therapy for tyrosinemia type II*

tyromedan INN *thyromimetic* [also: thyromedan HCl]

tyromedan HCl [see: thyromedan HCl]

Tyromex-1 powder OTC *formula for infants with tyrosinemia type I* ② Trimox

tyropanoate sodium USAN, USP *oral radiopaque contrast medium for cholecystography (57.4% iodine)* [also: sodium tyropanoate]

tyrosine (L-tyrosine) USAN, USP, INN *nonessential amino acid; symbols: Tyr, Y* ② Terocin; Trisan

L-tyrosine & L-serine & L-leucine *investigational (orphan) for hepatocellular carcinoma*

Tyrosum Cleanser topical liquid, packets OTC *cleanser for acne* [isopropanol; acetone] 50%•10%

tyrothricin USP, INN *antibacterial*

Tysabri IV infusion ℞ *anti-inflammatory for the treatment of multiple sclerosis and Crohn disease; availability restricted due to an increased risk of progressive multifocal leukoencephalopathy (PML)* [natalizumab] 20 mg/mL

Tyvaso solution for inhalation ℞ *peripheral vasodilator for pulmonary arterial hypertension (PAH)* [treprostinil (as sodium)] 0.6 mg/mL ② Toviaz

Tyzeka film-coated tablets, oral solution ℞ *once-daily antiviral for chronic hepatitis B virus (HBV) infection* [telbivudine] 600 mg; 100 mg/5 mL

Tyzine nasal spray, nose drops, pediatric nose drops ℞ *nasal decongestant* [tetrahydrozoline HCl] 0.1%; 0.1%; 0.05%

TZDs (thiazolidinediones) *a class of antidiabetic agents that increase cellular response to insulin without increasing insulin secretion* ② Tussi-D S

UAA sugar-coated tablets ℞ *urinary antibiotic; analgesic; antispasmodic; acidifier* [methenamine; phenyl salicylate; atropine sulfate; methylene blue; hyoscyamine sulfate; benzoic acid] 40.8•18.1•0.03•5.4•0.03•4.5 mg

ubenimex INN

ubidecarenone USAN, INN

Ubi-Q-Gel; Ubi-Q-Nol *natural enzyme cofactor; investigational (orphan) for Huntington disease, pediatric CHF, and mitochondrial cytopathies* [coenzyme Q10]

ubiquinol; ubiquinone [see: coenzyme Q10]

ubisindine INN

Ucephan oral solution (discontinued 2011) ℞ *adjunctive therapy (rescue agent) to prevent and treat hyperammonemia due to urea cycle enzymopathy (orphan)* [sodium benzoate; sodium phenylacetate] 10•10 g/100 mL ⅀ Acephen; Asaphen

UCG Beta Slide Monoclonal II slide tests for professional use ℞ *in vitro diagnostic aid; urine pregnancy test*

UCG Slide tests for professional use ℞ *in vitro diagnostic aid; urine pregnancy test* [latex agglutination test]

U-Cort cream ℞ *corticosteroidal anti-inflammatory* [hydrocortisone acetate] 1%

Udamin film-coated caplets ℞ *vitamin/mineral supplement* [multiple vitamins & minerals; folic acid; lycopene] ≐•2•5 mg

Udamin SP film-coated caplets ℞ *vitamin/mineral supplement; natural remedy for prostatic hyperplasia* [multiple vitamins & minerals; folic acid; lycopene; saw palmetto extract] ≐• 1•2.5•320 mg

Udderly Smooth cream OTC *moisturizer; emollient* [lanolin; mineral oil]

UDIP (trademarked packaging form) *unit-dose identification package*

Udo's Choice Oil oral liquid OTC *a blend of natural seed oils that supply a balance of essential fatty acids* [omega-3 oils; omega-6 oils; omega-9 oils; medium-chain triglycerides] 6.4•3.2•3•0.231 g/15 mL

Uendex *investigational (orphan) inhalant for cystic fibrosis* [dextran sulfate]

ufenamate INN

ufiprazole INN

U·Ject (trademarked delivery form) *prefilled disposable syringe*

Ulcerease mouth rinse OTC *mild mucous membrane anesthetic; antipruritic; counterirritant* [phenol] 0.6%

uldazepam USAN, INN *sedative*

Ulefsa lotion ℞ *antiseptic* [benzyl alcohol] 5% ⅀ Elevess; Eliphos

ulinastatin INN

ulipristal acetate *selective progesterone receptor modulator; emergency postcoital ("morning after") contraceptive that is effective when taken up to 5 days after unprotected sex*

Ulmus fulva; U. rubra *medicinal herb* [see: slippery elm]

ulobetasol INN *topical corticosteroidal anti-inflammatory* [also: halobetasol propionate]

Uloric tablets ℞ *xanthine oxidase inhibitor for gout-associated hyperuricemia* [febuxostat] 40, 80 mg

Ultane liquid for vaporization ℞ *inhalation general anesthetic* [sevoflurane]

Ultesa *investigational (Phase III) corticosteroidal anti-inflammatory for the remission of active ulcerative colitis* [budesonide]

Ultiva powder for IV infusion ℞ *short-acting narcotic analgesic for general anesthesia* [remifentanil HCl] 1, 2, 5 mg/vial

Ultra Freeda tablets OTC *vitamin/mineral supplement* [multiple vitamins & minerals; folic acid; biotin] ≐• 0.27•0.1 mg

Ultra Freeda with Iron tablets OTC *vitamin/mineral/calcium/iron supplement* [multiple vitamins & minerals; calcium (as carbonate, ascorbate, and citrate); iron (as ferrous fumarate); folic acid; biotin] ≜•83.3•6•0.27• 0.1 mg

Ultra KLB6 tablets OTC *dietary supplement* [vitamin B₆; multiple food supplements] 16.7•≜ mg

Ultra Mide 25 lotion OTC *moisturizer; emollient; keratolytic* [urea] 25%

Ultra NatalCare tablets ℞ *prenatal vitamin/mineral/calcium/iron supplement; stool softener* [multiple vitamins & minerals; calcium; iron (as carbonyl); folic acid; docusate sodium] ≜•200•90•1•50 mg

Ultra Strength D-2000 capsules OTC *vitamin D supplement* [cholecalciferol (vitamin D₃)] 2000 IU

Ultra Strength Vitamin D3 oral drops OTC *vitamin D supplement* [cholecalciferol (vitamin D₃)] 5000 IU/mL

Ultra Tears eye drops (discontinued 2010) OTC *moisturizer/lubricant* [hydroxypropyl methylcellulose] 1%

Ultra Vent (trademarked delivery device) *jet nebulizer*

Ultra Vita Time tablets (discontinued 2008) OTC *dietary supplement* [multiple vitamins & minerals; multiple food products; iron; folic acid; biotin] ≜•6•0.4•1 mg

UltraBag Dianeal PD-2 with Dextrose [see: Dianeal]

UltraBrom extended-release capsules ℞ *decongestant; antihistamine* [pseudoephedrine HCl; brompheniramine maleate] 120•12 mg

UltraBrom PD extended-release pediatric capsules (discontinued 2007) ℞ *decongestant; antihistamine* [pseudoephedrine HCl; brompheniramine maleate] 60•6 mg

Ultracal oral liquid OTC *enteral nutritional therapy* [lactose-free formula]

Ultra-Care solution + tablets OTC *two-step chemical disinfecting system for soft contact lenses* [hydrogen peroxide–based]

Ultracet film-coated caplets ℞ *opioid analgesic for acute pain; antipyretic* [tramadol HCl; acetaminophen] 37.5•325 mg

UltraJect prefilled syringe ℞ *narcotic analgesic* [morphine sulfate]

Ultralan oral liquid OTC *enteral nutritional therapy* [lactose-free formula]

Ultralytic 2 topical foam (discontinued 2009) ℞ *moisturizer; emollient; keratolytic* [urea; ammonium lactate] 20%•12%

Ultram film-coated caplets ℞ *opioid analgesic for moderate to severe pain; also used for premature ejaculation* [tramadol HCl] 50 mg

Ultram ER extended-release tablets ℞ *opioid analgesic for moderate to severe pain; also used for premature ejaculation* [tramadol HCl] 100, 200, 300 mg

Ultrase; Ultrase MT 12; Ultrase MT 18; Ultrase MT 20 capsules containing enteric-coated microspheres ℞ *porcine-derived digestive enzymes* [pancrelipase (lipase; protease; amylase)] 4500•25 000•20 000; 12 000•39 000•39 000; 18 000• 58 500•58 500; 20 000•65 000• 65 000 USP units

Ultravate ointment, cream ℞ *corticosteroidal anti-inflammatory* [halobetasol propionate] 0.05%

Ultravate PAC cream + lotion ℞ *corticosteroidal anti-inflammatory + antipruritic; emollient* [halobetasol propionate (cream) + ammonium lactate (lotion)] 0.05% + 12%

Ultravist 150; Ultravist 240; Ultravist 300; Ultravist 370 IV injection ℞ *radiopaque contrast medium for imaging of the head, heart, peripheral vascular system, and genitourinary tract* [iopromide (39% iodine)] 311.7 mg/mL (150 mg/mL); 498.72 mg/mL (240 mg/mL); 623.4 mg/mL (300 mg/mL); 768.86 mg/mL (370 mg/mL)

Ultrazyme Enzymatic Cleaner effervescent tablets OTC *enzymatic cleaner for soft contact lenses* [subtilisin A]

Ultrex gel in unit-dose packs OTC *hydrogel wound dressing* [acemannan]

Umecta emulsion, topical suspension, aerosol ℞ *moisturizer; emollient; keratolytic* [urea] 40% ⊡ Emoquette

Umecta 40% nail film, topical suspension ℞ *moisturizer; emollient; keratolytic* [urea] 40% ⊡ Emoquette

Umecta PD emulsion, topical suspension ℞ *moisturizer; emollient; keratolytic* [urea] 40%

umespirone INN

uña de gato *medicinal herb* [see: cat's claw]

UN-Aspirin caplets OTC *analgesic; antipyretic* [acetaminophen] 500 mg

Unasyn powder for IV or IM injection ℞ *aminopenicillin antibiotic plus synergist* [ampicillin sodium; sulbactam sodium] 1•0.5, 2•1, 10•5 g ⊡ Anacin; Enzone; inosine

Uncaria guianensis; U. tomentosa medicinal herb [see: cat's claw]

10-undecenoic acid [see: undecylenic acid]

10-undecenoic acid, calcium salt [see: calcium undecylenate]

undecoylium chloride-iodine

undecylenic acid USP *antifungal*

unfractionated heparin [see: heparin, unfractionated]

Unguentine cream OTC *anesthetic; antifungal* [benzocaine; resorcinol] 5%•2%

Unguentine ointment OTC *minor burn treatment* [phenol; zinc oxide; eucalyptus oil] 1%•⅟₂•⅟₂

Unguentine Plus cream OTC *anesthetic; antiseptic; antipruritic; counterirritant* [lidocaine HCl; chloroxylenol; phenol] 2%•2%•0.5%

Uni-Ace drops (discontinued 2008) OTC *analgesic; antipyretic* [acetaminophen] 100 mg/mL ⊡ anise

Uni-Amp (trademarked delivery form) *single-dose ampule*

Unibase cream OTC *nontherapeutic base for compounding various dermatological preparations* [a proprietary blend of emulsifiers plus a preservative]

Unibase ointment (discontinued 2010) OTC *nontherapeutic base for compounding various dermatological preparations* [a proprietary blend of emulsifiers plus a preservative]

Unicap capsules, tablets (discontinued 2008) OTC *vitamin supplement* [multiple vitamins; folic acid] ±•0.4 mg

Unicap Jr. chewable tablets (discontinued 2008) OTC *vitamin supplement* [multiple vitamins; folic acid] ±•0.4 mg

Unicap M; Unicap T tablets (discontinued 2008) OTC *vitamin/mineral/iron supplement* [multiple vitamins & minerals; iron; folic acid] ±•18•0.4 mg

Unicap Plus Iron tablets (discontinued 2008) OTC *vitamin/iron supplement* [multiple vitamins; iron; folic acid] ±•22.5•0.4 mg

Unicap Sr. tablets (discontinued 2008) OTC *vitamin/mineral/iron supplement* [multiple vitamins & minerals; iron; folic acid] ±•10•0.4 mg

Unicomplex M tablets OTC *vitamin/mineral/calcium supplement* [multiple vitamins & minerals; calcium; folic acid] ±•60•0.4 mg

Unicomplex T & M tablets (discontinued 2008) OTC *vitamin/mineral/iron supplement* [multiple vitamins & minerals; iron; folic acid] ±•18•0.4 mg

Unifed oral liquid OTC *nasal decongestant* [pseudoephedrine HCl] 30 mg/5 mL ⊡ INFeD

Unifiber powder OTC *bulk laxative* [cellulose powder]

unifocon A USAN *hydrophobic contact lens material*

Unimatic (trademarked delivery form) *prefilled disposable syringe*

Uni-nest (trademarked delivery form) *ampule*

Unipak (packaging form) *dispensing pack*

Uniphyl timed-release tablets (discontinued 2010) ℞ *antiasthmatic; bronchodilator* [theophylline] 400, 600 mg

Uniquin (foreign name for U.S. product **Maxaquin**)

Uniretic tablets ℞ *combination angiotensin-converting enzyme (ACE) inhibitor and diuretic for hypertension*

[moexipril HCl; hydrochlorothiazide] 7.5•12.5, 15•12.5, 15•25 mg

Uni-Rx (trademarked packaging form) *unit-dose containers and packages*

Unisert (trademarked dosage form) *suppository*

Unisol; Unisol 4 solution OTC *rinsing/storage solution for soft contact lenses* [sodium chloride (saline solution)] ⧉ anise oil; Anusol; Enisyl; Enseal

Unisol Plus aerosol solution OTC *rinsing/storage solution for soft contact lenses* [sodium chloride (saline solution)]

Unisom Nighttime Sleep-Aid tablets OTC *antihistamine; sleep aid* [doxylamine succinate] 25 mg

Unisom PM Pain SleepCaps caplets OTC *antihistamine; sleep aid; analgesic; antipyretic* [diphenhydramine citrate; acetaminophen] 50•325 mg

Unisom SleepGels (capsules) OTC *antihistamine; sleep aid* [diphenhydramine HCl] 50 mg

Unisom SleepMelts (orally disintegrating tablets) OTC *antihistamine; sleep aid* [diphenhydramine HCl] 25 mg

Unisom with Pain Relief tablets OTC *antihistamine; sleep aid; analgesic; antipyretic* [diphenhydramine citrate; acetaminophen] 50•650 mg

Unistep hCG test kit for professional use ℞ *in vitro diagnostic aid; urine pregnancy test*

Unithroid Direct tablets (discontinued 2009) ℞ *synthetic thyroid hormone (T₄ fraction only)* [levothyroxine sodium] 25, 50, 75, 88, 100, 112, 125, 150, 175, 200, 300 mcg

Univasc tablets ℞ *antihypertensive; angiotensin-converting enzyme (ACE) inhibitor* [moexipril HCl] 7.5, 15 mg

Univial (trademarked packaging form) *single-dose vials*

Unna's boot [see: Dome-Paste bandage]

UpCal D chewable tablets OTC *vitamin/calcium/magnesium supplement* [vitamin D; calcium (as citrate); magnesium] 125 U•250 mg•40 mg

UpCal D powder for oral solution OTC *vitamin/calcium supplement* [vitamin D; calcium] 250 U•500 mg per packet

Uplyso ⓔⓤⓡ (available in the European Union, Israel, and Brazil) *investigational (Phase III, orphan) recombinant glucocerebrosidase (GCD) for Gaucher disease* [taliglucerase alfa]

Uracid capsules ℞ *urinary acidifier to control ammonia production* [racemethionine] 200 mg ⧉ Urised

uracil USAN *antineoplastic potentiator for tegafur (not available separately; combined with tegafur in a 1:4 ratio)* ⧉ Eryzole; Orasol

uracil mustard USAN, USP *nitrogen mustard–type alkylating antineoplastic* [also: uramustine]

uradal [see: carbromal]

uralenic acid [see: enoxolone]

Uramaxin cream, lotion, aerosol foam ℞ *keratolytic for the removal of dystrophic nails* [urea] 45%; 45%; 20%

Uramaxin GT topical liquid ℞ *keratolytic for the removal of dystrophic nails* [urea] 45%

uramustine INN, BAN *nitrogen mustard–type alkylating antineoplastic* [also: uracil mustard]

uranin [see: fluorescein sodium]

uranium *element (U)*

urapidil INN, BAN

urate oxidase, recombinant *investigational (orphan) for prevention of chemotherapy-induced hyperuricemia*

urea USP *osmotic diuretic; keratolytic; emollient* 35%, 40%, 42%, 45%, 50% *topical*

Urea 40 gel ℞ *moisturizer; emollient; keratolytic* [urea] 40%

Urea 45% Nail gel ℞ *keratolytic for the removal of dystrophic nails* [urea] 45% ⧉ Aranelle

Urea Nail Gel ℞ *keratolytic for the removal of dystrophic nails* [urea] 50%

Urea Nailstick 50% topical solution (discontinued 2011) ℞ *keratolytic for the removal of dystrophic nails* [urea] 50%

urea peroxide [see: carbamide peroxide]

Ureacin-10 lotion OTC *moisturizer; emollient; keratolytic* [urea] 10% 🔟 AeroZoin; Orasone

Ureacin-20 cream OTC *moisturizer; emollient; keratolytic* [urea] 20% 🔟 AeroZoin; Orasone

Urealac lotion (discontinued 2009) OTC *moisturizer; emollient; keratolytic* [urea] 35%

Ureaphil IV infusion (discontinued 2010) ℞ *osmotic diuretic* [urea] 40 g/ 150 mL

Urecholine tablets ℞ *cholinergic urinary stimulant for postsurgical and postpartum urinary retention* [bethanechol chloride] 5, 10, 25, 50 mg

uredepa USAN, INN *antineoplastic*

uredofos USAN, INN *veterinary anthelmintic*

urefibrate INN

***p*-ureidobenzenearsonic acid** [see: carbarsone]

Urelle sugar-coated tablets ℞ *urinary antibiotic; antiseptic; analgesic; antispasmodic* [methenamine; sodium phosphate; phenyl salicylate; methylene blue; hyoscyamine sulfate] 81•40.8•32.4•10.8•0.12 mg

urethan NF [also: urethane] 🔟 Uritin

urethane INN, BAN [also: urethan] 🔟 Uritin

urethane polymers [see: polyurethane foam]

Uretron D/S sugar-coated tablets ℞ *urinary antibiotic; antiseptic; analgesic; antispasmodic* [methenamine; sodium biphosphate; phenyl salicylate; methylene blue; hyoscyamine sulfate] 120•40.8•36.2•10.8•0.12 mg

Urex tablets ℞ *urinary antibiotic* [methenamine hippurate] 1 g 🔟 Eurax

Urginea indica; U. maritima; U. scilla *medicinal herb* [see: squill]

Uricult culture paddles for professional use ℞ *in vitro diagnostic aid for nitrate, uropathogens, or bacteria in the urine*

uridine 5′-triphosphate *investigational (Phase I/II, orphan) for cystic fibrosis and primary ciliary dyskinesia*

Uridon Modified sugar-coated tablets (discontinued 2007) ℞ *urinary antibiotic; analgesic; antispasmodic; acidifier* [methenamine; phenyl salicylate; atropine sulfate; methylene blue; hyoscyamine sulfate; benzoic acid] 40.8•18.1•0.03•5.4•0.03•4.5 mg

Urief (available in Japan) *investigational (NDA filed) alpha$_{1a}$ adrenoceptor antagonist for benign prostatic hyperplasia (BPH)* [silodosin]

Urimar-T tablets ℞ *urinary antibiotic; antiseptic; analgesic; antispasmodic* [methenamine; sodium biphosphate; phenyl salicylate; methylene blue; hyoscyamine sulfate] 120•40.8•36.2•10.8•0.12 mg

Urimax film-coated delayed-release tablets ℞ *urinary antibiotic; analgesic; antispasmodic; acidifier* [methenamine; phenyl salicylate; methylene blue; hyoscyamine sulfate; sodium biphosphate] 81.6•36.2•10.8•0.12•40.8 mg

Urinary Antiseptic No. 2 tablets ℞ *urinary antibiotic; analgesic; antispasmodic; acidifier* [methenamine; phenyl salicylate; atropine sulfate; methylene blue; hyoscyamine sulfate; benzoic acid] 40.8•18.1•0.03•5.4•0.03•4.5 mg

Urised sugar-coated tablets (discontinued 2008) ℞ *urinary antibiotic; analgesic; antispasmodic; acidifier* [methenamine; phenyl salicylate; atropine sulfate; methylene blue; hyoscyamine sulfate; benzoic acid] 40.8•18.1•0.03•5.4•0.03•4.5 mg 🔟 Uracid

Urisedamine tablets ℞ *urinary antibiotic; antispasmodic* [methenamine mandelate; hyoscyamine] 500•0.15 mg

Uriseptic film-coated tablets ℞ *urinary antibiotic; antiseptic; analgesic; antispasmodic* [methenamine; phenyl salicylate; methylene blue; benzoic acid; atropine sulfate; hyoscyamine sulfate] 40.8•18.1•5.4•4.5•0.03•0.03 mg

Urispas film-coated tablets ℞ *urinary antispasmodic* [flavoxate HCl] 100 mg (200 mg available in Canada)

Uristat tablets ℞ *urinary analgesic* [phenazopyridine HCl] 95 mg

Uristix; Uristix 4 reagent strips OTC *in vitro diagnostic aid for multiple urine products*

UriSym capsules (discontinued 2008) ℞ *urinary antibiotic; antiseptic; analgesic; antispasmodic* [methenamine; sodium biphosphate; phenyl salicylate; methylene blue; hyoscyamine sulfate] 100•40.8•40•10.8•0.12 mg

Uritact DS caplets ℞ *urinary antibiotic; analgesic; antispasmodic; acidifier* [methenamine; phenyl salicylate; atropine sulfate; methylene blue; hyoscyamine sulfate; benzoic acid] 81.6•36.2•0.06•10.8•0.06•9 mg

Uritin tablets ℞ *urinary antibiotic; analgesic; antispasmodic; acidifier* [methenamine; phenyl salicylate; atropine sulfate; methylene blue; hyoscyamine sulfate; benzoic acid] 40.8•18.1•0.03•5.4•0.03•4.5 mg

Uro Blue sugar-coated tablets ℞ *urinary antibiotic; antiseptic; analgesic; antispasmodic* [methenamine; sodium biphosphate; phenyl salicylate; methylene blue; hyoscyamine sulfate] 120•40.8•36.2•10.8•0.12 mg

Urocit-K tablets ℞ *urinary alkalizer for nephrolithiasis and hypocitruria prevention (orphan)* [potassium (as citrate)] 5, 10, 15 mEq

urofollitrophin BAN *follicle-stimulating hormone (FSH)* [also: urofollitropin]

urofollitropin USAN, INN *follicle-stimulating hormone (FSH); ovulation stimulant for polycystic ovary disease (orphan) and assisted reproductive technologies (ART); investigational (orphan) for spermatogenesis in hormone-deficient males* [also: urofollitrophin]

urogastrone *investigational (orphan) to accelerate corneal regeneration following corneal transplant surgery*

Urogesic tablets ℞ *urinary tract analgesic for relief of pain, burning, urgency, and frequency due to mucosal irritation from surgery, catheterization, endoscopic procedures, or trauma; adjunct to antibacterial agents for urinary tract infection (UTI)* [phenazopyridine HCl] 100 mg ⑨ Ear-Gesic

Urogesic Blue sugar-coated tablets ℞ *urinary antibiotic; antiseptic; antispasmodic* [methenamine; sodium biphosphate; methylene blue; hyoscyamine sulfate] 81.6•40.8•10.8•0.12 mg

urokinase USAN, INN, BAN, JAN *plasminogen activator; thrombolytic enzyme*

urokinase alfa USAN *plasminogen activator; thrombolytic enzyme*

Uro-KP-Neutral film-coated caplets ℞ *urinary acidifier; phosphorus supplement* [sodium phosphate; potassium phosphate; monobasic sodium phosphate] 250 mg (14.25 mEq) P

Urolene Blue tablets (discontinued 2010) ℞ *urinary anti-infective and antiseptic; antidote to cyanide poisoning* [methylene blue] 65 mg

Uro-Mag capsules OTC *antacid; magnesium supplement* [magnesium oxide] 140 mg (84.5 mg Mg)

uronal [see: barbital]

Uro-Phosphate film-coated tablets ℞ *urinary antibiotic; acidifier* [methenamine; sodium biphosphate] 300•434.78 mg

Uroqid-Acid No. 2 film-coated tablets ℞ *urinary antibiotic; acidifier* [methenamine mandelate; sodium acid phosphate] 500•500 mg

Uroxatral extended-release tablets ℞ *alpha$_1$-adrenergic blocker for benign prostatic hyperplasia (BPH)* [alfuzosin HCl] 10 mg

Urso 250; Urso Forte tablets ℞ *naturally occurring bile acid for primary biliary cirrhosis (orphan)* [ursodiol] 250 mg; 500 mg ⑨ Oracea; OROS

ursodeoxycholic acid INN, BAN *naturally occurring bile acid; anticholelithogenic* [also: ursodiol]

ursodiol USAN *naturally occurring bile acid for primary biliary cirrhosis (orphan); gallstone preventative and dissolving* agent; *investigational (orphan) for cystic fibrosis liver disease* [also: ursodeoxycholic acid] 250, 300, 500 mg oral

Ursofalk suspension *naturally occurring bile acid; investigational (orphan) for cystic fibrosis liver disease* [ursodiol]

ursulcholic acid INN

Urtica dioica; U. urens medicinal herb [see: nettle]

ustekinumab *human immunoglobulin G1 (IgG1) kappa monoclonal antibody; interleukin-12 (IL-12) and -23 (IL-23) blocker for moderate to severe plaque psoriasis*

Ustell capsules ℞ *urinary antibiotic; antiseptic; analgesic; antispasmodic* [methenamine; sodium phosphate; phenyl salicylate; methylene blue; hyoscyamine sulfate] 120•40.8•36•10•0.12 mg

Utac film-coated tablets ℞ *urinary antibiotic; acidifier* [methenamine mandelate; monobasic sodium phosphate] 500•500 mg

UTI Relief tablets ℞ *urinary tract analgesic for relief of pain, burning, urgency, and frequency due to mucosal irritation from surgery, catheterization, endoscopic procedures, or trauma; adjunct to antibacterial agents for urinary tract infection (UTI)* [phenazopyridine HCl] 97.2 mg

Uticap capsules ℞ *urinary antibiotic; antiseptic; analgesic; antispasmodic*

[methenamine; sodium phosphate; phenyl salicylate; methylene blue; hyoscyamine sulfate] 120•40.8•36•10•0.12 mg

Utira-C tablets ℞ *urinary antibiotic; antiseptic; analgesic; antispasmodic* [methenamine; sodium phosphate; phenyl salicylate; methylene blue; hyoscyamine sulfate] 81.6•40.8•36.2•10.8•0.12 mg

Utrona-C tablets ℞ *urinary antibiotic; antiseptic; analgesic; antispasmodic* [methenamine; sodium phosphate; phenyl salicylate; methylene blue; hyoscyamine sulfate] 81.6•40.8•36.2•10.8•0.12 mg

uva ursi *(Arbutus uva ursi; Arctostaphylos uva ursi)* leaves *medicinal herb for bladder and kidney infections, Bright disease, constipation, diabetes, gonorrhea, nephritis, spleen disorders, urethritis, and uterine ulcerations*

Uvadex extracorporeal solution (leukocytes are collected, photoactivated with the UVAR Photopheresis System, then reinfused) ℞ *palliative treatment for cutaneous T-cell lymphoma (CTCL); investigational (orphan) treatment of diffuse systemic sclerosis and to prevent rejection of cardiac allografts* [methoxsalen] 20 mcg/mL

Uvidem *investigational (Phase II) theraccine (therapeutic vaccine) for melanoma* [melanoma vaccine]

VAB-6 (vinblastine, actinomycin D, bleomycin, cyclophosphamide, cisplatin) *chemotherapy protocol for testicular cancer*

VAC (vincristine, Adriamycin, cyclophosphamide) *chemotherapy protocol for small cell lung cancer (SCLC)* [also known as: CAV]

VAC pediatric (vincristine, actinomycin D, cyclophosphamide)

[with or without mesna rescue and filgrastim hematopoietic] *chemotherapy protocol for pediatric sarcomas*

VAC pulse; VAC standard (vincristine, actinomycin D, cyclophosphamide) *chemotherapy protocol for sarcomas*

VACAdr; VACA (vincristine, actinomycin D, cyclophosphamide, Adriamycin) *chemotherapy protocol* *for pediatric bone and soft tissue sarcomas*

vaccines *a class of drugs used for active immunization that consist of antigens that induce the endogenous production of antibodies*

vaccinia immune globulin (VIG) USP *passive immunizing agent; treatment for severe complications arising from smallpox vaccination (orphan)*

vaccinia immune human globulin [now: vaccinia immune globulin]

vaccinia virus, recombinant [now: human papillomavirus, recombinant]

Vaccinium edule; V. erythrocarpum; V. macrocarpon; V. oxycoccos; V. vitis medicinal herb [see: cranberry]

Vaccinium myrtillus medicinal herb [see: bilberry]

VAD (vincristine, Adriamycin, dactinomycin) *chemotherapy protocol for pediatric Wilms tumor*

VAD (vincristine, Adriamycin, dexamethasone) *chemotherapy protocol for multiple myeloma and acute lymphocytic leukemia (ALL)*

Vademin-Z capsules (discontinued 2008) OTC *vitamin/mineral supplement* [multiple vitamins & minerals]

vadocaine INN

Vagifem film-coated vaginal tablets ℞ *synthetic estrogen for postmenopausal atrophic vaginitis* [estradiol (as hemihydrate)] 10 mcg

Vagi-Gard; Vagi-Gard Advanced Sensitive Formula vaginal cream OTC *anesthetic; keratolytic; antifungal* [benzocaine; resorcinol] 20%•3%; 5%•2%

Vaginex vaginal cream (discontinued 2008) OTC *antihistamine* [tripelennamine HCl]

Vaginorm intravaginal cream *investigational (Phase III) natural hormone for vaginal atrophy and sexual dysfunction* [dehydroepiandrosterone (DHEA)]

Vagisec Douche vaginal solution ℞ *cleanser and deodorizer*

Vagisec Plus vaginal suppositories ℞ *antiseptic* [aminacrine HCl] 6 mg

Vagisil vaginal cream OTC *anesthetic; keratolytic; antifungal* [benzocaine; resorcinol] 5%•2%, 20%•3%

Vagisil vaginal powder OTC *moisture absorbent* [cornstarch; aloe]

Vagisil wipes OTC *local anesthetic* [pramoxine HCl] 1%

Vagistat-1 vaginal ointment in prefilled applicator OTC *antifungal* [tioconazole] 6.5%

Vagistat-3 Combination Pack vaginal inserts + cream OTC *antifungal* [miconazole nitrate] 200 mg + 2%

valaciclovir INN *oral antiviral for herpes simplex virus types 1 and 2 (HSV-1, cold sores; HSV-2, genital herpes) and herpes zoster (shingles) infections; suppressive therapy for recurrent outbreaks* [also: valacyclovir HCl]

valacyclovir HCl USAN *oral antiviral for herpes simplex virus types 1 and 2 (HSV-1, cold sores; HSV-2, genital herpes) and herpes zoster (shingles) infections; suppressive therapy for recurrent outbreaks* [also: valaciclovir] 0.5, 1 g oral

valconazole INN ② fluconazole

Valcyte tablets, powder for oral solution ℞ *nucleoside analogue antiviral for AIDS-related cytomegalovirus (CMV) retinitis; CMV prevention in organ transplants* [valganciclovir HCl] 450 mg; 50 mg/mL

valdecoxib USAN *COX-2 inhibitor; nonsteroidal anti-inflammatory drug (NSAID) for osteoarthritis (OA), rheumatoid arthritis (RA), and primary dysmenorrhea* (withdrawn from the market in 2005 due to safety concerns)

valdetamide INN

valdipromide INN

Valdoxan ⓔⓤⓡ (available in Europe) *investigational (Phase III) oral treatment for major depressive disorder (MDD)* [agomelatine]

valepotriate [see: valtrate]

valerian (*Valeriana officinalis*) root *medicinal herb for convulsions, hypertension, hysteria, hypochondria, nervousness, pain, and sedation*

valerian, false *medicinal herb* [see: life root]

valethamate bromide NF

valganciclovir HCl USAN *nucleoside analogue antiviral for AIDS-related cytomegalovirus (CMV) retinitis; CMV prevention in organ transplants; oral prodrug of ganciclovir* 450 mg oral

valine (L-valine) USAN, USP, INN, JAN *essential amino acid; symbols: Val, V*

valine & isoleucine & leucine *investigational (orphan) for hyperphenylalaninemia*

Valisone ointment, cream, lotion ℞ *corticosteroidal anti-inflammatory* [betamethasone valerate] 0.1%

Valisone Reduced Strength cream ℞ *corticosteroidal anti-inflammatory* [betamethasone valerate] 0.01%

Valium tablets ℞ *benzodiazepine sedative; anxiolytic; skeletal muscle relaxant; anticonvulsant; alcohol withdrawal aid; also abused as a street drug* [diazepam] 2, 5, 10 mg

valnoctamide USAN, INN *tranquilizer*

valofane INN ② Voluven

valomaciclovir stearate USAN *DNA polymerase inhibitor; antiviral for herpes zoster infections*

Valorin tablets OTC *analgesic; antipyretic* [acetaminophen] 325, 500 mg ② Florone

valperinol INN

valproate pivoxil INN

valproate semisodium INN *anticonvulsant for complex partial seizures and simple or complex absence seizures; treatment for manic episodes of a bipolar disorder; migraine headache prophylaxis* [also: divalproex sodium; semisodium valproate]

valproate sodium USAN *anticonvulsant for complex partial seizures and simple or complex absence seizures; valproic acid derivative* 500 mg injection

valproic acid USAN, USP, INN, BAN *anticonvulsant for complex partial seizures and simple or complex absence seizures* 125, 250, 500 mg oral; 250 mg/5 mL oral

valpromide INN

valrubicin USAN *anthracycline antibiotic antineoplastic for bladder cancer (orphan)*

valsartan USAN, INN *angiotensin receptor blocker (ARB) for hypertension, heart failure, and myocardial infarction*

valspodar USAN, INN *cyclosporine-derived P-glycoprotein (P-gp) inhibitor*

Valstar intravesical instillation solution ℞ *anthracycline antibiotic antineoplastic for bladder cancer* [valrubicin] 40 mg/mL

valtrate INN

Valtrex film-coated caplets ℞ *antiviral for herpes simplex virus types 1 and 2 (HSV-1, cold sores; HSV-2, genital herpes) and herpes zoster (shingles) infections; suppressive therapy for recurrent outbreaks* [valacyclovir HCl] 500, 1000 mg

Valturna tablets ℞ *combination direct renin inhibitor and angiotensin receptor blocker (ARB) for hypertension* [aliskiren (as hemifumarate); valsartan] 150•160, 300•320 mg

Vanacof Dx oral liquid OTC *antitussive; expectorant* [chlophedianol HCl; guaifenesin] 12.5•100 mg/5 mL

vanadium *element* (V)

Vanamide cream ℞ *keratolytic for the removal of dystrophic nails* [urea] 40% ② fenimide

Vancocin powder for oral solution, powder for IV or IM injection (discontinued 2009) ℞ *tricyclic glycopeptide antibiotic* [vancomycin HCl] 1, 10 g; 0.5, 1 g

Vancocin Pulvules (capsules) ℞ *tricyclic glycopeptide antibiotic* [vancomycin HCl] 125, 250 mg

Vancoled powder for IV or IM injection (discontinued 2009) ℞ *tricyclic glycopeptide antibiotic* [vancomycin HCl] 0.5, 1, 5 g

vancomycin INN, BAN *tricyclic glycopeptide antibiotic* [also: vancomycin HCl]

vancomycin HCl USP *tricyclic glycopeptide antibiotic* [also: vancomycin] 0.5, 0.75, 1, 5, 10 g/vial injection

Vandazole vaginal gel ℞ *antibacterial for bacterial vaginosis* [metronidazole] 0.75%

vandetanib *vascular endothelial growth factor regulator (VEGFR); tyrosine kinase inhibitor; oral antineoplastic for medullary thyroid cancer (orphan); investigational (NDA filed) for advanced or metastatic non–small cell lung cancer* 100, 300 mg oral

vaneprim INN

Vanex-HD oral liquid ℞ *narcotic antitussive; antihistamine; decongestant* [hydrocodone bitartrate; chlorpheniramine maleate; phenylephrine HCl] 1.7•2•5 mg/5 mL

Vanicream OTC *nontherapeutic base for compounding various dermatological preparations*

vanilla (Vanilla fragrans; V. planifolia; V. tahitensis) NF bean *medicinal herb for CNS stimulation, fever, and flatulence; flavoring agent; also used as an aphrodisiac*

vanillin NF *flavoring agent*

N-vanillylnonamide [see: nonivamide]

N-vanillyloleamide [see: olvanil]

Vaniqa cream ℞ *hair growth inhibitor for unwanted facial hair on women* [eflornithine HCl] 13.9%

vanitiolide INN

Vanocin lotion ℞ *antibiotic and keratolytic for acne* [sulfacetamide sodium; sulfur] 10%•5%

Vanos cream ℞ *corticosteroidal anti-inflammatory* [fluocinonide] 0.1%

Vanoxide-HC lotion ℞ *keratolytic and corticosteroidal anti-inflammatory for acne* [benzoyl peroxide; hydrocortisone] 5%•0.5%

Vanquish caplets OTC *analgesic; antipyretic; anti-inflammatory* [acetaminophen; aspirin (buffered with magnesium hydroxide and aluminum hydroxide); caffeine] 194•227•(50•25)•33 mg

Vantas once-yearly subcu implant ℞ *gonadotropin suppressant for the palliative treatment of advanced prostate cancer* [histrelin acetate] 50 mg

Vantin film-coated tablets ℞ *broad-spectrum third-generation cephalosporin antibiotic* [cefpodoxime proxetil] 100, 200 mg

Vantin granules for suspension (discontinued 2008) ℞ *broad-spectrum third-generation cephalosporin antibiotic* [cefpodoxime proxetil] 50, 100 mg/5 mL

vanyldisulfamide INN

vapiprost INN, BAN *antagonist to thromboxane* A_2 [also: vapiprost HCl]

vapiprost HCl USAN *antagonist to thromboxane* A_2 [also: vapiprost]

Vapor Lemon Sucrets lozenges (discontinued 2008) OTC *mucous membrane anesthetic* [dyclonine HCl] 2 mg

vapreotide USAN *antineoplastic; synthetic octapeptide analogue of somatostatin*

vapreotide acetate *antineoplastic; synthetic octapeptide analogue of somatostatin; investigational (Phase III, orphan) treatment for acute esophageal variceal bleeding due to portal hypertension; investigational (orphan) for GI and pancreatic fistulas, acromegaly, and carcinoid tumors*

Vaprisol IV infusion (discontinued 2011) ℞ *diuretic for euvolemic and hypervolemic hyponatremia in hospitalized patients; treatment for syndrome of inappropriate antidiuretic hormone (SIADH)* [conivaptan HCl] 5 mg/mL ② fuprazole

Vaprisol Premixed in Dextrose 5% IV infusion in bag ℞ *diuretic for euvolemic and hypervolemic hyponatremia in hospitalized patients; treatment for syndrome of inappropriate antidiuretic hormone (SIADH)* [conivaptan HCl; dextrose] 0.2 mg/mL•5%

Vaqta adult IM injection, pediatric/adolescent IM injection ℞ *immunization against hepatitis A virus (HAV)* [hepatitis A vaccine, inactivated] 50 U/mL; 25 U/0.5 mL

vardenafil HCl USAN *phosphodiesterase type 5 (PDE-5) inhibitor; selective vasodilator for erectile dysfunction (ED)* (base=84%)

varenicline tartrate *nicotine receptor agonist/antagonist; a non-nicotine smoking cessation aid; also used to reduce alcohol cravings* (base=59%)

Varibar Honey; Varibar Nectar; Varibar Pudding; Varibar Thin Honey; Varibar Thin Liquid *oral suspension* ℞ *radiopaque contrast medium for gastrointestinal imaging* [barium sulfate] 40%

varicella virus vaccine *live, attenuated vaccine for chickenpox*

varicella-zoster immune globulin (VZIG) USP *passive immunizing agent for chickenpox or zoster in infants, children, pregnant women, and immunocompromised adults* 10%–18% IgG (125 U/dose)

varicella-zoster virus vaccine, live *vaccine for adults* ≥ *50 years to prevent herpes zoster infections*

Varidin Forte *capsules* OTC *vitamin/ herbal supplement* [vitamins C and E; zinc; mixed bioflavonoids; multiple herbs] 125 mg•25 IU• ² •50 mg• ±

Varisan Vitality *tablets* OTC *vitamin/ herbal supplement* [multiple vitamins; multiple bioflavonoids; multiple herbs]

Varivax *powder for subcu injection* ℞ *vaccine for chickenpox* [varicella virus vaccine, live attenuated] 1350 PFU/ 0.5 mL

Varoniscastrum virgincum medicinal herb [see: Culver root]

vascular endothelial growth factor 165, human (hVEGF165) *investigational (Phase II, orphan) gene-based therapy for neointimal hyperplasia disease*

vascular serotonin 5-HT₁ receptor agonists *a class of antimigraine agents that constrict cranial blood vessels and inhibit the release of inflammatory neuropeptides*

Vaseretic 5-12.5; Vaseretic 10-25 *tablets* ℞ *combination angiotensin-converting enzyme (ACE) inhibitor and diuretic for hypertension* [enalapril maleate; hydrochlorothiazide] 5• 12.5 mg; 10•25 mg

vasoactive intestinal polypeptide (VIP) *investigational (orphan) for acute esophageal food impaction, pulmonary arterial hypertension, and acute respiratory distress syndrome (ARDS)*

Vasocidin *eye drops (discontinued 2009)* ℞ *corticosteroidal anti-inflammatory; antibiotic* [prednisolone sodium phosphate; sulfacetamide sodium] 0.25%•10%

VasoClear A *eye drops (discontinued 2011)* OTC *decongestant; astringent* [naphazoline HCl; zinc sulfate] 0.02%•0.25%

Vasocon-A *eye drops (discontinued 2011)* ℞ *decongestant; antihistamine* [naphazoline HCl; antazoline phosphate] 0.05%•0.5% ⃝ Visken

vasoconstrictors *a class of cardiovascular drugs that narrow the blood vessels*

Vasodilan *tablets* ℞ *peripheral vasodilator* [isoxsuprine HCl] 10, 20 mg

vasodilators *a class of cardiovascular drugs that dilate the blood vessels*

Vasolex *ointment* ℞ *proteolytic enzyme for débridement of necrotic tissue; vulnerary* [trypsin; Peruvian balsam; castor oil] 90 U•87 mg•788 mg per g

vasopressin (VP) USP, INN *pituitary antidiuretic hormone for diabetes insipidus or prevention of abdominal distention* 20 U/mL injection

vasopressin tannate USP *pituitary antidiuretic hormone for diabetes insipidus or prevention of abdominal distention*

vasopressors *a class of posterior pituitary hormones that raise blood pressure by causing contraction of capillaries and arterioles; a class of sympathomimetic agents that raise blood pressure by increasing myocardial contractility* [also called: vasopressins]

Vasoprost *investigational (orphan) prostaglandin for severe peripheral arterial occlusive disease* [alprostadil]

Vasosulf *eye drops (discontinued 2009)* ℞ *antibiotic; decongestant* [sulfacetamide sodium; phenylephrine HCl] 15%•0.125%

Vasotate HC ear drops ℞ *corticoster-oidal anti-inflammatory; antiseptic* [hydrocortisone; acetic acid] 1%•2%

Vasotec tablets ℞ *antihypertensive; angiotensin-converting enzyme (ACE) inhibitor; treatment for congestive heart failure (CHF)* [enalapril maleate] 2.5, 5, 10, 20 mg

Vasovist IV injection ℞ *contrast agent for vascular enhancement in magnetic resonance angiography (MRA)* [gado-fosveset trisodium] 224 mg/mL

VATH (vinblastine, Adriamycin, thiotepa, Halotestin [fluoxymes-terone]) *chemotherapy protocol for breast cancer*

VaxSyn HIV-1 *investigational (orphan) antiviral (therapeutic, Phase II) and vaccine (preventative, Phase I) for HIV and AIDS* [gp160 antigens]

VazoBID oral suspension ℞ *decongestant; antihistamine* [phenylephrine tannate; brompheniramine tannate] 20•12 mg/5 mL

VaZol oral liquid ℞ *antihistamine* [brompheniramine tannate] 2 mg/5 mL ☒ Feosol; PhosLo; VSL

VaZol-D oral liquid ℞ *decongestant; antihistamine* [phenylephrine HCl; brompheniramine maleate] 7.5•4 mg/5 mL

Vazotab chewable tablets ℞ *decongestant; antihistamine* [phenylephrine HCl; brompheniramine maleate] 15•6 mg

VazoTan Tannate oral suspension ℞ *antitussive; antihistamine; decongestant* [carbetapentane tannate; brompheniramine tannate; phenylephrine tannate] 50•12•20 mg/5 mL

Vazotuss HC Tannate oral suspension (discontinued 2009) ℞ *narcotic antitussive; antihistamine; decongestant* [hydrocodone tannate; chlorphenir-amine tannate; phenylephrine tannate] 10•12•20 mg/5 mL

VBAP (vincristine, BCNU, Adria-mycin, prednisone) *chemotherapy protocol for multiple myeloma*

VBCMP (vincristine, BCNU, cyclo-phosphamide, melphalan, pred-nisone) *chemotherapy protocol for multiple myeloma*

VC (vincristine) [q.v.]

VC (vinorelbine, cisplatin) *chemo-therapy protocol for cervical and non–small cell lung cancer* [also: cisplatin + vinorelbine]

VCAP (vincristine, cyclophospha-mide, Adriamycin, prednisone) *chemotherapy protocol for multiple myeloma*

VCF (vaginal contraceptive film) OTC *spermicidal contraceptive* [nonoxynol 9] 28%

VCMP (vincristine, cyclophospha-mide, melphalan, prednisone) *chemotherapy protocol for multiple myeloma* [also: VMCP]

V-Cof oral suspension ℞ *antitussive; antihistamine; decongestant* [carbeta-pentane citrate; brompheniramine maleate; phenylephrine HCl] 25•6•10 mg/5 mL ☒ VCF

VCR (vincristine) [q.v.]

VD (vinorelbine, doxorubicin) *che-motherapy protocol for breast cancer*

V-Dec-M sustained-release tablets (discontinued 2007) ℞ *decongestant; expectorant* [pseudoephedrine HCl; guaifenesin] 120•500 mg

Vectibix IV infusion ℞ *monoclonal antibody antineoplastic for metastatic colorectal cancer* [panitumumab] 20 mg/mL

Vectical ointment ℞ *vitamin D therapy for mild-to-moderate plaque psoriasis* [calcitriol (vitamin D_3)] 3 mcg/g (0.0003%)

vecuronium bromide USAN, INN, BAN *nondepolarizing neuromuscular blocker; muscle relaxant; adjunct to anesthesia* 10, 20 mg injection

Veetids film-coated tablets, powder for oral solution ℞ *natural penicillin anti-biotic* [penicillin V potassium] 250, 500 mg; 125, 250 mg/5 mL

vegetable oil, hydrogenated NF *tab-let and capsule lubricant*

vegetable tallow; vegetable wax *medicinal herb* [see: bayberry]

VEGF (vascular endothelial growth factor) inhibitor *angiogenesis inhibitor for various cancers and wet age-related macular degeneration (AMD)* [see: aflibercept; bevacizumab; pazopatinib; pegapatanib; ranibizumab; vandetanib]

VEGF Trap; VEGF Trap-Eye [see: aflibercept]

Vehicle/N; Vehicle/N Mild lotion OTC *nontherapeutic base for compounding various dermatological preparations*

VeIP (Velban, ifosfamide, Platinol) [with mesna rescue] *chemotherapy protocol for genitourinary and testicular cancer*

velaglucerase alfa *enzyme replacement therapy for Gaucher disease type 1*

Velban powder for IV injection ℞ *antineoplastic for Hodgkin disease, lymphoma, mycosis fungoides, testicular carcinoma, Kaposi sarcoma, and Letterer-Siwe disease* [vinblastine sulfate] 10 mg/vial

Velcade powder for IV injection ℞ *antineoplastic for multiple myeloma (orphan) and mantle cell (non-Hodgkin) lymphoma; investigational for rheumatoid arthritis* [bortezomib] 3.5 mg/vial

Velivet tablets (in packs of 28) ℞ *triphasic oral contraceptive; emergency postcoital contraceptive* [desogestrel; ethinyl estradiol] 🄽 Folvite
Phase 1 (7 days): 0.1 mg•25 mcg;
Phase 2 (7 days): 0.125 mg•25 mcg;
Phase 3 (7 days): 0.15 mg•25 mcg;
Counters (7 days)

velnacrine INN, BAN *cholinesterase inhibitor* [also: velnacrine maleate]

velnacrine maleate USAN *cholinesterase inhibitor for Alzheimer disease* [also: velnacrine]

Veltin gel ℞ *antibiotic and keratolytic for acne* [clindamycin phosphate; tretinoin] 1.2%•0.025%

Velvachol cream OTC *nontherapeutic base for compounding various dermatological preparations*

vemurafenib *kinase inhibitor antineoplastic for metastatic melanoma*

Venelex ointment ℞ *wound treatment for decubitus ulcers* [castor oil; Peruvian balsam] 788•87 mg

Venice turpentine *medicinal herb* [see: larch]

venlafaxine INN, BAN *antidepressant; anxiolytic; selective serotonin and norepinephrine reuptake inhibitor (SSNRI)* [also: venlafaxine HCl]

venlafaxine HCl USAN *antidepressant; anxiolytic; selective serotonin and norepinephrine reuptake inhibitor (SSNRI) for major depressive disorder (MDD), generalized anxiety disorder (GAD), social anxiety disorder (SAD), and panic disorder* [also: venlafaxine] 25, 37.5, 50, 75, 100, 150, 225 mg oral

Venofer IV injection ℞ *hematinic for iron deficiency in patients with non-dialysis-dependent chronic kidney disease (NDD-CKD), hemodialysis-dependent chronic kidney disease (HDD-CKD), and peritoneal dialysis-dependent chronic kidney disease (PDD-CKD)* [iron (as sucrose)] 20 mg/mL (100 mg/vial)

Venomil subcu or IM injection (discontinued 2010) ℞ *venom sensitivity testing (subcu); venom desensitization therapy (IM)* [extracts of honeybee, yellow jacket, yellow hornet, white-faced hornet, mixed vespid, and wasp venom] 🄽 fenamole

Ventavis solution for inhalation in single-dose ampules, for use with an adaptive aerosol delivery (AAD) system ℞ *vasodilator for pulmonary arterial hypertension (PAH) (orphan); investigational (orphan) intravenous treatment for thrombocytopenia and Raynaud phenomenon associated with systemic sclerosis* [iloprost] 10, 20 mcg

Venticute *investigational (orphan) for adult respiratory distress syndrome (ARDS)* [rSP-C lung surfactant]

Ventolin HFA inhalation aerosol with a CFC-free propellant ℞ *sympathomimetic bronchodilator* [albuterol] 90 mcg/dose

VePesid IV injection, capsules (discontinued 2009) ℞ *antineoplastic for testicular and small cell lung cancers* [etoposide] 20 mg/mL; 50 mg

veradoline INN *analgesic* [also: veradoline HCl]

veradoline HCl USAN *analgesic* [also: veradoline]

veralipride INN

Veramyst nasal spray in a metered-dose pump ℞ *once-daily corticosteroidal anti-inflammatory for seasonal or perennial allergic rhinitis* [fluticasone furoate] 27.5 mcg/dose

verapamil USAN, INN, BAN *coronary vasodilator; calcium channel blocker*

verapamil HCl USAN, USP *antianginal; antiarrhythmic; antihypertensive; calcium channel blocker* 40, 80, 100, 120, 180, 200, 240, 300, 360 mg oral; 2.5 mg/mL injection

verapamil HCl & trandolapril *combination calcium channel blocker and angiotensin-converting enzyme (ACE) inhibitor for hypertension* 180•2, 240•1, 240•2, 240•4 mg oral

Veratrum **species** *medicinal herb* [see: hellebore]

veratrylidene-isoniazid [see: verazide]

verazide INN, BAN

Verazinc capsules OTC *zinc supplement* [zinc sulfate] 220 mg

Verbascum nigrum; V. phlomoides; V. thapsiforme; V. thapsus *medicinal herb* [see: mullein]

Verbena hastata *medicinal herb* [see: blue vervain]

Verdeso foam ℞ *corticosteroidal anti-inflammatory* [desonide] 0.05%

Veregen ointment ℞ *topical treatment for external genital and perianal warts (condyloma acuminatum) in immunocompromised adults* [sinecatechins] 15%

Verelan sustained-release capsules ℞ *antihypertensive; antianginal; antiarrhythmic; calcium channel blocker* [verapamil HCl] 120, 180, 240, 360 mg ⊚ Furalan; Virilon

Verelan PM delayed-onset, extended-release capsules ℞ *antihypertensive; calcium channel blocker* [verapamil HCl] 100, 200, 300 mg

Veridate (trademarked packaging form) *patient compliance package for oral contraceptives*

verilopam INN *analgesic* [also: verilopam HCl]

verilopam HCl USAN *analgesic* [also: verilopam]

Veripred 20 oral solution ℞ *corticosteroid; anti-inflammatory* [prednisolone] 20 mg/5 mL

verlukast USAN, INN *bronchodilator; antiasthmatic*

Verluma technetium Tc 99 prep kit ℞ *monoclonal antibody imaging agent for small cell lung cancer* [nofetumomab merpentan]

vermicides; vermifuges *a class of drugs effective against parasitic infections* [also called: anthelmintics]

Vermox chewable tablets ℞ *anthelmintic for trichuriasis, enterobiasis, ascariasis, and uncinariasis* [mebendazole] 100 mg

vernakalant *investigational (NDA filed) selective ion channel blocker for the acute conversion of atrial fibrillation*

verofylline USAN, INN *bronchodilator; antiasthmatic*

veronal [see: barbital]

veronal sodium [see: barbital sodium]

Veronate *investigational (orphan) agent to reduce or prevent staphylococci-induced nosocomial bacteremia in very low birthweight infants* [INH-A00021 (code name—generic name not yet assigned)]

veronica, tall *medicinal herb* [see: Culver root]

Veronica beccabunga *medicinal herb* [see: brooklime]

Veronica officinalis *medicinal herb* [see: speedwell]

Versa Alcohol Base; Versa Aqua Base; Versa PLO20 gel OTC *non-therapeutic base for compounding various dermatological preparations*

Versa HRT Base Botanical; Versa HRT Base Heavy; Versa HRT Base Natural; Versa LipoBase Heavy; Versa LipoBase Regular; Versa VaniBase cream OTC *non-therapeutic base for compounding various dermatological preparations*

Versacaps sustained-release capsules (discontinued 2007) ℞ *decongestant; expectorant* [pseudoephedrine HCl; guaifenesin] 60•300 mg

Versed IV or IM injection, Tel-E-Ject syringes, pediatric syrup (discontinued 2005) ℞ *short-acting benzodiazepine general anesthetic adjunct for preoperative sedation* [midazolam HCl] 1, 5 mg/mL; 2 mg/mL

versetamide USAN *stabilizer; carrier agent for gadoversetamide*

Versiclear lotion ℞ *antifungal; keratolytic; antipruritic; anesthetic* [sodium thiosulfate; salicylic acid; alcohol 10%] 25%•1%

verteporfin USAN *light-activated treatment for subfoveal choroidal neovascularization (CNV) due to age-related macular degeneration (AMD), pathologic myopia, or ocular histoplasmosis*

vervain *medicinal herb* [see: blue vervain]

Vesanoid capsules (discontinued 2010) ℞ *antineoplastic for acute promyelocytic leukemia (orphan)* [tretinoin] 10 mg

vesicants *a class of agents that cause blisters*

VESIcare film-coated tablets ℞ *once-daily urinary antispasmodic for overactive bladder with urinary incontinence, urgency, and frequency* [solifenacin succinate] 5, 10 mg

vesnarinone USAN, INN *cardiotonic; inotropic for congestive heart failure*

vesperal [see: barbital]

vetrabutine INN, BAN

Vexol eye drop suspension ℞ *corticosteroidal anti-inflammatory for uveitis and ocular surgery* [rimexolone] 1%

Vfend film-coated tablets, powder for oral suspension, powder for IV injection ℞ *antifungal for invasive aspergillosis, candidemia of the skin and internal organs, esophageal candidiasis, and other serious fungal infections* [voriconazole] 50, 200 mg; 40 mg/mL; 200 mg/vial

V-Go (trademarked delivery device) *disposable insulin delivery device for* **NovoLog** *and* **Humalog**

Viactiv caplets OTC *vitamin/mineral/calcium/iron supplement* [multiple vitamins & minerals; calcium (as carbonate); iron (as ferrous fumarate); folic acid] ±•200•18•0.4 mg ▣ Factive

Viactiv Calcium Flavor Glides tablets (discontinued 2010) OTC *calcium supplement* [calcium; vitamins D and K] 500 mg•200 IU•40 mcg

Viactiv for Teens chewable tablets OTC *calcium supplement* [calcium (as carbonate); vitamin D; vitamin K; hydrogenated oil] 500 mg•100 IU•40 mcg

Viactiv Multi-Vitamin Flavor Glides caplets OTC *vitamin/mineral/calcium/iron supplement* [multiple vitamins & minerals; calcium; iron; folic acid; biotin] ±•200•18•0.4•0.03 mg

Viadur DUROS (once-yearly subcu implant) (discontinued 2008) ℞ *antihormonal antineoplastic for the palliative treatment of advanced prostate cancer* [leuprolide acetate] 72 mg (120 mcg/day)

Viaflex (trademarked packaging form) *ready-to-use IV bag*

Viagra film-coated tablets ℞ (available OTC in the U.K.) *selective vasodilator for erectile dysfunction (ED); also used for antidepressant- or antipsychotic-induced sexual dysfunction* [sildenafil citrate] 25, 50, 100 mg

Viagra Jet orally dissolving tablets (available in Mexico) *investigational*

doseform for erectile dysfunction (ED) [sildenafil citrate] 25, 50, 100 mg

Vianain investigational (orphan) proteolytic enzymes for débridement of severe burns [ananain; comosain; bromelains]

Vibativ powder for IV infusion ℞ antibiotic for drug-resistant gram-positive complicated skin and skin structure infections (cSSSI) [telavancin (as HCl)] 250, 750 mg

Vibramycin capsules ℞ tetracycline antibiotic [doxycycline hyclate] 100 mg

Vibramycin powder for oral suspension ℞ tetracycline antibiotic [doxycycline monohydrate] 25 mg/5 mL

Vibramycin syrup ℞ tetracycline antibiotic [doxycycline calcium] 50 mg/5 mL

Vibra-Tabs film-coated tablets ℞ tetracycline antibiotic [doxycycline hyclate] 100 mg

Viburnum opulus medicinal herb [see: cramp bark]

VIC (VePesid, ifosfamide, carboplatin) [with mesna rescue] chemotherapy protocol for non–small cell lung cancer [also known as: CVI]

Vicam injection (discontinued 2008) ℞ parenteral vitamin therapy [multiple B vitamins; vitamin C] ± • 50 mg/mL

Vicap Forte capsules ℞ vitamin/mineral supplement [multiple vitamins and minerals; folic acid] ± • 1 mg

Vicks Cough Drops; Vicks Menthol Cough Drops OTC mild anesthetic; antipruritic; counterirritant [menthol] 10 mg; 8.4 mg

Vicks DayQuil products [see: DayQuil]

Vicks Formula 44 products [see: Formula 44]

Vicks NyQuil products [see: NyQuil]

Vicks Sinex products [see: Sinex; DayQuil Sinex; NyQuil Sinex]

Vicks Vapor inhaler OTC nasal decongestant [levmetamfetamine] 50 mg

Vicks VapoRub cream OTC mild anesthetic; antipruritic; counterirritant; antiseptic [camphor; menthol; eucalyptus oil] 5.2% • 2.8% • 1.2%

Vicks VapoRub vaporizing ointment OTC mild anesthetic; antipruritic; counterirritant; antiseptic [camphor; menthol; eucalyptus oil] 4.8% • 2.6% • 1.2%

Vicks Vitamin C Drops (lozenges) OTC vitamin C supplement [ascorbic acid and sodium ascorbate] 25 mg

Vicodin; Vicodin ES; Vicodin HP tablets ℞ narcotic analgesic; antipyretic [hydrocodone bitartrate; acetaminophen] 5 • 500 mg; 7.5 • 750 mg; 10 • 660 mg

Vicon Forte capsules (discontinued 2008) ℞ vitamin/mineral supplement [multiple vitamins & minerals; folic acid] ± • 1 mg

Vicon Plus capsules (discontinued 2008) OTC vitamin/mineral supplement [multiple vitamins & minerals]

Vicon-C capsules (discontinued 2010) OTC vitamin/mineral supplement [multiple B vitamins & minerals; vitamin C] ± • 300 mg

Vicoprofen film-coated tablets ℞ narcotic analgesic & antitussive; antipyretic [hydrocodone bitartrate; ibuprofen] 7.5 • 200 mg

vicotrope [see: cosyntropin]

vicriviroc cellular chemokine receptor 5 (CCR5) inhibitor; investigational (Phase III) antiretroviral for HIV infections

Victoza subcu injection in a prefilled self-injector ℞ antidiabetic for type 2 diabetes; investigational (Phase III) for weight loss [liraglutide] 0.6, 1.2, 1.8 mg/dose (18 mg/3 mL injector)

Victrelis capsules ℞ hepatitis C virus (HCV) protease inhibitor for chronic hepatitis C infections [boceprevir] 200 mg

vidarabine USAN, USP, INN, BAN antiviral

vidarabine monohydrate [see: vidarabine]

vidarabine phosphate USAN antiviral

vidarabine sodium phosphate USAN antiviral

Vi-Daylin ADC drops (discontinued 2008) OTC vitamin supplement [vita-

mins A, C, and D] 1500 IU•35 mg•
400 IU per mL

Vi-Daylin ADC Vitamins + Iron
drops (discontinued 2008) oTc *vitamin/iron supplement* [vitamins A, C, and D; ferrous gluconate] 1500 IU•35 mg•400 IU•10 mg per mL

Vi-Daylin Multivitamin oral liquid, drops (discontinued 2008) oTc *vitamin supplement* [multiple vitamins]

Vi-Daylin Multivitamin + Iron oral liquid, drops (discontinued 2008) oTc *vitamin/iron supplement* [multiple vitamins; ferrous gluconate] ±•10 mg/5 mL; ±•10 mg/mL

Vi-Daylin/F ADC pediatric oral drops (discontinued 2008) ℞ *vitamin supplement; dental caries preventative* [vitamins A, C, and D; sodium fluoride] 1500 IU•35 mg•400 IU•0.25 mg per mL

Vi-Daylin/F ADC + Iron pediatric oral drops (discontinued 2008) ℞ *vitamin/iron supplement; dental caries preventative* [vitamins A, C, and D; sodium fluoride; ferrous sulfate] 1500 IU•35 mg•400 IU•0.25 mg•10 mg per mL

Vi-Daylin/F Multivitamin drops (discontinued 2008) ℞ *pediatric vitamin supplement and dental caries preventative* [multiple vitamins; sodium fluoride] ±•0.25 mg/mL

Vi-Daylin/F Multivitamin + Iron pediatric chewable tablets (discontinued 2008) ℞ *vitamin/iron supplement; dental caries preventative* [multiple vitamins; sodium fluoride; ferrous sulfate; folic acid] ±•1•12•0.3 mg

Vi-Daylin/F Multivitamin + Iron pediatric oral drops (discontinued 2008) ℞ *vitamin/iron supplement; dental caries preventative* [multiple vitamins; sodium fluoride; ferrous sulfate] ±•0.25•10 mg/mL

Vidaza suspension for subcu injection or IV infusion ℞ *antineoplastic for myelodysplastic syndrome (orphan); also used for acute lymphocytic leukemia and acute myelogenous leukemia* [azacitidine] 100 mg/vial

Videx chewable/dispersible tablets, powder for oral solution (discontinued 2009) ℞ *antiviral for advanced HIV infection* [didanosine] 25, 50, 100, 200 mg; 100, 250 mg/pkt.

Videx powder for oral solution ℞ *antiviral for advanced HIV infection* [didanosine] 2, 4 g/bottle

Videx EC enteric-coated delayed-release beads in capsules ℞ *antiviral for advanced HIV infection* [didanosine] 125, 200, 250, 400 mg

vifilcon A USAN *hydrophilic contact lens material*

vifilcon B USAN *hydrophilic contact lens material*

Vi-Flor [see: Poly-Vi-Flor; Tri-Vi-Flor]

VIG (vaccinia immune globulin) [q.v.]

vigabatrin USAN, INN, BAN *anticonvulsant for infantile spasms (orphan) and complex partial seizures; investigational (Phase II) treatment for cocaine and methamphetamine addictions*

Vigamox Drop-Tainer (eye drops) ℞ *broad-spectrum fluoroquinolone antibiotic* [moxifloxacin (as HCl)] 0.5%

Vigomar Forte tablets oTc *vitamin/mineral/iron supplement* [multiple vitamins & minerals; iron (as ferrous fumarate)] ±•12 mg

Vigortol oral liquid (discontinued 2011) oTc *vitamin/mineral/iron supplement* [multiple B vitamins & minerals; iron (as amino acid chelate); alcohol 18%] ±•2.5 mg

Viibryd tablets ℞ *once-daily antidepressant for major depressive disorder* [vilazodone HCl] 10, 20, 40 mg

Viibryd Patient Starter Kit tablets (in packs of 30) ℞ *once-daily antidepressant for major depressive disorder* [vilazodone HCl] 10 mg × 7 days + 20 mg × 7 days + 40 mg × 16 days

VIL *investigational (orphan) for hyperphenylalaninemia* [valine; isoleucine; leucine]

vilazodone HCl *oral selective serotonin reuptake inhibitor (SSRI) and partial 5-*

HT_{1A} *agonist for major depressive disorder (MDD)*

vildagliptin *investigational (NDA filed) dipeptidyl peptidase-4 (DPP-4) inhibitor oral antidiabetic that enhances the function of the body's incretin system to increase insulin production in the pancreas and reduce glucose production in the liver*

ViloFane-Dp tablets ℞ *hematinic* [folic acid (as L-methylfolate)] 7.5 mg

viloxazine INN, BAN *bicyclic antidepressant* [also: viloxazine HCl]

viloxazine HCl USAN *bicyclic antidepressant; investigational (orphan) for cataplexy and narcolepsy* [also: viloxazine]

Viminate oral liquid (discontinued 2008) OTC *geriatric vitamin/mineral supplement* [multiple B vitamins & minerals]

viminol INN

Vimovo delayed-release tablets ℞ *combination nonsteroidal anti-inflammatory drug (NSAID) and proton pump inhibitor for osteoarthritis, rheumatoid arthritis, and ankylosing spondylitis* [naproxen; esomeprazole (as magnesium)] 375•20, 500•20 mg

Vimpat tablets, oral solution, IV injection ℞ *adjunctive therapy for adults with partial-onset seizures* [lacosamide] 50, 100, 150, 200 mg; 10 mg/mL; 10 mg/mL

vinafocon A USAN *hydrophobic contact lens material*

Vinate II film-coated tablets ℞ *prenatal vitamin/mineral/calcium/iron supplement* [multiple vitamins & minerals; calcium; iron (as ferrous bisglycinate); folic acid] ±•200•29•1 mg

Vinate Calcium film-coated tablets ℞ *prenatal vitamin/mineral/calcium/iron supplement; stool softener* [multiple vitamins & minerals; calcium; iron (as carbonyl and ferrous gluconate); folic acid; docusate sodium] ±• 125•27•1•50 mg

Vinate Good Start Prenatal Formula chewable tablets (discontinued 2009) ℞ *prenatal vitamin/mineral/calcium/*

iron supplement [multiple vitamins & minerals; calcium; iron; folic acid] ± •200•29•1 mg

Vinate GT tablets ℞ *prenatal vitamin/mineral/calcium/iron supplement; stool softener* [multiple vitamins & minerals; calcium; iron (as carbonyl); folic acid; biotin; docusate sodium] ±• 200•90•1•0.03•50 mg

Vinate M tablets ℞ *prenatal vitamin/mineral/calcium/iron supplement* [multiple vitamins & minerals; calcium; iron (as ferrous fumarate); folic acid; biotin] ±•200•27•1•0.03 mg

vinbarbital NF, INN [also: vinbarbitone] ⊠ phenobarbital

vinbarbital sodium NF ⊠ phenobarbital sodium

vinbarbitone BAN [also: vinbarbital] ⊠ phenobarbitone

vinblastine INN *vinca alkaloid antineoplastic* [also: vinblastine sulfate]

vinblastine sulfate USAN, USP *vinca alkaloid antineoplastic for Hodgkin disease, lymphoma, mycosis fungoides, testicular carcinoma, Kaposi sarcoma, and Letterer-Siwe disease* [also: vinblastine] 10, 25 mg/vial injection

vinburnine INN

vinca alkaloids *a class of natural antineoplastics*

Vinca major; V. minor medicinal herb [see: periwinkle]

vincaleukoblastine sulfate [see: vinblastine sulfate]

vincamine INN, BAN

vincanol INN

vincantenate [see: vinconate]

vincantril INN

Vincasar PFS IV injection ℞ *antineoplastic* [vincristine sulfate] 1 mg/mL

vincofos USAN, INN *anthelmintic*

vinconate INN

vincristine (VC; VCR) INN, BAN *antineoplastic* [also: vincristine sulfate]

vincristine sulfate USAN, USP, JAN *antineoplastic* [also: vincristine] 1 mg/mL injection

vindeburnol INN

vindesine USAN, INN, BAN *synthetic vinca alkaloid antineoplastic*

vindesine sulfate USAN, JAN *synthetic vinca alkaloid antineoplastic*

vinegar [see: acetic acid]

vinepidine INN *antineoplastic* [also: vinepidine sulfate]

vinepidine sulfate USAN *antineoplastic* [also: vinepidine]

vinformide INN

vinglycinate INN *antineoplastic* [also: vinglycinate sulfate]

vinglycinate sulfate USAN *antineoplastic* [also: vinglycinate]

vinleurosine INN *antineoplastic* [also: vinleurosine sulfate]

vinleurosine sulfate USAN *antineoplastic* [also: vinleurosine]

vinmegallate INN

vinorelbine INN *antineoplastic* [also: vinorelbine tartrate]

vinorelbine + cisplatin *chemotherapy protocol for cervical and non–small cell lung cancer (NSCLC)* [also known as: VC; also: cisplatin + vinorelbine]

vinorelbine + doxorubicin *chemotherapy protocol for breast cancer* [also known as: NA]

vinorelbine + gemcitabine *chemotherapy protocol for non–small cell lung cancer (NSCLC)* [also known as: G+V; also: gemcitabine + vinorelbine (for lung and other cancers)]

vinorelbine tartrate USAN *antineoplastic* [also: vinorelbine] 10 mg/mL injection

vinpocetine USAN, INN *natural derivative of vincamine, an extract of the periwinkle plant; increases ATP levels in the brain, which increases memory and mental function by increasing the neuronal firing rate; also increases serotonin levels in the brain*

vinpoline INN

vinrosidine INN *antineoplastic* [also: vinrosidine sulfate]

vinrosidine sulfate USAN *antineoplastic* [also: vinrosidine]

vintiamol INN

vintoperol INN

vintriptol INN

vinyl alcohol polymer [see: polyvinyl alcohol]

vinyl ether USP

vinyl gamma-aminobutyric acid [see: vigabatrin]

vinylbital INN [also: vinylbitone]

vinylbitone BAN [also: vinylbital]

vinylestrenolone [see: norgesterone]

vinymal [see: vinylbital]

vinyzene [see: bromchlorenone]

vinzolidine INN *antineoplastic* [also: vinzolidine sulfate]

vinzolidine sulfate USAN *antineoplastic* [also: vinzolidine]

Viogen-C capsules OTC *vitamin/mineral supplement* [multiple B vitamins & minerals; vitamin C] ≛ • 300 mg ⑨ Vicon-C

Viokase powder (discontinued 2010) ℞ *porcine-derived digestive enzymes* [pancrelipase (lipase; protease; amylase)] 16 800 • 70 000 • 70 000 USP units per ¼ tsp.

Viokase 8; Viokase 16 tablets ℞ *porcine-derived digestive enzymes* [pancrelipase (lipase; protease; amylase)] 8000 • 30 000 • 30 000 USP units; 16 000 • 60 000 • 60 000 USP units

Viola odorata **medicinal herb** [see: violet]

Viola tricolor **medicinal herb** [see: pansy]

violet *(Viola odorata)* flowers and leaves *medicinal herb for asthma, bronchitis, cancer, colds, cough, sinus congestion, tumors, and ulcers*

violet, garden *medicinal herb* [see: pansy]

violetbloom *medicinal herb* [see: bittersweet nightshade]

viomycin INN [also: viomycin sulfate]

viomycin sulfate USP [also: viomycin]

viosterol in oil [see: ergocalciferol]

VIP (VePesid, ifosfamide, Platinol) [with mesna rescue; with or without filgrastim hematopoietic] *chemotherapy protocol for genitourinary cancers, testicular cancer, small cell lung cancer (SCLC), non–small cell lung cancer (NSCLC), and thymoma*

Viprinex Ⓒᴬᴺ subcu injection, IV infusion *anticoagulant for deep vein thrombosis (DVT) and severe chronic peripheral circulatory disorders; investigational (orphan) for cardiopulmonary bypass in heparin-intolerant patients; investigational (Phase III) for acute ischemic stroke* [ancrod] 70 IU/mL

viprostol USAN, INN, BAN *hypotensive; vasodilator*

viprynium embonate BAN *anthelmintic* [also: pyrvinium pamoate]

Vi-Q-Tuss syrup (discontinued 2007) ℞ *narcotic antitussive; expectorant* [hydrocodone bitartrate; guaifenesin] 5•100 mg/5 mL

viqualine INN

viquidil INN

Viracept film-coated tablets, powder for oral solution ℞ *antiretroviral; protease inhibitor for HIV-1 infection* [nelfinavir mesylate] 250, 650 mg; 50 mg/g

Viramune tablets, oral suspension ℞ *antiviral non-nucleoside reverse transcriptase inhibitor (NNRTI) for HIV-1 infections* [nevirapine] 200 mg; 50 mg/5 mL

Viramune XR extended-release tablets ℞ *once-daily antiviral non-nucleoside reverse transcriptase inhibitor (NNRTI) for HIV-1 infections* [nevirapine] 400 mg

Virasal topical liquid ℞ *keratolytic* [salicylic acid] 27.5% ② vorozole

ViraTan-DM B.I.D. chewable tablets, oral suspension ℞ *antitussive; antihistamine; sleep aid; decongestant* [dextromethorphan tannate; pyrilamine tannate; phenylephrine tannate] 25•30•25 mg; 12•30•12.5 mg/5 mL

Viravan-DM oral suspension, chewable tablets (discontinued 2007) ℞ *antitussive; antihistamine; sleep aid; decongestant; for children 2–12 years* [dextromethorphan tannate; pyrilamine tannate; phenylephrine tannate] 25•30•12.5 mg/5 mL; 25•30•25 mg

Viravan-P oral suspension ℞ *decongestant; antihistamine; sleep aid* [pseudoephedrine HCl; pyrilamine tannate] 30•20 mg/5 mL

Viravan-PDM oral suspension ℞ *antitussive; antihistamine; sleep aid; decongestant* [dextromethorphan hydrobromide; pyrilamine maleate; pseudoephedrine HCl] 15•15•15 mg/5 mL

Viravan-T chewable tablets (discontinued 2007) ℞ *decongestant; antihistamine; sleep aid* [phenylephrine tannate; pyrilamine tannate] 25•30 mg

Virazole powder for inhalation aerosol ℞ *antiviral for severe lower respiratory tract infections caused by respiratory syncytial virus (RSV); also used for influenza and herpes simplex virus infections* [ribavirin] 6 g/vial (20 mg/mL reconstituted) ② vorozole

Viread film-coated tablets ℞ *antiviral; nucleotide reverse transcriptase inhibitor (NRTI) for HIV-1 and chronic hepatitis B infections; investigational gel form for vaginal use to prevent HIV transmission to women during sex* [tenofovir disoproxil fumarate] 300 mg

Virginia mountain mint; Virginia thyme *medicinal herb* [see: wild hyssop]

Virginia silk *medicinal herb* [see: milkweed]

virginiamycin USAN, INN *antibacterial; veterinary food additive*

virginiamycin factor M₁ [see: virginiamycin]

virginiamycin factor S [see: virginiamycin]

virgin's bower *medicinal herb* [see: woodbine]

viridofulvin USAN, INN *antifungal*

Virilon capsules ℞ *synthetic androgen for hypogonadism or testosterone deficiency in men, delayed puberty in boys, and metastatic breast cancer in women; hormone replacement therapy (HRT) for postandropausal symptoms; also abused as a street drug* [methyltestosterone] 10 mg ② Verelan

Virogen Herpes slide test for professional use ℞ *in vitro diagnostic aid for*

herpes simplex virus antigen in lesions or cell cultures [latex agglutination test]

Virogen Rotatest slide test for professional use ℞ *in vitro diagnostic aid for fecal rotavirus* [latex agglutination test]

Viroptic Drop-Dose (eye drops) ℞ *antiviral for keratoconjunctivitis and epithelial keratitis due to herpes simplex virus infection* [trifluridine] 1%

viroxime USAN, INN *antiviral*

viroxime component A [see: zinviroxime]

viroxime component B [see: enviroxime]

Viroxyn oral gel OTC *germicide for cold sores/fever blisters* [benzalkonium chloride; isopropyl alcohol] 0.13%•70% ☑ Furoxone

Virulizin *investigational (Phase III) macrophage activator for AIDS-related lymphomas and Kaposi sarcoma; investigational (Phase III, orphan) for pancreatic cancer*

Viscoat prefilled syringes ℞ *viscoelastic agent for ophthalmic surgery* [hyaluronate sodium; chondroitin sulfate sodium] 30•40 mg/mL

Viscum album *medicinal herb* [see: mistletoe]

Visicol tablets ℞ *saline laxative; pre-procedure bowel evacuant* [sodium phosphate (monobasic and dibasic)] 1.5 g

visilizumab USAN *monoclonal antibody to CD3; investigational immunosuppressant for organ transplants, autoimmune diseases, and other T lymphocyte disorders*

visiluzumab [now: visilizumab]

Visine eye drops OTC *decongestant; vasoconstrictor* [tetrahydrozoline HCl] 0.05% ☑ Vision; Vusion

Visine A.C. eye drops OTC *decongestant; vasoconstrictor; astringent* [tetrahydrozoline HCl; zinc sulfate] 0.05%•0.25%

Visine Advanced Relief eye drops OTC *decongestant; vasoconstrictor; moisturizer/lubricant* [tetrahydrozoline HCl; polyethylene glycol 400; povidone] 0.05%•1%•1%

Visine All Day Eye Itch Relief eye drops OTC *antihistamine and mast cell stabilizer for allergic conjunctivitis* [ketotifen (as fumarate)] 0.025%

Visine L.R. eye drops OTC *decongestant; vasoconstrictor* [oxymetazoline HCl] 0.025%

Visine Maximum Redness Relief eye drops OTC *decongestant; vasoconstrictor; moisturizer/lubricant* [tetrahydrozoline HCl; hypromellose] 0.05%•0.36%

Visine Pure Tears; Visine Tears; Visine Tears Preservative Free eye drops OTC *moisturizer/lubricant* [polyethylene glycol 400; glycerin; hypromellose] 1%•0.2%•0.2%

Visine Tears Lasting Relief eye drops OTC *moisturizer/lubricant*

Visine Tired Eye Relief eye drops OTC *moisturizer/lubricant* [glycerin; hypromellose] 0.2%•0.36%

Visine Totally Multi-Symptom Relief eye drops OTC *decongestant; astringent; moisturizer/lubricant* [tetrahydrozoline HCl; zinc sulfate; hypromellose] 0.05%•0.25%•0.36%

Visine-A eye drops OTC *decongestant; vasoconstrictor* [naphazoline HCl; pheniramine maleate] 0.025%•0.3% ☑ Vision; Vusion

Vision (trademarked delivery device) *needle-free insulin injection system* ☑ Visine; Vusion

Vision Care Enzymatic Cleaner tablets (discontinued 2010) OTC *enzymatic cleaner for soft contact lenses* [pork pancreatin]

Vision Clear eye drops (discontinued 2008) OTC *decongestant; vasoconstrictor* [tetrahydrozoline HCl] 0.05%

VisionBlue ophthalmic injection in prefilled syringes ℞ *surgical aid for staining the anterior capsule of the lens* [trypan blue] 0.06%

Visipak (trademarked packaging form) *reverse-numbered package*

Visipaque 270; Visipaque 320 intra-arterial or IV injection ℞ *radiopaque contrast medium for CT, x-ray, and*

visceral digital subtraction angiography [iodixanol (49.1% iodine)] 550 mg/mL (270 mg/mL); 652 mg/mL (320 mg/mL)

Visken tablets ℞ *beta-blocker for hypertension; also used for fibromyalgia* [pindolol] 5, 10 mg ⬚ Vasocon

visnadine INN, BAN

visnafylline INN

Vi-Sol [see: Poly-Vi-Sol; Tri-Vi-Sol]

Visonex film-coated, extended-release tablets ℞ *decongestant; expectorant* [phenylephrine HCl; guaifenesin] 30•900 mg

Vistaril capsules ℞ *anxiolytic; minor tranquilizer; antihistamine for allergic pruritus* [hydroxyzine pamoate] 25, 50, 100 mg

Vistaril deep IM injection ℞ *anxiolytic; antiemetic; antihistamine for allergic pruritus; adjunct to preoperative or prepartum analgesia* [hydroxyzine HCl] 25 mg/mL

Vistaril oral suspension (discontinued 2007) ℞ *anxiolytic; minor tranquilizer; antihistamine for allergic pruritus* [hydroxyzine pamoate] 25 mg/5 mL

vistatolon INN *antiviral* [also: statolon]

Vistide IV infusion ℞ *nucleoside antiviral for AIDS-related cytomegalovirus (CMV) retinitis* [cidofovir] 75 mg/mL

Visual-Eyes ophthalmic solution (discontinued 2010) OTC *extraocular irrigating solution* [sterile isotonic solution]

Visudyne powder for IV infusion ℞ *treatment for subfoveal choroidal neovascularization (CNV) due to age-related macular degeneration (AMD), pathologic myopia, or ocular histoplasmosis; activated with the Opal Photoactivator laser* [verteporfin] 2 mg/mL (15 mg/vial)

Vita Drops OTC *vitamin supplement* [multiple vitamins]

Vita Drops with Iron OTC *vitamin/iron supplement* [multiple vitamins; iron (as ferrous sulfate)] ≛•10 mg/mL

Vitaball Vitamin gumballs OTC *vitamin supplement* [multiple vitamins; folic acid; biotin] ≛•400•45 mcg

Vita-bee with C Captabs (capsule-shaped tablets) (discontinued 2008) OTC *vitamin supplement* [multiple B vitamins; vitamin C] ≛•300 mg

Vita-Bob softgel capsules (discontinued 2008) OTC *vitamin supplement* [multiple vitamins; folic acid] ≛•0.4 mg

Vita-C crystals for oral liquid OTC *vitamin C supplement* [ascorbic acid] 4 g/tsp.

Vitafol film-coated tablets ℞ *hematinic; vitamin/calcium supplement* [iron (as ferrous fumarate); multiple vitamins; calcium (as carbonate); folic acid] 65•≛•125•1 mg

Vitafol syrup ℞ *hematinic* [iron (as ferric pyrophosphate and elemental iron); multiple B vitamins; folic acid] 100•≛•0.25 mg/5 mL

Vitafol OB+DHA caplets + gelcaps ℞ *prenatal vitamin/mineral/calcium/iron/omega-3 supplement* [multiple vitamins & minerals; calcium; iron (as ferrous fumarate); folic acid + docosahexaenoic acid (DHA)] ≛• 100•65•1 mg (tablets) + 250 mg (capsules)

Vitafol-OB; Vitafol-PN caplets ℞ *hematinic; vitamin/mineral/calcium supplement* [iron (as ferrous fumarate); multiple vitamins & minerals; calcium; folic acid] 65•≛•100•1 mg; 65•≛•125•1 mg

Vitafol-One softgels ℞ *prenatal vitamin/mineral/iron/omega-3 supplement* [multiple vitamins & minerals; iron; folic acid + docosahexaenoic acid (DHA)] ≛•29•1•200 mg

Vitagen Advance film-coated caplets ℞ *hematinic* [iron; vitamin B₁₂; vitamin C; desiccated stomach substance; succinic acid] 70•0.01•152•50•75 mg

Vita-Kid chewable wafers (discontinued 2008) OTC *vitamin supplement* [multiple vitamins; folic acid] ≛•0.3 mg

Vital B-50 timed-release tablets (discontinued 2008) OTC *vitamin supplement* [multiple B vitamins; folic acid; biotin] ± • 100 • 50 mcg

Vital High Nitrogen powder OTC *enteral nutritional therapy* [lactose-free formula] 79 g

Vital·D tablets OTC *vitamin/mineral supplement* [multiple vitamins and minerals; folic acid; biotin] ± • 1 • 0.3 mg

Vitalets chewable tablets OTC *vitamin/mineral/calcium/iron supplement* [multiple vitamins & minerals; calcium (as dicalcium phosphate); iron (as ferrous fumarate); folic acid; biotin] ± • 80 • 10 • 0.2 • 0.025 mg

Vitaline Biotin Forte tablets OTC *vitamin supplement* [multiple B vitamins; vitamin C; folic acid; biotin] ± • 200 • 0.8 • 3 mg, ± • 100 • 0.8 • 5 mg

Vitaline Maximum Blue; Vitaline Maximum Green tablets OTC *vitamin/mineral supplement* [multiple vitamins and minerals; folic acid; biotin] ± • 133 • 50 mcg

Vitaline Total Formula 3 tablets OTC *vitamin/mineral supplement* [multiple vitamins and minerals; folic acid; biotin] ± • 400 • 300 mcg

Vitalize SF oral liquid (discontinued 2008) OTC *vitamin/iron/amino acid supplement* [multiple B vitamins; iron (as ferric pyrophosphate); lysine] ± • 66 • 300 mg/15 mL

vitamin A USP *fat-soluble vitamin; antixerophthalmic; topical emollient; essential for vision, dental development, growth, cortisone synthesis, epithelial tissue differentiation, embryonic development, reproduction, and mucous membrane maintenance* 10 000, 15 000, 25 000 IU oral

vitamin A acid [see: tretinoin]

vitamin A palmitate

vitamin A₁ [see: retinol]

Vitamin B Complex 100 injection ℞ *parenteral vitamin therapy* [multiple B vitamins]

vitamin B₁ [see: thiamine HCl]

vitamin B₁ mononitrate [see: thiamine mononitrate]

vitamin B₂ [see: riboflavin]

vitamin B₃ [see: niacin; niacinamide; nicotinamide; nicotinic acid]

vitamin B₅ [see: calcium pantothenate; pantothenic acid]

vitamin B₆ [see: pyridoxine HCl]

vitamin B₈ [see: adenosine phosphate]

vitamin B₁₂ [see: cyanocobalamin; hydroxocobalamin]

vitamin B₁₅ [see: dimethylglycine HCl]

vitamin Bc [see: folic acid]

vitamin Bt [see: carnitine]

vitamin C [see: ascorbic acid; calcium ascorbate; sodium ascorbate]

vitamin D *a family of fat-soluble vitamins consisting of ergocalciferol (vitamin D₂) and cholecalciferol (vitamin D₃), that is converted to calcitriol (the active form) in the body; considered a non-endogenous hormone* [see also: calcifediol; dihydrotachysterol; doxercalciferol; paricalcitol]

Vitamin D Supplement Drops OTC *vitamin supplement* [cholecalciferol (vitamin D₃)] 400 U/drop

vitamin D₁ [see: dihydrotachysterol]

vitamin D₂ [see: ergocalciferol]

vitamin D₃ [see: cholecalciferol]

vitamin E USP *fat-soluble vitamin; antioxidant; platelet aggregation inhibitor; topical emollient; also used for reducing the toxic effects of oxygen therapy in premature infants, for preeclampsia, and for various cardiac and autoimmune conditions* [note relative potencies at alpha tocopherol, et seq.] 100, 200, 400, 500, 800, 1000 IU oral; 15 IU/30 mL oral

Vitamin E with Mixed Tocopherols tablets OTC *vitamin supplement* [vitamin E] 100, 200, 400 U

vitamin E-TPGS (tocopheryl polyethylene glycol succinate) [see: tocophersolan]

vitamin G [see: riboflavin]

vitamin H [see: biotin]

vitamin K₁ [see: phytonadione]

vitamin K$_2$ [see: menaquinone]
vitamin K$_3$ [see: menadione]
vitamin K$_4$ [see: menadiol sodium diphosphate]
Vitamin Liquid OTC *vitamin supplement* [multiple vitamins]
vitamin M [see: folic acid]
vitamin P [see: bioflavonoids]
vitamin P$_4$ [see: troxerutin]
Vitamin-Mineral Supplement oral liquid (discontinued 2008) OTC *vitamin/mineral supplement* [multiple B vitamins & minerals; alcohol 18%]
Vitamins To Go Maximum tablets OTC *vitamin/mineral/calcium/iron/herbal supplement* [multiple vitamins & minerals; calcium (as carbonate and dicalcium phosphate); iron (as carbonyl iron); folic acid; herbal blend] ≛•777•18•0.4•≛ mg
Vitaneed oral liquid OTC *enteral nutritional therapy* [lactose-free formula]
VitaPhil caplets ℞ *prenatal vitamin/mineral/calcium/iron supplement* [multiple vitamins & minerals; calcium; iron (as ferrous bisglycinate chelate); folic acid; biotin; choline bitartrate; hydrogenated oil] ≛•100•25•1•0.03•55 mg
Vita-Plus E softgels OTC *vitamin supplement* [vitamin E (as *d*-alpha tocopheryl acetate)] 400 IU
Vita-Plus G softgel capsules (discontinued 2008) OTC *geriatric vitamin/mineral supplement* [multiple vitamins & minerals]
Vita-Plus H softgel capsules (discontinued 2008) OTC *vitamin/mineral/iron supplement* [multiple vitamins & minerals; iron] ≛•13.4 mg
Vita-PMS tablets OTC *vitamin/mineral/calcium/iron supplement; digestive enzymes* [multiple vitamins & minerals; calcium (as carbonate); iron (as amino acid chelate); folic acid; biotin; betaine acid HCl; amylase; protease; lipase] ≛•20.8 mg•2.5 mg•0.33 mg•10.4 mcg•16.7 mg•2500 U•2500 U•200 U

Vita-PMS Plus tablets OTC *vitamin/mineral/calcium/iron supplement; digestive enzymes* [multiple vitamins & minerals; calcium (as carbonate); iron (as amino acid chelate); folic acid; biotin; betaine acid HCl; amylase; protease; lipase] ≛•166.7 mg•2.5 mg•0.33 mg•10.4 mcg•16.7 mg•2500 U•2500 U•200 U
Vita-Respa tablets ℞ *vitamin B supplement* [vitamins B$_6$ and B$_{12}$; folacin] 25•0.0013•2.2 mg
Vitarex tablets (discontinued 2008) OTC *vitamin/mineral/iron supplement* [multiple vitamins & minerals; iron] ≛•15 mg
Vita-Zinc capsules OTC *vitamin/zinc supplement* [multiple vitamins; zinc]
Vitazol cream ℞ *antibiotic for rosacea* [metronidazole] 0.75%
Vite E cream OTC *emollient* [vitamin E] 50 mg/g
Vitec cream OTC *emollient* [vitamin E]
Vitelle Irospan capsules OTC *vitamin/iron supplement* [iron (as ferrous sulfate, dried); ascorbic acid] 65•150 mg
Vitelle Lurline PMS tablets OTC *analgesic; antipyretic; diuretic; vitamin B$_6$* [acetaminophen; pamabrom; pyridoxine HCl] 500•25•50 mg
Vitelle Nesentials tablets OTC *vitamin/mineral supplement* [multiple vitamins & minerals]
Vitelle Nestabs OTC tablets (discontinued 2008) OTC *prenatal vitamin/calcium/iron supplement* [multiple vitamins; calcium; iron; folic acid] ≛•200•29•0.8 mg
Vitelle Nestrex tablets (discontinued 2008) OTC *vitamin B$_6$ supplement* [pyridoxine HCl] 25 mg
vitellin *natural remedy* [see: lecithin]
Vitex agnus-castus *medicinal herb* [see: chaste tree]
Vitis coigetiae; V. vinifera *medicinal herb* [see: grape seed]
Vitrase powder for injection, solution for injection ℞ *adjuvant to increase the absorption and dispersion of injected drugs, hypodermoclysis, and subcuta-*

neous urography; investigational (NDA filed) agent to clear vitreous hemorrhage; also used for diabetic retinopathy [hyaluronidase (ovine)] 6200 U; 200 U/mL

Vitrasert intraocular implant (5–8 months' duration) ℞ *antiviral for AIDS-related CMV retinitis (orphan)* [ganciclovir] 4.5 mg

Vitron-C tablets OTC *vitamin/iron supplement* [iron (as ferrous fumarate); ascorbic acid] 66•125 mg

Vitussin syrup (discontinued 2011) ℞ *narcotic antitussive; expectorant* [hydrocodone bitartrate; guaifenesin] 5•100 mg/5 mL

Vivactil film-coated tablets ℞ *tricyclic antidepressant* [protriptyline HCl] 5, 10 mg

Viva-Drops eye drops OTC *moisturizer/lubricant*

Vivaglobin subcu injection ℞ *passive immunizing agent for primary (inherited) immune deficiency (PID) (orphan)* [immune globulin (IGSC)] 16% (0.48, 1.6, 3.2 g/dose)

Vivarin tablets OTC *CNS stimulant; analeptic* [caffeine] 200 mg

Vivelle; Vivelle-Dot transdermal patch ℞ *estrogen replacement therapy for the treatment of postmenopausal symptoms and prevention of postmenopausal osteoporosis* [estradiol] 37.5, 50, 75, 100 mcg/day; 25, 37.5, 50, 75, 100 mcg/day

Viviant *second-generation selective estrogen receptor modulator (SERM); investigational (NDA filed) for the prevention and treatment of postmenopausal osteoporosis* [bazedoxifene]

Vivitrol powder for extended-release IM injection ℞ *once monthly narcotic antagonist for opiate dependence (orphan) and alcoholism* [naltrexone HCl] 380 mg

Vivonex T.E.N. powder OTC *enteral nutritional therapy* [lactose-free formula]

Vivotif Berna enteric-coated capsules ℞ *typhoid fever vaccine* [typhoid vaccine (Ty21a), live attenuated] 2–6 × 10⁹ viable CFU + 5–50 × 10⁹ nonviable cells

Vi-Zac capsules (discontinued 2008) OTC *vitamin/zinc supplement* [vitamins A, C, and E; zinc] 5000 IU•500 mg•50 mg•18 mg

VM (vinblastine, mitomycin) *chemotherapy protocol for breast cancer*

VM-26 [see: teniposide]

VMCP (vincristine, melphalan, cyclophosphamide, prednisone) *chemotherapy protocol for multiple myeloma* [also: VCMP]

vofopitant dihydrochloride USAN *tachykinin NK₁ receptor antagonist; antiemetic*

voglibose USAN, INN *alpha-glucosidase inhibitor that delays the digestion of dietary carbohydrates*

volatile nitrites *amyl nitrite, butyl nitrite, and isobutyl nitrite vapors that produce coronary stimulant effects, abused as street drugs* [see also: nitrous oxide; petroleum distillate inhalants]

volazocine USAN, INN *analgesic* ⍰ fluacizine

Vol-Tab Rx tablets ℞ *vitamin/mineral/calcium/iron supplement* [multiple vitamins & minerals; calcium; iron; folic acid; biotin] ≟•200•29•1•0.03 mg

Voltaren delayed-release tablets ℞ *analgesic; nonsteroidal anti-inflammatory drug (NSAID) for osteoarthritis, rheumatoid arthritis, and ankylosing spondylitis* [diclofenac (as sodium)] 75 mg ⍰ Foltrin

Voltaren eye drops ℞ *analgesic; nonsteroidal anti-inflammatory drug (NSAID) for cataract extraction and corneal refractive surgery* [diclofenac sodium] 0.1% ⍰ Foltrin

Voltaren gel ℞ *anti-inflammatory for osteoarthritis of the hands and knees* [diclofenac sodium] 1% ⍰ Foltrin

Voltaren-XR extended-release tablets ℞ *once-daily analgesic; nonsteroidal anti-inflammatory drug (NSAID) for osteoarthritis, rheumatoid arthritis, and*

ankylosing spondylitis [diclofenac (as sodium)] 100 mg

Voluven IV infusion ℞ *plasma volume expander for blood loss due to trauma or surgery* [hetastarch] 6% ⊡ valofane

von Willebrand factor (VWF) *antihemophilic for von Willebrand disease (orphan)*

Vopac caplets ℞ *narcotic antitussive; analgesic; antipyretic* [codeine phosphate; acetaminophen] 30•650 mg

vorapaxar *investigational (NDA filed) agent to prevent blood clots*

voriconazole *triazole antifungal for invasive aspergillosis, candidemia of the skin and internal organs, esophageal candidiasis, and other serious fungal infections* 50, 200 mg oral

vorinostat *histone deacetylase (HDAC) inhibitor; antineoplastic for cutaneous T-cell lymphoma (CTCL; orphan); investigational (orphan) for multiple myeloma, and mesothelioma*

vorozole USAN, INN, BAN *antineoplastic; aromatase inhibitor* ⊡ Virasal

vortel [see: clorprenaline HCl]

VōSol HC ear drops ℞ *corticosteroidal anti-inflammatory; antiseptic* [hydrocortisone; acetic acid] 1%•2%

VoSpire ER extended-release tablets ℞ *sympathomimetic bronchodilator* [albuterol sulfate] 4, 8 mg

Votrient film-coated caplets ℞ *antineoplastic for advanced renal cell carcinoma; investigational for thyroid tumors* [pazopanib (as HCl)] 200 mg

votumumab USAN *monoclonal antibody for cancer imaging and therapy*

voxergolide INN

Voxsuprine tablets ℞ *peripheral vasodilator* [isoxsuprine HCl] 10, 20 mg

VP (vasopressin) [q.v.]

VP (VePesid, Platinol) *chemotherapy protocol for small cell lung cancer (SCLC)*

VP-16 [see: etoposide]

Vpriv powder for IV infusion ℞ *enzyme replacement therapy for Gaucher disease type 1* [velaglucerase alfa] 200, 400 IU/vial

VSL#3 capsules ℞ *natural intestinal bacteria; probiotic; dietary supplement* [Lactobacillus sp.; Bifidobacterium sp.; Streptococcus thermophilus] ≥ 225 billion cells ⊡ Feosol; VaZol

VSL#3; VSL#3 DS powder for oral solution ℞ *natural intestinal bacteria; probiotic; dietary supplement* [Lactobacillus sp.; Bifidobacterium sp.; Streptococcus thermophilus] ≥ 450 billion cells; ≥ 900 billion cells ⊡ Feosol; VaZol

V-TAD (VePesid, thioguanine, ara-C, daunorubicin) *chemotherapy protocol for acute myelocytic leukemia (AML)*

V-Tann oral suspension (discontinued 2008) ℞ *decongestant; antihistamine; sleep aid* [phenylephrine tannate; pyrilamine tannate] 12.5•30 mg/5 mL ⊡ Vytone

vulneraries *a class of agents that promote wound healing*

Vumon IV infusion ℞ *antineoplastic for refractory childhood acute lymphoblastic leukemia (orphan); also used for adult acute lymphocytic leukemia and non-Hodgkin lymphoma* [teniposide; alcohol 42.7%] 10 mg/mL

Vusion ointment ℞ *diaper rash treatment; antifungal for candidiasis* [miconazole nitrate; zinc oxide] 0.25%•15% ⊡ Fuzeon; Visine; Vision

VWF (von Willebrand factor) [q.v.]

Vytone cream ℞ *corticosteroidal anti-inflammatory; antimicrobial* [hydrocortisone; iodoquinol] 1%•1% ⊡ V-Tann

Vytorin 10/10; Vytorin 10/20; Vytorin 10/40; Vytorin 10/80 caplets ℞ *combination intestinal cholesterol absorption inhibitor plus HMG-CoA reductase inhibitor to lower serum levels of LDL and total cholesterol* [ezetimibe; simvastatin] 10•10 mg; 10•20 mg; 10•40 mg; 10•80 mg

Vyvanse capsules ℞ *once-daily treatment for attention-deficit/hyperactivity disorder (ADHD)* [lisdexamfetamine dimesylate] 20, 30, 40, 50, 60, 70 mg

VZIG (varicella-zoster immune globulin) [q.v.]

wahoo (Euonymus atropurpureus) bark *medicinal herb used as a diuretic, expectorant, and laxative*

wakerobin *medicinal herb* [see: birth-root]

Wallette (trademarked packaging form) *patient compliance package for oral contraceptives* ② violet; Wilate

wallflower; western wallflower *medicinal herb* [see: dogbane]

walnut (Juglans spp.) *medicinal herb* [see: black walnut; butternut; English walnut]

walnut, lemon; white walnut *medicinal herb* [see: butternut]

Walpole tea *medicinal herb* [see: New Jersey tea]

wandering milkweed *medicinal herb* [see: dogbane]

warfarin INN, BAN *coumarin-derivative anticoagulant* [also: warfarin potassium]

warfarin potassium USP *coumarin-derivative anticoagulant* [also: warfarin]

warfarin sodium USP *coumarin-derivative anticoagulant for myocardial infarction, thromboembolic episodes, venous thrombosis, and pulmonary embolism* 1, 2, 2.5, 3, 4, 5, 6, 7.5, 10 mg oral

Wart Remover topical liquid OTC *keratolytic* [salicylic acid in flexible collodion] 17%

Wart-Off topical liquid OTC *keratolytic* [salicylic acid in flexible collodion] 17%

water, purified USP *solvent*

water, tritiated [see: tritiated water]

water cabbage *medicinal herb* [see: white pond lily]

water dock (Rumex aquaticus) *medicinal herb* [see: yellow dock]

water eryngo (Eryngium aquaticum) root *medicinal herb used as a diaphoretic, diuretic, emetic, expectorant, and stimulant*

water fern *medicinal herb* [see: buckhorn brake]

water flag *medicinal herb* [see: blue flag]

water hemlock; water parsley *medicinal herb* [see: poison hemlock]

water lily *medicinal herb* [see: blue flag; white pond lily]

water lily, sweet; sweet-scented water lily; white water lily *medicinal herb* [see: white pond lily]

water moccasin snake antivenin [see: antivenin (Crotalidae) polyvalent]

water O 15 USAN *radioactive diagnostic aid for vascular disorders*

water pepper *medicinal herb* [see: knotweed]

water pimpernel; water purslain *medicinal herb* [see: brooklime]

water shamrock *medicinal herb* [see: buckbean]

water smartweed *medicinal herb* [see: knotweed]

[¹⁵O] water [see: water O 15]

watercress (Nasturtium officinale) plant *medicinal herb for anemia, cramps, kidney and liver disorders, nervousness, and rheumatism*

water-d₂ [see: deuterium oxide]

wax, carnauba NF *tablet-coating agent*

wax, emulsifying NF *emulsifying and stiffening agent*

wax, microcrystalline NF *stiffening and tablet-coating agent*

wax, white NF *stiffening agent* [also: beeswax, white]

wax, yellow NF *stiffening agent* [also: beeswax, yellow]

wax cluster *medicinal herb* [see: wintergreen]

wax myrtle *medicinal herb* [see: bayberry]

Wee Care oral suspension OTC *iron supplement* [carbonyl iron] 15 mg/1.25 mL ② agar; Icar

weeping spruce *medicinal herb* [see: hemlock]

Welchol tablets, powder for oral suspension ℞ *nonabsorbable cholesterol-lowering polymer for hyperlipidemia and to improve glycemic control in type*

2 diabetes [colesevelam HCl] 625 mg; 1.875, 3.75 g/packet

Wellbutrin film-coated tablets ℞ *antidepressant for major depressive disorder (MDD); also used for attention-deficit/ hyperactivity disorder (ADHD), neuropathic pain, and weight loss* [bupropion (as HCl)] 75, 100 mg

Wellbutrin SR sustained-release (12-hour) film-coated tablets ℞ *antidepressant for major depressive disorder (MDD); also used for attention-deficit/ hyperactivity disorder (ADHD), neuropathic pain, and weight loss* [bupropion (as HCl)] 100, 150, 200 mg

Wellbutrin XL sustained-release (24-hour) tablets ℞ *antidepressant for major depressive disorder (MDD) and seasonal affective disorder (SAD); also used for attention-deficit/hyperactivity disorder (ADHD), neuropathic pain, and weight loss* [bupropion (as HCl)] 150, 300 mg

Wellements Organic Gripe Water oral liquid OTC *natural product to relieve colic, stomach cramps, hiccups, and gas in infants* [ginger; fennel; chamomile]

WellTuss EXP syrup (discontinued 2007) ℞ *narcotic antitussive; decongestant; expectorant* [dihydrocodeine bitartrate; pseudoephedrine HCl; guaifenesin] 7.5•15•100 mg/5 mL

Welltuss HC oral liquid (discontinued 2009) ℞ *narcotic antitussive; antihistamine; decongestant* [hydrocodone bitartrate; chlorpheniramine maleate; pseudoephedrine HCl] 3•2•15 mg/5 mL

Westcort ointment, cream ℞ *corticosteroidal anti-inflammatory* [hydrocortisone valerate] 0.2%

western wallflower *medicinal herb* [see: dogbane]

Westhroid tablets ℞ *natural thyroid replacement for hypothyroidism or thyroid cancer* [thyroid, desiccated (porcine)] 16.25, 32.4, 48.75, 64.8, 81.25, 97.5, 113.75, 129.6, 146.25, 162.5, 194.4, 260, 325 mg (64.8 mg=1 gr.)

Wet-N-Soak solution (discontinued 2010) OTC *rewetting solution for rigid gas permeable contact lenses*

Wet-N-Soak Plus solution (discontinued 2010) OTC *disinfecting/wetting/ soaking solution for rigid gas permeable contact lenses* [note: RGP contact indication is different from hard contact indication for same product]

Wet-N-Soak Plus solution (discontinued 2010) OTC *wetting/soaking solution for hard contact lenses* [note: hard contact indication is different from RGP contact indication for same product]

Wetting solution (discontinued 2010) OTC *wetting solution for hard contact lenses*

Wetting & Soaking solution OTC *disinfecting/wetting/soaking solution for rigid gas permeable contact lenses* (note: multiple products with the same name)

Wetting & Soaking solution OTC *wetting/soaking solution for hard contact lenses* (note: multiple products with the same name)

wheat germ oil (octacosanol) *natural dietary supplement for increasing muscle endurance*

WHF Lubricating Gel (discontinued 2010) OTC *vaginal antiseptic; moisturizer/lubricant* [chlorhexidine gluconate; glycerin]

white bay *medicinal herb* [see: magnolia]

white beeswax [see: beeswax, white]

White Cloverine Salve ointment OTC *skin protectant* [white petrolatum] 97%

White Cod Liver Oil Concentrate capsules, chewable tablets (discontinued 2008) OTC *vitamin supplement* [vitamins A, D, and E] 10 000•400• ≜ IU; 4000•200• ≜ IU

White Cod Liver Oil Concentrate with Vitamin C chewable tablets (discontinued 2008) OTC *vitamin supplement* [vitamins A, C, and D] 4000 IU•50 mg•200 IU

white cohosh *(Actaea alba; A. pachypoda; A. rubra)* plant and root *medicinal herb for arthritis, bowel evacuation, colds, cough, itching, promoting labor, reviving those near death, rheumatism, stimulating menses, stomach disorders, and urogenital disorders*
white endive *medicinal herb* [see: dandelion]
white fringe *medicinal herb* [see: fringe tree]
white hellebore *(Veratrum album)* [see: hellebore]
white horehound *medicinal herb* [see: horehound]
white lotion USP *astringent; topical protectant*
white mineral oil [see: petrolatum, white]
white mustard; white mustard seed *medicinal herb* [see: mustard]
white nettle *medicinal herb* [see: blind nettle]
white oak *(Quercus alba)* bark *medicinal herb for internal and external bleeding, menstrual disorders, mouth sores, skin irritation, toothache, strep throat, ulcers, and urinary bleeding*
white ointment [see: ointment, white]
white petrolatum [see: petrolatum, white]
white phenolphthalein [see: phenolphthalein]
white pine *(Pinus strobus)* bark *medicinal herb for bronchitis, dysentery, laryngitis, and mucous build-up*
white pond lily *(Nymphaea odorata)* root *medicinal herb used as an antiseptic, astringent, demulcent, discutient, and vulnerary*
white root *medicinal herb* [see: pleurisy root]
white sorrel *medicinal herb* [see: wood sorrel]
white walnut *medicinal herb* [see: butternut]
white water lily *medicinal herb* [see: white pond lily]
white wax [see: wax, white]
white willow *(Salix alba)* *medicinal herb* [see: willow]
whitethorn *medicinal herb* [see: hawthorn]
Whitfield's Ointment OTC *antifungal; keratolytic* [benzoic acid; salicylic acid] 6%•3%
Whitfield's ointment [see: benzoic & salicylic acids]
whole blood [see: blood, whole]
whole root rauwolfia [see: rauwolfia serpentina]
whole-cell pertussis vaccine [see: diphtheria & tetanus toxoids & whole-cell pertussis (DTwP) vaccine, adsorbed]
whorlywort *medicinal herb* [see: Culver root]
Wibi lotion OTC *moisturizer; emollient*
widow spider species antivenin [now: antivenin (Latrodectus mactans)]
Wilate powder for IV injection ℞ *antihemophilic for von Willebrand disease* [antihemophilic factor (AHF); von Willebrand factor (VWF)] 450•450, 900•900 U/vial ⊡ violet; Wallette
wild bergamot *(Monarda fistulosa)* leaves *medicinal herb used as a carminative and stimulant*
wild black cherry *(Prunus serotina)* bark *medicinal herb used as an astringent, pectoral, sedative, and stimulant*
wild carrot *medicinal herb* [see: carrot]
wild cherry *(Prunus virginiana)* bark *medicinal herb for asthma, bronchitis, cough, fever, hypertension, and mucosal inflammation with discharge; also used as an expectorant*
wild cherry syrup USP
wild chicory *medicinal herb* [see: chicory]
wild clover *medicinal herb* [see: red clover]
wild cranesbill *medicinal herb* [see: alum root]
wild daisy *(Bellis perennis)* flowers and leaves *medicinal herb used as an analgesic, antispasmodic, demulcent, digestive, expectorant, laxative, and purgative*

wild endive *medicinal herb* [see: dandelion]

wild fennel *medicinal herb* [see: fennel]

wild geranium *medicinal herb* [see: alum root]

wild ginger (Asarum canadense) root *medicinal herb used as a carminative, diaphoretic, expectorant, and irritant; sometimes used as a substitute for ginger (Zingiber)*

wild hydrangea *medicinal herb* [see: hydrangea]

wild hyssop *medicinal herb* [see: blue vervain]

wild hyssop (Pycnanthemum virginianum) plant *medicinal herb used as an antispasmodic, carminative, diaphoretic, and stimulant*

wild indigo (Baptisia tinctoria) plant *medicinal herb used as an antiseptic, astringent, emetic, purgative, and stimulant*

wild jalap (Ipomoea pandurata) root *medicinal herb used as a strong cathartic*

wild lemon *medicinal herb* [see: mandrake]

wild lettuce (Lactuca virosa) leaves, flowers, and seeds *medicinal herb for asthma, bronchitis, chronic pain, circulatory disorders, cramps, laryngitis, nervous disorders, stimulating lactation, swollen genitals, and urinary tract infections*

wild marjoram *medicinal herb* [see: marjoram]

wild Oregon grape *medicinal herb* [see: Oregon grape]

wild pepper *medicinal herb* [see: mezereon; eleuthero]

wild potato; wild scammony; wild sweet potato vine *medicinal herb* [see: wild jalap]

wild red raspberry *medicinal herb* [see: red raspberry]

wild senna *medicinal herb* [see: senna]

wild snowball *medicinal herb* [see: New Jersey tea]

wild strawberry *medicinal herb* [see: strawberry]

wild tobacco *medicinal herb* [see: lobelia]

wild turkey pea *medicinal herb* [see: turkey corn]

wild valerian, great *medicinal herb* [see: valerian]

wild woodbine *medicinal herb* [see: American ivy]

wild yam (Dioscorea villosa) root *medicinal herb for arthritis, bilious colic, bowel spasms, gas, menstrual cramps, morning sickness, and spasmodic asthma*

Willard water *natural remedy for acne, alopecia, anxiety, arthritis, hypertension, and stomach ulcers*

willow (Salix alba; S. caprea; S. nigra; S. purpurea) bark and buds *medicinal herb for analgesia, diuresis, eczema, fever, inducing diaphoresis, headache, nervousness, rheumatism, and ulcerations; also used as an anaphrodisiac, antiseptic, and astringent*

wind root *medicinal herb* [see: pleurisy root]

wineberry *medicinal herb* [see: currant]

winged elm *medicinal herb* [see: slippery elm]

WinRho SDF liquid for IV or IM injection ℞ *immunizing agent for antenatal or postpartum prophylaxis of Rh hemolytic disease of the newborn; treatment for immune thrombocytopenic purpura (orphan)* [Rh$_O$(D) immune globulin, solvent/detergent treated] 300, 500, 1000, 3000 mcg (1500, 2500, 5000, 15 000 IU)

WinRho SDF powder for IV or IM injection (discontinued 2007) ℞ *immunizing agent for antenatal or postpartum prophylaxis of Rh hemolytic disease of the newborn; treatment for immune thrombocytopenic purpura (orphan)* [Rh$_O$(D) immune globulin, solvent/detergent treated] 600, 1500, 5000 IU (120, 300, 1000 mcg)

winter bloom *medicinal herb* [see: witch hazel]

winter clover *medicinal herb* [see: squaw vine]

winter marjoram; winter sweet
medicinal herb [see: marjoram]

winter savory (*Calamintha montana; Satureja montana; S. obovata*)
leaves and stems *medicinal herb for diarrhea, nausea, promoting expectoration, relieving gas and flatulence, and stimulation of menstruation; also used as an aphrodisiac*

winterberry (*Ilex verticillata*) bark and fruit *medicinal herb used as an astringent, bitter tonic, and febrifuge*

wintergreen (*Gaultheria procumbens*) leaves and oil *medicinal herb for aches and pains, colds, gout, lumbago, and migraine headache; also used topically as an astringent and rubefacient*

wintergreen, bitter; false wintergreen *medicinal herb* [see: pipsissewa]

wintergreen oil [see: methyl salicylate]

winterlein *medicinal herb* [see: flaxseed]

Wintersteiner's compound F [see: hydrocortisone]

winterweed *medicinal herb* [see: chickweed]

witch hazel (*Hamamelis virginiana*) bark *medicinal herb for bruises, burns, colds, colitis, diarrhea, dysentery, eye irritations, hemorrhoids, internal and external bleeding, mucous membrane inflammation of mouth, gums, and throat, tuberculosis, and varicose veins*

withania (*Withania somnifera*) fruit and roots *medicinal herb for diuresis, inducing emesis, liver disorders, inflammation, sedation, tuberculosis, and tumors*

withe; withy *medicinal herb* [see: willow]

Wobe-Mugos *investigational (orphan) enzyme combination adjunct to chemotherapy for multiple myeloma* [papain; trypsin; chymotrypsin]

wolf claw *medicinal herb* [see: club moss]

Women's Daily Formula capsules (discontinued 2008) OTC *vitamin/calcium/iron supplement* [multiple vitamins; calcium; iron; folic acid] ±•450•25•0.4 mg

Women's Gentle Laxative enteric-coated tablets OTC *stimulant laxative* [bisacodyl] 5 mg

Wonder Ice gel OTC *mild anesthetic; antipruritic; counterirritant* [menthol] 5.25%

Wondra lotion OTC *moisturizer; emollient* [lanolin]

wood betony *medicinal herb* [see: betony]

wood creosote [see: creosote carbonate]

wood sanicle *medicinal herb* [see: sanicle] track entire entry at -4.3

wood sorrel (*Oxalis acetosella*) plant *medicinal herb used as an anodyne, diuretic, emmenagogue, irritant, and stomachic*

wood strawberry *medicinal herb* [see: strawberry]

woodbine (*Clematis virginiana*) leaves *medicinal herb for bowel evacuation, cancer, edema, fever, hypertension, inflammation, insomnia, itching, kidney disorders, skin cuts and sores, tuberculous cervical lymphadenitis, tumors, and venereal eruptions; not generally regarded as safe and effective*

woodbine; American woodbine; wild woodbine *medicinal herb* [see: American ivy]

woodruff *medicinal herb* [see: sweet woodruff]

woody nightshade *medicinal herb* [see: bittersweet nightshade]

Woolley's antiserotonin [see: benanserin HCl]

wooly parsnip *medicinal herb* [see: masterwort]

wormwood (*Artemisia absinthium*) plant and leaves *medicinal herb for aiding digestion, constipation, debility, fever, intestinal worms, jaundice, labor pains, menstrual cramps, and stomach and liver disorders; not generally regarded as safe and effective*

wound weed *medicinal herb* [see: goldenrod]

woundwort (*Prunella vulgaris*) plant *medicinal herb used as an antispas-*

modic, astringent, bitter tonic, diuretic, hemostatic, vermifuge, and vulnerary
woundwort, soldier's *medicinal herb* [see: yarrow]
WOWtabs (trademarked dosage form) *quickly dissolving "without water" tablets*
Wyanoids Relief Factor rectal suppositories OTC *emollient* [cocoa butter; shark liver oil] 79%•3%

Wycillin IM injection ℞ *natural penicillin antibiotic* [penicillin G procaine] 600 000, 1 200 000 U/vial
wymote *medicinal herb* [see: marsh mallow]
Wyseal (trademarked dosage form) *film-coated tablet* ⑦ Iosal; VaZol; VSL
Wytensin tablets ℞ *antihypertensive* [guanabenz acetate] 4, 8 mg

Xalatan eye drops ℞ *prostaglandin agonist for glaucoma and ocular hypertension* [latanoprost] 0.005% ⑦ zileuton
Xalkori capsules ℞ *antineoplastic for non–small cell lung cancer (NSCLC) in nonsmokers caused by a defective ALK gene* [crizotinib] 200, 250 mg ⑦ Salkera
xamoterol USAN, INN, BAN *cardiac stimulant* ⑦ cimaterol; Symmetrel
xamoterol fumarate USAN *cardiac stimulant*
Xanax tablets ℞ *benzodiazepine anxiolytic; sedative; treatment for panic disorders and agoraphobia* [alprazolam] 0.25, 0.5, 1, 2 mg
Xanax XR extended-release tablets ℞ *benzodiazepine anxiolytic for panic disorder and agoraphobia* [alprazolam] 0.5, 1, 2, 3 mg
xanomeline USAN *cholinergic agonist for Alzheimer disease* ⑦ xinomiline
xanomeline tartrate USAN *cholinergic agonist for Alzheimer disease*
xanoxate sodium USAN *bronchodilator*
xanoxic acid INN
xanthan gum NF *suspending agent*
xanthines, xanthine derivatives *a class of bronchodilators*
xanthinol niacinate USAN *peripheral vasodilator* [also: xantinol nicotinate]
xanthiol INN ⑦ Santyl
xanthiol HCl [see: xanthiol]
xanthocillin BAN [also: xantocillin]

Xanthorhiza simplicissima *medicinal herb* [see: yellow root]
xanthotoxin [see: methoxsalen]
Xanthoxylum americanum; X. fraxineum *medicinal herb* [see: prickly ash]
xantifibrate INN
xantinol nicotinate INN *peripheral vasodilator* [also: xanthinol niacinate]
xantocillin INN [also: xanthocillin]
xantofyl palmitate INN
Xarelto film-coated tablets ℞ *once-daily antithrombotic for the prevention of deep vein thrombosis (DVT) following knee or hip replacement surgery; investigational (NDA filed) for venous thromboembolism (VTE) and stroke prevention; investigational (Phase III) for acute coronary syndrome (ACS)* [rivaroxaban] 10 mg
Xatral (foreign name for U.S. product **Uroxatral**)
Xclair cream ℞ *moisturizer; emollient*
Xcytrin injection *investigational (NDA filed, orphan) radiosensitizer for non–small cell lung cancer patients with brain metastases* [motexafin gadolinium]
^{127}Xe [see: xenon Xe 127]
^{133}Xe [see: xenon Xe 133]
Xebcort gel (discontinued 2009) ℞ *corticosteroidal anti-inflammatory* [hydrocortisone] 1%
Xedec; Xedec II extended-release tablets (discontinued 2009) ℞ *decongestant; expectorant* [phenylephrine

HCl; guaifenesin] 20•800 mg; 30•
1100 mg ℞ Cydec; Zodeac

Xeloda film-coated tablets ℞ *antineo-plastic for metastatic breast and colo-rectal cancer; also used for pancreatic cancer* [capecitabine] 150, 500 mg

Xelox film-coated tablets + IV injection *investigational (Phase III) antineoplastic combination for colorectal cancer* [capecitabine (tablets) + oxaliplatin (IV)]

xemilofiban HCl USAN *antianginal*

Xenaderm ointment ℞ *proteolytic enzyme for débridement of necrotic tissue; vulnerary* [trypsin; Peruvian balsam; castor oil] 250–700 U•87 mg•788 mg per g

xenalamine [see: xenazoic acid]

xenaldial [see: xenygloxal]

xenalipin USAN, INN *hypolipidemic*

Xenazine tablets ℞ *selective dopamine depletor for chorea associated with Huntington disease (orphan)* [tetrabenazine] 12.5, 25 mg

xenazoic acid INN

xenbucin USAN, INN *antihypercholesterolemic*

xenbuficin [see: xenbucin]

Xenical capsules ℞ *lipase inhibitor for weight loss in obese patients with a body mass index (BMI) of 27 or more; preventative for type 2 diabetes* [orlistat] 120 mg ℞ sanicle

xenipentone INN

xenogeneic hepatocytes *investigational (orphan) for severe liver failure*

xenon element (Xe)

xenon (^{133}Xe) INN *radioactive agent* [also: xenon Xe 133]

xenon Xe 127 USP *diagnostic aid; medicinal gas; radioactive agent*

xenon Xe 133 USAN, USP *radioactive agent* [also: xenon (^{133}Xe)]

xenthiorate INN

xenygloxal INN

xenyhexenic acid INN

xenysalate INN, BAN *topical anesthetic; antibacterial; antifungal* [also: biphenamine HCl]

xenysalate HCl [see: biphenamine HCl]

xenytropium bromide INN ℞ *sintropium bromide*

Xeomin powder for injection ℞ *neurotoxin complex for blepharospasm and cervical dystonia; also used for achalasia, Frey syndrome, palmar hyperhidrosis, and Tourette syndrome* [incobotulinumtoxin A] 50, 100 IU/vial ℞ Cyomin; Zymine

Xerac AC topical liquid ℞ *cleanser for acne* [aluminum chloride; alcohol] 6.25%•96%

Xerecept *investigational (Phase I/II, orphan) agent for peritumoral brain edema* [corticotropin-releasing factor]

Xerese cream ℞ *antiviral and corticosteroidal anti-inflammatory for recurrent herpes labialis* [acyclovir; hydrocortisone] 5%•1% ℞ Cerisa

Xgeva subcu injection ℞ *monthly treatment to increase bone density and reduce fractures in patients with bone metastases from solid tumors* [denosumab] 70 mg/mL (120 mg/vial)

Xiaflex injection ℞ *enzyme therapy for Dupuytren contracture and Peyronie disease; investigational to reduce the appearance of cellulite* [collagenase Clostridium histolyticum] 0.9 mg

xibenolol INN

xibornol INN, BAN

Xibrom eye drops ℞ *long-acting (twice daily) nonsteroidal anti-inflammatory drug (NSAID) for pain and inflammation following cataract extraction surgery* [bromfenac (as sodium)] 0.09% ℞ ZyPram

Xifaxan film-coated tablets ℞ *broad-spectrum rifamycin antibiotic for traveler's diarrhea and hepatic encephalopathy; also used for irritable bowel syndrome (IBS)* [rifaximin] 200, 550 mg

Xigris powder for IV infusion ℞ *thrombolytic/fibrinolytic for severe sepsis* [drotrecogin alfa] 5, 20 mg/vial ℞ sucrose

xilobam USAN, INN *muscle relaxant*

ximoprofen INN

xinafoate USAN, INN, BAN *combining name for radicals or groups*

xinidamine INN

xinomiline INN ⊠ xanomeline

xipamide USAN, INN *antihypertensive; diuretic*

xipranolol INN

XiraHist DM Pediatric oral drops ℞ *antitussive; antihistamine; decongestant; for children 3–24 months* [dextromethorphan hydrobromide; carbinoxamine maleate; phenylephrine HCl] 3•2•2 mg/mL

XiraHist Pediatric oral drops ℞ *decongestant; antihistamine; for children 3–24 months* [phenylephrine HCl; carbinoxamine maleate] 2•2 mg/mL

Xiral sustained-release caplets (discontinued 2007) ℞ *decongestant; antihistamine; anticholinergic to dry mucosal secretions* [pseudoephedrine HCl; chlorpheniramine maleate; methscopolamine nitrate] 120•8•2.5 mg ⊠ sorrel

XiraTuss caplets ℞ *antitussive; antihistamine; decongestant* [carbetapentane tannate; chlorpheniramine tannate; phenylephrine tannate] 60•5•10 mg

Xodol caplets ℞ *narcotic analgesic; antipyretic* [hydrocodone bitartrate; acetaminophen] 5•300, 7.5•300, 10•300 mg ⊠ Sudal

Xolair powder for subcu injection ℞ *immunoglobulin E (IgE) blocker for moderate to severe asthma* [omalizumab] 150 mg/1.2 mL dose ⊠ Sular

Xolegel gel ℞ *antifungal for seborrheic dermatitis in immunocompromised patients* [ketoconazole; dehydrated alcohol] 2%•34%

Xolegel CorePak gel ℞ *antifungal + corticosteroidal anti-inflammatory* [Xolegel (q.v.) + Xebcort (q.v.)]

Xolegel Duo Convenience Pack gel + shampoo ℞ *antifungal for seborrheic dermatitis in immunocompromised patients* [(ketoconazole; dehydrated alcohol) + (pyrithione zinc)] 2%•34% + 1%

Xolox caplets ℞ *narcotic analgesic; antipyretic* [oxycodone HCl; aceta-

minophen] 2.5•500, 10•500 mg ⊠ Celexa; Cylex; Salex

XomaZyme-791 *investigational (orphan) for metastatic colorectal adenocarcinoma* [anti-TAP-72 immunotoxin]

XomaZyme-H65 *investigational (orphan) for graft vs. host disease following bone marrow transplants* [CD5-T lymphocyte immunotoxin]

Xopenex inhalation solution, inhalation solution concentrate ℞ *sympathomimetic bronchodilator* [levalbuterol (as HCl)] 0.31, 0.63, 1.25 mg/3 mL dose; 1.25 mg/0.5 mL dose

Xopenex HFA inhalation aerosol ℞ *sympathomimetic bronchodilator* [levalbuterol (as tartrate)] 45 mcg/actuation

xorphanol INN *analgesic* [also: xorphanol mesylate]

xorphanol mesylate USAN *analgesic* [also: xorphanol]

Xoten lotion OTC *analgesic; mild anesthetic; antipruritic; counterirritant* [methyl salicylate; menthol] 6.25%• 12.5%

Xoten-C lotion OTC *analgesic; mild anesthetic; antipruritic; counterirritant* [methyl salicylate; menthol; capsaicin] 20%•10%•0.001%

XPect-AT extended-release caplets ℞ *antitussive; expectorant* [carbetapentane citrate; guaifenesin] 60•600 mg

XPect-HC extended-release tablets (discontinued 2007) ℞ *narcotic antitussive; expectorant* [hydrocodone bitartrate; guaifenesin] 5•600 mg

X-Prep oral liquid (discontinued 2009) OTC *pre-procedure bowel evacuant* [senna extract] 74 mL

X-Prep Bowel Evacuant Kit-1 oral liquid + 2 tablets + suppository (discontinued 2009) OTC *pre-procedure bowel evacuant* [X-Prep (liquid); Senokot-S (tablets); Rectolax (suppository)]

XRT (x-ray therapy) *adjunct to chemotherapy* [not a pharmaceutical agent]

X-Seb shampoo OTC *antiseborrheic; keratolytic* [salicylic acid] 4%

X-Seb Plus shampoo OTC *antiseborrheic; keratolytic; antibacterial; antifungal* [salicylic acid; pyrithione zinc] 2%•1%

X-Seb T shampoo OTC *antiseborrheic; antipsoriatic; keratolytic* [coal tar; salicylic acid] 10%•4%

X-Seb T Plus shampoo OTC *antiseborrheic; antipsoriatic; keratolytic* [coal tar; salicylic acid] 10%•0.4%

xylamidine tosilate INN *serotonin inhibitor* [also: xylamidine tosylate]

xylamidine tosylate USAN *serotonin inhibitor* [also: xylamidine tosilate]

Xylarex oral solution OTC *daily non-antibiotic dietary supplement for the management of recurrent acute otitis media (AOM) in children ≥ 6 months* [xylitol]

xylazine INN *analgesic; veterinary muscle relaxant* [also: xylazine HCl] ⊘ psilocin

xylazine HCl USAN *analgesic; veterinary muscle relaxant* [also: xylazine]

xylitol NF *sweetened vehicle; non-antibiotic dietary supplement for the management of recurrent acute otitis media (AOM) in children ≥ 6 months*

Xylocaine ointment (discontinued 2007) OTC *anesthetic* [lidocaine] 2.5% ⊘ silicon; Solaquin

Xylocaine subcu and IV injection Ŗ *local anesthetic (subcu); antiarrhythmic for acute ventricular arrhythmias (IV)* [lidocaine HCl] 0.5%, 1%, 2% ⊘ silicon; Solaquin

Xylocaine topical liquid, oral ointment (discontinued 2007) Ŗ *mucous membrane anesthetic* [lidocaine HCl] 5%; 2.5%, 5% ⊘ silicon; Solaquin

Xylocaine topical solution, oral jelly Ŗ *mucous membrane anesthetic* [lidocaine HCl] 4%; 2% ⊘ silicon; Solaquin

Xylocaine 10% Oral throat spray (discontinued 2007) Ŗ *mucous membrane anesthetic* [lidocaine HCl] 10%

Xylocaine HCl injection Ŗ *local anesthetic* [lidocaine HCl; dextrose] 1.5%•7.5%

Xylocaine HCl injection Ŗ *local anesthetic* [lidocaine HCl; epinephrine] 0.5%•1:200 000, 1%•1:100 000, 1%•1:200 000, 2%•1:50 000, 2%•1:100 000, 2%•1:200 000

Xylocaine HCl IV for Cardiac Arrhythmias IV injection, IV admixture Ŗ *antiarrhythmic* [lidocaine HCl] 1%, 2%, 4%, 20%

Xylocaine MPF injection Ŗ *local anesthetic* [lidocaine HCl] 0.5%, 1%, 1.5%, 2%, 4%

Xylocaine MPF injection Ŗ *local anesthetic* [lidocaine HCl; epinephrine] 1%•1:200 000, 1.5%•1:200 000, 2%•1:200 000

Xylocaine MPF injection Ŗ *local anesthetic* [lidocaine HCl; glucose] 5%•7.5%

Xylocaine Viscous topical solution (discontinued 2010) Ŗ *mucous membrane anesthetic* [lidocaine HCl] 2%

xylocoumarol INN

xylofilcon A USAN *hydrophilic contact lens material* ⊘ silafilcon A

xylometazoline INN, BAN *vasoconstrictor; nasal decongestant* [also: xylometazoline HCl]

xylometazoline HCl USP *vasoconstrictor; nasal decongestant* [also: xylometazoline]

xylose (D-xylose) USP *diagnostic aid for intestinal function* ⊘ Cialis; Salese; Silace

xyloxemine INN

Xyntha powder for IV infusion Ŗ *systemic hemostatic; antihemophilic for the prevention and control of bleeding in classical hemophilia (hemophilia A)* [antihemophilic factor] 250, 500, 1000, 2000, 3000 IU/dose

Xyotax (name changed to **Opaxio** while in Phase III trials) ⊘ Zotex

Xyralid cream Ŗ *local anesthetic; corticosteroidal anti-inflammatory* [lidocaine HCl; hydrocortisone acetate] 3%•1%

Xyralid LP lotion Ŗ *local anesthetic; corticosteroidal anti-inflammatory* [lidocaine HCl; hydrocortisone acetate] 3%•0.5%

Xyralid RC anorectal cream ℞ *local anesthetic and corticosteroidal antiinflammatory for hemorrhoids* [lidocaine HCl; hydrocortisone acetate] 3%•1%

Xyrem oral solution ℞ *CNS depressant for narcolepsy (orphan), cataplexy, and excessive daytime sleepiness; investigational (Phase III) for fibromyalgia; also used for fatigue* [sodium oxybate] 500 mg/mL

Xyzal film-coated tablets, oral solution ℞ *second-generation piperazine antihistamine for allergic rhinitis and chronic idiopathic urticaria* [levocetirizine dihydrochloride] 5 mg; 2.5 mg/5 mL ⑨ Zazole

yam *medicinal herb* [see: wild yam]

yarrow (Achillea millefolium) flower *medicinal herb for bowel hemorrhage, colds, fever, flu, hypertension, inducing sweating, measles, mucosal inflammation with discharge, nosebleed, reducing heavy menstrual bleeding and pain, thrombosis, and topical hemostasis*

Yasmin film-coated tablets (in packs of 28) ℞ *monophasic oral contraceptive* [drospirenone; ethinyl estradiol] 3 mg•30 mcg × 21 days; counters × 7 days

yatren [see: chiniofon]

Yaz film-coated tablets (in packs of 28) ℞ *monophasic oral contraceptive in a novel 24-day regimen; also approved to treat premenstrual dysphoric disorder (PMDD) and acne vulgaris* [drospirenone; ethinyl estradiol] 3 mg•20 mcg × 24 days; counters × 4 days

169Yb [see: pentetate calcium trisodium Yb 169]

169Yb [see: ytterbium Yb 169 pentetate]

Y-Cof DM extended-release caplets ℞ *antitussive; antihistamine; decongestant* [dextromethorphan hydrobromide; dexbrompheniramine maleate; phenylephrine HCl] 30•6•20 mg

yeast, dried NF

yeast cell derivative *claimed to promote wound healing*

Yeast-Gard vaginal suppositories (discontinued 2010) OTC *for irritation, itching, and burning* [pulsatilla 28x; Candida albicans 28x]

Yeast-Gard Medicated Disposable Douche Premix vaginal solution OTC *antifungal cleanser and deodorizer; acidity modifier* [sodium benzoate; lactic acid]

Yeast-Gard Medicated Douche; Yeast-Gard Medicated Disposable Douche vaginal solution OTC *antiseptic/germicidal cleanser and deodorizer* [povidone-iodine] 10%; 0.3%

Yeast-X vaginal suppositories OTC *for irritation, itching, and burning* [pulsatilla 28x]

Yelets Teenage Formula tablets OTC *vitamin/mineral/calcium/iron supplement* [multiple vitamins & minerals; calcium (as carbonate and ascorbate); iron (as ferrous fumarate); folic acid] ≛•60•18•0.4 mg

yellow bedstraw; yellow cleavers *medicinal herb* [see: bedstraw]

yellow beeswax [see: beeswax, yellow]

yellow dock (Rumex crispus) root *medicinal herb for anemia, blood cleansing, constipation, itching, liver congestion, rheumatism, skin problems, and eyelid ulcerations; also used as a dentifrice*

yellow ferric oxide [see: ferric oxide, yellow]

yellow fever vaccine USP *active immunizing agent for yellow fever*

yellow gentian *medicinal herb* [see: gentian]

yellow ginseng *medicinal herb* [see: blue cohosh]

yellow Indian paint *medicinal herb* [see: goldenseal]

yellow jessamine *medicinal herb* [see: gelsemium]

yellow mercuric oxide [see: mercuric oxide, yellow]

yellow ointment [see: ointment, yellow]

yellow paint root; yellow root *medicinal herb* [see: goldenseal]

yellow petrolatum JAN *ointment base; emollient/protectant* [also: petrolatum]

yellow phenolphthalein [see: phenolphthalein, yellow]

yellow precipitate [see: mercuric oxide, yellow]

yellow puccoon *medicinal herb* [see: goldenseal]

yellow root *(Xanthorhiza simplicissima) medicinal herb used for diabetes and hypertension*

yellow root; yellow paint root *medicinal herb* [see: goldenseal]

yellow wax [see: wax, yellow]

yellow wood; yellow wood berries *medicinal herb* [see: prickly ash]

yerba maté *(Ilex paraguariensis)* leaves *medicinal herb used as a CNS stimulant, diuretic, and purifier*

yerba santa *(Eriodictyon californicum)* leaves *medicinal herb for asthma, bronchial congestion, colds, hay fever, inducing expectoration, inflammation, rheumatic pain, and tuberculosis*

Yervoy IV infusion ℞ *antineoplastic for unresectable or metastatic melanoma; investigational (NDA filed) for non–small cell lung cancer (NSCLC)* [ipilimumab] 3, 5 mg/mL

yew *(Taxus bacatta and other species)* leaves *medicinal herb for liver disorders, rheumatism, and urinary tract disorders*

YF-Vax powder for subcu injection ℞ (available from designated Yellow Fever Vaccination Centers only) *active immunizing agent for yellow fever* [yellow fever vaccine] 0.5 mL

Yocon tablets ℞ *alpha$_2$-adrenergic blocker for impotence and orthostatic hypotension; sympatholytic; mydriatic;* *may have aphrodisiac activity; no FDA-approved indications* [yohimbine HCl] 5.4 mg ☑ Acanya; A.C.N.

Yodoxin tablets, powder ℞ *amebicide for intestinal amebiasis* [iodoquinol] 210, 650 mg; 25 g

yohimbe *(Corynanthe johimbe; Pausinystalia johimbe)* bark *medicinal herb for angina, hypertension, and impotence and other sexual dysfunction; also used as an aphrodisiac*

yohimbic acid INN

yohimbine HCl *alpha$_2$-adrenergic blocker for impotence and orthostatic hypotension; sympatholytic; mydriatic; may have aphrodisiac activity; no FDA-approved indications* 5.4 mg oral

Yondelis ℰ℧℞ (available in Europe) *investigational (NDA filed, orphan) antineoplastic for soft tissue sarcoma and relapsed ovarian cancer; investigational (Phase III) for breast cancer; investigational (Phase II) for prostate cancer, advanced liposarcoma, and leiomyosarcoma* [trabectedin]

Your Choice Non-Preserved Saline solution (discontinued 2010) OTC *rinsing/storage solution for soft contact lenses* [sodium chloride (saline solution)]

Your Choice Sterile Preserved Saline solution (discontinued 2010) OTC *rinsing/storage solution for soft contact lenses* [sodium chloride (preserved saline solution)]

youthwort *medicinal herb* [see: masterwort]

ytterbium *element (Yb)*

ytterbium Yb 169 pentetate USP *radioactive agent*

yttrium *element (Y)*

yttrium Y 90 ibritumomab tiuxetan *radioimmunotherapy for non-Hodgkin B-cell lymphoma (orphan)*

yttrium Y 90 labetuzumab *monoclonal antibody to carcinoembryonic antigen (CEA); investigational (orphan) for ovarian cancer*

yucca (*Yucca glauca*) root *medicinal herb for arthritis, colitis, hypertension,* *migraine headache, and rheumatism*

yuma *medicinal herb* [see: wild yam]

zabicipril INN

zacopride INN *antiemetic; peristaltic stimulant* [also: zacopride HCl]

zacopride HCl USAN, INN *antiemetic; peristaltic stimulant* [also: zacopride]

Zactima tablets ℞ *antineoplastic for medullary thyroid cancer (orphan); investigational (NDA filed) for advanced or metastatic non–small cell lung cancer* [vandetanib] 300 mg

Zadaxin ⓔ *(approved in Italy) vaccine enhancer for hepatitis C, cancer, and infectious diseases; investigational (Phase III, orphan) for chronic active hepatitis B; investigational (orphan) for DiGeorge syndrome with immune defects and hepatocellular carcinoma* [thymalfasin]

Zaditor eye drops OTC *antihistamine and mast cell stabilizer for allergic conjunctivitis* [ketotifen (as fumarate)] 0.025%

zafirlukast USAN, INN, BAN *leukotriene receptor antagonist (LTRA) for prevention and long-term treatment of asthma* 10, 20 mg oral

zafuleptine INN

zalcitabine USAN *nucleoside reverse transcriptase inhibitor (NRTI); antiviral for advanced HIV infection (orphan)*

zaleplon USAN *pyrazolopyrimidine hypnotic for the short-term treatment of insomnia* 5, 10 mg oral

zalospirone INN *anxiolytic* [also: zalospirone HCl] ② Salazopyrin

zalospirone HCl USAN *anxiolytic* [also: zalospirone]

zaltidine INN, BAN *antagonist to histamine H_2 receptors* [also: zaltidine HCl]

zaltidine HCl USAN *antagonist to histamine H_2 receptors* [also: zaltidine]

Zaltrap injection *investigational (NDA filed) angiogenesis inhibitor for various solid tumors* [aflibercept]

Zamicet oral solution ℞ *narcotic analgesic; antipyretic* [hydrocodone bitartrate; acetaminophen; alcohol 6.7%] 3.3•108.3 mg/5 mL oral

zamifenacin INN, BAN *treatment for irritable bowel syndrome*

Zamyl *investigational (orphan) for acute myelogenous leukemia* [lintuzumab]

Zanaflex tablets, capsules ℞ *skeletal muscle relaxant; antispasmodic for multiple sclerosis and spinal cord injury (orphan)* [tizanidine] 2, 4 mg; 2, 4, 6 mg

zanamivir USAN *influenza neuraminidase inhibitor for the prophylaxis and treatment of acute influenza A and B virus infections; also used for H1N1 swine flu*

Zanfel cream, wash OTC *poison ivy treatment* [polyethylene granules]

zankiren HCl USAN *antihypertensive*

Zanosar powder for IV injection ℞ *nitrosourea-type alkylating antineoplastic for metastatic islet cell carcinoma of pancreas* [streptozocin] 1 g (100 mg/mL)

zanoterone USAN *antiandrogen*

Zantac film-coated tablets, syrup, IV or IM injection ℞ *histamine H_2 antagonist for gastric and duodenal ulcers* [ranitidine HCl] 150, 300 mg; 15 mg/mL; 1, 25 mg/mL ② Zinotic

Zantac 75; Zantac 150 tablets OTC *histamine H_2 antagonist for episodic heartburn* [ranitidine HCl] 75 mg; 150 mg ② Zinotic

Zantac EFFERdose effervescent tablets ℞ *histamine H_2 antagonist for gastric and duodenal ulcers* [ranitidine HCl] 25 mg

Zanthorhiza apiifolia *medicinal herb* [see: yellow root]

Zanzibar aloe *medicinal herb* [see: aloe]

zapizolam INN

zaprinast INN, BAN

Zarah film-coated tablets (in packs of 28) ℞ *monophasic oral contraceptive* [drospirenone; ethinyl estradiol] 3 mg•30 mcg × 21 days; counters × 7 days

zardaverine INN

Zarnestra *investigational (NDA filed, orphan) antineoplastic for acute myeloid leukemia (AML)* [tipifarnib]

Zarontin capsules, syrup ℞ *succinimide anticonvulsant* [ethosuximide] 250 mg; 250 mg/5 mL

Zaroxolyn tablets ℞ *antihypertensive; diuretic for congestive heart failure and renal disease; also used for osteoporosis and diabetes insipidus* [metolazone] 2.5, 5 mg

zatosetron INN, BAN *antimigraine* [also: zatosetron maleate]

zatosetron maleate USAN *antimigraine* [also: zatosetron]

Zavesca capsules ℞ *treatment for type I Gaucher disease (orphan); investigational (NDA filed) for Niemann-Pick type C (NP-C) dementia* [miglustat] 100 mg

Zazole vaginal cream (discontinued 2010) ℞ *antifungal* [terconazole] 0.4%, 0.8% ☒ Xyzal

Z-Bec caplets OTC *vitamin/zinc supplement* [multiple vitamins; zinc sulfate; folic acid; biotin] ±•22.5•0.4•0.3 mg ☒ Z-Pak

Z-Cof 8 DM; Z-Cof 12 DM oral suspension ℞ *antitussive; decongestant; expectorant* [dextromethorphan tannate; pseudoephedrine tannate; guaifenesin] 15•30•175 mg/5 mL; 30•60•175 mg/5 mL

Z-Cof HCX oral liquid (discontinued 2011) ℞ *narcotic antitussive; expectorant* [hydrocodone bitartrate; guaifenesin] 7.5•200 mg/5 mL

Z-Cof I oral suspension ℞ *antitussive; decongestant; expectorant* [dextromethorphan hydrobromide; pseudoephedrine HCl; guaifenesin] 15•30• 211 mg/5 mL

Z-Dex syrup ℞ *antitussive; decongestant; expectorant* [dextromethorphan hydrobromide; phenylephrine HCl; guaifenesin] 20•10•100 mg/5 mL ☒ Cedax; ciadox; Cidex; Sudex

Z-Dex 12D caplets ℞ *antitussive; antihistamine; decongestant* [dextromethorphan hydrobromide; chlorpheniramine maleate; phenylephrine HCl] 30•8•20 mg

Z-Dex Pediatric oral drops ℞ *antitussive; decongestant; expectorant; for children 6–18 months* [dextromethorphan hydrobromide; phenylephrine HCl; guaifenesin] 3•2.5•35 mg/mL

ZDV (zidovudine) [q.v.]

ZE Caps soft capsules (discontinued 2008) OTC *dietary supplement* [vitamin E; zinc gluconate] 200•9.6 mg

Zea mays *medicinal herb* [see: Indian corn]

Zeasorb powder OTC *absorbent; anhidrotic* [microporous cellulose; talc]

Zeasorb-AF powder, gel OTC *antifungal for tinea pedis, tinea cruris, and tinea corporis* [miconazole nitrate] 2%

zeaxanthin *natural carotenoid used to prevent and treat age-related macular degeneration (AMD), retinitis pigmentosa (RP), and other retinal dysfunction*

Zebeta film-coated tablets ℞ *beta-blocker for hypertension* [bisoprolol fumarate] 5, 10 mg

Zecnil *investigational (orphan) for secreting cutaneous gastrointestinal fistulas* [somatostatin]

Zee-Seltzer effervescent tablets OTC *antacid; analgesic; antipyretic* [sodium bicarbonate; citric acid; aspirin] 1916•1000•325 mg

Zefazone powder or frozen premix for IV injection (discontinued 2007) ℞ *second-generation cephalosporin antibiotic* [cefmetazole sodium] 1, 2 g ☒ Cefzon

Zeftera *investigational (NDA filed) broad-spectrum cephalosporin antibiotic for complicated skin and skin structure infections (SSSIs) and community-acquired pneumonia (CAP)* [ceftobiprole]

Zegerid capsules, powder for oral suspension ℞ *combination proton pump inhibitor and antacid for gastric and duodenal ulcers, erosive esophagitis, gastroesophageal reflux disease (GERD), upper GI bleeding, and other gastroesophageal disorders* [omeprazole; sodium bicarbonate] 20•1100, 40•1100; 20•1680, 40•1680 mg/pkt. ⍰ Sucraid

Zegerid OTC capsules OTC *combination proton pump inhibitor and antacid for acid indigestion and heartburn* [omeprazole; sodium bicarbonate] 20•1100 mg

Zegerid with Magnesium Hydroxide chewable tablets ℞ *combination proton pump inhibitor and antacid for gastric and duodenal ulcers, erosive esophagitis, gastroesophageal reflux disease (GERD), upper GI bleeding, and other gastroesophageal disorders* [omeprazole; sodium bicarbonate; magnesium hydroxide] 20•600•700, 40•600•700 mg

zein NF *coating agent*

Zelapar orally disintegrating tablets ℞ *monoamine oxidase inhibitor (MAOI); dopaminergic for Parkinson disease* [selegiline (as HCl)] 1.25 mg

Zelboraf film-coated tablets ℞ *antineoplastic for metastatic melanoma* [vemurafenib] 240 mg

Zelnorm tablets (discontinued 2007 due to safety concerns; limited availability through the manufacturer for specific cases) ℞ *selective serotonin receptor antagonist for irritable bowel syndrome (IBS) with chronic constipation in women and chronic idiopathic constipation in all* [tegaserod maleate] 2, 6 mg

Zelrix transdermal patch *investigational (NDA filed) vascular serotonin 5-HT₁ receptor agonist for the acute treatment of migraine headaches; the patch uses a novel on-board microprocessor to control the transfer of medication to the skin* [sumatriptan]

Zemaira powder for IV infusion ℞ *enzyme replacement therapy for heredi-*tary *alpha₁-proteinase inhibitor deficiency, which leads to progressive panacinar emphysema* [alpha₁-proteinase inhibitor] 50 mg/mL (1000 mg/vial) ⍰ Swim-Ear; Zymar

Zema-Pak 10 Day; Zema-Pak 13 Day tablets ℞ *corticosteroidal anti-inflammatory* [dexamethasone] 1.5 mg

Zemplar capsules, bolus injection during dialysis ℞ *vitamin D therapy for hyperparathyroidism secondary to chronic kidney disease (CKD)* [paricalcitol] 1, 2, 4 mcg; 2, 5 mcg/mL

Zemuron IV injection ℞ *nondepolarizing neuromuscular blocking agent; muscle relaxant; adjunct to general anesthesia* [rocuronium bromide] 10 mg/mL

Zenapax injection (discontinued 2010) ℞ *immunosuppressant; monoclonal antibody (MAb) to prevent acute rejection of kidney and bone marrow transplants (orphan)* [daclizumab] 25 mg/5 mL

zenarestat USAN *aldose reductase inhibitor*

Zenate, Advanced Formula film-coated tablets (discontinued 2008) ℞ *hematinic* [multiple vitamins; iron (as ferrous fumarate); folic acid] ≛• 65•1 mg

zenazocine mesylate USAN *analgesic*

Zenchent tablets (in packs of 28) ℞ *monophasic oral contraceptive* [norethindrone; ethinyl estradiol] 0.4 mg• 35 mcg × 21 days; counters × 7 days

Zencia soap ℞ *antibiotic and keratolytic for acne* [sulfacetamide sodium; sulfur] 9%•4% ⍰ Senna-S

Zenieva topical emulsion ℞ *moisturizer; emollient* [glycerin; olive oil; squalane; vegetable oil]

Zenpep delayed-release capsules ℞ *digestive enzymes* [pancrelipase (lipase; protease; amylase)] 5•17•27, 10•34•55, 15•51•82, 20•68•109 thousand USP units

Zenvia (name changed to **Nuedexta** upon marketing release in 2010)

zepastine INN

Zephiran Chloride aqueous solution (discontinued 2010) OTC *antiseptic* [benzalkonium chloride] 1:750

Zephiran Chloride tincture, tincture spray, towelettes, disinfectant concentrate OTC *antiseptic* [benzalkonium chloride] 1:750; 1:750; 1:750; 17%

zephirol [see: benzalkonium chloride]

Zephrex film-coated tablets (discontinued 2007) ℞ *decongestant; expectorant* [pseudoephedrine HCl; guaifenesin] 60•400 mg ② sfericase; Zovirax

Zephrex LA extended-release tablets (discontinued 2007) ℞ *decongestant; expectorant* [pseudoephedrine HCl; guaifenesin] 120•600 mg

zeranol USAN, INN *anabolic*

Zerit capsules, powder for oral solution ℞ *antiretroviral for HIV-1 infection* [stavudine] 15, 20, 30, 40 mg; 1 mg/mL ② XRT

Zerit XR extended-release capsules (discontinued 2011) ℞ *antiretroviral for HIV-1 infection* [stavudine] 37.5, 50, 75, 100 mg

Zertane ⓔ *opioid analgesic investigational (Phase III) for premature ejaculation* [tramadol HCl]

Zestoretic tablets ℞ *combination angiotensin-converting enzyme (ACE) inhibitor and diuretic for hypertension* [lisinopril; hydrochlorothiazide] 10•12.5, 20•12.5, 20•25 mg

Zestra oil OTC *natural sexual lubricant; claimed to "increase female sexual sensation, arousal, and pleasure" when topically applied to the vaginal area* [borage oil; evening primrose oil; angelica seed oil; coleus extract; vitamins C and E]

Zestril tablets ℞ *antihypertensive; angiotensin-converting enzyme (ACE) inhibitor; adjunctive treatment for congestive heart failure (CHF)* [lisinopril] 2.5, 5, 10, 20, 30, 40 mg

Zetacet topical suspension, wash (discontinued 2010) ℞ *antibiotic and keratolytic for acne* [sulfacetamide sodium; sulfur] 10%•5%

Zetar shampoo OTC *antiseborrheic; antipsoriatic; antipruritic; antibacterial* [coal tar] 1%

Zetia caplets ℞ *antihyperlipidemic for primary hypercholesterolemia and mixed hyperlipidemia; intestinal cholesterol absorption inhibitor* [ezetimibe] 10 mg

zetidoline INN, BAN

Zevalin powder for IV infusion ℞ *radioimmunotherapy carrier; monoclonal antibody to treat non-Hodgkin B-cell lymphoma (orphan)* [indium In 111 ibritumomab tiuxetan; yttrium Y 90 ibritumomab tiuxetan] 3.2 mg

Zevalin therapeutic regimen "kit" (complete package for a one-week course of treatment) ℞ *multistep treatment protocol for non-Hodgkin B-cell lymphoma* [rituximab; indium In 111 ibritumomab tiuxetan; yttrium Y 90 ibritumomab tiuxetan]

ZFlex tablets ℞ *analgesic; antipyretic; antihistamine; sleep aid* [acetaminophen; phenyltoloxamine citrate] 500•55 mg ② Soflax

Z-Gen tablets OTC *vitamin/zinc supplement* [multiple vitamins; zinc] ≟•22.5 mg ② Cecon; Ziagen

Zhuzishen (Panax pseudoginseng) *medicinal herb* [see: ginseng]

Ziac tablets ℞ *combination beta-blocker and diuretic for hypertension* [bisoprolol fumarate; hydrochlorothiazide] 2.5•6.25, 5•6.25, 10•6.25 mg

Ziagen film-coated caplets, oral solution ℞ *antiviral nucleoside reverse transcriptase inhibitor for HIV infection* [abacavir (as sulfate)] 300 mg; 20 mg/mL ② Cecon; Z-Gen

Ziana gel ℞ *antibiotic and keratolytic for acne* [clindamycin phosphate; tretinoin] 1.2%•0.025%

ziconotide USAN *non-narcotic analgesic; calcium channel blocker*

ziconotide acetate *calcium-channel blocker; non-narcotic analgesic for intractable pain of cancer or AIDS*

zidapamide USAN, INN

zidometacin USAN, INN *anti-inflammatory*

zidovudine (ZDV) USAN, INN, BAN *nucleoside reverse transcriptase inhibitor (NRTI); antiretroviral for AIDS* *and AIDS-related complex (orphan), HIV-1 infection, and the prevention of maternal-fetal HIV-1 transmission* 100, 300 mg oral; 50 mg/5 mL oral; 10 mg/mL injection

zidovudine & abacavir sulfate & lamivudine *nucleoside reverse transcriptase inhibitor (NRTI) combination for HIV and AIDS* 300•300•150 mg oral

zidovudine & lamivudine *nucleoside reverse transcriptase inhibitor (NRTI) combination for HIV and AIDS* 60•30, 200•200, 300•150 mg oral

zidovudine & nevirapine & lamivudine *combination nucleoside reverse transcriptase inhibitor (NRTI) and non-nucleoside reverse transcriptase inhibitor (NNRTI) for HIV and AIDS* 60•50•30, 300•200•150 mg oral

zifrosilone USAN *acetylcholinesterase inhibitor for Alzheimer disease*

Ziks cream OTC *analgesic; mild anesthetic; antipruritic; counterirritant* [methyl salicylate; menthol; capsaicin] 12%•1%•0.025% ⧆ Ziox

Zilactin oral gel OTC *antimicrobial throat preparation* [benzyl alcohol] 10%

Zilactin Medicated oral gel OTC *astringent and antiseptic for oral canker and herpes lesions* [tannic acid; alcohol 80%] 7%

Zilactin-B Medicated oral gel OTC *mucous membrane anesthetic; antiseptic* [benzocaine; alcohol 76%] 10%

Zilactin-L topical liquid OTC *antiseptic; anesthetic* [benzyl alcohol] 10%

zilantel USAN, INN *anthelmintic* ⧆ salantel

zileuton USAN, INN, BAN *5-lipoxygenase inhibitor; leukotriene formation inhibitor for the prophylaxis and chronic treatment of asthma* ⧆ Xalatan

zilpaterol INN

zimeldine INN, BAN *antidepressant* [also: zimeldine HCl]

zimeldine HCl USAN *antidepressant* [also: zimeldine]

zimelidine HCl [now: zimeldine HCl]

zimidoben INN

Zinacef powder or frozen premix for IV or IM injection ℞ *second-generation cephalosporin antibiotic* [cefuroxime sodium] 0.75, 1.5, 7.5 g

zinc *element (Zn)*

Zinc 15 tablets OTC *zinc supplement* [zinc sulfate] 66 mg

zinc acetate USP *copper blocking/complexing agent for Wilson disease (orphan); topical antiseptic; poison ivy treatment*

zinc acetate, basic INN

zinc acetate dihydrate [see: zinc acetate]

zinc bacitracin [see: bacitracin zinc]

zinc caprylate *antifungal*

zinc carbonate USAN *dietary zinc supplement*

zinc chloride USP *astringent; dentin desensitizer; dietary zinc supplement*

zinc chloride Zn 65 USAN *radioactive agent*

zinc citrate *dietary zinc supplement; sore throat treatment (34% elemental zinc)*

zinc complex bacitracins [see: bacitracin zinc]

zinc DTPA [see: pentetate zinc trisodium]

zinc gelatin USP

zinc gluconate USP *dietary zinc supplement; sore throat treatment* 10, 15, 50, 78 mg oral

zinc oleate NF

zinc oxide USP, JAN *astringent; topical protectant; emollient; antiseptic* 20%, 25% topical

zinc peroxide, medicinal USP

zinc phenolsulfonate NF *not generally regarded as safe and effective as an antidiarrheal*

zinc propionate *antifungal*

zinc pyrithione [see: pyrithione zinc]

zinc stearate USP *dusting powder; tablet and capsule lubricant; antifungal*

zinc sulfate USP, JAN *ophthalmic astringent; dietary zinc supplement; additive to IV solutions for total parenteral nutrition (41% elemental zinc)* 200, 220, 250 mg oral; 1, 5 mg/mL injection

zinc sulfate heptahydrate [see: zinc sulfate]

zinc sulfate monohydrate [see: zinc sulfate]

zinc sulfocarbolate [see: zinc phenol-sulfonate]

zinc trisodium pentetate [see: pentetate zinc trisodium]

zinc undecylenate USP *antifungal*

zinc valerate USP

Zinc-220 capsules OTC *zinc supplement* [zinc sulfate] 220 mg ☒ Cena-K; senega

Zinca-Pak IV injection (discontinued 2011) ℞ *intravenous nutritional therapy* [zinc sulfate] 1, 5 mg/mL

Zincate capsules ℞ *zinc supplement* [zinc sulfate] 220 mg

zinc-eugenol USP

Zincfrin Drop-Tainers (eye drops) (discontinued 2010) OTC *decongestant; astringent* [phenylephrine HCl; zinc sulfate] 0.12%•0.25%

Zincon shampoo OTC *antiseborrheic; antibacterial; antifungal* [pyrithione zinc] 1% ☒ Sinequan

Zincvit capsules (discontinued 2008) ℞ *vitamin/mineral supplement* [multiple vitamins & minerals; folic acid] ±•1 mg

zindotrine USAN, INN *bronchodilator*

zindoxifene INN

Zinecard powder for IV drip or push ℞ *cardioprotectant for doxorubicin-induced cardiomyopathy (orphan)* [dexrazoxane (as HCl)] 250, 500 mg/vial

Zingiber officinale *medicinal herb* [see: ginger]

Zingo intradermal powder in a prefilled, needle-free delivery system (discontinued 2009) ℞ *fast-acting local anesthetic to reduce the pain of injections and blood draws in children 3–18 years* [lidocaine HCl] 0.5 mg ☒ senega

zinoconazole INN *antifungal* [also: zinoconazole HCl]

zinoconazole HCl USAN *antifungal* [also: zinoconazole]

zinostatin USAN, INN *antineoplastic*

Zinotic; Zinotic ES ear drops ℞ *local anesthetic; antiseptic; emollient* [pramoxine HCl; chloroxylenol; zinc acetate dihydrate; glycerin] 0.5%•0.1%•0.1%•1%; 1%0.1%•1%•1% ☒ Zantac

zinterol INN *bronchodilator* [also: zinterol HCl] ☒ Center-Al

zinterol HCl USAN *bronchodilator* [also: zinterol]

zinviroxime USAN, INN *antiviral*

Zinx Chlor-D extended-release capsules ℞ *decongestant; antihistamine* [pseudoephedrine HCl; chlorpheniramine maleate] 120•8 mg

Zinx D-Tuss oral suspension ℞ *antitussive; decongestant* [carbetapentane tannate; phenylephrine tannate] 30•25 mg/5 mL

Zinx GCP oral solution ℞ *antitussive; decongestant; expectorant* [carbetapentane citrate; phenylephrine HCl; guaifenesin] 20•10•100 mg/5 mL

Zinx GP extended-release caplets ℞ *decongestant; expectorant* [phenylephrine HCl; guaifenesin] 30•1000 mg

Zinx PCM oral solution ℞ *decongestant; antihistamine; anticholinergic to dry mucosal secretions* [phenylephrine HCl; chlorpheniramine maleate; methscopolamine nitrate] 10•2•1.25 mg/5 mL

Ziox 405 ointment ℞ *proteolytic enzyme for débridement of necrotic tissue; vulnerary; wound deodorant* [papain; urea; chlorophyllin copper complex] 405 900 IU/g•10%•0.5% ☒ Ziks

zipeprol INN

ziprasidone HCl *oral novel (atypical) benzisoxazole antipsychotic for schizophrenia and manic episodes of a bipolar disorder; serotonin 5-HT₂ and dopamine D₂ antagonist*

ziprasidone mesylate USAN *novel (atypical) benzisoxazole antipsychotic injection for rapid control of acute agitation in schizophrenic patients; serotonin 5-HT₂ and dopamine D₂ antagonist*

Zipsor capsules ℞ *analgesic; nonsteroidal anti-inflammatory drug (NSAID) for* *osteoarthritis, rheumatoid arthritis, anky-losing spondylitis, and dysmenorrhea* [diclofenac (as potassium)] 25 mg

Ziradryl lotion OTC *antihistamine; astringent; protectant; antiseptic* [diphenhydramine HCl; zinc oxide; alcohol 2%] 1%•2%

zirconium *element (Zr)*

zirconium oxide *astringent*

Zirgan ophthalmic gel ℞ *antiviral for AIDS-related CMV retinitis (orphan); investigational (NDA filed) for herpetic keratitis* [ganciclovir] 0.15%

Zithranol-RR cream ℞ *antipsoriatic* [anthralin] 1.2%

Zithromax film-coated tablets, Tri-Pak (3 tablets), Z-Pak (6 tablets), powder for oral suspension, powder for IV or IM injection ℞ *macrolide antibiotic* [azithromycin (as dihydrate)] 250, 500, 600 mg; 500 mg; 250 mg; 100, 200 mg/5 mL, 1 g/pkt.; 500 mg

Zixoryn *investigational (orphan) agent for neonatal hyperbilirubinemia* [flumecinol]

Zmax powder for extended-release oral suspension ℞ *macrolide antibiotic* [azithromycin (as dihydrate)] 167 mg/5 mL (2 g/dose)

65Zn [see: zinc chloride Zn 65]

Zn-DTPA (zinc pentetate) [see: pentetate zinc trisodium]

ZNP cleansing bar OTC *antiseborrheic; antibacterial; antifungal* [pyrithione zinc] 2%

zocainone INN ⍰ *siccanin*

Zocor film-coated tablets ℞ *HMG-CoA reductase inhibitor for hyperlipidemia, hypertriglyceridemia, and coronary heart disease (CHD)* [simvastatin] 5, 10, 20, 40, 80 mg

Zocor Heart-Pro film-coated tablets ℞ (available OTC in England) *HMG-CoA reductase inhibitor for hyperlipidemia, hypertriglyceridemia, and coronary heart disease* [simvastatin] 10 mg

Zodeac-100 tablets (discontinued 2008) ℞ *hematinic; vitamin/mineral/iron supplement* [multiple vitamins & minerals; iron (as ferrous fumarate);

folic acid; biotin] ≐•60•1•0.3 mg ⍰ Cydec; Xedec

ZoDen DM oral drops ℞ *antitussive; antihistamine; decongestant; for children 6–12 years* [dextromethorphan hydrobromide; chlorpheniramine maleate; phenylephrine HCl] 3•1•1.5 mg/mL

Zoderm gel, cream, liquid cleanser ℞ *keratolytic for acne* [benzoyl peroxide (in a urea base)] 4.5%, 5.75%, 6.5%, 8.5% ⍰ Zyderm

Zodryl AC 25; Zodryl AC 30; Zodryl AC 35; Zodryl AC 40; Zodryl AC 50; Zodryl AC 60; Zodryl AC 80 oral drops ℞ *narcotic antitussive; antihistamine* [codeine phosphate; chlorpheniramine maleate] 1•0.333 mg/mL; 1•0.286 mg/mL; 1•0.25 mg/mL; 1•0.222 mg/mL; 1•0.4 mg/mL; 1•0.267 mg/mL; 1•0.2 mg/mL

Zodryl DAC 25; Zodryl DAC 30; Zodryl DAC 35; Zodryl DAC 40; Zodryl DAC 50; Zodryl DAC 60; Zodryl DAC 80 oral liquid ℞ *narcotic antitussive; antihistamine; decongestant* [codeine phosphate; chlorpheniramine maleate; pseudoephedrine HCl] 5•1.665•25 mg/5 mL; 5•1.43•21.43 mg/5 mL; 5•1.25•18.75 mg/5 mL; 5•1.11•16.665 mg/5 mL; 5•2•30 mg/5 mL; 5•1.43•20 mg/5 mL; 5•1•15 mg/5 mL

Zodryl DEC 25; Zodryl DEC 30; Zodryl DEC 35; Zodryl DEC 40; Zodryl DEC 50; Zodryl DEC 60; Zodryl DEC 80 oral suspension ℞ *narcotic antitussive; decongestant; expectorant* [codeine phosphate; pseudoephedrine HCl; guaifenesin] 5•25•100 mg/5 mL; 5•21.43•100 mg/5 mL; 5•18.75•100 mg/5 mL; 5•16.7•100 mg/5 mL; 5•30•100 mg/5 mL; 5•20•100 mg/5 mL; 5•15•100 mg/5 mL

zofenopril INN, BAN *antihypertensive; angiotensin-converting enzyme (ACE) inhibitor* [also: zofenopril calcium]

zofenopril calcium USAN *antihypertensive; angiotensin-converting enzyme (ACE) inhibitor* [also: zofenopril]

zofenoprilat INN *antihypertensive* [also: zofenoprilat arginine]

zofenoprilat arginine USAN *antihypertensive* [also: zofenoprilat]

zoficonazole INN

Zofran film-coated tablets, oral solution, IM injection ℞ *antiemetic to prevent nausea and vomiting following chemotherapy, radiation, or surgery* [ondansetron HCl] 4, 8, 24 mg; 4 mg/5 mL; 2 mg/mL ⊡ saffron; Zophren

Zofran IV infusion (discontinued 2009) ℞ *antiemetic to prevent nausea and vomiting following chemotherapy, radiation, or surgery* [ondansetron HCl] 32 mg/50 mL ⊡ saffron; Zophren

Zofran ODT (orally disintegrating tablets) ℞ *antiemetic to prevent nausea and vomiting following chemotherapy, radiation, or surgery* [ondansetron] 4, 8 mg

Zohydro timed-release tablets *investigational (Phase III) narcotic analgesic* [hydrocodone]

Zoladex subcu implant in preloaded syringe ℞ *hormonal antineoplastic for palliative treatment of prostatic carcinoma, breast cancer, and endometriosis* [goserelin acetate] 3.6 mg (1-month implant), 10.8 mg (3-month implant) ⊡ Zeldox

zolamine INN *antihistamine; topical anesthetic* [also: zolamine HCl]

zolamine HCl USAN *antihistamine; topical anesthetic* [also: zolamine]

zolazepam INN, BAN *sedative* [also: zolazepam HCl] ⊡ sulazepam

zolazepam HCl USAN *sedative* [also: zolazepam]

zoledronate disodium USAN *bone resorption inhibitor for osteoporosis*

zoledronate trisodium USAN *bone resorption inhibitor for osteoporosis*

zoledronic acid USAN *bisphosphonate bone resorption inhibitor for hypercalcemia of malignancy (HCM; orphan), multiple myeloma, bone metastases,* *and metabolic bone disorders such as Paget disease; annual or biannual treatment for osteoporosis*

zolenzepine INN

zolertine INN *antiadrenergic; vasodilator* [also: zolertine HCl]

zolertine HCl USAN *antiadrenergic; vasodilator* [also: zolertine]

Zolicef powder for IV or IM injection (discontinued 2007) ℞ *first-generation cephalosporin antibiotic* [cefazolin sodium] 1 g

zolimidine INN

zolimomab aritox USAN *monoclonal antibody to pan T lymphocyte; investigational (orphan) for in vivo and ex vivo treatment of bone marrow transplants*

Zolinza capsules ℞ *antineoplastic for cutaneous T-cell lymphoma (CTCL; orphan)* [vorinostat] 100 mg

zoliprofen INN

zoliridine [see: zolimidine]

zolmitriptan USAN *vascular serotonin 5-HT$_{1B/1D}$ receptor agonist for the acute treatment of migraine*

Zoloft film-coated tablets, oral drops ℞ *selective serotonin reuptake inhibitor (SSRI) for depression, obsessive-compulsive disorder (OCD), panic disorder, post-traumatic stress disorder (PTSD), premenstrual dysmorphic disorder (PMDD), and social anxiety disorder* [sertraline HCl] 25, 50, 100 mg; 20 mg/mL

zoloperone INN

zolpidem INN, BAN *imidazopyridine sedative/hypnotic* [also: zolpidem tartrate]

zolpidem tartrate USAN *imidazopyridine sedative/hypnotic for the short-term treatment of insomnia* [also: zolpidem] 5, 6.25, 10, 12.5 mg oral

ZolpiMist metered oral spray, metered dose inhaler ℞ *sedative/hypnotic for the short-term treatment of insomnia* [zolpidem tartrate] 5 mg/actuation; 10 mg/actuation

zomebazam INN

zomepirac INN, BAN *analgesic; anti-inflammatory* [also: zomepirac sodium]

zomepirac sodium USAN, USP *analgesic; anti-inflammatory* [also: zomepirac]

Zometa IV infusion ℞ *bone resorption inhibitor for hypercalcemia of malignancy (orphan), multiple myeloma, and bone metastases from solid tumors* [zoledronic acid] 4 mg

zometapine USAN *antidepressant*

Zomig film-coated tablets, nasal spray ℞ *vascular serotonin receptor agonist for the acute treatment of migraine* [zolmitriptan] 2.5, 5 mg; 5 mg/dose ⊘ Sea-Omega

Zomig-ZMT orally disintegrating tablets ℞ *vascular serotonin receptor agonist for the acute treatment of migraine* [zolmitriptan] 2.5, 5 mg

Zonalon cream ℞ *antihistamine; antipruritic* [doxepin HCl] 5%

Zonatuss capsules ℞ *antitussive* [benzonatate] 150 mg

Zone-A Forte lotion ℞ *corticosteroidal anti-inflammatory; anesthetic* [hydrocortisone acetate; pramoxine] 2.5%•1%

Zonegran capsules ℞ *sulfonamide anticonvulsant for partial seizures* [zonisamide] 25, 50, 100 mg

zoniclezole INN *anticonvulsant* [also: zoniclezole HCl]

zoniclezole HCl USAN *anticonvulsant* [also: zoniclezole]

zonisamide USAN, INN, BAN *sulfonamide anticonvulsant for partial seizures* 25, 50, 100 mg oral

Zonite Douche vaginal solution concentrate OTC *antiseptic cleanser and deodorizer; mild anesthetic; antipruritic; counterirritant* [benzalkonium chloride; menthol; thymol]

zopiclone INN, BAN, JAN *sedative; hypnotic*

zopolrestat USAN *antidiabetic; aldose reductase inhibitor*

zorbamycin USAN *antibacterial*

Zorbtive powder for subcu injection ℞ *treatment for short bowel syndrome (SBS) in children (orphan)* [somatropin (rDNA)] 8.8 mg (24.6 IU) per vial

ZORprin Zero Order Release tablets ℞ *analgesic; antipyretic; anti-inflammatory; antirheumatic* [aspirin] 800 mg

Zortress tablets ℞ *immunosuppressant to prevent rejection of kidney transplants* [everolimus] 0.25, 0.5, 0.75 mg

zorubicin INN *antineoplastic* [also: zorubicin HCl]

zorubicin HCl USAN *antineoplastic* [also: zorubicin]

Zostavax powder for subcu injection ℞ *vaccine for adults ≥ 50 years to prevent herpes zoster infections* [varicella-zoster virus vaccine, live attenuated (Oka/Merck strain)] 19 400 PFU/0.65 mL dose

zoster vaccine, live [see: varicella-zoster virus vaccine, live]

Zostrix; Zostrix Diabetic Foot Pain; Zostrix-HP cream OTC *counterirritant; topical analgesic for muscle and joint pain* [capsaicin] 0.025%, 0.075%; 0.075%; 0.075%

Zostrix Neuropathy cream (discontinued 2011) OTC *counterirritant; topical analgesic for muscle and joint pain* [capsaicin] 0.25%

Zosyn powder or frozen premix for IV injection ℞ *extended-spectrum penicillin antibiotic plus synergist* [piperacillin sodium; tazobactam sodium] 2•0.25, 3•0.375, 4•0.5, 36•4.5 g ⊘ Saizen; Susano

zotepine INN, JAN *antipsychotic* ⊘ cetaben

Zotex; Zotex-D syrup ℞ *antitussive; decongestant; expectorant* [dextromethorphan hydrobromide; phenylephrine HCl; guaifenesin] 20•10•100 mg/5 mL; 15•8.5•100 mg/5 mL ⊘ Xyotax

Zotex-C syrup ℞ *narcotic antitussive; antihistamine; sleep aid; decongestant* [codeine phosphate; pyrilamine maleate; phenylephrine HCl] 10•5•5 mg/5 mL ⊘ Xyotax

Zotex-EX caplets ℞ *antitussive; decongestant; expectorant* [dextromethorphan hydrobromide; phenylephrine HCl; guaifenesin] 15•10•350 mg

Zotex-G syrup (discontinued 2007) ℞ *antitussive; decongestant; expectorant* [dextromethorphan hydrobromide; phenylephrine HCl; guaifenesin] 15•10•133 mg/5 mL

Zotex-GPX extended-release tablets ℞ *decongestant; expectorant* [phenylephrine HCl; guaifenesin] 8.5•550 mg

Zotex-PE extended-release tablets ℞ *decongestant; antihistamine* [phenylephrine HCl; brompheniramine maleate] 30•6 mg

Zotex Pediatric oral drops ℞ *antitussive; decongestant; expectorant; for children 6–18 months* [dextromethorphan hydrobromide; phenylephrine HCl; guaifenesin] 3•2.5•35 mg/mL

Zoto-HC ear drops ℞ *corticosteroidal anti-inflammatory; antiseptic; anesthetic* [hydrocortisone; chloroxylenol; pramoxine HCl] 10%•1%•10% ⊡ Zytiga

Zovia 1/35E; Zovia 1/50E tablets (in packs of 21 or 28) ℞ *monophasic oral contraceptive* [ethynodiol diacetate; ethinyl estradiol] 1 mg•35 mcg; 1 mg•50 mcg

Zovirax capsules, tablets, oral suspension ℞ *antiviral for herpes simplex, herpes zoster, and adult-onset chickenpox* [acyclovir] 200 mg; 400, 800 mg; 200 mg/5 mL ⊡ sfericase; Zephrex

Zovirax cream ℞ *antiviral for recurrent herpes labialis* [acyclovir] 5% ⊡ sfericase; Zephrex

zoxazolamine NF, INN

Z-Pak (trademarked packaging form) ℞ *6-tablet pack of* **Zithromax** ⊡ Z-Bec

Z-Tuss AC oral liquid ℞ *narcotic antitussive; antihistamine* [codeine phosphate; chlorpheniramine maleate] 9•2 mg/5 mL ⊡ Cytuss HC

Z-Tuss Expectorant oral liquid ℞ *narcotic antitussive; decongestant; antihistamine; expectorant* [hydrocodone bitartrate; pseudoephedrine HCl; chlorpheniramine maleate; guaifenesin] 2.5•15•2•100 mg/5 mL

Z-Tuss ZT caplets (discontinued 2007) ℞ *narcotic antitussive; expectorant* [hydrocodone bitartrate; guaifenesin] 5•300 mg

Zucapsaicin *investigational (orphan) agent for postherpetic neuralgia of the trigeminal nerve* [civamide]

zucapsaicin USAN *topical analgesic*

zuclomifene INN

zuclomiphene USAN

zuclopenthixol INN, BAN *thioxanthene antipsychotic*

Zuplenz PharmFilm (orally disintegrating film) ℞ *antiemetic to prevent nausea and vomiting following chemotherapy, radiation, or surgery* [ondansetron] 4, 8 mg

Zurase *investigational (orphan) agent for cancer-related tumor lysis syndrome and hyperuricemia due to cancer or severe gout* [pegloticase]

Zutripro oral solution ℞ *narcotic antitussive; antihistamine; decongestant* [hydrocodone bitartrate; chlorpheniramine maleate; pseudoephedrine HCl] 5•4•60 mg/5 mL

Z-Xtra lotion OTC *anesthetic; antihistamine; emollient* [pyrilamine maleate; benzocaine; zinc oxide] 2.07•2.08•41.35 mg/mL

Zyban sustained-release film-coated tablets ℞ *non-nicotine aid to smoking cessation* [bupropion (as HCl)] 150 mg

Zyclara cream ℞ *immunomodulator for actinic keratoses* [imiquimod] 3.75% ⊡ Ceclor; Sochlor

Zycose tablets ℞ *vitamin B supplement* [folic acid; benfotiamine; Benzamine (q.v.)] 1•150•850 mg

Zyderm gel for subcu injection ℞ *dermal filler for fine-to-moderate scars and wrinkles* [collagen, purified bovine] 35, 65 mg/mL ⊡ Zoderm

Zydis (trademarked dosage form) *orally disintegrating tablets*

Zydone tablets, capsules ℞ *narcotic analgesic; antipyretic* [hydrocodone bitartrate; acetaminophen] 5•400, 7.5•400, 10•400 mg; 5•500 mg

Zyflo film-coated tablets ℞ *leukotriene formation inhibitor for the prophylaxis*

and chronic treatment of asthma [zileuton] 600 mg ⑨ Cefol

Zyflo CR extended-release film-coated tablets ℞ *twice-daily leukotriene receptor antagonist (LTRA) for the prophylaxis and chronic treatment of asthma* [zileuton] 600 mg

Zylet eye drop suspension ℞ *corticosteroidal anti-inflammatory; aminoglycoside antibiotic* [loteprednol etabonate; tobramycin] 0.5%•0.3%

zylofuramine INN

Zyloprim tablets ℞ *xanthine oxidase inhibitor for gout and hyperuricemia; antineoplastic adjunct for reducing uric acid levels following chemotherapy for leukemia, lymphoma, and solid-tumor malignancies (orphan)* [allopurinol] 100, 300 mg

Zymacap capsules (discontinued 2008) OTC *vitamin supplement* [multiple vitamins; folic acid] ±•0.4 mg

Zymar eye drops ℞ *broad-spectrum fluoroquinolone antibiotic* [gatifloxacin] 0.3% ⑨ Swim-Ear; Zemaira

Zymaxid eye drops ℞ *broad-spectrum fluoroquinolone antibiotic* [gatifloxacin] 0.5%

Zymine oral liquid ℞ *antihistamine* [triprolidine HCl] 1.25 mg/5 mL ⑨ Cyomin; Xeomin

Zymine DXR oral suspension ℞ *decongestant; antihistamine* [pseudoephedrine HCl; triprolidine HCl] 45•2.5 mg/5 mL

Zymine HC oral liquid (discontinued 2008) ℞ *narcotic antitussive; antihistamine; decongestant* [hydrocodone bitartrate; triprolidine HCl; pseudoephedrine HCl] 2.5•1.25•30 mg/5 mL

Zymine XR oral suspension ℞ *antihistamine* [triprolidine HCl] 2.5 mg/5 mL

Zyplast gel for subcu injection ℞ *dermal filler for deep scars and wrinkles* [collagen, purified bovine, cross-linked] 35 mg/mL

ZyPram cream ℞ *corticosteroidal anti-inflammatory; local anesthetic* [hydrocortisone acetate; pramoxine HCl] 2.35%•1% ⑨ Xibrom

Zyprexa film-coated tablets ℞ *rapid-acting novel (atypical) antipsychotic for schizophrenia, treatment-resistant depression, and manic or depressive episodes of a bipolar disorder; also used for obsessive-compulsive disorder (OCD)* [olanzapine] 2.5, 5, 7.5, 10, 15, 20 mg ⑨ Sprix; Suprax

Zyprexa Adhera (name changed to **Zyprexa Relprevv** upon marketing release in 2009)

Zyprexa IntraMuscular powder for IM injection ℞ *novel (atypical) antipsychotic for rapid control of psychomotor agitation due to schizophrenia or bipolar disorder* [olanzapine] 10 mg/vial

Zyprexa Relprevv long-acting (2 to 4 weeks) suspension for IM injection ℞ *novel (atypical) antipsychotic for schizophrenia* [olanzapine (as pamoate monohydrate)] 210, 300, 405 mg

Zyprexa Zydis orally disintegrating tablets ℞ *rapid-acting novel (atypical) antipsychotic for schizophrenia, treatment-resistant depression, and manic or depressive episodes of a bipolar disorder* [olanzapine] 5, 10, 15, 20 mg

Zyrtec chewable tablets, syrup (name changed to **Zyrtec Children's Allergy** upon status change to OTC in 2007) ⑨ Psoriatec

Zyrtec film-coated tablets (name changed to **Zyrtec Allergy** upon status change to OTC in 2007) ⑨ Psoriatec

Zyrtec liquid-filled capsules OTC *nonsedating antihistamine for allergic rhinitis and chronic idiopathic urticaria; also used for bronchial asthma* [cetirizine HCl] 10 mg ⑨ Psoriatec

Zyrtec Allergy tablets, orally disintegrating tablets, liquid-filled gelcaps OTC *nonsedating antihistamine for allergic rhinitis; also used for bronchial asthma* [cetirizine HCl] 10 mg

Zyrtec Children's Allergy chewable tablets, syrup OTC *nonsedating antihistamine for allergic rhinitis; also used for bronchial asthma* [cetirizine HCl] 5, 10 mg; 1 mg/mL

Zyrtec Children's Hives Relief oral solution OTC *nonsedating antihistamine for hives* [cetirizine HCl] 1 mg/mL

Zyrtec Hives Relief tablets, liquid-filled gelcaps OTC *nonsedating antihistamine for chronic idiopathic urticaria* [cetirizine HCl] 10 mg

Zyrtec Itchy Eye Drops OTC *antihistamine and mast cell stabilizer for allergic conjunctivitis* [ketotifen (as fumarate)] 0.025%

Zyrtec-D 12 Hour extended-release tablets OTC *nonsedating antihistamine and decongestant for allergic rhinitis* [cetirizine HCl; pseudoephedrine HCl] 5•120 mg

Zytiga tablets ℞ *testosterone antagonist antineoplastic for late-stage metastatic prostate cancer* [abiraterone acetate] 250 mg

Zyvox film-coated caplets, powder for oral suspension, IV infusion ℞ *antibiotic for gram-positive bacterial infections* [linezolid] 600 mg; 100 mg/5 mL; 200, 400, 600 mg/bag

APPENDIX **A**
Sound-Alikes

Below are 1312 drug names that may be confused in transcription, followed by one or more possible "sound-alike" names. The list below includes only ℞, oTc, and generic drugs available in the U.S. The main section of the book includes all of these, plus sound-alikes on 1394 additional entries, including chemotherapy protocols, medicinal herbs and natural remedies, foreign drugs, and more. Look for the "ear" icon (🔊) on over 2700 entries in the main list.

A1cNOW+ 🔊 Acanya; A.C.N.
Abstral 🔊 epiestriol
Acanya 🔊 A1cNOW; A.C.N.
Accolate 🔊 Equilet
Aceon 🔊 Aczone; Ocean
aceperone 🔊 aspirin; azaperone; Easprin; esuprone
Acephen 🔊 Asaphen; Ucephan
acetone 🔊 Istin
acifran 🔊 Isovorin
aconitine 🔊 Akineton
ACT 🔊 AZT
ActHIB 🔊 AK-Tob
actisomide 🔊 octazamide
Aczone 🔊 Aceon; Ocean
Adoxa 🔊 ADEKs; Edex; Iodex
ADT 🔊 ACT; AZT
Advantage 🔊 ADD-Vantage
Advate 🔊 Adavite
AeroBid; AeroBid-M 🔊 EryPed
Aerofreeze 🔊 OraVerse
AeroSpan 🔊 erizepine
Aerotrol 🔊 Urotrol
AeroTuss 🔊 Artiss
AeroZoin 🔊 Orasone; Ureacin
A/G Pro 🔊 AKPro
agar 🔊 Icar
Agoral 🔊 Aquoral
Airacof 🔊 Ercaf
Akineton 🔊 aconitine
aklomide 🔊 iogulamide
AK-Spore 🔊 Exubera
AK-Sulf 🔊 Ocusulf
AK-Ten 🔊 Accutane
Ala-Quin 🔊 Alcaine; Aloquin; Elocon; elucaine

AlaSTAT 🔊 Elestat
Alasulf 🔊 alusulf
Alcaine 🔊 Ala-Quin; Aloquin; Elocon; elucaine
Alcare 🔊 Allegra
Aleve 🔊 Aluvia; ELF; olive
alexidine 🔊 aloxidone
Alimta 🔊 Elimite
Alinia 🔊 aloin; ellaOne
Allegra 🔊 agar; Alcare; Icar
Allergy 🔊 Uloric
AlleRx 🔊 Alrex
aloin 🔊 ellaOne
Aloquin 🔊 Ala-Quin; Alcaine; Elocon; elucaine
alosetron 🔊 Elestrin
Aloxi 🔊 I-L-X; Olux
aloxidone 🔊 alexidine
Alphanate 🔊 Alfenta
Alrex 🔊 AlleRx
Altazine 🔊 Ilotycin
alusulf 🔊 Alasulf
Aluvia 🔊 Aleve; ELF; olive
amalgucin 🔊 imiloxan
ambazone 🔊 ampyzine
Ambi 🔊 AMPA
amedalin 🔊 imidoline; omidoline
Amicar 🔊 Omacor
amikhelline 🔊 Amoclan
Aminosyn 🔊 amanozine
amiperone 🔊 Empirin
amipizone 🔊 ampyzine
amiterol 🔊 Emetrol
amitivir 🔊 emitefur
amixetrine 🔊 amogastrin
Amoclan 🔊 amikhelline

amogastrin ⧉ amixetrine
AMPA ⧉ Ambi
ampyrimine ⧉ embramine; imipramine
ampyzine ⧉ amipizone
Anacin ⧉ Enzone; inosine; Unasyn
Anadrol ⧉ Inderal
Anatrofin ⧉ Entrophen
ancitabine ⧉ enocitabine
Androxy ⧉ Ondrox
Angeliq ⧉ one.click
anisatil ⧉ inositol
Antizol ⧉ Entsol
Aosept ⧉ Azopt
Apetigen ⧉ aptocaine; Opti-gen
Aphrodyne ⧉ avridine
Aphthasol ⧉ efetozole
Apokyn ⧉ Opcon
Aquabase ⧉ Equipoise
AquADEKs ⧉ Ocudox
Aquasol ⧉ Ixel
Aquavit-E ⧉ Ocuvite
Aquoral ⧉ Agoral
ara-G ⧉ ARC; Eryc
Aranelle ⧉ Urea Nail
argon ⧉ AeroCaine; Ircon
Aricept ⧉ Orasept
arsenic ⧉ Orazinc
Artiss ⧉ AeroTuss
Arzerra ⧉ OraSure
Asacol ⧉ Isocal; Os-Cal
Ascor ⧉ ozagrel
asparagine ⧉ esproquine
aspirin ⧉ aceperone; azaperone;
    Easprin; esuprone
AspirLow ⧉ Isuprel
atevirdine ⧉ etofuradine
atosiban ⧉ etazepine
Atralin ⧉ iotrolan
A/T/S ⧉ oats
Attain ⧉ 8 in 1
Auro Ear Drops ⧉ E-R-O Ear Drops
Auro-Dri ⧉ Ear-Dry
Aurolate ⧉ Oralet
Avelox ⧉ Euflex; I-Valex
Aviane ⧉ Iophen
Avidoxy ⧉ Efudex
avridine ⧉ Aphrodyne
azabon ⧉ Isopan
azaconazole ⧉ isoconazole
azamulin ⧉ azumolene

azaperone ⧉ aceperone; aspirin;
    Easprin; esuprone
azapetine ⧉ Aseptone; isobutane
azaprocin ⧉ isoprazone
azaquinzole ⧉ isoconazole
azarole ⧉ acerola
azithromycin ⧉ astromicin
Azopt ⧉ Aosept
azumolene ⧉ azamulin
BAL in Oil ⧉ bolenol
Balneol ⧉ bolenol
bamifylline ⧉ pimefylline
Banzel ⧉ Panasal
Baricon ⧉ Paracaine; Puregon
Baridium ⧉ Pyridium
barium ⧉ broom
batoprazine ⧉ butaperazine
befunolol ⧉ pafenolol
befuraline ⧉ bufrolin
benaxibine ⧉ pinoxepin
Bencort ⧉ Penecort
Benicar ⧉ Penecare
berkelium ⧉ brooklime
Betagen ⧉ butacaine
Bidex-A ⧉ Pediox
Bidhist-D ⧉ PD-Hist D
binedaline ⧉ pinadoline
binifibrate ⧉ ponfibrate
Biogil ⧉ Bo-Cal
BioThrax ⧉ Bite Rx
biotin ⧉ betony; Bitin; butane
bisobrin ⧉ buspirone
Bite Rx ⧉ BioThrax
bizelesin ⧉ pecilocin
bleomycin (BLM) ⧉ peliomycin
Blue Ice ⧉ Boil-Ease
Boil-Ease ⧉ Blue Ice
bolenol ⧉ BAL in Oil
Boost ⧉ Bucet
boric acid ⧉ BrachySeed
BrachySeed ⧉ boric acid
Bravelle ⧉ Prefill
Brevicon ⧉ parvaquone
brimonidine ⧉ bromindione
bromazepam ⧉ premazepam
bromazine ⧉ promazine
bromindione ⧉ brimonidine
bufrolin ⧉ befuraline
bulaquine ⧉ Bellacane
buramate ⧉ PowerMate

buspirone 🔊 bisobrin
butane 🔊 betony; biotin; Bitin
butaperazine 🔊 batoprazine
butikacin 🔊 Betaxon
butoprozine 🔊 batoprazine
Caduet 🔊 Duet
caffeine 🔊 C-Phen; Kuvan
Calafol 🔊 clove oil
calamine 🔊 Chlo-Amine; gallamine
Cal-C-Caps 🔊 gelcaps
Cal-Cee 🔊 Colace
Calcet 🔊 Glyset
Calcibon 🔊 clozapine
Caldesene 🔊 clodazon
Calphosan 🔊 clofezone
Calphron 🔊 Claforan; Kolephrin
Camila 🔊 COMLA
camphor 🔊 comfrey
Candin 🔊 quinidine
Capex 🔊 Copegus
caplet 🔊 cobalt
Capsin 🔊 Cubicin
capuride 🔊 Key-Pred
Carac 🔊 Coreg; Kuric
Carafate 🔊 Geravite
caramel 🔊 Gerimal
caraway oil 🔊 coral; Kerol
carazolol 🔊 Kerasal AL
carfimate 🔊 crufomate
Carmol 🔊 Gerimal
CarraFoam 🔊 Kerafoam
Carrasyn 🔊 chrysin; garcinia
carticaine 🔊 Corticaine
carumonam 🔊 germanium
CAST 🔊 Cocet
cathine 🔊 Kao-Tin; K-Tan
cathinone 🔊 cotinine
Cayston 🔊 guaisteine
Ceclor 🔊 Sochlor; Zyclara
Cedax 🔊 ciadox; Cidex; Sudex; Z-Dex
cefixime 🔊 Zyvoxam
ceforanide 🔊 Zofran ODT
cefpiramide 🔊 sevopramide
Celestone 🔊 sulisatin
Celexa 🔊 Cylex; Salex; Xolox
Cena-K 🔊 senega; zinc
Center-Al 🔊 zinterol
Ceprotin 🔊 sparteine
Cerebyx 🔊 Surbex
Cerisa 🔊 Xerese

Ceron 🔊 Sereine
cetaben 🔊 zotepine
Cetacort 🔊 S-T Cort
Cetafen; Cetafen Extra 🔊 Cytovene
cetiedil 🔊 Stadol
cetrimide 🔊 sweet wormwood
Cevi-Bid 🔊 Cefobid
Chlo-Amine 🔊 calamine; gallamine
chloramphenicol 🔊 cloramfenicol
chloramphenicol palmitate 🔊 cloramfenicol pantotenate
chloramphenicol sodium succinate 🔊
   cloramfenicol
chlorine 🔊 Klaron
chloroquine 🔊 Klor-Con
Chronosule 🔊 Granisol
ciadox 🔊 Cedax; Cidex; Sudex; Z-Dex
Cialis 🔊 Salese; Silace; xylose
ciamexon 🔊 Sumaxin
cicliomenol 🔊 cyclomenol
cideferron 🔊 Pseudofrin
Cidex 🔊 Cedax; ciadox; Sudex; Z-Dex
cilostamide 🔊 salacetamide
cimaterol 🔊 Symmetrel; xamoterol
cioteronel 🔊 citronella; soterenol;
   SteriNail
Cipro I.V. 🔊 Spiriva
ciprofloxacin 🔊 sparfloxacin
Ciprofloxacin 🔊 sparfloxacin
Citralax 🔊 Starlix
citric acid 🔊 stearic acid
Claforan 🔊 Calphron; Kolephrin
Claravis 🔊 Klorvess
Claris 🔊 Clerz
clazuril 🔊 Clozaril; glycerol
clemastine 🔊 galamustine
Clenia 🔊 Calan; Gilenya; kaolin;
   khellin
Cleocin 🔊 Quelicin
clodazon 🔊 Caldesene
clofezone 🔊 Calphosan
clomocycline 🔊 colimecycline
cloprothiazole 🔊 glyprothiazol
cloramfenicol pantotenate complex 🔊
   chloramphenicol palmitate
clostebol 🔊 colestipol
clove oil 🔊 Calafol
clozapine 🔊 Calcibon
Clozaril 🔊 clazuril; glycerol
coal tar 🔊 Caltro; Kaletra

Coartem ▯ Cort-Dome
cobalt ▯ caplet
Cocet ▯ CAST
codeine ▯ Kadian; Quad Tann
Cognex ▯ Kionex
Colace ▯ Cal-Cee
Colazal ▯ Gelseal
colestipol ▯ clostebol
colimecycline ▯ clomocycline
colistin ▯ glycitein
collagen ▯ Glyquin; Qualaquin
colterol ▯ glutaral
CoLyte ▯ Klout; K-Lyte
Copegus ▯ Capex
copper ▯ Keppra
Coreg ▯ Carac; Kuric
Corque ▯ Carac; Kuric
Cort-Dome ▯ Coartem
Corzall ▯ cresol; Cryselle; Kerasal
Cotab ▯ CTAB; K-Tab; Q-Tapp
C-Phen ▯ caffeine; Kuvan
C-Phen DM ▯ G Phen DM; Guaifen DM
cresol ▯ Corzall; Cryselle; Kerasal
crufomate ▯ carfimate
Cryselle ▯ Corzall; cresol; Kerasal
CTAB ▯ Cotab; K-Tab; Q-Tapp
Cubicin ▯ Capsin; quipazine
Cyanokit ▯ Senokot
Cyclessa ▯ Sequels
cyclizine ▯ seclazone
cyclomenol ▯ cicliomenol
Cylex ▯ Celexa; Salex; Xolox
Cymbalta ▯ Simplet
cyromazine ▯ Seromycin
cystine ▯ Sustain; Systane
Cytovene ▯ Cetafen
Cytra ▯ Scytera; Zetar
dacemazine ▯ duazomycin
Daily-Vite ▯ Dialyvite
Dairy Ease ▯ Dry Eyes; DUROS
Dayhist ▯ Duohist
Daypro ▯ Dopar
DDAVP ▯ DVP
decil ▯ Dicel
Deconsal ▯ doconazole
Delazinc ▯ Dalacin C
Denaze ▯ Doan's
Depacon ▯ dibucaine
Depakene ▯ dibucaine

deprodone ▯ diperodon
deprostil ▯ dipyrocetyl
Derifil ▯ Duraflu
Dermolin ▯ Dramilin
desipramine ▯ diisopromine
Desogen ▯ Diascan
Despec ▯ Dosepak
Dexodryl ▯ dioxadrol
Dex-Tuss DM ▯ docusate sodium
DHC Plus ▯ DOK-Plus
D-Hist ▯ Dosette; Duocet
Dialyvite ▯ Daily-Vite
Diamox ▯ DMax
dibucaine ▯ Depacon
Dicel ▯ decil
diethazine ▯ Detussin
Difil-G ▯ Duphalac
Di-Gel ▯ Dical
diisopromine ▯ desipramine
dimethazan ▯ duometacin
dinsed ▯ Donna-Sed
diolamine ▯ Dalmane; Dilomine
diotyrosine ▯ dotarizine
Diovan ▯ D-Phen
dioxadrol ▯ Dexodryl
diperodon ▯ deprodone
dipyrocetyl ▯ deprostil
dipyrone ▯ duoperone
Diskus ▯ Dacex; Desoxi
dithranol ▯ deterenol
Diuril ▯ Doral
Doan's ▯ Denaze
doconazole ▯ Deconsal
docusate sodium ▯ Dex-Tuss DM
DOK-Plus ▯ DHC Plus
Dolacet ▯ Dulcet
Donna-Sed ▯ dinsed
Doral ▯ Diuril
Doryx ▯ Droxia
Dosepak ▯ Despec
Dosette ▯ Duocet
dotarizine ▯ diotyrosine
D-Phen ▯ Diovan
Dramilin ▯ Dermolin
DroTuss ▯ Duratuss
Droxia ▯ Doryx
Dry Eyes ▯ Dairy Ease; DUROS
Drysol ▯ Durasal
Drytex ▯ diuretics
D-Tann AT ▯ Dinate; Duonate

Duac CS ▣ Degas
duazomycin ▣ dacemazine
Dulcet ▣ Dolacet
Duocet ▣ Dosette
Duohist ▣ Dayhist
duoperone ▣ dipyrone
Duraflu ▣ Derifil
DuraGen ▣ Diurigen
Duratuss ▣ DroTuss
Durezol ▣ Drysol
DUROS ▣ Dairy Ease; Dry Eyes
Dytan ▣ Detane
Ear-Dry ▣ Auro-Dri
Ear-Gesic ▣ Urogesic
Easprin ▣ aceperone; azaperone;
  esuprone
ebastine ▣ epostane
ebselen ▣ epicillin
Ed-Spaz ▣ Ed Spaz
Edex ▣ ADEKs; Adoxa; Iodex
elanzepine ▣ olanzapine
Elestat ▣ AlaSTAT
Elestrin ▣ alosetron
Elevess ▣ Eliphos; Ulefsa
Eligard ▣ Allegra
Elimite ▣ Alimta
Eliphos ▣ Elevess; Ulefsa
Elocon ▣ Ala-Quin; Alcaine; Alo-
  quin; elucaine
elucaine ▣ Ala-Quin; Alcaine; Alo-
  quin; Elocon
embramine ▣ ampyrimine; imipramine
Emend ▣ Immun-Aid
emetine ▣ iometin
Emetrol ▣ amiterol
emitefur ▣ amitivir
EMLA ▣ Emollia; emu oil
Emollia ▣ EMLA; emu oil
emonapride ▣ Omnipred
Emoquette ▣ Umecta
Empirin ▣ amiperone
EndaRoid ▣ Android; Inderide
Enduret ▣ woundwort
Enfalyte ▣ Infalyte
Enisyl ▣ anise oil; Anusol; Enseal;
  Unisol
Enlive! ▣ One-Alpha
Enlon ▣ inulin
enocitabine ▣ ancitabine

Enseal ▣ anise oil; Anusol; Enisyl;
  Unisol
Entsol ▣ Antizol
Enzone ▣ Anacin; inosine; Unasyn
Eovist ▣ Evista
eperisone ▣ euprocin
Epi-C ▣ APC; Apo-K; EPOCH
epicillin ▣ ebselen
epiestriol ▣ Abstral
epioestriol ▣ Abstral
Epitol ▣ Apetil
Epogen ▣ Apokyn; Opcon-A
epostane ▣ ebastine
Equilet ▣ Accolate
Equipoise ▣ Aquabase
erbium ▣ europium
Ercaf ▣ Airacof
erizepine ▣ AeroSpan
E-R-O Ear Drops ▣ Auro Ear Drops
Errin ▣ iron
Eryc ▣ ara-G; ARC
Erygel ▣ Orajel
EryPed ▣ AeroBid
esilate ▣ Isolyte
Estra-L ▣ Ezetrol
Estring ▣ Oestring
estriol ▣ Ezetrol
esuprone ▣ aceperone; aspirin; azaperone; Easprin
esylate ▣ Isolyte E
etafenone ▣ etifenin
etasuline ▣ etozolin
etazepine ▣ atosiban
ethisterone ▣ itasetron
Ethrane ▣ ATryn
ethylene ▣ Atolone
etifenin ▣ etafenone
etofuradine ▣ atevirdine
etorphine ▣ Etrafon; Otrivin
etozolin ▣ etasuline
Etrafon ▣ etorphine; Otrivin
Euflexxa ▣ Avelox; I-Valex
euprocin ▣ eperisone
Eurax ▣ Urex
europium ▣ erbium
Evista ▣ Eovist
E-Vitamin ▣ iofetamine
Evoclin ▣ ivoqualine
Exact ▣ Oxecta
Exelon ▣ ioxilan

Eye-Lube-A ▯ Albay
Factive ▯ Viactiv
farnesil ▯ Fer-In-Sol
felypressin ▯ fluprazine
fenamole ▯ Venomil
fendosal ▯ Vandazole
fenethazine ▯ phenothiazine
fenethylline ▯ phenythilone; Ventolin
fenetylline ▯ Ventolin
fenharmane ▯ pheniramine
fenimide ▯ Vanamide
fenoterol ▯ Phentrol
fenquizone ▯ Vancocin
fenthion ▯ phenytoin
Feosol ▯ PhosLo; VaZol; VSL
Ferretts ▯ Fortaz
Filmseal ▯ flumizole
Finac ▯ FNC
Flagyl ▯ Ful-Glo
Flarex ▯ Fluarix
flazalone ▯ flusalan
Flexon ▯ Floxin; fluquazone
Flo-Pack ▯ Folbic
Florone ▯ fluorine; valerian
floverine ▯ Fluvirin
Floxin ▯ Flexon; fluquazone
fluacizine ▯ volazocine
Fluarix ▯ Flarex
fluconazole ▯ valconazole
flumizole ▯ Filmseal
fluorine ▯ Florone
fluprazine ▯ felypressin
fluquazone ▯ Flexon; Floxin
Flurox ▯ Flarex
flusalan ▯ flazalone
Fluvirin ▯ floverine
Folbic ▯ Flo-Pack
Folotyn ▯ Veltin
Folpace ▯ Phillips'
Foltrin ▯ Voltaren
Foltx ▯ Flutex
Folvite ▯ Velivet
fomocaine ▯ Foamicon
Forane ▯ 4-N-1
Fortaz ▯ Ferretts
fosfosal ▯ Phosphasal
4-N-1 ▯ Forane
FreAmine ▯ furomine
Freezone ▯ Furacin
fungimycin ▯ vancomycin

Fungi-Nail ▯ vincanol
fuprazole ▯ Vaprisol
furomine ▯ FreAmine
Fuzeon ▯ Visine; Vusion
Gabitril ▯ Capitrol
galamustine ▯ clemastine
gallamine ▯ calamine; Chlo-Amine
gallic acid ▯ Gly-Oxide
gallium ▯ Kolyum
galosemide ▯ Calcium
Galzin ▯ glycine
Gas-Ban ▯ Kao-Spen
GaviLAX ▯ Keflex
Gelseal ▯ Colazal
Gelusil ▯ Colazal
Genac ▯ Gonak; Kank-a
Genaphed ▯ Confide
Genasal ▯ Goniosol; Gynazole; Konsyl
Genasoft ▯ Goniosoft
Gentex ▯ Cognitex
Gentran ▯ Contrin
Geodon ▯ codeine; Kadian; Quad Tann
gepirone ▯ Gabarone
Geridium ▯ Karidium
Gerimal ▯ caramel
Geri-Vite ▯ Carafate
germanium ▯ carumonam
GFN/DM ▯ C-Phen DM; G Phen
  DM; Guaifen DM
Gianvi ▯ Januvia
Gilenya ▯ Calan; Clenia; Jalyn; kao-
  lin; khellin
giparmen ▯ Cuprimine
gitalin ▯ guaietolin
Gleevec ▯ Glivec
glucalox ▯ GlycoLax
Glucerna ▯ glycerin
glucose ▯ Caelyx
glutaral ▯ colterol
Glutarex ▯ Klotrix
Glutose ▯ Giltuss
glycerin ▯ Glucerna
glycerol ▯ clazuril; Clozaril
glycine ▯ Cleocin; Galzin
GlycoLax ▯ glucalox
Gly-Oxide ▯ gallic acid
glyprothiazol ▯ cloprothiazole
Glyset ▯ Calcet
Gonak ▯ Kank-a
Goniosol ▯ Gynazole; Konsyl

Granisol ⃞ Chronosule
guaiacol ⃞ guggul
Guaifed ⃞ CVD
Guaifen DM ⃞ C-Phen DM; G Phen DM
guaimesal ⃞ Kemsol
guaisteine ⃞ Cayston
guanisoquine ⃞ quinisocaine
guar gum ⃞ karaya gum
Gynazole ⃞ Genasal; Goniosol; Konsyl
Gy-Pak ⃞ K-Pek
heliox ⃞ Hyalex
Hemopad ⃞ Humibid
Hiberix ⃞ Hiprex
Hiprex ⃞ Hiberix
homatropine ⃞ HumatroPen
Humalog ⃞ hemlock
Humatin ⃞ Hemotene
HumatroPen ⃞ homatropine
Humibid ⃞ Hemopad
Humibid E ⃞ Hemopad
Hyalex ⃞ heliox
Hyophen ⃞ Hy-Phen
Ibudone ⃞ Iopidine
Icar ⃞ agar; Wee Care
icospiramide ⃞ oxiperomide
Igel ⃞ OCL
imafen ⃞ Imovane
Imdur ⃞ imidurea
imidoline ⃞ amedalin; omidoline
imidurea ⃞ Imdur
imipramine ⃞ ampyrimine; embramine
Immun-Aid ⃞ Emend
Inderal ⃞ Anadrol
Infalyte ⃞ Enfalyte
INFeD ⃞ Unifed
inosine ⃞ Anacin; Enzone; Unasyn
inositol ⃞ anisatil
Intergel ⃞ Antrocol
inulin ⃞ Enlon
Iodex ⃞ ADEKs; Adoxa; Edex
iofetamine ⃞ E-Vitamin
iometin ⃞ emetine
Iophen ⃞ Aviane
iopydone ⃞ Ibudone
Iosal ⃞ Ocella; Wyseal
Iosat ⃞ Aceta; ICE-T
iotrolan ⃞ Atralin
ioxilan ⃞ Exelon
IPOL ⃞ apple

Ircon ⃞ AeroCaine; argon
Iressa ⃞ Aerius; Ear-Eze; Oracea; OROS; Urso
iron ⃞ Errin
Irrigate ⃞ ergot
isobutane ⃞ azapetine
Isocal ⃞ Asacol; Os-Cal
isoconazole ⃞ azaconazole
Isolyte ⃞ esilate; esylate
Isomil ⃞ Esimil
Isopan ⃞ azabon
isoprazone ⃞ azaprocin
Isovorin ⃞ acifran
I-Valex ⃞ Avelox; Euflex
ivoqualine ⃞ Evoclin
Ixiaro ⃞ OxyIR
Jalyn ⃞ Alinia; aloin; ellaOne
Januvia ⃞ Gianvi
Jay-Phyl ⃞ Avail
Jets ⃞ A/T/S; oats
Jevity ⃞ Avita
Jinteli ⃞ Intal
Jolessa ⃞ Alesse
J-Tan ⃞ Attain
Junel Fe ⃞
Just Tears ⃞ Estrace
Kadian ⃞ codeine; Quad Tann
Kaletra ⃞ Caltro; coal tar
Kao-Spen ⃞ Gas-Ban
Kao-Tin ⃞ K-Tan
Karidium ⃞ Geridium
kasal ⃞ Kay Ciel; KCl
Keflex ⃞ GaviLAX
Keppra ⃞ copper
Kerafoam ⃞ CarraFoam
Keralac ⃞ garlic
Kerasal ⃞ Corzall; cresol; Cryselle
Kerasal AL ⃞ carazolol
Kerodex ⃞ cardiacs; Kredex
Kerol ⃞ caraway oil; coral
ketocaine ⃞ quatacaine
khellin ⃞ Calan; Clenia; Gilenya; kaolin
khelloside ⃞ Colazide
Kionex ⃞ Cognex
Klaron ⃞ chlorine
Klor-Con ⃞ chloroquine
Klorvess ⃞ Claravis
Klotrix ⃞ Glutarex
Klout ⃞ CoLyte; K-Lyte

K-Lyte 🔊 CoLyte; Klout
Kof-Eze 🔊 Coughtuss
Konsyl 🔊 Goniosol; Gynazole
K-Pek 🔊 Gy-Pak
K-Tab 🔊 Cotab; CTAB; Q-Tapp
Kuvan 🔊 caffeine; C-Phen
Lac-Dose 🔊 Liqui-Doss
Lagesic 🔊 Luxiq
Lanacane 🔊 lignocaine
Lanacort 🔊 lungwort
Lanoxin 🔊 Lincocin
Latisse 🔊 lettuce
Lessina 🔊 leucine; lysine
Letairis 🔊 LTRAs
leucine 🔊 Lessina; lysine
Levall 🔊 Livalo
levamisole 🔊 lofemizole
levamisole HCl 🔊 lofemizole HCl
Levolet 🔊 Lypholyte
liarozole 🔊 Lioresal
Librax 🔊 Loprox
Librium 🔊 Lipram
lignocaine 🔊 Lanacane
Lincocin 🔊 Lanoxin
Lioresal 🔊 liarozole
Lipram 🔊 Librium
Liqui-Doss 🔊 Lac-Dose
Listerine 🔊 Loestrin
litracen 🔊 Lotrisone
Livalo 🔊 Levall
Locoid 🔊 Liquadd
Loestrin 🔊 Listerine
lofemizole 🔊 levamisole
lofemizole HCl 🔊 levamisole HCl
Loprox 🔊 Librax
Lotrisone 🔊 litracen
Lubrin 🔊 Lupron
Lufyllin 🔊 Levlen
Lypholyte 🔊 Levlite
Macugen 🔊 Mycogen
mafilcon A 🔊 mefloquine
Magan 🔊 Makena
Magnacal 🔊 Monocal
Magnacet 🔊 Menest
Magnox 🔊 Minox
Mag-SR 🔊 Maxair
Makena 🔊 Magan
Malarone 🔊 Myleran
malathion 🔊 Miltown
malotilate 🔊 Multilyte

mannitol 🔊 Mynatal
Maox 🔊 Megace; M-oxy
Māpap 🔊 MOBP
Marezine 🔊 morazone
Marinol 🔊 Moranyl
Mavik 🔊 MVAC
Maxair 🔊 Mag-SR
Maxidone 🔊 mixidine
meclocycline 🔊 meglucycline
meclozine 🔊 Miacalcin
Medrol 🔊 Mydral
mefloquine 🔊 mafilcon
Megace 🔊 Maox
megestrol 🔊 Maxitrol
meglucycline 🔊 meclocycline
meglutol 🔊 miglitol
menadione 🔊 Minidyne
Menest 🔊 Magnacet
Mentax 🔊 Metanx; Mintox
menthol 🔊 mannitol; Mynatal
Meprozine 🔊 mupirocin
mequinol 🔊 Micanol; Myconel
Mersol 🔊 Murocel
mesalamine 🔊 mezilamine; muzolimine
Metanx 🔊 Mentax
metetoin 🔊 mitotane
methazolamide 🔊 mitozolomide
methetoin 🔊 mitotane
mezilamine 🔊 mesalamine; muzolimine
Miacalcin 🔊 meclozine
Midrin 🔊 Mudrane
miglitol 🔊 meglutol
Migrazone 🔊 Myochrysine
minaprine 🔊 Magnaprin
Minidyne 🔊 menadione
Mintox 🔊 Mentax
Mirena 🔊 Murine
mitotane 🔊 metetoin
mixidine 🔊 Maxidone
Mobic 🔊 MBC
Modicon 🔊 Medicone
Monocal 🔊 Magnacal
monteplase 🔊 Mynate Plus
morazone 🔊 Marezine
morphine 🔊 myrophine
M-oxy 🔊 Maox
MSIR 🔊 mouse ear
Multilyte 🔊 malotilate
mupirocin 🔊 Meprozine
Murine 🔊 Mirena

Murocel ▢ Mersol
muzolimine ▢ mesalamine; mezilamine
Mycogen ▢ Macugen
Myconel ▢ mequinol; Micanol
Mydral ▢ Medrol
Myleran ▢ Malarone
Myochrysine ▢ Migrazone
Myolin ▢ mullein
Myozyme ▢ MSM; MZM
myrophine ▢ morphine
nafcillin ▢ naphazoline
nafomine ▢ Novamine
naloxone ▢ Nyloxin
naphazoline ▢ nafcillin
Naphcon ▢ nefocon; Novocain
Naprosyn ▢ niaprazine
naproxen ▢ nibroxane
naranol ▢ Norinyl
NāSal ▢ Neosol
Nasotuss ▢ NiaStase
Natazia ▢ NeoTuss
Naturalyte ▢ Nutrilyte
Naturvus ▢ Neutra-Phos
nefocon ▢ Naphcon; Novocain
Neocate ▢ nicotine
Neo-fradin ▢ nifuradene
Neofrin ▢ Nephron
neomycin ▢ nimazone; Numoisyn
Neoral ▢ Norel
Neosalus ▢ Neusalus
Neosol ▢ NāSal
NeoTuss ▢ Natazia
Nephrox ▢ Niferex
nequinate ▢ Nu-knit
Nesacaine ▢ New-Skin
Neulasta ▢ Nulecit
Neusalus ▢ Neosalus
Neutra-Caine ▢ Nutricon
NeutraSal ▢ Nutr-E-Sol
Neutrogena Moisture ▢ nitrogen mustard
New-Skin ▢ Nesacaine
niaprazine ▢ Naprosyn
Niaspan ▢ NuSpin
nibroxane ▢ naproxen
Nicorette ▢ NuCort
nicotine ▢ Neocate One
Niferex ▢ Nephrox
nifuradene ▢ Neo-fradin
nimazone ▢ neomycin; Numoisyn

niometacin ▢ Pneumotussin
nitrogen ▢ Neutra-Caine; Nutricon
nitrogen mustard ▢ Neutrogena Moisture
Nitrolan ▢ Nutrilan
nivazol ▢ Novasal
Nizoral ▢ Nasarel
NoHist ▢ Nuhist
Norinyl ▢ naranol
Novamine ▢ nafomine
Novocain ▢ Naphcon; nefocon
NuCort ▢ Nicorette
Nu-knit ▢ nequinate
Nulecit ▢ Neulasta
Numoisyn ▢ neomycin; nimazone
NuOx ▢ Nix
NuSpin ▢ Niaspan
Nu-Tears ▢ Neotrace
Nutr-E-Sol ▢ NeutraSal
Nutrilan ▢ Nitrolan
Nutrilyte ▢ Naturalyte
Nytol ▢ nettle
Ocean ▢ Aceon; Aczone
Ocella ▢ Iosal
ocrase ▢ Eucrease
octazamide ▢ actisomide
Ocudox ▢ AquADEKs
Ocufen ▢ Aquavan
Ocuvite ▢ Aquavit
Ogestrel ▢ Oxytrol
olanzapine ▢ elanzepine
Olux ▢ Aloxi; I-L-X
omidoline ▢ amedalin; imidoline
Omnipred ▢ emonapride
One Touch ▢ Ontak
Ontak ▢ One Touch
Opcon ▢ Apokyn
Opti-gen ▢ Apetigen; aptocaine
Optigene ▢ Apetigen; aptocaine
Oracea ▢ Aerius; Ear-Eze; Iressa; OROS; Urso
Orajel ▢ Erygel
Oralet ▢ Aurolate
Orasept ▢ Aricept
Orasol ▢ Eryzole; uracil
OraSure ▢ Arzerra
OraVerse ▢ Aerofreeze
Orazinc ▢ arsenic
Orencia ▢ Orinase
Orinase ▢ errhines; Orencia

ornithine 🔊 aranotin
OROS 🔊 Aerius; Ear-Eze; Iressa; Oracea; Urso
Orsythia 🔊 Oracit
osalmid 🔊 iosulamide
Os-Cal 🔊 Asacol; Isocal
Oticin 🔊 Otozin
Otozin 🔊 Oticin
Otrivin 🔊 etorphine; Etrafon
Ovide 🔊 Ovoid
Ovoid 🔊 Ovide
oxazorone 🔊 oxisuran
Oxecta 🔊 Exact
oxethazaine 🔊 oxytocin
oxiperomide 🔊 icospiramide
oxisuran 🔊 oxazorone
Oxycel 🔊 Oxizole
OxyIR 🔊 Ixiaro
ozagrel 🔊 Ascor L
pafenolol 🔊 befunolol
Paladin 🔊 belladonna; Polydine
Panafil 🔊 PenFill
Panokase 🔊 Pain-X; Pin-X
Paracaine 🔊 procaine; pyrrocaine
paraffin 🔊 Preven; Privine
Parafon Forte 🔊 Profen Forte
paramethasone 🔊 perimetazine; promethazine
parbendazole 🔊 propenidazole
parconazole 🔊 pirquinozol
Paremyd 🔊 PerioMed; ProMod
pargolol 🔊 pyrogallol
paridocaine 🔊 piridocaine
Parnate 🔊 burnet
parvaquone 🔊 porofocon
Patanol 🔊 Botanol
paulomycin 🔊 peliomycin
Paxil 🔊 piquizil
pecazine 🔊 Bicozene
pecilocin 🔊 bizelesin
peliomycin 🔊 bleomycin
Penecare 🔊 Benicar
Penecort 🔊 Bencort
PenFill 🔊 Panafil
pentaquine 🔊 Pontocaine
perastine 🔊 prazitone; Prosteon
Percocet 🔊 Pyrroxate
Perdiem 🔊 Prodium
perhexiline 🔊 pyroxylin
Periguard 🔊 Procardia

PerioMed 🔊 Paremyd; ProMod
Periostat 🔊 Pro-Stat
Perlane 🔊 Prelone; proline
Perloxx 🔊 Pyrlex
Permapen 🔊 prampine
phanquone 🔊 phenacaine
phenacaine 🔊 phanquone
pheniramine 🔊 fenharmane
phenobarbital 🔊 vinbarbital
phenobarbital sodium 🔊 vinbarbital sodium
phenobarbitone 🔊 vinbarbitone
phenol 🔊 fennel
phenothiazine 🔊 fenethazine
Phentrol 🔊 fenoterol
phenythilone 🔊 fenethylline
Phillips' 🔊 Folpace
PhosLo 🔊 Feosol; VaZol
Phosphasal 🔊 fosfosal
piberaline 🔊 piperylone
pifexole 🔊 pivoxil
pimefylline 🔊 bamifylline
pinadoline 🔊 binedaline
pinoxepin 🔊 benaxibine
Pin-X 🔊 Pain-X
piperylone 🔊 piberaline
piquizil 🔊 Paxil
pirenzepine 🔊 Principen
piribedil 🔊 Prepidil
piridocaine 🔊 paridocaine
pirolate 🔊 Prialt
piroximone 🔊 pyroxamine
pirquinozol 🔊 parconazole
pivoxil 🔊 pifexole
platinum 🔊 plutonium
plutonium 🔊 platinum
Polocaine 🔊 Bellacane
Polydine 🔊 Paladin
ponfibrate 🔊 binifibrate
porofocon A 🔊 parvaquone
PR Natal 🔊 Prenatal; pyrantel
pramocaine 🔊 primaquine
Pramosone 🔊 primycin; promazine
prampine 🔊 Permapen
prazepine 🔊 prozapine
Prefill 🔊 Bravelle
Pregnyl 🔊 proguanil
Prelone 🔊 Perlane; proline
Prelu 🔊 Paral; perilla; Prolia
Premarin 🔊 Primorine

premazepam ⅀ bromazepam
Prenatal ⅀ PR Natal; pyrantel
Prenatal Plus ⅀ Par-Natal Plus
Pre-Pen ⅀ propane
Prepidil ⅀ piribedil
Pretz ⅀ protease
Prialt ⅀ pirolate
pridefine ⅀ proadifen
prifelone ⅀ Prophyllin
primaquine ⅀ pramocaine
primycin ⅀ Pramosone; promazine; puromycin
Principen ⅀ pirenzepine
Privigen ⅀ Brevicon
Privine ⅀ paraffin; Preven; Profen
proadifen ⅀ pridefine
procaine ⅀ Paracaine; Puregon; pyrro-caine
procaine HCl ⅀ pyrrocaine HCl
Procardia ⅀ Periguard
Pro-Clear ⅀ PruClair
Prodium ⅀ Perdiem
Prolia ⅀ Paral; perilla; Prelu
proline ⅀ Perlane; Prelone
promazine ⅀ bromazine; Pramosone; primycin
promethazine ⅀ paramethasone; perimetazine
propane ⅀ Pre-Pen
propenidazole ⅀ parbendazole
Prophyllin ⅀ prifelone
Pro-Stat ⅀ Periostat
Prostin ⅀ perastine; prazitone
Provigil ⅀ Pravachol
prozapine ⅀ prazepine
PruClair ⅀ Pro-Clear
Prudoxin ⅀ pyridoxine
psilocin ⅀ Salacyn; Selsun; xylazine
psilocybin ⅀ Soluspan
psilocybine ⅀ Soluspan
psyllium husk ⅀ Sulmasque
Purinethol ⅀ PR Natal; Prenatal; pyrantel
puromycin ⅀ primycin
pyrantel ⅀ PR Natal; Prenatal
Pyridium ⅀ Baridium; Perdiem; Prodium
pyridoxine ⅀ Prudoxin
pyrogallol ⅀ pargolol
pyroxamine ⅀ piroximone

pyroxylin ⅀ perhexiline
pyrrocaine ⅀ Paracaine; procaine
pyrrocaine HCl ⅀ procaine HCl
Pyrroxate ⅀ Percocet
Q-Pap ⅀ cubeb
Q-Tapp ⅀ Cotab; CTAB; K-Tab
quatacaine ⅀ ketocaine
Quelicin ⅀ Cleocin
quinisocaine ⅀ guanisoquine
quipazine ⅀ Cubicin
radium ⅀ rhodium
Ralix ⅀ RuLox
Ranexa ⅀ Renax
Refludan ⅀ rofelodine
Rēgain ⅀ Rogaine
RenAmin ⅀ Ranamine
Renax ⅀ Ranexa
Repan ⅀ Riopan
Repetab ⅀ Ribatab; Robitab
Rescon ⅀ risocaine
Resol ⅀ rose oil
Re-Tann ⅀ R-Tanna; rutin; Ry-Tann
Retin-A ⅀ R-Tanna; rutin; Ry-Tann
R-Gen ⅀ Rēgain; Rogaine
R-Gene ⅀ Rēgain; Rogaine
Rhinall ⅀ ronnel
rhodium ⅀ radium
Rid-A-Pain ⅀ riodipine
Rimso ⅀ RMS
riodipine ⅀ Rid-A-Pain
Riopan ⅀ Repan
risocaine ⅀ Rescon
Robitab ⅀ Repetab; Ribatab
rofelodine ⅀ Refludan
Rogaine ⅀ Rēgain
ronnel ⅀ Rhinall
rose oil ⅀ Resol
Rosula ⅀ Resol
R-Tanna ⅀ Re-Tann; rutin; Ry-Tann
RuLox ⅀ Ralix
rutin ⅀ Re-Tann; R-Tanna; Ry-Tann
Ryna-X ⅀ Ranexa; Renax
Ry-Tann ⅀ Re-Tann; R-Tanna; rutin
Saizen ⅀ Susano; Zosyn
salacetamide ⅀ cilostamide
Salacyn ⅀ psilocin; Selsun; xylazine
Salagen ⅀ silicon; Solaquin; Xylocaine
salantel ⅀ zilantel
Salese ⅀ Cialis; Silace; xylose
Salex ⅀ Celexa; Cylex; Xolox

Salflex ⊡ Sulfolax
salicin ⊡ psilocin; Selsun
Salkera ⊡ Xalkori
Sal-Tropine ⊡ sulotroban
Sani-Pak ⊡ Cinobac
Saphris ⊡ sfRowasa
Scytera ⊡ Cytra; Zetar
Sea-Omega ⊡ Zomig
seclazone ⊡ cyclizine
Secule ⊡ squill
Selenos ⊡ "cillins"
Selsun ⊡ psilocin; Salacyn
Senna-Gen ⊡ Sinequan; Zincon
Senna-S ⊡ Zencia
Senokot ⊡ Cyanokit
Sequels ⊡ Cyclessa
Sereine ⊡ Ceron
serine ⊡ Ceron
Seromycin ⊡ cyromazine
Serutan ⊡ Soriatane
sevopramide ⊡ cefpiramide
sfericase ⊡ Zephrex; Zovirax
sfRowasa ⊡ Saphris
shellac ⊡ Cholac
siccanin ⊡ zocainone
Silace ⊡ Cialis; Salese; xylose
silafilcon A ⊡ xylofilcon A
silicon ⊡ silicone; Solaquin; Xylocaine
silicone ⊡ silicon; Solaquin; Xylocaine
Simuc ⊡ sumach; Zomig
Sina-X ⊡ Xanax
Sinequan ⊡ Zincon
sintropium bromide ⊡ xenytropium
   bromide
Sinuhist ⊡ Sonahist
Sitrex ⊡ storax
Sochlor ⊡ Ceclor; Zyclara
Sof-lax ⊡ ZFlex
Solaquin ⊡ silicon; Xylocaine
Soluspan ⊡ psilocybin
Sonahist ⊡ Sinuhist
Soriatane ⊡ Serutan
soterenol ⊡ cioteronel; citronella;
   SteriNail
Soyalac ⊡ SalAc
sparfloxacin ⊡ ciprofloxacin
spirazine ⊡ Sprayzoin
Sprayzoin ⊡ spirazine
Sprix ⊡ Suprax; Zyprexa
S-T Cort ⊡ Cetacort

Starlix ⊡ Citralax
Staxyn ⊡ Cytoxan
stearic acid ⊡ citric acid
subathizone ⊡ sopitazine
sucrose ⊡ Xigris
Sular ⊡ celery; Xolair
sulazepam ⊡ zolazepam
sulfalene ⊡ Slo-phyllin
Sulfolax ⊡ Salflex
sulisatin ⊡ Celestone
Sulmasque ⊡ psyllium husk
sulotroban ⊡ Sal-Tropine
Sulpho-Lac ⊡ Salofalk
Sumaxin ⊡ ciamexon
Supprette ⊡ soapwort
Suprane ⊡ Syprine
Suprax ⊡ Sprix; Zyprexa
Suprep ⊡ X-Prep
Surbex ⊡ Cerebyx
Surgel ⊡ Seroquel
Surpass ⊡ Ser-Ap-Es
Sustagen ⊡ Cystagon
Sustain ⊡ cystine; Systane
Symmetrel ⊡ cimaterol
Synagis ⊡ Xanax
Syprine ⊡ Suprane
Systane ⊡ cystine; Sustain
TachoSil ⊡ Taxol; Tygacil
Tannic S ⊡ TNKase; tonics
Tarka ⊡ Tri-K
Tarlene ⊡ triolein
tauromustine ⊡ trimustine
Tazidime ⊡ Tusso-DM
Tearisol ⊡ Terazol
Tears Again ⊡ triaziquone
tebuquine ⊡ Topicaine
tefazoline ⊡ tofisoline
teprenone ⊡ tiopronin
Tera-Gel ⊡ Trocal
Terazol ⊡ Tearisol
terguride ⊡ TearGard
terizidone ⊡ trazodone
Terocin ⊡ Trisan; tyrosine
teroxalene ⊡ trixolane
Terrell ⊡ Touro LA
Tessalon ⊡ tiosalan
T-Gen ⊡ Tigan
thallium ⊡ thulium
thebacon ⊡ tebuquine; Topicaine
thenalidine ⊡ tenylidone

Theochron ⊘ tacrine
TheraDerm ⊘ Triderm
Thermazene ⊘ Trimo-San
thiamiprine ⊘ timiperone
thiamylal ⊘ timolol
thiosalan ⊘ Tessalon
thiouracil ⊘ Tearisol
thiram ⊘ thorium; Triam
thorium ⊘ thiram; Triam
Thrive ⊘ Theravee
thulium ⊘ thallium
Thyrogen ⊘ tarragon; Torecan; Treagan; Trocaine
thyroid ⊘ Triad
thyroxine ⊘ TriOxin
Tikosyn ⊘ toquizine
tinazoline ⊘ Tensilon; Tonsaline
tiopronin ⊘ teprenone
tiosalan ⊘ Tessalon
tiospirone ⊘ tisopurine
TiSol ⊘ Tussall
tisopurine ⊘ tiospirone
tisoquone ⊘ Tussigon
Tisseal ⊘ Tussall
TL Icon ⊘ tolycaine
TNKase ⊘ tonics
tofisoline ⊘ tefazoline
tolycaine ⊘ TL Icon
Tonsaline ⊘ Tensilon; tinazoline
Topicaine ⊘ tebuquine
toquizine ⊘ Tikosyn
Touro LA ⊘ Terrell
Toviaz ⊘ Tyvaso
Travasol ⊘ Triphasil
trazitiline ⊘ trestolone
trazodone ⊘ terizidone
Treagan ⊘ tarragon; Torecan; Trocaine
trestolone ⊘ trazitiline
Trexall ⊘ Tricosal
Triacet ⊘ Trycet
triaziquone ⊘ Tears Again
Tri-Biozene ⊘ Trobicin
tribuzone ⊘ Trobicin
Tri-Chlor ⊘ Tracleer
Tricosal ⊘ Trexall
Tri-K ⊘ Tarka
Trimo-San ⊘ Terramycin
Trimox ⊘ Tyromex
trimustine ⊘ tauromustine
triolein ⊘ Tarlene

Triphasil ⊘ Travasol
Tri-Vi-Sol ⊘ Travasol
trixolane ⊘ teroxalene
Trocaine ⊘ tarragon; Torecan; Treagan
Tronothane HCl ⊘ trientine HCl
Trugene ⊘ tarragon; Teargen; Torecan; Treagan; Trocaine
Tussall ⊘ TiSol
Tussigon ⊘ tisoquone
Tusso-DM ⊘ Tazidime
Tygacil ⊘ TachoSil; Taxol
tylosin ⊘ Talacen
Tylox ⊘ Taloxa
Tyromex ⊘ Trimox
tyrosine ⊘ Terocin; Trisan
Tyvaso ⊘ Toviaz
Ulefsa ⊘ Elevess; Eliphos
Umecta ⊘ Emoquette
Unasyn ⊘ Anacin; Enzone; inosine
Unifed ⊘ INFeD
Unisol ⊘ anise oil; Anusol; Enisyl; Enseal
Uracid ⊘ Urised
uracil ⊘ Eryzole; Orasol
Urea Nail ⊘ Aranelle
Ureacin ⊘ AeroZoin; Orasone
urethan ⊘ Uritin
urethane ⊘ Uritin
Urex ⊘ Eurax
Urogesic ⊘ Ear-Gesic
Urso ⊘ Oracea; OROS
valconazole ⊘ fluconazole
valofane ⊘ Voluven
Valorin ⊘ Florone
Vanamide ⊘ fenimide
Vanocin ⊘ phenazone
Vanos ⊘ Phenazo
VaZol ⊘ Feosol; PhosLo; VSL
V-Cof ⊘ VCF
Velban ⊘ filipin; fleabane
Velivet ⊘ Folvite
Veltin ⊘ Folotyn
Verelan ⊘ Furalan; Virilon
Viactiv ⊘ Factive
viloxazine ⊘ Flexzan
vinbarbital ⊘ phenobarbital
vinbarbital sodium ⊘ phenobarbital sodium
vinbarbitone ⊘ phenobarbitone
Viogen-C ⊘ Vicon-C

Virasal 🔊 vorozole
Virazole 🔊 FeroSul; vorozole
Virilon 🔊 Verelan
Viroxyn 🔊 Furoxone
Visine 🔊 Vision; Vusion
Vision 🔊 Visine; Vusion
Visken 🔊 Vasocon
volazocine 🔊 fluacizine
Voltaren 🔊 Foltrin
Voluven 🔊 valofane
vorozole 🔊 Virasal
Vusion 🔊 Fuzeon; Visine; Vision
Vytone 🔊 V-Tann
Wallette 🔊 violet; Wilate
Wee Care 🔊 agar; Icar
Wilate 🔊 violet; Wallette
Wyseal 🔊 Feosol; Iosal; VaZol; VSL
Xalatan 🔊 zileuton
Xalkori 🔊 Salkera
xamoterol 🔊 cimaterol; Symmetrel
xanomeline 🔊 xinomiline
xanthiol 🔊 Santyl
Xenical 🔊 sanicle
xenytropium bromide 🔊 sintropium bromide
Xeomin 🔊 Cyomin; Zymine
Xerese 🔊 Cerisa
Xibrom 🔊 ZyPram
Xigris 🔊 sucrose
xinafoate 🔊 SunVite
xinomiline 🔊 xanomeline
XiraTuss 🔊 Sortis
Xodol 🔊 Sudal
Xolair 🔊 Sular
Xolox 🔊 Celexa; Cylex; Salex
xylazine 🔊 psilocin
Xylocaine 🔊 silicon; Solaquin
xylofilcon A 🔊 silafilcon A
xylose 🔊 Cialis; Salese; Silace
Xyzal 🔊 Zazole
Yocon 🔊 Acanya; A.C.N.

zalospirone 🔊 Salazopyrin
Zantac 🔊 Zinotic
Z-Bec 🔊 Z-Pak
Z-Dex 🔊 Cedax; ciadox; Cidex; Sudex
Zegerid 🔊 Sucraid
Zemaira 🔊 Swim-Ear; Zymar
Zencia 🔊 Senna-S
Zerit 🔊 XRT
ZFlex 🔊 Soflax
Z-Gen 🔊 Cecon; Ziagen
Ziagen 🔊 Cecon; Z-Gen
Ziks 🔊 Ziox
zilantel 🔊 salantel
zileuton 🔊 Xalatan
Zinc 🔊 Cena-K; senega
Zincon 🔊 Sinequan
Zinotic; Zinotic ES 🔊 Zantac
zinterol 🔊 Center-Al
Ziox 🔊 Ziks
zocainone 🔊 siccanin
Zoderm 🔊 Zyderm
Zofran 🔊 saffron; Zophren
Zoladex 🔊 Zeldox
zolazepam 🔊 sulazepam
Zomig 🔊 Sea-Omega
Zosyn 🔊 Saizen; Susano
zotepine 🔊 cetaben
Zotex 🔊 Xyotax
Zotex-C 🔊 Xyotax
Zoto-HC 🔊 Zytiga
Zovirax 🔊 sfericase; Zephrex
Z-Pak 🔊 Z-Bec
Z-Tuss AC 🔊 Cytuss HC
Zyclara 🔊 Ceclor; Sochlor
Zyderm 🔊 Zoderm
Zyflo 🔊 Cefol
Zymar 🔊 Swim-Ear; Zemaira
Zymine 🔊 Cyomin; Xeomin
ZyPram 🔊 Xibrom
Zyprexa 🔊 Sprix; Suprax
Zyrtec 🔊 Psoriatec

Abbreviations Used with Medications and Dosages

Abbreviation/Term	Literally	Meaning
a.c.	ante cibum	before meals or food
ad	ad	to, up to
A.D., AD*	auris dextra	right ear
ad lib.	ad libitum	at pleasure
A.L.	auris laeva	left ear
a.m., A.M.	ante meridiem	morning
Aq.	aqua	water
A.S., AS*	auris sinistra	left ear
A.U., AU*†	auris uterque	each ear
b.i.d.	bis in die	twice daily
b.m.	bowel movement	
cc, cm³*	cubic centimeter; use mL or milliliter(s)	
CFU	colony-forming unit(s)	
d.	die	day
EL.U.	ELISA unit(s)	
et	et	and
g	gram(s)	
gt. (plural gtt.)	gutta (plural guttae)	a drop (drops)
h.	hora	hour
HAU	hemagglutinating unit(s)	
h.s.*	hora somni	at bedtime/half strength
IM‡	intramuscular	
IU*	international unit(s)	units
IV‡	intravenous	
LfU	limes flocculating unit(s) limit of flocculation unit(s)	
mcg	microgram(s)	
mg	milligram(s)	
mEq	milliequivalent(s)	
mkat	millikatal unit(s)	
mL, ml	milliliter(s)	
mU, mIU	milliunit(s)	
MU, MIU	megaunit(s)	one million (10^6) IU
μg*	microgram(s)	use mcg
nkat	nanokatal unit(s)	
O.D.*	oculus dexter	right eye
O.L.	oculus laevus	left eye
O.S.*	oculus sinister	left eye
O.U.*§	oculus uterque	each eye

Abbreviation/Term	Literally	Meaning
p.c.	post cibum	after meals
p.m., P.M.	post meridiem	afternoon or evening
p.o.	per os	by mouth
p.r.n.	pro re nata	as needed
q.d.*	quaque die	every day
q.h.	quaque hora	every hour
q.i.d.	quater in die	four times a day
q.o.d.*		every other day
q.s.	quantum satis	sufficient quantity
q.s. ad	quantum satis ad	a sufficient quantity to make
℞, Rx	recipe	take; a recipe
Sig.	signetur	label
s.o.s.	si opus sit	if there is need
stat	statim	at once, immediately
subcu, subq, SQ*	subcutaneous	beneath the skin
t.i.d.	ter in die	three times a day
tsp.	teaspoonful	
μg*	microgram(s)	use mcg

---

* Error-prone abbreviation. If dictated, translate as shown in the third column. For more information, contact the Institute for Safe Medication Practices (ISMP), Huntington Valley, PA; www.ismp.org

† Although some references have aures unitas (Latin, both ears), this cannot be justified by classical Latin.

‡ Some references suggest that IM and IV be typed with periods to distinguish from Roman numerals, but we believe context is sufficient to make this distinction.

§ Although some references have oculi unitas (Latin, both eyes), this cannot be justified by classical Latin.

Therapeutic Drug Levels

Drug	Class	Serum Levels metric units (SI units)
amantadine	antiviral	300 ng/mL
amikacin	aminoglycoside	16–32 mcg/mL
aminophylline	bronchodilator	10–20 mcg/mL
amiodarone	antiarrhythmic	0.5–2.5 mcg/mL
amitriptyline	antidepressant	110–250 ng/mL
amoxapine	antidepressant	200–500 ng/mL
amrinone	cardiotonic	3.7 mcg/mL
bretylium	antiarrhythmic	0.5–1.5 mcg/mL
bupropion	antidepressant	25–100 ng/mL
carbamazepine	anticonvulsant	4–12 mcg/mL (17–51 mcmol/L)
chloramphenicol	antibiotic	10–20 mcg/mL (31–62 mcmol/L)
chlorpromazine	antipsychotic	30–500 ng/mL
clomipramine	antidepressant	80–100 ng/mL
cyclosporine	immunosuppressive	250–800 ng/mL (whole blood, RIA*)
trough values:		50–300 ng/mL (plasma, RIA*)
desipramine	antidepressant	125–300 ng/mL
digitoxin	antiarrhythmic	9–25 mcg/L (11.8–32.8 mcmol/L)
digoxin	antiarrhythmic	0.5–2.2 ng/mL (0.6–2.8 nmol/L)
disopyramide	antiarrhythmic	2–8 mcg/mL (6–18 mcmol/L)
doxepin	antidepressant	100–200 ng/mL
ethosuximide	anticonvulsant	40–100 mcg/mL
flecainide	antiarrhythmic	0.2–1 mcg/mL
fluphenazine	antipsychotic	0.13–2.8 ng/mL
gentamicin	aminoglycoside	4–8 mcg/mL
haloperidol	antipsychotic	5–20 ng/mL
hydralazine	antihypertensive	100 ng/mL
imipramine	antidepressant	200–350 ng/mL
kanamycin	aminoglycoside	15–40 mcg/mL
lidocaine	antiarrhythmic	1.5–6 mcg/mL (4.5–21.5 mcmol/L)
lithium	antipsychotic	0.5–1.5 mEq/L (0.5–1.5 mmol/L)
maprotiline	antidepressant	200–300 ng/mL

Drug	Class	Serum Levels *metric units (SI units)*
methotrexate	antineoplastic	> 0.01 mcmol
mexiletine	antiarrhythmic	0.5–2 mcg/mL
netilmicin	aminoglycoside	6–10 mcg/mL
nortriptyline	antidepressant	50–150 ng/mL
perphenazine	antipsychotic	0.8–1.2 ng/mL
phenobarbital	anticonvulsant	15–40 mcg/mL (65–172 mcmol/L)
phenytoin	anticonvulsant	10–20 mcg/mL (40–80 mcmol/L)
primidone	anticonvulsant	5–12 mcg/mL (25–46 mcmol/L)
procainamide	antiarrhythmic	4–8 mcg/mL (17–34 mcmol/L)
propranolol	antiarrhythmic	50–200 ng/mL (190–770 nmol/L)
protriptyline	antidepressant	100–200 ng/mL
quinidine	antiarrhythmic	2–6 mcg/mL (4.6–9.2 mcmol/L)
salicylate	analgesic	100–200 mg/L (725–1448 mcmol/L)
streptomycin	aminoglycoside	20–30 mcg/mL
sulfonamide	antibiotic	5–15 mg/dL
terbutaline	bronchodilator	0.5–4.1 ng/mL
theophylline	bronchodilator	10–20 mcg/mL (55–110 mcmol/L)
thiothixene	antipsychotic	2–57 ng/mL
tobramycin	aminoglycoside	4–8 mcg/mL
tocainide	antiarrhythmic	4–10 mcg/mL
trazodone	antidepressant	800–1600 ng/mL
valproic acid	anticonvulsant	50–100 mcg/mL (350–700 mcmol/L)
vancomycin	antibiotic	30–40 ng/mL (peak)
verapamil	antiarrhythmic	0.08–0.3 mcg/mL

* radioimmunoassay

The Most Prescribed Drugs

Drug	Class/Indication(s)
Abilify (aripiprazole)	quinolinone antipsychotic, antimanic
acetaminophen with codeine	analgesic, anti-inflammatory
Aciphex (rabeprazole sodium)	proton pump inhibitor for GERD
Actonel (risedronate sodium)	osteoporosis prevention and treatment
Actos (pioglitazone HCl)	oral antidiabetic
acyclovir	antiviral
Adderall XR (mixed amphetamines)	CNS stimulant for ADHD
Advair Diskus (salmeterol xinafoate, fluticasone propionate)	bronchodilator and corticosteroidal anti-inflammatory for asthma
albuterol; albuterol sulfate	bronchodilator for asthma
alendronate sodium	postmenopausal osteoporosis treatment
allopurinol	treatment for gout and hyperuricemia
alprazolam	anxiolytic, sedative
Ambien CR (zolpidem tartrate)	sedative, hypnotic
amitriptyline HCl	tricyclic antidepressant
amlodipine besylate	antianginal, antihypertensive
amlodipine besylate & benazepril HCl	antihypertensive, ACE inhibitor, calcium channel blocker
amoxicillin	aminopenicillin antibiotic
amoxicillin & clavulanate potassium	aminopenicillin antibiotic
amphetamines, mixed	CNS stimulant for ADHD
Aricept (donepezil HCl)	cognition enhancer for dementia
aspirin, enteric coated	analgesic, antipyretic, NSAID
atenolol	β-blocker for hypertension
atenolol & chlorthalidone	β-blocker and diuretic for hypertension
Avalide (irbesartan, hydrochlorothiazide)	antihypertensive, angiotensin II blocker, diuretic
Avapro (irbesartan)	antihypertensive
Avelox (moxifloxacin HCl)	fluoroquinolone antibiotic
Aviane (levonorgestrel, ethinyl estradiol)	monophasic oral contraceptive
Avodart (dutasteride)	α-blocker for BPH
azithromycin	macrolide antibiotic
baclofen	skeletal muscle relaxant
benazepril HCl	antihypertensive, ACE inhibitor
Benicar (olmesartan medoxomil)	antihypertensive, angiotensin II blocker
Benicar HCT (olmesartan medoxomil, hydrochlorothiazide)	antihypertensive, angiotensin II blocker, diuretic
benzonatate	antitussive
benztropine mesylate	Parkinson disease treatment
bisoprolol & hydrochlorothiazide	β-blocker and diuretic for hypertension
Boniva (ibandronate sodium)	osteoporosis prevention and treatment

Drug	*Class/Indication(s)*
Budeprion XL or SR (bupropion HCl)	aminoketone antidepressant
bupropion HCl [sustained-release form]	aminoketone antidepressant
buspirone HCl	anxiolytic
butalbital & acetaminophen & caffeine	barbiturate sedative, analgesic
Bystolic (nebivolol HCl)	β-blocker for hypertension
carisoprodol	skeletal muscle relaxant
carvedilol	α- and β-blocker for hypertension and congestive heart failure
cefdinir	cephalosporin antibiotic
cefuroxime axetil	cephalosporin antibiotic
Celebrex (celecoxib)	antiarthritic, NSAID, COX-2 inhibitor
cephalexin	cephalosporin antibiotic
Chantix (varenicline tartrate)	non-nicotine smoking cessation aid
Cheratussin AC (codeine phosphate, guaifenesin)	narcotic antitussive, expectorant
chlorhexidine gluconate	broad-spectrum antimicrobial, antiseptic
Cialis (tadalafil)	vasodilator for erectile dysfunction
ciprofloxacin HCl	fluoroquinolone antibiotic
citalopram hydrobromide	SSRI antidepressant
clarithromycin	macrolide antibiotic
clindamycin	lincosamide antibiotic
clobetasol propionate	topical steroidal anti-inflammatory
clonazepam	anticonvulsant
clonidine	antihypertensive
clotrimazole & betamethasone dipropionate	broad-spectrum antifungal, cortico-steroidal anti-inflammatory
colchicine	gout suppressant
Combivent (ipratropium bromide, albuterol sulfate)	bronchodilator for COPD
Concerta (methylphenidate HCl)	CNS stimulant for ADHD
Cozaar (losartan potassium)	antihypertensive, angiotensin II blocker
Crestor (rosuvastatin potassium)	antihyperlipidemic
cyclobenzaprine HCl	skeletal muscle relaxant
Cymbalta (duloxetine HCl)	SSRI antidepressant
Detrol LA (tolterodine tartrate)	treatment for urinary frequency
diazepam	anxiolytic, skeletal muscle relaxant
diclofenac sodium	antiarthritic, analgesic, NSAID
dicyclomine HCl	anticholinergic, GI antispasmodic
digoxin	antiarrhythmic
diltiazem HCl	antihypertensive, antianginal
Diovan (valsartan)	antihypertensive, angiotensin II blocker
Diovan HCT (valsartan, hydrochloro-thiazide)	antihypertensive, angiotensin II blocker, diuretic
divalproex sodium	anticonvulsant
doxazosin mesylate	α-blocker for hypertension and BPH
doxycycline hyclate	tetracycline antibiotic
Effexor XR (venlafaxine)	SSNRI antidepressant, anxiolytic
enalapril maleate	antihypertensive, ACE inhibitor

Drug	*Class/Indication(s)*
Endocet (oxycodone HCl, APAP)	narcotic analgesic
estradiol	oral estrogen for postmenopausal HRT
Evista (raloxifene HCl)	postmenopausal osteoporosis treatment
famotidine	histamine antagonist for gastric ulcers
fenofibrate	antihyperlipidemic
fentanyl [transdermal form]	narcotic analgesic
ferrous sulfate	hematinic, iron supplement
fexofenadine HCl	nonsedating antihistamine for allergy
finasteride	androgen hormone inhibitor for BPH
Flomax (tamsulosin HCl)	benign prostatic hypertrophy treatment
Flovent HFA (fluticasone propionate)	steroidal anti-inflammatory
fluconazole	systemic antifungal
fluocinonide	corticosteroidal anti-inflammatory
fluoxetine HCl	SSRI antidepressant
fluticasone propionate	steroidal anti-inflammatory
folic acid	hematopoietic, prevents birth defects
furosemide	diuretic, antihypertensive
gabapentin	anticonvulsant
gemfibrozil	antihyperlipidemic
glimepiride	oral antidiabetic
glipizide	oral antidiabetic
glyburide	oral antidiabetic
Humalog (insulin lispro)	parenteral antidiabetic
hydralazine HCl	antihypertensive, peripheral vasodilator
hydrochlorothiazide	diuretic, antihypertensive
hydrocodone & acetaminophen	antitussive, analgesic
hydrocortisone [topical forms]	corticosteroidal anti-inflammatory
hydroxychloroquine sulfate	antimalarial
hydroxyzine HCl; hydroxyzine pamoate	anxiolytic, minor tranquilizer
ibuprofen	analgesic, antiarthritic, NSAID
isosorbide mononitrate	coronary vasodilator, antianginal
Januvia (sitagliptin phosphate)	oral antidiabetic
ketoconazole [topical forms]	broad-spectrum antifungal
Klor-Con (potassium chloride)	potassium supplement
labetalol	α- and β-blocker for hypertension
lamotrigine	anticonvulsant, antimanic
lansoprazole	antisecretory, antiulcer
Lantus (insulin glargine)	parenteral antidiabetic
levetiracetam	anticonvulsant
Levaquin (levofloxacin)	fluoroquinolone antibiotic
levothyroxine sodium	thyroid hormone
Levoxyl (levothyroxine sodium)	thyroid hormone
Lexapro (escitalopram oxalate)	SSRI antidepressant
Lidoderm (lidocaine) [transdermal]	anesthetic for post-herpetic neuralgia
Lipitor (atorvastatin calcium)	antihyperlipidemic
lisinopril	antihypertensive, ACE inhibitor
lisinopril & hydrochlorothiazide	antihypertensive, ACE inhibitor, diuretic

Drug	Class/Indication(s)
Loestrin 24 Fe (norethindrone acetate, ethinyl estradiol, ferrous fumarate)	monophasic oral contraceptive, iron supplement
lorazepam	anxiolytic, tranquilizer
losartan potassium	antihypertensive, angiotensin II blocker
lovastatin	antihyperlipidemic
Lovaza (omega-3 fatty acids)	antihyperlipidemic
Lunesta (eszopiclone)	nonbarbiturate sedative and hypnotic
Lyrica (pregabalin)	anticonvulsant; neuropathy agent
meclizine HCl	antiemetic for motion sickness, vertigo
meloxicam	analgesic, antiarthritic, NSAID
metformin HCl	oral antidiabetic
metformin HCl & glyburide	oral antidiabetic
methadone HCl	narcotic analgesic; addiction detoxicant
methocarbamol	skeletal muscle relaxant
methotrexate	antineoplastic, antipsoriatic, anti-rheumatic
methylprednisolone	corticosteroidal anti-inflammatory
metoclopramide HCl	antiemetic for chemotherapy
metoprolol tartrate/succinate	antianginal, antihypertensive
metronidazole	oral antibiotic, antiprotozoal
minocycline HCl	broad-spectrum antibiotic
mirtazapine	tetracyclic antidepressant
morphine sulfate [extended-release form]	narcotic analgesic
mupirocin	topical antibiotic
nabumetone	analgesic, antiarthritic, NSAID
Namenda (memantine HCl)	cognition enhancer for dementia
naproxen; naproxen sodium	analgesic, antiarthritic, NSAID
Nasonex (mometasone furoate)	nasal steroid for allergic rhinitis
Nexium (esomeprazole magnesium)	proton pump inhibitor for GERD
Niaspan (niacin)	vasodilator, antihyperlipidemic
nifedipine [extended-release form]	antianginal, antihypertensive
nitrofurantoin	urinary antibiotic
nitroglycerin	antianginal, coronary vasodilator
nortriptyline HCl	tricyclic antidepressant
NovoLog (insulin aspart)	parenteral antidiabetic
NuvaRing (ethinyl estradiol, etonogestrel)	contraceptive vaginal insert
nystatin [topical and systemic forms]	broad-spectrum antifungal
Ocella (drospirenone, ethinyl estradiol)	monophasic oral contraceptive
omeprazole	proton pump inhibitor for GERD
ondansetron	post-procedure antiemetic
Ortho Tri-Cyclen Lo (norgestimate, ethinyl estradiol)	triphasic oral contraceptive
oxybutynin chloride	treatment for urinary frequency
oxycodone HCl	narcotic analgesic
oxycodone HCl & acetaminophen	narcotic analgesic, NSAID
OxyContin (oxycodone HCl)	narcotic analgesic
pantoprazole sodium	proton pump inhibitor for GERD

Drug	*Class/Indication(s)*
paroxetine HCl	SSRI antidepressant
penicillin VK (penicillin V potassium)	natural antibiotic
phenazopyridine HCl	urinary analgesic
phentermine HCl	CNS stimulant for weight loss
phenytoin sodium	anticonvulsant
Plavix (clopidogrel bisulfate)	platelet aggregation inhibitor
polyethylene glycol	laxative, pre-procedure bowel evacuant
potassium chloride	potassium supplement
pravastatin sodium	antihyperlipidemic
prednisolone sodium phosphate	corticosteroidal anti-inflammatory
prednisone	corticosteroidal anti-inflammatory
Premarin (conjugated estrogens)	estrogen replacement
Prempro (conjugated estrogens, medroxyprogesterone acetate)	estrogen/progestin replacement
Pristiq (desvenlafaxine succinate)	SSNRI antidepressant
ProAir HFA (albuterol sulfate)	bronchodilator for asthma
promethazine HCl	antihistamine, antiemetic
promethazine with codeine	narcotic antitussive, antihistamine
propoxyphene napsylate/acetaminophen	narcotic analgesic, NSAID
propranolol HCl	antihypertensive, antiarrhythmic
Protonix (pantoprazole sodium)	proton pump inhibitor for GERD
Proventil HFA (albuterol sulfate)	bronchodilator for asthma
quinapril HCl	antihypertensive, ACE inhibitor
ramipril	antihypertensive, ACE inhibitor
ranitidine HCl	histamine antagonist for gastric ulcers
risperidone	antipsychotic, antimanic
ropinirole	Parkinson disease treatment
Seroquel (quetiapine fumarate)	antipsychotic
sertraline HCl	SSRI antidepressant
simvastatin	antihyperlipidemic
Singulair (montelukast sodium)	antiasthmatic
Spiriva (tiotropium bromide)	bronchodilator for emphysema, COPD
spironolactone	antihypertensive, diuretic
Sprintec (norgestimate, ethinyl estradiol)	monophasic oral contraceptive
Suboxone (buprenorphine HCl, naloxone HCl)	narcotic agonist-antagonist for opiate dependence
sulfamethoxazole & trimethoprim	anti-infective, antibacterial
sumatriptan	migraine headache treatment
Symbicort (formoterol fumarate, budesonide)	bronchodilator and corticosteroidal anti-inflammatory for asthma
Synthroid (levothyroxine sodium)	thyroid replacement
tamsulosin	benign prostatic hypertrophy treatment
temazepam	tranquilizer, hypnotic
terazosin HCl	α-blocker for hypertension and BPH
tizanidine HCl	skeletal muscle relaxant
topiramate	anticonvulsant
Toprol XL (metoprolol succinate)	antihypertensive, antianginal
tramadol HCl	central analgesic

Drug	Class/Indication(s)
trazodone HCl	tetracyclic antidepressant
triamcinolone acetonide	topical steroidal anti-inflammatory
triamterene & hydrochlorothiazide	diuretic, antihypertensive
Tricor (fenofibrate)	antihyperlipidemic
Trilipix (fenofibrate)	antihyperlipidemic
Trinessa (norgestimate, ethinyl estradiol)	triphasic oral contraceptive
Tri-Sprintec (norgestimate, ethinyl estradiol)	triphasic oral contraceptive
valacyclovir HCl	antiviral for herpes infections
venlafaxine [extended-release form]	SSNRI antidepressant, anxiolytic
Ventolin HFA (albuterol)	bronchodilator for asthma
verapamil HCl [sustained-release form]	antianginal, antiarrhythmic, calcium channel blocker
VESIcare (solifenacin succinate)	treatment for urinary frequency
Viagra (sildenafil citrate)	vasodilator for erectile dysfunction
Vigamox (moxifloxacin HCl)	fluoroquinolone antibiotic
vitamin D	fat-soluble vitamin
Vivelle-Dot (estradiol)	oral estrogen for postmenopausal HRT
Vytorin (simvastatin, ezetimibe)	antihyperlipidemic
Vyvanase (lisdexamfetamine dimesylate)	CNS stimulant for ADHD
warfarin sodium	anticoagulant
Xalatan (latanoprost)	topical antiglaucoma agent
Yaz (drospirenone, ethinyl estradiol)	monophasic oral contraceptive
Zetia (ezetimibe)	antihyperlipidemic
zolpidem tartrate	sedative, hypnotic
Zyprexa (olanzapine)	antipsychotic, antimanic

Dropped from the previous year's list:

Armour Thyroid (thyroid, desiccated)	thyroid hormone
felodipine [sustained-release form]	antihypertensive, calcium channel blocker
Fluvirin (influenza virus vaccine)	vaccine for influenza A and B
Hyzaar (losartan potassium, hydro-chlorothiazide)	antihypertensive, angiotensin II blocker, diuretic
Levitra (vardenafil HCl)	vasodilator for erectile dysfunction
Mirapex (pramipexole dihydrochloride)	Parkinson disease treatment
Prenatal 1+1 (vitamins & minerals)	prenatal vitamin/mineral supplement
Prevacid (lansoprazole)*	antisecretory, antiulcer
Strattera (atomoxetine HCl)	nonstimulant ADHD treatment
Tamiflu (oseltamivir phosphate)	antiviral for influenza A and B
Topamax (topiramate)*	anticonvulsant
Tussionex (hydrocodone polistirex, chlorpheniramine polistirex)	narcotic antitussive, antihistamine
Valtrex (valacyclovir HCl)*	antiviral for herpes infections
Xopenex HFA (levalbuterol tartrate)	bronchodilator for asthma

*On this list as a generic drug.